Terry

OBSOLETE

Handbook of Nonprescription Drugs

Seventh Edition

APhA Staff

Publication Development

Richard P. Penna, Pharm.D., *Director of Professional Affairs*
Dorothy L. Smith, Pharm.D., *Project Director*
Sigrid C. Laitin, *Project Editor*

Publication Production

Edward G. Feldmann, Ph.D., *Acting Director of Publications*
Kristi Brown, *Production Editor*
Joyce Duncan, *Editorial Production Coordinator*
Marlene Povich, *Designer and Graphics Manager*

Anatomical Drawings

Walter Hilmers, Jr. and Judith M. Guenther, with Alexa L. Chun

Illustrations

Dean Williams

Photography

Robert Llewellyn

Index

Winfield Swanson

Library of Congress Cataloging in Publication Data
Main entry under title:

Handbook of nonprescription drugs.

Bibliography: p.
Includes index.
1. Drugs, Nonprescription—Handbooks, manuals, etc.
2. Therapeutics—Handbooks, manuals, etc.   I. American Pharmaceutical
Association. [DNLM: 1. Drugs—Period. W1 HA513]
RM671.A1H35 1982   615'.1   82–3994
ISBN 0–917330–40–4   AACR2

Handbook of Nonprescription Drugs

Seventh Edition

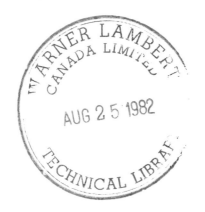

Published by

American Pharmaceutical Association
The National Professional Society of Pharmacists
2215 Constitution Avenue, N.W.
Washington, DC 20037

Contents

Project Advisory Committee

Howard C. Ansel, Ph.D
Dean, School of Pharmacy
University of Georgia
Athens, Georgia

Richard W. Brady, B.S.
Department of Pharmacy
H. H. Raulerson Jr. Memorial Hospital
Okeechobee, Florida

James P. Caro, B.S.
Manager, Special Publications
American Society of Hospital Pharmacists
Washington, D.C.

Robert K. Chalmers, Ph.D.
Professor and Head
Department of Pharmacy Practice
School of Pharmacy and Pharmacal Sciences
Purdue University
West Lafayette, Indiana

William E. Gilbertson, Pharm.D.
Director, Division of OTC Drug Evaluation
Food and Drug Administration
Rockville, Maryland

George B. Griffenhagen, M.S.
Director, Communications Division
American Pharmaceutical Association
Washington, D.C.

Richard P. Penna, Pharm.D.
Director of Professional Affairs
American Pharmaceutical Association
Washington, D.C.

David S. Roffman, Pharm.D.
Associate Professor and Chief
Inpatient Clinical Pharmacy Services
School of Pharmacy/University Hospital
University of Maryland
Baltimore, Maryland

Joseph Suárez, B.S.
Community Pharmacy Practitioner
Clinical Instructor of Pharmacy
School of Pharmacy
Medical College of Virginia
Virginia Commonwealth University
Richmond, Virginia

Linwood F. Tice, D.Sc.
Dean Emeritus
Philadelphia College of Pharmacy and Science
Philadelphia, Pennsylvania

Sara J. White, M.S.
Associate Director of Pharmacy
University of Kansas Medical Center
Kansas City, Kansas

Senior Reviewers

Color Plate Contributors

Jean A. Borger, B.A.
Manager of Special Services
Bureau of Communications
American Dental Association
Chicago, Illinois

Richard C. Childers, M.D., P.A.
Diplomate, American Board of Dermatology
Associate Professor of Dermatology
University of Florida
College of Medicine
Gainesville, Florida

Stanley Cullen, M.D.
Diplomate, American Board of Dermatology
Fellow, American Academy of Dermatology
Associate Professor of Medicine (Dermatology)
University of Florida
College of Medicine
Gainesville, Florida

Harold L. Hammond, D.D.S., M.S.
Associate Professor of Oral Pathology and Diagnosis
Director, Surgical Oral Pathology Laboratory
College of Dentistry
University of Iowa
Iowa City, Iowa

**R. Gary Sibbald, M.D., F.R.C.P.(C), (Med),
F.R.C.P.(C), (Dermatology), M.A.C.P.**
Diplomate, American Board of Dermatology
Department of Medicine
Toronto General Hospital
Toronto, Ontario, Canada

Authors and Reviewers

1 The FDA's OTC Drug Review

Author

William E. Gilbertson, Pharm.D.
Director, Division of OTC Drug Evaluation
Food and Drug Administration
Rockville, Maryland

2 Patient Assessment and Consultation

Authors

Wendy Klein-Schwartz, Pharm.D.
Assistant Director, Maryland Poison Information Center
Assistant Professor
School of Pharmacy
University of Maryland
Baltimore, Maryland

John M. Hoopes, Pharm.D.
Assistant Professor
School of Pharmacy
University of Maryland
Baltimore, Maryland

Reviewers

Daniel E. Baker, Pharm.D.
Assistant Professor, College of Pharmacy, University of Oklahoma, Oklahoma City, Oklahoma

Alan Cheung, Pharm.D., M.P.H.
Deputy Director, Pharmacy Service Central Office, Veterans Administration Department of Medicine and Surgery, Washington, D.C.

Daniel A. Hussar, Ph.D.
Dean of Faculty, Remington Professor of Pharmacy, Philadelphia College of Pharmacy and Science, Philadelphia, Pennsylvania

O. James Inashima, Ph.D.
Professor of Pharmacology and Pharmacy, Preceptor in Clinical Pharmacy Practice, College of Pharmacy and Allied Health, Northeastern University, Boston, Massachusetts

David A. Knapp, Ph.D.
Professor of Pharmacy, School of Pharmacy, University of Maryland, Baltimore, Maryland

Michael Montagne, Ph.D.
Assistant Professor, College of Pharmacy, University of Kentucky, Lexington, Kentucky

Judith M. Ozbun, M.S.
Associate Professor of Pharmacy Practice, College of Pharmacy, North Dakota State University, Fargo, North Dakota

Robert L. Snively, B.S.
Pharmacist, Georgetown, Delaware

John F. Stegeman, M.D.
Special Lecturer (Disease States and Therapeutics), School of Pharmacy, University of Georgia, Athens, Georgia

Gilbert N. Weise, B.S.
Pharmacist and Owner, Weise Prescription Shop, Jacksonville, Florida

3 Antacid Products

Author

William R. Garnett, Pharm.D.
Associate Professor
School of Pharmacy
Virginia Commonwealth University
Richmond, Virginia

Reviewers

Stephen M. Caiola, M.S.
Associate Professor of Pharmacy Practice, School of Pharmacy, University of North Carolina, Chapel Hill, North Carolina; Director of Pharmacy Services, Orange-Chathem Comprehensive Health Services, Inc., Carrboro, North Carolina

Bruce C. Carlestedt, Ph.D.
Associate Professor of Clinical Pharmacy, School of Pharmacy and Pharmacal Sciences, Purdue University; Indiana University Hospitals, Indianapolis, Indiana

Thomas E. Lackner, Pharm.D.
Assistant Professor of Clinical Pharmacy, St. Louis College of Pharmacy, St. Louis, Missouri

Buford T. Lively, Ph.D.
Assistant Professor of Pharmacy and Pharmacy Administration, School of Pharmacy, Northeast Louisiana University, Monroe, Louisiana

Robert S. Mosser, M.D., F.A.C.P.
Chairman, Department of Medicine, Kern Medical Center, Bakersfield, California

Francis L. Tse, Ph.D.
Unit Head, Pharmacokinetics, Pharmaceutical Division, Research and Development, Sandoz, Inc., East Hanover, New Jersey; Visit-

ing Assistant Professor of Pharmacy, College of Pharmacy, Rutgers University, The State University of New Jersey, Piscataway, New Jersey

C. Wayne Weart, Pharm.D.
Director, Pharmacy Education in Family Medicine, Associate Professor of Pharmacy, Assistant Professor of Family Medicine, Medical University of South Carolina, Charleston, South Carolina

4 Anthelmintic Products

Author

Frank A. Pettinato, Ph.D.
Professor, Pharmaceutical Chemistry
University of Montana
Missoula, Montana

Reviewers

J. Fred Bennes, B.S.
Clinical Assistant Professor of Pharmacy, State University of New York at Buffalo; Chief of Pharmacy Services, The Health Care Plan, Inc., Buffalo, New York

Timothy S. Johnston, Pharm.D.
Assistant Professor of Clinical Pharmacy, Family Practice Clinic, College of Pharmacy, University of New Mexico, Albuquerque, New Mexico

Kent E. Lieginger, Pharm.D.
Assistant Clinical Professor, Department of Family Practice, University of California at Davis; Clinical Pharmacist, Family Practice Clinic, Sacramento, California

Richard H. Meade III, M.D.
Professor of Pediatrics, New England Medical Center, Boston, Massachusetts

C. Kirk Phares, Ph.D.
Associate Professor of Biochemistry and Medical Microbiology, Department of Biochemistry, University of Nebraska Medical Center, Omaha, Nebraska

David E. Stewart, Pharm.D.
Pharmacist and Vice President, Stewart's Pharmacy, McMinnville, Tennessee; Assistant Professor, College of Pharmacy, University of Tennessee, Memphis, Tennessee

5 Antidiarrheal and Other Gastrointestinal Products

Author

R. Leon Longe, Pharm.D.
Assistant Professor of Clinical Pharmacy
Medical College of Georgia
Augusta, Georgia

Reviewers

Timothy R. Covington, Pharm.D.
Associate Professor of Clinical Pharmacy and Chairman, Clinical Programs and Services, School of Pharmacy, West Virginia University, Morgantown, West Virginia

Stuart Feldman, Ph.D.
Associate Professor of Pharmaceutics and Chairman, Department of Pharmaceutics, College of Pharmacy, University of Houston, Houston, Texas

Walter D. Hadley, B.S.
Community Practitioner, Corner Drug Store, Noblesville, Indiana

Wayne A. Kradjan, Pharm.D.
Associate Professor of Pharmacy Practice, School of Pharmacy, University of Washington, Seattle, Washington

Richard K. Ogden, D.O.
Lakeside Hospital, Kansas City, Missouri

Rosalie Sagraves, Pharm.D.
Assistant Professor of Pharmacy, College of Pharmacy, University of Texas at Austin, Austin, Texas

Thomas S. Sisca, Pharm.D.
Director, Drug Information and Clinical Pharmacy Services, Memorial Hospital, Easton, Maryland

6 Laxative Products

Author

Clarence E. Curry Jr., Pharm.D.
Assistant Professor of Clinical Pharmacy
College of Pharmacy and Pharmacal Sciences
Howard University
Washington, D.C.

Reviewers

Michael M. Alexander, Pharm.D.
Clinical Assistant Professor of Pharmacy, College of Pharmacy, University of Iowa, Iowa City, Iowa

R. Randolph Beckner, Pharm.D.
Senior Clinical Pharmacist, Department of Pharmacy and Clinical Pharmacy, University of Massachusetts Medical Center, Worcester, Massachusetts

Eddie L. Boyd, Pharm.D.
Associate Professor, College of Pharmacy, University of Michigan, Ann Arbor, Michigan

Anthony T. Buatti, B.S., M.B.A.
Assistant Professor of Health Care Administration, College of Pharmacy and Allied Health Professions, St. John's University, Jamaica, New York

Thomas W. Campbell, B.S.
Pharmacist and President, Capitol Pharmacy, Inc., Seaford, Delaware

Donald M. Vickery, M.D.
President, The Center for Consumer Health Education, Vienna, Virginia; Associate Clinical Professor of Family Medicine, Medical College of Virginia, Richmond, Virginia; Assistant Professor of Community and Family Medicine, Georgetown University, School of Medicine, Washington, D.C.

Victor A. Yanchick, Ph.D.
Professor and Assistant Dean, College of Pharmacy, The University of Texas at Austin, Austin, Texas

7 Emetic and Antiemetic Products

Authors

Gary M. Oderda, Pharm.D., M.P.H.
Director, Maryland Poison Information Center
Assistant Professor
School of Pharmacy
University of Maryland
Baltimore, Maryland

Sheila West, Pharm.D.
USAID American Embassy
Manilla, Phillipines
APO San Francisco, California

Reviewers

Robert L. Day, Pharm.D.
Associate Dean for Professional Affairs, School of Pharmacy, University of California, San Francisco, California

Metta Lou Henderson, Ph.D.
Associate Professor of Pharmacy, Raabe College of Pharmacy and Allied Health Sciences, Ohio Northern University; Assistant to the Vice President for Academic Affairs, Ohio Northern University, Ada, Ohio

Gary A. Holt, B.S.
Pharmacist, Oklahoma Memorial Hospital; Adjunct Professor of Pharmacology, Allied Health and Consumer Drug Education, South Oklahoma City Junior College, Oklahoma City, Oklahoma

Alan H. Lau, Pharm.D.
Assistant Professor of Pharmacy Practice, College of Pharmacy, University of Illinois at the Medical Center, Chicago, Illinois

Anthony J. Silvagni, Pharm.D.
Clinical Pharmacist, Thomas Jefferson University Hospital, Philadelphia, Pennsylvania

Anthony R. Temple, M.D.
Director, Medical Affairs, McNeil Consumer Products Company, Fort Washington, Pennsylvania; Adjunct Associate Professor of Pediatrics, University of Pennsylvania; Adjunct Faculty, Philadelphia College of Pharmacy and Science, Philadelphia, Pennsylvania

8 Ostomy Care Products

Authors

Michael L. Kleinberg, M.S.
Associate Director, Department of Pharmacy
University of California Medical Center, San Diego
San Diego, California

Melba C. Connors, R.N., B.S.
Enterostomal Therapist
Enterostomal Therapy Department;
Program Director
School of Enterostomal Therapy
University of California Medical Center, San Diego
San Diego, California

Reviewers

George B. Browning, B.S.
Pharmacist and Owner, Medical Arts Building Pharmacy, Melbourne, Florida

Theodore Eisenstat, M.D.
Associated Colon-Rectal Surgeons PA, Plainfield, New Jersey

K. Richard Knoll, Pharm.D.
Assistant Professor, Department of Pharmaceutics, College of Pharmacy, University of Arkansas Medical Center, Little Rock, Arkansas

Mary M. Losey, M.S.
Associate Professor of Clinical Pharmacy, School of Pharmacy and Pharmacal Sciences, Purdue University, West Lafayette, Indiana

Richard Y. Miller, B.S.
Pharmacist and President, Millers Pharmacy and Surgical Supply, Wyckoff, New Jersey

Joan L. Selekof, R.N.
Enterostomal Therapist, Med.-Surg. II Division, University of Maryland Hospital, Baltimore, Maryland

9 Cold and Allergy Products

Authors

Bobby G. Bryant, Pharm.D.
Associate Professor of Clinical Pharmacy
School of Pharmacy and Pharmacal Sciences
Purdue University
West Lafayette, Indiana

John F. Cormier, Pharm.D., M.S.
Associate Professor of Clinical Pharmacy
Acting Chairman, Department of Clinical and
Institutional Pharmacy
College of Pharmacy
Medical University of South Carolina
Charleston, South Carolina

Reviewers

David E. Domann, M.S.
Assistant Professor of Pharmacy Practice, University of Kansas Medical Center, College of Health Sciences and Hospital, Kansas City, Kansas

Renee J. Goldberg, Pharm.D.
Assistant Professor of Clinical Pharmacy, Arnold and Marie Schwartz College of Pharmacy and Health Sciences, Long Island University, Brooklyn, New York

Leslie Hendeles, Pharm.D.
Associate Professor of Clinical Pharmacy, College of Pharmacy, University of Florida, Gainesville, Florida

H. Won Jun, Ph.D.
Associate Professor of Pharmaceutics, School of Pharmacy, University of Georgia, Athens, Georgia

H. William Kelly, Pharm.D.
Associate Professor of Pharmacy and Assistant Professor of Pediatrics, College of Pharmacy and School of Medicine, University of New Mexico; Clinical Pharmacist, University of New Mexico Pediatric Pulmonary Center, Albuquerque, New Mexico

James H. Ralstin, M.D.
Shawnee Mission, Kansas

Raymond W. Roberts, Pharm.D.
Director of Pharmacy, Riverside Hospital, Jacksonville, Florida

D. Barry Smith, Pharm.D.
President, Medical Dental Pharmacy, Inc., Fresno, California

10 Asthma Products

Authors

J. Robert Powell, Ph.D.
Associate Professor
School of Pharmacy
University of North Carolina
Chapel Hill, North Carolina

Lawrence J. Hak, Pharm.D.
Associate Professor of Pharmacy
School of Pharmacy
University of North Carolina
Chapel Hill, North Carolina

Reviewers

William H. Jeffery, Pharm.D.
Associate Professor of Pharmacy, Coordinator of Clinical Pharmacy, College of Pharmacy, University of New Mexico, Albuquerque, New Mexico

Kenneth R. Keefner, Ph.D.
Director, Division of Clinical Pharmacy, Associate Professor of Clinical Pharmacy, St. Louis College of Pharmacy, St. Louis, Missouri

Lloyd Kennon, Ph.D.
Associate Professor of Industrial Pharmacy, Arnold and Marie Schwartz College of Pharmacy and Health Sciences, Long Island University, Brooklyn, New York

Bernie R. Olin, Pharm.D.
Director, Xavier University Drug Information Center at Tulane Medical Center; Assistant Professor of Pharmacy, Xavier College of Pharmacy; Adjunct Instructor, Tulane University School of Medicine, New Orleans, Louisiana

Peter M. Penna, Pharm.D.
Chief Hospital Pharmacist, Eastside Hospital and Specialty Center of Group Health Cooperative of Puget Sound, Redmond, Washington

Gary D. Smith, Pharm.D.
Clinical Assistant Professor of Pharmacy, College of Pharmacy, and Clinical Pharmacist, Pediatric Allergy and Pulmonary Division, University of Iowa, Iowa City, Iowa

Miles Weinberger, M.D.
Chairman, Pediatric Allergy and Pulmonary Division, and Professor of Pediatrics, Department of Pediatrics, University of Iowa Hospitals and Clinics, Iowa City, Iowa

11 Internal Analgesic Products

Author
W. Kent Van Tyle, Ph.D.
Associate Professor of Pharmacology
College of Pharmacy
Butler University
Indianapolis, Indiana

Reviewers

George E. Francisco, Pharm.D.
Assistant Professor of Pharmacy Practice, School of Pharmacy, University of Georgia; Clinical Pharmacist, St. Mary's Hospital, Athens, Georgia

Joseph Greensher, M.D., F.A.A.P.
Chief, Department of Pediatrics, Nassau Hospital, Mineola, New York; Associate Director, Poison Control Center, and Attending Pediatrician, Nassau County Medical Center, East Meadow, New York; Associate Professor of Clinical Pediatrics, State University of New York at Stony Brook, New York; Associate Professor of Clinical Pediatrics, School of Nursing, Adelphi University, Garden City, New York

Arthur G. Lipman, Pharm.D.
Professor and Chairman, Department of Pharmacy Practice, College of Pharmacy, University of Utah, Salt Lake City, Utah

James K. Martilla, Pharm.D.
Consultant, Pharmaceutical Consultant Services, PA; Assistant Professor, College of Pharmacy, University of Minnesota, Minneapolis, Minnesota

Joel Owerbach, Pharm.D.
Associate Director of Pharmacy for Clinical and Educational Services, Rochester Medical Group Associates, P.C., Rochester, New York

Gary M. Thudium, B.S., Phm.
President, Wright Pharmacy, Vinton, Iowa; President, Associated Druggists, Wichita, Kansas

12 Nutritional Supplement, Mineral, and Vitamin Products

Authors
Marianne Ivey
Associate Director, Clinical and Ambulatory
Pharmacy Services
University Hospital and Harborview Medical Center;
Acting Associate Clinical Professor
School of Pharmacy
University of Washington
Seattle, Washington

Gary Elmer, Ph.D.
School of Pharmacy
University of Washington
Seattle, Washington

Reviewers

Lester G. Bruns, Ph.D.
Professor of Biochemistry and Nutritional Biochemistry, and Director, Division of Physical Sciences, St. Louis College of Pharmacy, St. Louis, Missouri

Donald R. Gronewold
President and Owner, Don's Pharmacy; Pharmacy Consultant, Washington Nursing Center, Washington, Illinois

Carl J. Malanga, Ph.D.
Professor of Biopharmacy, and Chairman, Basic Pharmaceutical Science, School of Pharmacy, West Virginia University Medical Center, Morgantown, West Virginia

William A. Miller, Pharm.D., M.Sc.
Professor of Pharmacy Practice, College of Pharmacy, University of Tennessee Center for the Health Sciences, Memphis, Tennessee

Debra V. Naccarto
Assistant Director for Nutritional Services, Department of Pharmacy, University of Maryland Hospital; Clinical Pharmacy and Pharmacy Practice and Administration, School of Pharmacy, University of Maryland, Baltimore, Maryland

Robert M. Russell, M.D.
Associate Professor of Medicine, Tufts University School of Medicine; Director, Clinical Studies, USDA Human Nutrition Research Center on Aging at Tufts University, Boston, Massachusetts

B. Blackburn Thompson, Ph.D.
Associate Professor of Medicinal Chemistry, School of Pharmacy, University of Georgia, Athens, Georgia

J. Ken Walters Jr., Pharm.D.
Assistant Director for Clinical Services, Department of Pharmacy Service, Hartford Hospital; Associate Clinical Professor, School of Pharmacy, University of Connecticut, Storrs, Connecticut

13 Diabetes Care Products

Author
R. Keith Campbell, M.S.
College of Pharmacy
Washington State University
Pullman, Washington

Reviewers

Roland P. Galley, B.S.
Pharmacist and President, Galley's Prescription Center, Inc., Arlington, Virginia

John A. Gans, Pharm.D.
Professor of Clinical Pharmacy, Philadelphia College of Pharmacy and Science, Philadelphia, Pennsylvania

Charles Y. McCall, Pharm.D.
Assistant Professor of Pharmacy Practice, School of Pharmacy, University of Georgia, Clinical Pharmacist, Athens General Hospital, Athens, Georgia

James M. Moss, M.D., F.A.C.P.
Clinical Professor of Medicine, Georgetown University School of Medicine, Washington, D.C.; Active Staff, Circle Terrace Hospital, Alexandria, Virginia, and Georgetown University Hospital, Washington, D.C.

George Narinian, D.Sc.
Professor of Pharmacy, Director, Ambulatory Health Care Programs, and Chairman, Department of Pharmacy, Massachusetts College of Pharmacy and Allied Health Sciences, Boston, Massachusetts

Michael S. Torre, M.S.
Assistant Clinical Professor, College of Pharmacy and Allied Health Professions, St. John's University, Jamaica, New York

Thomas Wiser, Pharm.D.
Associate Professor of Clinical Pharmacy, School of Pharmacy, University of Maryland; Associate Director, Pharmacy Programs, Office for Coordination of Primary-Care Programs, University of Maryland School of Medicine, Baltimore, Maryland

14 Infant Formula Products

Authors

Michael W. McKenzie, Ph.D.
Associate Professor of Clinical Pharmacy
J. Hillis Miller Health Center
College of Pharmacy
University of Florida
Gainesville, Florida

Kenneth J. Bender, Pharm.D.
Director of Pharmacy Services
Truckee Meadows Hospital
Reno, Nevada

A. Jeanece Seals
Director, Health and Wellness Program
Tennessee Department of Public Health
Nashville, Tennessee

Reviewers

Tery L. Baskin, B.S.
Manager, Williamson Drug, North Little Rock, Arkansas

Gary C. Cupit, Pharm.D.
Associate Professor of Clinical Pharmacy, Philadelphia College of Pharmacy and Science; Assistant Director of Education, Department of Pharmacy, Children's Hospital of Philadelphia, Philadelphia, Pennsylvania

F. James Grogan, Pharm.D.
Clinical Pharmacist, St. Louis State Hospital; Assistant Professor of Clinical Pharmacy, St. Louis College of Pharmacy, St. Louis, Missouri

Donald E. Letendre, Pharm.D.
Assistant Director, Department of Pharmacy, University of Kansas Medical Center; Assistant Professor, Department of Pharmacy Practice, School of Pharmacy, University of Kansas, Kansas City, Kansas

Howard C. Mofenson, M.D.
Director, Long Island Regional Poison Control Center, and Director, Pediatric Pharmacology, Nassau County Medical Center, East Meadow, New York; Professor of Clinical Pediatrics, State University of New York at Stony Brook, New York

Lawrence E. Schreiber Jr., B.S.
Instructor in Clinical Pharmacy, St. Louis College of Pharmacy, St. Louis, Missouri

15 Weight Control Products

Author

Glenn D. Appelt, Ph.D.
Professor of Pharmacology
Assistant Dean for Student Affairs
School of Pharmacy
University of Colorado
Boulder, Colorado

Reviewers

Robert L. Beamer, Ph.D.
Professor of Medicinal Chemistry and Biochemistry, College of Pharmacy, University of South Carolina, Columbia, South Carolina

Thomas H. Chin, Pharm.D.
Assistant Clinical Professor of Pharmacy, and Director, Drug Information Center, College of Pharmacy and Allied Health Professions, St. John's University, Jamaica, New York

Michael D. Kimminau, M.S.
Assistant Professor of Pharmacy, School of Pharmacy, University of Missouri–Kansas City, Kansas City, Missouri

William S. Lackey, B.S.
Community Pharmacy Practitioner, Green Valley Pharmacy, Green Valley, Arizona

Alan M. Siegal, M.D.
Professor of Medicine, Department of Internal Medicine, University of South Alabama, College of Medicine, Mobile, Alabama

Dennis D. Williams, Pharm.D.
Chief, Pharmacy Service, Veterans Administration Medical Center, Cleveland, Ohio

16 Sleep Aid, Sedative, and Stimulant Products

Authors

James P. Caro, B.S.
Manager, Special Publications
American Society of Hospital Pharmacists
Washington, D.C.

Charles A. Walker, Ph.D.
Dean and Professor of Toxicology
and Pharmacology
School of Pharmacy
Florida A & M University
Tallahassee, Florida

Reviewers

Kenneth A. Bachmann, Ph.D.
Associate Professor of Pharmacology, College of Pharmacy, The University of Toledo, Toledo, Ohio

W. Ray Burns, Pharm.D.
Executive Director, Palmetto Family Health Care Center, Inc., Pacolet, South Carolina

Elizabeth F. Crichton, B.Sc. Pharm.
Pharmacist, Ambulatory Patient Pharmacy, Sunnybrook Medical Center, University of Toronto, Toronto, Ontario, Canada

Gary E. Greiner, Pharm.D.
Chief, Pharmacy Services, Veterans Administration Medical Center, Cincinnati, Ohio

Arthur J. McBay, Ph.D.
Chief Toxicologist, Office of the Chief Medical Examiner, State of North Carolina; Professor of Pathology, University of North Carolina, School of Medicine; Professor of Pharmacy, School of Pharmacy, University of North Carolina, Chapel Hill, North Carolina

17 Menstrual Products

Authors

Barbara H. Korberly, Pharm.D.
Associate Professor of Clinical Pharmacy
Philadelphia College of Pharmacy and Science
Philadelphia, Pennsylvania

Catherine A. Sohn, Pharm.D.
Assistant Professor of Clinical Pharmacy
Philadelphia College of Pharmacy and Science
Philadelphia, Pennsylvania

Renee P. Tannenbaum, Pharm.D.
Assistant Professor of Clinical Pharmacy
Philadelphia College of Pharmacy and Science
Philadelphia, Pennsylvania

Reviewers

Francoise Abrams, M.D.
Resident in Obstetrics and Gynecology, St. Agnes Hospital, Baltimore, Maryland

Rinaldo A. Brusadin, M.S.
Pharmacist and Owner, The Apothecary, Inc.; Assistant Professor, College of Pharmacy, The Ohio State University, Columbus, Ohio

Kathleen B. Kennedy, Pharm.D.
Assistant Professor of Clinical Pharmacy, College of Pharmacy, Xavier University of Louisiana, New Orleans, Louisiana

Charma A. Konnor, B.S.
Pharmacist/Interdisciplinary Scientist, Division of OTC Drug Evaluation, Food and Drug Administration, Rockville, Maryland; Practitioner/Teacher, School of Pharmacy, Medical College of Virginia, Virginia Commonwealth University, Richmond, Virgina

Gae M. Ryan, Ph.D.
Assistant Director, Ambulatory Care Pharmacy, Department of Pharmacy and Clinical Pharmacy, University of Massachusetts Medical Center, Worcester, Massachusetts

Kenneth A. Skau, Ph.D.
Research Assistant Professor of Pharmacology, College of Pharmacy, University of Utah, Salt Lake City, Utah

Karam F. A. Soliman, Ph.D.
Professor of Pharmacology, School of Pharmacy, Florida A & M University, Tallahassee, Florida

18 Contraceptive Methods and Products

Author

Luis Hernandez, M.Sc.
Director of Pharmacy
Norfolk General Hospital
Norfolk, Virginia

Reviewers

Emily C. Bennett, M.S., O.G.N.P.
Department of Obstetrics and Gynecology, Medical College of Virginia, Virginia Commonwealth University, Richmond, Virginia

Sandra H. Hak, B.S.
Pharmacist, University of North Carolina, Student Health Service, Pharmacy Department; Clinical Instructor, School of Pharmacy, The University of North Carolina, Chapel Hill, North Carolina

Peter P. Lamy, Ph.D.
Professor and Director, Institutional Pharmacy Program; Chairman, Pharmacy Practice and Administrative Science, School of Pharmacy, University of Maryland, Baltimore, Maryland

David M. Margulies, M.D.
Assistant Professor of Obstetrics and Gynecology, George Washington University Medical Center, Washington, D.C.

John B. Modrak, Ph.D.
Associate Professor, Department of Pharmacodynamics and Toxicology, College of Pharmacy, University of Nebraska Medical Center, Omaha, Nebraska

Timothy D. Moore, M.S.
Associate Director, Department of Pharmacy, The Ohio State University Hospitals; Assistant Professor, Department of Family Medicine, Clinical Assistant Professor, Division of Pharmacy Practice, College of Pharmacy, Ohio State University, Columbus, Ohio

Thomas P. Reinders, Pharm.D.
Associate Professor of Pharmacy, School of Pharmacy, Medical College of Virginia, Virginia Commonwealth University, Richmond, Virginia

19 Personal Care Products

Authors

Donald R. Miller, Pharm.D.
Assistant Professor of Pharmacy
Director, Drug Information Center
College of Pharmacy
North Dakota State University
Fargo, North Dakota

Stephen G. Hoag, Ph.D.
Associate Dean of Pharmacy
College of Pharmacy
North Dakota State University
Fargo, North Dakota

Reviewers

George M. Hocking, Ph.D.
Professor Emeritus, Pharmacognosy, School of Pharmacy, Auburn University, Auburn, Alabama

Linda Hogan, M.S.
Assistant Professor of Pharmacy Practice, University of Kansas School of Pharmacy; Coordinator of Drug Information Services, Department of Pharmacy, University of Kansas Medical Center, College of Health Sciences and Hospital, Kansas City, Kansas

Alan W. Hopefl, Pharm.D.
Assistant Professor of Clinical Pharmacy, St. Louis College of Pharmacy; Assistant Professor of Pharmacy in Internal Medicine, St. Louis University, School of Medicine, St. Louis, Missouri

Lawrence A. Lemchen, B.S.
Pharmacist, Western Pharmaceutical Services, Bellevue, Washington

Reid A. Nishikawa, Pharm.D.
Assistant Professor of Pharmacy, Clinical Pharmacist, Renal Transplant, University of Illinois Medical Center, Chicago, Illinois

Linda Gore Sutherland, B.S., M.B.A.
Pharmacist and Director, Drug Information Services, School of Pharmacy, University of Wyoming, Laramie, Wyoming

20 Otic Products

Author

Keith O. Miller, Pharm.D., M.S.
Associate Professor of Clinical Pharmacy
Department of Clinical and Institutional Pharmacy
Medical University of South Carolina
Charleston, South Carolina

Reviewers

Jerry L. Bauman, Pharm.D.
Assistant Professor of Pharmacy Practice, College of Pharmacy, University of Illinois, Chicago, Illinois

Robert A. Curtis, Pharm.D.
Assistant Professor of Pharmacy Practice, College of Pharmacy, University of Illinois; Clinical Pharmacist, Department of Emergency Services, University of Illinois Hospital, Chicago, Illinois

Carl F. Emswiller Jr., B.S.
Consultant Pharmacist, The National Childrens Rehabilitation Center and Heritage Hall Health Care Nursing Home, Leesburg, Virginia

Michael S. Madux, Pharm.D.
Clinical Associate, College of Pharmacy, University of Illinois; Clinical Pharmacist, Department of Hospital Pharmacy, University of Illinois, Chicago, Illinois

Joseph J. Mitala, Ph.D.
Research Scientist, Reproduction Toxicology, Adria Laboratories, Inc., Research Park, Plain City, Ohio

Dennis Richmond, M.D.
Family Practitioner in Private Practice, Lafayette, Indiana

21 Ophthalmic Products

Authors

Dick R. Gourley, Pharm.D.
Professor and Chairman of Pharmacy Practice
College of Pharmacy
University of Nebraska
University of Nebraska Medical Center
Omaha, Nebraska

Michael C. Makoid, Ph.D.
Assistant Dean and Associate Professor of
Pharmaceutical Sciences
School of Pharmacy
Creighton University
Omaha, Nebraska

Reviewers

George Asadourian, M.D.
Acting Chief, Department of Ophthalmology, University of Massachusetts Medical Center; Assistant Professor and Acting Chairman, Department of Ophthalmology, University of Massachusetts Medical School, Worcester, Massachusetts

Alexander F. Demetro
Pharmacist, Westwood Pharmaceuticals, San Jose, California

Eugene I. Isaacson, Ph.D.
Professor of Pharmaceutical Chemistry, College of Pharmacy, Idaho State University, Pocatello, Idaho

Raymond W. Jurgens Jr., Ph.D.
Manager, Optical Products, Alcon Laboratories, Fort Worth, Texas

Diane S. Kitt, M.S.
Associate Professor of Clinical Pharmacy, Department of Clinical Pharmacy, School of Pharmacy and Pharmacal Sciences, Purdue University, West Lafayette, Indiana

Michael D. Thompson, Pharm.D.
Assistant Professor of Clinical Pharmacy, School of Pharmacy, Florida A & M University, Tallahassee, Florida

22 Contact Lens Products

Author

James W. Sieg, Ph.D.
Assistant Professor of Pharmacy
College of Pharmacy
University of Kentucky
Lexington, Kentucky

Reviewers

Bryon A. Barnes, Ph.D.
Dean and Professor of Pharmacy, St. Louis College of Pharmacy, St. Louis, Missouri

David W. Love, M.S.
Assistant Director of Pharmacy for Ambulatory Care Services, Pharmacy Central Supply Department, University Hospital; Associate Professor, College of Pharmacy, University of Kentucky, Lexington, Kentucky

Susan C. Miller, Ph.D.
Assistant Professor, Department of Pharmaceutics, College of Pharmacy, University of Minnesota, Minneapolis, Minnesota

Thomas F. Patton, Ph.D.
Associate Professor of Pharmaceutical Chemistry and Pharmacy Practice, School of Pharmacy, Department of Pharmaceutical Chemistry, University of Kansas, Lawrence, Kansas

John B. Ward, Ph.D.
Manager of Product Development, Ives Laboratories, Inc., New York, New York

23 Oral Health Products

Authors

John A. Walker, B.S.
Clinical Instructor
Division of Clinical/Hospital Pharmacy
College of Pharmacy
Clinical Instructor/Clinical Pharmacist
College of Dentistry
University of Iowa
Iowa City, Iowa

Dennis K. Helling, Pharm.D.
Associate Professor and Head
Division of Clinical/Hospital Pharmacy
College of Pharmacy
University of Iowa
Iowa City, Iowa

Reviewers

George E. Dukes Jr., Pharm.D.
Assistant Professor of Clinical Pharmacy, College of Pharmacy, University of Utah, Salt Lake City, Utah

Jefferey G. Garber, D.M.D.
Assistant Professor of Anesthesia, School of Medicine; Assistant Professor of Pharmacology, School of Dental Medicine, University of Pennsylvania; Staff Appointment, Department of Anesthesia, Hospital of the University of Pennsylvania and Graduate Hospital, Philadelphia, Pennsylvania

Lawrence W. Lubick, B.S.
Pharmacist and Co-owner, Northtown Pharmacy, Inc., Amherst, New York

Roger H. Scholle, D.D.S.
Editor-in-Chief, American Dental Association, Chicago, Illinois

Stewart B. Siskin, Pharm.D.
Assistant Director of Medical Services, Bristol Laboratories, Syracuse, New York

Kenneth W. Witte, Pharm.D.
Assistant Professor, Department of Pharmacy Practice, University of Illinois, College of Pharmacy; Assistant Professor, Department of Family Practice, Abraham Lincoln School of Medicine, Chicago, Illinois

24   Insect Sting and Bite Products

Authors

Farid Sadik, Ph.D.
Professor and Associate Dean
College of Pharmacy
University of South Carolina
Columbia, South Carolina

Jeffrey C. Delafuente, M.S.
Assistant Professor, Department of Clinical Pharmacy
St. Louis College of Pharmacy
Assistant Professor, Department of Medicine
St. Louis University School of Medicine
St. Louis, Missouri

Reviewers

Abdul Khan, Ph.D.
Entomologist, San Francisco, California

Howard I. Maibach, M.D.
Professor of Dermatology, University of California Medical School, University of California Hospital, San Francisco, California

James R. Morse, M.S.
Lecturer, Department of Pharmacy Practice, College of Pharmacy, The University of Arizona, Tucson, Arizona

Bernard P. Romano, B.S.
Owner and Pharmacist, Pacific Pharmacy, San Francisco, California

Kathleen Tierno, B.S.
Pharmacist, Eckerd Drugs, Wilmington, Delaware

Ralph W. Trottier Jr., Ph.D.
Associate Professor, Department of Pharmacology, Morehouse College, School of Medicine, Atlanta, Georgia

25   Burn and Sunburn Products

Author

Chester A. Bond, Pharm.D.
Clinical Associate Professor
School of Pharmacy
University of Wisconsin
Center for the Health Sciences
Madison, Wisconsin

Reviewers

Robert W. Bennett, M.S.
Associate Professor of Clinical Pharmacy, Department of Clinical Pharmacy, Purdue University, School of Pharmacy and Pharmacal Sciences, West Lafayette, Indiana

Ray E. Marcrom, Pharm.D.
Assistant Professor, College of Pharmacy, University of Tennessee, Memphis, Tennessee; Owner and Pharmacist, Marcrom's Pharmacy, P.C., Manchester, Tennessee

John W. Mauger, Ph.D.
Professor of Pharmacy, West Virginia University Medical Center, Morgantown, West Virginia

Joseph A. Romano, Pharm.D.
Associate Dean and Associate Professor of Pharmacy Practice, School of Pharmacy, University of Washington, Seattle, Washington

Charles F. Ryan, Ph.D.
Deputy Dean, Faculty of Pharmacy, College of Pharmacy and Allied Health Professions, Wayne State University, Detroit, Michigan

Joseph Witkowski, M.D.
Clinical Associate Professor of Dermatology, School of Medicine, University of Pennsylvania; Professor of Dermatology, Pennsylvania College of Podiatric Medicine, Philadelphia, Pennsylvania

26   Sunscreen and Suntan Products

Author

Edward M. DeSimone II, Ph.D.
Assistant Professor of Pharmacy
College of Pharmacy
Butler University
Indianapolis, Indiana

Reviewers

M. Lynn Crismon, Pharm.D.
Assistant Professor of Pharmacy, College of Pharmacy, The University of Texas at Austin, Austin, Texas

Martin S. Jinks, Pharm.D.
Associate Professor of Clinical Pharmacy, College of Pharmacy, Washington State University, Pullman, Washington

Linda McCoy, Pharm.D.
Coordinator of Clinical Pharmacy Services, Department of Pharmacy, Good Samaritan Hospital, Phoenix, Arizona

Shirley P. McKee, B.S.
Pharmacist and Department Manager, Foley's Pharmacies, Houston, Texas

E. William Rosenberg, M.D.
Professor and Chairman, Division of Dermatology, University of Tennessee, Center for Health Sciences; Consultant in Dermatology, Veterans Administration Hospital, Memphis, Tennessee

J. Alan Scoggin, Pharm.D.
Associate Professor of Pharmacy Practice, College of Pharmacy, University of Tennessee, Memphis, Tennessee

27   External Analgesic Products

Authors

Paul Skierkowski, Ph.D.
Associate Professor
School of Pharmacy
University of Mississippi
University, Mississippi

Nancy Lublanezki, B.S.
Instructor of OTC Drugs
School of Pharmacy
University of Mississippi
University, Mississippi

Reviewers

Lowell J. Anderson
Pharmacist, Falcon Heights, Minnesota

Neta A. Hodge, Pharm.D.
Assistant Professor of Clinical Pharmacy, Philadelphia College of Pharmacy and Science, Philadelphia, Pennsylvania

Arthur I. Jacknowitz, Pharm.D.
Associate Professor of Clinical Pharmacy, Director, Drug Information Center, School of Pharmacy, West Virginia University, Morgantown, West Virginia

Gary L. Prah, M.D.
Staff Physician, Department of Internal Medicine, Purdue University Hospital; Team Physician, Purdue University, School of Medicine, West Lafayette, Indiana

Randall L. Vanderveen, M.S.
Director of Clinical Education, Associate Professor of Clinical Pharmacy, School of Pharmacy, Ferris State College, Big Rapids, Michigan

Richard L. Yost, Pharm.D.
Associate Professor of Pharmacy Practice, Coordinator of the Doctor of Pharmacy Program, College of Pharmacy, University of Florida, Gainesville, Florida

28 Topical Anti-infective Products

Authors

Paul Zanowiak, Ph.D.
Chairman, Department of Pharmacy
School of Pharmacy
Temple University of the Commonwealth
System of Higher Education
Philadelphia, Pennsylvania

Michael R. Jacobs, Pharm.D.
Assistant Professor of Clinical Pharmacy
School of Pharmacy
Temple University of the Commonwealth
System of Higher Education
Philadelphia, Pennsylvania

Reviewers

Andrew T. Canada, Pharm.D.
Director, Department of Pharmacy and Clinical Pharmacy, University of Massachusetts Medical Center, Worcester, Massachusetts

Robert J. Cluxton Jr., Pharm.D.
Associate Professor of Clinical Pharmacy, Director of Clinical Programs, College of Pharmacy, University of Cincinnati, Cincinnati, Ohio

Kenneth F. Crahan, M.D.
Associate Professor of Pharmacy Administration, Director, Clinical Experience Program, College of Pharmacy, North Dakota State University, Fargo, North Dakota

Irwin I. Lubowe, M.D., F.A.C.A.
Professor Emeritus, Department of Dermatology, New York Medical College, New York, New York

Larry R. Reis, B.S.
President and Pharmacist, Day Care, Inc.; Director of Pharmacy Services, Fowler Municipal Hospital, Fowler, California

Marilyn Speedie, Ph.D.
Associate Professor of Pharmacology, Department of Medicinal Chemistry and Pharmacognosy, School of Pharmacy, University of Maryland, Baltimore, Maryland

Janet L. Wagner-Willig, Pharm.D.
Assistant Professor of Clinical Pharmacy, College of Pharmacy, University of Cincinnati, Cincinnati, Ohio

29 Acne Products

Authors

Joye A. Billow, Ph.D.
Associate Professor of Pharmacy
College of Pharmacy
South Dakota State University
Brookings, South Dakota

Raymond E. Hopponen, Ph.D.
Dean, College of Pharmacy
South Dakota State University
Brookings, South Dakota

Reviewers

Angele Carabillo D'Angelo, M.S.
Assistant Dean, College of Pharmacy and Allied Health Professions, St. John's University, Jamaica, New York

Peggy S. Heinz, M.D.
Department of Dermatology, Yale University School of Medicine, New Haven, Connecticut

Jeff M. Jellin, Pharm.D.
Assistant Professor of Health Care Practices Coordinator, Preceptor–Extern Program, School of Pharmacy, University of the Pacific Stockton, California

Donald W. Moore, B.S.
Pharmacist and President, Professional Pharmacy, Inc., Wichita, Kansas

Henry A. Palmer, Ph.D.
Associate Clinical Professor, Assistant Dean for Clinical Affairs, School of Pharmacy, University of Connecticut, Storrs, Connecticut

J. Richard Wuest, Pharm.D.
Director, Professional Experience Programs, Associate Professor of Clinical Pharmacy, College of Pharmacy, University of Cincinnati, Cincinnati, Ohio

30 Dermatitis, Dry Skin, Dandruff, Seborrhea, and Psoriasis Products

Authors

Joseph R. Robinson, Ph.D.
Professor of Pharmacy
School of Pharmacy
Center for Health Sciences
University of Wisconsin
Madison, Wisconsin

Laura J. Gauger, B.S.
Pharmacist
Madison General Hospital
Madison, Wisconsin

Reviewers

Emery W. Brunett, Ph.D.
Associate Professor of Pharmacy, School of Pharmacy, University of Wyoming, Laramie, Wyoming

Ronald Goldner, M.D., F.A.C.P.
Pharmacist, Dermatologist, and Head, Division of Dermatology, Maryland General Hospital; Assistant Professor of Medicine in Dermatology, School of Medicine; Clinical Assistant Professor of Pharmacy, School of Pharmacy, University of Maryland, Baltimore, Maryland

Anthony J. Lamonica, B.S.
President and Pharmacist, Prescription Shoppe, Inc., Everett, Massachusetts

Janet Landau, M.S.
Clinical Instructor, Arnold and Marie Schwartz College of Pharmacy and Health Sciences, Long Island University, Brooklyn, New York

David M. Scott, B.S.
Pharmacy Director, Community University Health Care Center Pharmacy; Instructor, Clinical Sciences Unit, College of Pharmacy, University of Minneapolis, Minneapolis, Minnesota

Helen E. Spencer, Pharm.D.
Assistant Professor of Pharmacy, School of Pharmacy, University of the Pacific, Stockton, California

31 Poison Ivy and Poison Oak Products

Author

Henry Wormser, Ph.D.
Professor of Pharmacy Chemistry
College of Pharmacy and Allied Health Professions
Wayne State University
Detroit, Michigan

Reviewers

Andrew J. Bartilucci, Ph.D.
Dean, College of Pharmacy and Allied Health Professions, Vice President of Health Professions, St. Johns University, Jamaica, New York

David C. Beck, M.D.
Dermatologist, West Lafayette, Indiana

Darrell F. Bennett, Pharm.D.
Director of Pharmacy, Student Health Center, California Polytechnic State University, San Luis Obispo, California

Thomas A. Gossel, Ph.D.
Associate Professor of Pharmacology, and Chairman, Department of Pharmacology and Biomedical Sciences, College of Pharmacy, Ohio Northern University, Ada, Ohio

Jerry D. Karbeling, B.S.
Pharmacist and Manager, Big Creek Pharmacy, Polk City, Iowa

Robert B. Sause, Ph.D.
Assistant Professor, Department of Clinical Sciences and Professional Practice, College of Pharmacy and Allied Health Professions, St. John's University, Jamaica, New York

Joel L. Zatz, Ph.D.
Professor of Pharmacy, College of Pharmacy, Rutgers University, The State University of New Jersey, Busch Campus, Piscataway, New Jersey

32 Diaper Rash and Prickly Heat Products

Author

Gary H. Smith, Pharm.D.
Associate Professor of Pharmacy Practice
Assistant Department Head and Director,
Drug Information Center
College of Pharmacy
University of Arizona
Tucson, Arizona

Reviewers

John A. Bosso, Pharm.D.
Associate Professor of Clinical Pharmacy, College of Pharmacy, University of Utah; Adjunct Associate Professor of Pediatrics, School of Medicine, University of Utah; Coordinator of Clinical Pharmacy Services, University Hospital, University of Utah, Salt Lake City, Utah

Nancy B. Esterly, M.D.
Head, Division of Dermatology, Department of Pediatrics, The Children's Memorial Hospital; Professor of Pediatrics and Dermatology, Northwestern University Medical School, Chicago, Illinois

Donald O. Fedder, Pharm.B.S., M.P.H.
Assistant Professor in Pharmacy Practice and Administrative Science; Director, Community Pharmacy, and Professional Experience Programs, School of Pharmacy, University of Maryland, Baltimore, Maryland

Dennis P. Hays, Pharm.D.
Senior Clinical Pharmacist, Department of Clinical Pharmacy, and Instructor, Department of Pediatrics, University of Massachusetts, Medical Center, Worcester, Massachusetts; Assistant Clinical Professor of Pharmacy, Massachusetts College of Pharmacy and Allied Health Professions, Boston, Massachusetts

Elaine O. Reale, Pharm.D.
Assistant Clinical Professor and Clinical Pharmacist (Pediatrics), Division of Clinical Pharmacy, School of Pharmacy, University of California, San Francisco, California

Debra Ricciatti-Sibbald, M.S.
Pharmacist, Toronto General Hospital, Toronto, Ontario, Canada

33 Foot Care Products

Author

Nicholas G. Popovich, Ph.D.
Associate Professor of Clinical Pharmacy
School of Pharmacy and Pharmacal Sciences
Purdue University
West Lafayette, Indiana

Reviewers

Sandra M. Gawchik, D.O.
Co-Director, Allergy and Clinical Immunology, Crozer-Chester Medical Center, Division of Allergy and Clinical Immunology, Chester, Pennsylvania

Thomas J. Holmes Jr., Ph.D.
Assistant Professor of Medicinal Chemistry, College of Pharmacy, University of Minneapolis, Minneapolis, Minnesota

Nean Molthan, B.S.
Pharmacist, McCutchen Health Sciences, Ft. Smith, Arkansas

Victoria A. Serrano, Pharm.D.
Supervisor, Pediatric Pharmacy Practice Area, Department of Pharmaceutical Services, University of California Hospitals and Clinics, Los Angeles, California

Brian R. Wright, D.P.M.
Staff Member, Stuart Circle Hospital, Richmond, Virginia

34 Hemorrhoidal Products

Author

Benjamin Hodes, Ph.D.
Assistant Dean
School of Pharmacy
Duquesne University
Pittsburgh, Pennsylvania

Reviewers

Thomas D. Decillis, B.S.
Retired Officer, U.S. Public Health Service and Retired Consultant, Bethany Beach

Ross L. Egger, M.D.
Director, Family Practice Residency Program, Director, Department of Family Practice, Ball Memorial Hospital, Muncie, Indiana

Sidney Fish, B.S.
Owner and Pharmacist, Northtown Pharmacy, Inc., Amherst, New York

Nancy C. MacDonald, Pharm.D.
Manager of Scientific Services, Johnson & Johnson Baby Products Company, Guelph, Ontario, Canada

Anthony Palmieri III, Ph.D.
Associate Professor of Pharmaceutics, School of Pharmacy, University of Wyoming, Laramie, Wyoming

Quentin M. Srnka, Pharm.D.
Associate Professor, Department of Pharmacy Practice, Director, Family Pharmacy Practice Program, College of Pharmacy, University of Tennessee, Memphis, Tennessee; Owner and Pharmacist, Moscow Apothecary, Moscow, Tennessee

Peter H. Vlasses, Pharm.D.
Assistant Director, Clinical Programs, Division of Clinical Pharmacology, Department of Medicine, Thomas Jefferson University, Philadelphia, Pennsylvania

Preface

The American Pharmaceutical Association is pleased to introduce the Seventh Edition of the *Handbook of Nonprescription Drugs.* Since the first edition of this publication in 1967, the American Pharmaceutical Association has been committed to providing pharmacists with a reliable and practical reference source. The *Handbook of Nonprescription Drugs* remains the most widely used reference source on nonprescription drugs by pharmacy practitioners, pharmacy educators and students, and other health professionals. The book is becoming well-known in consumer circles and has been quoted and commended by numerous consumer magazines, as well as by radio, newspaper, and television reporters.

The Seventh Edition of the *Handbook of Nonprescription Drugs* has been prepared to assist pharmacists in advising patients about the proper use of nonprescription drugs. The text will also be of value to pharmacists as they monitor the medication profiles of their patients for the influence of nonprescription drug use on the medical progress of patients and/or the possibility of drug interactions with prescription drugs.

Special Features

The Seventh Edition of the *Handbook of Nonprescription Drugs* has been completely updated and several new features have been added.

FDA's OTC Drug Review

A new chapter entitled *FDA's OTC Drug Review* has been added. In addition, every chapter in the Seventh Edition has been reviewed by a staff member of the Food and Drug Administration to ensure accuracy of the regulatory status of various nonprescription drugs and drug categories as the book goes to print.

Patient Assessment and Consultation

A new chapter entitled *Patient Assessment and Consultation* has been added. Emphasis has been placed on the decision-making process, which should be utilized in counseling patients who are self-medicating. Several communication techniques are suggested to assist the pharmacist who wants to become more active in self-

care. Special attention is given to the principles of therapy to be considered in advising elderly patients, parents of pediatric patients, and pregnant women about nonprescription drugs.

Questions to Ask the Patient

The section, "*Questions to Ask the Patient,*" which appears at the beginning of each chapter, has been carefully reviewed by a panel of experts. These questions are general in nature and the reader is cautioned that the specific questions may have to be revised depending upon the specific patient situation. In some cases, it may not be appropriate to ask a patient a certain question or more detailed questioning may be required and pharmacists will have to use their professional judgment.

Personal Care Products

A new chapter, *Personal Care Products,* replaces the Sixth Edition chapter, *Feminine Cleansing and Deodorant Products.* Information has been added on skin bleaching products, antiperspirants and underarm deodorants, depilatories, and nonmedicated shampoos.

Expanded Clinical Information

Every chapter contains expanded clinical information to assist the pharmacist in assessing the complaints of a patient who requests advice on self-medication, as well as information regarding methods of counseling a self-diagnosing or a self-medicating patient. This new information has been carefully reviewed by pharmacy and medical practitioners so that the information is both accurate and practical.

Color Plates

A new section containing color plates of common dermatologic, dental, and oral conditions has been added to the Seventh Edition. The color plates have been carefully selected by three dermatologists, a dentist, and a staff member of the American Dental Association. Each plate is accompanied by a brief description and is cross-referenced to the appropriate chapter in the book. The purpose of the color plates is to assist the reader in visualizing many of the dermatologic, dental, and oral conditions described in the *Handbook of Nonprescription Drugs*. It is important that the pharmacist be able to recognize these common conditions to counsel a patient most appropriately regarding self-treatment or referral to a physician or dentist.

Product Tables

The product tables continue to be a very useful element of this book. Every effort has been made to expand the tables to include more products and more information on the quantitative amounts of active and inactive ingredients. Information in the tables has been obtained directly from product manufacturers. However, the rate at which nonprescription drug products are reformulated is very high, especially in those drug classes that are being reviewed by the FDA advisory review panels on nonprescription drug products. As information regarding reformulated products reaches the editorial staff, tables in subsequent printings of this edition will reflect these new data. In the meantime, pharmacists are encouraged to refer to the drug product tables for the most up-to-date information on active ingredients.

The product table format follows the one established in the previous editions. A concerted effort has been made to make the product tables consistent throughout. Because of the diverse nature of the product classes, however, consistency has not been possible in all cases. All products are listed alphabetically by trade name. Generally, column headings are identified by pharmacologic class. Whenever a large number of products contain a particular drug entity, the specific drug heads the column. Rarely, when there is substantial diversity in the product contents, the column heading is simply "active ingredients." Most product tables contain an "other ingredients" column classification that identifies additional active and/or inactive ingredients (no distinction is made between the two categories).

In columns specified by pharmacologic class, entries are listed as either the name of the drug entity and the quantitative amount (when supplied) or a blank space. A blank space indicates the product contains no ingredients in that class. Columns that specify a drug entity are identified by

- Quantitative data (the amount of drug entity in the product);
- NS (amount not specified);
- A blank space (indicating that the product does not contain the ingredient).

A blank space in the "other ingredients" column signifies that the manufacturer did not supply additional information; it should not be interpreted to mean that no other ingredients are contained in the product.

Information regarding sodium content has been expanded. This information was obtained from product manufacturers. In most cases, sodium content is expressed as milliequivalents (mEq). This measure was chosen since electrolyte concentrations are frequently expressed in terms of equivalent weight. When a manufacturer indicated that its product contained no sodium or was sodium-free, the term *free* is included in the approximate space. In all other cases the amounts of sodium supplied by the manufacturers are included even though some of the amounts may be very small.

Expanded Index

To make the book a handy reference tool for practicing pharmacists, the Seventh Edition contains an expanded index of drug entities by their generic names and drug products by their trade names, as well as their indications in specific disease states. Wherever possible, common names of disease states and symptoms are given along with the medical nomenclature. Trade names of products included in the product tables appear in italics. Page numbers referring to products and ingredients listed in the product tables are also italicized. Generic names and all other main entries appear in bold face.

Organization and Review Process

The APhA Board of Trustees appointed an Advisory Committee in 1980 to provide general direction and guidance in designing and implementing the revision process for the Seventh Edition. The Advisory Committee determined the chapters to be included in this edition, developed content guidelines for each chapter, appointed authors and review panels, and reviewed each chapter during its various draft states.

The authors were appointed on the basis of their expertise in the specific subject matters. To help standardize the content of each chapter, detailed guidelines were provided to each author. Each chapter contains the following basic information:

- Description of the conditions in the chapter considered for self-medication;
- Anatomy and normal physiology of the affected systems;
- Etiology of the conditions;
- Pathophysiology of the affected systems;
- Signs and symptoms that patients could present with;
- Assessment criteria;
- Primary pharmacologic agents contained in the nonprescription products;
- Secondary formulation ingredients and specialized dosage forms;
- Rationale for label warnings on products;
- Considerations in product selection;
- Practical patient advice;
- Summary and conclusions.

The review process was expanded and every chapter was reviewed by a panel of approximately 6 to 10 experts. Every chapter was also reviewed by at least two pharmacists who specialized in the subject area, a pharmacy educator, and a physician, dentist, podiatrist, and/or dietician whenever appropriate. To ensure that the information was pertinent to the practice situation, every chapter was reviewed by a community pharmacy practitioner and a hospital pharmacy practitioner. In total, there were 221 reviewers for the Seventh Edition.

The reviewers were requested to review the manuscripts from the standpoint of accuracy, completeness, and practicality of the information. The initial comments were reviewed by a senior reviewer and/or the author(s). The revised second drafts of the manuscripts were reviewed again by the review panels to provide acceptable manuscripts that reflected a consensus of scientific thought.

The comments and recommendations made by the reviewers were constructive and extremely valuable. By expanding the number of reviewers, and selecting reviewers from a wide variety of specialty areas, the comments covered a wide range of topics, and several authors have commented on the usefulness of the information. Every chapter was also reviewed through each stage by a staff member of the FDA Division of OTC Drug Evaluation.

Utilize This Book: Your Patients Need You

Within every health care system, there are certain essential levels of care characterized by specific responsibilities: self-care, primary professional care, general specialist care, and subspecialist care. Self-care is a very important level of care, and pharmacists have an exciting and unique opportunity to motivate and assist patients in the proper selection and use of nonprescription drug products.

The Seventh Edition of the *Handbook of Nonprescription Drugs* has been designed to provide the pharmacist with both the clinical and product information that is needed to assess a specific situation and make an appropriate professional judgment. The decision to refer a patient to a physician or to recommend a nonprescription drug product carries a great professional responsibility. The pharmacist must consider every potential complicating factor before recommending self-medication to a patient.

The Seventh Edition is offered to pharmacists with the anticipation that it will help them fulfill their professional responsibilities to the self-medicating public.

Dorothy L. Smith, Pharm.D.
Project Director

Acknowledgments

Grateful appreciation is expressed to the authors who dedicated many hours of their time in the preparation of their chapters as well as during the several stages of review. A special thanks is also extended to the 221 reviewers and senior reviewers who critiqued the manuscripts and offered invaluable constructive comments. The assistance of William E. Gilbertson, Pharm.D., and Dennis L. Myers, B.Sc., Pharm.D., of the FDA Division of OTC Drug Evaluation in the review of every chapter is gratefully acknowledged.

The generosity of the five health professionals who loaned color slides from their private collections to the American Pharmaceutical Association has made the new section containing color plates a reality. Appreciation is also expressed to Alfred C. Griffin, D.D.S., for his assistance in providing illustrative materials.

The Proprietary Association was very helpful during the initial stages of obtaining the addresses of several manufacturers of nonprescription products. Appreciation is also expressed to the many product manufacturers who have cooperated by supplying the information for the product tables.

This book would not have been possible without the dedication and participation of the many APhA staff members, including pharmacist Charlene Celano, and Karen L. Mrak, who were involved at certain stages of its publication. Appreciation is also expressed to pharmacist Fred Figa for his assistance in reviewing the Product Tables. The assistance of Gloria N. Francke is greatly appreciated for her contribution to the preparation of the index.

1

The FDA's OTC Drug Review

William E. Gilbertson

Our society has a highly developed system of professional health care and a medical technology that sometimes appears to advance by quantum leaps. However, even with available resources for skilled professional treatment, there are still instances in which it is quicker, easier, and just as effective for the consumer to resort to self-diagnosis and treatment. A wide variety of medications are available without a physician's prescription to carry out self-treatment.

Over-the-counter (OTC) drugs are intended to be used to treat symptoms of minor discomfort, illness, or injury. Usually, their aim is to make the consumer more comfortable for as long as the condition lasts, although they include some prophylactic ingredients and some ingredients capable of treating and curing certain minor conditions. They include the analgesic tablets taken for headache; the first-aid preparation applied to a skinned knee; the cough suppressant that soothes a nagging cough accompanying a cold; antifungal agents that are capable of clearing up an attack of athlete's foot; and even antiperspirants to prevent excessive underarm wetness.

But how can a consumer or pharmacist be sure that an OTC medication will work or that it is safe? Obviously, self-medication with drugs not proven safe and effective poses undue risks to the individual. As a result, FDA has been involved since 1972 in a massive review of nonprescription drug products to ensure that they contain safe and effective ingredients and bear fully informative labeling.

Background and Structure of the OTC Drug Review

Safety, effectiveness, and proper labeling have not always been characteristic of medications used in the United States. The history and evolution of our federal laws is a fascinating and complex story in itself, and is far beyond the scope of this chapter. It suffices to note that the first major legislation regulating drugs was the Pure Food and Drug Act passed in 1906. "Unsafe" and "nonefficacious" drug products were not dealt with directly. Rather, drugs were only required to meet standards of strength and purity claimed by manufacturers. Drug safety was not required by law until the passage

of the 1938 Federal Food, Drug, and Cosmetic Act. The act was precipitated by the tragic deaths of many individuals using elixir of sulfanilamide, which contained the toxic solvent ethylene glycol. The 1938 law required that all drugs entering the marketplace after that date be shown to be safe for human use before they could be marketed.

In addition, the 1962 Drug Amendments to the act required that all drugs be shown effective for their intended uses. However, a review in the mid-1960's of drug products that had been approved for safety only since 1938 included 512 nonprescription drugs, only 25% of which were shown to be effective for their intended uses. Clearly, it was time for FDA to take a further look at the marketplace.

It is estimated that over 300,000 individual nonprescription drug products are marketed, but only some 700 active ingredients are claimed in the labeling of these products. The number of individual products may seem large, but it must be recognized that each manufacturer's or distributor's labeled product is considered a separate marketed drug. In determining the logistics of the review, FDA decided that a product-by-product review would not be feasible because of the sheer volume of nonprescription pharmaceuticals. Practicality dictated a review that focused on the ingredients used in these products broken down by therapeutic category (Table 1). Thus, instead of examining individual antacid products, of which there are estimated to be more than 8,000, it was deemed more practical to evaluate their active ingredients, such as aluminum hydroxide and magnesium carbonate. Clearly, FDA's review of nonprescription drugs is different from that applied to prescription drugs, a review of finished dosage forms. For most nonprescription drugs there need not be an affirmative demonstration that specific formulations of active and inactive ingredients are safe and effective. In some cases, however, a specific vehicle for the active ingredient may be identified.

The Advisory Panel Review

The OTC drug review program is a three-phase rulemaking process culminating in the establishment of

Table 1. Product categories by which FDA is reviewing OTC ingredients

Acne Products
Alcohol (topical) First Aid Products
Ammonia Inhalants
Antacid Products
Anorectal Products
Anthelmintic Products
Antibiotic (topical) First Aid Products
Anticaries Products
Antidiarrheal Products
Antidotes (acute toxic ingestion)
Antiemetic Products
Antimicrobial First Aid Products
Antimicrobials (hospital use)
Antimicrobials (soaps and skin cleansers)
Antiflatulent Products
Antifungal Products
Antiperspirant Products
Aphrodisiac Products
Astringent Products
Boil Relief Products
Cholecystokinetic Products
Corn and Callus Removers
Cough/Cold Products
  Anticholinergics
  Antihistamines
  Antitussives
  Bronchodilators
  Expectorants
  Nasal Decongestants
Dandruff Relief Products
Daytime Sedatives
Deodorants (internal use)
Diaper Rash Products
Digestive Aids
Diuretic Products
Emetic Products
Exocrine Pancreatic Insufficiency Products
External Analgesic Products

Fever Blister/Cold Sore Remedies
Hair Grower Products
Hair Loss Prevention Products
Hormone Products (topical)
Hyperphosphatemia Products
Hypophosphatemia Products
Ingrown Toenail Relief Products
Insect Repellents (internal use)
Insect Sting and Bite Products
Internal Analgesic Products
Laxatives
Male Genital Desensitizers
Menstrual Products
Mercurial First Aid Products (topical)
Nailbiting/Thumbsucking Deterrents
Night-time Sleep-Aids
Ophthalmic Products
Oral Discomfort Relief Products
Oral Health Care Products
Oral Mucosal Injury Products
Otic Products (topical)
Overindulgence Remedies
Pediculicides
Poison Ivy and Poison Oak Prevention
  Products
Psoriasis Relief Products
Seborrheic Dermatitis Relief Products
Skin Bleaching Products
Skin Protectants
Smoking Deterrent Products
Stimulant Products
Stomach Acidifier Products
Sunscreen Products
Vaginal Contraceptives
Vaginal Drug Products
Vitamin and Mineral Products
Wart Removers
Weight Control Products

standards for the different nonprescription therapeutic drug categories. The first phase was accomplished by advisory review panels, each of which included as voting members a pharmacist, a pharmacologist or toxicologist, physicians, and other scientifically qualified individuals, as well as nonvoting technical liaison members representing consumer and drug industry interests. The panels were charged with reviewing the ingredients in nonprescription drug products to determine whether these ingredients could be generally recognized as safe and effective for use in self-treatment. They were also charged with reviewing claims and recommending appropriate labeling, including therapeutic indications, dosage instructions, and warnings about side effects and preventing misuse.

According to the terms of the review, the panels classified ingredients in three categories as follows:

- **Category I**—generally recognized as safe and effective for the claimed therapeutic indication;

- **Category II**—not generally recognized as safe and effective or unacceptable indications;
- **Category III**—insufficient data available to permit final classification.

Originally, the regulations provided a period of time after publication of the final monograph for the testing of Category III ingredients. During this period, products containing such ingredients would be allowed to remain on the market. However, the concept of Category III was legally challenged. In the court decision, *Cutler* v. *Kennedy*, [475 F. Supp. 838 (D.D.C. 1979)], the court held that the OTC drug review regulations were unlawful to the extent that they authorized the marketing of Category III drugs after a final monograph. Accordingly, the agency has revised the regulations to require that any necessary testing be done and the data resulting from such testing be submitted before the final monograph is published (see *Federal Register*, Sept. 9, 1981 [46 FR 47730]). A manufacturer would have 12 months following publication of the tentative final monograph to complete any necessary studies and submit the data to the agency. During this time the agency will assist the manufacturer in developing testing guidelines and will provide interim feedback on data submitted.

The panel phase of the OTC drug review extended over a period of almost 10 years, with over 300 individuals participating in this unprecedented project. The first panel meeting was held in February 1972, by the panel convened to review nonprescription antacid ingredients. The last meeting convened in October 1981, at which time the panel charged with reviewing ingredients for miscellaneous internal use finished its review of menstrual products. Between 1972 and 1981, an initial determination was made of the safety and effectiveness of over 700 ingredients for therapeutic claims ranging from antiflatulents to antimicrobials, and from hair restorers to pinworm remedies. These findings were based on a review of 14,000 volumes of data submitted largely by manufacturers, but also by concerned consumers, pharmacists, and other interested parties. The panels' judgments were also based on their own clinical experience and expertise, on marketing experience of ingredients, and on both controlled and uncontrolled clinical trials. The panels also relied on the published literature, but isolated case reports, random experience, testimonials, and reports lacking sufficient details to permit scientific evaluation were not considered.

Overall, FDA received nearly 60 reports from the panels. These reports and monographs summarizing the panels' recommendations to the Commissioner of Food and Drugs were published in the *Federal Register*. With each publication, public comment was invited.

FDA's Review and Proposal

The second phase of the OTC drug review is the agency's review of the ingredients in each class of drugs, based on the panel's findings, on public comment, and on new data that may have become available. The agency, in turn, publishes its conclusions in the form of a tentative final monograph. This tentative final monograph is actually FDA's proposal and offers the first clear signal of the agency's ultimate intentions. After publication of a tentative final monograph, a period of time is allotted for objections to the agency's proposal, or for requests to be submitted for a hearing before the commissioner. New data may also be submitted during this period. This is a lengthy but necessary public process, involving both scientific and legal forces. After carefully considering objections, new data, and processing hearing requests, the agency issues a final monograph.

Establishment of OTC Drug Monographs

This publication of final regulations in the form of drug monographs is the third and last phase of the review process. The monographs represent the regulatory stan-

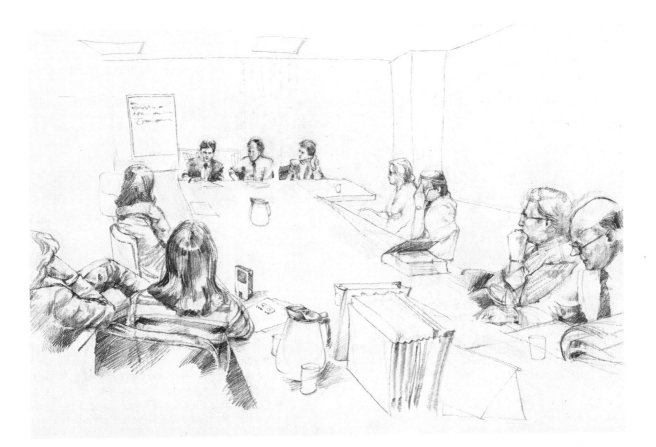

dards for the marketing of nonprescription drug products not covered by new drug applications. Marketing preclearance by FDA is not required if these standards are followed. Few final monographs have thus far been established, and it may well be that further changes in the structure and content will occur, but monographs generally will contain the following components: general provisions, active ingredients, and labeling. In some cases procedures for testing final dosage forms are also included.

Subpart A: General Provisions

This section specifies pertinent regulations detailing conditions that must be met that are common to all nonprescription drug categories, such as manufacturing practices, drug registration, suitable inactive ingredients, product container specifications, and the requirement for all OTC drug labeling to contain the general warning: "Keep this and all drugs out of reach of children."

Subpart B: Active Ingredients

Subpart B identifies the specific ingredients and the concentrations of these ingredients that can be used in nonprescription products. Details will be provided concerning ingredients that may be combined with other active ingredients, not only from that particular monograph but also from other monographs. Any stipulations on the number of active ingredients that may be combined in one product will be set forth, and specific combinations of active ingredients that are permitted will be identified. These permitted combinations will include active ingredients combined with other active ingredients that are from the same monograph and from other monographs. An example of the latter would be the combination of an antacid with an analgesic. In this case, combinations of specific antacid and analgesic ingredients judged to be safe and effective will be identified under the pertinent subsections of the monograph.

Subpart C: Testing Procedures

Any testing of finished dosage forms necessary before marketing of the product will be identified. An example is the battery of tests required for all antacid products. Each antacid ingredient must be included in the product at a level that contributes at least 25% of the total acid-neutralizing capacity of the product. In addition, the finished product must contain at least 5 mEq of acid-neutralizing capacity and result in a pH of 3.5 or greater at the end of a specified test period of 10 minutes.

Subpart D: Labeling

This section contains the indications for the product; warnings against misuse, which may also include drug interaction precautions; directions for use, including the time interval (frequency) and amount for use for specific age groups; and any specialized labeling. The monographs may also contain professional labeling, that is, labeling of the product provided to health professionals, but not to the general public.

Impact of the Review on the Nonprescription Market

Although the review is still probably several years away from completion in terms of final regulations, it has already had an impact on the public's attitude toward self-medication and on the marketplace. Publicity given the review by the news media has resulted in a heightened public awareness of nonprescription drugs and their usefulness in health care.

The review has also generated substantial scientific research that has produced impressive amounts of new data on nonprescription drugs. Approximately one-third of the ingredients reviewed by the panels were shown to be safe and effective for their intended uses. Additional data are being developed on many of the ingredients in the balance in an effort to demonstrate their safety or effectiveness. However, ingredients that cannot be shown to be both safe and effective for their intended uses have been and are continuing to be dropped from formulations and will eventually disappear from the marketplace.

A few ingredients were found to be so unsafe by the panels that they were removed from the market before completion of the full rulemaking process. In these special cases, the panels' recommendations were published as the agency's proposals to expedite market removal. For example, the antimicrobial ingredient hexachlorophene was removed from the nonprescription drug market in 1972 because of potential neurologic toxicity. The drug is still available, but by prescription only. In 1975, other antimicrobials, including tribromsalan and similar halogenated salicylanilides that were found to be photosensitizing ingredients, were removed from the market; and, in 1977, zirconium, widely used in antiperspirants, was removed from "aerosolized" drug and cosmetic products because of the potential for particulate zirconium to cause granuloma formation in the lungs.

In 1980, the agency acted to remove sweet spirits of nitre from the marketplace. The ingredient had been sold for many years as a diaphoretic to reduce fevers in children, as a diuretic, and as an intestinal antispasmodic to treat flatulent colic in infants. The agency acted on the basis of a panel's conclusions that sweet spirits of nitre is not effective for any nonprescription medicinal use and, moreover, posed a considerable risk to infants because of their undeveloped enzyme systems and the drug's potential for causing severe methemoglobinemia.

In addition, in 1980 the agency supported a panel's recommendation to remove camphorated oil (camphor liniment) from the market because of the reported toxicity and the large number of accidental ingestions that have occurred because camphorated oil has been mistaken for either castor oil or cod liver oil. This action was largely attributable to the efforts of a pharmacist who for several years collected statistics on camphorated oil poisoning from poison control centers and pediatricians throughout the United States. The panel responsible for reviewing these products concluded that the benefit-to-risk ratio of camphorated oil was an adverse one and that this ingredient should be removed from the market.

Drugs Switched from Prescription to Nonprescription Marketing Status

It becomes apparent that all drugs that have been marketed as nonprescription drugs cannot meet the requirement of demonstrated safety and effectiveness for their labeled use. Therefore, the future holds a nonprescription drug market with fewer ingredients. However, the number of OTC drug ingredients is being augmented; several panels have recommended changing the marketing status of particular ingredients from prescription use to nonprescription drug availability.

Before passage of the 1951 Durham-Humphrey Amendment to the U.S. Food, Drug, and Cosmetic Act, there was no clear-cut distinction between prescription and nonprescription drugs. This amendment requires that drugs that cannot be used safely without medical supervision be dispensed only on the prescription of a practitioner licensed by law to administer them. Such drugs include those that are habit-forming, toxic or have potential for harmful effects, and drugs limited by new drug applications approved for use under the supervision of a practitioner licensed by law to prescribe them. In effect, all other drugs in the marketplace are nonprescription.

Panels that have recommended changing the marketing status of ingredients from prescription to nonprescription thereby judged that these ingredients could be safely used by consumers in self-treatment without professional supervision.

The FDA's policy, with respect to such recommendations, has been to permit the marketing change to take place upon publication of the panel report unless it found compelling reason to dissent. However, these reports merely represent recommendations to the agency. Unfortunately, it takes many months or even years to establish final regulations. Where the consumer can clearly benefit, the agency has allowed prescription drugs to be changed to nonprescription status at this earlier stage.

Even when the agency does not dissent from the nonprescription marketing of prescription ingredients during the rulemaking process, it should be recognized that it does not reach a final decision until publication of the final monograph. Should new data become available indicating that nonprescription use of these drugs is not appropriate, their marketing status could revert to prescription only. The reverse situation may also exist in which the agency may initially disagree with a panel recommendation but ultimately conclude that the ingredient may be marketed as a nonprescription drug. In any event, only the final regulation will establish each drug's marketing status.

As of December 1980, panel reports published in the *Federal Register* recommended that the active ingredients shown in Table 2 be switched from prescription to nonprescription drug status.

Moreover, because of the panel recommendations, many nonprescription drugs are now being marketed at concentrations that were previously restricted to prescription use. For example, chlorpheniramine maleate, formerly available as a nonprescription drug in a 2-mg dosage form as an antihistamine, became available in a 4-mg dosage form upon publication in September 1976 of the report from the panel evaluating cough and cold medications. The Commissioner of Food and Drugs indicated that he did not disagree with the panel's recommendations, but was concerned that consumers accustomed to purchasing products containing this ingredient at the lower strength would not be aware of the increased amount of active ingredient per dosage unit. He therefore recommended that all manufacturers electing to reformulate their products at the higher strength should indicate the higher dosage level on the principal display panel of the package. He also recommended that if these ingredients were marketed in tablet form, the tablet should be scored to assist the consumer in achieving a lower dosage if desired.

Drug Information—Labeling and Advertising

To ensure safe and effective self-medication, the labeling of a nonprescription drug product should inform the consumer how to use the product for best results and how to avoid misusing it. The panels took seriously their charge to ensure that the products under their review had fully informative labeling, and in many instances, they developed new labeling.

New warnings against misuse were recommended for a number of products, including analgesic and antipyretic products containing salicylates and acetaminophen. In an effort to prevent toxic overdose of salicylates, a panel recommended the warning, "Stop taking this product if ringing in the ears or other symptoms occur." The panel was also concerned that individuals using salicylates might not be aware of possible interactions between these drugs, particularly aspirin, and some prescription drugs. It therefore recommended the warning, "Do not take this product if you are presently taking a prescription drug for anticoagulation (thinning the blood), diabetes, gout, or arthritis except under the advice and supervision of a physician." The agency is presently reviewing these warnings, and, if it concurs with the panel that they are necessary, they will be implemented on publication of the final monograph for these products.

Panels also recommended informative labeling statements related to product effectiveness. For example, the panel reviewing sunburn prevention products included a particularly useful innovation for the consumer in its recommended labeling for nonprescription sunscreen products. The panel recommended a sunscreen protection factor (SPF) for these products along with an explanation of the amount of protection a consumer may expect from a product with a particular SPF. Some manufacturers have already implemented this product labeling without waiting for publication of the final monograph.

Obviously, the language in which information is presented in the labeling of a nonprescription product is

Table 2. Prescription to OTC drug status recommended by panels' published reports

Panel report	Active ingredients	Indication
External Analgesic (published 12/4/79)	Hydrocortisone (topical) 0.25–0.5% Hydrocortisone acetate (topical) 0.25–0.5%	Anti-inflammatory (for itching)
Cold, Cough, Allergy, Bronchodilator and Anti-asthmatic (published 9/9/76)	Brompheniramine maleate (oral) (4 mg/4–6 hours)	Antihistamine
	Chlorpheniramine maleate (oral) (4 mg/4–6 hours)	Antihistamine
	*Diphenhydramine hydrochloride (oral) (25–50 mg/4–6 hours)	Antihistamine
	Doxylamine succinate (oral) (7.5–12.5 mg/4–6 hours)	Antihistamine
	*Promethazine hydrochloride (oral) (6.25–12.5 mg/8–12 hours)	Antihistamine
	*Diphenhydramine hydrochloride (oral) (25 mg/4 hours)	Antitussive
	Methoxyphenamine hydrochloride (oral) (100 mg/4–6 hours)	Bronchodilator
	*Theophylline ingredients (oral) aminophylline theophylline calcium salicylate theophylline sodium glycinate theophylline equivalent (100–200 mg/6 hours)	Bronchodilator
	Oxymetazoline hydrochloride (topical) 0.05% aqueous solution	Nasal decongestant
	Pseudoephedrine hydrochloride (oral) (60 mg/4 hours)	Nasal decongestant
	Pseudoephedrine sulfate (oral) (60 mg/4 hours)	Nasal decongestant
	Xylometazoline hydrochloride (topical) 0.1% aqueous solution	Nasal decongestant
Anthelmintic (published 10/3/80)	Pyrantel pamoate (oral) 11 mg/kg	Anthelmintic (for pinworm)
Anorectal (published 5/27/80)	Epinephrine hydrochloride 2–25% aqueous solution	Vasoconstrictor
	Phenylephrine hydrochloride 100–200 μg aqueous solution	Vasoconstrictor
	Ephedrine sulfate 0.5 mg aqueous solution	Vasoconstrictor
Night-time Sleep-Aid (published 12/8/75)	*Diphenhydramine hydrochloride (oral) 50–100 mg	Night-time sleep-aid
	*Doxylamine succinate (oral) 25–50 mg	Night-time sleep-aid
	*Phenyltoloxamine dihydrogen citrate (oral) 100–200 mg	Night-time sleep-aid
Anticaries (published 3/28/80)	Sodium fluoride rinse (0.05%)	Anticaries
	Stannous fluoride rinse (0.1%)	Anticaries
	Stannous fluoride gel (0.4%)	Anticaries
	Acidulated phosphate fluoride rinse (0.02% fluoride)	Anticaries

*The agency dissented from OTC marketing at the time of publication.

important. The OTC drug regulations require that labeling be stated in terms that are likely to be read and understood by the average consumer, including those of low comprehension, under customary conditions of purchase and use. In addition to evaluating the content of the labeling recommended by the panels, the agency is also evaluating the language used in order to ensure that it is in fact likely to be understandable to the consumer.

One heavily criticized policy of the OTC drug review is the limitation of labeling terms to those listed in the OTC drug monographs. Attention has focused mainly on the terms used to describe a product's intended uses and results, that is, its indication for use. The agency's position is that the limitation of labeling terminology to language developed and approved through the review process ensures proper and safe use of nonprescription drugs by the public.

A drug is only effective in its ability to achieve a therapeutic result. This therapeutic result, in turn, is an indication for use of the drug. For example, the FDA OTC antacid panel found that antacid ingredients neutralize gastric acid. Their therapeutic effectiveness, then, is their ability to relieve symptoms associated with excess gastric acid. The panel found that these symptoms were commonly described as "heartburn," "sour stomach," and "acid indigestion." Therefore, these terms were chosen for use in antacid labeling because they accurately reflect symptoms the drugs relieve. In response to a petition, the agency has since proposed that the terms "heartburn," "sour stomach," and "acid indigestion" may, alone or in combination, be followed by the phrase "and upset stomach associated with this symptom" (or "these symptoms").

The FDA does not contend that the terms selected for monograph labeling exhaust all the possibilities. If there are additional terms that can appropriately be used, manufacturers can present them to FDA, as in the case of antacid labeling, and they will be carefully considered. The agency will modify monograph labeling when there is a proper basis for such change.

FDA does not regulate or have authority over nonprescription drug advertising. Authority rests with the Federal Trade Commission (FTC), which, until recently, was proposing to allow in nonprescription drug advertising only those indications allowed in the FDA final monographs. The FTC, however, has rejected this across-the-board approach to regulation of nonprescription drug advertising. It will instead use a case-by-case approach, giving support to FDA's findings on the safety and effectiveness of nonprescription drugs in weighing advertising claims for them.

The Pharmacist as a Source of Health Information

Pharmacists have made a major contribution to the work of the OTC drug review. As noted, they participated in the advisory review panels, and they make up over half the staff of the FDA Division of OTC Drug Evaluation. They have contributed knowledge and expertise that has greatly benefited the review. The pharmacist represents a direct communications link to the consumer. Labeling is a communications tool that FDA is working to refine and improve; however, there is no guarantee that all consumers will read the labeling on nonprescription drug products. The pharmacist can perform a real service at the time of a nonprescription drug purchase by calling the consumer's attention to labeling, particularly to important directions or warnings. Pharmacists can also explain labeling when it is not understood by consumers and provide helpful supplementary information in the process. The result is a positive one: If a person knows why a nonprescription drug bears particular directions or warnings, the information is more likely to be remembered.

Beyond the OTC Drug Review

The agency anticipates that, once the last OTC drug monograph is published in final form, there still will be new conditions to review that are not spelled out in the final regulations, including ingredients, combinations of ingredients, and labeling. Manufacturers can take either of two approaches to gain marketing clearance: submit supportive data in the form of a petition to amend a final monograph to include the new marketing conditions, or submit a new drug application for nonprescription use.

The goal of the OTC review is to achieve a set of products that are fully rational in their composition and accurately labeled for the consumer. To help achieve this goal, the agency counts on a better informed public, the strengthened science base and research capacity of the nonprescription drug industry, and the assistance of pharmacists in promoting the rational and safe use of all drug products, especially those sold over the counter.

2

Patient Assessment and Consultation

Wendy Klein-Schwartz and John M. Hoopes

Self-diagnosis and self-medication are important components of the health care system in the United States. Many people do not seek the attention of a physician but self-diagnose and treat their symptoms with nonprescription drugs and home remedies (1).

It is estimated that there were more than 350,000 nonprescription products available in the United States with more than 8 billion dollars spent on them in 1980 (Table 1). An 84% increase in nonprescription drug sales in the United States has been projected over the next 5 years (2).

Nonprescription products are invaluable, allowing the individual to manage relatively minor medical problems rapidly, inexpensively, and conveniently without unnecessary visits to the physician. However, appropriate use of these products, like any other medication, requires certain restrictions and limitations. In recognition that no drug is harmless, warnings are required on the labels of nonprescription products. However, labeling alone will never safeguard the public, and the consumer needs assistance in the selection and the proper use of nonprescription medications.

Many consumers do not appreciate the need for professional assistance in the selection of nonprescription products. This attitude has recently become more evident by the large number of nonprescription products that are being purchased in nonpharmacy outlets, such as food supermarkets (3). Some investigators have stated that "the only thing that differentiates the nonprescription department in a pharmacy from a similar department in a food store is the pharmacist" (3). Similarly, it is inappropriate for nonprofessional pharmacy personnel such as technicians or clerks to provide advice on nonprescription products. These inquiries should always be referred to the pharmacist. It is essential to increase the consumer's awareness of the importance of consulting the pharmacist, especially when considering a given product for the first time. Just as industry is promoting the product, pharmacists must emphasize the value of the pharmacist's opinion during the process of purchasing a nonprescription drug.

The decision as to which nonprescription product to use is usually based upon prior use of the product, advice received from pharmacists, neighbors, and/or relatives as well as commercial advertisements by manufacturers. Even though consumers usually first hear about a new nonprescription drug remedy from several of the above sources, the pharmacist is most frequently mentioned as the most important factor in influencing the product chosen (4).

One study showed that consumers chose a particular pharmacist because he or she discussed instructions for using a nonprescription drug with them, was available to give advice on health problems, and recommended certain nonprescription products for minor health problems. Friendliness, courtesy, and neatness were also cited by consumers to be influencing factors in their choice of a pharmacist. In 95% of the cases, consumers used the medication recommended by the pharmacist, and 92% said that they were satisfied with the purchase. Eighty-seven percent either bought the item again or said that they would do so. Sixty-nine percent of consumers said that their pharmacist supplied information and advice when they sought it, and 9 out of 10 consumers said they would follow the pharmacist's advice, particularly if the pharmacist advised seeking medical help for a possible serious medical disorder (5).

According to the 1979 Schering report, the friendliness of the pharmacist was more important than the atmosphere of the pharmacy (6). However, only 34% felt that the pharmacist was easy to approach. Even though the pharmacist's advice is frequently followed, over one-half the consumers do not seek their pharmacists' advice regularly (5).

Advising patients on self-medication is an important part of pharmacy practice, providing an opportunity for the pharmacist to act in a primary-care role. Additionally, in this role the pharmacist can perform a triage function (7). Since the pharmacist is frequently the initial point of contact with the health care system, the pharmacist is in the position to assess the situation and recommend a course of action. The course of action may include self-medication with a nonprescription drug, dissuading the patient from buying a nonprescription drug in those instances where drug therapy is not indicated, recommending a nondrug modality of treatment, or referring the person to another health care practitioner. If self-medication is warranted, the pharmacist must select the most appropriate product as well as give the patient specific recommendations for its correct use. To successfully educate a patient to self-medicate safely, the pharmacist must have effective communication and counseling skills.

Patient Interview

Communication Skills

The establishment of a positive pharmacist-patient relationship is important and can be accomplished by being aware of those factors that facilitate or inhibit communication (7, 8). Poor communication often exists between patients and health care professionals, resulting in frustration for both and in part for poor compliance by the patient (9, 10). As the role of the pharmacist in patient care continues to expand, the pharmacist will be expected to communicate even more extensively with patients and other health professionals. Since communication is part of everyday interaction, it is often assumed that communication is effective and individual factors, which can markedly affect the communication process and ultimately patient care, may be overlooked.

Communication is the process of exchanging information. During an interaction, the participants change roles as sender and receiver. Effective communication is achieved when what the sender wishes to communicate matches what is received. What is received is influenced by the content of the message as well as the process used to convey the message. Communication, therefore, may be improved by paying attention to both what is said and how it is said. One can be certain of the message sent by obtaining feedback from the receiver. There are certain skills that can be developed to improve communication, which, when combined with an understanding of the physical and psychological barriers found in the pharmacy itself, will optimize the patient-pharmacist interaction.

An effective pharmacist-patient relationship can only be established if the pharmacist conveys the impression of being a capable, empathetic information source and if the patient feels that he or she needs the information. The past experience of the patient with pharmacists may influence his or her attitude toward the pharmacist as an information source (7). The pharmacist should feel confident in this role and should put the patient at ease. Since patients will resent being told what they already know, the pharmacist should first determine what the patient knows and then fill in the gaps (4). In counseling a consumer, the pharmacist should speak in language that the person can understand and should avoid complex medical terminology (7).

An awareness of those factors that inhibit positive communication and a conscious effort to eliminate them should improve the pharmacist-patient interaction (8). The pharmacist's underlying attitude toward the patient will influence the quality of the communication (11). The effective pharmacist must eliminate psychosocial barriers by avoiding bias related to attitude, interest, or the patient's level of education or socioeconomic or cultural background. Listening is an important component of communication. After the pharmacist has asked a question, he or she should be alert and receptive to the patient's response.

Listening to the patient requires that he or she be allowed to state the problem completely and the pharmacist give his or her undivided attention. The patient must be given feedback that conveys empathy and clarifies the details of the patient's problem. Empathy can be conveyed by paraphrasing the patient's words or by reflecting on what was said in terms of one's own experience. For instance, after having listened to a complaint of pain from a patient, the pharmacist should in his or her own words describe the pain just told by the patient ending with a statement such as "that must be very uncomfortable." This tells the patient that more was heard than just the details of the complaint. Interrupting the patient or expressing disinterest or disapproval may inhibit expression of the patient's problems and concerns.

Table 1. Expenditures for nonprescription drugs: 1980 (in thousands)

Category	Total expenditures	Expenditures in pharmacies	Expenditures in pharmacies (%)
Dental products	1,635,201	490,475	30
Internal analgesics	1,309,326	558,946	43
Cough and cold	1,006,709	657,777	65
Vitamins	915,594	583,399	64
Baby needs	562,830	168,476	30
Antacids	508,388	242,222	48
Laxatives	337,047	229,627	68
Diet aids	310,997	156,242	50
Skin care	222,492	77,872	35
Eye care	219,128	122,820	56
Suntan lotions and screens	204,542	88,824	43
First aid	192,674	131,763	68
External analgesics	160,060	93,660	59
Acne preparations	135,317	97,428	72
Anti-diarrheals	111,846	64,860	58
Foot care	91,946	61,875	67
Contraceptives	68,495	60,460	88
Hemorrhoidal preparations	63,960	53,726	84
Feminine hygiene (douches)	63,750	30,600	48
Other OTC's	630,878	479,349	76
Total	8,751,180	4,450,401	51

Compiled from D. A. Knapp, *Drug Topics, 125,* 13 (1981).

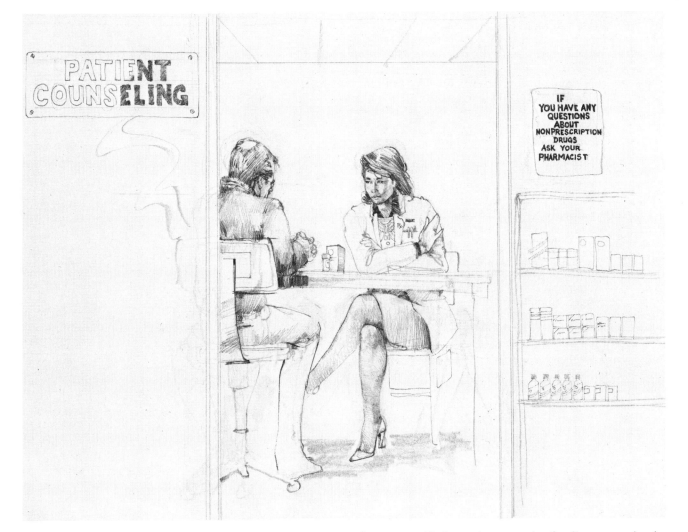

Alternatively, encouraging the patient to talk, exploring the patient's comments, and expressing understanding will facilitate communication. The pharmacist should reinforce correct decisions the patient has made. The pharmacist should also be nonjudgmental and communicate with warmth, feeling, and interest in the patient's concerns.

Every effort should be taken to phrase questions carefully. The patient should understand that the questions the pharmacist is asking are reflective of a genuine interest and desire to be of assistance. A patient may refuse to cooperate if he or she feels that questions are being asked merely out of superficial curiosity. To help prevent a negative initial reaction from a patient, the pharmacist should explain the reason for asking personal questions. An explanation such as "For me to select a product for your specific problem, I need some additional information," may be helpful in obtaining the consumer's cooperation.

Two types of questions are generally asked. Open-ended questions are useful in gathering information regarding the medical problem. An example of an open-ended question is: "Can you tell me more about the symptoms you have?" Open-ended questions allow more flexibility and provide more information than questions that can be answered with yes or no. Direct questions are useful when information is required about a specific item. An example of a direct question is "How long have you had this pain?" It is important to ask one question at a time. The use of two questions in rapid succession or multiple choice questions will only result in confusion and restriction of communication.

Nonverbal communication skills are also important in counseling people about nonprescription drugs (12, 13). Since what the communicator does with his or her body is as important as what is said, the pharmacist must be aware of nonverbal behavior (12). Posture, body orientation, and distance from the patient influences the effectiveness with which the pharmacist gets the message across. Interpretation by the pharmacist of the patient's nonverbal communications is also important.

Physical barriers to communication should be eliminated. High counters, glass separators, and elevated platforms inhibit information exchange, and the pharmacist should make every effort to be at the same eye-level as the patient (12). Discussions between the patient and pharmacist should be as private and uninterrupted as possible (7). If the pharmacist anticipates or perceives that a patient is embarrassed or uncomfortable discussing the problem, a quiet or private counseling area should be used. Ideally, a specific relatively private area of the pharmacy should be designated for patient consultation. Information obtained from a patient should remain confidential.

Special communications techniques may be required with some patients (14, 15). Writing down the information may be necessary if the patient is deaf or is hearing impaired. If the person can read lips or has poor hearing, the pharmacist should be positioned physically close to and directly in front of the patient. A quiet well-lighted environment is essential since background noise can markedly diminish the hearing-impaired individual's ability to communicate and since visual cues greatly facilitate the process. The pharmacist should face the patient, speak directly to him or her, and maintain eye contact. In addition, the pharmacist should speak slowly and distinctly in a low-pitched moderately toned voice and should avoid turning his or her head while speaking. Yelling only serves to further distort the sound. If the patient is blind it is important to initially identify yourself to the patient as the pharmacist. Since the patient cannot be aware of visual nonverbal communication the pharmacist should depend upon touching and tone of voice as well as verbal feedback to convey empathy and interest in the patient's problem.

The response of the patient can be used to assess the effectiveness of the pharmacist's advice and communication skills. A willingness to accept the advice of the pharmacist and other positive verbal and nonverbal feedback will indicate patient respect and satisfaction.

The discussion with the patient should be concluded with encouragement for follow-up with a statement such as "Please let me know whether you feel better in a couple of days," or "If your cough is not better in a few days, you should see your physician. Be sure that you tell him you have been taking this medicine." A patient will sense a feeling of caring on the part of the pharmacist. The concern expressed by the pharmacist for the correct use of the nonprescription drugs will also reinforce to the patient that these products are drugs and must be used carefully. In addition, follow-up provides feedback to the pharmacist, which allows self-evaluation of one's own advice as well as communication skills. Based on this feedback, pharmacists can assess whether or not their communication skills require modification and whether they have provided useful information to the patient.

If an effective pharmacist-patient relationship is established, it is likely the patient will return to that particular pharmacist for further self-medication advice and for the dispensing of any prescriptions he or she may need. In other words, an effective patient counseling service for nonprescription drugs can indirectly contribute to increased prescription activities.

Problem-Oriented History

Self-medication counseling is a primary-care activity that carries with it a great professional responsibility. The initial interaction between the patient and the pharmacist is frequently initiated by the patient (Figure 1). The patient may approach the pharmacist with a symptom, often in the form of a question such as, "What do you recommend for . . . ?" On the other hand, the patient may ask a product-related question such as, "Which of these two products do you recommend?"

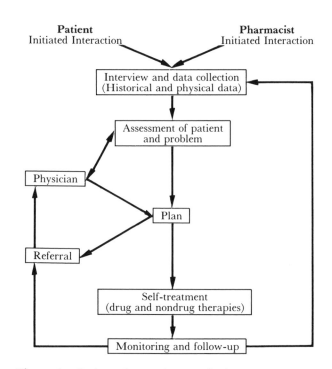

Figure 1. Patient-pharmacist consultation process.

The pharmacist should also assist a patient who is deliberating over nonprescription products and intervene when a patient selects a product that is contraindicated or has a significant potential for causing problems.

The pharmacist must concentrate on the history and accumulate a subjective data base from which an assessment can be made. The history is a very powerful tool available to the pharmacist in assessing the clinical situation presented by a given patient. The community pharmacist is limited almost exclusively to the history. Therefore, the pharmacist must develop good history-taking skills.

When evaluating the problem, it is important for the pharmacist to view the patient and the disease as a whole rather than keying in only on the drug therapy aspects. This enables the pharmacist to make the most appropriate recommendation, which may or may not include a drug product.

The first step in the decision-making process is identification of the problem that the patient is seeking to treat. Patients may initially present incomplete and vague information. By delving deeper into the problem, the pharmacist should be able to determine the patient's real needs. Asking questions, the pharmacist elicits a problem-oriented and patient-oriented history. The objective is to determine the specific symptoms and whether they are amenable to self-medication.

Symptom analysis requires obtaining the following information:

- **Onset**—When did the symptom start?
- **Duration**—How long does it last? Does it come and go or is it continuous?
- **Severity**—How severe is the symptom?
- **Description**—How does the patient describe the symptom?

- **Acute versus chronic**—Is this a new problem or the recurrence or continuation of an old one?
- **Associated symptoms**—Are there any other symptoms that occur concurrently?
- **Exacerbating factors**—Does anything make the symptoms worse?
- **Relieving factors**—Does anything relieve the symptom? What has relieved it in the past?
- **Previous therapy**—What has been done so far to treat the symptoms?

The next step in the process is to gather patient-related data. The pharmacist must consider the individual's characteristics before an assessment of the situation can be made. The pharmacist should therefore selectively elicit the following information:

- **Patient**—Is the consumer the patient or someone else?
- **Age**—How old is the patient? Is the patient an infant, a child, or an elderly person?
- **Sex**—Is the patient male or female? If the patient is a woman, is she pregnant or breast feeding?
- **Other illnesses**—Does the patient have any other diseases that may alter the expected effects of a given nonprescription drug or be aggravated by the drug's effects? Is the complaint related to chronic disease?
- **Special diets**—Is the patient on any special diet?
- **Other medication**—Is the patient on any prescription, nonprescription, or social drugs (caffeine, nicotine, alcohol, or marijuana)?
- **Allergies**—Does the patient have any allergies?
- **Adverse drug reactions**—Has the patient experienced adverse drug reactions in the past?

After gathering the patient's history, the pharmacist should determine if there are any absolute or relative contraindications to the drug being considered for recommendation. In addition, the pharmacist should ascertain if the patient is in a high-risk group on the basis of age, other illnesses, or pregnancy. Similarly, the situation should be evaluated to determine whether the patient has confused the situation, done any harm by waiting to seek advice, or worsened the condition by previous self-treatment.

The pharmacist must ask questions to obtain enough information to identify and assess the problem before a plan can be formulated. Obviously the pharmacist must do this within certain time constraints. Therefore, the problem must be approached logically, keeping the line of questioning direct and to the point. The pharmacist must use judgment when obtaining a history, since all of the given questions will not be necessary or appropriate in all discussions. With experience, the pharmacist should be able to acquire the necessary information to assess a particular circumstance within a few minutes. If the situation is more complex, requiring more time, the pharmacist must decide whether to request that the patient come back at a mutually agreeable time or to refer the patient to a physician.

Physical Data

In addition to specific information obtained through questioning techniques, physical data are extremely helpful in assessing the medical problem. Physical data include information such as pulse rate, heart sounds, respiration rate, age, and weight. Depending on the training and skill of the health care practitioner, physical data are collected through the application of all or some of the following techniques: observation or inspection, palpation or manipulations, percussion, and auscultation. The importance of each in the process of data collection depends upon the system involved. For example, the skin is easily assessed by inspection and palpation. The lung requires percussion and auscultation. All four skills are essential in examining the abdomen.

Collection of some physical data may be easily done by the pharmacist. Physical data have been collected routinely for years and some pharmacists have acquired additional skills, which in appropriate settings have greatly expanded their ability to assess and monitor patients. However, the majority of pharmacists obtain physical data exclusively through the use of observational skills.

Observational skills can be extremely valuable. Many clues as to the overall state of health of a patient and the seriousness of a problem can come from simply observing the patient. The degree of discomfort due to pain may be judged from the facial expressions or lack of use of a particular limb. Toxicity from an infectious process may be manifested by lethargy and pallor. Many an error has been made because such data were ignored. Inspection of the skin in a patient with a dermatologic condition is a very useful skill, especially with the availability of hydrocortisone as a nonprescription item. Skin rashes, for example, may result from a simple contact phenomenon or may be indicative of significant systemic disease. If a serious disease is suspected, accurate diagnosis by a physician should not be delayed and the pharmacist should be able to facilitate this process.

Assessment

Assessment is the evaluation of all the data (historical and physical) collected from the patient. Basically, the pharmacist must make an assessment as to the etiology and severity of the condition. Etiology refers to the cause of the problem. Determining this may assist in selecting a particular type of therapy. Severity refers to the relative significance of the event.

Assessment of severity will vary depending upon the problem. Problems may be considered severe only when they accumulate to a certain level, such as in diabetics with glucosuria. The higher the level, the more severe the problem, and the greater the potential for referral. Some problems may be considered severe only when they become symptomatic or the symptoms begin to impair the functional activity of the patient. For instance, the pharmacist may elect not to recommend a cough suppressant for a patient with an intermittent cough, although the cough should be treated if it is keeping the patient awake at night. Finally, other problems should be considered severe whenever they are present. Such is the case when ketonuria is noted by a diabetic or when an insulin-dependent diabetic is unable to take in calories because of vomiting.

Determining etiology and severity is essential to ensure appropriate conclusions regarding treatment and need for referral. Many times this is not definitive since certain data may not be accessible. Action may be required in such situations because the information suggests that a certain etiology is responsible or the condition is particularly severe. An acute inflammatory joint, one that is swollen, warm to touch, tender, and painful, may be due to a number of causes such as trauma, bacterial infection, gout, or rheumatoid arthritis. This may require that the joint fluid be examined and should be referred immediately for proper evaluation. Finally, there are certain groups of patients that require more careful evaluation because they are at greater risk of complications. These groups include the elderly; infants and children; those with certain chronic diseases, such as diabetes or renal or heart disease; those with multiple medical conditions; those taking multiple medications; those recently hospitalized; and those being treated by several physicians.

The Plan

The plan of action is the most critical step in advising the self-medicating patient. At this point in the interaction with the patient, the pharmacist recommends a course of action, and something can be done to or for the patient. All concerned desire this to have a beneficial outcome. Proper data collection and assessment will not ensure good outcome. Even in an uncertain situation, a well-considered plan can ensure proper patient management.

A sound plan of action requires careful attention to six specific areas:

- Additional information needs;
- Selection of therapeutic modality (drug and/or nondrug);
- Referral;
- Selection of monitoring indices;
- Patient education;
- Follow-up interval and methods.

Additional data may be needed to enable proper assessment and this may require specific action, such as talking to a parent or calling a physician. If enough information is available to assess the problem, the pharmacist then must decide to advise referral or self-treatment.

The pharmacist may need to contact the patient's physician for additional information for assessment of the situation or to act in a more direct role in the referral process. Communication between pharmacists and physicians is essential to avoid conflict in the overall management of the patient and to overcome the problem of overlapping responsibilities between these two health practitioners.

Situations in which communication between the pharmacist and physician may be necessary include the following:

- To obtain additional data needed on pre-existing medical conditions to determine whether self-treatment is appropriate;
- To seek the physician's assistance in evaluating the problem;
- To determine if the physician wants to see the patient or patient should go to the emergency room;
- To determine if the physician wants to deal with the problem over the phone;
- To provide information on the reason for referral.

If the plan involves referral to a physician, consideration must be given to the treatment center to which the patient will be referred (private office or emergency care facility) as well as the urgency. Some conditions do not require immediate attention or extensive evaluation offered by emergency care facilities personnel. A proper referral will reflect consideration of these two factors.

Whenever the pharmacist advises a patient to see a physician, it is important to use tact and firmness so that the patient will not be unnecessarily frightened, and yet will be convinced of the value of the advice. Whenever a referral is made, the pharmacist should tell the patient to whom and why referral is being made.

The pharmacist should refer the patient to the physician in any of the following situations:

- The symptoms are too severe to be endured by the patient without definitive diagnosis and treatment;
- The symptoms are minor but have persisted and do not appear to be due to some easily identifiable cause;
- The symptoms have returned repeatedly for no readily recognizable cause;
- The pharmacist is in doubt about the patient's condition.

When the decision is to advise self-treatment, consideration of several factors is required. A therapeutic objective should be identified based upon a consideration of the problem and the patient. The objective should be measurable and achievable. As a result of this decision, a therapeutic modality, either drug or nondrug, may be recommended. Final selection of a specific modality requires reviewing drug variables (dosage forms, ingredients, side effects, adverse reactions, and relative effectiveness) and matching with patient variables (age, sex, drug history, and other physiologic problems).

Self-treatment may be indicated with a nondrug modality. Selection of the nondrug modality will be modified based on patient variables. For example, in a patient with vomiting and diarrhea, the pharmacist may recommend that the person limit oral intake to fluids only for a 24-hour period to provide bowel rest. However, if the patient is an insulin-dependent diabetic this recommendation will have to be modified since caloric intake must be maintained. Communication with the physician is a must in this situation.

Selection of monitoring indices is influenced by the therapeutic objective, toxicities of the treatment selected, and the nature of the problem itself. The objective in treating sinusitis with decongestants for example is to facilitate drainage and relieve symptoms such as headache. The first can be measured by observing or asking about the nature of nasal discharge (quantity, color, and viscosity); the second objective by simply asking about the headache. Indices of toxicity are those symptoms indicative of too high dosing or of an untoward reaction. Finally, indices that indicate the disease may be worsening and may require special attention should be identified.

The patient education plan should be short, concise, and very specific. Patients need to be advised so they can participate in their own care. Such information should include what to do for the problem and what to observe to determine if the agent is working or causing adverse effects. They must be informed of symptoms that may indicate worsening of their condition and when to seek a physician's advice.

Follow-up is critical and may take many forms. Simply advising patients to call or return if symptoms fail to resolve is a method of ensuring follow-up in responsible patients. Other problems or situations may require a telephone call, letter, or monitoring by a third party. The length of time between follow-up intervals should be considered in the final recommendation. The interval would also be influenced by both the type of problem and the patient involved.

High-Risk Groups

It is difficult and often misleading to generalize about patients, particularly in regard to any predictable response to therapy. Therapy for every patient must be individualized. This includes an assessment of the particular variables involving the drug used that may predispose or otherwise place the patient at risk for adverse effects.

Three groups of patients (elderly, very young, and pregnant patients) are often identified as generally experiencing a higher incidence of adverse drug effects. Adverse effects may also have dire consequences in certain patients. These patients require special attention. Awareness of their physiologic state, the existence of pathologic conditions, and the special social context of these patients is necessary for proper assessment and recommendation.

Elderly and Pediatric Patients

In many respects, elderly and pediatric patients require surprisingly similar considerations. Both groups share differences in dose requirements because of altered pharmacokinetic parameters; decreased ability to cope with illness or drug side effects because of changes associated with normal aging or child development; patterns of impaired judgment because of immaturity or altered sensory function; different drug effects unique to their age groups and uncommonly seen in other ages; adverse effects that are unique to them and are not seen otherwise; and needs for special dosage consideration not usually required by other adults. Since each of these groups is heterogeneous, it is important to consider each of these factors on an individual basis.

Normal or physiologic aging is associated with changes that alter the pharmacokinetics of certain drugs (16–18). There are documented significant decreases in renal function, total body water, lean body mass, concentration of plasma albumin, organ perfusion, hepatic microsomal enzyme activity, and increased proportion of body fat. This may lead to altered absorption, distri-

bution, metabolism, and elimination of certain drugs. The result is often an unexpected accumulation of the drug to toxic levels. Only a few drugs have been studied extensively in this patient population, leaving the kinetic parameters for most drugs poorly characterized. Thus continuous caution in dosing the elderly is required.

The pediatric patient is in a continuous state of development of body and organ functions. Data on pharmacokinetics in neonates, infants, and children have been more extensively studied for prescription medicines than for nonprescription medications. In the neonate, factors such as decreased gastric acidity, prolonged gastric emptying, irregular peristalsis, immature biliary function, and altered intestinal enzyme systems are responsible for alterations in the oral absorption of drugs (19–21). Continuous changes in body weight and relative body composition (lipid content and body water compartments) as well as differences in protein binding account for distribution differences. Drug metabolism is usually slower in the neonate and young infant followed by an increase in infants and children. Similarly, renal drug elimination is impaired early but improves rapidly over the first year of life.

Illness in the young and old is potentially more serious because their physiologic state is less tolerant of changes. Both are very susceptible to fluid loss; therefore, fever, vomiting, or diarrhea represents a greater potential risk to them. Pulmonary function is decreased in the elderly, which predisposes them to the complications of respiratory tract infections. Similar changes are found in each body system and may be quite varied among individual patients, making the elderly a very heterogeneous group. The common cold can be serious in the first few years of life since children are more susceptible to infections such as otitis media and pneumonia. These examples more than amply demonstrate the need for plans that differ according to the age of the patient, and in general, indicate more careful and closer monitoring in the very young and elderly.

Assessment of pediatric and elderly patients requires recognition that patient judgment may be altered. In the young, immaturity requires that others provide information and carry out parts of the plan. The elderly may require special consideration when an organic brain syndrome has developed. Subtle changes in mental status, such as confusion, should be anticipated in situations where an illness has caused anxiety over the patient's overall state of health. Additionally, CNS depressants should be anticipated to have more effect on judgment in the elderly than in the nonelderly adult.

Drugs may have unusual yet predictable effects in the elderly and the young patient. Antihistamines and central nervous system depressants may cause excitation. Paradoxical reactions of this type are rare in the adult population.

Certain adverse effects are more often seen in the young and old. Elderly patients frequently have altered urinary bladder function and require a more conscious effort to maintain good bladder control. Incontinence may be precipitated in such patients by administration of antihistamines, and because of their sedative properties, may reduce this voluntary control (22).

Children have different diseases or frequently have differing causes of similar problems. For example, rashes in children are frequently the result of common viral illnesses such as measles or chickenpox, which are rarely a cause in adults. Other problems such as otitis media and febrile seizures occur more frequently in children. Certain symptoms have particular significance in children. Fever in any infant less than 6 weeks of age is a very serious sign, requiring immediate attention since there is an increased risk of serious infection such as bacterial septicemia.

The elderly differ too in several ways. They tend to have serious and multiple diseases, such as coronary artery disease, chronic renal failure or congestive heart failure, and other similar conditions. These conditions can be aggravated by concurrent therapy for other acute problems. Their nutritional status is often marginal and hence more easily affected. Social supports are often lacking to supply the aid required by an illness. Lastly, physiologic changes associated with aging may alter the presentation of certain illnesses and confuse the assessment. The elderly do not mount fevers to the same degree as younger patients and altered pain perception may cause very significant pathology to be unrecognized by the patient.

Finally, special dosage considerations may be necessary. Since infants and children are unable to swallow tablets and capsules, chewable tablets and liquid preparations are required. To assist in accurate delivery of liquid preparations, devices such as calibrated droppers and spoons will be needed. Parents may need assistance in using these devices to measure dosages accurately as well as advice on how to facilitate drug administration to reluctant or struggling children.

The Pregnant Patient

Pregnancy introduces a very important variable. Since most drugs penetrate the placenta to some extent, administration of these substances to the mother can potentially result in exposure of the fetus to the drug. Drug therapy during pregnancy may be necessary to treat pre-existing medical conditions or may be considered for the management of common complaints related to the pregnancy such as vomiting or constipation. There is concern for the developing fetus as well as a desire to ease the discomfort of the mother.

Unequivocal evidence of teratogenesis is available for some drugs such as thalidomide, androgens, cancer chemotherapeutic agents, tetracyclines, hydantoins, oral anticoagulants, and others (23). Many more are suspect and each year additional drugs are shown to be potentially harmful if used during pregnancy. A major problem faced by the pregnant patient, her physician, and her pharmacist is the lack of readily available information on the teratogenic effects of various drugs. A survey of the *Physicians Desk Reference* found that for 80.2% of the drugs there was either no statement on use in pregnancy or a statement that data on use in pregnancy are not available (24). This lack of consultation on prescription drugs will be partly remedied by a new regulation

of the FDA labeling revision program that began on November 1, 1980. The FDA program will place all prescription drugs in one of five categories (A, B, C, D, X) according to the level of risk to the fetus (25, 26). Although this regulation may increase the amount of information readily available on prescription drugs, there is still a paucity of data on nonprescription preparations. Therefore, a constant awareness of the potential danger of the use of many nonprescription drugs in pregnant patients is essential and will help to avoid unnecessary exposure.

Animal studies and epidemiologic human studies are the methods available for determining potential teratogens. There are difficulties associated with interpreting either of these types of studies. Although animal data can be useful, caution must be used in evaluating animal data because of marked species variability in the susceptibility to the teratogenic effect of a drug. The animal may be more or less susceptible to teratogenicity than humans. For example, rats and mice are relatively insensitive to thalidomide, the prototype human teratogen. On the other hand, meclizine, an antiemetic available both by prescription and without a prescription, is teratogenic in some strains of mice and rats but appears to be safe in humans (27, 28, 29). Retrospective human studies are often inaccurate because of differences in the ability to recall drug use during the pregnancy by mothers of malformed infants compared with mothers of normal infants. Prospective studies are difficult because of the need to follow a very large number of subjects.

Drug use during pregnancy is very common. A prospective study of 186 women found that the average number of drug products used during the pregnancy was 11.0 (30). Another study of drug use in the last trimester of pregnancy found that each mother took an average of 8.7 drugs (31). An average of 6.9 (80%) of these were taken without medical supervision or knowledge. The most commonly used drugs were prenatal vitamins (86%), aspirin (69%), and antacids (60%).

Several factors are important in determining whether a drug taken by a pregnant woman will produce an adverse effect in the fetus (29). The ability of the drug to pass from the maternal circulation via the placenta to the fetal circulation and the stage of pregnancy are important in determining the teratogenic susceptibility. The first trimester, when organogenesis occurs, is the period of greatest teratogenic susceptibility for the embryo and is the critical period for induction of major anatomical malformations. However, exposure at other times may be no less important since the exact critical period is dependent upon the specific drug in question.

Generally, it is prudent to avoid the use of any drug during pregnancy. Evidence has even implicated products such as aspirin and caffeine. Aspirin is available in a variety of prescription and nonprescription products and is frequently taken during pregnancy. Conflicting data are available on the teratogenicity of aspirin (29, 32). Although animal studies and retrospective studies in humans have found aspirin to be teratogenic, prospective human studies have not found a difference in malformation rates between aspirin-exposed infants and those not exposed to aspirin in utero. Similarly, there are conflicting reports on the relationship between prenatal aspirin and the incidence of stillbirths, neonatal deaths, or reduced birth weight. Use of aspirin late in the pregnancy has been associated with an increase in the length of gestation and an increase in the duration of labor (33). These effects are related to inhibition of prostaglandin synthesis by aspirin. In addition, because of the effect of aspirin on platelet function, perinatal aspirin ingestion has been found to increase the incidence of hemorrhage in both the pregnant woman and the newborn infant during and following delivery (33–36). Therefore, aspirin should be avoided if possible during the last trimester. Since acetaminophen is generally considered safe for use in pregnancy, it is the nonprescription drug of choice for antipyresis and analgesia.

Caffeine has recently been implicated as a potential teratogen (37–39). Studies in rats demonstrate that caffeine produces missing toes or parts of toes and delayed skeletal development at doses that could be potentially consumed on a daily basis by humans in beverages and drugs. In addition, high caffeine intake in both males and females may increase the risk of spontaneous abortion, stillbirths, and premature births (40). It is not known whether caffeine is a human teratogen, although one retrospective study did not find any increased risk (41). Rats metabolize caffeine differently than humans and were given the drug by gavage. However, it is known that caffeine crosses the placenta and, although there is no conclusive evidence that caffeine produces birth defects in humans, the FDA has recommended removal of caffeine from the GRAS (generally regarded as safe) list and is recommending that women who are or may become pregnant avoid or limit consumption of foods and drugs containing caffeine. Caffeine is found in coffee, tea, cola drinks, some other soft drinks, cocoa, and chocolate. Caffeine is also in many nonprescription drugs such as headache, cold, allergy, and stimulant (stay-awake) drugs as well as in prescription drugs. Studies are being performed to assess the safety or lack of safety of caffeine in humans. However, it would be prudent to recommend that pregnant women avoid or limit their use of caffeine-containing products. For example, cola syrup, which is often taken for morning sickness, contains caffeine and probably should be avoided.

A possible link between the use of nonprescription vaginal spermicides and the birth of infants with congenital disorders has been reported (42). Cigarette smoking and alcohol have also been associated with increased risk to the fetus and congenital abnormalities (43–46).

The potential for adverse effects on the fetus exists with a variety of agents that are widely used and that have not been considered a problem in the past. The decision to use a drug must be based on an up-to-date knowledge of the literature and a very critical risk/benefit evaluation to both the mother and the fetus.

The assessment and management of the pregnant patient requires observation of the following basic principles:

- Maintain a high index of suspicion for the presence of pregnancy in women of child-bearing age with certain key symptoms of early pregnancy. Such symptoms include nausea, vomiting, and urinary frequency. All women in the child-bearing age group may be pregnant and they should also be given the warning "don't take if you're pregnant."
- Avoid the use of drugs, in general, at any state of pregnancy.
- Increase the reliance upon nondrug modalities as treatment alternatives.

For example, the first approach to nausea and vomiting should be small, frequent meals and avoiding foods, smells, or situations that lead to vomiting (47). Next, an effervescent glucose or buffered carbohydrate solution may be effective. Only if these are ineffective should an antihistamine or antiemetic be considered. Refer the patient to a physician for certain problems that carry increased risk of poor outcomes in pregnancy (vaginal bleeding, urinary tract infections, rapid weight gain, and edema).

The pharmacist can aid the self-medicating woman in the decision as to which drug or nondrug modalities to consider as well as when self-medication may be harmful to the mother or her unborn child.

Summary

Nonprescription drugs are an important component of the health care system. Properly used, these products can help relieve minor physical complaints of patients and permit physicians to concentrate their time on more serious illnesses.

Improperly used nonprescription drugs can create a multitude of problems. Many people diagnose their own symptoms, prescribe their own nonprescription product, and monitor their own therapeutic response. As pharmacists continue to expand their patient counseling services, and patients learn of this expertise that is available to them, they will begin to seek the assistance of the pharmacist whenever they are in doubt.

To be of the greatest service to the patient, pharmacists must continually update their therapeutic knowledge as well as their interpersonal communication skills. The benefit will be a healthier patient who will utilize the professional services and recognize the contributions of the pharmacist to patient health care.

References

1. D. Mechanic, "Medical Sociology, A Selective View," Free Press, University of Wisconsin, Madison, Wisc., 1968.
2. M. C. Inhorn, *Drug Topics, 125,* 27 (1981).
3. D. A. Knapp and R. S. Beardsley, *Am. Pharm., NS19* (1979).
4. D. E. Knapp, P. D. Oeltien, and D. A. Knapp, *Med. Market. Media, 10,* 28 (1975).
5. *J. NARD, 10,* 22–23 (1980).
6. Schering report, 1979.
7. T. R. Covington, presentation at 120th Annual Meeting of the American Pharmaceutical Association, Academy of General Practice, Boston, Mass., July 23, 1973.
8. B. J. Andrew, *Am. J. Pharm. Ed., 37,* 290 (1973).
9. B. M. Korsch, E. K. Gozzi, and V. Francis, *Pediatrics, 42,* 855 (1968).

10. V. Francis, B. M. Korsch, and M. J. Morris, *N. Engl. J. Med.,* *280*, 535 (1969).
11. P. W. Keys, and M. J. Manolios, *Drug Intell. Clin. Pharm., 32,* 828 (1975).
12. P. L. Ranelli, *Soc. Sci. Med., 13A,* 733 (1979).
13. M. R. DiMatteo, A. Taranta, H. S. Friedman et al., *Med. Care, 18,* 376 (1980).
14. G. Chermak and M. Jinks, *Drug Intell. Clin. Pharm., 15,* 377 (1981).
15. D. L. Smith, "Medication Guide for Patient Counseling," Lea and Febiger, Philadelphia, Pa., 1977, pp. 1–25.
16. R. E. Vestal, *Drugs, 16,* 358 (1978).
17. D. P. Richey and A. D. Bender, *Ann. Rev. Pharmacol. Toxicol., 17,* 49 (1977).
18. P. P. Lamy and R. E. Vestal, *Hosp. Prac., 11,* 111 (1976).
19. P. O. Morselli, *Clin. Pharmacokinet., 1,* 81 (1976).
20. G. Udkow, *Am. J. Dis. Child., 132,* 1025 (1978).
21. A. Rane and J. T. Wilson, *Clin. Pharmacokinet., 1,* 2 (1976).
22. F. L. Willington, *Geriatrics, 35,* 41 (1980).
23. T. H. Shepard, *Curr. Prob. Ped., 10,* 5 (1979).
24. D. P. Hays, *Drug Intell. Clin. Pharm., 15,* 444 (1981).
25. *Federal Register, 44,* 37434 (1980).
26. *Federal Register, 45,* 32550 (1980).
27. J. F. Tourville, *Hosp. Pharm., 12,* 386 (1977).
28. L. Millcovich and B. J. VanDenBerg, *Am. J. Obstet. Gynecol., 125,* 244 (1976).
29. D. P. Hays, *Drug Intell. Clin. Pharm., 15,* 542 (1981).
30. P. L. Doering and R. B. Stewart, *J. Am. Med. Assoc., 239,* 843 (1978).
31. W. A. Blyer, W. Y. W. Au, W. A. Lange et al., *J. Am. Med. Assoc., 213,* 2046 (1970).
32. D. G. Corby, *Pediatrics, 62* (suppl), 930 (1978).
33. R. B. Lewis and J. D. Schulman, *Lancet, 2,* 1159 (1973).
34. E. Collins and G. Turner, *Lancet, 2,* 335 (1975).
35. W. A. Bleyer and R. T. Breckenridge, *J. Am. Med. Assoc., 213,* 2049 (1970).
36. R. R. Haslam, H. Ekert, and G. L. Gillam, *J. Ped., 84,* 556 (1974).
37. FDA EDRO Talk Paper, January 18, 1980.
38. J. E. Goyan, HHS news release, September 4, 1980.
39. *FDA Drug Bulletin, 11,* 19 (1980).
40. P. W. Weathersbee, L. K. Olsen, and J. R. Lodge, *Postgrad. Med., 62,* 64 (1977).
41. S. Linn, S. C. Schoenbaum, R. R. Monson et al., *N. Engl. J. Med., 306,* 141 (1982).
42. H. Jick, A. M. Walker, K. J. Rothman et al., *J. Am. Med. Assoc., 245,* 1329 (1981).
43. American Academy of Pediatrics Committee on Environmental Hazard, *Pediatrics, 57,* 411 (1976).
44. J. E. Fielding, *N. Engl. J. Med., 298,* 337 (1978).
45. S. K. Clarren and D. W. Smith, *N. Engl. J. Med., 298,* 1063 (1978).
46. S. E. Shaywitz, D. J. Cohen, and B. A. Shaywitz, *J. Ped., 96,* 978 (1980).
47. J. S. G. Biggs and J. A. Allan, *Drugs, 21,* 69 (1981).

3

Antacid Products

William R. Garnett

Questions to Ask the Patient

How long have you had this pain?

Where and when does the pain occur? Do you get the pain immediately after meals or several hours after meals?

Is the pain relieved by food? Do certain foods, coffee, or carbonated beverages make the pain worse?

Have you vomited blood or black material that looks like coffee grounds?

Have you noticed blood in the stool or have the stools been black or tarry?

What medicines are you currently taking?

Are you taking aspirin or aspirin-containing products? Do you smoke? How much? Do you drink alcoholic beverages? How much?

Have you used any antacids before to treat this pain? Which ones? Did they relieve the pain?

Are you on any special diet such as a low-salt diet?

Are you currently under a physician's care for other medical conditions?

Do you have any medical conditions such as diabetes, kidney, or heart disease?

Every year Americans spend one-quarter billion dollars on antacid products for the relief of upper GI distress (1). These products may be used without a prescription for short-term treatment of indigestion, excessive eating and drinking, heartburn, and for long-term treatment of chronic peptic ulcer disease. The pharmacist should be able to evaluate, on an individual patient basis, the need for a medical examination before antacid therapy and be able to select an antacid for either short-term or chronic use.

Anatomy of the Gastrointestinal System

The GI system can be divided into upper and lower regions. The esophagus, the stomach, the duodenum, the jejunum, and the ileum comprise the upper GI tract. Although peptic ulcer disease may occur at any site in the upper GI tract exposed to the digestive action of acid and pepsin, it usually affects the stomach and/or duodenum (2).

Esophagus

The esophagus conducts ingested materials from the mouth to the stomach. The esophagus is relaxed basally but contracts to deliver materials to the stomach. The

proximal part is composed of striated muscle. The distal portion is different physiologically and anatomically from the rest of the esophagus and is made up of smooth muscle (3, 4).

Following the ingestion and mastication of food, swallowing initiates a progressive wave of alternate contraction and relaxation (peristalsis) of the esophageal musculature to propel the contents to the stomach. Gravity, to a lesser extent, also promotes the delivery of food to the stomach. Liquids are conducted without peristalsis. A region of elevated intraluminal pressure exists approximately 2–5 cm above the gastroesophageal junction. This physiologic barrier, the lower esophageal sphincter (LES), results from tonic, but variable, constriction of the muscular esophageal wall (5). It is now recognized that the lower esophageal sphincter is the major determinant of competence of the gastroesophageal barrier (6). The lower esophageal sphincter is innervated by the autonomic nervous system and becomes relaxed after either beta-adrenoreceptor stimulation or cholinergic blockade. Thus, anticholinergics or drugs that stimulate beta-receptors may predispose individuals to episodes of gastroesophageal reflux.

The lower esophageal sphincter allows the passage of food into the stomach and prevents gastric contents from refluxing up into the esophagus. This is critical since resting pressure in the esophagus is lower than that in the stomach. It relaxes in the basal state and contracts with swallowing (7). The pressure can change in response to a number of stimuli. Gastrin and motilin increase pressure, and secretin, cholecystokinin, and glucagon decrease the pressure (8–12). Alcohol, smoking, and fatty foods decrease the lower esophageal sphincter pressure and increase the likelihood of reflux (13–15). However, many factors can influence the integrity of the lower esophageal sphincter, making reflux possible.

Stomach

The stomach is divided anatomically and functionally. Anatomically, the stomach consists of the cardia, the fundus, the body (corpus), and the antrum. Functionally, the stomach is divided into proximal and distal areas concerned with gastric emptying.

Each anatomical area has a different type of mucosa and contributes different secretions to the gastric juice. The cardia, consisting of cardiac mucosa, is the smallest area of the stomach, occupying only a 0.5–3.0-cm strip that begins at the esophagogastric sphincter. Little is known about the function of cardiac mucosa (16).

Gastric mucosa has a total surface area of about 900 sq m and contains surface mucous cells, mucous neck cells, argentaffin cells, parietal cells, and chief cells. It lines both the fundus and the body and is responsible for most of the components of gastric juice. The parietal cells secrete hydrochloric acid and intrinsic factor. The active proteolytic enzyme pepsin is formed from pepsinogen secreted from chief cells in the presence of hydrochloric acid. The mucosal cells of the epithelium protect the stomach from the acid-pepsin complex by releasing an alkaline mucous secretion (17). The pyloric mucosa and the surface mucous cells that line the antrum and the prepyloric canal secrete gastrin and a protective mucus.

The vagus nerve provides parasympathetic innervation to the stomach. The vagus fibers synapse with the intrinsic plexus and postganglionic fibers leading to the secretory glands and to muscle. However, only a small portion of the intrinsic plexus fibers, which are related to local reflexes, such as secretion, synapse with the vagus (18). Thus, vagotomy either by chemical or surgical means will not totally eliminate local reflexes.

Functionally, the proximal stomach (fundus) is responsible for the emptying of liquids, and the distal stomach (antrum) is responsible for the emptying of solids (19). A pacemaker in the greater curvature initiates peristaltic waves, and the resistance of the pyloric sphincter determines the gastric emptying rate (20).

Gastric Secretion

The stomach releases secretions at different rates depending on whether it is in the basal state or has been stimulated. The three phases of gastric secretion are cephalic, gastric, and intestinal. Initiated by food, they proceed simultaneously and continue for several hours. The cephalic and gastric phases are stimulatory and synergistic. The intestinal phase is weakly stimulatory but primarily provides negative feedback (21).

Cephalic Phase

Only small amounts of gastric secretions are produced during the fasting state in the healthy individual. However, the thought, smell, taste, chewing, and swallowing of food set off a parasympathetic response through the vagus nerve (the cephalic phase) (22). The precise site in the brain in which this occurs is uncertain since changes in acid secretion may be found when medullary, hypothalmic, limbic, or cortical areas of the brain are stimulated (23). The vagus nerve postsynaptic transmitter, acetylcholine (the "first messenger"), then stimulates the release of hydrochloric acid, pepsinogen, and gastrin (24). The exact method of stimulation is unknown but may involve activation of a second messenger such as cyclic adenosine $3':5'$-monophosphate (cyclic AMP) (25). Cyclic AMP in turn may activate a protein kinase that releases gastric secretions (26). Although it is thought that cholinergic receptors exist as well as histamine receptors (27), their exact relationship is unclear (23). Vagotomy or large doses of anticholinergics may block this phase.

Gastric Phase

The presence of food in the stomach stimulates secretion directly and indirectly (28). The physical presence of food distends the gastric mucosa and causes a direct release of gastric secretions that require no intermediate mechanisms. Amino acids and peptides found in protein also cause the release of gastrin, which is a major humoral mediator for acid and pepsinogen secretion (29). The direct and indirect processes are synergistic (16). The gastric phase is also mediated by cholinergic innervation.

Food stimulates the release of gastrin by mechanical distention of the antrum, by vagal stimulation, and by a direct action on the G-cells of the antrum and the duodenum (30). G-cells are specialized endocrine cells that contain gastrin and respond to chemical changes. They are shaped like a flask with a broad base and a narrow neck that extends to the mucosa surface. Gastrin release may also be stimulated by epinephrine and calcium, but this process requires amounts above physiologic concentrations (31). Gastrin release is inhibited by acid, secretin, glucagon, vasoactive intestinal peptide, gastric inhibitory peptide, and calcitonin (30, 31).

There are several gastrin molecules. They vary in molecular weight, site of release, and potency (32). "Little" gastrin is secreted by the antrum and is the most potent; "big" gastrin, which has a longer half-life, is released from the duodenum; and "big-big" gastrin is released from the jejunum (33). All gastrins stimulate the same receptor. The gastric mucosa makes no distinction between the gastrins and responds by secreting hydrochloric acid and pepsinogen (30). "Big-big" gastrin is believed to be responsible for basal acid secretion.

Gastrin mediates physiologic functions other than acid and pepsinogen release. It may protect the stomach from the proteolytic action of acid and pepsin by stimulating gastric mucosal cell proliferation (34) and by tightening the gastric mucosal cell barrier (35). There are conflicting reports about gastrin's effect on increasing lower esophageal sphincter tone (36, 37). Because its chemical structure resembles pancreozymin and cholecystokinin, gastrin increases pancreatic enzyme secretions, bile flow, and gastric and intestinal motility (16).

The mechanism by which gastrin mediates acid and pepsinogen release is unknown. Separate receptors for histamine and gastrin have been postulated, but a sequential process seems more likely (26). Gastrin may release histamine, which in turn may cause acid and pepsinogen release. Histamine receptors are classified as H_1 and H_2. H_2 receptors are responsible for acid release (38). Selective H_2 antihistamines are capable of blocking pentagastrin-mediated gastric secretion (39), suggesting that gastrin acts via histamine (40). Histamine may act by releasing cyclic AMP as a second messenger (41), which activates a protein kinase (26). The interrelationships among acetylcholine, gastrin, and histamine are unknown.

Intestinal Phase

The third phase of gastric secretion, the intestinal phase, involves both stimulation and inhibition. As long as chyme, or partly digested food, is in the intestine, there is continued gastric secretion. The mediators are "big" gastrin, cholecystokinin, and pancreozymin (21). Stimulation is weak, and the main function of the intestinal phase seems to be a negative feedback to further secretion.

Inhibition is mediated by an enterogastrone, which can be any substance secreted from the small intestine that inhibits gastric secretion. An enterogastrone may inhibit gastric secretion by direct inhibition of either acid and pepsinogen release, or gastrin, or both. Cholecystokinin, pancreozymin, and glucagon inhibit gastrin release (42, 43). Gastric inhibitory peptide has been isolated from cholecystokinin. At pharmacologic doses, it acts similarly to glucagon. There is some doubt as to what it does at physiologic doses (44). Secretin blocks acid secretion and inhibits glucagon release (45, 46). Vasoactive intestinal peptide can be extracted from the gastric mucosa and has pharmacologic effects similar to secretin (44). The stimulus for the release of enterogastrones is the presence of acid, fat, protein breakdown products, or hyperosmolar substances in the duodenum (22). Acid in the antrum also diminishes gastrin release (47).

Factors Influencing Gastric Secretion

The endogenous stimulants of gastric acid secretion are acetylcholine, gastrin, histamine, cyclic AMP, and protein kinase. The release of these endogenous substances is stimulated by exogenous substances. Amino acids and peptides are the main exogenous sources of stimuli. They are probably responsible for the increase in gastrin secretion after meals. While digested proteins stimulate acid production, they also buffer gastric contents to decrease the fall in pH (44). Although coffee is a stimulant for gastric secretion, this effect is primarily due to its amino acid and peptide components and not to the caffeine, which is a very weak stimulant to gastric secretion (48). Calcium also promotes gastric secretion

by stimulating gastrin release (49). Alcohol has a much greater gastric stimulatory effect in dogs than in humans (50).

In addition to the previously described enterogastrones, there are a number of factors that inhibit gastric secretion. A lowering of the pH in both the stomach and duodenum initiates responses that decrease gastric secretion. Acid inhibits the release of gastrin in the antrum (51) and releases enterogastrones in the duodenum. Fat, hypertonic solutions, and hyperglycemia also inhibit gastric secretion (52–55).

The amount of gastric acid secreted depends on the balance of the stimulatory and inhibitory factors.

Gastric Motility

The proximal stomach receives and stores ingested foods. By slow, sustained contractions, it releases its contents into the distal stomach, where peristaltic contractions mix the contents with gastric juice before allowing them to pass through the pyloric sphincter into the duodenum. The contraction rate is regulated by a pacemaker under vagal control (22).

Gastric emptying rate depends on the resistance of the pyloric sphincter, which is controlled by many stimuli (20). Hormones (secretin, cholecystokinin, and motilin), hyperosmolar solutions, acid solutions, and fats delay gastric emptying; gastric distention increases the emptying rate (56). Distention is the only factor known to stimulate gastric emptying (57).

The stomach is considered to be exposed to the outside environment; it receives anything capable of entering the mouth and passing down the esophagus. The stomach must respond to and act on agents that are hot or cold, acid or alkaline, polar or nonpolar, liquid or solid, digestible or nondigestible. Occasionally, the protective mechanisms fail to cope with these agents, and inflammation occurs in the form of acute or chronic upper GI distress (58).

Types of GI Disorders

Acute Upper GI Distress

Acute upper GI disorders develop very quickly but usually are self-limiting. They usually respond very quickly to symptomatic treatment with acid neutralization. With the exception of hemorrhagic gastritis, they are not usually life-threatening. Chronic acid suppression is not required for treatment.

Gastroesophageal Reflux

Gastroesophageal reflux is the retrograde flow of gastric or duodenal contents across the gastroesophageal junction into the esophagus. The effects depend on the mixture of gastric acid, pepsin, bile salts, and pancreatic enzymes refluxing onto the esophageal mucosa (4). Although gastroesophageal reflux may be asymptomatic (59), the most common patient complaint is retrosternal discomfort, which radiates upward and is aggravated in the recumbent position (4). Reflux esophagitis is also aggravated by obesity, tight garments about the abdomen, and pregnancy. The patient may refer to these symptoms as "heartburn," "indigestion," or "sour stomach." The regurgitation of fluid while sleeping or bending over is conclusive evidence of gastroesophageal reflux. Other less common symptoms include painful or difficult swallowing, hemorrhage, and pulmonary complaints (6). These may also represent more serious GI disorders including carcinomas. Although gastroesophageal reflux may exist simultaneously with a hiatal hernia, the terms are not synonymous. Gastroesophageal reflux and hiatal hernia are two separate clinical entities, and one has no effect on the other (6).

The exact explanation for gastroesophageal reflux is not known. There is general agreement that dysfunction of the lower esophageal sphincter is the cause of reflux (4). Symptoms have been associated with unexplained, inappropriate, and transient relaxation of the lower esophageal sphincter (60). However, there is no explanation for the lower esophageal sphincter dysfunction. Other factors that may be associated with reflux are disordered peristalsis and delayed gastric emptying (61, 62).

An appropriate history and prompt relief by acid neutralization usually indicate gastroesophageal reflux. Diagnostic testing may be necessary if cardiac, biliary, or gastroduodenal disorders are suspected. The techniques used to diagnose gastroesophageal reflux include barium esophagography with fluoroscopy, esophageal endoscopy, esophageal mucosal biopsy, esophageal manometry, acid perfusion test, esophageal pH monitoring, and gastroesophageal scintiscanning (4). Acid perfusion and esophageal biopsy are the most sensitive tests.

Treatment of gastroesophageal reflux is multifactoral. Although most pharmacologic therapy is aimed at improving the tone of the lower esophageal sphincter and/or neutralizing gastric acid, some very effective results can be obtained if the patient changes his or her life-style (6). Smoking, and the ingestion of fatty foods, coffee, and chocolate, which can decrease LES tone, should be discouraged. Individuals should eat slowly and not recline after meals. Carbonated beverages will also increase intragastric pressure and should be avoided. Perhaps the most effective treatment is to utilize gravity to diminish the gastroesophageal pressure gradient by elevating the head of the patient's bed with 6-inch (15-cm) blocks (63, 64). Weight loss is also successful in decreasing symptoms. Bethanechol and antacids have been used to increase competence of the lower esophageal sphincter. Alginic acid has been used to provide a physical barrier that will be neutral if refluxed, although there is controversy regarding efficacy of this agent (61). If nonpharmacologic measures and antacids or cimetidine are not effective, bethanechol or metoclopramide may be tried. However, bethanechol has the therapeutic disadvantage of increasing gastric acidity through its cholinergic action (65). Metoclopramide is reported to strengthen the lower esophageal sphincter and to increase the gastric emptying rate (64).

Gastritis

Gastritis implies an inflammation of the gastric mucosa. Acute gastritis has occurred after the ingestion of aspirin and alcohol, in uremia, following gastric freezing, during treatment with antitumor agents, during an infection, after ingestion of caustic substances, and as a complication of stress (67). The disease mechanism appears to be a break in the normal gastric mucosal barrier allowing hydrochloric acid to enter the mucosa, injure vessels, and cause inflammation, erosion, and hemorrhage (68). The lesions are usually superficial, but more severe lesions may develop (67).

The primary manifestation of gastritis is acute GI bleeding. Acute gastritis may account for as much as 30% of all GI bleeding episodes. Radiologic examination is of no use in acute gastritis. Diagnosis is best made by endogastroscopy (58).

The process is usually self-limiting and the bleeding stops spontaneously in 2–5 days if the initiating cause is removed. Patients require intensive antacids for a short period of time, but chronic therapy is not required. Occasionally, lavage or surgery may be required to stop the bleeding. If antacids fail to relieve the symptoms quickly, the possibility of a hiatal hernia or gallbladder disease should be considered (33).

Drug-Induced Ulceration

Alcohol, aspirin, caffeine, glucocorticosteroids, reserpine, colchicine, nonsteroidal anti-inflammatory agents, and tobacco smoke are often reported as being ulcerogenic. The amino acids and peptides in coffee stimulate gastric secretion (69). Coffee has a greater effect on stimulating gastric secretion and on lowering esophageal sphincter pressure than an equivalent amount of caffeine. Caffeine alone produces no change or only a slight decrease in LES pressure (70). Decaffeinated and instant coffee and whole coffee beans seem equipotent (71). Aspirin and alcohol cause breaks in the mucosal barrier, resulting in acute gastritis. Corticosteroids may prevent the manifestation of the symptoms of a peptic ulcer before perforation occurs. However, they do not cause peptic ulcer disease (72). Indomethacin causes inconsistent breaks, and the other drugs apparently are not involved (69). In evaluating drug-induced ulcers, it must be remembered that some diseases such as rheumatoid arthritis and systemic lupus erythematosus are associated with a higher incidence of ulcers even without drug therapy.

Stress Ulcer

Stress ulcers occur frequently in critically ill patients and in patients undergoing physical stress. They may be considered as a subclassification of hemorrhagic gastritis. Stress ulcers are acute ulcerations that occur mainly in the stomach but may also be found in the duodenum and esophagus. They are usually multiple, shallow, small, superficial erosions but may be associated with wider ulcers if there is bleeding. The destruction and scarring seen in peptic ulcers are lacking in stress ulcers. The real incidence is unknown, since many heal as rapidly as gastritis, but they may be the most common cause of upper GI bleeding (73). The cause is usually identifiable, and they have been associated with CNS lesions, trauma, burns (Curling's ulcer), sepsis, uremia, cerebrovascular accidents, surgery, and endocrine tumors producing gastrin (74).

Painless GI bleeding is the major, and often only, clinical manifestation of stress ulceration. There is usually a delay between the development of lesions and overt hemorrhage. There may be signs of subtle blood loss, such as guaiac-positive stools, nasogastric aspirates, and a decreasing hemoglobin and hematocrit before the patient develops the signs of hemorrhagic shock. Lesions begin in the body and fundus but can progress to the antrum and duodenum. The primary method of diagnosing stress ulcerations is gastroduodenoscopy (75).

The mechanism of stress ulcers seems to depend on an interaction among acid, changes in mucosal circulation, excretion of glycoproteins in the mucus, and mitotic rate of mucosal stomach lining. Mucosal ischemia seems to be the ultimate mediator of stress ulcers (76). Cold, starvation, increased acidity, bile reflux, adrenalectomy, and hemorrhage favor ulceration. Vagotomy, anticholinergics, antacids, elemental diets, vitamin A, prevention of bile reflux, epinephrine, norepinephrine, serotonin antagonists, and immediate replacement of blood loss are inhibiting factors (77). The major treatment is removing the precipitating event; long-term antacid therapy is rarely required.

Prophylaxis of stress ulceration can be achieved by neutralization of gastric acid by frequent administration of antacids (every hour) through a nasogastric tube. One study showed that antacids offered consistent protection against gastric acidity and prevented significant gastrointestinal bleeding in critically ill patients (78).

Chronic Upper GI Distress

Chronic Gastritis

Chronic gastritis refers to a variety of gastric lesions that persist over long periods of time. There is a variation in effect on gastric function. In chronic superficial gastritis gastric secretion remains normal. In atrophic gastritis there is a variable loss of function, and in gastric atrophy there is a complete loss of gastric glands.

Indirect evidence tends to corroborate the suggestion that there is a strong correlation between chronic gastritis and smoking. However, it is still not known whether smoking per se is a definite cause of chronic gastritis. In addition, it has long been suspected that inheritance plays a role in the pathogenesis of chronic gastritis, because pernicious anemia, a disease associated with atrophic gastritis, tends to run in families.

There are no specific symptoms associated with chronic gastritis. There may be bleeding and there may be symptoms that correspond with deficiencies in secretion (cyanocobalamin deficiency due to deficient intrinsic factor). Although diagnosis can be made by endoscopy in severe cases, it is best made by performing multiple biopsies.

Although it is suggested that repeated attacks of acute gastritis can lead to chronic gastritis, no firm data substantiate this. An association with bile salt reflux and atrophic gastritis has been made.

Management of chronic gastritis primarily involves treating pernicious anemia if it develops and monitoring for occult blood (67).

Peptic Ulcer Disease

Peptic ulcers are chronic but may have acute exacerbations. They are most often solitary and occur at any level of the GI tract exposed to the proteolytic action of acid and pepsin. They are truly peptic. If acid and pepsin are diverted from an established ulcer, the ulcer will heal and not recur (79). In decreasing order of incidence, they occur in the duodenum, stomach (gastric), esophagus, stoma of a gastroenterostomy, Meckel's diverticulum, and jejunum (2). However, the most significant sites of peptic ulcer disease are the duodenum and stomach. Peptic ulcers are caused by an increase in acid and pepsin, a decrease in the mucosal resistance, or a combination of the two (79). Chronic peptic ulcers differ from acute gastritis or stress ulcers by the presence of fibrosis in the ulcer wall. They tend to be deep, burrowing through the mucosa and submucosa to the muscularis (80). Although they are often considered together, duodenal and gastric ulcers have different symptoms and etiologies. However, both types may be induced by acid and pepsin stimulation (81).

Before World War I, gastric ulcers were more common, but today, duodenal ulcers predominate (82). The incidence of both types seems to have peaked and is on the decline (83). Men have a higher incidence of the disease than women, but the predominance is decreasing (84).

Although there is a decline in the overall incidence of peptic ulcer disease, there has been an increase in the percentage of patients over the age of 60 who have been hospitalized for both gastric and duodenal ulcer disease (85). Ulcers may recur even after surgical removal of the diseased tissue (86). Both types have a low mortality but may cause morbidity. The disease does not occur in primitive tribes or lower primates until they live in conditions of "civilization."

Gastric Ulcer

Approximately 600,000 persons experience gastric ulceration each year (87). Gastric ulcers occur most often as single lesions along the lesser curvature and adjacent posterior wall of the antrum up to within 4–5 cm of the pyloric sphincter (Figure 1). They may occur occasionally in the cardia, pyloric canal, and greater curvature of the body and fundus (80). Hyperacidity is a less frequent observation in gastric ulcers than in duodenal ulcers. Gastric ulcer patients may have low or normal acid secretion. However, there are local mucosal pH differences in the stomach and duodenum, and most gastric ulcers occur in areas adjacent to acid-secreting mucosa where the local pH is more acidic (88). Primary gastric ulcers are characterized by low-acid secretion, whereas gastric ulcers secondary to duodenal ulcers are characterized by hypersecretion (89). Acid seems more important in determining where, rather than when, a gastric ulcer will occur, so that lesser curvature ulcers are frequently associated with diminished acid production. Gastric ulcers associated with duodenal ulcers are frequently associated with normal acid production and prepyloric gastric ulcers are often associated with increased acid production.

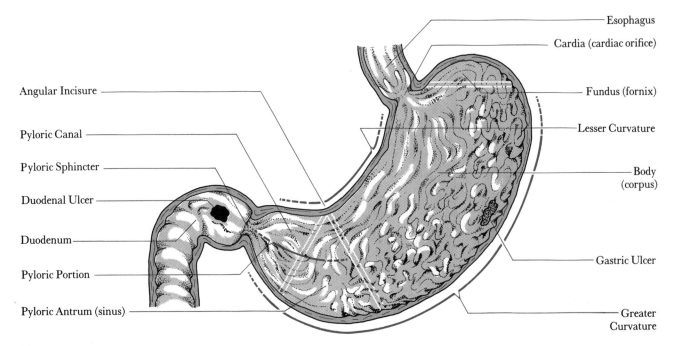

Figure 1. Sites of duodenal and gastric ulcers. Adapted from F. H. Netter, *The Ciba Collection of Medical Illustrations*, Ciba Pharmaceutical Company, New York, N.Y., 1962, p. 49, 52. Vol. 3, Part II.

Etiology   Several theories have been proposed for the etiology of gastric ulcer disease (79, 87, 89–92). Among these are delayed gastric emptying and distention accompanied by increased gastric secretions (93). Although this hypothesis is based on experimental and clinical observations, there are reasons to question its accuracy since some patients with gastric ulcers have normal gastric emptying times and low-acid secretion in the presence of high-gastrin levels (90).

Many gastric ulcer patients have chronic gastritis, which may damage the mucosa and make it more susceptible to peptic ulceration. However, gastritis may persist after the ulcer heals (91). Chronic gastritis may increase back diffusion of hydrogen ions that break down the gastric mucosal barrier; this process may continue even after resolution of the ulcer (35).

One theory holds that reflux of duodenal contents, especially bile acids, is due to pyloric sphincter dysfunction (94). Smoking, which is associated with an increased incidence of gastric ulcer, induces duodenogastric reflux (95). Bed rest improves ulcer healing and decreases reflux (96). Hypergastrinemia occurs in gastric ulcer patients, and gastrin has been reported to inhibit the pyloric sphincter (97). Pyloric sphincter dysfunction has been shown in patients with gastric ulcer, whereas control subjects and duodenal ulcer patients have normal pyloric sphincter pressure (98, 99). A reflux of bile salts may cause gastritis in the distal portion of the stomach and a break in the mucosal barrier. The damaged mucosa next to the acid-secreting mucosa is more susceptible to ulceration. Bile salts occur more frequently and in higher concentrations in the stomachs of gastric ulcer patients than in normal persons or patients

with duodenal ulcers (94). As attractive as this theory is, reflux has not been shown to precede either gastritis or gastric ulceration (100).

Gastric ulcers may result from an abnormality in the gastric mucosa. Normally, there is a relatively impermeable barrier called the gastric mucosal barrier that prevents the back diffusion of certain ions. If the barrier is impaired and allows the back diffusion of hydrogen ions, bleeding and ulceration could occur (92).

Other factors may be involved. A genetic factor is implied by the association of gastric ulcer in patients with blood group type O and nonsecretor status (101). Smoking is associated with both gastric and duodenal ulcer. The use of aspirin on 4 or more days/week for at least 3 months is associated with a higher incidence of gastric but not duodenal ulcer (75). Unknown environmental factors may cause ulcers, or the disease may be a heterogeneous group of disorders that requires the interrelation of several factors in a predisposed individual.

Symptoms   Although gastric mucosal erosion may be asymptomatic, the most common complaints are pain and GI bleeding. Gastric ulcer pain occurs within 30–60 minutes after eating and lasts 60–90 minutes. The pain may be described as "aching," "nagging," "cramplike," or "dull." Its relationship to food intake results from distention of inflamed areas and acid release. The patient may associate the pain with eating and may stop eating, with resultant weight loss. Rhythm or chronicity associated with the pain is rare, and the pain covers a wide area of the midepigastrium. Somatic pain radiating into the back indicates penetration, perforation, or obstruction. These three conditions constitute a medical emergency and referral is indicated. If there is GI bleeding, the vomitus or stool may contain blood (the stool is black and tarry). Nausea, bloating, anorexia, vomiting, and weight loss may also occur.

Diagnosis Five to ten percent of gastric ulcers are carcinomas of the stomach; therefore definitive diagnosis is needed for chronic or recurring symptoms. Bleeding, either acute or chronic, requires medical evaluation. Although a patient history is helpful, it is not as definitive for gastric ulcers as it is for duodenal ulcers. Physical examination rarely helps to locate the ulcer. Definitive gastric ulcer diagnosis is made by gastroscopy, X-ray with radiopaque contrast media, gastric analysis for acid and cytogenic cells, and testing for blood (occult or frank) in the feces.

The mortality from nonmalignant gastric ulcers is low, but the morbidity is high. The most frequent complications are bleeding and perforation (87). Gastric ulcers are less responsive to medical management than duodenal ulcers and require surgery more often.

Duodenal Ulcer

About 2,400,000 people experience symptoms of duodenal ulcer each year. Of these, an estimated 200,000 are new cases (102). Duodenal ulcers are mucosal lesions in the anterior wall of the duodenum's proximal end just beyond the pyloric channel through which gastric contents enter the duodenum (Figure 1). Ulcers also may occur distal to the duodenal bulb or spread back into the pyloric channel or antrum. These ulcers may recur frequently or infrequently, hence the term "duodenal ulcer diathesis" (103). Duodenal ulcer is caused by excessive acid and pepsin (89). The role of mucosal resistance has been incompletely evaluated (90).

Etiology Several abnormalities may explain increased acid and pepsin delivery from the stomach to the duodenum (89–92). There may be an increased capacity to secrete due to a large parietal cell mass, an increased response to agents that normally stimulate secretion, an increased vagal or hormonal drive to secrete, a defective inhibition to secretion, or an increased gastric emptying rate (104–108). Conflicting data exist for each of these theories and there is question as to whether they should be evaluated using maximal secretory capacity or physiologic secretory rates (109). There seems to be less supporting data for an increased vagal or gastrin stimulus to secrete and an impaired feedback (109, 110).

Other factors may be interrelated. Familial or genetic influence is evidenced by the three-fold increase in the incidence of duodenal ulcer in first-degree or primary relatives of patients with duodenal ulcer (111). In addition, there is a higher concordance in monozygotic than dizygotic twins, and a greater incidence in those with type O blood who are nonsecretors of blood group substances (90). Persons with elevated plasma pepsinogen I are eight times more likely to experience duodenal ulceration (112). Persons who smoke cigarettes are twice as likely to have duodenal ulceration (113). With regard to smoking, this difference may be due to a nicotine-induced decrease in pancreatic bicarbonate secretion, allowing a lower duodenal pH (114). Emotional and psychological factors are believed to contribute to the disease but have never been documented (84). Patients with other diseases such as arthritis, chronic pancreatitis, chronic pulmonary disease, hyperthyroidism, and cirrhosis also seem to have an increased incidence of duodenal ulcers (115). It has been suggested that duodenal ulcer disease represents a mixture of disorders with different etiologies but a common pathologic expression (116).

Symptoms As in gastric ulcer, the primary symptoms of duodenal ulcer are pain and GI bleeding. However, key differences occur in the way the patient describes the symptoms (117). Duodenal ulcer pain is rhythmical, periodic, and chronic. The rhythmical nature corresponds to the release of gastric acid. The pain usually begins 2–3 hours after meals and may continue until the next meal. It occurs when the stomach is empty and is relieved by food. The sensation is described as gnawing, burning, pressing, aching, or resembling hunger pain. The patient is often awakened at night by the pain. It is usually located in an area in the midepigastrium between the xiphoid and the umbilicus that the patient can indicate with one finger. Typically the pain does not radiate. The pain is prone to exacerbation and remission with or without therapy. Exacerbations are most common in the spring and fall and may last for days or months (103).

If there is bleeding, stool color and consistency may change. The stools become black and tarry because of the blood (melena). Other GI symptoms include retrosternal burning, alteration in bowel habits, and rarely, nausea and vomiting. The patient's appetite is good; frequently, weight gain results from the increased food intake to allay pain (115).

The major complications of duodenal ulcer are bleeding, perforation, and obstruction. The bleeding may cause anemia, iron deficiency, and hypotension. Iron deficiency anemia is characterized by weakness, easy fatiguability, tachycardia, and dyspnea on exertion. More specifically, inflammation of the tongue (glossitis), brittleness and deformity of the nails (koilonychia), inflammation of the corners of the mouth, and stomatitis can also occur. Perforation and obstruction are indications for acute surgical intervention and are manifested by acute changes in symptoms. Perforation is accompanied by a sudden, severe, generalized abdominal pain, prostration, abdominal rigidity, and pneumoperitoneum (air or gas in the abdominal cavity). Vomiting is the most common symptom of gastric outlet obstruction (103).

Diagnosis A good patient history is essential in recognizing duodenal ulcer. As in gastric ulcer, physical assessment helps localize the site of pain but does little to make the diagnosis. Definitive diagnosis is made by X-ray following ingestion of radiocontrast media and by duodenoscopy. Endoscopy of either the stomach or the duodenum involves passing fiberscopes down the upper GI tract and is the most sensitive method of detecting ulcers (119, 120).

Patient Assessment

The most valuable service that the pharmacist can provide in consulting with a patient is to help the patient decide whether the ailment is amenable to self-therapy or requires medical attention. In upper GI complaints, only acute gastritis without bleeding and gastroesophageal reflux should be treated without medical intervention. Careful patient interviewing is the only method for the pharmacist to evelute the type, severity, and duration of patient complaint.

When recommending an antacid, the pharmacist should ascertain that the complaint is acute in onset and can be related to overeating, dietary indiscretion, alcohol consumption, or tension. If the pain is acute but suggestive of perforation, the patient should be referred. If the pain is chronic or resembles ulcer disease, the patient should have endoscopic evaluation (4) because symptoms of more serious diseases, such as hiatal hernia, ulcerating gastric carcinoma, duodenal neoplasm, pancreatitis, coronary artery disease, pancreatic carcinoma, and radiating pleuritic chest pain, may mimic ulcer pain (115, 119). Patients returning frequently with complaints of acute gastritis should receive a medical examination because repeated gastritis may be associated with gastric ulcer. Chronic gastroesophageal reflux should also be medically evaluated. If relief is not obtained promptly and sustained, the pharmacist should refer the patient to a physician for evaluation.

The pharmacist should look for patient symptoms suggesting bleeding, vomiting, or obstruction that are life threatening and require immediate medical evaluation. Bleeding may be suspected in a patient complaining of black tarry stools or "coffee ground" vomitus. A blood loss of 50–100 ml will result in black tarry stools, whereas a blood loss of 500 ml will result in systemic symptoms of anemia. Prolonged vomiting may lead to fluid and electrolyte abnormalities. If perforation or obstruction is suspected, the patient should be referred for surgical evaluation.

Treatment

Antacids are useful in the treatment of acute and chronic upper GI disorders. In addition, they may be useful in the prophylaxis of GI bleeding, stress ulcers, and aspiration pneumonitis. Ulcer treatment is unique in that nonprescription medications are a mainstay in its medical management. A patient may find that the physician alters only the dose or dosing interval. In addition to the use of antacids, careful dietary habits, H_2-receptor antagonists, sucralfate, anticholinergics, rest, removal from a stressful environment, and discontinuing smoking or alcohol ingestion may prevent the need for surgery.

Antacids

Antacids have been used in the treatment of GI distress for more than 2,000 years, but until the modern era of intensive antacid therapy, their use was mainly empirical and subjective (121). Only recently have the actions of antacids been evaluated closely and objectively.

Pharmacology

Antacids are compounds that raise the pH of gastric contents. Most are not classical alkalis in that they do not contain the OH radical (122). The primary action of antacids is to neutralize gastric acid, resulting in an increase in the pH in the stomach and duodenal bulb (123). They do not neutralize all of the stomach acid, nor do they bring the pH to 7.0. At a pH of 2.3, 90% of the acid has been neutralized, and at a pH of 3.3, 99% has been neutralized (124). Since the optimal proteolytic range of pepsin is at a pH of 1.5–2.5, raising the pH inhibits the action of pepsin with resultant progressive proteolytic neutralization. Above the pH of 4.0, pepsin activity is completely inhibited (125). The main antipepsin effect of antacids is attributed to altered pH. A secondary effect may be the adsorption of pepsin by the antacid; however, this is controversial (126–128). Antacids containing aluminum are more likely to adsorb pepsin (122).

In one study, aluminum hydroxide-magnesium hydroxide gel was shown to increase the volume of postprandial acid secretion primarily in the 2–4-hour period immediately following meals. However, more than one-half of the acid secreted was neutralized, leading to a marked decrease in the net gastric acid. Neutralization was incomplete because of the formation of aluminum trichloride. Antacids did not modify the rate of postprandial gastric emptying, but increased the dilution of gastric contents expanding the intragastric volume (129).

Antacids do not coat the mucosal lining (130). A possible protective effect is the tightening of the mucosal barrier (131). Antacids increase the lower esophageal sphincter tone, and this action may be responsible for their effectiveness in esophageal reflux (heartburn) (132, 133). Raising intragastric pH leads to elevated serum gastrin levels and may explain the antacid effect on the gastric mucosa and lower esophageal sphincter (134). The effect of antacids on gastrin release is not uniform (134). Calcium-containing antacids have the greatest effect. Many factors including alkalization, distention, vagal mechanism, and hypercalcemia are thought to be involved (135). Of the cations in antacids, only aluminum seems to delay gastric emptying time in animals (136). In humans, this effect is related to the concentration of aluminum in solution in the stomach (137). Aluminum hydroxide binds bile acids more strongly than magnesium hydroxide or aluminum phosphate (138). The potential therapeutic benefit that may result from the binding of bile salts by antacids has not been studied, but it may be useful in gastric ulcers where a reflux of bile salts has been seen.

The ideal antacid should be:

- **Efficient**—Only small amounts of the drug should be required to control large amounts of gastric acid.
- **Effective**—The drug should exert a prolonged effect without a secondary increase in gastric secretion and should be void of carbon dioxide release after reacting with hydrochloride.
- **Safe**—It should not interfere with electrolyte balance or blood glucose, or cause diarrhea or constipation

when administered in therapeutic amounts. It should not interfere with absorption or excretion of other drugs the patient may be taking.

- **Inexpensive**—Treatment with the drug may be prolonged.
- **Palatable.**

All antacid products contain at least one of the four primary neutralizing ingredients: sodium bicarbonate, calcium carbonate, aluminum salts, and magnesium salts.

Sodium Bicarbonate Sodium bicarbonate is a potent, rapid-acting, effective antacid of short duration for relief of symptoms of occasional overeating or indigestion. It reacts with gastric acid to form sodium chloride, water, and carbon dioxide. The loss of carbon dioxide makes the reaction irreversible. Ingestion of sodium bicarbonate results in a base excess equivalent to the amount ingested because sodium chloride will not react with carbonate, phosphate, or hydroxide ions in the GI tract (139). It is contraindicated for chronic or prolonged therapy, since large doses or prolonged therapy may lead to sodium overload or systemic alkalosis (124).

Each gram of sodium bicarbonate contains 12 mEq of sodium. This high quantity may cause problems for individuals on low-salt diets, patients receiving diuretic therapy, pregnant patients, or those with a tendency toward fluid overload. The suggested daily maximum intake is 200 mEq of sodium bicarbonate for patients under 60 years old and 100 mEq for those 60 years old and over (140).

Since the bicarbonate ion is readily absorbable, it can cause systemic alkalosis. Chronic administration with milk or calcium leads to an increase in calcium absorption and may precipitate the milk-alkali syndrome (141, 142), a possibility enhanced by a salt-losing nephropathy (143). The syndrome is characterized by hypercalcemia, renal insufficiency, and metabolic alkalosis; it improves when the antacid and calcium are discontinued (144). Symptoms include nausea, vomiting, headache, mental confusion, and anorexia (145). This may be particularly important in pregnancy where milk or calcium intake is emphasized (146).

Gastric distension and flatulence leading to perforation may occur with effervescent sodium bicarbonate. A rebound gastric hypersecretion of acid has been postulated but has not been shown in humans, even with sodium bicarbonate doses of 4–8 g (147). Some commercial forms of sodium bicarbonate contain aspirin. Ingesting such products after heavy alcohol intake may lead to hematemesis and melena (148).

Calcium Carbonate Calcium carbonate exerts rapid, prolonged, and potent neutralization of gastric acid. It reacts with gastric acid to form carbon dioxide, water, and calcium chloride. However, the calcium chloride will react in the GI tract to form calcium carbonate or phosphate. Acid neutralization is reversible and systemic alkalosis is of a lesser magnitude than sodium bicarbonate (139). It may be used safely in small doses (0.5 g) for relief of occasional gastritis, but it is not recommended for chronic use. Constipation has been thought to be a limiting factor. A literature search indicated that calcium carbonate may not only be nonconstipating, but it may even occasionally act as a laxative. There is some evidence that the constipation seen in patients taking calcium carbonate for peptic ulcer disease may be caused by the ulcer rather than calcium (149). Although there has been much enthusiasm for calcium carbonate as the antacid of choice, the recognition of its systemic side effects has prompted a re-evaluation of the agent.

Calcium carbonate reacts with hydrochloric acid to form calcium chloride, which is highly soluble and available for absorption while in the stomach. The absorption is limited because about 90% of the calcium chloride is reconverted to insoluble calcium salts, mainly calcium carbonate, when it reaches the small intestine (150). However, enough calcium may be absorbed after several days of antacid ingestion to induce hypercalcemia, which in turn may induce neurologic symptoms, renal calculi, and decreased renal function (144, 151).

Although rare, the milk-alkali syndrome is more common with sodium bicarbonate, but it also occurs after calcium carbonate therapy. The risk of developing this syndrome is increased by prolonged administration of calcium carbonate or the concomitant administration of sodium bicarbonate and/or homogenized milk containing vitamin D. It is presumed that patients who absorb large amounts of calcium develop alkalosis because the net loss of hydrogen ions in the stomach is no longer balanced by the binding of bicarbonate ions in the upper small intestine by unabsorbed calcium. When marked hypercalcemia occurs, increased epigastric pain, nausea, vomiting, polyuria, alkalosis, and eventually azotemia may result. Patients with renal impairment or dehydration and electrolyte imbalance are predisposed to developing the milk-alkali syndrome.

Calcium carbonate may induce gastric hypersecretion, an action markedly enhanced by food (147, 152, 153). Gastric secretory volume and acidity were found to be greater after calcium carbonate ingestion than after aluminum hydroxide or food ingestion (154). In a study of 24 patients with chronic duodenal ulcer disease, 4–8 g of calcium carbonate induced gastric hypersecretion 3–5.5 hours after ingestion, whereas 30–60 ml of aluminum hydroxide or 4–8 g of sodium bicarbonate did not (147). This mechanism may be mediated by the calcium ion action in the GI tract.

To determine the effect of various antacids on gastric secretion, four equivalent neutralizing doses of calcium carbonate, sodium bicarbonate, and magnesium hydroxide were administered to 20 duodenal ulcer patients. The mean gastric output in the 60-minute period beginning 2 hours after the last dose of antacid and 30 minutes after the insertion of a nasogastric tube was twice as great with calcium carbonate as it was in the basal state or with the other antacids (155). Thus, calcium carbonate itself, rather than a nonspecific action of antacids, may be responsible for the effects.

Observance of increased gastric secretion after calcium infusion indicates that calcium may increase serum gastrin and that hypergastrinemia may be responsible for the hypersecretion (156). A dose as small as 0.5 g of calcium carbonate (the usual dose recommended as an antacid) may increase acid secretion in male subjects with or without duodenal ulcers (157). Although several theories have been presented to explain this acid rebound, it seems most likely that the mechanism is a local effect of calcium on the gastrin-producing cells (152).

Aluminum   Aluminum is administered most often as the hydroxide, but also may be given as the carbonate, phosphate, or aminoacetate. Of these, aluminum hydroxide has the greatest neutralizing capacity but still less than magnesium hydroxide, calcium carbonate, or sodium bicarbonate. Products that contain large quantities of anhydrous aluminum oxide react too slowly to be useful as antacids. After aluminum antacids interact with gastric acid to form $AlCl_3$, a series of chlorohydroxides is formed. This along with the formation of insoluble $AlPO_4$ reduces the anticipated neutralizing capacity to about 80% (139). Liquid preparations that lose their water content lose their neutralizing effect, and it cannot be regained by resuspending the dried powder in water (124). The drying procedure needed to convert the aluminum hydroxide gel into a powder or tablet alters the structure and results in a less reactive antacid (158).

The main side effect of aluminum antacids is constipation. Intestinal obstruction may occur in the elderly and in patients with decreased bowel motilities, dehydration, or fluid restrictions (124). Impaction may be increased by agents such as sodium polystyrene sulfonate resin (Kayexalate) (159). The constipative effect may be avoided by combining aluminum with magnesium salts or by administering laxatives and stool softeners.

It was thought that aluminum was not absorbed and did not cause systemic toxicity. However, several studies reported elevated serum or bone levels of aluminum in patients receiving chronic aluminum hydroxide therapy (160–162). Systemic aluminum toxicity was postulated after elevated aluminum levels were found in brain gray matter of uremic patients who died of a neurologic syndrome of unknown causes (163). These patients had taken aluminum hydroxide as a phosphate binder for 3 years or longer. Aluminum is known to be toxic to the nervous system, and an encephalopathy was reported in an aluminum flake powder factory worker (164–165). It was shown recently that aluminum is absorbed in small quantities and excreted readily in the urine (166). In patients with little or no renal function who chronically ingest aluminum salts, aluminum may accumulate and possibly be neurotoxic. The time needed for this side effect to appear is usually longer than the treatment time of either acute gastritis or peptic ulcer.

Aluminum binds with and decreases dietary phosphate absorption in the gut. This effect is useful in patients with chronic renal failure who have hyperphosphatemia, but it can cause phosphate depletion in others. Doses of 30 ml of aluminum hydroxide 3 times/day can have adverse effects on phosphate and calcium

metabolism (167). Hypophosphatemia is manifested by anorexia, malaise, and muscle weakness (124). Phosphate depletion causes release of calcium from bone with resulting hypercalciuria leading to osteomalacia and osteoporosis (168). Serum phosphate levels may need to be monitored bimonthly during chronic therapy with aluminum-containing antacids (169). The syndrome may occur as early as the second week of therapy and is complicated by a low-phosphate diet, diarrhea, or restoration of renal function after a renal transplant, and is particularly likely to occur in the elderly (170–173). Effects may be reversed by aluminum phosphate or by increasing phosphate in the diet, so that 300 mg of phosphate is excreted in the urine daily (168, 174).

Magnesium   The magnesium salts with antacid properties are the oxide, carbonate, hydroxide, and trisilicate. (Magnesium oxide is converted to hydroxide in water.) Of these, the hydroxide, carbonate, and oxide are the most potent.

Their potencies are somewhat greater than that of aluminum hydroxide but somewhat less than that of sodium bicarbonate and calcium carbonate.

Magnesium antacids react with gastric acid to form $MgCl_2$ and water (139). Magnesium forms insoluble salts that are responsible for its major side effect, which is osmotic diarrhea. This may cause systemic effects of fluid and electrolyte depletion (150). This side effect may lead to patient noncompliance; it may be minimized by using a combination of magnesium salts and aluminum salts. If this fails, alternating an aluminum-magnesium product with an aluminum product may be of benefit.

After hydrochloric acid is neutralized by magnesium salts, magnesium chloride is formed. It is partly absorbed and is rapidly eliminated by the kidneys; but in the presence of renal disease, magnesium may accumulate, causing hypermagnesemia (150). Hypermagnesemia is manifested by hypotension, nausea, vomiting, depressed reflexes, muscle paralysis, respiratory depression, and coma (175, 176). Significant increases in magnesium levels may be seen 3–5 days after starting therapy (177). This condition may be complicated by the administration of other magnesium-containing products and may occur after renal transplant (178).

Magnesium is a strong CNS depressant, and toxicity may cause severe cardiac depression leading to coma and death.

Manifestations of magnesium cardiotoxicity do not usually occur until there is severe hypermagnesemia (10–15 mEq/liter) in the presence of depressed renal function. However, junctional bradyarrhythmia occurred in a patient with chronic renal failure receiving 30 ml of a magnesium-aluminum combination antacid every 2 hours, although the patient's blood magnesium level never rose above 4.8 mEq/liter (179).

An infrequent side effect of magnesium trisilicate is the formation of renal stones. When this antacid is taken daily for long periods (several years), silica renal stones may develop (180–182).

Caution should be used if more than 50 mEq of magnesium is given daily to a patient with renal disease

(140). Magnesium should be avoided in patients with severe renal failure.

Magnesium-Aluminum Combinations The total neutralizing capacity of magnesium and aluminum combinations appear to be roughly equivalent to the sum of the capacities of its constituents, though the pH value at which buffering occurs may be altered (183). A mixture of magnesium and aluminum hydroxide gels is a less potent acid buffer than an equal volume of magnesium hydroxide if a pH higher than 4.5 is desired. However, if a pH less than 3.5 is desired, it is a more potent buffer. One report indicated that a mixture of aluminum hydroxycarbonate gel and magnesium hydroxide failed to meet the sum of the acid neutralization of each antacid (184). It has been hypothesized that the aluminum hydroxycarbonate forms a coating on the magnesium hydroxide due to electrostatic attraction. The coating reduces the neutralizing capacity of the magnesium hydroxide (184). Because of the presence of both salts, magnesium-aluminum combinations have the potential for any of the adverse effects of either agent. They may cause hypermagnesemia in patients with chronic renal failure, hypophosphatemia, or aluminum retention.

Magaldrate is a chemical entity of aluminum and magnesium hydroxides, not a physical mixture, and has a lower neutralizing capacity than a physical mixture (185). The magnesium and aluminum ions are balanced to prevent any alteration in bowel function, but diarrhea or constipation may occur. Diarrhea seems to be more common.

Additional Ingredients

Many ingredients are added to antacid preparations that have no basic antacid properties but give the preparation a degree of uniqueness and added basis for advertising claims.

Sugars Some antacid preparations contain considerable amounts of sugars and hexitols. When taken in large quantities or for an extended period of time, these ingredients could result in various clinical problems, especially in diabetes. Ingestion of large amounts of sugars and hexitols could complicate the control of diabetes. With prolonged use, tooth decay may also be accelerated.

Simethicone Simethicone, an inert silicon polymer, is a gastric defoaming agent. By reducing their surface tension, it causes gas bubbles to be broken or coalesced into a form that can be eliminated more easily by belching or passing flatus. It has no activity as an antacid. In a randomized, double-blind, placebo-controlled trial, statistically significant improvement in symptoms treated with simethicone was measured by patients and physicians (186). The FDA considers simethicone safe and effective (140). It is rational to administer simethicone for acute symptoms that have components related to gas, but there is no indication for chronic use of simethicone in peptic ulcer disease. In addition, one report indicated that simethicone's defoaming activity was greatly reduced when combined with aluminum hydroxide. The observed low activity suggested that the defoaming agent had been adsorbed onto the antacid, rendering both substances less available (187). The combination of simethicone with aluminum-containing antacids is questionable.

Oxethazaine Oxethazaine is a local anesthetic combined with antacids as a prescription antacid. It has been claimed to be more effective than an antacid alone since it is said to add to the action of the antacids by exerting an analgesic effect on the gastric mucosa (188). Carefully controlled trials have not proved increased efficacy over adequate doses of antacid for gastroesophageal reflux, acute gastritis, or peptic ulcer. Toxicity and absorption data have not been reported.

Because the combination of oxethazaine and antacid requires a prescription, physicians prescribe it for patients whose insurance will not pay for nonprescription drugs. The requirement of a prescription precludes recommendation by the pharmacist directly to patients.

Alginic Acid Some antacid products contain alginic acid with sodium bicarbonate and other antacid ingredients. In the presence of saliva in the buccal cavity, alginic acid reacts with sodium bicarbonate to form a highly viscous solution of sodium alginate. A tablet containing alginic acid is chewed and followed by a glass of water to wash the sodium alginate into the stomach, where it floats on top of the gastric contents. If there is esophageal reflux, the esophageal mucosa comes into contact with the sodium alginate rather than the acidic gastric contents (189). Alginic acid has been shown not to have any effect on the lower esophageal sphincter pressure and that its entire effect is due to its foaming, floating, and viscous properties (190). Although one study showed no effect (64), other studies have shown a decreased exposure of the esophagus to acid (189–194). Contact was decreased by 39% in one study (189). Effectiveness of the preparation in esophageal reflux depends on the patient's remaining in a vertical position (191–193). The patient should be instructed to sleep on pillows or to elevate the head of the bed with 15-cm blocks. The FDA considers the drug safe (140). Products containing alginic acid should be restricted to treatment of esophageal reflux and hiatal hernia and should not be used for acute gastritis or peptic ulcer disease. There is insufficient bicarbonate, aluminum hydroxide, or magnesium trisilicate in the commercial preparations containing alginic acid to buffer gastric acid effectively. Alginic acid is regarded as useful in mild to moderate symptomatic disease but is probably not adequate for patients with severe disease (61).

Bismuth Bismuth compounds have been used for gastric distress since the 1850's but have declined in popularity in recent years since they were shown to have little antacid activity (195). In addition, bismuth absorption from preparations such as the subgallate, subnitrate, or oxychloride leading to reversible encephalopathy has limited its use (196). There has been renewed interest in bismuth since the introduction in Europe of a new bismuth salt, tripotassium dicitratbismuthate, which is poorly soluble and insignificantly absorbed (197). This new stable colloidal complex acts by chelating protein and amino acids produced by necrotic ulcer tissue to form a protective layer at the site of the ulcer crater, thereby protecting the ulcer from acid-pepsin digestion (198). This is a different compound and mechanism of action from the bismuth salts available in the United States.

The effectiveness of the compound in the treatment of both duodenal and gastric ulceration has been verified by a number of endoscopically controlled studies of 4–6 weeks duration (199).

Colloidal bismuth is safe and is available in liquid form, but has the disadvantages of causing black stools and occasionally a black tongue and of having an unpleasant odor of ammonia.

Bismuth compounds, available in the United States, are being reviewed by the FDA advisory review panel on miscellaneous external analgesic drug products for various conditions such as overindulgence and intestinal distress. Though still under review by the FDA for treatment of intestinal distress and overindulgence, the bismuth compounds that are available in the United States are categorized as antacids and are not recognized as gastric mucosal protectants.

Evaluation   No commercially available product fulfills the criteria previously mentioned for an ideal antacid. Therefore, their evaluation must include the formulation, neutralizing capacity, sodium content, sugar content, intended use, palatability, and cost-effectiveness.

Formulation   Antacids are available as chewing gums, tablets, lozenges, powders, and liquids. Insoluble antacids depend on particle size for acid neutralization. A smaller particle size increases the surface area; the greater surface area increases the wettability and ease of mixing with gastric contents. Therefore, an increased surface area means an increased antacid effect. Many solid dosage forms must be masticated before they will disintegrate and react with acid in the stomach. Chewable antacid tablets must be chewed thoroughly before swallowing for the patient to receive the greatest therapeutic benefit. Liquid suspensions of antacids are milled to a fine particle size and provide a greater surface area. Tablet antacids are not equal to liquid antacids on a milligram-for-milligram basis (150). While in-vitro effects of liquid and tablet antacids have been described as equal, one in-vivo test showed that a chewable antacid tablet was inferior to a liquid suspension in neutralizing capacity (200, 201). Although equal neutralizing capacity can be obtained with tablets and liquids, the difference is in the extraordinarily large number of tablets needed to reach the desired neutralizing capacity (202). This difference may be due to the desiccation process used in manufacturing. Tablets that do not disintegrate may lodge in the bowel and cause obstruction (203). Powders must be suspended in water before ingestion. Liquids (suspensions) generally are easier to ingest and have a greater neutralizing capacity. Tablets should be

reserved for people who find liquids awkward or inconvenient and subsequently are noncompliant.

Potency   Several in-vitro comparisons showed that all antacids are not equally potent (179, 204–207). A 17-fold difference in acid-neutralizing capacity was found in commercial antacids following a standard test meal. This difference is even more pronounced with the new high-potency or concentrated antacids (208, 202). One test (the Fordtran test) correlated in-vivo potency with in-vitro potency and this has been used to compare the newer concentrated antacids (Table 1) and also tablet antacids (Table 2) (185, 202). The neutralizing capacity in independent tests are less than those capacities quoted by individual companies (209).

The FDA defines antacids in terms of minimal buffering capacity. To be called an antacid, the ingredient must contribute 25% of the total acid neutralization of the product. The product must neutralize at least 5 mEq of acid and must maintain a pH of 3.5 for 10 minutes in an in-vitro test.

The potencies listed in Tables 1 and 2 are the most clinically useful guidelines to antacid neutralizing capacity. Antacids that contain calcium carbonate and concentrated antacids are the most potent. However, as was previously discussed, calcium carbonate should be avoided for chronic intensive therapy. Aluminum-magnesium hydroxide gels generally offer adequate neutralizing capacity with the least toxicity potential. An initial attempt to correlate the FDA test to the Fordtran test used a limited number of antacids. The neutralizing capacity results for both tests were less than the values stated by the manufacturers. The modified FDA test closely approximated the data from the Fordtran test, but the modified FDA test was faster (210).

Efficacy

Gastroesophageal Reflux   As discussed, the treatment of gastroesophageal reflux includes bethanechol, metoclopramide, alginic acid, and acid neutralization. Adjunctive measures such as ingestion of small meals, exclusion of individual food intolerances and cigarette smoking, a low-fat diet, weight reduction, and avoidance of tight fitting garments are measures that can be taken to prevent gastroesophageal reflux. In addition, the elevation of the head of the bed increases the gravity factor or pressure gradient between the stomach and esophagus, thereby facilitating clearance of refluxed material and reducing the duration of reflux. According to one review, the mainstay of management of esophageal reflux has been antacid therapy. Antacids neutralize hydrogen ions present in gastric secretion, thereby reducing their concentration in the refluxed material (211). In addition to neutralizing gastric acid, antacids have been reported to increase the lower esophageal sphincter pressure (4), although this observation has not been confirmed (212). Antacids appear to be a logical treatment; however, much of the data on their effectiveness in gastroesophageal reflux is empiric (61).

In a recent double-blind, cross-over study of patients with scleroderma and reflux esophagitis, cimetidine was found to be superior to antacids in relief of heart-

Table 1. Various antacids listed in order of decreasing in-vitro neutralizing capacity

Antacid[a]	Capacity (mEq/ml)	Equivalent volume[b] (ml)
Maalox TC†	4.2	19.0
Mylanta II*	4.14	19.3
Delcid†	4.1	19.5
Titralac*	3.87	20.7
Mylanta II†	3.6	22.2
Camalox*	3.59	22.3
Gelusil II†	3.0	26.7
Basaljel ES†	2.9	27.6
Aludrox*	2.81	28.5
Maalox*	2.58	31.0
Creamalin*	2.57	31.1
Di-Gel*	2.45	32.7
Mylanta*	2.38	33.6
Silain-Gel*	2.31	34.6
Maalox Plus†	2.3	34.8
Marblen*	2.28	35.1
WinGel*	2.25	35.6
Riopan*	2.21	36.2
Gelusil†	2.2	36.4
Amphojel*	1.93	41.5
Riopan Plus†	1.8	44.4
A.M.T.*	1.79	44.7
Kolantyl Gel*	1.69	47.3
Trisogel*	1.65	48.5
Robalate*	1.13	70.8
Phosphaljel*	0.42	190.5

Adapted from J. S. Fordtran et al., *N. Engl. J. Med.*, *288*, 923 (1973), and D. Drake and D. Hollander, *Ann. Intern. Med.*, *94*, 215 (1981).

[a]For antacid components, see product table.

[b]Based on a desired 80mEq of neutralizing capacity. To determine the amount of antacid to use for a desired neutralizing capacity, divide the milliequivalents per milliliter capacity into the desired milliequivalents of antacid. For example, the neutralizing capacity of Maalox is 2.58 mEq/ml. To achieve 156 mEq of antacid activity, 60 ml of Maalox must be given; to achieve the same antacid potency using Trisogel, 94.5 ml must be given.

*A mEq of antacid is defined by the mEq of HCl that is required to keep antacid suspension at pH=3 for 2 hours in vitro (Fordtran).

†A mEq of antacid is defined by the mEq of HCl that is required to keep antacid suspension at pH=3 for 1 hour in vitro (Drake and Hollander).

burn and endoscopic improvement in the esophageal mucosa (213). This syndrome represents a chronic condition and suggests that antacids may give acute relief but no long-term benefit. Therefore, the use of H_2-receptor antagonists such as cimetidine may supplement or even replace antacids in the treatment of gastroesophageal reflux.

Acute Gastritis, Stress Ulceration, and GI Bleeding   The treatment goal for acute gastritis and stress ulceration is the prevention of GI bleeding (73). Although histamine H_2 antagonists, anticholinergics, vitamin A, steroids, and gastric lavage have been tried, there is no conclusive evidence of their efficacy, and acid neutralization with antacids is the treatment of choice (75).

In a placebo-controlled study, one group of patients was administered antacids hourly to maintain the gastric pH above 3.5. Findings revealed a significant decrease in the number of patients who experienced bleeding, compared with a control group (214). In another group, neither GI bleeding nor perforation could be demonstrated in patients treated with either antacids or cimetidine (215). Others have shown that fewer patients treated with cimetidine achieved the desired pH compared with those treated with antacids (216). One study found no treatment failures in 37 patients treated with antacids, but 7 of 38 cimetidine-treated patients developed GI bleeding (217). The findings suggest that the secretory rate and intracellular buffering capacity may be more important than the actual pH. Antacids have less effect on the secretory rate and do not affect mucosal buffering capacity and may be more useful in preventing GI bleeds than cimetidine. Nutritional supplementation may enhance the effects of antacids (218).

Peptic Ulcer Disease   Antacids have a long history of empiric use in the treatment of peptic ulcer disease. However, only in the last few years have antacids been tested for efficacy in peptic ulcer disease (219, 220). These trials have shown mixed results, possibly due to study design (221–225). In one study, statistically significant improvement in healing and pain relief was reported in patients with gastric ulcers treated with calcium carbonate tablets (221). However, other studies (222–224) using small doses of liquid antacids failed to

Table 2. Various tablet antacids listed in order of decreasing in-vitro neutralizing capacity

Antacids[a]	Acid neutralizing capacity	Dose equivalent in tablets[b]
Camalox	16.7	5
Basaljel	15.4	6
Mylanta II	11.0	8
Tums	10.5	8
Alka II	10.5	8
Riopan Plus	10.0	8
Titralac	9.5	9
Gelusil II	8.2	10
Rolaids	6.9	12
Maalox Plus	5.7	14
Digel	4.7	17
Amphojel	2.0	40

Adapted from D. Drake and D. Hollander, *Ann. Intern. Med.*, *94*, 215 (1981).

[a]For antacid components see product table.

[b]Based on a desired 80 mEq of neutralizing capacity. For method of calculation see Table 1.

show significant improvement when compared with placebo in either healing or pain relief for gastric or duodenal ulcers. A formulation identical to Mylanta II, a liquid antacid, but containing less simethicone, was given in seven divided doses [1 and 3 hours after each meal and at bedtime (30 ml/dose, 1,008 mEq/day)] for 28 days to patients with duodenal uclers (225). Patients showed significant improvement in ulcer healing but no difference in symptomatic relief compared with a placebo group.

There is agreement that intensive antacid therapy will promote healing of duodenal ulcer (225–228). Ulcer healing has no reliable association with pain relief (229). One study showed that antacids were significantly superior to placebo in relieving pain associated with duodenal ulcer (230). Although the placebo effect is very important (231, 232), it is rational to give something for pain relief. It has been suggested that asymptomatic patients with an ulcer may not need treatment (229).

Double-blind clinical studies using endoscopy to measure healing and pain relief in gastric ulcer are lacking. Although acid secretion is diminished in gastric ulcers, antacids will reduce the diffusion of acid into vulnerable areas (228). Though the evidence supporting the efficacy of antacids in the treatment of gastric ulcer is less clear than for duodenal ulcer (226, 227), clinical experience would support the use of antacids for gastric ulcer (228). There is no other FDA-approved medical therapy for gastric ulcers.

Studies proclaiming no benefits for antacids in peptic ulcer disease generally have been too sweeping in their conclusions. They have summarized all antacids in all forms and in any dose when only one antacid in one form and one dose was studied. Antacids continue to be the standard of practice. However, practitioners should consider higher doses than have been traditionally used and should constantly re-evaluate efficacy. Also, the placebo response should not be forgotten for both healing and pain relief.

Palatability   Patients frequently complain about the taste of antacids and are noncompliant. They should be questioned about palatability as a guide to compliance. The pharmacist should consider recommending to the physician that the patient be switched to another antacid if the patient develops a taste aversion to one particular product. Refrigerating the antacid may help improve the flavor. Care should be taken to avoid freezing suspensions. Freezing causes particles to become coarse and less reactive to acid, particularly magnesium hydroxide (233). Mylanta II has been the most accepted antacid in taste tests, although there is much individual variation (234, 235). The newer high-potency antacids allow ingestion of a smaller volume of antacid while still achieving the same amount of acid neutralization.

Dosage Recommendations

Dosage recommendations depend on intended use (acute or chronic), antacid neutralizing capacity, dosage interval, and temporal relationship to meals. Antacids ingested in the fasting state reduce acidity for only ap-

proximately 30 minutes. This short duration of action is caused by rapid gastric emptying of the antacid. On the other hand, antacids ingested 1 hour after meals reduce gastric acidity for at least 3 hours (236). The dose of liquid antacids is best expressed in terms of milliequivalents (mEq) of neutralizing capacity. As has already been discussed, equal volumes are not equipotent.

Gastroesophageal Reflux   The dosing for gastroesophageal reflux may be different than for other disorders especially if the gastroesophageal reflux is chronic. In acute incidences of gastroesophageal reflux 40–80 mEq of liquid antacid or 2–4 g of sodium bicarbonate or calcium carbonate is often effective. Acute incidences are usually self-limiting and will resolve spontaneously.

In chronic gastroesophageal reflux, more frequent treatment, ideally frequent daily dosing, is indicated. A noncalcium-containing antacid should be used, since hypercalcemia may result from long-term high-dose usage. It has been suggested that a dose be given immediately after each meal and repeated in 2 hours, and at bedtime (61). Because of patient intolerance, smaller, more frequent doses may be used (237). Although no studies have been done to document an effective dose, a dose of 80–160 mEq of antacids would seem appropriate. A lower dose may be used if adequate documentation is available to demonstrate that a patient is a hyposecretor of gastric acid, as may be found in many of these patients (238).

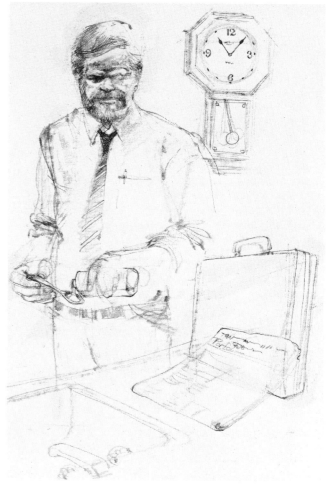

Prevention of Gastric Bleeding The treatment goal in the prophylaxis of GI bleeding is to keep the gastric pH above 3.5. Therapy may be started with 120 mEq of antacid and doubled every hour until the subsequent gastric aspirate has a pH greater than 3.5 (217).

Peptic Ulcer Disease Recommended regimens for antacids in peptic ulcer disease range from taking the antacid only when there is pain to taking as much antacid as can reasonably be tolerated (239). The latter protocol is favored because there are objective data to support it (225). Intensive antacid therapy for hospitalized patients who are not eating begins with 40 mEq/hour during waking hours for gastric ulcer patients and 80 mEq/hour for duodenal ulcer patients (150). These individuals should be closely monitored for side effects and adverse reactions.

Hourly dosing is neither practical nor necessary when the patient resumes eating. Food acts as a buffer to stomach acid for about 60 minutes, and then gastric acidity increases (240, 241). Antacids taken on an empty stomach have a duration of action of only 20–40 minutes (242). However, if they are taken 1 hour after meals, their duration of action is increased to up to 3 hours (185). For chronic therapy, antacids should be given 1 and 3 hours after meals and at bedtime.

Therapy should be continued for 6–8 weeks (243). The recommended dose is 80 mEq of antacid for gastric ulcer and 160 mEq of antacid for duodenal ulcer given 1 and 3 hours after meals and at bedtime (92, 244).

Other Therapy for Peptic Ulcer Disease

Diet

If food is withheld from the patient during the acute phase of a peptic ulcer, the main stimulus to acid secretion is removed. This will promote pain relief. For chronic treatment, bland diets or ulcer diets are ineffective in treating peptic ulcers (245). Conversely, there is no evidence that pepper or other spices are ulcerogenic (220). Milk increases gastric acid production and has no antacid properties. Therefore, diets that alternate milk and antacids have been or should be abandoned. Bland diets are monotonous, unpalatable, have a poor patient compliance, and are ineffective (246). Coffee (both caffeinated and decaffeinated), caffeine-containing beverages, such as cola, and alcohol are the only items that should be withheld from an ulcer patient. The patient should also be encouraged to stop smoking (245). Patients should be advised to have regular meals and to avoid irritants and foods known to cause symptoms.

Anticholinergics

Anticholinergics are prescription ingredients that have been used to reduce acid secretion and to prolong the duration of action of antacids. If they are used, the dose of both the antacid and the anticholinergic should be individualized; side effects from the anticholinergic may occur if it is administered in fixed combination with antacids. The FDA considers fixed-dose combinations of antacids and anticholinergics unsafe (140). Anticholinergic agents should not be administered simultaneously with antacids because antacids reduce absorption of anticholinergics.

Of the controlled clinical trials that have studied the use of anticholinergics in peptic ulcer disease, most have shown no significant benefit (220), although most of these studies were done before endoscopy was available. Not all anticholinergics have been shown to reduce gastric acid (248). The benefit from these drugs seldom justifies the side effects they cause. Recent evidence suggests that the side effects have been caused by excessive dosage. Though it is customary to dose to the precipitation of side effects, some studies have reported no difference in food-stimulated acid secretion after a 15-mg dose of propantheline compared with the accepted "optimal-effective dose" of 15–90 mg (249). The smaller dose would prevent many of the side effects. This dose also augmented the effect of cimetidine to reduce gastric acid. The main indications for anticholinergics in peptic ulcer disease are for duodenal ulcer patients who have persistent pain, especially nocturnal pain not responding to routine measures, patients whose ulcers fail to heal after an adequate trial of standard therapy, and for those with a high incidence of recurrence (250). This technique has been shown to accelerate healing of duodenal ulcer (251). Anticholinergics should be considered adjunctive therapy to antacids or H_2 antagonists and should not be used as the major basis of therapy.

H_2 Antagonists

The discovery of histamine H_2-receptors and the development of H_2-receptor antagonists have done much to explain gastric physiology. The presence of an ultimate mediator has been postulated by the ability of H_2 antagonists to block the release of gastric acid from multiple stimuli (vagal stimulation, gastrin, or calcium). Cimetidine, a prescription-only drug, is the only commercially available H_2 antagonist. It has been impressive in promoting healing in duodenal ulcer and looks promising for gastric ulcer (252). Cimetidine has produced healing rates in duodenal and gastric ulcers that are greater than placebos and comparable to antacids (253–255). The acid-reducing effects of cimetidine and antacids are equal (256). The combination of cimetidine and antacid delivers a more alkaline load to the duodenum (257). However, there is no evidence that combining antacid therapy with cimetidine will produce an additive or synergistic effect. In a multicenter study, patients receiving cimetidine 3 times/day before meals and at bedtime, combined with 15 ml of Mylanta II, 1 and 3 hours after meals, at bedtime, and as needed for pain showed no statistical differences in healing when compared with patients treated with cimetidine alone or antacid alone (258).

In addition, preliminary data obtained from nine patients with peptic ulcer disease indicate that the concomitant administration of an antacid suspension and cimetidine on a fasting stomach can lower the amount of cimetidine absorbed by a mean value of 22% (259). Cimetidine and antacids are equal therapeutically; however, they have markedly different side effects.

Cimetidine may be the treatment of choice to prevent aspirin-induced ulcers (260, 261), anastomotic ulcers after partial gastrectomy (262), and for chronic prophylaxis of duodenal ulcers (263).

Although cimetidine was originally thought to have very few side effects, significant side effects have been identified with more widespread use. The mental status changes are particularly significant (264) and are related to altered hepatic and renal function (265). Disturbingly, they often go unnoticed and untreated in geriatric patients (266). When severe, the mental confusion induced by cimetidine can be rapidly reversed by physostigmine (267). Discontinuing the drug will improve mental impairment within 48 hours (264). In most cases, antacids can be substituted. In those patients who require combined treatment with cimetidine and antacids, cimetidine can be restarted at half the previous dosage after mental status returns to normal (265). Further dosage adjustments are dependent upon continued surveillance of mental status and gastric pH. The more extensive use of cimetidine has also resulted in a number of drug interactions. It is believed that cimetidine is a microsomal enzyme inhibitor. Additional interactions may be anticipated.

Sucralfate

Sucralfate (Marion Laboratories) has been approved for use in the treatment of duodenal ulcer. Sucralfate binds directly to the ulcer crater to form a protective barrier that inhibits gastric acid and enhances healing. Sucralfate has a healing rate equivalent to that of cimetidine or antacid therapy.

Combination Therapy for Peptic Ulcer Disease

The benefit of combination therapy has been suggested (257, 249). One study demonstrated that intensive antacids plus one-half the dose of trimipramine or cimetidine gave comparable healing rates to full doses of trimipramine or cimetidine alone (268). The ideal combination therapy has not been evaluated in clinical trials. In one group of patients with inactive duodenal ulcers, the most convenient regimen was cimetidine, an anticholinergic, and antacids at the end of each meal (269). The most effective regimen was cimetidine with antacids 1 and 3 hours after meals. None of the combination regimens was more effective than cimetidine for decreasing nocturnal acid.

Miscellaneous

Drugs under investigation for the treatment of peptic ulcer disease include pirenzepine, carbenoxolone sodium, tripotassium dicitrate bismuthate, anisotropine methylbromide, anitidine, tiotidine, amylopectin, benzimidazole, prostaglandin E_2, trimipramine, sulpiride, and pepstatin (270–279). No comparisons to antacids or cimetidine can be made at this time.

Drug Interactions due to Antacids
General Mechanisms

The GI tract may be the site of clinically important drug interactions. Antacids may interfere with other drugs by forming insoluble complexes or altering GI absorption or renal elimination. Raising the gastric pH with antacids may alter disintegration, dissolution, solubility, ionization, and gastric emptying time of other drugs and as a result may either increase or decrease absorption (279, 280). Enteric coating dissolves more readily in an alkaline medium, exposing acid labile drugs to digestion and exposing the upper GI tract to irritating drugs. Weakly acidic drugs have a decreased absorption because ionization is increased. Conversely, weakly basic drugs are absorbed at a faster rate.

Weakly acidic drugs include isoniazid, pentobarbital, nalidixic acid, nitrofurantoin, penicillin, sulfonamides, and salicylates. Weakly basic drugs include pseudoephedrine. Antacids may bind or adsorb other drugs to their surfaces. Magnesium trisilicate and magnesium hydroxide have the greatest adsorption potential, calcium carbonate and aluminum hydroxide have an intermediate potential, and kaolin and bismuth have the least potential (281).

Antacid-induced changes in the urinary pH may alter drug elimination (282). Readily absorbed antacids such as sodium bicarbonate have the most pronounced effect. Studies in which various doses of commercial antacids were administered 4 times/day found that aluminum hydroxide and dihydroxyaluminum aminoacetate had no effect on urinary pH. Magnesium hydroxide and calcium carbonate suspensions raised urinary pH by 0.4 and 0.5 unit, respectively, and magnesium-aluminum hydroxide gel raised urinary pH by 0.9 unit (283). A follow-up study revealed that both 15 and 30 ml of magnesium-aluminum hydroxide gel increased the urinary pH significantly compared with the increase resulting from 5 ml of the antacid. However, the increase resulting from 30 ml was not significantly different from the increase resulting from 15 ml. The effect on the urine persisted for 1 day after the antacid was stopped (284). The effect of antacids does not change the circadian sine-wave nature of urinary pH but does shift it in a more alkaline direction (285). The effect is enough to enhance the excretion of acidic drugs and inhibit the excretion of basic drugs (282).

Significant Interactions

Tetracyclines exert their therapeutic effect by a bacteriostatic mechanism of action. Therefore, it is important that serum levels not fall below the minimum inhibitory concentration. Since antacids inhibit the absorption of tetracyclines by chelation with polyvalent cations (aluminum, calcium, and magnesium), clinical response to the antibiotic would be expected to vary depending on the extent of chelation (286). Antacids incapable of causing chelates (sodium bicarbonate) may also decrease absorption of tetracycline capsules by increasing gastric pH and thereby decreasing the dissolution rate (287). The effect is not based totally on raising the gastric pH, however (288). A 90% reduction in tetracycline absorption was demonstrated in one group of patients when given concomitantly with magnesium-aluminum hydroxide gel, but there was no decrease in absorption when tetracycline was given with cimetidine. Pharmacists should advise patients on appropriate spacing of doses of antacids when taken with tetracycline, calcium-containing foods such as milk, or iron supplements (289). If antacids are indicated they should be administered at least 3 hours after tetracycline administration. Likewise, iron salts should not be given with antacids because antacids decrease iron absorption (290).

Digoxin and digitoxin are adsorbed to antacids in vitro (291) and in vivo (292). Since variable bioavailability of cardiac glycerides is recognized as a factor in possible therapeutic failures with these drugs, pharmacists should advise patients on the proper spacing of doses when these drugs must be taken concurrently.

The administration of a magnesium trisilicate-aluminum hydroxide antacid caused a decrease in plasma chlorpromazine levels after oral administration (293). Decreased absorption may also occur when chlorpromazine is given with magnesium-aluminum hydroxide gel (294). Antacids and chlorpromazine should not be given concurrently. Dosing at alternate times may reduce the probability of this interaction.

Antacids do not alter quinidine absorption (295); however, since quinidine excretion varies inversely with urinary pH, a potentially dangerous interaction could result through alteration of urinary pH by antacids (296). In fact, a single case report documenting quinidine toxicity due to an alteration in urinary pH has appeared in the literature (296). Concurrent use of these drugs should be avoided or monitored closely.

In vitro, indomethacin is adsorbed by magnesium trisilicate, magnesium oxide, aluminum hydroxide, bismuth oxycarbonate, calcium carbonate, and kaolin (297). The peak concentration is delayed, and the bioavailability is reduced (298, 299). Although antacids frequently are suggested for patients taking indomethacin, concurrent dosing should be avoided. Again, alternating doses may decrease the probability of this interaction.

Buffering agents added to aspirin tablets result in a faster rate of dissolution, which results in earlier and higher peaks. However, the extent of absorption between buffered and unbuffered tablets is the same (300). The absorption rate may increase if aspirin is given in an enteric-coated form (301–303). Although the separate ingestion of antacids has not been extensively studied, renal elimination of aspirin may be increased by 30–70% by an antacid-induced increase in urinary pH (303). If aspirin and aluminum-magnesium hydroxide gel are given together and sustained levels are important, as in rheumatoid arthritis and systemic lupus erythematosus, it is advisable to monitor serum levels and to observe symptoms.

Levodopa absorption is increased as much as three times when antacids are taken concurrently (304). Alkalinization accelerates gastric emptying and delivers more levodopa to the small intestine, where it is more rapidly absorbed (305). There may be individual variation in response (306). The addition of antacids to a well-controlled parkinsonian patient may result in toxicity. Relapse may occur if the patient is well controlled on levodopa and antacid and the antacid is removed.

One in-vivo study confirmed an in-vitro interaction between magnesium trisilicate and dexamethasone. Measurement of urinary excretion of 11-hydroxycorticosteroids revealed a significant decrease in the effect of dexamethasone on 11-hydroxycorticosteroids when the steroid was given with the antacid (307). However, in seven healthy subjects, a magnesium-aluminum hydroxide antacid, when given as either tablets or liquid, had no effect on cortisone absorption (308). Therefore, further studies of corticosteroid-antacid interactions are needed.

The in-vitro adsorption of nitrofurantoin to magnesium trisilicate has been confirmed in vivo. Both the rate and extent of absorption were decreased. In addition, the time during which the drug concentration in the urine was above the minimum effective concentration was also significantly reduced (309).

Potentially Significant Interactions

Isoniazid absorption is more inhibited by aluminum hydroxide than by magaldrate. The mechanism is probably due to decreased gastric emptying rate and caused primarily by aluminum. It has been reported, however, that isoniazid is adsorbed in vitro by magnesium oxide (310). Although the clinical significance is not known, isoniazid probably should be given 1 hour before the antacid (311).

A potentially significant interaction between antacids and anticoagulants can be avoided by selecting the proper anticoagulant. The absorption of a single oral dose of dicumarol was increased by 50% by 15 ml of magnesium hydroxide and 30 ml of aluminum hydroxide (312). The absorption or the effect of warfarin is not altered by antacids (313, 314). Thus only patients taking dicumarol need cautioning about antacids. Patients who require both anticoagulants and antacids should be given warfarin (314).

Different antacids affect naproxen differently. Sodium bicarbonate administered with naproxen resulted in earlier and higher peak concentrations of naproxen, while magnesium oxide and aluminum hydroxide delayed absorption and decreased peak plasma concentrations. Aluminum-magnesium hydroxide gel tended to decrease the time required to reach peak plasma concentrations and slightly increased the total area under the curve (315). The clinical significance of this effect is unknown. It would seem best not to administer antacids simultaneously with naproxen.

Urinary excretion of amphetamine is decreased with sodium bicarbonate (316). Because of the potential for retention and subsequent intoxication due to urinary pH alteration with all antacids, antacids and amphetamines should not be given concurrently.

Benzodiazepines react differently with antacids. When chlordiazepoxide was administered with magnesium-aluminum hydroxide gel, the absorption rate of chlordiazepoxide was slowed, but the total amount absorbed and the apparent rate of elimination remained unchanged (317). Thus the interaction would be significant only for acute anxiety states where single doses of chlordiazepoxide are used. It would not be significant for chronic therapy. The absorption of diazepam has been reported to be increased by administration with aluminum hydroxide (318). Administration of diazepam with either aluminum-magnesium hydroxide gel or aluminum hydroxide trisilicate decreased the rate of absorption but not the extent of absorption (319).

The simultaneous administration of an unspecified antacid and phenytoin resulted in low nontherapeutic phenytoin levels in three patients. When the same dose of phenytoin was given 2–3 hours before the antacid, plasma levels increased two- to threefold (320). Additional studies using specified doses of specific antacids have provided conflicting results. Studies showing no effect of antacids used small doses (321, 322), while studies using larger doses of antacid showed decreased bioavailability of phenytoin (323, 324). A large inter-subject variability has been shown (325). The effect may be related to the dose of the antacid.

The absorption rate of pseudoephedrine was increased in the first 4 hours in six volunteers. The antacid increased the portion of the drug that was in the nonionized, more soluble form. Total absorption was not changed, and the clinical significance was unknown (325).

Administration of a single dose of aluminum hydroxide decreased the bioavailability of a single dose of propranolol in four of five subjects (326). What effect the concomitant administration of antacids and propranolol will have on prolonged therapy has not been assessed. Likewise, the clinical significance of this interaction remains to be determined.

Aluminum magnesium hydroxide antacid has been shown to decrease the rate and extent of aminophylline absorption at 40 and 60 minutes. However, at other sampling times, while the rate was decreased, the extent of absorption was not significantly different. For chronic administration this would not be clinically significant (327).

The administration of single doses of valproic acid with aluminum magnesium hydroxide, calcium carbonate, and aluminum hydroxide magnesium trisilicate resulted in a significant increase in total absorption with aluminum magnesium hydroxide and an insignificant trend toward increased absorption with the other two (328).

Magnesium trisilicate has been found to adsorb both estrogen and progestogen components of oral contraceptives in vitro (329). Although this interaction has not been reported in vivo, it may be important and can be avoided if patients are counseled not to take antacids and oral contraceptives concomitantly.

Product Selection Guidelines

The label of an antacid product as defined by the FDA, may contain the following indications: "upset stomach associated with heartburn, sour stomach, or acid indigestion." The label must contain caution if constipation or diarrhea occurs in more than 5% of the population and if there are more than 25 mEq of potassium, 50 mEq of magnesium, or 5 g of lactose/daily dose. If the product contains more than 0.2 mEq (5 mg) of sodium per dosage unit, the content must be on the label. Directions for time intervals between doses must be given, and a limit of 2 weeks of self-therapy is stated. A listing of the quantity of active ingredients is voluntary (140, 330).

The panel does not make specific dosage recommendations or give any comparative data. The label is an aid to product selection, but final selection and dosage must be based on individual evaluation and patient history. Antacids containing little or no sodium should be selected for individuals on low-salt diet (patients who are pregnant or who have congestive heart failure, hypertension, edema, or renal failure). Sodium content should be compared for equipotent volumes of drug to be administered. Magnesium-containing antacids should be avoided in patients with chronic renal failure. Antacids that cause constipation or diarrhea should not be given to a patient who already has these complaints. However, a magnesium antacid may be appropriate for an elderly patient who complains of chronic constipation.

The patient's current medications should be reviewed so that a product or a dosage schedule can be selected that does not interfere with any other medications.

Although cost is not a major consideration in the initial selection of a product, there is great variability when acid-neutralizing capacity is compared. These differences are reflected in the wholesome costs of 1 month of therapy, which varies from $35.00 to $55.00 with the five most potent antacids, and from $61.00 to $498.00 with the five least effective antacids (331). Cost should be computed for equipotent, not equivolume, quantities.

Patient Counseling

Specific advice for the patient should include:

- Antacids for relief of indigestion symptoms should not be taken longer than 2 weeks. If relief is not obtained, a physician should be contacted. If the antacid is being taken for peptic ulcer disease, it should be taken 1 and 3 hours after meals and at bedtime to provide a maximum duration of action.
- To prevent self-medication of an iatrogenic condition, the patient should understand that the antacid may cause diarrhea or constipation.
- Patients with restricted salt intake should be informed of the amount of sodium in the medications and advised of those products with a low-sodium content. Patients with medical problems that could be influenced by potassium or magnesium should be told of the content of these ions.
- The lesser effectiveness of tablets should be made clear. If liquid antacids are unacceptable, tablets should be chewed thoroughly and followed with a full glass of water to help dissolution and dispersion in the stomach. Effervescent tablets should be dissolved in water and most of the bubbles allowed to subside before they are swallowed.
- Additional medication that the patient is taking should be identified to enable the pharmacist to monitor for drug interactions.

Summary

Before recommending an antacid for self-therapy, the pharmacist must ensure that the use is appropriate. If the patient's history is indicative of peptic ulcer, or if there is evidence of bleeding, the patient should be referred to a physician for a medical evaluation.

Self-medication may be recommended if the history is indicative of acute gastritis, indigestion, heartburn, or upset stomach. Subjectively, any antacid will be effective, and therapy may be initiated with 40–80 mEq of a liquid antacid or 2–4 g of sodium bicarbonate or calcium carbonate. A product with simethicone should be recommended for the patient with gas. The pharmacist should caution against frequent use and monitor the patient for effectiveness and toxicity. If the discomfort is not relieved after 2 weeks or recurs frequently, medical help is indicated.

Since antacids constitute the mainstay of peptic ulcer therapy, the pharmacist may be asked to recommend an antacid for the physician-supervised management of peptic ulcer disease. Aluminum-magnesium hydroxide gel is the agent of choice for initial therapy in the absence of other complications. Other agents would be more appropriate for patients with renal failure, those on low-salt diets, and those with abnormal bowel function.

All antacids are not equal. Care should be taken to select one with good buffering capacity, and a taste acceptable to the patient. Equipotent volumes should be used if side effects necessitate switching to another product. Failure of antacid therapy may be due to poor selection, too infrequent or poorly timed administration, inadequate doses, or noncompliance due to unpalatability or disagreeable side effects.

References

1. *Drug Topics*, July 3, 68 (1981).
2. S. L. Robbins, "Pathologic Basis of Disease," W. B. Saunders, Philadelphia, Pa., 1974.
3. R. Fisher and S. Cohen, *Med. Clin. North Am.*, 62, 3 (1978).
4. J. Christensen, *Clin. Gastroenterol.*, 5, 15 (1976).
5. A. C. Guyton, "Textbook of Medical Physiology," W. B. Saunders, Philadelphia, Pa., 1981.
6. Charles E. Pope, in "Gastrointestinal Disease: Pathophysiology, Diagnosis, Management," M. H. Sleisenger and J. S. Fordtran, Eds., 2nd ed., W. B. Saunders, Philadelphia, Pa., 1978, pp. 541–568.
7. J. Christensen, J. L. Conklin, and B. W. Freeman, *Am. J. Physiol.*, 225, 1265 (1973).
8. G. R. Freeland, R. H. Higgins, D. O. Castell et al., *Gastroenterology*, 71, 570 (1976).
9. D. O. Castell and L. D. Harris, *N. Engl. J. Med.*, 282, 886 (1970).
10. W. H. Lipshutz and S. Cohen, *Am. J. Physiol.*, 222, 775 (1972).
11. H. Resin, D. H. Stern, R. A. L. Sturdevant et al., *Gastroenterology*, 64, 946 (1973).
12. H. M. Jennewein, F. Waldeck, R. Siewert et al., *Gut*, 14, 861 (1973).
13. W. J. Hogan, S. R. Viegas de Andrade, and D. H. Winship, *J. Appl. Physiol.*, 36, 755 (1972).
14. G. W. Dennis and D. O. Castell, *N. Engl. J. Med.*, 284, 1136 (1971).
15. O. T. Nebel and D. O. Castell, *Gut*, 14, 270 (1973).
16. A. C. Guyton, "Textbook of Medical Physiology," W. B. Saunders, Philadelphia, Pa., 1976, p. 858.
17. "Peptic Ulcer," H. M. Spiro, Ed., Rorer, Fort Washington, Pa., 1971.
18. M. I. Grossman, in "Gastrointestinal Disease: Pathophysiology, Diagnosis, Management," M. H. Sleisenger and J. S. Fordtran, Eds., 2nd ed., W. B. Saunders, Philadelphia, Pa., 1978, pp. 640–659.
19. K. A. Kelley, "Surgery Annual," Appleton-Century-Crofts, New York, N.Y., 1974, p. 103.
20. A. M. Cooperman and S. A. Cook, *Surg. Clin. N. Am.*, 56, 1277 (1976).
21. K. J. Ivey, *Am. J. Med.*, 58, 389 (1975).
22. R. R. Dozois and K. A. Kelley, *Surg. Clin. N. Am.*, 56, 1267 (1975).
23. F. P. Brooks, "Handbook of Physiology," Vol. II, Sec. 6, C. F. Code, Ed., Washington, D.C., American Physiological Society, 1967, p. 805.
24. H. T. Debas, *Am. Surg.*, 42, 498 (1976).
25. J. H. Eichhorn, E. W. Salzman, and W. Silen, *Nature*, 248, 238 (1974).
26. J. H. Wyllie, "Surgery Annals," L. M. Nyhus, Ed., Appleton-Century-Crofts, New York, N.Y., 1979, p. 207.
27. B. Schofield, B. L. Tepperman, and F. S. Tepperman, *Gastroenterology*, 68, A-125 (1975).
28. T. Scratcherd, *Clin. Gastroenterol.*, 2, 259 (1973).
29. J. E. McGuigan, *Am. J. Dig. Dis.*, 22, 712 (1977).
30. A. M. Ebeid and J. E. Fischer, *Surg. Clin. N. Am.*, 56, 1249 (1976).
31. J. H. Walsh and M. I. Grossman, *N. Engl. J. Med.*, 292, 1324 (1975).
32. J. E. McGuigan, *Gastroenterology*, 64, 497 (1973).
33. D. H. Stern and J. H. Walsh, *Gastroenterology*, 64, 363 (1973).
34. S. Cohen and W. Lipshutz, *J. Clin. Invest.*, 50, 449 (1971).
35. M. L. Chapman, J. L. Werther, J. Rudick, and H. D. Janowitz, *Gastroenterology*, 63, 962 (1972).
36. I. W. McCall, R. F. Harvey, C. J. Owens, and B. G. Clendinren, *Br. J. Surg.*, 62, 15 (1975).
37. W. J. Dodds, W. J. Hogan, W. N. Miller, R. F. Barreras, R. C. Arndorfer, and J. J. Stef, *Am. J. Dig. Dis.*, 20, 201 (1976).
38. J. W. Black, W. A. Duncan, and C. J. Durant, *Nature*, 236, 385 (1972).
39. S. J. Konturek, J. Biernat, and J. Olesky, *Am. J. Dig. Dis.*, 19, 609 (1974).
40. J. H. Wyllie, T. Hesselbo, and J. W. Black, *Lancet*, 2, 1117 (1972).
41. R. R. Dozois, A. Wollin, and R. D. Rettmann, *Physiologist*, 18, 196 (1975).
42. A. M. Brooks and M. I. Grossman, *Gastroenterology*, 59, 114 (1970).
43. D. E. Wilson, B. Ginsberg, R. A. Levine, and A. Washington, *Gastroenterology*, 63, 45 (1972).
44. E. Straus, *Med. Clin. North Am.*, 62, 21 (1978).
45. K. G. Wormsley, *Gastroenterology*, 62, 156 (1972).
46. J. Hansky, C. Soveny, and M. G. Korman, *Gastroenterology*, 61, 62 (1971).
47. M. H. Wheeler, *Gut*, 15, 420 (1974).
48. R. Cano, J. I. Isenberg, and M. Grossman, *Gastroenterology*, 70, 1055 (1976).
49. R. F. Barberas, *Gastroenterology*, 64, 1168 (1973).
50. H. D. Becker, D. D. Reeder, and J. C. Thompson, *Ann. Surg.*, 179, 906 (1974).
51. J. H. Walsh, C. T. Richardson, and J. S. Fordtran, *J. Clin. Invest.*, 55, 462 (1975).
52. R. A. Gross, D. L. Hogan, and J. I. Isenberg, *Gastroenterology*, 70, 891 (1976).
53. A. S. Ward, R. A. Wilkins, R. Cockel et al., *Gut*, 10, 1020 (1969).
54. R. K. Teichmann, J. S. Swierczek, P. L. Rayford et al., *World J. Surg.*, 3, 623 (1979).
55. I. L. MacGregor, C. Deveney, L. W. Way et al., *Gastroenterology*, 70, 197 (1976).
56. A. R. Cooke, *Gastroenterology*, 68, 804 (1975).
57. S. Moberg, *Scand. J. Gastroenterol.*, 15(80), 17 (1980).
58. S. H. Danovitch, in "Disorders of the Gastrointestinal Tract, Disorders of the Liver, Nutritional Disorders," J. M. Dietschy, Ed., Grune and Stratton, New York, N.Y., 1976, p. 111.
59. R. S. Fisher, L. S. Malmua, G. S. Roberts et al., *Gastroenterology*, 70, 301 (1976).
60. J. Dent et al., *J. Clin. Invest.*, 65, 256 (1980).
61. C. S. Winans, *Drug Ther.*, 10, 33 (1980).
62. M. D. Kaye and J. P. Showalter, *J. Lab. Clin. Med.*, 83, 198 (1974).

63. R. S. Fisher, G. S. Roberts, I. F. Lobis et al., *Gastroenterology*, *68*, 893 (1975).

64. L. F. Johnson and R. R. Demuster, *Am. J. Gastroenterol.*, *62*, 325 (1974).

65. D. W. Piper, *Gastroenterology*, *52*, 1009 (1967).

66. R. M. Pinder et al., *Drugs*, *12*, 81–131 (1976).

67. G. H. Jeffries, in "Gastrointestinal Disease: Pathophysiology, Diagnosis, Management," M. H. Sleisenger and J. S. Fordtran, Eds., 2nd ed., W. B. Saunders, Philadelphia, Pa., 1978, pp. 733–743.

68. B. S. Wolf, *J. Am. Med. Assoc.*, *235*, 1244 (1976).

69. A. R. Cooke, *Am. J. Dig. Dis.*, *21*, 155 (1976).

70. G. W. Dennish and D. O. Castell, *Am. J. Dig. Dis.*, *17*, 993 (1972).

71. *Nutrition Reviews*, *34*, 167 (1976).

72. A. R. Cooke, in "Gastrointestinal Disease: Pathophysiology, Diagnosis, Management," M. H. Sleisenger and J. S. Fordtran, Eds., 2nd ed., W. B. Saunders, Philadelphia, Pa., 1978, pp. 807–826.

73. C. E. Lucas, C. Sugawa, J. Riddle, F. Rector, B. Rosenberg, and A. J. Walt, *Arch. Surg.*, *102*, 266 (1971).

74. W. C. Butterfield, *Surg. Annu.*, *7*, 261 (1975).

75. M. Levy, *N. Engl. J. Med.*, *290*, 1158–1162 (1979).

76. W. T. Wightkin, *Am. J. Hosp. Pharm.*, *37*, 1651 (1980).

77. P. H. Guth, *Gastroenterology*, *64*, 1187 (1973).

78. J. C. Stothert, D. A. Simonowitz, E. R. Dellinger et al., *Surgery*, *192*, 169–174 (1980).

79. M. I. Grossman, *Scand. J. Gastroenterol.*, *15*(58), 7 (1980).

80. J. E. McGuigan, in "Disorders of the Gastrointestinal Tract, Disorders of the Liver, Nutritional Disorders," J. M. Dietschy, Ed., Grune and Stratton, New York, N.Y., 1976, p. 88.

81. M. I. Grossman, K. I. Isenberg, and J. H. Walsh, *Gastroenterology*, *69*, 1071 (1975).

82. M. J. S. Langman, *Clin. Gastroenterol.*, *2*, 219 (1973).

83. R. C. Brown, M. J. S. Langman, and P. M. Lambert, *Br. Med. J.*, *1*, 35 (1976).

84. R. A. L. Sturdevant, *Am. J. Epidemiol.*, *104*, 9 (1976).

85. J. D. Elashoff and M. I. Grossman, *Gastroenterology*, *78*, 280 (1980).

86. B. E. Stabile and E. Passaro, *Gastroenterology*, *70*, 124 (1976).

87. C. T. Richardson, in "Gastrointestinal Disease: Pathophysiology, Diagnosis, Management," M. H. Sleisenger and J. S. Fordtran, Eds., 2nd ed., Saunders, Philadelphia, Pa., 1978, pp. 875–891.

88. Y. Nagamachi and S. C. Skoryna, *Am. J. Surg.*, *133*, 593 (1977).

89. L. Olbe, *Scand. J. Gastroenterol.*, *14*(55), 49 (1979).

90. M. I. Grossman, P. H. Guth, J. I. Isenberg, E. P. Passaro, Jr., B. E. Roth, R. A. L. Sturdevant, and J. H. Walsh, *Ann. Intern. Med.*, *84*, 57 (1976).

91. A. Ippoliti and J. Walsh, *Surg. Clin. N. Am.*, *56*, 1479 (1976).

92. M. L. Chapman, *Med. Clin. N. Am.*, *62*, 39 (1978).

93. L. R. Dragstedt and E. R. Woodward, *Scand. J. Gastroenterol.*, *5*(6), 243 (1970).

94. J. Rhodes and B. Calcraft, *Clin. Gastroenterol.*, *2*, 227 (1973).

95. N. W. Read and P. Grech, *Br. Med. J.*, *3*, 313 (1973).

96. F. J. Flint and P. Grech, *Gut*, *11*, 735 (1970).

97. R. S. Fisher and G. Boden, *Gastroenterology*, *66*, 839 (1974).

98. R. S. Fisher and S. Cohen, *N. Engl. J. Med.*, *288*, 273 (1973).

99. J. E. Valenzuela and C. Defilippi, *Am. J. Dig. Dis.*, *21*, 229 (1976).

100. R. A. Roverstad, *Am. J. Dig. Dis.*, *21*, 165 (1976).

101. J. I. Rotter and D. L. Rimoin, *Gastroenterology*, *73*, 604 (1977).

102. R. Sturdevant and J. H. Walsh, in "Gastrointestinal Disease: Pathophysiology, Diagnosis, Management," M. H. Sleisenger and J. S. Fordtran, Eds., 2nd ed., Saunders, Philadelphia, Pa., 1978, pp. 840–860.

103. G. A. Hallenbeck, *Surg. Clin. N. Am.*, *56*, 1235 (1976).

104. A. J. Cox, *Arch. Pathol.*, *54*, 407 (1952).

105. J. I. Isenberg, M. I. Grossman, V. Maxwell, and J. Walsh, *J. Clin. Invest.*, *55*, 330 (1975).

106. J. E. McGuigan and W. L. Trudeau, *N. Engl. J. Med.*, *228*, 64 (1973).

107. J. Walsh, C. Richardson, and J. Fordtran, *J. Clin. Invest.*, *55*, 462 (1975).

108. J. S. Fordtran and J. H. Walsh, *J. Clin. Invest.*, *52*, 645 (1973).

109. J. R. Malagelada, *Scand. J. Gastroenterol.*, *14*(55), 39 (1979).

110. W. Creutzfeldt and R. Arnold, *World J. Surg.*, *3*, 605 (1979).

111. J. I. Isenberg, *Postgrad. Med.*, *57*, 163 (1975).

112. J. I. Rotter, J. Q. Sones, I. M. Samloff et al., *N. Engl. J. Med.*, *300*, 66 (1979).

113. A. Harrison, J. Elashoff, and M. I. Grossman, "Surgeon General's Report on Smoking and Health," 1979.

114. W. H. Taylor and A. Walker, *J. Roy. Soc. Med.*, *73*, 159 (1980).

115. "Harrison's Principles of Internal Medicine," 9th ed., G. W. Thorn, R. D. Adams, E. Braunwald, K. J. Isselbacher, and R. G. Petersdorf, Eds., McGraw-Hill, New York, N.Y., 1980.

116. J. I. Rotter and D. L. Rimoin, *Gastroenterology*, *73*, 604 (1977).

117. R. Earlam, *Gastroenterology*, *71*, 314 (1976).

118. H. Susser, *J. Chron. Dis.*, *20*, 435 (1967).

119. H. Colcher, *N. Engl. J. Med.*, *293*, 1129 (1975).

120. M. C. Sheppard, G. R. T. Holmes, and R. Cockel, *Gut*, *18*, 524 (1977).

121. H. M. Pollard and N. A. Augar, *Practitioner*, *201*, 139 (1968).

122. D. W. Piper and J. Kang, *Drugs*, *17*, 124 (1979).

123. S. Hannibal, L. Remvig, and S. J. Rune, *Scand. J. Gastroenterol.*, *15*(58), 29 (1980).

124. M. D. Korenmen, M. B. Stubbs, and J. C. Fish, *J. Am. Med. Assoc.*, *240*, 54 (1978).

125. D. W. Piper and B. H. Fenton, *Gut*, *5*, 506 (1964).

126. J. T. Kuruvilla, *Gut*, *12*, 897 (1971).

127. H. A. Holm, *Scand. J. Gastroenterol.*, *2*(42), 119 (1976).

128. D. W. Piper and B. H. Fenton, *Am. J. Dig. Dis.*, *6*, 134 (1961).

129. T. B. Deering, G. L. Carlson, J. R. Malagelada et al., *Gastroenterology*, *77*, 986 (1979).

130. J. F. Morrissey, T. Honda, Y. Tanaka, and G. Perna, *Arch. Intern. Med.*, *119*, 510 (1967).

131. J. E. Dill, *Gastroenterology*, *62*, 697 (1972).

132. R. H. Higgs, R. D. Smyth, and D. O. Castell, *N. Engl. J. Med.*, *291*, 486 (1974).

133. D. O. Castell and S. M. Levine, *Ann. Intern. Med.*, *74*, 223 (1971).

134. G. E. Feurle, *Gastroenterology*, *68*, 1 (1975).

135. E. Schrumpf, *Scand. J. Gastroenterol.*, *15*(58) 97 (1980).

136. A. Hurwitz and M. B. Sheehan, *J. Pharmacol. Exp. Ther.*, *179*, 124 (1971).

137. A. Hurwitz, R. G. Robinson, T. S. Vats, F. C. Whittier, and W. F. Herrin, *Gastroenterology*, *71*, 268 (1976).

138. J. E. Clain, J. R. Malagelada, V. S. Chadwick, and A. F. Hofmann, *Gastroenterology*, *73*, 556 (1977).

139. J. R. Malagelada and G. L. Carlson, *Scand. J. Gastroenterol.*, *14*(55), 67 (1977).

140. A. M. Schmidt, *Federal Register*, *39*, 19862 (1974).

141. C. H. Barnett, R. R. Commons, F. Albright, and J. E. Howard, *N. Engl. J. Med.*, *240*, 787 (1949).

142. C. J. Riley, *Practitioner*, *205*, 657 (1970).

143. A. Ansari and J. A. Vennes, *Minn. Med.*, *54*, 611 (1971).

144. D. W. Piper, *Clin. Gastroenterol.*, *2*, 361 (1973).

145. F. W. Green, R. A. Norton, and M. M. Kaplan, *Am. J. Hosp. Pharm.*, *32*, 425 (1975).

146. R. E. Barry, *J. Intern. Med. Res.*, *6*(1), 11 (1978).

147. J. S. Fordtran, *N. Engl. J. Med.*, *279*, 900 (1968).

148. *Medical Letter on Drugs and Therapeutics*, *15*(8), 36 (1973).

149. J. D. Clemens and N. Feinstein, *Gastroenterology*, *72*, 957 (1977).

150. J. S. Fordtran, in "Gastrointestinal Disease: Pathophysiology, Diagnosis, Management," M. H. Sleisenger and J. S. Fordtran, Eds., 2nd ed., W. B. Saunders, Philadelphia, Pa., 1973, p. 718.

151. J. Stiel, C. A. Mitchell, F. J. Radcliff, and D. W. Piper, *Gastroenterology*, *53*, 900 (1967).

152. R. F. Barreras, *Gastroenterology*, *64*, 1168 (1973).

153. R. M. Case, *Digestion*, *8*, 269 (1973).

154. H. Breuhaus, O. H. Akre, and J. B. Eyeler, *Gastroenterology*, *16*, 172 (1950).

155. R. F. Barreras, *N. Engl. J. Med.*, *282*, 1402 (1970).

156. D. D. Reeder, B. M. Jackson, J. Ban, B. G. Clendinnen, W. D. Davidson, and J. C. Thompson, *Ann. Surg.*, *172*, 540 (1970).

157. J. A. Levant, J. H. Walsh, and J. I. Isenberg, *N. Engl. J. Med.*, *289*, 555 (1973).

158. S. L. Hem, *J. Chem. Educ.*, *52*, 383 (1975).
159. C. M. Townsend, A. R. Remmers, H. E. Sarles, and J. C. Fish, *N. Engl. J. Med.*, *288*, 1058 (1973).
160. E. M. Clarkson, V. A. Luck, W. V. Hynson, R. R. Bailey, J. B. Eastwood, J. S. Woodhead, V. R. Clements, J. L. H. O'Riordan, and H. E. De Wardener, *Clin. Sci.*, *43*, 519 (1972).
161. G. M. Berlyne, J. Ben-Ari, D. Pest, J. Weinberger, M. Stern, G. R. Gilmore, and R. Levine, *Lancet*, *2*, 494 (1970).
162. V. Parsons, C. Davies, C. Goode, C. Ogg, and J. Siddiqui, *Br. Med. J.*, *4*, 273 (1971).
163. A. C. Alfrey, G. R. LeGendre, and W. D. Kaehny, *N. Engl. J. Med.*, *294*, 184 (1976).
164. C. A. Miller and E. M. Levine, *J. Neurochem.*, *22*, 751 (1974).
165. A. I. McLaughlin, G. Kazantzis, E. King, D. Teare, R. J. Porter, and R. Owen, *Br. J. Ind. Med.*, *19*, 253 (1962).
166. W. D. Kaehny, A. P. Hegg, and A. C. Alfrey, *N. Engl. J. Med.*, *296*, 1389 (1977).
167. *Journal of the American Medical Association*, *238*, 1017 (1977).
168. H. Spencer and M. Lender, *Gastroenterology*, *76*, 603 (1979).
169. D. E. Abrams, R. B. Silcott, R. Terry, T. V. Berne, and B. H. Barbour, *West. J. Med.*, *120*, 157 (1974).
170. H. M. Shields, *Gastroenterology*, *75*, 1137 (1978).
171. M. Lotz, E. Zisman, and F. C. Bartter, *N. Engl. J. Med.*, *278*, 409 (1968).
172. R. E. Chojnacki, *Ann. Intern. Med.*, *74*, 297 (1971).
173. K. L. Insogna, D. R. Bordley, J. F. Caro et al., *J. Am. Med. Assoc.*, *244*, 2544 (1980).
174. H. Spencer and M. Lender, *Gastroenterology*, *76*, 603 (1979).
175. R. E. Randall, M. D. Cohen, C. C. Spray, and E. C. Rossmeisl, *Ann. Intern. Med.*, *61*, 73 (1964).
176. F. J. Goodwin and F. P. Vince, *Br. J. Urol.*, *42*, 586 (1970).
177. S. Jameson, *Scand. J. Urol. Nephrol.*, *6*, 260 (1972).
178. A. C. Alfrey, D. S. Terman, L. Brettschneider, K. M. Simpson, and D. A. Ogden, *Ann. Intern. Med.*, *73*, 367 (1970).
179. A. S. Berns and K. R. Kollmeyer, *Ann. Intern. Med.*, *85*, 760 (1976).
180. J. R. Herman and A. S. Goldbert, *J. Am. Med. Assoc.*, *174*, 1206 (1960).
181. C. Lagergren, *J. Urol.*, *87*, 994 (1962).
182. A. M. Joekes, G. A. Rose, and J. Sutor, *Br. Med. J.*, *1*, 146 (1973).
183. F. W. Green, R. A. Norton, and M. M. Kaplan, *Am. J. Hosp. Pharm.*, *32*, 425 (1975).
184. R. K. Vanderlaan, J. L. White, and S. L. Hem. *J. Pharm. Sci.*, *68*, 1498 (1979).
185. M. D. Korenmen, M. B. Stubbs, and J. C. Fisk, *J. Am. Med. Assoc.*, *240*, 54 (1978).
186. J. E. Bernstein and A. M. Kasich, *J. Clin. Pharmacol.*, *14*, 617 (1974).
187. J. A. Stead, R. A. Wilkins, and J. J. Ashford, *J. Pharm. Pharmacol.* *30*, 350 (1978).
188. J. F. Pontes, D. J. Richards, and J. N. Sartoretto, *Curr. Ther. Res. Clin. Exp.*, *18*, 315 (1975).
189. C. Stanciu and J. R. Bennet, *Lancet*, *1*, 109 (1974).
190. L. S. Malmud, N. D. Charles, J. Littlefield et al., *J. Nucl. Med.*, *20*, 1023 (1979).
191. M. Beeley and J. O. Warner, *Curr. Med. Res. Opin.*, *1*, 63 (1972).
192. *South African Medical Journal*, *48*, 2239 (1974).
193. G. L. Beckloff, J. H. Chapman, and P. Shiverdecker, *J. Clin. Pharmacol.*, *12*, 11 (1972).
194. D. E. Barnardo, M. Lancaster-Smith, I. D. Strickland et al., *Curr. Med. Res. Opin.*, *3*, 388 (1975).
195. *Lancet*, *1*, 1290 (1975).
196. R. Burns, D.W. Thomas, and U. J. Baron, *Br. Med. J.*, *1*, 220 (1974).
197. *Postgraduate Medical Journal*, *51*(5) (1975).
198. R. N. Brogden, R. M. Pinder, P. R. Sawyer, T. M. Speight, and G. S. Avery, *Drugs*, *12*, 401 (1976).
199. I. N. Marks, *Drugs*, *20*, 283 (1980).
200. G. Ekeved and A. Walan, *Scand. J. Gastroenterol.*, *10*, 267 (1975).
201. J. R. B. J. Brouwers and G. N. J. Tytgat, *J. Pharm. Pharmacol.*, *30*, 148 (1978).
202. D. Drake and D. Hollander, *Ann. Intern. Med.*, *94*, 215 (1981).
203. D. Patyk, *N. Engl. J. Med.*, *283*, 134 (1970).
204. D. W. Piper and B. H. Fenton, *Gut*, *5*, 585 (1964).
205. E. W. Packman and A. R. Gennaro, *Am. J. Pharm.*, *145*, 162 (1973).
206. J. E. Clain, J. P. Wright, R. N. Price et al., *South Afr. Med. J.*, *57*, 158 (1980).
207. R. E. Barry and J. Ford, *Br. Med. J.*, *1*, 413 (1978).
208. W. L. Peterson and J. S. Fordtran, in "Gastrointestinal Disease: Pathophysiology, Diagnosis, Management," M. H. Sleisenger and J. S. Fordtran, Eds., 2nd ed., W. B. Saunders, Philadelphia, Pa., 1978.
209. M. P. Dutro and A. B. Amerson, *Colo. Pharm.*, *8*, Sept.–Oct. (1980).
210. G. D. Rudd, *Ann. Intern. Med.*, *95*, 120 (1981).
211. S. Fox and J. Behar, *Clin. Gastroenterol.*, *8*, 37 (1979).
212. M. M. Kline, R. W. McCallum, W. Curry, and R. A. Sturdevant, *Gastroenterology*, *68*, 1137 (1975).
213. R. J. Petrokubi and G. H. Jeffries, *Gastroenterology*, *77*, 69 (1979).
214. P. R. Hastings, J. J. Skillman, L. S. Bushnell et al., *N. Engl. J. Med.*, *298*, 1041 (1978).
215. H. P. McElwee, K. R. Sirinek, B. A. Levine et al., *Surgery*, *86*, 620 (1979).
216. L. F. Martin, M. H. May, H. C. Polk, *Surgery*, *88*, 59 (1980).
217. H. J. Priebe, J. J. Skillman, L. S. Bushnell et al., *N. Engl. J. Med.*, *302*, 426 (1980).
218. L. D. Solem, R. G. Strate, and R. P. Fischer, *Surg. Gynecol. Obstet.*, *148*, 367 (1979).
219. E. Christensen, E. Juhl, and N. Tygstrup, *Gastroenterology*, *73*, 1170 (1977).
220. J. H. Meyer, A. Schwabe, J. I. Isenberg, R. A. L. Sturdevant, M. I. Grossman, and E. Passaro, *West. J. Med.*, *126*, 273 (1977).
221. D. Hollander and J. Harlan, *J. Am. Med. Assoc.*, *226*, 1181 (1973).
222. M. L. Butler and H. Gersh, *Am. J. Dig. Dis.*, *20*, 803 (1975).
223. R. A. L. Sturdevant, J. I. Isenberg, D. Secrist, and J. Ansfield, *Gastroenterology*, *72*, 1 (1977).
224. A. Littman, R. Welch, R. C. Fruin, and A. R. Aronson, *Gastroenterology*, *73*, 6 (1977).
225. W. L. Peterson, R. A. L. Sturdevant, H. D. Frank, C. T. Richardson, J. I. Isenberg, J. D. Elashoff, J. Q. Sones, R. A. Gross, R. W. McCallum, and J. S. Fordtran, *N. Engl. J. Med.*, *297*, 341 (1977).
226. M. I. Grossman, *Scand. J. Gastroenterol.*, *15*(58), 37 (1980).
227. T. Morris and J. Rhodes, *Gut*, *20*, 538 (1979).
228. D. M. McCarthy, *Hosp. Pract.*, *14*, 52 (1979).
229. A. Ippoliti and W. Peterson, *Clin. Gastroenterol.*, *8*, 53 (1979).
230. S. J. Rune and A. Zachariassen, *Scand. J. Gastroenterol.*, *15*(58), 41 (1980).
231. E. Gudjonsson and H. Spiro, *Am. J. Med.*, *65*, 399 (1978).
232. H. Sarles, R. Camatte, and J. Sahel, *Digestion*, *16*, 289 (1977).
233. J. I. Warbick and A. N. Martin, in "American Pharmacy," J. B. Sprowls and H. B. Beal, Eds., J. B. Lippincott, Philadelphia, Pa., 1972, p. 176.
234. R. P. Schneider and A. C. Roach, *South. Med. J.*, *69*, 1312 (1976).
235. D. Sklar, M. H. Liang, and J. Porta, *N. Engl. J. Med.*, *296*, 1007 (1977).
236. J. S. Fordtran and J. A. H. Collyns, *N. Engl. J. Med.*, *274*, 921 (1966).
237. R. F. Barreras, J. L. Allen, and C. M. Thoreson, *Gastroenterology*, *72*, 1027 (1977).
238. S. Cohen and W. J. Snape, *Arch. Intern. Med.*, *138*, 1398 (1978).
239. M. J. S. Langman, *Drugs*, *14*, 105 (1977).
240. J. S. Fordtran and J. H. Walsh, *J. Clin. Invest.*, *52*, 645 (1973).
241. J. R. Malagelada, G. F. Longstreth, W. H. Summerskill, and V. L. W. Go, *Gastroenterology*, *70*, 203 (1976).
242. J. S. Fordtran and J. A. H. Collyns, *N. Engl. J. Med.*, *274*, 921 (1966).
243. A. Littman, *Gastroenterology*, *61*, 567 (1971).
244. D. E. Wilson and J. D. Siegfried, *Drug Therap. (hosp.)*, *9*, 22 (1979).
245. H. Peterson, *Scand. J. Gastroenterol.*, *14*(55), 56 (1979).
246. H. S. Caron and H. P. Roth, *Am. J. Med. Sci.*, *261*, 61 (1971).
247. J. D. Welsh, *Gastroenterology*, *72*, 740 (1977).

248. A. Walan, *Scand. J. Gastroenterol.*, *14*(55), 84 (1979).
249. M. Feldman, C. T. Richardson, W. L. Peterson et al., *N. Engl. J. Med.*, *297*, 1427 (1977).
250. K. J. Ivey, *Gastroenterology*, *68*, 154 (1975).
251. J. Bowers, J. Forbes, and J. Freston, *Gastroenterology*, *72*, 1032 (1977).
252. J. W. Freston, *Gastroenterology*, *74*, 426–430 (1978).
253. A. Berstad, *Scand. J. Gastroenterol.*, *15*(Suppl. 58), 79 (1980).
254. A. F. Ippoliti, R. A. L. Sturdevant, J. I. Isenberg et al., *Gastroenterology*, *74*, 393 (1978).
255. G. Fedeli, M. Anti, G. L. Rapaccini et al., *Dig. Dis. Sciences*, *24*, 758 (1979).
256. T. B. Deering and J. R. Malagelada, *Gastroenterology*, *73*, 11 (1977).
257. J. H. B. Saunders, S. Drummond, and K. G. Wormsley, *Br. Med. J.*, *1*, 418 (1977).
258. E. Englert, J. W. Freston, and D. Y. Graham, *Gastroenterology*, *74*, 416 (1978).
259. G. Bodemar, B. Norlander, and A. Walan, *Lancet 1*, 444, (1979).
260. P. A. MacKercher, K. J. Ivey, W. N. Baskin et al., *Ann. Intern. Med.*, *87*, 676 (1977).
261. G. L. Kauffman and M. I. Grossman, *Gastroenterology*, *75*, 1099 (1978).
262. R. Gugler, H. Lindstaedt, S. Miederer et al., *N. Engl. J. Med.*, *301*, 1077 (1979).
263. J. I. Isenberg, *Hosp. Pract.*, *15*, 63 (1980).
264. J. E. McGuigan, *Gastroenterology*, *80*, 181 (1981).
265. D. Sawyer, C. S. Conner, R. Scalley, *Am. J. Hosp. Pharm.*, *38*, 188 (1981).
266. R. E. Small, D. R. Atwell, and W. R. Garnett, "Abstracts of Contributed Papers," 128th APhA Meeting, 1981.
267. S. R. Mogelnicki, J. L. Waller, and D. C. Finlayson, *J. Am. Med. Assoc.*, *241*, 826 (1979).
268. A. Berstad, K. Bjerke, E. Carlsen et al., *Scand. J. Gastroenterol.*, *15*(58), 46 (1980).
269. W. L. Peterson, C. Barnett, M. Feldman et al., *Gastroenterology*, *77*, 1015 (1979).
270. G. S. Wagby, *Gastroenterology*, *74*, 7 (1978).
271. H. Abrahamsson and G. Dotevall, *Scand. J. Gastroenterol.*, *14*(55), 17 (1979).
272. K. F. R. Sewing, A. Billian, and M. Malchan, *Gut*, *21*, 750 (1980).
273. S. Kaojarern, M. Feldman, C. T. Richardson, and D. C. Brater, *Clin. Pharmacol. Ther.*, *29*, 198 (1981).
274. *British Medical Journal*, *3*, 95 (1980).
275. L. Olbe, T. Berglindh, B. Elander et al., *Scand. J. Gastroenterol.*, *14*(55), 131 (1979).
276. C. Johansson and B. Kollberg, *Scand. J. Gastroenterol.*, *14*(55), 126 (1979).
277. S. Wetterhas, K. Valnes, and J. Myren, *Scand. J. Gastroenterol.*, *14*(55), 124 (1979).
278. S. K. Lam, K. C. Lam, C. L. Lai et al., *Gastroenterology*, *76*, 322 (1979).
279. A. Hurwitz, *Clin. Pharmacokinet.*, *2*, 269 (1977).
280. J. A. Romankiewicz, *Primary Care*, *3*, 537 (1976).
281. S. Khalil and M. Moustafa, *Pharmazie*, *28*, 116 (1973).
282. *British Medical Journal*, *2*, 405 (1975).
283. M. Gibaldi, B. Grundhofer, and G. Levy, *Clin. Pharmacol. Ther.*, *16*, 520 (1974).
284. M. Gibaldi, B. Grundhofer, and G. Levy, *J. Pharm. Sci.*, *64*, 2003 (1975).
285. J. W. Ayres, D. J. Weidler, J. Mackichan et al., *Eur. J. Clin. Pharmacol.*, *12*, 415 (1977).
286. S. K. Khalil, N. A. Daabis, V. F. Naggar, and M. M. Motawi, *Pharmazie*, *31*, 105 (1976).
287. W. H. Barr, J. Adir, and L. Garrettson, *Clin. Pharmacol. Ther.*, *12*, 779 (1971).
288. M. Garty and A. Hurwitz, *Clin. Pharmacol. Ther.*, *28*, 203 (1980).
289. "Evaluations of Drug Interactions," 2nd ed., American Pharmaceutical Association, Washington, D.C., 1976, pp. 227–230.
290. G. Ekenved, L. Halvorsen, and L. Solvell, *Scand. J. Haematol. Suppl.*, *28*, 65 (1976).
291. S. A. Khalil, *J. Pharm. Pharmacol.*, *26*, 961 (1974).
292. D. D. Brown and R. P. Juhl, *N. Engl. J. Med.*, *295*, 1034 (1976).
293. W. E. Fann, J. M. Davis, D. S. Janowsky, H. J. Sekerke, and D. M. Schmidt, *J. Clin. Pharmacol.*, *13*, 388 (1973).
294. F. M. Forrest, I. S. Forrest, and M. T. Serra, *Biol. Psychiatry*, *2*, 53 (1970).
295. J. A. Romankiewicz, M. Reidenberg, D. Drayer, and J. E. Franklin, *Am. Heart J.*, *96*, 518 (1978).
296. M. B. Zinn, *Tex. Med.*, *66*, 64 (1970).
297. V. F. Naggar, S. A. Khalil, and N. A. Daabis, *Pharmazie*, *31*, 461 (1976).
298. H. W. Emori, H. Paulus, R. Bluestone, G. D. Champion, and C. Pearson, *Ann. Rheum. Dis.*, *35*, 333 (1976).
299. R. L. Galeazzi, *Euro. J. Clin. Pharmacol.*, *12*, 65 (1977).
300. R. K. Nayak, R. D. Smyth, A. Polk et al., *J. Pharmacokin. Biopharm.*, *5*, 597 (1977).
301. B. Strickland-Hodge, T. R. Thomas, W. A. Gould, and I. Haslock, *Rheumatol. Rehabil.*, *15*, 148 (1976).
302. S. Feldman and B. C. Carlstedt, *J. Am. Med. Assoc.*, *227*, 660 (1974).
303. G. Levy, T. Lampman, B. L. Kamath, and L. K. Garrettson, *N. Engl. J. Med.*, *293*, 323 (1975).
304. L. Rivera-Calimlim, C. A. Dujovne, J. P. Morgan, L. Lasagna, and J. R. Bianchine, *Eur. J. Clin. Invest.*, *1*, 313 (1971).
305. G. B. T. Pocelinko and H. M. Solomon, *Clin. Pharmacol. Ther.*, *13*, 149 (1972).
306. A. S. Leon and H. E. Spiegel, *J. Clin. Pharmacol.*, *12*, 263 (1972).
307. V. F. Naggar, S. A. Khalil, and M. W. Gouda, *J. Pharm. Sci.*, *67*, 1029 (1978).
308. R. L. Galleazzi, N. Berber, H. W. Iff, *Schweiz. Mediz. Wochen.*, *103*, 1021 (1973).
309. V. F. Naggar and S. A. Khalil, *Clin. Pharmacol. Ther.*, *25*, 857 (1979).
310. W. H. Wu, T. F. Chin, and J. L. Lack, *J. Pharm. Sci.*, *59*, 1234 (1970).
311. A. Hurwitz and D. L. Scholozman, *Am. Rev. Respir. Dis.*, *109*, 41 (1974).
312. J. J. Ambre and L. J. Fischer, *Clin. Pharmacol. Ther.*, *14*, 231 (1973).
313. D. S. Robinson, M. B. David, and J. J. McCormack, *Clin. Pharmacol. Ther.*, *12*, 491 (1971).
314. P. D. Hansten, "Drug Interactions," 4th ed., Lea & Febiger, Philadelphia, Pa., 1979, p. 36.
315. E. J. Segre, H. Sevelius, and J. Varady, *N. Engl. J. Med.*, *291*, 582 (1974).
316. A. H. Beckett, M. Rowland, and P. Turner, *Lancet*, *1*, 302 (1965).
317. D. J. Greenblatt, R. I. Shader, and J. S. Harmatz, *Clin. Pharmacol. Ther.*, *19*, 234 (1976).
318. S. G. Nair, J. A. S. Gamble, J. W. Dundee, and P. J. Howard, *Br. J. Anaesth.*, *48*, 1175 (1976).
319. D. J. Greenblatt, M. D. Allen, D. S. MacLaughlin et al., *Clin. Pharmacol. Ther.*, *24*, 600 (1978).
320. H. L. Kutt, *Epilepsia*, *16*, 393 (1975).
321. D. J. Chapron, P. A. Kramer, S. L. Mariano et al., *Arch. Neurol.*, *36*, 436 (1979).
322. L. S. O'Brien, M. L. E. Orme, and A. M. Breckenridge, *Br. J. Clin. Pharmacol.*, *6*, 176 (1978).
323. V. K. Kulshrestha, M. Thomas, J. Wadsworth et al., *Br. J. Clin. Pharmacol.*, *6*, 177 (1978).
324. B. L. Carter, W. R. Garnett, J. M. Pellock et al., *Ther. Drug Monitor*, *3*, 333 (1981).
325. R. Lucarotti, J. L. Colaizzi, H. Barry, and R. L. Poust, *J. Pharm. Sci*, *61*, 903 (1972).
326. J. H. Dobbs, V. A. Skoutakis, S. R. Acchiardo, and B. R. Dobbs, *Curr. Ther. Res.*, *21*, 887 (1977).
327. L. A. Arnold, G. H. Spurbeck, W. H. Shelver et al., *Am. J. Hosp. Pharm.*, *36*, 1059 (1979).
328. C. A. May, W. R. Garnett, J. M. Pellock et al., *Clin. Pharm.*, (in press).
329. S. A. H. Khalil and M. Iwragwr, *J. Pharm. Pharmacol.*, *28*, 47 (1976).
330. *FDA Consumer* July–Aug., 1974. (DHEW Publication No. FDA-75-3003.).
331. D. Drake and D. Hollander, *Ann. Intern. Med.*, *94*, 215 (1981).

Antacid Product Table

Product (Manufacturer)	Dosage Form	Calcium Carbonate	Aluminum Hydroxide	Magnesium Oxide or Hydroxide	Magnesium Trisilicate	Other Ingredients	Sodium Content
Alka-2 Chewable Antacid (Miles)	chewable tablet	500 mg					NS[a]
Alka-Seltzer Effervescent Antacid (Miles)	tablet					sodium bicarbonate, 1.008 g citric acid, 800 mg potassium bicarbonate, 300 mg	12.8 mEq/tablet
Alkets (Upjohn)	tablet	780 mg		65 mg		magnesium carbonate, 130 mg	<0.04 mEq/dose
Allimin (Health Care Industries)	tablet					garlic powder, 309 mg parsley powder	NS[a]
ALternaGel (Stuart)	suspension		120 mg/ml				0.02 mEq/ml
Aludrox (Wyeth)	tablet suspension		233 mg/tablet 61.4 mg/ml	84 mg/tablet 20.6 mg/ml			0.07 mEq/tablet 0.01 mEq/ml
Aluminum Hydroxide Gel USP (Philips Roxane)	suspension		70.4 mg/ml			sorbitol, 15% peppermint sucrose, 15%	0.07 mEq/ml
Alurex (Rexall)	tablet suspension		NS[a]	NS[a] (hydroxide)			NS[a]
Amitone (Norcliff Thayer)	tablet	350 mg				mint flavor	<0.09 mEq/tablet
Amphojel (Wyeth)	tablet suspension		300 or 600 mg/tablet 64 mg/ml				0.06 or 0.12 mEq/tablet 0.1 mEq/ml
A.M.T. (Wyeth)	tablet suspension		164 mg/tablet 61 mg/ml		250 mg/tablet 125 mg/ml		0.15 mEq/tablet 0.06 mEq/ml
Antacid Powder (DeWitt)	powder		dried gel, 15%		31%	sodium bicarbonate, 25% magnesium carbonate (heavy), 10%	NS[a]
Banacid (Buffington)	tablet		NS[a]	NS[a] (hydroxide)	NS[a]		free
Basaljel (Wyeth)	suspension capsule tablet					aluminum carbonate, equiv. to: 80 mg aluminum hydroxide/ ml; 500 mg aluminum hydroxide/ capsule or tablet	0.02 mEq/ml 0.12 mEq/capsule 0.09 mEq/tablet

Antacid Product Table, continued

Product (Manufacturer)	Dosage Form	Calcium Carbonate	Aluminum Hydroxide	Magnesium Oxide or Hydroxide	Magnesium Trisilicate	Other Ingredients	Sodium Content
Basaljel Extra Strength (Wyeth)	suspension		200 mg/ml				0.2 mEq/ml
Bell-Ans (Dent)	tablet					sodium bicarbonate, 527 mg wintergreen ginger	NS[a]
BiSoDol (Whitehall)	tablet powder	195 mg/tablet		178 mg/tablet		sodium bicarbonate, 644 mg/tsp (powder) magnesium carbonate, 475 mg/tsp (powder) peppermint oil	0.001 mEq/ tablet 6.8 mEq/tsp. (powder)
Camalox (Rorer)	suspension tablet	50 mg/ml 250 mg/tablet	45 mg/ml 225 mg/tablet	40 mg/ml 200 mg/tablet (hydroxide)			0.02 mEq/ml 0.07 mEq/ tablet
Chooz (Plough)	gum tablet	500 mg					0.14 mEq/ tablet
Citrocarbonate (Upjohn)	suspension powder					sodium bicarbonate, 200 mg/g (suspension) 208 mg/g (powder) sodium citrate, anhydrous, 467 mg/g (suspension), 261 mg/g (powder)	6.09 mEq/ml (suspension)
Creamalin (Winthrop)	tablet		248 mg	75 mg		mint flavor	1.78 mEq
Delcid (Merrell-Dow)	suspension		120 mg/ml	133 mg/ml (hydroxide)			0.13 mEq/ml
Dialume (Armour)	tablet		dried gel, 500 mg				0.05 mEq
Dicarbosil (Arch)	tablet	500 mg				peppermint oil	0.12 mEq
Di-Gel (Plough)	tablet liquid		codried with magnesium carbonate, 282 mg/ tablet 56.2 mg/ml (liquid)	85 mg/tablet 17.4 mg/ml		simethicone, 25 mg/tablet 5 mg/ml	0.46 mEq/ tablet 0.07 mEq/ml
Dimacid (Otis Clapp)	tablet	NS[a]				magnesium carbonate	free

Antacid Product Table, continued

Product (Manufacturer)	Dosage Form	Calcium Carbonate	Aluminum Hydroxide	Magnesium Oxide or Hydroxide	Magnesium Trisilicate	Other Ingredients	Sodium Content
Eno (Beecham Products)	powder					sodium tartrate, 1.6 g/tsp sodium citrate, 1.2 g/tsp	35.6 mEq/tsp
Enzymet (O'Neal, Jones & Feldman)	tablet					pancreatin, 300 mg pepsin, 200 mg sucrose, 50 mg	free
Estomul-M (Riker)	tablet liquid		codried with magnesium carbonate, 500 mg/ tablet, 183.6 mg/ml	45 mg/tablet (oxide)			0.7 mEq/ tablet 0.1 mEq/ml
Flacid (Amfre-Grant)	tablet		282 mg			simethicone, 25 mg magnesium carbonate, 282 mg	NS[a]
Gaviscon (Marion)	tablet		80 mg		20 mg	sodium bicarbonate, 70 mg alginic acid, 200 mg	0.83 mEq
Gaviscon (Marion)	suspension		6.3 mg/ml			magnesium carbonate, 27.5 mg/ml sodium alginate, 26.7 mg/ml	0.1 mEq/ml
Gaviscon-2 (Marion)	tablet		160 mg		40 mg	sodium bicarbonate, 140 mg alginic acid, 400 mg	1.7 mEq
Gelusil (Parke-Davis)	tablet suspension		200 mg/tablet 40 mg/ml	200 mg/tablet 40 mg/ml		simethicone, 25 mg/tablet 5 mg/ml mint flavor	0.03 mEq/ tablet 0.006 mEq/ ml
Gelusil II (Parke-Davis)	tablet suspension		400 mg/tablet 80 mg/ml	400 mg/tablet 80 mg/ml		simethicone, 30 mg/tablet 6 mg/ml orange flavor citrus flavor	0.09 mEq/ tablet 0.01 mEq/ml
Gelusil M (Parke-Davis)	tablet suspension		300 mg/tablet 60 mg/ml	200 mg/tablet 40 mg/ml		simethicone, 25 mg/tablet 5 mg/ml mint flavor	0.07 mEq/ tablet 0.01 mEq/ml
Glycate (O'Neal, Jones & Feldman)	tablet	300 mg				glycine, 150 mg	NS[a]
Gustalac (Geriatric Pharmaceutical)	tablet	300 mg				defatted skim milk powder, 200 mg	0.06 mEq/ tablet

Antacid Product Table, continued

Product (Manufacturer)	Dosage Form	Calcium Carbonate	Aluminum Hydroxide	Magnesium Oxide or Hydroxide	Magnesium Trisilicate	Other Ingredients	Sodium Content
Kessadrox (McKesson)	suspension		67 mg/ml	11 mg/ml (hydroxide)		peppermint oil sorbitol	0.08 mEq/ml
Kolantyl (Merrell-Dow)	gel tablet wafer		10 mg/ml 300 mg/tablet (dried gel) 180 mg/wafer (dried gel)	10 mg/ml (hydroxide) 185 mg/tablet (oxide) 170 mg/wafer (hydroxide)		mint flavor	< 0.04 mEq/ml ≤ 0.65 mEq/tablet ≤ 0.22 mEq/wafer
Krem (Mallinckrodt)	tablet	400 mg				magnesium carbonate, 200 mg milk base mint or cherry flavor	NSª
Kudrox (Kremers-Urban)	liquid		113 mg/ml	36 mg/ml		sorbitol solution, 0.2 ml/ml	≤ 0.13 mEq/ml
Liquid Antacid (McKesson)	liquid		67 mg/ml	11 mg/ml (hydroxide)		peppermint oil sorbitol	0.08 mEq/ml
Maalox (Rorer)	suspension		dried gel, 45 mg/ml	40 mg/ml (hydroxide)			0.01 mEq/ml
Maalox #1 (Rorer)	tablet		dried gel, 200 mg	200 mg (hydroxide)			0.04 mEq
Maalox #2 (Rorer)	tablet		dried gel, 400 mg	400 mg (hydroxide)			0.08 mEq
Maalox Plus (Rorer)	tablet suspension		dried gel, 200 mg/tablet 45 mg/ml	200 mg/tablet (hydroxide) 40 mg/ml (hydroxide)		simethicone, 25 mg/tablet 5 mg/ml	0.04 mEq/tablet 0.01 mEq/ml
Maalox TC (Rorer)	suspension		120 mg/ml (dried gel)	60 mg/ml (hydroxide)			0.007 mEq/ml
Magna Gel (North American)	suspension		NSª	NSª (hydroxide)		peppermint flavor	NSª
Magnatril (Lannett)	tablet suspension		260 mg/tablet 52 mg/ml	130 mg/tablet 26 mg/ml	454 mg/tablet 52 mg/ml		NSª
Magnesia and Alumina Oral Suspension (Philips Roxane)	suspension			0.41 g/ml		aluminum oxide, 24 mg/ml sorbitol, 16% saccharin sodium peppermint	0.07 mEq/ml
Marblen (Fleming)	tablet suspension	520 mg (tablet) 104 mg/ml (suspension)				magnesium carbonate, 800 mg (tablet) 80 mg/ml (suspension) peach or apricot flavor	≤ 0.03 mEq/ml

Antacid Product Table, continued

Product (Manufacturer)	Dosage Form	Calcium Carbonate	Aluminum Hydroxide	Magnesium Oxide or Hydroxide	Magnesium Trisilicate	Other Ingredients	Sodium Content
Mylanta (Stuart)	tablet suspension		200 mg/tablet 40 mg/ml	200 mg/tablet (hydroxide) 40 mg/ml (hydroxide)		simethicone, 20 mg/tablet 4 mg/ml	0.067 mg/ mEq of acid-neutralizing capacity (tablet) 0.054 mg/ mEq of acid-neutralizing capacity (suspension)
Mylanta II (Stuart)	tablet suspension		400 mg/tablet 80 mg/ml	400 mg/tablet (hydroxide) 80 mg/ml (hydroxide)		simethicone, 30 mg/tablet 6 mg/ml	0.057 mg/ mEq of acid-neutralizing capacity (tablet) 0.045 mg/ mEq of acid-neutralizing capacity (suspension)
Nephrox (Fleming)	suspension		64 mg/ml			mineral oil, 10%	0.03 mEq/ml
Noralac (North American)	tablet		codried with magnesium carbonate, 300 mg		100 mg	bismuth aluminate, 100 mg alginic acid, 50 mg	NS[a]
Nutramag (Cenci)	suspension			NS[a] (hydroxide)		aluminum oxide	NS[a]
Pama (North American)	tablet	420 mg				glycine, 180 mg	NS[a]
Phillips' Milk of Magnesia (Glenbrook)	suspension tablet			76–87 mg/ml 311 mg/tablet			0.1 mEq/ tablet
Ratio (Warren-Teed)	tablet	400 mg				magnesium carbonate, 50 mg	0.03 mEq
Riopan (Ayerst)	tablet chewable tablet suspension					magaldrate, 400 mg/tablet 80 mg/ml	0.01 mEq/ tablet 0.003 mEq/ ml
Riopan Plus (Ayerst)	tablet suspension					simethicone, 20 mg/tablet 4 mg/ml magaldrate, 480 mg/tablet 80 mg/ml	≤ 0.03 mEq/ tablet ≤ 0.006 mEq/ml
Robalate (Robins)	tablet					dihydroxy-aluminum aminoacetate, 500 mg	< 0.04 mEq/ tablet

Antacid Product Table, continued

Product (Manufacturer)	Dosage Form	Calcium Carbonate	Aluminum Hydroxide	Magnesium Oxide or Hydroxide	Magnesium Trisilicate	Other Ingredients	Sodium Content
Rolaids (Warner-Lambert)	tablet					dihydroxy-aluminum sodium carbonate, 334 mg	2.3 mEq
Silain-Gel (Robins)	suspension tablet		gel, 56.4 mg/ml codried with magnesium carbonate, 282 mg/tablet	57 mg/ml 85 mg/tablet		simethicone, 5 mg/ml 25 mg/tablet	0.04 mEq/ml 0.33 mEq/tablet
Simeco (Wyeth)	suspension		60 mg/ml	60 mg/ml (hydroxide)		simethicone, 6 mg/ml	0.09 mEq/ml
Soda Mint (Lilly)	tablet					sodium bicarbonate, 324 mg peppermint oil	3.9 mEq/tablet
Spastosed (North American)	tablet	precipitated, 226 mg				magnesium carbonate, 162 mg	NSa
Syntrogel (Reed & Carnrick)	tablet		codried with magnesium carbonate, 220 mg	120 mg (hydroxide)			0.33 mEq
Titralac (Riker)	tablet suspension	420 mg/tablet 200 mg/ml				glycine, 180 mg/tablet 60 mg/ml	0.01 mEq/tablet 0.09 mEq/ml
Tralmag (O'Neal, Jones & Feldman)	suspension		30 mg/ml	30 mg/ml (hydroxide)		dihydroxy-aluminum aminoacetate, 40 mg/ml sucrose, 300 mg/ml	free
Trimagel (Columbia Medical)	tablet		dried gel, 250 mg		500 mg		NSa
Trisogel (Lilly)	capsule		100 mg/capsule		300 mg/capsule		<0.04 mEq/ml
Tums (Norcliff Thayer)	tablet	500 mg				peppermint oil	0.12 mEq
WinGel (Winthrop)	tablet suspension		180 mg/tablet 36 mg/ml	160 mg/tablet 32 mg/ml		mint flavor	0.1 mEq/tablet 0.02 mEq/ml

aQuantity not specified.

4 Anthelmintic Products

Frank A. Pettinato

Questions to Ask the Patient

Have worms appeared in the stools?

Have you had any nausea, diarrhea, or abdominal pain recently?

Have you been bothered by itching in the anal area?

Are other members of your family or close contacts also affected?

Have you lost weight or do you become fatigued easily?

How long have the symptoms been present?

Has the problem occurred in the past? How was it treated? Did the treatment work?

If the patient is not an adult, what is the age and approximate weight of the patient?

Have you seen a physician?

Have you traveled out of the country? If so, where and when?

Anthelmintics are used to treat worm (helminth) infections. It has been estimated that approximately 3.5 billion humans harbor helminths (1). The incidence of helminth infection exceeds 90% in primitive areas where sanitation is insufficient, economic conditions are poor, and preventive medicine practices are inadequate. Worm infections are a serious health problem, particularly in tropical regions, and result in a general debilitation of large populations. Resistance to disease, physical development in children, and productivity are reduced by these infections. In the United States and other temperate-zone countries, these infections are considered to be more an annoyance than a major health problem.

Helminth infections encountered in the United States are trichinosis, enterobiasis (pinworm infection), ascariasis (roundworm infection), and hookworm infection. Pinworms are one of the most frequently encountered human helminthic parasites in the United States. There are no effective nonprescription drugs available for helminth infections; consequently, self-medication should be discouraged. Human helminth infections and their symptoms are listed in Table 1.

Other parasitic worms that infect humans include the cestodes (tapeworms) and the trematodes (flukes). Approximately 3% of the school-aged children in the Southern United States are infected with dwarf tapeworm (*Hymenolepsis nana*). Various types are included in Table 1. No nonprescription drugs are available to treat tapeworm infections.

Trichinosis

Trichinosis is caused by a small nematode (*Trichinella spiralis*). Although pork is the principal source of infection, about 10% of the cases reported in the United States during the last decade were attributed to bear meat (2). In Idaho and California, 23 people were involved in an outbreak of trichinosis from this source in 1970 (3). When infected meat is eaten, the action of the gastric juices frees the larvae, which penetrate the small intestinal wall. When they develop into sexually mature adults, the males and females mate, and the female deposits larvae in the intestinal mucosa. These larvae enter the bloodstream, are carried throughout the body, and enter striated muscle fibers, where they complete their development. The muscles of the diaphragm, tongue, and eye and the deltoid pectoral and intercostal muscles are affected most often. Larvae that reach other tissues, such as the heart and brain, disintegrate and are absorbed. This can cause marked inflammation and result in encephalitis and myocarditis.

The incidence of trichinosis in the United States fell from an estimated 12% in 1940 to 2.2% in 1970. There are now approximately 100 cases/year in the United States. This decline is directly attributed to laws requiring that garbage fed to hogs be cooked thoroughly and meat be stored at low temperatures. In addition, public education programs were developed on the need to cook pork thoroughly (4).

Table 1. Human helminth infections

	Common name	Source of infection	Symptoms
Nematode			
Ancylostoma duodenale, Necator americanus	Hookworm	Contact with contaminated soil; larvae are ingested or penetrate the skin on contact	Anemia caused by blood loss (0.5 ml/worm/day); indigestion, anorexia, headache, cough, vomiting, diarrhea, weakness; urticaria at the site of entry into the skin
Ascaris lumbricoides	Roundworm	Ingestion of eggs through contact with fecally contaminated soil	Mild cases may be asymptomatic; GI discomfort, pain, and diarrhea; intestinal obstruction in severe cases; occasionally, bile or pancreatic duct may be obstructed; allergic reactions
Enterobius (Oxyuris) vermicularis	Pinworm, seatworm, threadworm	Ingestion of eggs by fecal contamination of hands, food, clothing, and bedding; reinfection is common; the most common worm infestation in the United States, especially in school children	Indigestion, intense perianal itching, especially at night, resulting in loss of sleep; scratching may cause infection; irritability and fatigue in children
Trichinella spiralis	None	Ingestion of poorly cooked pork; particularly prevalent in the United States	Adult worms in intestinal tract cause vomiting, nausea, and diarrhea; migrating larvae cause malaise, weakness, fever, sweating, dermatitis, and cardiac and respiratory distress; can be fatal
Cestode			
Taenia saginata	Beef tapeworm	Eating poorly cooked infected beef	No characteristic symptoms; digestive upset, diarrhea, anemia, and dizziness vary with the degree of infestation
Diphyllobothrium latum	Fish tapeworm	Eating raw or inadequately cooked fish	Similar to beef tapeworm infestation
Hymenolepis nana	Dwarf tapeworm	Eating food contaminated with human feces	Similar to beef tapeworm infestation

Symptoms

Symptoms of trichinosis are extremely variable, depending on the severity of the infection. If the meat is heavily infected, larval invasion into the intestinal mucosa 1–4 days after ingestion may cause nausea, vomiting, and diarrhea. In some cases, no symptoms are evident. After the seventh day, migration of the larvae may produce muscle weakness, stiffness or pain, and irregular, persistent fever of 100–105°F (37.7–40.5°C). These symptoms may be accompanied by an urticarial rash and respiratory symptoms such as cough and bronchospasm. Skeletal muscle invasion produces muscular pain, tenderness, and often severe weakness. There may be pain on chewing, swallowing, breathing, or moving the eyes or limbs. Another common symptom is edema, usually manifested as a puffiness around the eyes. Once the larvae are encysted, the only symptom may be a vague aching in the muscles.

Clinical diagnosis of trichinosis is difficult because most mild infections are asymptomatic and the nature of the symptoms may vary and change. A combination of irregular fever, periorbital edema, GI disturbances, muscle soreness, hypereosinophilia, and hemorrhages in the nail beds may suggest trichinosis. The pharmacist should refer patients with these symptoms to a physician for evaluation and diagnosis. Self-diagnosis is unwise, since many diseases, such as sinusitis, influenza, and rheumatoid arthritis, mimic the symptoms of trichinosis (5).

Treatment

Treatment includes mild analgesics (for pain relief), sedatives, adequate diet, and anti-inflammatory steroids. Thiabendazole has been shown to kill the larvae in experimental animals; results in humans have been variable. It also has been effective in reducing the fever and relieving the muscle pain, tenderness, and edema of trichinosis (6). For severe symptoms, corticosteroids in addition to thiabendazole, constitute the current recommended therapy (7). There are no nonprescription drugs for the mitigation of the disease.

Enterobiasis

Enterobiasis is commonly called pinworm, seatworm or threadworm infection, or oxyuriasis. The intestinal infection in humans is caused by *Enterobius vermicularis*. Unlike many helminth infections, enterobiasis is not limited to rural and poverty-stricken areas but occurs in urban communities of every economic status. *Enterobius vermicularis* is common in temperate climates and is especially prevalent among school children. The female adult worm is about 10 mm long, and the adult male is about 3 mm. The adult worms inhabit the first portion of the large intestine. The mature female usually does not pass her eggs into the intestinal lumen but stores them in her body until several thousand accumulate, at which time she migrates down the colon and out the anus and deposits the eggs in the perianal region. Within a few hours, infective larvae develop. Ingestion of the larvae releases them in the small intestine. Within 15–43 days from the time of ingestion, newly developed gravid females migrate to the anal area and discharge eggs, and the cycle continues.

The most common way of transmitting pinworm infection in children is probably direct anus-to-mouth transfer of eggs by contaminated fingers and eating food that has been handled by soiled hands. Reinfection may occur readily because eggs frequently are found under the fingernails of infected children after scratching anal areas. The eggs may be dislodged from the perianal region into the environment and may enter the mouth via hands, food, or swallowing of airborne eggs.

Symptoms

Slight infections of enterobiasis may be asymptomatic. The most important and most frequent symptom is usually an irritating itching in the perianal and perineal regions. This itching normally occurs at night when the gravid female deposits her eggs in these areas. Scratching to relieve the itching may lead to bacterial infection of the area. Nervousness, inability to concentrate, lack of appetite, and unusual dark circles around the eyes frequently are observed in pinworm-infected children. Worms occasionally enter the female genital tract and become encapsulated within the uterus or fallopian tubules or they may migrate into the peritoneal cavity, resulting in the formation of granulomas in these areas.

The physical symptoms are not the sole misery-inducing effects of pinworms. Parents are often dismayed to find worms near the anus of a child, and this psychological trauma or "pinworm neurosis" also must be considered one of the harmful effects of enterobiasis (8). Patients need to be assured that pinworms are common and there is no stigma attached to their occurrence.

Perianal itching is a symptom of many other conditions mistakenly attributed to pinworm infection (9). Seborrheic dermatitis, atopic eczema, psoriasis, lichen planus, and neurodermatitis may produce severe itching when the perianal region is involved. An allergic or contact dermatitis may result from soaps or ointments used by the patient in an attempt to alleviate the initial mild symptoms. Ointments containing local anesthetics are well-known sensitizers and should be suspected as contributing to the problem. Other parasitic infestations that induce itching, such as scabies and pediculosis pubis, may involve the perianal skin in addition to the larger areas of the body. Monilial infection may be the cause of pruritus ani especially in patients with diabetes mellitus. Other causes of pruritus include excessive vaginal discharge and urinary incontinence in women and excessive sweating during hot weather. When mineral oil is used as a cathartic, it tends to leak and may produce increased moisture and itching unless appropriate anal hygiene is practiced.

Treatment of pinworm infection should begin with an accurate diagnosis. This can be done by either of two methods (10). One method is to cover the end of a swab or tongue depressor with scotch tape (sticky side out) and apply this end to the perianal area. The presence or absence of eggs is confirmed by examining the tape under the microscope. Collection of eggs can be done at home but inspection and evaluation must be done in a laboratory or physician's office. Another detection method used frequently in children is to visually inspect the anal site using a flashlight an hour or so after the child has gone to bed. Female pinworms, which are ¼–½ inch in length, can be seen emerging from the perianal region after depositing their eggs.

Treatment

Gentian violet is the only nonprescription drug available for treatment of pinworm infections. Genetic toxicity data indicate that gentian violet interacts with DNA in cultured cells, suggesting a potential carcinogenic effect (11–13). Even though the evidence is not conclusive, the FDA intends to place gentian violet in Category II (14). However, in light of the potential carcinogenicity of gentian violet and the availability of more effective prescription agents, the drug should not be recommended as an anthelmintic.

Prescription-only drugs, such as piperazine salts, pyrvinium pamoate, pyrantel pamoate, and mebendazole, may cure 80–95% of pinworm infections. Pyrantel pamoate and mebendazole are the drugs of choice because of easy administration and patient tolerance (15).

The FDA has made a tentative decision to accept the recommendation to move pyrantel pamoate from prescription-only status to nonprescription status for the treatment of pinworms (16). Pyrantel pamoate is effective against a variety of helminth infections, but only pinworm infections will be recommended for self-treatment. All others should be treated by a physician.

Pyrantel pamoate first was used in veterinary practice as a broad-spectrum drug effective against pinworms, roundworms, and hookworms. Because of its effectiveness and lack of toxicity, it became an important drug for treating certain helminth infections in humans (17). To treat pinworm infections, the recommended dosage (as the pamoate) is 5 mg/lb or 11 mg/kg, not to exceed 1 g. Pyrantel is a depolarizing neuromuscular agent that results in paralysis of the helminths contractile hold onto the intestinal wall so that the worm is eliminated readily.

The FDA panel has recommended the following labeling for Category I nonprescription anthelmintic drug products:

Indication

- For the treatment of pinworms.

Warnings

- If upset stomach, diarrhea, nausea, or vomiting occurs with this medication, discontinue using it and consult a physician.
- Do not take this product if you are pregnant or ill, without first consulting a physician.
- Do not give to infants under 2 years of age or children who weigh less than 25 pounds without first consulting a physician.

Directions

- When one individual in a household has pinworms, the entire household should be treated. Persons who are ill or pregnant, infants under 2 years of age, or children who weigh less than 25 pounds should not be treated without first consulting a physician.
- Take only according to directions.
- Do not exceed the recommended dosage.
- If any worms other than pinworms are present before or after treatment, consult a physician.

The following additional measures are recommended to prevent reinfections (15):

- Wash bed linens, bed clothes, and underwear of entire family.
- Take a daily morning shower to remove eggs deposited in the perianal region during the night.
- Use disinfectants daily on the toilet seat and bathtub.
- Apply antipruritic ointment regularly over the perianal region at bedtime (avoid contaminating the ointment) to decrease itching and prevent secondary bacterial infection. Discontinue use if sensitization occurs.
- Wear close-fitting shorts under one-piece pajamas to prevent scratching at night and migration of worms.
- Trim an infected child's nails regularly and scrub the fingers with a brush after going to the bathroom.
- Wash hands frequently, especially before meals and after using the toilet.

Ascarid Infection

Ascarid infection is caused by *Ascaris lumbricoides* (roundworm). The adult ascarides are 15–35-cm long and live in the small intestine, where they receive their nourishment. The female lays eggs, which are passed in the feces and develop into infective larvae in the soil. Although the mature larvae in the shell remain viable in the soil for many months, the eggs do not hatch until they are ingested by humans. Upon ingestion, the larvae are released in the small intestine. They penetrate the intestinal wall and migrate via the bloodstream to the lungs, travel up the respiratory tree to the epiglottis, where they are swallowed, and develop into male and female adults in the small intestine.

Symptoms

The larvae and adults are capable of extensive migration and therefore induce diverse symptoms involving the respiratory and GI tracts in particular. Although many patients are asymptomatic, the most common symptoms caused by ascarid infections are vague abdominal discomfort and abdominal colic (18). Occasionally diarrhea is present. Children characteristically have fever and may lose weight or fail to grow. The symptoms may suggest abdominal tumor or peptic ulcer disease. Migration of the worms may cause intestinal obstruction that may lead to perforation, appendicitis, and peritonitis. Light infestations may be asymptomatic; heavy infestations present symptoms that may be mistaken for a variety of respiratory and GI diseases.

Cough is produced during migration of the larvae through the lungs; the larvae may be coughed up and seen in the sputum. Fever and a pulmonary infiltrate also may accompany this pulmonary syndrome.

Allergic reactions such as asthma, hay fever, urticaria, and conjunctivitis also may result from absorption of toxins from the worm.

Treatment

There are no nonprescription drugs for treating ascarid infections. Cure rates of more than 90% are achieved with mebendazole, piperazine salts, and pyrantel pamoate, which are available only by prescription (17). Pyrantel pamoate may be available as a nonprescription drug in the future for treating ascarid infections. Piperazine is contraindicated in the presence of convulsive disorders, or impaired renal or hepatic functions.

Hookworm Infection

In the United States, hookworm infections in humans is caused by *Necator americanus*. The adult worms, which are about 10 mm long, attach themselves to the small intestine. Their eggs are excreted in the feces, hatch in warm, moist soil, and develop into active filariform larvae. On contact with humans, the larvae rapidly penetrate the skin, enter the bloodstream, and are carried to the lungs. They then enter the alveoli, ascend the trachea to the throat, are swallowed, and pass into the small intestine, where they develop into mature adults.

Symptoms

When the larvae penetrate the exposed skin, there may be an erythematous maculopapular rash and edema with severe itching. These symptoms may persist for several days. The lesions occur most commonly on the feet, particularly between the toes, and have been termed "ground itch."

Heavy infections may produce a cough and fever when the larvae migrate through the lungs. Mild intestinal infections may be asymptomatic; moderately severe infections may result in indigestion, dizziness, headache, weakness, fatigue, nausea, and vomiting. In advanced cases, there is epigastric pain, abdominal tenderness, chronic fatigue, and alternating constipation and diarrhea. The epigastric pain is relieved by eating foods high in bulk or fiber (19). As with ascariasis, these symptoms may be mistaken for those of some respiratory and GI disorders.

A major clinical manifestation is iron deficiency anemia resulting from the loss of as much as 0.67 ml of blood/worm/day, which the adult worm extracts while it is attached to the intestinal mucosa (20). Malnourished children and some menstruating women are especially prone to anemia, depending on the severity of the infection. Even people with adequate iron intake may become anemic if the hookworm infection is severe enough to cause a blood loss that the normal body erythropoietic mechanisms cannot handle.

Treatment

The drugs of choice to treat hookworm infections are mebendazole and pyrantel pamoate.

Summary

The pharmacist should be familiar with the common helminth infections and their effects to discourage self-diagnosis and treatment. The clinical manifestations of these parasitic diseases are so general and characteristic of so many other illnesses that attempts at self-diagnosis of helminthiasis not only is difficult, but could lead to the neglect of a more serious condition. Diagnosis should be based on clinical and laboratory evidence.

Self-medication should be discouraged at every opportunity. The availability of effective, relatively safe, easy-to-take prescription drugs that can eradicate many infections in one or two doses should be reason enough to avoid self-medication. The pharmacist is the most available and capable person to encourage the patient to consult a physician for treatment.

References

1. "Foundations of Parasitology," G. D. Schmidt and L. S. Roberts, C. V. Mosby, St. Louis, Mo., 1977, p. 2.
2. "Harrison's Principles of Internal Medicine," 9th ed., K. J. Isselbacher, R. D. Adams, E. Braunwald, R. G. Petersdorf, and J. D. Wilson, Eds., McGraw-Hill, New York, N.Y., 1980, p. 894.
3. M. Wand and D. Lyman, *J. Am. Med. Assoc.*, *220*, 245 (1972).
4. *Morbidity and Mortality Weekly Report*, *29*, 482 (Oct. 10, 1980).
5. S. E. Gould, "Trichinosis in Man and Animals," Charles C Thomas, Springfield, Ill., 1970, pp. 307–321.
6. W. C. Campbell and A. C. Cuckler, *Tex. Rep. Biol. Med.*, 27 (2), 665 (1969).
7. *Medical Letter on Drugs and Therapeutics*, 21, (26), 111 (1979).
8. H. C. Wormser and H. N. Abramson, *U.S. Pharm.*, 2, 46 (1977).
9. T. L. Schrock, in "Gastrointestinal Disease," M. H. Sleisinger and J. S. Fordtran, Eds., W. B. Saunders, Philadelphia, Pa., 1978, pp. 1882–1884.
10. *Federal Register*, *45*, 59543 (1980).
11. H. R. Rosencranz and H. S. Carr, *Br. Med. J.*, 3, 702 (1971).
12. W. Au, S. Pathak, C. J. Collie, and T. C. Hsu, *Mutation Res.*, *58*, 269 (1978).
13. T. C. Hsu, C. J. Collie, A. F. Lusby, and D. A. Johnston, *Mutation Res.*, 45, 233 (1977).
14. *Federal Register*, *45*, 59441 (1980).
15. "Drugs of Choice 1978/1979," W. Modell, Ed., C. V. Mosby, St. Louis, Mo., 1978, p. 378.
16. *Federal Register*, *45*, 59445 (1980).
17. "The Pharmacological Basis of Therapeutics," 6th ed., A. G. Gilman, L. S. Goodman, and A. Gilman, Eds., Macmillan, New York, N.Y., 1980, p. 1024.
18. L. L. Brandborg, in "Gastrointestinal Diseases," M. H. Sleisinger and J. S. Fordtran, Eds., W. B. Saunders, Philadelphia, Pa., 1978, p. 1164.
19. L. L. Brandborg, in "Gastrointestinal Diseases," M. H. Sleisinger and J. S. Fordtran, Eds., W. B. Saunders, Philadelphia, Pa., 1978, p. 1169.
20. "Clinical Parasitology," 8th ed., E. Faust, P. Russell, and R. Jung, Eds., Lea and Febiger, Philadelphia, Pa., 1970, p. 312.

5

Antidiarrheal and Other Gastrointestinal Products

R. Leon Longe

Questions to Ask the Patient

Is the diarrhea associated with other symptoms such as fever, vomiting, or pain?

How long have you had diarrhea? Was it sudden in onset? How often do you have a bowel movement?

Are the stools foul smelling, light in color, or greasy?

Is there blood or mucus present in the stool?

What is your age?

Can you relate the onset of diarrhea to a specific cause such as a particular food (milk products) or drug? Have you traveled recently to a foreign country?

Have other members of your family experienced similar symptoms?

Have you changed your diet recently?

Are you currently taking or have you recently stopped taking any prescription or nonprescription medications? Which ones?

Do you have diabetes or any other chronic disease?

Have you tried any antidiarrheal products? Which ones? How effective were they?

Diarrhea is the abnormally frequent passage of watery stools. The frequency of bowel movements varies with the individual. Some healthy adults may have as many as three stools per day; others may defecate once in 2 or more days (1). The mean daily fecal weight is 100–150 g. An increase of from 150–300 g is interpreted as diarrhea. The major factor contributing to diarrhea is excretion of excess water that normally is reabsorbed from the gut. Disruption in the water absorption process resulting in accumulation in the gut of even a few hundred milliliters of water may cause diarrhea (2, 3).

Diarrhea usually is viewed and treated as a symptom of an undiagnosed and presumed minor and transient GI disorder. More than 50 conditions, including major diseases involving the kidneys, heart, liver, thyroid, and lungs are associated with diarrhea. Additionally, numerous drugs may induce diarrhea. Often, diarrhea is only one of many symptoms associated with a major illness (4–6).

Physiology of Digestive System

The small intestine originates at the pylorus and terminates at the cecum of the ascending colon (Figure 1). It is a convoluted tube, approximately 6.4 meters long, made up of the duodenum, jejunum, and ileum. The small intestine is the site of digestion, absorption of nu-

trients, and retention of waste material; these activities depend on normal musculature, nerve tone, and digestive enzymes.

The alimentary tract is basically a long, hollow tube surrounded by layers of smooth muscle: a thick, circular layer on the mucosal side of the intestine; a thinner, longitudinal layer on the serosal side; and a third layer of both circular and longitudinal muscle fibers. The active contractions of the various muscles control tone, or tension, of the intestinal wall. Normally, this tone is maintained with little expenditure of energy so that the muscles remain generally free from fatigue and capable of continued performance.

A mucous layer protects and lubricates the walls of the intestine. The mucus, composed of glycoproteins and sulfated aminopolysaccharides, is released from goblet cells interspersed among the columnar epithelial cells in the intestine. Secretion of mucus is increased by local irritation caused by foods or cathartics and by psychic trauma, which suggests control by the autonomic nervous system. The mucus is more viscous in the upper part of the small intestine than in the colon and forms a protective physical barrier to the intestinal lining, reducing contact with irritating substances and bacteria. The alkalinity of the mucus contributes further to the protection of the intestinal lining by neutralizing acidic bacterial products.

Normal intestinal motility and peristalsis are maintained by the smooth muscles and the intrinsic nerves (Auerbach's and Meissner's plexuses). The vagus and parasympathetic pelvic nerves stimulate intestinal motility; sympathetic innervation inhibits intestinal motility and secretion. Extrinsic autonomic innervation influences the strength and frequency of these movements and mediates reflexes by which activity in one part of the intestine influences another.

After eating, the lumen of the intestine is distended, causing the smooth muscle layers to contract. Normally, the segmental contractions of the circular muscles are accompanied by a decrease in the propulsive activity of the gut. The process retains the food in the lumen and increases the duration of its exposure to the digestive elements, enhancing digestion and absorption.

Normally, about 7 liters of digestive fluid are secreted into the GI tract each day. This is made up of about 1 liter of saliva, 2 liters of gastric juice, 2 liters of pancreatic juice, about 1 liter of fluid from the liver, and 1 liter from the small bowel. An additional 2 liters enter the GI tract with food and drinks. Of these 9 liters, all but one are reabsorbed in the small intestine. The large bowel reabsorbs about 850 ml of the remaining 1 liter, leaving about 150 ml to be excreted in the stool each day (2).

Approximately 3 liters of fluid containing electrolytes and nutrients enters the small intestine every 24 hours (5). Reabsorption reduces the quantity that reaches the large intestine to 1,000 ml of an isotonic semiliquid substance (chyme) consisting in part of nonabsorbed, undigested food residue, nutrients, electrolytes, water, and bacteria. Chyme has an average electrolyte content of 83 mEq of sodium, 20 mEq of bicarbonate, 6 mEq of potassium, and 60 mEq of chloride (7).

The large intestine, which is about 1.5 meters long extends from the cecum to the rectum. It is composed of

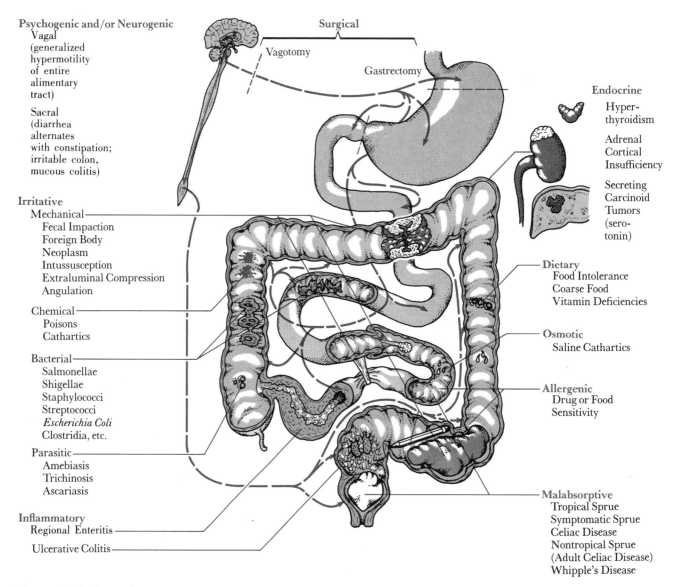

Figure 1. The lower digestive tract showing the induction of diarrhea by various causes. Adapted from F. H. Netter, *The Ciba Collection of Medical Illustrations*, Ciba Pharmaceutical Company, New York, N.Y., 1962, p. 99, Vol. 1.

the cecum, ascending colon, transverse colon, descending colon, sigmoid colon, and rectum. The colon has two primary functions: absorption and storage. The first two-thirds of the colon facilitates absorption, and the remainder functions as a storage area. The proximal half (ascending and transverse parts) of the colon reduces chyme to a semisolid substance called feces, or stool. Feces are 75% water and 25% solid material consisting of nonabsorbed food residue, bacteria, desquamated epithelial cells, unabsorbed minerals, and a small quantity of electrolytes (Table 1). The stool is stored in the descending colon until defecation.

The colon is structured like the small intestine with both circular and longitudinal muscles. The longitudinal muscles are shorter than the underlying colonic tissue and tend to draw the colon into sacs. The segmented contractions of the circular musculature further cause the division of the colon into sausage-like units, known as haustra, that facilitate churning of the colonic contents and the absorption of water. Thus, a decrease in the occurrence or intensity of the segmental contractions and the predominance of the propulsive force of the longitudinal muscles may lead to diarrhea. In the absence of circular muscle contractions, mass colonic movements may occur during which the colon may contract to half its length and may resemble a smooth, hollow tube devoid of segmented units. Colonic activity is increased by parasympathetic stimulation while sympathetic stimulation inhibits colonic motor activity.

The normal bowel movement, or defecation, begins with the stimulation of stretch receptors in the rectum by feces. Peristaltic waves propel the feces to the anal canal where the voluntarily controlled external anal sphincter controls defecation (8).

In the colon, nonpathogenic bacterial flora produce enzymes necessary for degradataion of waste products, synthesize certain vitamins, and generate ammonia. *Bacteroides* and anaerobic *Lactobacilli* make up the majority of the colonic flora. Pathogenic organisms such as Enterobacteriaceae (*Escherichia coli*), hemolytic *Streptococci*, *Clostridia*, and yeasts also are found in the colon, but are only a small proportion of the normal flora. Many factors such as diet, pH, GI disease, and drugs, such as antibiotics, influence the proportion of the population of these organisms. If these potential pathogens are allowed to grow uncontrolled, their increased proportion can present serious complications (9).

Types of Diarrhea

Acute diarrhea is characterized by a sudden onset of frequent, liquid stools accompanied by weakness, flatulence, pain, and often fever and vomiting. Chronic diarrhea is the persistent or recurrent passage of unformed stools and usually is the result of multiple factors.

The variability in the origins of diarrhea make identification of the pathophysiologic mechanism difficult and may make a complete physical examination necessary, including supportive clinical laboratory tests. The etiology of diarrhea can be psychogenic, neurogenic, surgical, endocrine, irritant, osmotic, dietary, allergenic, malabsorptive, infectious, and/or inflammatory.

Table 1. Electrolyte and water content of normal and diarrheal feces

Component	Normal[a]	Diarrheal[b]
Bicarbonate, mEq/24 hours	30	135–450
Chloride, mEq/24 hours	60	120–400
Potassium, mEq/24 hours	11.3	105–350
Sodium, mEq/24 hours	6.5	130–500
Water, ml/24 hours	111	3,000–10,000

[a]Adapted with kind permission from CIBA-GEIGY, from *Documenta GEIGY, Scientific Tables*, 7th ed., K. Diem and C. Lentner, Eds., CIBA-GEIGY Ltd., Basel, Switzerland, 1970, pp. 657–658.

[b]Adapted from "Manual of Medical Therapeutics," 23rd ed., J. J. Freitag and L. W. Miller, Eds., Little, Brown, Boston, Mass., 1980.

Etiology of Diarrhea

Acute Diarrhea

Acute diarrhea may be infectious, toxic, drug-induced, or dietary in origin. It may also be the result of acute or chronic illness. Infectious diarrhea in adults is usually bacterial while viral diarrhea is more commonly seen in pediatric patients (Table 2).

Two general pathophysiologic mechanisms may be involved in the development of diarrhea: decreased absorption and increased secretion. The gut maintains a balance between absorption and secretion of GI fluids. Historically, diarrhea has been thought of as a malabsorption syndrome. However, evidence supports the theory that diarrhea, characterized by large-volume stools, is a hypersecretory disease (10). Hypersecretion into the intestinal lumen is a common response to infectious organisms in the gut (11). Diarrhea also may be provoked by stimulating adenyl cyclase and this in turn causes a rise in cyclic AMP, which leads to hypersecretion (12, 13).

Infectious Diarrhea Although the causative agent is not readily identified in most cases of acute diarrhea, the bacterial pathogens most commonly responsible in the United States are *E. coli*, *Shigella*, *Salmonella*, and *Staphylococci* species (14–17). Some organisms cause diarrhea through an enterotoxin (toxigenic *E. coli* and *Staphylococcus aureus*). Others (*Shigella*, *Salmonella*, and invasive *E. coli*) directly invade the mucosal epithelial cells. Patients with diarrhea caused by toxin-producing agents clinically present with a "cholera-like" syndrome, which primarily involves the small bowel. The patient experiences an abrupt onset of large volumes of watery stools, variable nausea, vomiting, and cramps, possibly with a low-grade fever. Invasive organisms produce a "dysentery-like" syndrome if the large bowel is the site of attack. This type is characterized by fever, abdominal crampy pain, tenesmus (straining), and frequent small-volume stools that may contain blood and pus.

When the patient is first seen, a careful history is essential in identifying a cause. For example, staphylococci grow rapidly in food (ham and milk) producing a toxin. Upon ingestion, the toxin quickly (within 1–2 hours) provokes the diarrhea attack. In contrast, the incubation period for *Salmonellae* is 12–24 hours. Fever, malaise, muscle aching, and profound epigastric or periumbilical discomfort with severe anorexia suggest an infectious, inflammatory disease of the bowel. Severe periumbilical pain and vomiting commonly are experienced with viral gastroenteritis and are acute for 2–3 days before gradually subsiding (18).

The treatment of infectious diarrhea is based upon treating the spread of the pathogen, generally with a prescribed antibiotic or other anti-infective agent and fluid support. In many instances the illness is self-limiting, and normal function of the alimentary tract is restored with or without treatment in 24–48 hours. If the patient has a persistent *Salmonella* fecal flora and is a food handler, a 10–14-day course of ampicillin, chloramphenicol, or trimethoprim-sulfamethoxazole may be indicated.

Infantile Diarrhea   Diarrhea in infants and young children is a common pediatric problem, and the etiology often is difficult to identify, although it is frequently caused by a viral infection of the intestinal tract. Diet and systemic and local infections, such as otitis media, are other known etiologies of acute diarrheal episodes in children.

Rotaviruses have been implicated as the cause of about 50% of all infantile diarrhea (19, 20). Clinical features include a 12–48-hour incubation period, vomiting, watery diarrhea, and a low-grade fever. The illness usually is self-limiting, lasting 5–8 days. Generally, it requires only symptomatic therapy. Evidence has demonstrated that breast feeding is effective in preventing viral diarrhea (21). Parvoviruses (Norwalk-like viruses) also have been implicated, with signs and symptoms resembling those of rotaviruses (22).

In children, particularly infants, severe acute diarrhea may cause severe, and possibly dangerous, dehydration and electrolyte imbalance. In the newborn water may comprise 75% of the total body weight; water loss in severe diarrhea may be 10% or more of body weight. After 8–10 bowel movements in 24 hours, a 2-month-old infant could lose enough fluid to cause circulatory collapse and renal failure. For this reason, moderate to severe diarrhea in infants should receive a physician's evaluation. The pharmacist must be cautious in recommending treatment for all pediatric patients (23–27).

Traveler's Diarrhea (Turista)   The acute diarrhea that frequently develops among tourists visiting foreign countries with warm climates and relatively poor sanitation usually cannot be traced to known pathogens. However, a study conducted during the Fifth World Congress of Gastroenterology found that enterotoxigenic *E. coli* was the most common cause of traveler's diarrhea in Mexico (28). It probably results from an extensive alteration in the bacterial flora of the gut caused by exposure, through food and drink, to a markedly different microbial population. Traveler's diarrhea

Table 2. Causes of acute diarrhea in infants and children
Infection
Parenteral
Urinary
Respiratory
Enteral
Viruses—Rotaviruses, others
Bacterias—*Escherichia coli, Shigella, Salmonella, Yersinia*
Protozoa— *Giardia lamblia*
Other inflammatory disorders
Food allergy
Idiopathic ulcerative colitis
Crohn's disease
Necrotizing enterocolitis (in the newborn)
Pseudomembranous enterocolitis
Hirschsprung's enterocolitis
Intra-abdominal sepsis—e.g., appendicitis
Iatrogenic
Diet—e.g., hypertonic formula
Drugs—e.g., antibiotics, laxatives

Reprinted with permission from Richard Hamilton, in "Gastrointestinal Disease," 2nd. ed., Vol. 1, W. B. Saunders, Philadelphia, Pa., 1978, p. 338.

is characterized by a sudden onset of loose stools, nausea, occasional vomiting, and abdominal cramping. Children seem particularly susceptible, and most cases develop during the first week of exposure to the new location.

Protozoal Diarrhea   *Giardia lamblia* and *Entamoeba histolytica* are protozoa associated with acute diarrhea. Giardiasis especially infests hikers, children, travelers, and institutionalized patients. Following a 1–3-day incubation, sudden onset of explosive watery stool begins along with abdominal cramps (29). Metronidazole, 250 mg orally 3 times/day for 7 days, is very effective (29, 30). The pediatric dose for metronidazole is 15 mg/kg/ 24 hours by mouth for 10 days (31).

Entamoeba histolytica causes amebiasis in areas with poor sanitation, in institutionalized patients, and among travelers and migrant workers. The illness is characterized by severe crampy pain, tenesmus, and disentery in 3–10 days. Metronidazole, 750 mg orally 3 times/day, is generally effective (32). The pediatric dose of metronidazole for amebic dysentery is 35–50 mg/kg/24 hours for 10 days orally.

Drug-Induced Diarrhea   Diarrhea is frequently a side effect of drug administration. All antibiotics can produce adverse GI symptoms including diarrhea, but severity depends largely on the specific antibiotic. Antibiotics that have a broad spectrum of activity against aerobic and anaerobic organisms frequently cause diarrhea. Ampicillin, clindamycin, erythromycin, lincomycin, neomycin, trimethoprim-sulfamethoxazole, and the tetracyclines are commonly prescribed broad-spectrum antibiotics (33).

Two processes may account for antibiotic-induced diarrhea. Diarrhea associated with the first few doses is attributed to mild irritant properties of the drug itself. Diarrhea beginning within a few days of the initial antibiotic therapy is due most likely to a disruption in the normal intestinal flora.

In general, orally administered antibiotics are not absorbed completely. The unabsorbed fraction of the dose may be irritating to the intestinal mucosa, cause alterations in intestinal motility, and induce diarrhea. Even the soluble antibiotics may cause irritation if they form strongly acidic solutions, such as tetracycline hydrochloride. Some antibiotics, (kanamycin and neomycin) affect intestinal absorption of nutrients, even at usual dosage levels (4).

The following antibiotics are reported to cause colitis (pseudomembranous colitis), a severe and persistent diarrhea (34):

* Chloramphenicol;
* Neomycin;
* Cephalosporins;
* Tetracyclines;
* Sulfonamides;
* Ampicillin;
* Lincomycin;
* Clindamycin;
* Trimethoprim-sulfamethoxazole, Metronidazole.

In many studies no distinction has been made between diarrhea and colitis as defined by proctosigmoidoscopy.

Antibiotic-induced diarrhea also may be caused by overgrowth of an antibiotic-resistant bacterial or fungal strain or a toxin-producing bacteria *Clostridium difficile.* Intestinal microorganisms that tend to proliferate during antibiotic therapy include *Staphylococcus aureus*, *Pseudomonas aeruginosa*, *Streptococcus faecalis*, *Candida albicans*, and species of *Salmonella* and *Proteus*. *Clostridium difficile*, a toxin-producing microbe, is reported to cause pseudomembranous colitis (35, 36). Except in cases of severe staphylococcal enterocolitis, a reduction in the drug dose, a change in parenteral administration, or the withdrawal of the antibiotic may relieve the problem. Oral vancomycin appears to be the treatment of choice for antibiotic-associated pseudomembranous colitis (36, 37). Cholestyramine may also be tried; however, agents that inhibit peristalsis, such as opiates, may prolong and worsen the condition (38).

Other drugs, such as cathartics, which are irritating to the intestinal mucosa, may precipitate diarrhea, as may drugs that cause the retention of salts and water in the intestinal lumen. Certain antacid preparations contain magnesium to prevent the constipating effects of aluminum and calcium. Depending on the dose taken and the individual, these types of antacid preparations may induce diarrhea. Drugs that alter autonomic control of intestinal motility also may cause diarrhea. For example, it is not uncommon for the antiadrenergic, antihypertensive agents such as guanethidine, methyldopa, and reserpine to produce diarrhea. Generalized cramping and diarrhea may follow the use of a parasympathomimetic drug, such as bethanecol, used as a urinary tract stimulant.

Food-Induced Diarrhea   Food intolerance, caused by allergy, or the ingestion of foods that are excessively fatty, spicy, or contain a high degree of roughage or a large number of seeds, can also provoke diarrhea. If diarrhea occurs in more than one person within 24 hours of ingestion of the same food, it is likely that a preformed toxin (food poison) has been ingested.

Food intolerance and diarrhea are associated with disaccharidase deficiency (lactase deficiency). Carbohydrates in the diet commonly include lactose and sucrose, which are hydrolyzed to monosaccharides. These enzymatic activities are reduced in intestinal disorders such as infectious diarrhea, congenital disaccharidase deficiency, and gastrointestinal allergy. When disaccharides such as sucrose and lactose are not hydrolyzed they pool in the lumen of the intestine where they ferment and produce an osmotic and pH change. The resulting osmolarity increase draws more fluid into the lumen, resulting in diarrhea.

Chronic Diarrhea

Chronic diarrhea is usually the result of multiple factors and therefore can be difficult to diagnose. The condition may be defined as recurring episodes of watery stools lasting more than 2 weeks. It may be caused by a disease of the bowel or may be a secondary manifestation of a systemic disease. Some investigators differentiate chronic diarrhea into functional or organic groups (39). The pharmacist should refer patients with persistent or recurrent diarrhea to a physician. Correct causative diagnosis usually can be made only after a physician studies the patient's history carefully and performs a physical examination and appropriate laboratory tests. Chronic diarrheal illness may be caused by one of many conditions but is generally related to GI diseases.

Determining chronic diarrhea can be very difficult because it does not always involve frequent daily passage of watery stools. Three categories of chronic diarrhea can be described: frequent, small, formed stools with tenesmus (straining); large, oily, malodorous, formed stools; and frequent, voluminous, loosely formed stools. The patient may complain of weight loss, fever, anxiety/depression, nausea, vomiting, or perianal tenderness.

Psychogenic factors are frequent causes of chronic diarrhea. Psychogenic diarrhea is usually characterized by small, frequent stools and abdominal pain. The stools may be watery and may follow a normal bowel movement or may appear shortly after eating. Psychogenic diarrhea is related to emotional stress that may periodically increase the parasympathetic nervous system impulses to the GI tract. The diarrhea may alternate with constipation. Patients complaining of chronic diarrhea that appears to be psychogenically related should be referred to a physician.

One drug-induced cause of chronic diarrhea is laxative abuse. Chronic laxative use may lead to serious electrolyte imbalance, steatorrhea, protein loss, and weight loss (40–43). These patients seek medical advice for long-standing complaints and undergo expensive work-ups. Usually the problem is resolved after other causes cannot be identified. Upon questioning, the patient will frequently deny laxative use. To avoid this problem, a very careful drug history should be taken.

Some people who suffer from persistent diarrhea are aware of the cause and can manage the condition symptomatically. For example, about 2.5% of adult diabetics and 22% of diabetics with evident neuropathy have chronic diarrhea. Individuals who have persistent or recurrent diarrhea and are unaware of its cause should seek prompt medical attention because conditions such as cancer of the stomach or colon or an endocrine tumor may be causing the diarrhea. One of the seven "danger signals" of cancer is a change in bowel habits. In both sexes, cancer of the colon and rectum is a frequently reported type of cancer. The American Cancer Society estimates that almost three of every four patients may be saved by early diagnosis and proper treatment (44). A follow-up study of patients who had been suffering from "unexplained" diarrhea revealed the risk of missing a diagnosis such as neoplasm (45).

Evaluation

The most common complaints voiced by patients with acute diarrhea are abrupt onset of frequent, watery, loose stools, abdominal cramping, flatulence, fever, muscle aches, vomiting, and malaise. In chronic diarrhea, the most significant finding usually is a history of previous bouts of diarrhea and complaints of anorexia, weight loss, and chronic weakness. These patients generally have histories of poor health.

In assessing the patient's complaint, the pharmacist should determine

- The patient's age;
- Mode of onset (events coincident, past episodes, acute or chronic onset, duration);
- The character and location of the symptom;
- Factors that precipitate or aggravate the complaint;
- The medications (including laxatives) the patient is taking;
- Factors that relieve the symptom;
- Past treatment of the problem.
- Other current illness or family history of diarrhea or GI disorders.

Evaluation of patient responses should enable the pharmacist to recommend an appropriate course of action.

The pharmacist should obtain a history of present illness before recommending self-treatment. The following four groups of patients with either acute or chronic diarrhea should be referred to a physician for a complete diagnostic evaluation:

- Children under 3 years of age;
- Patients over 60 years of age who have a poor medical history;
- Patients with a medical history of chronic illness such as asthma, peptic ulcer, diabetes, or heart disease;
- Pregnant patients.

Other medical conditions that necessitate physician referral include

- Bloody stools;
- Abdominal tenderness;
- High fever;
- Dehydration;
- Weight loss of greater than 5% of body weight;
- Diarrhea that has lasted 5–7 days.

Clinical judgment must be used in evaluating these patients. For example, access to medical treatment may not be readily available, and temporary self-treatment may be needed until a medical appointment can be arranged. When a drug is implicated as a cause of diarrhea, the pharmacist should refer the patient to a physician, since the patient may need to continue taking the drug even though it is causing problems.

The medication history helps rule out drug-induced diarrhea. With this background, the pharmacist should determine which self-treatments have already been tried, the patient's age, symptoms, date of onset, and characteristics of stools (number, consistency, odor, and appearance). Alcohol abuse, ankylosing spondylitis, diverticulosis, emotional problems, gastritis, irritable bowel, and ulcerative colitis or regional enteritis are some frequently reported past medical problems. Referral to a physician is the rule and not the exception in such patients.

The early signs of dehydration include sunken eyes, dry mucous membranes, and decreased skin turgor. The patient should be questioned about the nature and amount of fluid intake, occurrence of vomiting, and frequency of urination.

Stool character gives valuable information about diarrhea. For example, undigested food particles in the stool indicate small bowel irritation; black, tarry stools can indicate upper GI bleeding; and red stools suggest possible lower bowel bleeding or simply the recent ingestion of red-colored food such as beets or drug products such as Povan. Diarrhea originating from the small bowel probably is manifested as a marked outpouring of fluid high in potassium and bicarbonate. A paste-like or semisolid loose stool is indicative of colon-type diarrhea.

Treatment

Diarrhea is a symptom, and symptomatic relief must not be interpreted as being a cure for the underlying cause. Symptomatic relief generally suffices in simple functional diarrhea that is only temporary and relatively uncomplicated. More than 100 nonprescription products are available; however, the pharmacist should exercise caution in recommending their use in self-medication. Certain diseases that cause diarrhea might be serious or treated more effectively with agents specific for the underlying cause. Table 3 summarizes the causes of diarrhea and appropriate treatment. The following statement is required by the FDA on all nonprescription antidiarrheal preparations:

WARNING Do not use for more than 2 days or in the presence of high fever or in infants or children under 3 years of age unless directed by a physician.

Table 3. Diarrhea and its treatment

Type	History	Symptoms	Usual duration	Treatment	Prognosis
Acute					
Salmonella	Recent ingestion of contaminated food; affects all age groups	Sudden onset of abdominal cramps, watery diarrhea, nausea, vomiting, fever; onset of symptoms usually within 12–24 hours after ingestion; infects perineal ileum and cecum	1–5 days	Symptomatic; bed rest, fluid, and electrolyte replacement; antibiotics (ampicillin—if susceptible; chloramphenicol in life-threatening cases for 3–5 days)	Usually self-limiting
Shigella	Affects all age groups	Sudden onset of abdominal cramps, diarrhea containing shreds of mucus and specks of blood, tenesmus (frequently), fever; infects small bowel (early) and colon (later)	4–7 days	Symptomatic; bed rest, fluid, glucose, electrolyte replacement; antibiotics (ampicillin if susceptible)	Usually self-limiting
Escherichia coli	Affects children under 2 and the elderly in an overcrowded environment (e.g., hospital nursery or nursing home)	Abdominal cramps, fever, tenesmus; infects mostly small bowel	7–21 days	Fluid, glucose electrolyte replacement	Severe if not treated
Staphylococcus	Recent food ingestion	Sudden onset (1–2 hours) of nausea, vomiting, diarrhea	6–12 hours	Supportive; fluid replacement	Self-limiting
Viral, infantile	Predilection for children and infants; usually occurs in summer and autumn; very contagious	Abrupt onset of profuse, watery diarrhea, slight fever; frequent vomiting; upper respiratory symptoms	1–21 days	Symptomatic and supportive	Usually self-limiting
Traveler's diarrhea (caused by *Escherichia coli, Salmonella, Shigella, Giardia lamblia*)	Travel outside normal locus	Sudden onset of nausea, abdominal cramps, tenesmus, fever, prostration	5 days (onset is 6 days)	Symptomatic and supportive	Usually self-limiting
Drug-induced	Broad-spectrum antibiotics, autonomic drugs, laxative, nitrofurantoin, antacids, antineoplastics, antituberculins, ferrous sulfate, colchicine	Sudden onset of rectal urgency, abdominal cramps	Variable	Discontinue or change drug; vancomycin	Usually self-limiting; however, can be fatal
Chronic	History of repeated episodes; poor health history	Weight loss, anorexia, mucus and/or blood in feces	Weeks to years	Depends on etiology	Severe if not treated

From *Gastroenterology*, A. Bogoch, Ed., McGraw-Hill, New York, N.Y., 1973, pp. 33–38, 602–721; A. I. Mendeloff, in *Harrison's Principles of Internal Medicine*, 7th ed., McGraw-Hill, New York, N.Y., 1974, pp. 213–217; and S. M. Mellinkoff, *The Differential Diagnosis of Diarrhea*, New York, N.Y., 1964, pp. 310–325.

In many parts of the world, iodochlorhydroxyquin has been used prophylactically against traveler's diarrhea. However, the FDA recommends that the drug not be used for this purpose (46). The FDA conclusion is based on findings from Japan, Australia, and Sweden implicating iodochlorhydroxyquin as the cause of a severe, subacute myelo-opticoneuropathy (SMON) (47). As a result, oral iodochlorhydroxyquin and diiodohydroxyquin were removed from the U.S. market (48, 49). There is no acceptable evidence that iodochlorhydroxyquin or other halogenated oxyquinolines such as chiniofon, are effective in the treatment or prevention of traveler's diarrhea (50).

Many remedies have been tried for curing traveler's diarrhea. Antibiotics have not been effective in the treatment of this form of diarrhea (51); however, doxycycline has been effective in the prophylaxis of diarrhea. Extreme selectivity in the use of doxycycline is recommended, however. Antiperistaltic agents such as Lomotil, may prolong or enhance the severity of the symptoms of traveler's diarrhea because of the retention of the toxin in the intestine (52). Pepto-Bismol has been shown to be effective in treatment and prevention of symptoms (53, 54). The bismuth subsalicylate in Pepto-Bismol appears to inhibit intestinal secretions. The prophylactic dose is 60 ml taken 4 times/day during the first 2 weeks of travel. During acute illness, 30–60 ml should be taken every 30 minutes for a total of eight doses (55).

The salicylate in Pepto-Bismol may be a problem if patients are taking aspirin or other salicylate-containing drugs since toxic levels of salicylate may be reached even if the patient follows label directions for each drug. Patients who are sensitive to aspirin should not use Pepto-Bismol. Pepto-Bismol may interact adversely with oral anticoagulants, methotrexate, probenecid, and sulfinpyrazone or any drug that potentially interacts with aspirin. Also, high blood salicylate levels may exert an antiplatelet effect (56).

The FDA suggests that travelers to areas where hygiene and sanitation are poor may prevent diarrhea by eating only recently peeled and thoroughly cooked foods and by drinking only boiled or bottled water, bottled carbonated soft drinks, beer, or wine. Tap water used for brushing teeth or for ice in drinks may be a source of infection.

Nondrug Treatment

Mild to moderate acute diarrhea, possibly accompanied by vomiting, is usually self-limiting. Proper dietary measures can help replacement of lost fluids and electrolytes and thereby prevent dehydration. Children under 3 years of age should be referred to a physician. The following dietary management of mild to moderate diarrhea for children over 3 years old without a high fever or vomiting has been recommended as one method of treatment in cases of uncomplicated gastroenteritis (57):

- The stomach and intestines should be allowed to rest by not giving the child anything to eat or drink for 4–6 hours. (Significant water loss from concurrent diarrhea will modify this recommendation because of the potential for dehydration.)

- After the first 4–6 hours, small amounts of one of the following liquids at room temperature may be given to the child:

   Flat cola or ginger ale (all carbonation, or bubbles, should be removed by stirring in an open glass);
   Liquid gelatin dessert (Jell-O or Royal) that has not been allowed to gel and consists of twice the recommended amount of water;
   Gatorade (available in grocery stores);
   Pedialyte or Lytren (available in pharmacies).

- One teaspoon of one of these liquids should be given every 10–15 minutes for approximately 30 minutes; if the child retains this amount, 1 tablespoon should be given every 15–20 minutes, followed by 2 tablespoons (1 ounce) every half hour. If the child cannot retain the fluid, or if watery diarrhea persists, the physician should be notified.

- For the next 12 hours, ¼ cup of fluid should be given every 30 minutes; if diarrhea, vomiting, or "dry heaves" occur at this time, the physician should be notified.

- For the next 24 hours, easily digested foods (bananas, rice, and applesauce) should be given. Sweet, clear liquid fluids should continue to be given.

The normal diet should be reinstituted slowly. Milk should be avoided for 10 days. Other investigators have suggested adding milk, administered half strength, to the diet 12 hours after the patient has shown steady improvement by an appreciable reduction in number and volume of stools (58). This recommendation concerns acute infectious diarrhea in children when dehydration is not significant enough to require hospitalization. (Infants may receive soy-based formulas such as Isomil, Soyalac, Neo-Mull-Soy, or ProSobee.) Spicy and fatty foods also should be avoided for 5–6 days.

Pharmacologic Agents

Some antidiarrheal drugs are directed against the symptoms of diarrhea, some against the cause, and some against the effect of the disease such as loss of nutrients or electrolytes. The categories of drugs generally used are opiates, adsorbents, astringents, electrolytes, nutrients, bulk laxatives, anti-infectives, digestive enzymes, intestinal flora modifiers, sedatives, tranquilizers, smooth muscle relaxants, and anticholinergic drugs. Many of the drugs used to combat diarrhea (opiates, anti-infectives, and sedatives) are available by prescription only.

In 1975 the FDA advisory review panel on nonprescription laxative, antidiarrheal, emetic, and antiemetic drug products published its report on antidiarrheal agents (48). According to the panel, only opiates and polycarbophil were recognized as being safe and effective for nonprescription use. The panel concluded that "adequate and reliable scientific evidence is not available at this time to permit final classification" of other ingredients submitted, including alumina powder, attapulgite, belladonna alkaloids, bismuth salts, calcium carbonate, calcium hydroxide, carboxymethyl cellulose sodium, charcoal, kaolin, *Lactobacilli* species,

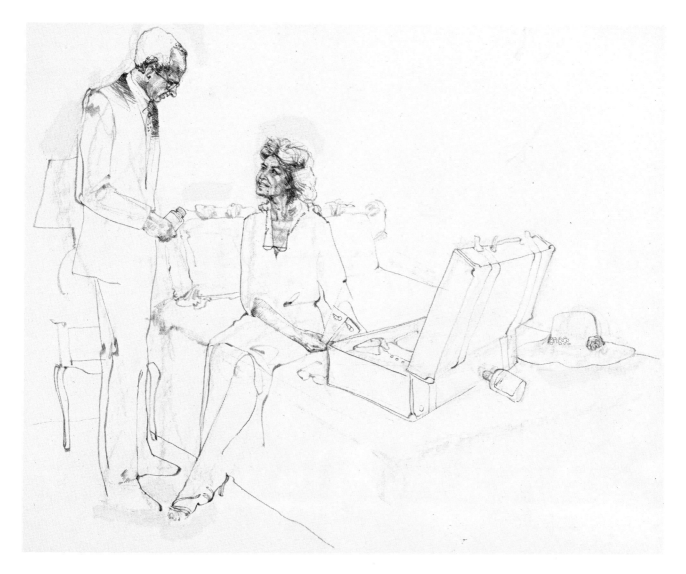

pectin, salol, and zinc phenolsulfonate. Generally, the panel agreed that the agents are safe in recommended doses but believed that there was a lack of acceptable clinical evidence to establish their effectiveness as antidiarrheal agents.

Opiates

The opiates (opium powder, tincture of opium, and paregoric) are safe and effective in doses of 15–20 mg of opium (1.5–2.0 mg of morphine) for adults and 5–10 mg of opium (0.5–1.0 mg of morphine) for children 6–12 years old taken 1–4 times/day, not to exceed 2 days (59). Most opiate-containing nonprescription antidiarrheals contain paregoric or its equivalent in the usual dose of 1 teaspoon (~5.0 ml) of paregoric containing 20 mg of powdered opium (2.0 mg of morphine). Several nonprescription products incorporate paregoric or its equivalent in a mixture with other ingredients.

Because of their morphine content, paregoric-containing products exert a direct musculotropic effect to inhibit effective propulsive movements in the small intestine and colon. Thus, hyperperistaltic movements decrease, and the passage of intestinal contents slows, resulting in absorption of water and electrolytes. In the usual oral antidiarrheal doses, addiction liability is low for acute diarrheal episodes because the morphine is not well absorbed orally. The low dose given produces an effective action in the GI tract but does not produce analgesia or euphoria. However, chronic use, as in ulcerative colitis (or acute overdose), increases the risk of physical dependency (60). Paregoric alone is a Schedule III prescription-only item, but it is a Schedule V item available for over-the-counter purchase in combination with antidiarrheals that contain no more than 100 mg of opium (5 teaspoons, or about 25 ml, of paregoric/100 ml of mixture). Opium derivatives are CNS depressants, and excessive sedation may be a problem in patients taking other CNS depressants concomitantly with the diarrhea remedy.

Antiperistaltic drugs (diphenoxylate, paregoric, and loperamide) are effective in relieving cramps and stool frequency. However, they do not appear to prevent fluid loss. In addition, they may worsen the effects of invasive bacterial infection and toxic megacolon in antibiotic-induced diarrhea. Therefore, these drugs should be used with caution in patients presenting with fecal leukocytes, fever, or recent history of antibiotic use (61, 62).

Polycarbophil

Polycarbophil is a calcium salt of a synthetic polyacrylic resin that acts as an absorbent. Because of its ability to absorb 60 times its original weight in water, it has been recommended in the treatment of both diarrhea and constipation (63). Clinical studies in patients with acute diarrhea and chronic diarrhea have shown polycarbophil to be safe and effective (64–69). The frequency of bowel movements decreased, and the consistency of stools improved. Polycarbophil is metabolically inert, and no systemic toxicity has been demonstrated. Local toxicities have been epigastric pain and bloating, which are dose related. The effective adult dose is 4.0–6.0 g/day taken orally. Adults should chew two 500-mg tablets 4 times/day. Children 6–12 years old should chew one 500-mg tablet 3 times/day, and children 3–6 years old should chew one 500 mg tablet 2 times/day. Dosage instructions are not commercially available for children under 3 years of age.

Adsorbents

The adsorbents are the most frequently used type of drug in nonprescription antidiarrheal preparations. Because large doses generally are used, most commercially available products are formulated as flavored liquid suspensions to improve palatability. Adsorbents generally are used in the treatment of mild diarrhea. The FDA panel determined that even though adsorbents are safe, there is insufficient evidence that these agents are effective in treating diarrhea (59).

Adsorption is not a specific action, and, when given orally, materials possessing this capability adsorb nutrients and digestive enzymes as well as toxins, bacteria, and various noxious materials in the GI tract. They also may have the effect of adsorbing drugs (lincomycin) from the GI tract. Although the systemic absorption of a drug from the GI tract during a diarrheal episode is expected to be poor, its absorption may be further hampered by the concomitant administration of an antidiarrheal adsorbent. Thus, a judgment must be made when drugs other than the antidiarrheal preparation are to be taken by the patient, perhaps for an unrelated condition. Depending on the medication involved, its usual rate and site of absorption, and the absolute necessity of attaining specific and consistent blood levels of the drug, an alteration of the dose or the dosage regimen may be required. In some cases, it might be better to administer the drug parenterally until the diarrheal episode is over and adsorbent drugs are discontinued.

Following the initial treatment, most antidiarrheal preparations containing adsorbents are taken after each loose bowel movement until the diarrhea is controlled. The total amount of adsorbent taken may be quite large if the diarrheal episodes occur in rapid succession and for several hours. Because there is negligible systemic absorption of the adsorbent drug, the usual consequence is constipation.

The main GI adsorbents used are activated charcoal, aluminum hydroxide, attapulgite, bismuth subsalts, kaolin, magnesium trisilicate, and pectin. Adsorbents used with ion-exchange resins combine their individual activities in relieving gastric distress and diarrhea. These agents are relatively inert and nontoxic except for possible interference with drugs and nutrient adsorption. Kaolin, which has long been used in the Orient against diarrhea and dysentery, is a native hydrated aluminum silicate. Attapulgite is a hydrous magnesium aluminum silicate. It is activated by thermal treatment and used in a finely powdered form. Although it is seldom used as an antidiarrheal today, activated charcoal, which in a single gram has a surface area of about 100 m², possesses excellent adsorption properties and has been used for conditions of various origin, including cholera and infantile and nervous diarrhea (70). In a study of the treatment of acute nonspecific diarrhea, eight children, 3–11 years old, were treated for 2 days with either kaolin-pectin concentrate (Kao-Con), kaolin suspension, pectin suspension, diphenoxylate-atropine liquid (Lomotil), or placebo. The treatments resulted in additional stool consistency, but the actual volume of water loss remained unchanged (71).

Pectin, a purified carbohydrate extracted from the rind of citrus fruit or from apple pomace, is used in the treatment of diarrhea, although its exact mechanism of action is not known. Pectin generally is found in combination with other adsorbents.

The bismuth subsalts such as the subnitrate and subsalicylates are used in antidiarrheal preparations as adsorbents, astringents, and protectives. However, subnitrate may form nitrate ion in the bowel which, upon absorption, may cause hypotension and methemoglobinemia. Bismuth subnitrate is contraindicated in infants under 2 years old. Stools may become dark with use of a bismuth compound. According to the FDA panel, bismuth salts are safe in amounts taken orally (0.6–2.0 g of bismuth subsalicylate every 6–8 hours), but at the time of the FDA panel report, there was insufficient data to establish the effectiveness of bismuth in diarrhea. However, more recent data indicate that bismuth may be effective in the treatment and prevention of symptoms of traveler's diarrhea (53, 54).

Anticholinergics

The formulations of adsorbents frequently are fortified by the addition of belladonna alkaloids (anticholinergics) in concentrations that make them prescription drugs. The primary effect of anticholinergic agents is relief of cramping through reduction of contractile activity. Their effectiveness in the reduction of diarrhea is negligible (72). When the diarrhea is due to an increase in intestinal tone and peristalsis, belladonna alkaloids are effective "when given in doses that are equivalent to 0.6–1.0 mg of atropine sulfate" (59). However, in some available combinations of nonprescription antidiarrheal products, the usual dose of belladonna alkaloids is less than the recognized effective dose. When these agents are combined with adsorbents, the possibility of inactivation by adsorption must be considered. Hence, the FDA panel recommends that "antidiarrheal products containing anticholinergics when given in doses that are equivalent to 0.6–1.0 mg of atropine sulfate be available only by prescription" (59).

Anticholinergics have a narrow margin of safety, especially in young children. Their containers carry the following warning statement that should be reviewed before dispensing:

> **WARNING** Not to be used by persons having glaucoma or excessive pressure within the eye, or by elderly persons (when undiagnosed glaucoma or excessive pressure within the eye occurs most frequently), or by children under 6 years of age, unless directed by physician. Discontinue use if blurring of vision, rapid pulse, or dizziness occurs. Do not exceed recommended dosage. Not for frequent or prolonged use. If dryness of the mouth occurs, decrease dosage. If eye pain occurs, discontinue use and see your physician immediately as this may indicate undiagnosed glaucoma.

Lactobacillus Preparations

One of the most controversial forms of diarrhea treatment is the use of *Lactobacillus* organisms. The bacteriology of the intestinal tract is extremely complex, and it is difficult to explain many changes in the numbers and types of microorganisms. The flora of the GI tract plays a significant role in maintaining bowel function, nutrition, and the overall well-being of the individual. Antibiotic therapy often disrupts the balance of intestinal microorganisms, resulting in abnormal intestinal and bowel function. Seeding the bowel with viable *Lactobacillus acidophilus* and *Lactobacillus bulgaricus* microorganisms has been suggested as effective treatment for functional intestinal disturbances, including diarrhea. These microorganisms are believed to be effective in suppressing the growth of pathogenic microorganisms and in re-establishing the normal intestinal flora. A diet of milk, yogurt, or buttermilk, containing 240–400 g of lactose or dextrin is equally effective in colonizing the intestine without supplemental lactobacilli (59). However, the FDA panel states that there are no controlled studies documenting the effectiveness of *Lactobacillus* preparations in treating diarrhea (59).

Other Active Ingredients

Various other active ingredients are blended in antidiarrheal products. These include drugs such as zinc phenolsulfonate (zinc sulfocarbolate), carboxymethyl cellulose sodium, zinc phenol, phenyl salicylate, and various digestive enzymes. The indications are myriad. Intestinal antiseptic and astringent action has been attributed to zinc phenolsulfonate; phenyl salicylate (salol) is reported to be hydrolyzed into phenol and salicylic acid and act as an antiseptic (73–75). Carboxymethyl cellulose sodium, a bulking agent, supposedly adds consistency to the watery diarrhea. In the small amounts in nonprescription products, these agents appear to be safe; however their efficacy has not been proven (59).

Fluid Therapy

Replacement of fluid loss and correction of electrolyte imbalance is very important. In mild to moderate diarrhea, oral fluids can be safely prescribed if the patient is not vomiting. The secretory and absorptive mechanisms appear to function separately; therefore, an oral sugar-electrolyte solution can be absorbed during severe diarrhea. This has saved many lives in third world countries (76). The World Health Organization recommends an oral replacement fluid that contains: 20 g of glucose/liter, 90 mEq of sodium/liter, 30 mEq of bicarbonate/liter, and 20 mEq of potassium/liter (77). No commercial product available fulfills WHO recommendations. The Center for Disease Control recommends a homemade solution (Table 4). In severe cases of diarrhea, fluid deficits must be replaced intravenously. In developed countries, commercial oral electrolyte replacement solutions are more convenient and potentially safer since they are premixed and there is less chance of error in preparation.

Other GI Disorders

The agents found in products recommended as GI "protectives" and antidiarrheal mixtures sometimes overlap. Gastrointestinal protectives are intended to soothe acutely irritated or inflamed gastric mucosa or intestinal lining resulting from ingestion of an irritant or the contraction of an illness affecting the digestive tract. The following acute disorders may be treated with nonprescription protectives:

- **Acute gastritis**—This is inflammation of the gastric mucosa. Acute gastritis occurs suddenly, occasionally violently, lasts for short periods, and involves inflammation and erosion of the mucosa of the stomach.
- **Acute erosive gastritis**—This common disorder is caused by acute alcohol ingestion, drugs (especially aspirin), hot spicy foods, allergenic foods in hypersensitive individuals (especially milk, eggs, and fish), bacteria or toxins in food poisoning, or an acute illness, such as viral infection.
- **Acute corrosive gastritis**—This more serious disorder is caused by swallowing corrosive materials such as strong acids or alkalis, iodine, potassium permanganate, or salts of heavy metals. Such ingestion requires hospitalization and immediate emergency treatment directed toward removing or neutralizing the offending agent and providing supportive measures (78). (See Chapter 7, *Emetic and Antiemetic Products*.)

Table 4. Home treatment of diarrhea

Glass No. 1	Glass No. 2
8 oz orange, apple, or other fruit juice (rich in potassium)	8 oz tap water (boiled or carbonated if purity of source is unknown)
½ tsp honey or corn syrup (rich in glucose necessary for absorption of essential salts)	¼ tsp baking soda (sodium bicarbonate)
1 pinch table salt (sodium chloride)	

Drink alternately from each glass. Supplement with carbonated beverages, water (boiled if necessary), tea, or coffee, as desired.

Adapted from J. J. Plorde, *Drug Ther. (hosp. ed.)*, August 1979, p. 62.

• **Acute gastroenteritis**—This condition is an acute inflammation of the lining of the stomach and intestine. It may be precipitated by excessive use of harsh cathartics, salicylates, and other irritant drugs.

The nonprescription products for relief of acute GI irritation and inflammation contain adsorbents, bulk formers, astringents (especially the bismuth subsalts), antacids, and GI analgesics. The commercial claims for some of these products refer to their ability to coat the stomach, reducing the irritation and inflammation. The report of the FDA advisory review panel on nonprescription antacids and antiflatulent drug products states that "the evidence currently available is inadequate to support the claim that such properties as . . . 'coating' . . . 'demulcent' . . . contribute to the relief of gastrointestinal symptoms" (79).

Patients also may be suffering from any of the following chronic or GI disorders:

• **Chronic gastritis**—Chronic gastritis is an inflammatory reaction of the gastric mucosa. It may be associated with serious underlying diseases such as gastric carcinoma, pernicious anemia, diabetes mellitus, and thyroid disease, or it may be the result of chronic drug ingestion (aspirin).
• **Colitis**—Colitis is inflammation and pain of the colon. It is classified as ulcerative, amebic, bacillary, or pseudomembranous.
• **Irritable colon**—Irritable colon ("spastic colon" or "mucous colitis") is a motor disorder of the colon, resulting in abdominal discomfort and pain, usually with alternating episodes of diarrhea and constipation (33).

Patients with chronic conditions should be under a physician's care. Treatment is based on managing the underlying cause and avoiding the ingestion of agents that contribute to the condition. The medications prescribed may include prescription-only drugs, such as antispasmodics and anti-inflammatory agents, and nonprescription products, such as bulk formers and mucilaginous products.

Many commercial products sold as protectives are thick, viscous suspensions that probably physically protect the mucous membranes from the irritating agents. The adsorbent drugs can bind certain offending agents. The drug substances that form bulk or thick mucilaginous fluids within the GI tract can dilute the concentration of the irritant, act as a physical barrier between it and the GI walls, and hasten the passage of the irritant toward the bowel.

Product Selection Guidelines

The information obtained during the patient interview and from the family medication record must be assessed before product selection. The treatment alternatives are an adsorbent such as kaolin-pectin mixture, a nonprescription opiate-containing antidiarrheal product, or physician referral.

It is better to undertreat than to overtreat diarrhea. No product should be recommended that the patient has taken previously and found unsatisfactory. Nonprescription antidiarrheal products usually can manage mild to moderate acute diarrhea. Severe acute diarrhea probably requires a prescription drug such as diphenoxylate, loperamide, or paregoric.

Medical care should be sought if control of uncomplicated diarrhea is not achieved in 24 hours. After this period a reassessment can be made and another treatment chosen. The pharmacist could recommend continuing treatment for another 24 hours with the same or more potent product or advise the patient to consult a physician. If control of the symptoms is not achieved within 48 hours a physician should be consulted. Immediate physician contact is required if the patient is an infant.

The pharmacist should review the label contents to determine the appropriate dosage schedule based on the patient's age, the maximum number of doses per 24 hours, proper storage, and auxiliary administration information such as shaking well before using. The patient must be informed about special precautions on the label such as contraindications to use. Adjunctive therapy includes rest, drinking appropriate fluids, and appropriate diet. Physical and GI tract rest should be encouraged by advising bed rest and discontinuation of all solid foods.

Fluid loss and electrolyte imbalance are a primary problem, especially in infants, young children, and elderly patients.

Summary

Diarrhea is often treated as a simple disorder, but it can be a symptom of a more serious underlying disease. The condition is either acute or chronic. Acute diarrhea is characterized by a sudden onset of loose stools in a previously healthy patient. Chronic diarrhea is characterized by persistent or recurrent episodes with anorexia, weight loss, and chronic weakness. Simple diarrhea usually can be treated by supportive care or with a nonprescription product.

The debilitating effect of persistent diarrhea is due largely to loss of water and resulting electrolyte imbalance through excretion. The replacement of these vital fluids and electrolytes is an integral part of diarrhea therapy, particularly in infants and children. This balance can be accomplished by the ingestion of the appropriate fluids or by the use of oral sugar-electrolyte formulations that provide a balanced formulation of important electrolytes and carbohydrates.

Complaints of GI irritation should be evaluated for their severity and nature (acute or chronic). For relatively minor acute problems, such as food or drink intolerance, relief may be provided by nonprescription protectives containing adsorbent, bulk-forming, or mucilaginous ingredients. All severely acute, uncontrolled, or chronic GI complaints should be referred promptly to a physician. The pharmacist can contribute to better patient care by being familiar with the disease processes involved in diarrhea and other GI illnesses and by assisting in appropriate selection and use of pharmacologic agents.

References

1. A. M. Connell, C. Helton, and G. Irvine, *Br. Med. J.*, 2, 1095 (1965).
2. E. Engler, "Dealing with Diarrhea," Science and Medical, Chicago, Ill., 1974.
3. S. F. Phillips, *Postgrad. Med.*, 57, 65 (1974).
4. H. L. Dupont and R. B. Hornick, "Disease a Month," Year Book Medical, Chicago, Ill., July 1969, pp. 1–40.
5. "The Macmillan Medical Cyclopedia," W. A. R. Thomas, Ed., Macmillan, New York, N.Y., 1955, p. 244.
6. W. C. Matousek, "Manual of Differential Diagnosis," Year Book Medical, Chicago, Ill., 1967, p. 76.
7. "Documenta Geigy: Scientific Tables," 7th ed., K. Diem and C. Lentner, Eds., Ciba-Geigy Limited, Basel, Switzerland, 1970, pp. 657–658.
8. A. C. Guyton, "Textbook of Medical Physiology," 5th ed., W. B. Saunders, Philadelphia, Pa., 1976, pp. 850–866.
9. "Gastroenterology," A. Bogoch, Ed., McGraw-Hill, New York, N.Y., 1973, pp. 33–38, 602–721.
10. R. A. Findlestein, *CRC Crit. Rev. Microbiol.*, 2, 563 (1973).
11. "Textbook of Medicine," 15th ed., Vol. 2, P. B. Beason, W. McDermot, and J. B. Wyngaarden, Eds., W. B. Saunders, Philadelphia, Pa., 1979, p. 1479.
12. M. Field, D. Fromm, and Q. Al-Aqwati, *J. Clin. Invest.*, 51, 796 (1972).
13. R. A. Frizzell and S. G. Schultz, *Gastrointest. Physiol.*, 19, 205 (1979).
14. L. K. Pickering, H. L. Dupont, and J. Olarte, *Am. J. Clin. Pathol.*, 68, 562 (1977).
15. R. B. Sack, *Ann. Intern. Med.*, 94, 129 (1981).
16. R. B. Hornick, *Adv. Intern. Med.*, 21, 349 (1976).
17. R. C. Patter, *Am. Fam. Phys.*, 23, 112 (1981).
18. "Harrison's Principles of Internal Medicine," 8th ed., G. W. Thorn, Ed., McGraw-Hill, New York, N.Y., 1977, pp. 210–214.
19. A. Z. Kapikian, *N. Engl. J. Med.*, 294, 965 (1976).
20. D. S. Schreiber, *Gastroenterology*, 73, 174 (1977).
21. A. Simhon and L. Mata, *Lancet*, 1, 39 (1978).
22. J. R. Hamilton, *Can. Med. Assoc. J.*, 12, 29 (1980).
23. S. M. Mellinkoff, "The Differential Diagnosis of Diarrhea," McGraw-Hill, New York, N.Y., 1964, pp. 310–325.
24. "Pediatric Therapy," 6th ed., H. C. Shirkey, Ed., C. V. Mosby, St. Louis, Mo., 1980, pp. 602–604.
25. S. Ware, *Lancet*, 1, 252 (1977).
26. *Lancet*, 2, 1126 (1976).
27. J. O. Sherman and J. D. Lloyd-Still, *Drug Ther. (hosp. ed.)*, 2, 52 (1977).
28. M. H. Merson, G. K. Morris, D. A. Sack, J. G. Wells, J. C. Feeley, R. B. Sack, W. B. Creech, A. Z. Kapikian, and E. J. Gangarosa, *N. Engl. J. Med.*, 294, 1299 (1976).
29. M. S. Wolf, *N. Engl. J. Med.*, 298, 319 (1978).
30. E. J. Eastham, A. P. Douglas, and A. J. Watson, *Lancet*, 2, 950 (1976).
31. "Problems in Pediatric Drug Therapy," L. Pagliats and R. Levin, Eds., Drug Intelligence, Hamilton, Ill., 1979.
32. A. A. F. Machmoud and K. S. Warren, *J. Infect. Dis.*, 134, 639 (1976).
33. W. L. George, V. L. Sutter, and S. M. Finegold, *J. Infect. Dis.*, 136, 822 (1977).
34. A. Jacknowitz, *Am. J. Hosp. Pharm.*, 37, 1635, (1980).
35. *FDA Drug Bulletin*, 5, 2 (Jan.-March 1975).
36. F. J. Tedesco, F. W. Barton, and D. H. Alpers, *Ann. Intern. Med.*, 81, 429 (1974).
37. F. J. Tedesco, M. Gurwith, and R. Markham, *Lancet*, 2, 226 (1978).
38. F. J. Tedesco, *J. Infect. Dis.*, 135, 95 (1977).
39. J. W. Matseshe and S. F. Phillips, *Med. Clin. N. Am.*, 62, 141 (1978).
40. J. H. Cummings, G. E. Sladen, and O. F. W. James, *Br. Med. J.*, 1, 537 (1974).
41. W. D. Heizer, A. L. Warshaw, T. A. Waldmann, and L. Laster, *Ann. Intern. Med.*, 68, 839 (1968).
42. L. S. Basser, *Med. J. Aust.*, 1, 47 (1979).
43. M. D. Rawson and M. B. Leeds, *Lancet*, 2, 1121 (1966).
44. "Cancer Facts and Figures," American Cancer Society, New York, N.Y., 1975.
45. C. F. Hawkins and R. Cockel, *Gut*, 12, 208 (1971).
46. *FDA Drug Bulletin*, 2 (May 1972).
47. G. P. Oakley, *J. Am. Med. Assoc.*, 225, 395 (1973).
48. *Medical Letter on Drugs and Therapeutics*, 17, 105 (1975).
49. G. H. Schneller, *J. Am. Pharm. Assoc.*, NS17, 234 (1977).
50. M. H. Merson and E. J. Gangarosa, *J. Am. Med. Assoc.*, 17, 105 (1975).
51. J. A. Lee and B. H. Kean, *J. Infect. Dis.*, 137, 335 (1978).
52. H. L. Dupont and R. B. Hornick, *J. Am. Med. Assoc.*, 226, 1525 (1973).
53. C. D. Ericsson, D. G. Evans, and H. L. Dupont, *J. Infect. Dis.*, 136, 693 (1977).
54. H. L. Dupont, P. Sullivan, and L. K. Pickering, *Gastroenterology*, 74, 829 (1978).
55. H. L. Dupont, *J. Am. Med. Assoc.*, 243, 237 (1980).
56. S. Feldman, *Clin. Pharmacol. Ther.*, 29, 788 (1981).
57. *Patient Care*, 12(9), 221 (1978).
58. R. Barker, *Postgrad. Med.*, 65, 173 (1979).
59. *Federal Register*, 40, 12924 (1975).
60. "Opium Preparations," American Hospital Formulary Service, American Society of Hospital Pharmacists, Washington, D.C., Section 28:08.
61. R. Wheeldon and H. J. Heggarty, *Arch. Dis. Child.*, 46, 562 (1971).
62. H. L. Dupont and R. B. Hornick, *J. Am. Med. Assoc.*, 226, 1525 (1973).
63. B. D. Pimparker, F. F. Paustan, J. L. A. Roth, and H. L. Bockus, *Gastroenterology*, 40, 397 (1961).
64. A. J. Grossman, R. C. Batterman, and P. Leifer, *J. Am. Geriatr. Soc.*, 5, 187 (1957).
65. M. L. Rutledge, M. M. Willner, and J. T. King, *Clin. Pediatr.*, 2, 61 (1963).
66. A. Winkelstein, *Curr. Ther. Res.*, 6, 572 (1964).
67. J. L. A. Roth, *Am. J. Dig. Dis.*, 5, 965 (1960).
68. W. S. Lacorte, *Clin. Pharmacol. Ther.*, 27, 263 (1980).
69. M. L. Rutledge, *Curr. Ther. Res.*, 23, 443 (1978).
70. J. A. Riese and F. Damrau, *J. Am. Geriatr. Soc.*, 12, 500 (1964).
71. B. L. Portnoy, H. L. Dupont, D. Pruitt, J. A. Abdo, and J. T. Rodriguez, *J. Am. Med. Assoc.*, 236, 844 (1976).
72. "AMA Drug Evaluations," 4th ed., 1980, p. 962.
73. "The Merck Index," 9th ed., M. Windholz, S. Budavari, L. Y. Stroumtsos, and M. N. Fertig, Eds., Merck, Rahway, N.J., 1976, pp. 1309, 951, 927.
74. "Clinical Toxicology of Commercial Products," 4th ed., R. E. Gosselin, H. C. Hodge, R. P. Smith, and M. N. Gleason, Eds., Williams and Wilkins, Baltimore, Md., 1976, pp. 99, 138.
75. "Martindale's The Extra Pharmacopeia," 26th ed., N. W. Blacow and A. Wade, Eds., The Pharmaceutical Press, London, 1972, pp. 893, 459, 931, 582.
76. N. Hirschhorn, *Am. J. Clin. Nutr.*, 33, 637 (1980).
77. A. Chatterjee, D. Mahalanabis, and K. N. Jalan, *Arch. Dis. Child.*, 53, 284 (1978).
78. "The Merck Manual of Diagnosis and Therapy," 13th ed., D. H. Holvey, Ed., Merck, Rahway, N.J., 1977, pp. 730–731.
79. *Federal Register*, 39, 19874 (1974).

Antidiarrheal Product Table

Product (Manufacturer)	Dosage Form	Opiates[a]	Adsorbents	Other Active Ingredients	Inactive Ingredients
Bacid (Fisons)	capsule			carboxymethyl cellulose sodium, 100 mg *Lactobacillus acidophilus* ≥500,000,000	
Corrective Mixture (Beecham Labs)	liquid		bismuth subsalicylate, 17 mg/ml	pepsin, 9 mg/ml phenyl salicylate, 4.4 mg/ml zinc sulfocarbolate, 2 mg/ml	alcohol, 1.5% carminatives demulcents flavoring
Corrective Mixture with Paregoric (Beecham Labs)	liquid	paregoric, 0.12 ml/ml	bismuth subsalicylate, 17 mg/ml	pepsin, 8 mg/ml phenyl salicylate, 4.4 mg/ml zinc sulfocarbolate, 2 mg/ml	alcohol, 2% carminatives demulcents flavoring
Diabismul (O'Neal, Jones & Feldman)	suspension	opium, 0.47 mg/ml	kaolin, 170 mg/ml pectin, 5.3 mg/ml		methylparaben propylparaben
Dia-eze (Central)	suspension		kaolin, 370 mg/ml bismuth subgallate, 10 mg/ml		eucalyptus oil menthol methyl salicylate preservatives thymol
DIA-quel (Marion Laboratories)	liquid	paregoric, 0.15 ml/ml	pectin, 4.8 mg/ml	homatropine methylbromide, 0.03 mg/ml	alcohol, 10%
Diatrol (Otis Clapp)	tablet		pectin	calcium carbonate	
Digestalin (North American)	tablet		activated charcoal, 5.30 mg bismuth subgallate, 3.80 mg	pepsin, 2.00 mg berberis, 1.20 mg papain, 1.20 mg pancreatin, 0.40 mg hydrastis, 0.08 mg	
Donnagel (Robins)	suspension		kaolin, 200 mg/ml pectin, 4.76 mg/ml	hyoscyamine sulfate, 0.0035 mg/ml atropine sulfate, 0.0006 mg/ml hyoscine hydrobromide, 0.0002 mg/ml	alcohol, 3.8% sodium benzoate, 2 mg/ml
Donnagel-PG (Robins)	suspension	powdered opium, 0.8 mg/ml	kaolin, 200 mg/ml pectin, 4.76 mg/ml	hyoscyamine sulfate, 0.0035 mg/ml atropine sulfate, 0.0006 mg/ml hyoscine hydrobromide, 0.0002 mg/ml	alcohol, 5% sodium benzoate, 2 mg/ml
Hydra-Lyte (Jayco)	packet			glucose dextrose sodium	
Infantol Pink (Scherer)	liquid	opium, 0.5 mg/ml	bismuth subsalicylate, 13.0 mg/ml pectin, 7.4 mg/ml	zinc phenolsulfonate, 3.5 mg/ml	calcium carrageenan, 3.6 mg/ml saccharin sodium, 0.27 mg/ml glycerin, 0.05 ml/ml alcohol, 2% peppermint oil, 0.00016 ml/ml

Antidiarrheal Product Table, continued

Product (Manufacturer)	Dosage Form	Opiates[a]	Adsorbents	Other Active Ingredients	Inactive Ingredients
Kaodene Non-Narcotic (Pfeiffer)	suspension		kaolin, 129.6 mg/ml pectin, 6.5 mg/ml		
Kaodene with Paregoric (Pfeiffer)	suspension	paregoric, 0.125 ml/ml	kaolin, 129.6 mg/ml pectin, 6.5 mg/ml		
Kaolin Pectin Suspension (Philips Roxane)	suspension		kaolin, 190 mg/ml pectin, 4.34 mg/ml	carboxymethyl cellulose sodium, 0.4%	glycerin, 1.75% lime mint flavor saccharin sodium, .025%
Kaopectate (Upjohn)	suspension		kaolin, 190 mg/ml pectin, 4.34 mg/ml		
Kaopectate Concentrate (Upjohn)	suspension		kaolin, 290 mg/ml pectin, 6.47 mg/ml		
Lactinex (Hynson, Westcott & Dunning)	tablet granules			*Lactobacillus acidophilus* *Lactobacillus bulgaricus*	
Pabizol with Paregoric (Rexall)	suspension	opium, 0.5 mg/ml	bismuth subsalicylate, 17.0 mg/ml	aluminum magnesium silicate, 8.83 mg/ml phenyl salicylate, 3.3 mg/ml zinc phenolsulfonate, 1.3 mg/ml hydroxypropyl methylcellulose, 6.7 mg/ml	alcohol, 9.6%
Parelixir (Purdue Frederick)	liquid	tincture of opium, 0.007 ml/ml	pectin, 4.83 mg/ml		alcohol, 18%
Parepectolin (Rorer)	suspension	paregoric, 0.12 ml/ml	kaolin, 186 mg/ml pectin, 5.5 mg/ml		alcohol, 0.69%
Pektamalt (Warren-Teed)	liquid		kaolin, 217 mg/ml pectin, 20 mg/ml		
Pepto-Bismol (Norwich)	tablet liquid		bismuth subsalicylate, 300 mg/tablet bismuth subsalicylate, 525 mg/30ml		
Percy Medicine (Merrick)	liquid		bismuth subnitrate, 96 mg/ml	calcium hydroxide, 0.22 mg/ml	alcohol, 5%
Quintess (Lilly)	suspension		activated attapulgite, 100 mg/ml colloidal attapulgite, 30 mg/ml		alcohol, 0.9%
Rheaban (Leeming)	tablet suspension		activated attapulgite, 600 mg/tablet 140 mg/ml		

[a]Schedule V drug: nonprescription sale forbidden in some states.

6

Laxative Products

Clarence E. Curry Jr.

Questions to Ask the Patient

Why do you feel you need a laxative?

Do you have any abdominal discomfort or pain, bloating, weight loss, nausea, or vomiting?

Are you currently being treated by a physician for any illness?

Have you had any abdominal surgery recently?

How often do you normally have a bowel movement?

How would you describe your bowel movements? Have they changed in any way recently?

Has the appearance of your stools changed? In what way?

How long has constipation been a problem?

Have you used laxatives previously to relieve constipation?

Are you currently taking any medicine other than laxatives?

Are you using a laxative now? How often and how long have you used a laxative?

Have you attempted to relieve the constipation by eating more cereals, bread with a high fiber content, fruits, or vegetables?

How much physical exercise do you get?

How many glasses of water do you drink each day?

Are you allergic to any medicines?

Have you had any unwanted effects from laxatives, such as diarrhea?

Extensive media advertising promotes the idea that having clockwork-like bowel movements in some way enhances well-being and social acceptability. With the general increase in consumer interest in natural products, specifically in treating constipation, overall sales of laxatives in the United States in 1980 increased 10% over the previous year and accounted for one-third of a billion dollars in sales (1). Obviously, not all laxatives are natural products in the pharmaceutical sense nor are "natural" products natural to normal body biochemical and physiologic processes.

Laxative products facilitate the passage and elimination of feces from the colon and rectum (2). There are few recognized medical indications for the use of laxatives, but many people misuse these products to alleviate what they consider to be constipation. Constipation has different meanings for different patients. However, it generally is defined as a decrease in the frequency of fecal elimination characterized by the difficult passage of hard dry stools. It usually results from the abnor-mally slow movement of feces through the colon with resultant accumulation in the descending colon.

Causes of Constipation

Causes of constipation are numerous (Table 1-5). The main disorders of the colon, ulcerative colitis and excessive parasympathetic stimulation, and the chronic misuse of irritant laxative drugs, may cause constipation or diarrhea. The etiology of colitis remains unknown. Constipation is often a problem in ulcerative colitis patients in whom the disease process is limited to the rectum. Indeed, in an ulcerative colitis patient with diarrhea, the use of antidiarrheal agents can result in colonic dilation or the accumulation of hard stool in an area of bowel not affected by disease (3).

Constipation of organic origin may be due to hypothyroidism, megacolon, stricture, or lesions (benign or malignant). Laxatives are contraindicated in such cases; proper diagnosis and medical treatment should be obtained.

Physiology of the Gastrointestinal Tract

The digestive and absorptive functions of the gastrointestinal (GI) system involve the intestinal smooth muscle, visceral reflexes, and GI hormones (Figure 1). (See Chapter 3, *Antacid Products.*) Nearly all absorption (>94%) occurs in the small intestine; relatively little absorption occurs in the stomach or duodenum. The function of the colon is to allow for the orderly elimination from the body of nonabsorbed food products,

---

Table 1. Drugs inducing constipation

Analgesics
Anesthetic agents
Antacids (calcium and aluminum compounds)
Anticholinergics
Anticonvulsants
Antidepressive agents
Barium sulfate
Bismuth
Diuretics
Drugs for parkinsonism
Ganglionic blockers
Hematinics (especially iron)
Hypotensives
MAO inhibitors
Metallic intoxication (arsenic, lead, mercury, phosphorus)
Muscle paralyzers
Opiates
Psychotherapeutic drugs
Laxative addiction

Adapted with permission from "Gastrointestinal Disease," J. S. Fordtran and M. Sleisenger, Eds., W. B. Saunders, Philadelphia, Pa., 1978, pp. 370–373.

Table 2. Metabolic and endocrine disorders inducing constipation

Metabolic disorders
Diabetes: acidosis, neuropathy
Porphyria
Type I (Portuguese) and type II (Indiana) amyloid neuropathy; sporadic primary amyloidosis
Uremia
Hypokalemia

Endocrine disorders and changes
Panhypopituitarism
Hypothyroidism
Hypercalcemia: hyperparathyroidism, milk-alkali syndrome, carcinomatosis
Pheochromocytoma
Pregnancy
Enteric glucagon excess

Adapted with permission from "Gastrointestinal Disease," J. S. Fordtran and M. Sleisenger, Eds., W. B. Saunders, Philadelphia, Pa., 1978, pp. 370–373.

---

desquamated cells from the gut lumen, and detoxified and metabolic end products. The colon functions to conserve fluid and electrolytes so that the quantity eliminated represents about 10% presented to it in a 24-hour time period. In addition to conserving fluid and electrolytes, the colon has the capacity (as does the kidney) to absorb certain electrolytes in a nonisotonic fashion (4). If approximately 6 liters of fluid/day are ingested and supplied by secretions of the GI tract, about 1.5%, or 90 ml, would be excreted with the feces (5).

Tonic contractions of the stomach churn and knead food, and large peristaltic waves start at the fundus and move food toward the duodenum. The rate at which the stomach contents are emptied into the duodenum is regulated by autonomic reflexes or a hormonal link between the duodenum and the stomach. Carbohydrates are emptied from the stomach most rapidly, proteins more slowly, and fats exhibit the slowest emptying rate. Vagotomy and fear tend to lengthen emptying time; excitement generally shortens it. Most factors that slow the stomach emptying rate also inhibit secretion of hydrochloric acid and pepsin. When the osmotic pressure of the stomach contents is higher or lower than that of the plasma, the gastric emptying rate is slowed until isotonicity is achieved.

The mixing and passage of the contents of the small and large intestines are the result of four muscular movements: pendular, segmental, peristaltic, and vermiform. Pendular movements result from contractions of the longitudinal muscles of the intestine, which pass up and down small segments of the gut at the rate of about 10 contractions/minute. Pendular movements mix, rather than propel, the contents. Segmental movements result from contractions of the circular muscles and occur at about the same rate as pendular movements. Their primary function also is mixing. Pendular and segmental movements are caused by the intrinsic contractility of smooth muscle and occur in the absence of innervation of intestinal tissue.

Peristaltic movements propel intestinal contents by circular contractions that form behind a point of stimulation and pass along the GI tract toward the rectum. The contraction rate ranges from 2 to 20 cm/second. These contractions require an intact myenteric (Auerbach's) nerve plexus, which apparently is located in the intestinal mucosa. Peristaltic waves move the intestinal contents through the small intestine in about 3.5 hours. Vermiform (worm-like) movements occur mainly in the large intestine (colon) and are caused by the contraction of several centimeters of the colonic smooth muscle at one time. In the cecum and ascending colon, the contents retain a fluid consistency, and peristaltic and antiperistaltic waves occur frequently. However, the activity of the transverse, descending, and sigmoid segments of the colon is very irregular, and here through further water absorption the contents become semisolid.

Three or four times per day, a strong peristaltic wave (mass movement) propels the contents about one-third (38 cm) the length of the colon. When initiated by a meal, the mass movement is referred to as the gastrocolic reflex. This normal reflex seems to be associated with the entrance of food into the stomach. The sigmoid colon serves as a storage place for fecal matter until defecation. Except for the fauces and anus, the entire alimentary canal normally functions involuntarily as a coordinated unit (6).

The act of defecation involves multiple physiologic processes, but basically amounts to the rectal passage of accumulated fecal material. The rectum is a passageway and a central "notification chamber." The fecal material from the sigmoid colon is propelled into the rectum by a mass peristaltic movement, which in normal persons with normal eating habits, usually occurs at breakfast time. This results in a desire to defecate due to the initiation of somatic impulses to the defecation center in the sacral spinal cord. The defecation center then sends impulses to the internal anal sphincter, causing it to relax. This causes an increase in interabdominal pressure produced by tightening the abdominal wall muscles and a Valsalva maneuver forces the stool down. Voluntary relaxation of the external anal sphincter occurs followed by elevation of the pelvic diaphragm, which lifts the anal sphincter over the fecal mass allowing it to be expelled. Defecation, a spinal reflex, is vol-

Table 3. Neurogenic constipation
Bowel abnormalities
Aganglionosis (Hirschsprung's disease)
"Hypoganglionosis"
"Hyperganglionosis"
Ganglioneuromatosis:
Primary
von Recklinghausen's disease
Multiple endocrine neoplasia, type 2B
Paraneoplastic autonomic neuropathy
Pseudobowel obstruction
Chagas' disease
Nerve abnormalities
Resection of nervi erigentes
Spinal abnormalities
Cauda equina tumor
Meningocele (anterior or posterior)
Destruction of lumbosacral cord
Paraplegia
Tabes dorsalis
Multiple sclerosis
Cerebral abnormalities
Parkinson's disease
Cerebral tumors
Cerebrovascular disturbance
Shy-Drager syndrome

Adapted with permission from "Gastrointestinal Disease," J. S. Fordtran and M. Sleisenger, Eds., W. B. Saunders, Philadelphia, Pa., 1978, pp. 370–373.

untarily inhibited by keeping the external sphincter contracted or is facilitated by relaxing the sphincter and contracting the abdominal muscles. Distention of the stomach by food initiates contractions of the rectum (gastrocolic reflex) and, frequently, a desire to defecate. Children usually defecate after meals; in adults, however, habits and cultural factors may determine the "proper" time for defecation.

Pathophysiology of the Lower GI Tract

Alteration in motor activities is responsible for disorders in the small intestine. Distention or irritation of the small intestine can cause nausea and vomiting; the duodenum is most sensitive to irritation. The motility in the small intestine is intensified when the mucosa is irritated by bacterial toxins, chemical or physical irritants, and mechanical obstruction.

Pain from various causes, including gallbladder disease, appendicitis, and regional ileitis, may inhibit gastrointestinal reflexes. As a result, functional obstruction often occurs in the small intestine, resulting in symptoms of acute intestinal blockage.

Often, large masses of fecal material accumulate in a greatly dilated rectum. This is especially true of older individuals. The loss of tonicity in the rectal musculature may be caused by ignoring or suppressing the urge

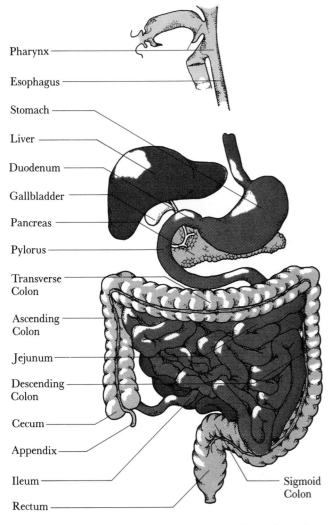

Pharynx

Esophagus

Stomach

Liver

Duodenum

Gallbladder

Pancreas

Pylorus

Transverse Colon

Ascending Colon

Jejunum

Descending Colon

Cecum

Appendix

Ileum

Rectum

Sigmoid Colon

Note: Portion of small intestine pulled aside for clarity.

Figure 1. Anatomy of the digestive system.

to defecate. It also may be caused by degeneration of nerve pathways concerned with defecation reflexes.

Painful lesions of the anal canal, such as ulcers, fissures, and thrombosed hemorrhoidal veins, impede defecation by causing a spasm of the sphincter and by promoting voluntary suppression of defecation to avoid pain.

The normal rectal mucosa is relatively insensitive to cutting or burning. However, when it is inflamed, it becomes highly sensitive to all stimuli, including those acting on the receptors mediating the stretch reflex. A constant urge to defecate in the absence of appreciable material in the rectum may occur with inflamed rectal mucosa (7).

Symptoms of Constipation

If constipation does occur, complex symptoms of varying degrees may develop. Typical symptoms include anorexia, dull headache, lassitude, low back pain, abdominal distention, and lower abdominal distress. Abdominal discomfort and inadequate response to increasing varieties and doses of laxatives are frequent complaints. Although only limited quantitative data are available, one study indicated that the range of bowel movement frequency in humans is from 3 times/day to 3 times/week (8). These latter individuals are usually symptom-free and do not have any specific abnormality related to their individual pattern of defecation. Therefore, constipation cannot be defined solely in terms of the number of bowel movements in any given period.

Patients have many different concepts of what constipation is (9) and many misconceptions concerning normal bowel functioning (10). Indeed, various definitions of constipation were expressed by participants in a study (9). Despite that, 75% of these persons indicated that they used a laxative when they were constipated. Regardless of how the patient defines constipation, it is likely that a laxative product will be considered to treat it.

Treatment

Constipation that does not have an organic etiology can often be alleviated without the use of a laxative product. The pharmacist should stress the importance of a high-fiber diet, plentiful fluid consumption, and exercise. However, treatment may require recommendation of a laxative.

Pharmacologic Agents

The ideal laxative would be nonirritating and nontoxic, would act only on the descending and sigmoid colon, and would produce a normally formed stool within a few hours. Its action would then cease, and normal bowel activity would resume. Since a laxative that meets these criteria is not presently available, proper selection of such an agent depends upon the etiology of the constipation.

Laxative drugs have been classified according to site of action, intensity of action, chemical structure, or mechanism of action. The most meaningful classification is the mechanism of action, whereby laxatives are

Table 4. Disorders of bowel structures associated with constipation

Colonic disorders
Obstruction
  Extraluminal
    Tumors
    Chronic volvulus
    Hernias
    Rectal prolapse
  Luminal
    Tumors
    Strictures
      Chronic diverticulitis
      Chronic amebiasis
      Lymphogranuloma venereum
      Syphilis
      Tuberculosis
      Ischemic colitis sequelae
      Endometriosis
      Corrosive enemas
      Surgery
Functional disorders
  Mucosal abnormalities
    Ulcerative proctitis
  Muscular abnormalities
    Diverticular disease, irritable colon syndrome
    Myotonic dystrophy
    Systemic sclerosis
    Dermatomyositis

Rectal disorders
Rectocele

Anal disorders
Mechanical disorders
  Stenosis
Functional disorders
  Puborectalis syndrome
  Anal fissure
  Anal fistulous abscess
  Mucosal prolapse

Adapted with permission from "Gastrointestinal Disease," J. S. Fordtran and M. Sleisenger, Eds., W. B. Saunders, Philadelphia, Pa., 1978, pp. 370–373.

classified as bulk forming, emollients, lubricants, saline, and stimulants (Table 6).

Bulk-Forming Laxatives

Because they approximate most closely the physiologic mechanism in promoting evacuation, bulk-forming products are the recommended choice as initial therapy for constipation. These laxatives are natural and semisynthetic polysaccharides and cellulose derivatives that dissolve or swell in the intestinal fluid, forming emollient gels that facilitate the passage of the intestinal contents and stimulate peristalsis. They are usually effective in 12–24 hours but may require as long as 3 days in some individuals. This type may be indicated for people on low-residue diets that cannot be corrected as well as in postpartum patients, elderly patients, and patients with irritable bowel syndrome or diverticular disease.

Since they are not absorbed systemically, the hydrophilic colloid laxatives do not seem to interfere with the absorption of nutrients. When given as a powder or granules, they should be mixed with pleasant tasting fluids, such as fruit juice, just before ingestion and administered with a full (8 oz) glass of fluid. Most patients prefer juices or soft drinks over water because they help to avoid the gritty, tasteless sensation of the bulk-forming laxatives. Failure to consume sufficient fluid with the laxative decreases drug efficacy and may result in intestinal or esophageal obstruction. These agents may be inappropriate for patients who must severely restrict their fluid intake, such as those with significant renal disease.

Esophageal obstruction has occurred in patients who have difficulty swallowing, such as those with strictures of the esophagus when these drugs are chewed or taken in dry form. In addition, there have been reports of acute bronchospasm associated with the inhalation of dry hydrophilic mucilloid (11). Because of the danger of fecal impaction or intestinal obstruction, the bulk-forming laxatives should not be taken by individuals with intestinal ulcerations, stenosis, or disabling adhesions. When administered properly, these agents are essentially free from systemic side effects because they are not absorbed.

Bulk-forming laxatives are derived from agar, plantago (psyllium) seed, kelp (alginates), and plant gums [tragacanth, chondrus, karaya (sterculia), and others]. The synthetic cellulose derivatives—methylcellulose and carboxymethyl cellulose sodium—are being used more frequently, and many preparations that contain these drugs also contain stimulant and/or fecal-softening laxative drugs. Although the natural product psyllium appears to be the most popular, the synthetic colloidal materials, including methylcellulose and carboxymethyl cellulose sodium, have a high degree of uniformity and can be readily compressed into tablets. Because they are more convenient to take, the use of these agents is increasing.

Calcium polycarbophil, the calcium salt of a synthetic polyacrylic resin that has a marked capacity for binding water, has been released for the treatment of constipation associated with irritable bowel syndrome and diverticular disease. Since the maximum calcium content of this agent is approximately 150 mg (7.6 mEq) the ingestion of recommended therapeutic dosages may increase the risk of hypercalcemia in suscepti-

ble patients. However, the maximum daily dosage limit for calcium adopted by the FDA is considerably higher than the 1,800 mg of calcium contained in the maximum daily dose of 12 calcium polycarbophil tablets (12).

A final member of the bulk forming laxatives is malt soup extract, which is obtained from barley and contains maltose protein and potassium as well as amylolytic enzymes. An interesting aspect of this agent is that it reduces fecal pH, which may contribute to its activity.

One study indicated that a mixture of cellulose and pectin (Phybrex), was equivalent to psyllium as a bulk laxative. The agent had the added advantage of not gelling when mixed with liquids, allowing its usage in baked foods, sauces, drinks, stews, and other recipes. Because of its wider range of methods of consumption, this agent may ensure better compliance over long periods of time (13).

It has been observed that making a specific choice among the different bulk products is relatively unimportant (14). It is more important that each dose be taken with a full glass of water (at least 240 ml, or 8 oz). The sodium and dextrose content of some of the commercial products should be evaluated in patients on sodium and carbohydrate-restricted diets. The dose should be adjusted until the required effect has been obtained. In addition to being relatively safe, bulk-forming laxatives are suitable should long-term therapy become necessary.

Patients with symptoms of cathartic colon from stimulant laxative overuse should be warned that the use of a bulk-forming laxative can result in intestinal obstruction.

Emollient Laxatives

Docusate, formerly known as dioctyl sodium sulfosuccinate, is a surfactant which, when administered orally, increases the wetting efficiency of intestinal fluid and facilitates admixture of aqueous and fatty substances to soften the fecal mass. Docusate does not retard absorption of nutrients from the intestinal tract. In many cases of fecal impaction, a solution of docusate is added to the enema fluid. Docusate and its congeners are claimed to be nonabsorbable, nontoxic, and pharmacologically inert.

Other fecal-softening laxatives are docusate calcium (anionic surfactant), docusate potassium (anionic surfactant), and poloxamer 188 (nonionic surfactant). The latter has no irritant properties and is compatible with electrolytes.

Emollient laxatives should be used only for short-term therapy (less than 1 week without physician consultation) where hard fecal masses are present: either in acute perianal disease in which elimination of painful stools is desired or in which the avoidance of straining at the stool is desirable (following rectal surgery or myocardial infarction).

Orally administered emollient laxatives are of no value in treating constipation of long-term duration, especially in elderly and debilitated patients. One study indicated that the prophylactic administration of doc-

---

Table 5. Dietary factors associated with constipation

Lack of sufficient bulk in the diet
Excessive ingestion of foods that harden stools, such as processed cheese
Inadequate fluid intake

Adapted with permission from "Gastrointestinal Disease," J. S. Fordtran and M. Sleisenger, Eds., W. B. Saunders, Philadelphia, Pa., 1978, pp. 370–373.

Table 6. Classification and properties of laxatives

Agent	Dosage form	Daily dosage range Adult	Pediatric (age in years)	Site of action	Approximate time required for action	Systemic absorption
Bulk-Forming						
Methylcellulose	Solid	4–6 g	1–1.5 g (>6)	Small and large intestines	12–72 hours	No
Carboxymethyl cellulose sodium	Solid	4–6 g	1–1.5 g (>6)	Small and large intestines	12–72 hours	No (laxative) Yes (sodium)
Malt soup extract	Solid, liquid, powder	12–64g	6–32 oz (1 month–2 year)	Small and large intestines	12–72 hours	—
Polycarbophil	Solid	4–6 g	0.5–1.0 g (<2) 1–1.5 g (2–5) 1.5–3.0 g (6–12)	Small and large intestines	12–72 hours	No
Plantago seeds	Solid	2.5–30 g	1.25–15 g (>6)	Small and large intestines	12–72 hours	No
Emollient						
Dioctyl calcium sulfosuccinate	Solid	0.05–0.36 g	0.025 g (<2) 0.05–0.150 g (≥2)	Small and large intestines	12–72 hours	Yes
Dioctyl sodium sulfosuccinate	Solid	0.05–0.36 g	0.02–0.05 g (<2) 0.05–0.15 g (≥2)	Small and large intestines	12–72 hours	Yes
Dioctyl potassium sulfosuccinate	Solid (rectal)	0.05–0.25 g	0.1 g (children)	Colon	2–15 min	—
Lubricant						
Mineral oil	Liquid (oral)	14–45 ml	10–15 ml (>6)	Colon	6–8 hours	Yes-minimal amount
Saline						
Magnesium citrate	Solid	11–18 g	2.5–5.0 g (2–5)	Small and large intestines	0.5–3 hours	Yes
Magnesium hydroxide	Solid	2.4–4.8 g	0.4–1.2 g (2–5) 1.2–2.4 g (≥6)	Small and large intestines	0.5–3 hours	
Magnesium sulfate	Solid	10–30 g	2.5–5.0 g (2–5) 5.0–10.0 g (6)	Small and large intestines	0.5–3 hours	Yes
Dibasic sodium phosphate	Solid (oral) Solid (rectal)	1.9–3.8 g 3.8 g	¼ adult dose (5–10) ½ adult dose (≥10) ½ adult dose (>2)	Small and large intestines colon (rectal)	0.5–3 hours 2–15 min	Yes
Monobasic sodium phosphate	Solid (oral) Solid (rectal)	8.3–16.6 g 16.6 g	¼ adult dose (5–10) ½ adult dose (≥10) ½ adult dose (>2)	Small and large intestines Colon	0.5–3 hours 2–15 min	Yes
Sodium biphosphate	Solid (oral) Solid (rectal)	9.6–19.2 g 19.2 g	¼ adult dose (5–10) ¼ adult dose (≥10) ½ adult dose (>2)	Small and large intestines Small and large intestines	0.5–3 hours 2–15 min	Yes —
Hyperosmotic						
Glycerin	Suppository	3 g	1–1.5 g (<6)	Colon	0.25–1 hour	
Stimulants						
Anthraquinones Aloe	Solid	0.12–0.25 g	Not recommended (<6) 0.04–0.08 g (6–8)	Colon	8–12 hours	Yes
Cascara sagrada	Fluidextract Aromatic Fluidextract Bark Extract Casanthranol	0.5–1.5 ml 2–6 ml 0.3–1.0 g 0.2–0.4 ml 0.03–0.09 ml	¼ adult dose (>2) ½ adult dose (2–12)	Colon — — —	6–8 hours — — —	Yes — — —

Table 6. continued

Agent	Dosage form	Daily dosage range		Site of action	Approximate time required for action	Systemic absorption
		Adult	Pediatric (age in years)			
Stimulants						
Danthron	Solid	0.075–0.15 g	Not recommended (<12)	Colon	8 hours	Yes
Senna	Powder	0.5–2.0 g	⅛ adult dose (>2)	Colon	6–10 hours	Yes
	Fluidextract	2.0 ml				
	Syrup	8.0 ml	¼ adult dose (1–6)			
	Fruit extract	3.4–4.0 ml	½ adult dose (6–12)			
	Suppository	1	½ adult dose (children over 60 lb)			
Sennosides A and B	Solid	0.012–0.036 g	0.0015–0.018 g 0.0015–0.1812 g	Colon	6–10 hours	—
Diphenyl methanes						
Bisacodyl	Tablet	0.005–0.015 g	0.005 g (>3)	Colon	6–10 hours	Yes
Phenolphthalein	Solid	0.03–0.27 g	Not recommended (<2) 0.015–0.020 g (2–6) 0.03–0.06 g (<6)	Colon	6–8 hours	Yes
Miscellaneous						
Castor oil	Liquid	15–60 ml	1–5 ml (<2) 5–15 ml (2–12)	Small intestines	2–6 hours	Yes

usate did not alter the incidence of constipation in a hospitalized geriatric population who received the drug for a 4-week period (17).

By facilitating the absorption of other poorly absorbed substances, such as danthron and mineral oil, the toxicity of the latter may be increased by concomitant administration of emollient laxatives (18, 19). A risk of hepatotoxicity exists when docusate is combined with danthron, although neither laxative by itself has been reported to cause this effect (20). It has been postulated that the detergent properties of docusate facilitates transport of other substances across cell membranes (21). Consequently, the FDA advisory review panel on nonprescription laxative, antidiarrheal, emetic, and antiemetic drug products recommended that these laxatives carry the following warning statement: "Do not take this product if you are presently taking a prescription drug or mineral oil" (16). Reports have indicated that daily use for 8 months or longer of preparations containing docusate sodium and oxyphenisatin acetate may produce chronic active liver disease with the attendant symptoms, including jaundice (22–25). As a result of these reports and other recommendations, laxatives containing oxyphenisatin acetate are no longer commercially available (26).

Patients with abdominal hernia, severe hypertension, or cardiovascular disease as well as those immediately post partum should not strain to defecate; neither should those who are about to undergo or have undergone surgery for hemorrhoids or other anorectal disorders. An emollient or fecal-softening laxative is indicated in such cases.

Lubricant Laxatives

Liquid petrolatum and certain digestible plant oils, such as olive oil, soften fecal contents by coating them and thus preventing colonic absorption of fecal water. Emulsified products are used to increase palatability. There is little difference in their cathartic efficacy, although emulsions of mineral oil penetrate and soften fecal matter more effectively than nonemulsified preparations. Liquid petrolatum is useful when it is used judiciously in cases that require the maintenance of a soft stool to avoid straining (after a hemorrhoidectomy or abdominal surgery, or in cases of hernia, aneurysm, hypertension, myocardial infarction, or cerebrovascular accident). However, routine use in these cases is probably not indicated. Stool softeners such as docusate sodium are probably better agents for these conditions.

The side effects and toxicity of mineral oil are associated with repeated and prolonged use. Significant absorption of mineral oil may occur, especially if emulsified products are used. The oil droplets may reach the mesenteric lymph nodes and may also be present in the intestinal mucosa, liver, and spleen, where they elicit a typical foreign body reaction.

Lipid pneumonia may result from the oral ingestion and subsequent aspiration of mineral oil, especially when the patient reclines. Therefore, it should not be taken at bedtime nor administered to debilitated patients. The pharynx becomes coated with the oil, and droplets gain access to the trachea and the posterior part of the lower lobes of the lungs.

The role of mineral oil in the absorption of fat-soluble nutrients is controversial, but there is apparently sufficient evidence to consider this effect significant. Absorption of vitamins A, D, E, and K may be impaired. Impaired vitamin D absorption may affect the absorption of calcium and phosphates.

In addition, mineral oil should not be taken with meals because it may delay gastric emptying. Mineral oil should not be given to pregnant patients since it can decrease the availability of vitamin K to the fetus. Those patients receiving oral anticoagulants should not receive mineral oil for the same reason (27).

Large doses of mineral oil may cause the oil to leak through the anal sphincter. This leakage may produce anal pruritus (pruritus ani), hemorrhoids, cryptitis, and other perianal disease and can be avoided by reducing the dose, dividing the dose, or using a stable emulsion of mineral oil. Prolonged use should be avoided. Because of the tendency of surfactants to increase the absorption of "nonabsorbable" drugs, mineral oil should not be taken with emollient fecal softeners. Mineral oil is not recommended for use in the very young or the elderly because of the greater possibility of aspiration into the lungs resulting in lipid pneumonia (28).

Saline Laxatives

The active constituents of saline laxatives are relatively nonabsorbable cations and anions such as magnesium and sulfate ions. Sulfate salts are considered to be the most potent of this category of laxatives. The wall of the small intestine, acting as a semipermeable membrane to the magnesium, sulfate, tartrate, phosphate, and citrate ions, retains the highly osmotic ions in the gut. The presence of these ions draws water into the gut causing an increase in intraluminal pressure. The increased intraluminal pressure exerts a mechanical stimulus that increases intestinal motility. However, reports suggest that different mechanisms, independent of the osmotic effect, also are responsible for the laxative properties of the salts. Saline laxatives have a complex series of actions, both secretory and motor, on the GI tract. For example, the action of magnesium sulfate on the GI tract is similar to that of cholecystokinin-pancreozymin. There is evidence that this hormone is released from the intestinal mucosa when saline laxatives are administered (29). This release in turn favors intraluminal accumulation of fluid and electrolytes. However, attempts at measuring cholecystokinin levels in patients before and after ingestion of magnesium-containing laxatives failed to demonstrate a change in serum cholecystokinin levels (30). One report indicated that magnesium sulfate is still useful in emergency situations as a cathartic (31).

Saline laxatives are indicated for use only in acute evacuation of the bowel (preparation for endoscopic examination and elimination of drugs in suspected poisonings) and in ridding the gut of blood in conditions such as hepatic coma. Saline laxatives do not have a place in the long-term management of constipation.

In cases of food or drug poisoning, the saline laxatives are sometimes used in purging doses. Magnesium sulfate is recommended except in cases of depressed CNS activity or renal dysfunction (32).

There are cases in which the unwise choice of a saline laxative results in serious side effects. As much as 20% of the administered magnesium ion may be absorbed from magnesium salts. If renal function is normal, the absorbed ion is excreted so rapidly that no change in the blood level of the ion can be detected. If the renal function is impaired, or if the patient is a newborn or elderly, toxic concentrations of the magnesium ion could accumulate in the extracellular body fluids. In addition, hypotension, muscle weakness, and EKG changes may indicate a toxic effect of magnesium. Magnesium exerts a depressant effect on the central nervous system and neuromuscular activity.

Phosphate salts are available both in oral and rectal dosage forms. The normal oral dose contains 96.5 mEq of sodium and therefore should be administered with caution to patients on sodium-restricted diets. The use of phosphate salts in children under the age of 2 can result in hypocalcemia, tetany, hypernatremia dehydration, and hyperphosphatemia (33, 34). When given in an enema, up to 10% or more of its sodium content may be absorbed. Barium enema preparations and elimination of fecal impaction are indications for the rectal use of phosphates. Cathartics that contain sodium may be toxic to individuals with edema and congestive heart disease. Since dehydration may occur from the repeated use of hypertonic solutions of saline cathartics, they should not be used by those who cannot tolerate fluid loss and should be followed by at least 1 full glass of water in normal patients to prevent dehydration.

Hyperosmotic Laxatives

Glycerin suppositories are available for infants and adults and usually produce a bowel movement within 30 minutes. Glycerin for many years was the main suppository used for lower bowel evacuation. In infants, the physical manipulation usually will initiate the reflex to defecate, and because of this property, adverse reactions and side effects are minimal (35). The laxative effect of glycerin suppositories is due to the combination of glycerin's osmotic effect with the local irritant effect of sodium stearate. However, rectal irritation may occur with its use. The customary rectal dosages of glycerin considered to be safe and effective for adults and children older than 6 years are 3 g as a suppository or 5–15 ml as an enema. For infants and children under 6 years of age, the dose is 1–1.5 g as a suppository or 2–5 ml as an enema (16). Claims have been made that suppositories may be equal in effectiveness to enemas (37).

Stimulant Laxatives

A comprehensive review of stimulant laxatives has been reported, and the structure–activity relationships of the anthraquinone or emodin-containing laxatives have been investigated (38–40). Stimulant laxatives increase the propulsive peristaltic activity of the intestine by local irritation of the mucosa or by a more selective action on the intramural nerve plexus of intestinal smooth muscle, thus increasing motility. Depending on the laxative, the site of action may be the small intestine, the large intestine, or both. Intensity of action is proportional to dosage, but individually effective doses vary. All stimulant laxatives produce gripping, increased mucus secretion, and, in some people, excessive evacuation of fluid.

Listed doses and dosage ranges are only guides to the correct individual dose. Stimulant laxatives should be used with caution when symptoms of appendicitis (abdominal pain, nausea, and vomiting) are present and should not be used at all when the diagnosis of appendicitis is made.

Stimulant laxatives are effective but should be recommended cautiously because they may produce undesirable and sometimes dangerous side effects (15). This property becomes more important when the agents are abused. It has been said that of all laxative products available, stimulant laxatives are the most widely abused (41). Chronic abuse can lead to "cathartic colon," a poorly functioning colon resembling ulcerative colitis.

In general, stimulant laxatives are not recommended as initial therapy in patients with constipation, and they should never be used for more than 1 week of regular treatment. The dose should be within the dosage range indicated as safe and effective (Table 6). These laxatives do not necessarily provide a good stimulus for the body to return to normal function. Major hazards of stimulant laxatives are severe cramping, electrolyte and fluid deficiencies, enteric loss of protein and malabsorption resulting from excessive catharsis, and hypokalemia. Since the intensity of stimulant laxative activity is proportional to the dose employed, if the dose is large enough, any of the stimulant laxatives can produce these unwanted side effects.

Stimulant laxatives, such as castor oil and bisacodyl, frequently are used before radiologic examination of the GI tract and before bowel surgery. Bisacodyl also is used orally or rectally instead of an enema for emptying the colon before proctologic examination.

Stimulant laxatives are classified according to their structure and activity.

Anthraquinones Anthraquinone laxative agents, also called anthracene laxatives, include aloe, cascara sagrada, danthron, and rhubarb. Also included in this category are senna, aloin, casanthranol, and frangula. The drugs of choice in this group are the cascara and senna compounds. Neither rhubarb, which contains an astringent (tannin), nor aloe, or aloin, which are very irritating, should be recommended. The properties of each of the anthraquinone laxatives vary, depending on the anthraquinone content and the speed of liberation of the active principles from their glycosidic combinations. The anthraquinone glycosides are hydrolyzed by colonic bacteria into active compounds. Crude drug formulation also may contain active constituents not found in extractive preparations or more highly purified compounds.

The precise mechanism by which peristalsis is increased is unknown. The cathartic activity of anthraquinones is limited primarily to the colon, which is reached by direct passage. Bacterial enzymes are partly responsible for the hydrolysis of the glycosides in the colon, making the drug more readily absorbed. Anthraquinones usually produce their action 6–12 hours after administration but may require up to 24 hours.

The active principles of anthraquinones are absorbed from the GI tract and subsequently appear in body secretions, including human milk. However, the practical significance of this finding in nursing infants is controversial.

After taking a senna laxative, postpartum women reported a brown discoloration of breast milk and subsequent catharsis of their nursing infants. A follow-up study indicated that the amount of senna laxative principles in breast milk was inadequate to stimulate defecation in the child (42). Another study with constipated postpartum breast-feeding women receiving a senna laxative reported that 17% of their infants experienced diarrhea (43).

Chrysophanic acid, a component of rhubarb and senna excreted in the urine, colors acidic urine yellowish-brown and alkaline urine reddish-violet.

The prolonged use of anthraquinone laxatives, especially cascara sagrada, can result in a melanotic pigmentation of the colonic mucosa, which is usually found on sigmoidoscopy or rectal biopsy. The shortest time observed for the appearance of melanosis coli in patients taking an anthraquinone cathartic in the presence of fecal stasis was 4 months and the longest was 13 months. In almost all cases, melanosis disappears within 5–11 months after discontinuation of the drug (44). Melanosis coli is virtually always due to prolonged use of anthraquinone laxatives (45). Pigment-containing macrophages appear in the mucosa, but staining reactions indicate that the pigment is not melanin but has many characteristics of lipofuscin. It may be a combination of a pigment of this type and either anthraquinone or one of its breakdown products. There is little evidence to suggest that laxatives other than anthraquinones lead to this pathologic feature.

The liquid preparations of cascara sagrada (fluidextracts) are more reliable than the solid dosage forms (extract and tablet). Aromatic cascara fluidextract is less active and less bitter than cascara sagrada fluidextract. This is reflected by the recommended dosages (Table 6). Magnesium oxide, used in the preparation of the former, removes some of the bitter and irritating principles from the crude drug.

Preparations of senna are more potent than those of cascara and produce considerably more gripping. Those that contain the crystalline glycosides of senna are more stable and reliable, and cause less gripping then those made from the crude drug. This difference is important in making a standardized senna product the logical choice among anthracene laxatives (46).

Danthron (1,8-dihydroxyanthraquinone), a breakdown product of the glycosides of senna, is a free anthraquinone rather than a glycoside. Its action, use, properties, and limitations are similar to those of the natural anthraquinone drugs. Like the glycosides, its site of action is the colon. Unlike the naturally occurring agents, it is partly absorbed from the small intestine, and much of the absorbed drug is metabolized by the liver. The metabolites are excreted by the kidneys, sometimes causing a pink to red discoloration of the urine.

Diphenylmethane Laxatives

The most common diphenylmethane laxatives are bisacodyl and phenolphthalein.

Bisacodyl   Bisacodyl was introduced as a cathartic as a result of structure-activity studies of phenolphthalein-related compounds. Practically insoluble in water or a saline medium, bisacodyl exerts its action in the colon on contact with the mucosal nerve plexus. Stimulation is segmented and axonal, producing contractions of the entire colon. Its action is independent of intestinal tone, and the drug is minimally absorbed systemically (approximately 5%) (27). Action on the small intestine is negligible. A soft, formed stool usually is produced 6–10 hours after oral administration and 15–60 minutes after rectal administration. Bisacodyl tablets are enteric coated to prevent irritation of the gastric lining and therefore should not be broken, chewed, or administered with alkaline materials such as antacid products.

The tablet and suppository combination have been recommended for cleaning the colon before and after surgery and before X-ray examination. Bisacodyl increases ileostomy water output and is effective in patients with colostomies and reduces or eliminates the need for irrigations (47). No systemic or adverse effects on the liver, kidney, or hematopoietic system have been observed following its administration. Side effects occur primarily from purgative action and include metabolic acidosis or alkalosis, hypocalcemia, tetany, and loss of enteric protein and malabsorption (48). Bisacodyl has not been detected in the milk of nursing women. The suppository form may produce a burning sensation in the rectum.

Phenolphthalein   This drug exerts its stimulating effect mainly on the colon, but the activity of the small intestine may be increased as well. Its exact mechanism of action is not known but phenolphthalein appears to alter multiple steps of the absorptive process. It is usually active 6–8 hours after administration.

Phenolphthalein is effective in small doses and is tasteless, making it desirable for marketing in candy and chewing gum forms. When ingested, it passes through the stomach unchanged and is dissolved by the bile salts and the alkaline intestinal secretions. As much as 15% of the dose is absorbed, and the rest is excreted unchanged in the feces. Some of the absorbed drug appears in the urine, which is colored pink to red if it is sufficiently alkaline. Similarly, the drug excreted in the feces causes a red coloration if the feces are sufficiently alkaline (soap suds enemas). This effect may alarm people who are not aware of this property.

Part of the absorbed phenolphthalein is excreted back into the intestinal tract with the bile. The resulting enterohepatic cycle may prolong the action of phenolphthalein for 3–4 days. Since bile must be present for it to be effective, phenolphthalein is ineffective in relieving constipation associated with obstructive jaundice.

Phenolphthalein is usually nontoxic. However, at least two types of allergic reactions may follow the use of phenolphthalein. In susceptible individuals, a large dose may cause diarrhea, colic, cardiac and respiratory distress, or circulatory collapse. The other reaction is a polychromatic rash that ranges from pink to deep purple. The eruptions may be pinhead-sized or as large as the palm of the hand. Itching and burning may be moderate or severe. If the rash is severe, it may lead to vesication and erosion, especially around the mouth and genital areas. Other skin reactions, including toxic epidermal necrosis and bullous eruptions, may occur and are related to sunlight exposure (49).

Osteomalacia due to impaired absorption of vitamin D and calcium is one untoward effect that has been attributed to excessive phenolphthalein ingestion (49, 50). Phenolphthalein abuse can mimic Bartter's syndrome by inducing juxtaglomerular cell hyperplasia with secondary aldosteronism. This is characterized by hypokalemic alkalosis and marked renin increase in the absence of hypertension (51).

Miscellaneous: Castor Oil

The laxative action of castor oil is due to ricinoleic acid, which is produced when castor oil is hydrolyzed in the small intestine by pancreatic lipase. Its mechanism of action is unknown. However, its laxative effect depends upon cyclic adenosine monophosphate mediated fluid secretion and not from increased peristalsis due to the irritant effect of ricinoleic acid (52).

Castor oil, a glyceride, may be absorbed from the GI tract and is probably metabolized like other fatty acids. Because the main site of action is the small intestine, its prolonged use may result in excessive loss of fluid, electrolytes, and nutrients. Castor oil is most effective when administered on an empty stomach and produces an evacuation within 2–6 hours after ingestion. Because of its unpleasant taste it should be administered with fruit juices or carbonated beverages. Although used in situations requiring a thorough evacuation of the GI tract, it is seldom used routinely for constipation.

Dosage Forms

Laxative products are available in a wide array of dosage forms. Most of these are given orally. Variety in dosage forms probably yields the most benefits when laxatives are needed in pediatric or geriatric patients. However, by no means are all of the available dosage forms necessary for effective laxative action. Many of the dosage forms enhance patient acceptability and perhaps, make laxative use pleasant. Laxatives available as chewing gum, effervescent granules, and chocolate tablets may certainly be associated with pleasantness but may not always be thought of as drug products because of this. Consequently, patients may use them indiscriminately. It is important to keep this fact in mind especially when considering laxative abuse.

Enemas and suppositories are dosage forms used extensively for laxative administration. Enemas are used routinely to prepare patients for surgery, child delivery, radiologic examination, and in certain cases of constipation. The enema fluid determines the mechanism by which evacuation is produced. Tap water and normal saline create bulk by an osmotic volume effect; vegetable oils lubricate, soften, and facilitate the passage of hardened fecal matter; soapsuds produce defecation by their irritant action. There have been reports of rectal irritation that has lasted as long as 3 weeks after soap enemas. In addition, there have been reports of anaphylaxis, rectal gangrene, and serious fluid loss secondary to acute colitis after soap enemas (52). Therefore, it is recommended that soap enemas not be used (54).

The popular sodium phosphate–sodium biphosphate preparations fall into the category of saline laxatives. They are usually effective evacuants in preparing patients for surgical, diagnostic, or other procedures involving the bowel. In a crossover study of healthy individuals, these drugs were more efficient and effective than tap water, soap-suds, or saline enemas (55). These agents can alter fluid and electrolyte balance significantly if they are used on a prolonged basis. Consequently, chronic use of these products in the control of constipation is not warranted.

A properly administered enema cleans only the distal colon, most nearly approximating a normal bowel movement (56). Proper administration requires that the diagnosis, the enema fluid, and the technique of administration be correct. Improperly administered, an enema can produce fluid and electrolyte imbalances. A misdirected or inadequately lubricated nozzle may cause abrasion of the anal canal and rectal wall or colonic perforation.

Enema fluids have caused mucosal changes or spasm of the intestinal wall. Water intoxication has resulted from the use of tap water or soap-suds enemas in the presence of megacolon (57).

To administer an enema properly, the patient should be placed on the left side with knees bent or in the knee-chest position. Using an enema in a sitting position clears only the rectum of fecal material. The container holding the fluid should be 2.5–5 cm above the buttocks to allow free but not forcible flow of the fluid from the tube. The solution should be allowed to flow in the rectum slowly; if the patient is uncomfortable, the flow is probably too fast. One pint (500 ml) of properly introduced fluid usually causes adequate evacuation, if it is retained until definite lower abdominal cramping is felt. As long as 1 hour may be needed for the entire procedure. Two or three pints of nonirritating fluid usually produce a clean bowel and a nonirritated mucosa.

Bisacodyl-, senna-, and carbon dioxide-releasing suppositories are promoted as replacements for enemas in cases where cleaning the distal colon is required. Suppositories that contain senna concentrate are advertised as effective in postsurgical and postpartum care; those that contain bisacodyl are promoted for postoperative, antepartum, and postpartum care and are adequate in the preparation for proctosigmoidoscopy. A suppository that exerts its action by the pressure of the released carbon dioxide is recommended for the same uses (58). Although bisacodyl suppositories are prescribed and used more frequently than others, some clinicians still employ enemas as agents for cleaning the lower bowel.

It has been suggested that the carbon dioxide-releasing suppository might serve as a replacement for some of the uses of the enema. One study reported that it was used successfully in institutionalized, spastic, and mentally retarded pediatric patients to replace enemas. It also replaced enemas in preparing these patients for intravenous pyelograms and for the instillation of rectal anesthetics (57).

Pediatric Laxative Use

The use of laxatives in pediatric patients occurs with reasonable frequency. Parents should be cautioned about the indiscriminant use of laxative products. Children can have numerous problems with constipation, and these problems are often difficult to manage. Often emotional factors may interplay in children and must be dealt with to bring about an appropriate change in bowel habits. Particular factors that may contribute to constipation in children include change in environment, diet, and the occurrence of a febrile illness (59).

In many instances, improvement in the bulk content of the child's diet may improve constipation. Simply increasing the amount of fluid or sugar in the formula may be corrective in the first few months of life. After this age, better results are obtained by adding or increasing the amounts of cereal, vegetables, and fruits. If medication is needed, stimulants should probably be avoided as should frequent use of enemas (60). Due to its relative safety, malt soup extract can be administered to infants less than 2 months of age. Dietary changes are usually necessary in addition to this type of laxative in infants. Glycerin suppositories are useful in initiating the defecation reflex. Docusate sodium also is useful in children and can be given in 3 divided doses during the day. Age should always be considered in recommendation of products. Route of administration may have added significance in this age group as will taste of products if the oral route is desired. Phosphate-type enemas are reserved primarily for use in cases of fecal impaction.

Geriatric Laxative Use

The aging process is accompanied by physiologic changes that may affect or be affected by drug therapy. In addition, geriatric patients tend to have multiple diseases and have to take multiple drugs.

It appears that laxative preparations may increase the rate at which other drugs pass through the gastrointestinal tract by increasing GI motility. As a result, there may be a decreased absorption of drugs if excessive motility is produced. When a patient is taking several drugs, there is always the likelihood that concurrent use of a laxative may pose a problem. Pharmacists advising each patient should be mindful of this. Elderly patients usually have decreased fluid volumes and are particularly sensitive to shifts in fluid with the accompanying shifts in electrolytes. Use of any type of laxative that alters fluid volume, particularly saline type laxatives, can be inappropriate to administer in an elderly patient.

Elderly patients often fall prey to the advertising claims made for laxative products. This emphasis causes elderly patients to use laxatives on a more routine basis, and as time goes by, they often develop dependence on the laxative. This becomes a difficult problem to cope with from a practitioner's point of view. Proper education and selection advice for the elderly patient is perhaps more crucial than with the general population.

In those geriatric patients who previously did not have a history of constipation, a thorough investigation should be carried out to determine if the acute case of constipation has resulted from new or old diseases or from the use of medicines. Many geriatric patients have an atonic colon resulting in loss of muscle tone and consequently rely on laxatives or enemas for bowel movements. In addition, a low-residue diet, poor chewing of food, or ill-fitting dentures can cause constipation in this age group. Finally, many geriatric patients receive drugs that can induce constipation. If any of these reasons are valid, corrective action in the patient's lifestyle or therapy should be advised instead of immediately recommending a laxative.

Geriatric patients should be approached individually because of the vulnerability these patients have to medicines in general. Even though bulk-forming agents have been used successfully in these patients, a complete and thorough history will probably provide the information needed to make an appropriate recommendation on an individualized basis (61).

Self-Medication in Pregnancy

Constipation is a fairly common occurrence in pregnancy. One study showed a 31% incidence, with 65% of these women treating themselves with either diet or laxatives without the benefit of professional advice (43). Constipation that develops during pregnancy is usually attributed to compression of the colon caused by increase in the size of the uterus. However, the primary reason is probably a reduction in muscle tone which contributes to a decrease in peristalsis (62). In addition, vitamin and mineral supplements that contain iron and calcium tend to be constipating.

Most types of laxatives appear to be effective in pregnancy. However, due to various effects such as possible loss of vitamins caused by mineral oil, premature labor due to the irritant effect of castor oil, or the possibility of dangerous electrolyte imbalance with osmotic agents, the laxatives used in pregnancy should probably be limited to an emollient or a bulk-former (63). Stimulant laxatives should probably be avoided during pregnancy and lactation period.

As with other types of patients, pregnant women should be counseled on proper diet, adequate fluid intake, and reasonable amounts of exercise (62). If these measures do not alleviate or prevent the development of constipation, the recommendation of a laxative preparation may be in order. The pharmacist should be in communication with the patient's physician, especially if any doubt exists regarding the patient's perceived problem and the physician's desire for the the patient to have a laxative. Laxatives may also have to be administered post partum to reestablish normal bowel function that may have been lost due to ileus secondary to colonic dilatation in a decompressed abdomen; perineal pain, laxness of the anal sphincter, and abdominal musculature; and low fluid intake and the administration of enemas during labor. In addition, hemorrhoids in the period after delivery are aggravated, if not caused by constipation (64).

Laxative Abuse

Regular use of most laxatives, particularly the stimu- lant preparations, can result in laxative abuse. The pharmacist should be aware of this possibility.

Excessive use of laxatives can cause diarrhea and vomiting, leading to fluid and electrolyte losses, especially hypokalemia, where there is a general loss of tone of smooth and striated muscle (65, 66). The clinical features of laxative abuse include (65):

- Factitious diarrhea;
- Electrolyte imbalance (hypokalemia, hypocalcemia, hypermagnesemia);
- Osteomalacia;
- Protein-losing enteropathy;
- Steatorrhea;
- Cathartic colon;
- Liver disease.

The "cathartic colon," which develops after years of laxative abuse is difficult to diagnose and may present symptoms similar to acute nephritis, diabetes insipidus, neurasthenia, ulcerative colitis, or Addison's disease. In a study of seven hospitalized female patients, 26–65 years old, the chief admitting complaints were abdominal pain and diarrhea, the number of hospital admissions ranged from 2 to 11, and the total number of days spent in the hospital ranged from 58 to 202 (65). The diagnosis of laxative abuse was difficult because the patients denied taking laxatives, and none of the colonic tissue characteristics usually associated with excessive laxative use was observed on sigmoidoscopy or radiologic examination. However, excessive laxative use was later revealed.

Diarrhea can be a serious consequence of the overuse of laxative products, especially irritant laxatives. The prolonged misuse of laxative drugs can cause morbid anatomical changes in the colon. In a study of 12 chronic laxative users, the primary anatomical changes were loss of intrinsic innervation, mucosal inflammation, atrophy of smooth muscle coats, and pigmentation of the colon (67). Most users had been taking laxatives regularly for 30–40 years; two were less than 30 years old when they had their colons removed and therefore had a much shorter history. In these cases, the myenteric plexus showed many swollen, but otherwise normal, neurons. This evidence suggests that the initial action of an irritant laxative is to stimulate neurons and that prolonged and continuous stimulation causes cell death. In such cases, the transverse colon is often pendulous, the sigmoid section is highly dilated, and the muscle coats are thin and contain excess adipose tissue, indicating some tissue atrophy. Psychiatric help should be sought for patients who are chronically abusing laxatives. It may be possible to wean the patient off the laxatives before permanent bowel damage occurs and to regularize the bowel habits with a high-fiber diet (45, 61, 68).

Product Selection Guidelines
Consultation Information

The most useful approach to the patient who requests a laxative product for self-medication should first include a discussion of dietary habits, exercise activities, fluid intake, and general emotional well-being. It is well known that these factors may be responsible to a large degree for problems associated with constipation. It cannot be assumed that patients understand the interplay of these factors in the development of constipation. For example, one study on self-medication showed that 65% of patients questioned about their use of laxative products were unable to associate the role of diet with the development of constipation (9). This indicates the lack of understanding of constipation and the kinds of normal factors that can have a larger effect on its development. The following factors are very important in returning a person to a relatively normal state without laxative intervention (69):

- Adequate fiber in the diet;
- Retraining the individual to respond to the urge to defecate;
- Physical exercise;
- Adequate fluid intake;
- Relaxation to reduce emotional stress and its effect on defecation.

A diet consisting of high-fiber foods and plenty of fluids (4–6 8-oz glasses of water/day) will help relieve chronic constipation. Caution regarding fluid intake must be used in patients on fluid restriction. Dietary fiber is that part of whole grain, vegetables, fruits, and nuts that resist digestion in the GI tract. It is composed of carbohydrates (cellulose, hemicelluloses, polysaccharides, and pectin) and a noncarbohydrate, lignin. Food fiber content, which is expressed in terms of crude fiber residue after treatment with dilute acid and alkali, has a significant effect on bowel habits. Because fiber holds water, in persons with a higher fiber intake, stools tend to be softer, bulkier, and heavier and probably pass through the colon more rapidly.

Along with a high-fiber diet, the pharmacist may encourage regular, mild exercise such as walking provided the patient's cardiovascular system is normal and the patient is under a physician's care. Physical activity is important in the propulsion mechanisms in the colon. Exercise in any form improves muscle tone, but exercise using the abdominal muscles is the most beneficial in improvement of intestinal muscle tone (70).

The patient should learn not to ignore the urge to defecate and should allow adequate time for elimination (46). A relaxed, unhurried atmosphere can be very important in aiding elimination. The patient should be encouraged to set a regular pattern for bathroom visits. Mornings, particularly after breakfast, seem to be a very good time. Having a specific time period set aside for elimination may help the body adjust itself to producing a regular stool.

The fact that normal defecation empties only the descending and sigmoid colon should always be remembered when considering the use of any preparation in a suspected situation of constipation. The preparation chosen should duplicate the normal process as much as possible. Clearly, stimulant products act more distantly to this process than most other types. Stimulant products cause emptying of the entire colon and thereby discourage the proper return to normal function. The laxative user who is unaware of this effect may take another laxative dose on the first or second postlaxative day, thereby maintaining a completely empty colon.

In counseling the patient on laxative use, the pharmacist should stress the following points:

- Laxative agents should not be used on a regular basis; more natural methods such as diet, exercise, and fluid intake should be sought to produce regular movements;
- The use of a laxative agent in the treatment of constipation should be only a temporary measure; once regularity has returned, the laxative product should be discontinued.

Indications for self-medication with a nonprescription laxative include preparation for diagnostic procedures and acute constipation. Treatment for perianal disease (preoperatively or postoperatively) or use during specific illnesses (postoperatively, postmyocardial infarction, or any other condition where straining is undesirable) or chronic constipation is best accomplished with the knowledge of the patient's physician (71). Because defecation has been found to alter hemodynamics, straining to defecate has resulted in death from emboli, ventricular rupture, and cardiogenic shock in patients who had experienced a myocardial infarction (72).

Specific advice to patients concerning laxative products should include these reminders:

- Laxatives are not designed for long-term use; if they are not effective after 1 week, a physician should be consulted.
- If a skin rash appears after the patient has taken a laxative containing phenolphthalein, the product should be discontinued and a physician should be contacted.
- Saline laxatives should not be used daily and should not be administered orally to children under 6 years or rectally to infants under 2 years.
- Mineral oil should not be given to children under 6 years or in conjunction with emollient laxatives; they should not be used during pregnancy and should be avoided in patients taking anticoagulants.
- Castor oil should not be used to treat constipation.
- Enemas and suppositories must be administered properly to be effective.
- Laxatives should not be used in the presence of abdominal pain, nausea, vomiting, bloating, or cramping.
- Laxatives containing phenolphthalein, rhubarb, or senna may discolor urine; laxatives containing phenolphthalein may discolor feces pink to red depending on the alkalinity.

Specific product notes for pharmacists include the following:

- Laxative products containing more than 15 mEq (345 mg) of sodium, more than 25 mEq (975 mg) of potassium, or more than 50 mEq (600 mg) of magnesium in the maximum daily dose should not be used if kidney disease or other conditions requiring sodium, potassium, or magnesium restriction are present.
- Caution should be used with any product containing

dextrose in diabetes as the possibility of the loss of control may result (73).

Patient Assessment

The pharmacist should try to obtain as much information about the patient as possible before making any recommendations for relief of constipation. The information gathered through the assessment process allows the pharmacist to make rational recommendations based on knowledge of the patient, the problem, and the product and his or her own judgment and experience. It should be kept in mind that laxative products are both widely used and abused. The pharmacist can provide a valuable service by educating patients on the appropriate use of laxatives.

The first question that the pharmacist should ask is for what purpose the patient intends to use a laxative product. Not all patients purchasing a laxative are constipated. The product might be needed as a result of an upcoming X-ray examination of the bowel, or the product may be purchased for a friend or a relative. It is important to know why the patient feels that a laxative product is necessary at the present time.

The pharmacist should determine the patient's symptoms and their duration. If symptoms have persisted for more than 2 weeks or have recurred after previous laxative use, the patient should be referred to a physician. Perhaps the patient has already attempted to alleviate symptoms by dietary measures such as increasing fruit and vegetable consumption. This, too, is important information for the pharmacist.

Any patient who has an established disease affecting the GI tract presents particular concern. It is quite possible that laxative products used by these patients may adversely affect their condition. The pharmacist should obtain accurate information regarding all diseases present. The patient should be referred to a physician when insufficient information or any doubt exists regarding disease states.

As previously suggested, the normal population experiences from three bowel movements per day to three bowel movements per week (8), and individuals who fall outside this range might be classed as unusual but not always abnormal. Thus, the frequency of movements may not be the most relevant concern; the consistency of the stool and accompanying symptoms are important characteristics of constipation as well (74).

When it is necessary to use a laxative for the treatment of constipation, the recommended choice is a bulk-forming product; however, the pharmacist should keep in mind the situations in which its use is inappropriate. Laxatives are not recommended to treat constipation associated with intestinal pathology or to treat constipation secondary to laxative abuse unless bowel retraining has been successful. They also are not a cure for functional constipation and therefore are of only secondary importance in its treatment.

The pharmacist should also be concerned about the patient's current and past use of laxative products. The patient already may be using one or more products, and improper use may be preventing the desired effect. The

possibility of laxative abuse also should be considered. Stimulant laxatives may be a cause of constipation in abusers due to tolerance development. An in-depth knowledge of the patient's history of laxative use provides the pharmacist with information about past patterns of drug use, effective or ineffective products, the incidence of constipation, and the use of home remedies. Depending on the pharmacist's findings, referral to a physician may be necessary.

Furthermore, all medication use by a patient is an important consideration of the pharmacist. Caution should be exercised when laxatives are recommended for use by patients receiving prescription drug products. Laxative preparations may increase the rate at which other drugs pass through the GI tract. The resulting effect could be decreased absorption of those drugs (75, 76). Drugs with constipating side effects (calcium or aluminum antacids, narcotic analgesics, and anticholinergic-type drugs) may counteract the effects of laxatives; drugs with laxative side effects, such as magnesium antacids and antiadrenergic-type drugs, may tend to intensify the effect of laxative ingredients. Pharmacists must investigate all drug use and provide guidance for the rational selection of appropriate laxatives.

In some cases, treatment for another ailment may relieve symptoms of constipation. In perianal disease, for example, constipation is usually the result of the patient's unwillingness to defecate due to the pain encountered. When medical and/or surgical treatment is given, the barrier to normal defecation is removed. Conditions such as hypothyroidism or depression may be responsible for a patient's complaint of constipation. Successful treatment of these disorders usually eliminates the constipation problems.

Summary

The widespread abuse of nonprescription laxatives is evidence of a greater need for professional consultation and patient education. Successful treatment of a patient with constipation depends on careful identification of the cause. To determine whether referral to a physician or self-therapy is indicated, the pharmacist requires a knowledge of the case history and current symptoms. If the case history discloses a sudden change in bowel habits that has persisted for 2 weeks, the pharmacist should refer the patient to a physician. However, if the constipation can be treated without physician intervention, knowledge of the many available products is essential.

For most cases of simple constipation, proper diet, exercise, and adequate fluid intake will promote alleviation of the condition. Therapy with any laxative product should be limited in most cases to short-term use (1 week). If after a 1-week period of proper laxative therapy no relief has been achieved, the product should be discontinued.

Pharmacists who successfully perform their professional responsibilities with nonprescription laxatives will lessen patient demand for these products and will establish themselves as important public health consultants.

References

1. *Drug Topics*, *125*, 75 (1980).
2. "New and Non-Official Drugs," Lippincott, Philadelphia, Pa., 1965, p. 615.
3. A. Jacknowitz, *Am. J. Hosp. Pharm.*, *38*, 1122 (1981).
4. W. D. Carey, *Cleveland Clin.*, *44*, 73 (1977).
5. J. R. DiPalma, "Drill's Pharmacology in Medicine," 4th ed., McGraw-Hill, New York, N.Y., 1971, p. 747.
6. W. F. Ganong, "Review of Medical Physiology," 6th ed., Lange Medical, Los Altos, Calif., 1971, p. 357.
7. F. H. Netter, "The Ciba Collection of Medical Illustrations," Vol. 3, Part II, Ciba Pharmaceutical Co., Summit, N.J., 1962, p. 98.
8. A. M. Connell, C. Hilton, G. Irvine, J. E. Lennard-Jones, and J. J. Misiewich, *Br. Med. J.*, *2*, 1095 (1965).
9. D. A. Matte and W. M. McLean, *Drug Intell. Clin. Pharm.*, *12*, 603 (1978).
10. G. E. Sladen, *Proc. Roy. Soc. Med.*, *65*, 289 (1972).
11. R. Gross, *J. Am. Med. Assoc.*, *241*, 1573 (1979).
12. *Federal Register*, *39*, 19874 (1974).
13. G. A. Spiler, E. A. Shipley, M. C. Chernoff et al., *J. Clin. Pharmacol.*, 19, 313 (1979).
14. T. P. Almy, *Ann. N.Y. Acad. Sci.*, *58*, 398 (1954).
15. K. Rutter and D. Maxwell, *Br. Med. J.*, *2*, 997 (1976).
16. *Federal Register*, *40*, 12907, 12911-12 (1975).
17. J. Goodman, J. Pang, and A. N. Bessman, *J. Chron. Dis.*, *29*, 59 (1976).
18. *Medical Letter on Drugs and Therapeutics*, *19*, 45 (1977).
19. K. Naess, *J. Am. Med. Assoc.*, *212*, 1961 (1970).
20. K. G. Tolman, S. Hammar, and J. J. Sannella, *Ann. Intern. Med.*, *84*, 290 (1976).
21. C. A. Dujoune, D. Shoeman, J. Bianchine et al., *J. Lab. Clin. Med.*, *79*, 832 (1972).
22. T. B. Reynolds, R. L. Peters, and S. Yamada, *N. Engl. J. Med.*, *285*, 813 (1971).
23. E. Gjone, J. P. Blumhoff, S. Ritland, E. Elgjo, and G. Husby, *Scand. J. Gastroenterol.*, *7*, 395 (1972).
24. O. Dietrichson, E. Juhl, J. O. Nielsen, J. J. Oxlund, and P. Christoffersen, *Scand. J. Gastroenterol.*, *9*, 473 (1974).
25. R. L. Willing and R. Hecker, *Med. J. Aust.*, *1*, 1179 (1971).
26. *Journal of the American Medical Association*, *211*, 114 (1970).
27. E. C. Rosenow, *Ann. Intern. Med.*, *77*, 977–991, (1972).
28. L. E. Nochmovitz, C. J. Vys, and S. Epstein, *S. Afr. Med. J.*, *49*, 2187 (1975).
29. G. Forbes, A. Bradley, *Br. Med. J.*, *2*, 1566–1568, (1958).
30. L. Sillin, J. Woods, D. Gentile et al., *Gastroenterology*, *74*, 1144 (1978).
31. D. G. Spoeke, *Am. J. Hosp. Pharm.*, *38*, 498 (1981).
32. "The Pharmacological Basis of Therapeutics," 6th ed., L. G. Goodman, L. S. Goodman, and A. Gilman, Eds., Macmillan, New York, N.Y., 1980, pp. 120, 513, 1002.
33. T. H. McConnell, *J. Am. Med. Assoc.*, *216*, 147 (1971).
34. R. W. Chisney and P. B. Haughton, *Am. J. Dis. Child.*, *127*, 684 (1974).
35. R. Salm, *Thorax*, *25*, 762 (1970).
37. M. R. Barnes, *Radiology*, *9*, 948 (1968).
38. "The Pharmacological Basis of Therapeutics," 6th ed., L. G. Goodman, L. S. Goodman, and A. Gilman, Eds., Macmillan, New York, N.Y., 1980, pp. 1006–1009.
39. "Textbook of Pharmacology," 2nd ed., W. C. Bowman and M. J. Rand, Eds., Blackwell Scientific, London, England, 1980, p. 25–33.
40. R. R. Harvey and A. E. Reed, *Lancet*, *2*, 185 (1973).
41. J. Travel, *Ann. N.Y. Acad. Sci.*, *58*, 416 (1954).
42. S. J. Loewe, *J. Pharmacol. Exp. Ther.*, *94*, 288 (1948).
43. L. Schmidt and E. Seeger, *Arzneim-Forsch.*, *b*, 22 (1965).
44. "Gastrointestinal Disease," 2nd ed., M. H. Sleisinger and J. S. Fordtran, Eds., W. B. Saunders, Philadelphia, Pa., 1978, p. 1862.
45. J. H. Cummings, *Gut*, *15*, 758 (1974).
46. T. D. McCaffery, *Drug Therapy*, *5*, 41 (1975).
47. D. G. Tracht and A. R. Clement, *Radiology*, *99*, 69 (1971).
48. F. Nahman and G. D. Cam, *South. Med. J.*, *66*, 724 (1973).
49. R. G. Pietrusko, *Am. J. Hosp. Pharm.*, *34*, 291 (1977).
50. H. W. Stein and D. G. Colin-Jones, *J. Pathol.*, *115*, 199-205, 1975.
51. N. Fleisher, H. Brown, D. Y. Graham et al., *Ann. Intern. Med.*, *70*, 791 (1969).
52. H. J. Binder, J. W. Dobbins, and D. S. Whiting, *Gastroenterology*, *72*, 1079 (1977).
53. B. F. Pike, P. J. Phillippi, and E. H. Lawson, *N. Engl. J. Med.*, *265*, 217 (1971).
54. "Applied Therapeutics for the Clinical Pharmacist," 2nd ed., M. A. Koda-Kimble, B. S. Katcher, and L. Y. Young, Eds., Applied Therapeutics, San Francisco, Calif., 1978, p. 119.
55. S. G. Page, C. R. Riley, and H. B. Hoag, *J. Am. Med. Assoc.*, *157*, 1208 (1955).
56. M. W. Werthmann and S. V. Krees, *Med. Ann. D.C.*, *42*, 4 (1973).
57. J. O. Greenhalf and H. S. Leonard, *Practitioner*, *210*, 259 (1973).
58. "Applied Therapeutics for Clinical Pharmacists," 2nd ed., M. A. Koda-Kimble, B. S. Katcher, and L. Y. Young, Eds., Applied Therapeutics, San Francisco, Calif., 1978, p. 117.
59. K. Goulston, *Drugs*, *14*, 128 (1977).
60. B. Frame, H. L. Guiang, H. M. Frost, and W. A. Reynolds, *Arch. Intern. Med.*, *128*, 794 (1971).
61. H. Cummings, G. E. Sladen, O. F. W. James, M. Sarner, and J. J. Misiewicz, *Br. Med. J.*, *1*, 537 (1974).
62. J. S. G. Biggs and E. J. Vesey, *Drugs*, *19*, 70 (1980).
63. L. L. Hart, in "Applied Therapeutics for the Clinical Pharmacist," 2nd ed., M. A. Koda-Kimble, B. S. Katcher, and L. Y. Young, Eds., Applied Therapeutics, San Francisco, Calif., 1978, p. 121.
64. L. Mundow, *Br. Med. J. Clin. Prac.*, *29*, 95 (1975).
65. R. R. Babb, *West. J. Med.*, *122*, 93 (1975).
66. L. S. Basser, *Med. J. Aust.*, *1*, 47 (1979).
67. B. Smith, *Dis. Colon Rectum*, *16*, 455 (1973).
68. M. D. Rawson, *Lancet*, *1*, 1121 (1966).
69. H. R. Erle, *Primary Care*, *3*, 301 (1976).
70. *Drug Therapy*, *5*, 41 (1975).
71. W. G. Thompson, *Drugs*, *19*, 49 (1980).
72. A. D. Dennison, *Am. J. Cardiol.*, *1*, 400 (1968).
73. J. Catellani and R. J. Collins, *Lancet*, *2*, 98 (1978).
74. W. G. Thompson, *Can. Med. Assoc. J.*, *114*, 927 (1976).
75. "Remington's Pharmaceutical Sciences," 16th ed., A. Osal, Ed., Mack, Easton, Pa., 1980, p. 1749.
76. "American Hospital Formulary Service," R. J. Reilly, Ed., American Society of Hospital Pharmacists, Washington, D.C., 1978, p. 56:12.

Laxative Product Table

Product (Manufacturer)	Dosage Form	Stimulant	Bulk	Emollient/ Lubricant	Other Laxatives	Other Ingredients
Adlerika (Alvin Last)	liquid				magnesium sulfate	
Afko-Lube (Amer. Pharm.)	capsule syrup			docusate sodium, 100 mg (capsule) 4 mg/ml (syrup)		
Afko-Lube Lax (Amer. Pharm.)	capsule	casanthranol, 30 mg		docusate sodium, 100 mg		
Agoral (Parke-Davis)	emulsion	phenolphthalein, 13.3 mg/ml	agar tragacanth acacia	mineral oil, 280 mg/ml		egg albumin glycerin sodium, 0.98 mEq/ 15 ml
Agoral Plain (Parke-Davis)	emulsion		agar tragacanth acacia	mineral oil, 280 mg/ml		egg albumin glycerin sodium, 0.98 mEq/15 ml
Alophen (Parke-Davis)	tablet	phenolphthalein, 60 mg				sodium free
Bisacodyl (Philips Roxane)	tablet suppository	bisacodyl, 5 mg/tablet, 10 mg/suppository				
Black Draught (Chattem)	tablet syrup granules	casanthranol, 30 mg/tablet, 6 mg/ml (syrup), 30 mg/g (granules)				sucrose, 54.6% anise peppermint cinnamon clove nutmeg (spices only in syrup)
Caroid Laxative Tablets (Winthrop)	tablet	cascara sagrada extract, 55 mg phenolphthalein, 32.4 mg				
Carter's Little Pills (Carter)	tablet	bisacodyl, 5 mg				
Cas-Evac (Parke-Davis)	liquid	cascara sagrada, 2 mg/ml				alcohol, 18% sodium saccharin, 1.45 mg/ml
Casyllium (Upjohn)	granules	cascara fluidextract, 0.5 ml/g	psyllium husk, 0.68 g/g prune powder, 0.2 g/g			sodium, 0.5 mEq/tsp
Colace (Mead Johnson)	capsule liquid syrup			docusate sodium, 50 and 100 mg/capsule, 1% (liquid), 4 mg/ml (syrup)		sucrose, 600 mg/ml (syrup) sodium, 0.11 mEq/50 mg (capsule), 0.015 mEq/ml
Coloctyl (Vitarine)	capsule			docusate sodium, 100 mg		

Laxative Product Table, continued

Product (Manufacturer)	Dosage Form	Stimulant	Bulk	Emollient/ Lubricant	Other Laxatives	Other Ingredients
Comfolax (Searle)	capsule			docusate sodium, 100 mg		sodium, 0.225 mEq
Comfolax Plus (Searle)	capsule	casanthranol, 30 mg		docusate sodium, 100 mg		sodium, 0.225 mEq
Concentrated Milk of Magnesia (Philips Roxane)	suspension				magnesium hydroxide, 0.233 g/ml	glycerin, 2.5% sorbitol, 29% sugar, 8% lemon sodium, 0.09 mEq/ml
Constiban (Columbia Medical)	capsule	casanthranol, 30 mg		docusate sodium, 100 mg		
Correctol (Plough)	tablet liquid	yellow phenolphthalein, 65 mg (tablet), 4.3 mg/ml (liquid)		docusate sodium, 100 mg (tablet)		sodium, 0.34 mEq peppermint flavor (liquid)
Dialose (Stuart)	capsule			docusate potassium, 100 mg		
Dialose Plus (Stuart)	capsule	casanthranol, 30 mg		docusate potassium, 100 mg		
Dioctyl Sodium Sulfosuccinate (Philips Roxane)	capsule syrup			docusate sodium, 50, 100, and 250 mg/capsule, 3.33 mg/ml (syrup)		propylene glycol, 20% (syrup) sucrose, 55% (syrup) peppermint (syrup) sodium, 0.06 mEq/ml
Dio Medicone (Medicone)	tablet			docusate sodium, 50 mg		
Dio-Sul (North American)	capsule			docusate sodium, 100 mg		
Diothron (North American)	capsule	casanthranol, 30 mg		docusate sodium, 100 mg		
Disanthrol (Lannett)	capsule	casanthranol, 30 mg		docusate sodium, 100 mg		
Disolan (Lannett)	capsule	phenolphthalein, 65 mg		docusate sodium, 100 mg		
Disolan Forte (Lannett)	capsule	casanthranol, 30 mg	carboxymethyl cellulose sodium, 400 mg	docusate sodium, 100 mg		
Disonate (Lannett)	capsule liquid syrup			docusate sodium, 60, 100, and 240 mg/capsule, 10 mg/ml (liquid), 4 mg/ml (syrup)		

Laxative Product Table, continued

Product (Manufacturer)	Dosage Form	Stimulant	Bulk	Emollient/ Lubricant	Other Laxatives	Other Ingredients
Disoplex (Lannett)	capsule		carboxymethyl cellulose sodium, 400 mg	docusate sodium, 100 mg		
Doctate (Glaxo)	capsule			docusate sodium, 100 and 300 mg		
Doctate-P (Glaxo)	capsule	danthron, 40 mg		docusate sodium, 60 mg		
Dorbane (Riker)	tablet	danthron, 75 mg				
Dorbantyl (Riker)	capsule	danthron, 25 mg		docusate sodium, 50 mg		
Dorbantyl Forte (Riker)	capsule	danthron, 50 mg		docusate sodium, 100 mg		
Doxan (Hoechst-Roussel)	tablet	danthron, 50 mg		docusate sodium, 60 mg		sodium, 0.15 mEq
Doxidan (Hoechst-Roussel)	capsule	danthron, 50 mg		docusate calcium, 60 mg		
Doxinate (Hoechst-Roussel)	capsule 5% solution			docusate sodium, 60 and 240 mg (capsule) 50 mg/ ml (sol.)		sodium, 0.13 mEq/60 mg 0.53 mEq/ 240 mg 1.1 mEq/dose (sol.)
Dr. Caldwell's Senna Laxative (Glenbrook)	liquid	senna, 77 mg/ml				alcohol, 4.5% peppermint oil, 0.19 mg/ml sodium free
Dual Formula Feen-A-Mint (Plough)	tablet	yellow phenolphthalein, 64.8 mg		docusate sodium, 100 mg		sodium, 0.34 mEq
Dulcolax (Boehringer-Ingelheim)	tablet suppository	bisacodyl, 5 mg/tablet, 10 mg/suppository				sodium free
Effersyllium (Stuart)	powder		psyllium hydrocolloid, 3 g/tsp			
Emulsoil (Paddock)	instant-mix liquid				castor oil, 30 and 60 ml	sodium free
Espotabs (Combe)	tablet	yellow phenolphthalein, 97.2 mg				
Evac-Q-Kit (Warren-Teed)	liquid tablet suppository	phenolphthalein, 130 mg (Evac Q-Tabs)			magnesium citrate (Evac-Q-Mag), 300 ml carbon dioxide releasing suppository (Evac-Q-Sert)	sodium, 0.84 mEq/dose (liq.) trace (tablet) 7.63 mEq/ suppos.

Laxative Product Table, continued

Product (Manufacturer)	Dosage Form	Stimulant	Bulk	Emollient/ Lubricant	Other Laxatives	Other Ingredients
Evac-Q-Kwik (Warren-Teed)	liquid tablet suppository	phenolphthalein, 130 mg (Evac-Q-Tabs)			magnesium citrate (Evac-Q-Mag), 300 ml bisacodyl (suppository), 10 mg	sodium, 0.84 mEq/dose (liq.), trace (tablet), trace (suppos.)
Evac-U-Gen (Walker Corp.)	tablet	yellow phenolphthalein, 97.2 mg				sodium, 0.004 mEq
Ex-Lax (Ex-Lax)	chocolate tablet unflavored pill	yellow phenolphthalein, 90 mg				sodium, 0.023 mEq/ tablet 0.001 mEq/ pill
Feen-A-Mint (Plough)	chewing gum mint	yellow phenolphthalein, 97.2 mg				
Fleet Bagenema (Fleet)	enema				liquid castile soap, 19.7 ml	
Fleet Bagenema #1105 (Fleet)	enema	bisacodyl, 10 mg				
Fleet Bisacodyl Enema (Fleet)	enema	bisacodyl, 10 mg				
Fleet Enema (Fleet)	enema				sodium biphosphate, 0.16 g/ml sodium phosphate, 0.06 g/ml	sodium, 193 mEq/ 120 ml
Fleet Enema Oil Retention (Fleet)	enema			mineral oil, 118 ml		
Fleet Pediatric Enema (Fleet)	enema				sodium biphosphate, 0.16 g/ml sodium phosphate, 0.06 g/ml	sodium, 96 mEq/ 60 ml
Fletcher's Castoria (Glenbrook)	liquid	senna, 135 mg/ml				alcohol, 3.5% sodium, 0.03 mEq/ml
Garfields Tea (Alvin Last)	cut and sifted botanical	senna				mixed botanicals
Gentlax B (Blair)	tablet granules	senna concentrate, 108.7 mg/tablet, 326.1 mg/tsp (granules)	guar gum, 333 mg/ tablet, 1 g/tsp (granules)			
Gentlax S (Blair)	tablet	senna concentrate, 187 mg		docusate sodium, 50 mg		

Laxative Product Table, continued

Product (Manufacturer)	Dosage Form	Stimulant	Bulk	Emollient/ Lubricant	Other Laxatives	Other Ingredients
Glysennid (Dorsey)	tablet	sennosides A and B (as calcium salt), 12 mg				sodium, 0.04 mEq
Haley's M-O (Winthrop)	emulsion			mineral oil, 25%	magnesium hydroxide, 6%	
Hydrocil Instant (Rowell)	powder		psyllium, 95%			sodium, <0.43 mEq/dose
Hydrolose (Upjohn)	syrup		methyl-cellulose, 0.019 g/ml			
Innerclean Herbal Laxative (Alvin Last)	cut and sifted botanical	senna leaves buckthorn bark	psyllium seed, husks			buchu leaves anise seed fennel seed
Innerclean Herbal Laxative (Alvin Last)	tablet	senna leaves buckthorn bark	psyllium seed, bark			buchu leaves anise seed fennel seed
Kasof (Stuart)	capsules			docusate potassium, 240 mg		sodium free
Kellogg's Tasteless Castor Oil (Beecham Products)	liquid				castor oil, 100%	sodium free
Kondremul (Fisons)	micro-emulsion		chondrus	heavy mineral oil, 55%		sodium, 0.09 mEq/15 ml
Kondremul with Cascara (Fisons)	micro-emulsion	cascara	chondrus	heavy mineral oil, 55%		sodium, 0.07 mEq/15 ml
Kondremul with Phenolphthalein (Fisons)	micro-emulsion	phenolphthalein	chondrus	heavy mineral oil, 55%		sodium, 0.10 mEq/15 ml
Konsyl (Burton Parsons)	powder		psyllium mucilloid, 100%			
L. A. Formula (Burton Parsons)	powder		psyllium mucilloid, 50%			dextrose, 50%
Lane's Pills (Alvin Last)	tablet	casanthranol, 45 mg				
Maltsupex (Wallace)	tablet		malt soup extract, 750 mg			
Metamucil (Searle)	powder		psyllium mucilloid, 50%			dextrose, 50% sodium, 0.06 mEq/dose
Metamucil Instant Mix (Searle)	powder in single-dose packets		psyllium mucilloid, 3.6 g/packet			sodium, 0.3 mEq/dose sucrose citric acid potassium bicarbonate

Laxative Product Table, continued

Product (Manufacturer)	Dosage Form	Stimulant	Bulk	Emollient/ Lubricant	Other Laxatives	Other Ingredients
Metamucil Orange Flavor (Searle)	powder		psyllium mucilloid, 32%			sucrose, 68% sodium, 0.06 mEq/dose
Metamucil Orange Flavor Instant Mix (Searle)	powder		psyllium mucilloid, 3.6 g/packet			sucrose citric acid potassium bicarbonate sodium, 0.24 mEq/dose
Milkinol (Kremers-Urban)	liquid			mineral oil, 0.95 ml/ml		emulsifiers
Milk of Magnesia USP (Philips Roxane)	suspension				magnesium hydroxide, 0.078 g/ml	sodium, 0.03 mEq/15 ml
Milk of Magnesia–Cascara Suspension (Philips Roxane)	suspension	cascara sagrada (equiv. to 5 ml USP fluidextract)			magnesium hydroxide, 0.078 g/ml	yellow 6 sodium, 0.12 mEq/ 15 ml
Mitrolan (A.H. Robins)	chewable tablet		calcium polycarbophil			
Modane (Warren-Teed)	tablet liquid	danthron, 75 mg/tablet 7.5 mg/ml				
Modane Mild (Warren-Teed)	tablet	danthron, 37.5 mg				
Modane Soft (Warren-Teed)	capsule			docusate sodium, 120 mg		sodium, 0.27 mEq/dose
Mucilose (Winthrop)	flakes granules		psyllium, 100% (flakes) 50% (granules)			dextrose, 50% (granules)
Nature's Remedy (Norcliff Thayer)	tablet	aloe, 100 mg cascara sagrada, 150 mg				
Neo-Cultol (Fisons)	suspension			refined mineral oil jelly		sodium, 0.03 mEq/ 15 ml chocolate flavor
Neoloid (Lederle)	emulsion				castor oil, 36.4% (w/w)	
Nuggets (Tayco)	granules		psyllium			
Nujol (Plough)	liquid			mineral oil		sodium free
Nytilax (Leeming)	tablet	sennosides A and B, 12 mg				
Occy-Chrystine Laxative (Alvin Last)	liquid				magnesium sulfate	sodium thiosulfate

Laxative Product Table, continued

Product (Manufacturer)	Dosage Form	Stimulant	Bulk	Emollient/ Lubricant	Other Laxatives	Other Ingredients
Peri-Colace (Mead Johnson)	capsule syrup	casanthranol, 30 mg/capsule, 2 mg/ml		docusate sodium, 100 mg/capsule, 4 mg/ml		sodium, 0.22 mEq/ capsule, 0.23 mEq/5 ml, 0.69 mEq/ 15 ml
Petrogalar (Wyeth)	emulsion			mineral oil, 65%		agar, 4% acacia glycerin sodium alginate, 0.006%
Petrogalar with Phenolphthalein	emulsion	phenolphthalein, 0.3%		mineral oil, 65%		acacia agar, 4% glycerin sodium alginate, 0.006% sodium, 0.33 mEq/15 ml
Petro-Syllium No. 1 Plain (Whitehall)	emulsion		psyllium seed, 0.75%	mineral oil, 47.5%		sodium, 0.004 mEq/ dose
Petro-Syllium No. 2 with Phenolphthalein (Whitehall)	emulsion	phenolphthalein, 8.126 mg/ml	psyllium seed, 0.75%	mineral oil, 47.5%		sodium, 0.004 m Eq/ dose
Phenolax (Upjohn)	wafer	phenolphthalein, 64.8 mg				sugar imitation hot cassia and safrol flavors methyl salicylate, 1.7 mg
Phillip's Milk of Magnesia (Glenbrook)	suspension tablet				magnesium hydroxide, 0.76–0.87 g/ml 311 mg/ tablet	peppermint oil, 0.038 mg/ml, 1.166 mg/ tablet sodium, 0.004 mEq/ml (unflavored), 0.007 mEq/ml, (flavored) 0.13 mEq/ tablet
Phospho-Soda (Fleet)	liquid				sodium biphosphate, 0.48 g/ml sodium phosphate, 0.18 g/ml	sodium, 217 mEq/ 45 ml sodium saccharin sodium benzoate glycerin flavors
Pleasant Pellets (Alvin Last)	tablet	stramonium podophyllin jalap resin aloin				

Laxative Product Table, continued

Product (Manufacturer)	Dosage Form	Stimulant	Bulk	Emollient/ Lubricant	Other Laxatives	Other Ingredients
Purge Evacuant (Fleming)	liquid					castor oil, 95%
Regul-Aid (Columbia Medical)	capsule syrup			docusate sodium, 100 mg/capsule, 4 mg/ml		
Regutol (Plough)	tablet			docusate sodium, 100 mg		sodium, 0.34 mEq
Saf-Tip Oil Retention Enema (Parke-Davis)	enema			light mineral oil		
Saf-Tip Phosphate Enema (Parke-Davis)	enema				sodium biphosphate, 0.16 g/ml sodium phosphate, 0.06 g/ml	sodium, 217.5 mEq/ 100 ml
Saraka (Plough)	powder		psyllium hydrophillic mucilloid, 3.4 g/5g			sodium, 0.04 mEq/5ml
Senokap DSS (Purdue Frederick)	capsule	senna concentrate, 163 mg		docusate sodium, 50 mg		sodium, 0.2 mEq
Senokot (Purdue Frederick)	granules tablet suppository syrup	senna concentrate, 326 mg/tsp (granules), 187 mg/tablet, 652 mg/ suppository, 43.6 mg extract/ml (syrup)				alcohol, 7% (syrup) sodium, 0.06 mEq/dose (granules) 0.007 mEq/ dose (tablet)
Senokot-S (Purdue Frederick)	tablet	senna concentrate, 187 mg		docusate sodium, 50 mg		sodium, 0.15 mEq
Senokot with Psyllium (Purdue Frederick)	powder	senna concentrate, 109 mg/g	psyllium, 333 mg/g			
Siblin (Parke-Davis)	granules		psyllium seed husks, 50%			sugar, 48% caramel sodium, 1.11 mEq/ml
Sodium Phosphate and Biphosphate Oral Solution USP (Philips Roxane)	solution				sodium biphosphate, 0.48 g/ml sodium phosphate, 0.18 g/ml	yellow 5 ginger/lemon saccharin, 0.265% sodium, 0.055 mEq/ml
Softenex (Alval Amco)	drops			docusate sodium		vitamin B_6 fructose
Stimulax (Geriatric Pharmaceutical)	capsule	cascara, 30 mg		docusate sodium, 250 mg		

Laxative Product Table, continued

Product (Manufacturer)	Dosage Form	Stimulant	Bulk	Emollient/ Lubricant	Other Laxatives	Other Ingredients
Surfak (Hoechst-Roussel)	capsule			docusate calcium, 50 and 240 mg		sodium free
Swiss Kriss (Modern Products)	powder tablet	senna, 52.5%				herbs flowers sodium free
Syllact (Wallace)	powder		psyllium seed husks, 50%			dextrose, 50%
Syllamalt (Wallace)	powder		malt soup extract, 50% psyllium seed husks, 50%			
Theralax (Beecham Labs)	tablet suppository	bisacodyl, 5 mg/ tablet, 10 mg/suppository				triglyceride base (suppository) sodium free
Tonelax (A.V.P.)	tablet	danthron, 75 mg				calcium pantothenate, 25 mg sodium free
Unilax (B.F. Ascher)	tablet	danthron, 75 mg		docusate sodium, 150 mg		

7

Emetic and Antiemetic Products

Gary M. Oderda and Sheila West

Questions to Ask the Patient

Emetics

Are you requesting the emetic for immediate emergency use or possible future use?

Who is the medicine for?

How old is the patient?

What has been taken?

How long ago did the ingestion occur?

How much was taken?

Has the patient already been given something for the ingestion?

What symptoms is the patient showing now?

Antiemetics

Do you know what has caused the nausea and vomiting?

Who is the medicine for?

How old is the patient? Is the patient pregnant?

How long have nausea and/or vomiting been problems?

Have you noted blood in the vomitus that resembles coffee grounds?

Have you noted other symptoms such as abdominal pain, headache, or diarrhea?

What medicines are currently being taken?

What other medical problems does the patient have?

Severe nausea and the realization that one is about to vomit are two of the more unpleasant symptoms an individual may have. However disagreeable the sensation, vomiting (emesis) is an important body defense mechanism for ridding itself of a variety of toxins and poisons; vomiting also may be an irritating accompaniment to travel or pregnancy.

The nonprescription antiemetics have been used to prevent or control the symptoms of nausea and vomiting primarily due to motion sickness, pregnancy, and mild infectious diseases. Some nonprescription antiemetics are promoted for the relief of such vague symptoms as "upset stomach," "indigestion," and "distention" associated with excessive food indulgence, although their value in treating these complaints is not well documented.

Nonprescription emetic drugs are used to induce vomiting primarily in the treatment of poisoning.

Nausea and vomiting associated with radiation therapy, cancer chemotherapy, and the more serious metabolic and endocrine disorders are not appropriate conditions for self-medication and are not covered in this chapter.

The Vomiting Process

Vomiting is a complex process involving both the CNS and the GI system (Figure 1). The reflex is mediated by a "vomiting center" located in the medulla oblongata. The vomiting center by itself does not carry out the function of vomiting but rather coordinates the activities of other neural structures in its vicinity to produce a patterned response. The vomiting center receives stimuli from peripheral areas, such as the gastric mucosa, in addition to stimuli from areas within the central nervous system itself, in part through the coordination of the chemoreceptor trigger zone (CTZ). Stimulation of the CTZ, which is the afferent pathway to the vomiting center, is responsible for its activation and may be involved in eliciting nausea and vomiting from a variety of causes (1, 2).

Centrally acting emetics work primarily by stimulating the CTZ, while centrally active antiemetics inhibit the CTZ. In addition to stimuli from the CTZ, impulses from the GI tract and the labyrinth apparatus in the ear are received at the vomiting center. Stimuli then are sent to the abdominal musculature, stomach,

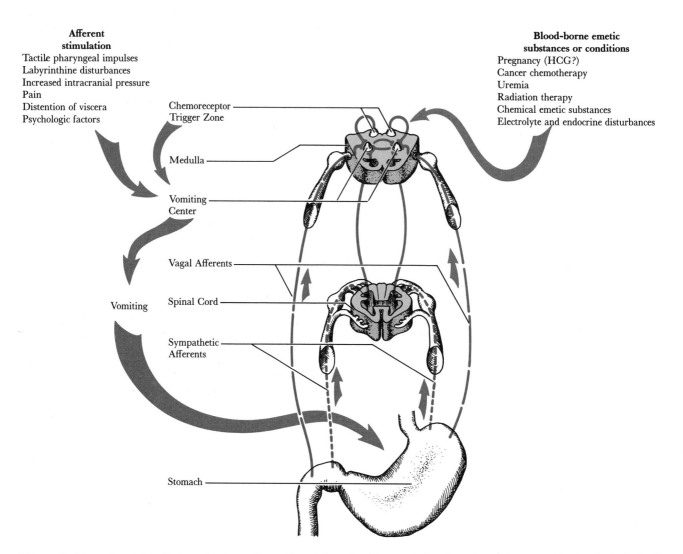

Afferent stimulation
Tactile pharyngeal impulses
Labyrinthine disturbances
Increased intracranial pressure
Pain
Distention of viscera
Psychologic factors

Blood-borne emetic substances or conditions
Pregnancy (HCG?)
Cancer chemotherapy
Uremia
Radiation therapy
Chemical emetic substances
Electrolyte and endocrine disturbances

Chemoreceptor Trigger Zone

Medulla

Vomiting Center

Vagal Afferents

Spinal Cord

Vomiting

Sympathetic Afferents

Stomach

Figure 1. Neural and chemical mechanisms of vomiting. Adapted with permission from A. C. Guyton, "Textbook of Medical Physiology," 5th ed., W. B. Saunders, Philadelphia, Pa., 1976, p. 899, and R. S. H. Wang, "Practical Drug Therapy, J. B. Lippincott, Philadelphia, Pa., 1979, p. 29.

and esophagus to initiate vomiting. (See Chapter 3, *Antacid Products.*)

Vomiting begins with a deep inspiration, closing of the glottis, and depression of the soft palate. A forceful contraction of the diaphragm and abdominal musculature occurs, producing an increase in intrathoracic and intra-abdominal pressure that compresses the stomach and raises esophageal pressure. The body of the stomach and the esophageal musculature relax. The positive intrathoracic and intra-abdominal pressure move stomach contents into the esophagus and mouth. Several cycles of reflux into the esophagus occur before the actual vomiting (3). Regurgitation is the casting up of stomach contents without oral expulsion. Vomitus is expelled from the esophagus by a combination of increased intrathoracic pressure and reverse peristaltic waves (4, 5). Normally, the glottis closes off the trachea and prevents the vomitus from entering the airway. Aspiration of the vomitus may occur in some cases (patients with severe CNS depression).

Vomiting is a symptom produced by benign processes as well as by significant, serious illnesses. The practitioner should be aware of the possibility that patients using nonprescription antiemetics may be self-treating the early stages of a serious illness. Nausea and vomiting may be symptomatic of digitalis toxicity, opiate use, or ingestion of other drugs and chemicals. Knowledge of the patient's drug history is important in assessing the cause of nausea and vomiting. Nausea and vomiting may also be symptoms of diverse disorders such as hypothyroidism, pyelonephritis, renal calculi, or conditions such as acute appendicitis, cholecystitis, migraine headache, food allergy, radiation, cancer chemotherapy, or pregnancy.

Overstimulation of the labyrinth apparatus produces the nausea and vomiting of motion sickness. The three semicircular canals on each side of the head in the inner ear (labyrinth) are responsible for maintaining equilibrium. Postural adjustments are made when the brain receives nervous impulses initiated by the movement of fluid in the semicircular canals. Some individuals are more tolerant than others to the effect of a particular type of motion, but no one is immune. Moreover, it appears that individuals can vary in their susceptibility to various kinds of motions, such as flying and boat riding (6). Motion sickness may be produced by unusual motion patterns in which the head is rotated in two axes simultaneously. Mechanisms other than the stimulation of the semicircular canals also are important. Erroneous interpretation of visual stimuli by stationary subjects watching a film taken from a roller coaster or an airplane doing aerobatics or simply extending the head upward while standing on a rotating platform can produce motion sickness. Regardless of the type of stimulus-producing event being considered, motion sickness is much easier to prevent than to treat once it has occurred.

The mechanism of vomiting, or "morning sickness," of pregnancy has not been established. One-half of all pregnant women experience nausea, and about one-third suffer vomiting (7). Increased levels of chorionic gonadotropin have been implicated as a cause of morning sickness; levels of this hormone are maximal during early pregnancy, when nausea and vomiting are most common (7, 8). Other work suggests that there is no relationship between chorionic gonadotropin levels and morning sickness (9). Nausea and vomiting of pregnancy are difficult symptoms to treat, partly because no agent seems to be completely effective, but more importantly because of the concern that drug use during pregnancy should be restricted whenever possible (8).

Acute transient attacks of vomiting, in association with diarrhea, are very common. Fever may be slight or absent. No precise figure is available for the incidence of this "viral gastroenteritis," although this usually harmless, self-limiting disorder may affect any age group and can occur in sizable outbreaks (7).

Emetics

Incidence of Poisoning

Emetics are used most commonly for the treatment of poisoning, both accidental and intentional. There were 3,300 accidental poisoning deaths from the ingestion of solids and liquids in the United States in 1979, of which 120 occurred in children 4 years old and younger (10). The number of poisoning fatalities is only a small percentage of total exposures. During 1978, poison centers reported 152,433 ingestions to the National Clearinghouse for Poison Control Centers. During 1980, mem-

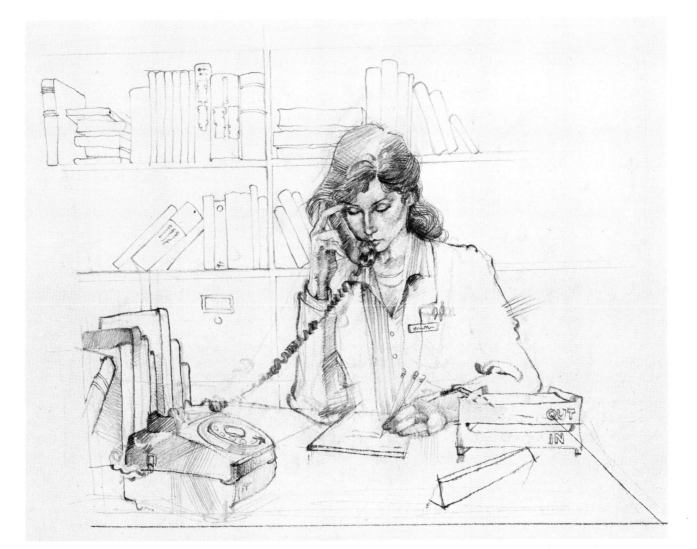

ber centers reported 187,315 exposures to the National Poison Center Network and of these, 67.3% involved children under 5 years of age (11). Approximately 148,580 patients were treated at home and 12.5% of these received syrup of ipecac. Of patients treated in an emergency room, 33.2% were given syrup of ipecac. Reporting to either the National Clearinghouse or the National Poison Center Network is voluntary and some large centers report to neither system. In addition, epidemiologists indicate that only 1 ingestion in 10 is reported to a poison center (12).

Emergency Treatment with a Nonprescription Emetic

Emetics remove potentially toxic agents from the stomach. It is often difficult to decide whether a patient should be referred directly to an emergency treatment facility or should be given nonprescription emetic and managed at home. Obtaining a reliable history, identifying the agent, and accurately assessing the patient's condition are critical in making this decision. Knowledge of the telephone number of the nearest poison center is also extremely important. All ingestions where moderate to severe toxicity is expected must be referred to an emergency treatment facility. If minimal toxicity (no serious or life-threatening symptoms) is anticipated, the administration of a nonprescription emetic at home by a competent adult may be all that is necessary. Many ingestions reported to poison centers fall into this category. For example, a child who ingests approximately 65–130 mg of aspirin/0.45 kg (1 lb) of body weight can usually be managed at home with syrup of ipecac-induced emesis and appropriate follow-up. To determine whether administration of a nonprescription emetic is appropriate or whether the patient should be referred, the following information must be obtained.

Name of Product Ingested

The ingredients and the amount of each ingredient can be determined once the name of the ingested agent is known. Then, the potential toxicity of each ingredient must be investigated. The product label or container, if available, may provide ingredients and the name of the manufacturer (13, 14).

Amount Ingested

This information frequently is unavailable or difficult to determine. For example, a child is found with an empty bottle of aspirin, and no one is quite sure how full the bottle was before ingestion. In addition, a parent often underestimates the amount consumed or provides unreliable information. For example, a parent reports that a child has taken two digoxin tablets. To substantiate the consumption of only two tablets, the parent may respond that the child was alone for a short period or that the tablets had an unpleasant taste.

It should be stressed that drugs can be both therapeutic agents and poisons, depending on the dose. Thus, a 2-year-old who takes two children's aspirin tablets would probably require no treatment; the same child who takes 15 adult aspirin tablets may be severely poisoned.

Time Since Ingestion

The time since ingestion is important because an emetic is useful only if a sufficient amount of the ingested substance remains in the stomach. Thus, an emetic would not be recommended for quickly absorbed agents, if several hours had elapsed after ingestion. The use of an emetic may be rational several hours after ingestion of some agents that are slow to leave the stomach. Drugs that slow gastric emptying and GI motility include anticholinergics, such as atropine and scopolamine, and drugs that have anticholinergic activity, such as antihistamines.

Symptoms

Certain symptoms are contraindications to the use of emetics. Whenever these or other significant symptoms of CNS depression, such as lethargy, ataxia, or hallucinations, or seizures are present, a nonprescription emetic at home should not be considered; the patient should be referred immediately for treatment by a physician or emergency room staff.

Patient's Age and Weight

Much toxicity information is given on a dose per body weight basis (mg/kg). Thus, knowledge of the patient's weight is needed to determine appropriate treatment. The patient's age may help to determine the appropriateness and dose of an emetic.

This information should assist in answering the following questions: Is an emetic indicated? Are there any contraindications to using an emetic? Can the emetic be administered safely outside an emergency treatment facility? Poison centers are available to help pharmacists answer these questions or handle referrals. Pharmacists should be aware of how to contact their nearest poison center. A list of poison centers is currently printed in the *Merck Index*, the *Physician's Desk Reference*, and the *Drug Topics Red Book*.

Treatment of Poisoning

The mainstay of treatment in poisoning cases is the provision of symptomatic and supportive care. Support of vital functions, especially respiratory and cardiovascular, is critical. Treatment of specific symptoms such as seizures also is important. Many patients will detoxify themselves and survive with symptomatic and supportive care alone. Other specific treatments, including emptying the stomach and administering agents such as adsorbents, cathartics, or antidotes, do not replace the need for symptomatic and supportive care.

Stomach contents may be removed by administering an emetic or by lavage. Gastric lavage is a procedure in which a tube is placed into the stomach through the mouth or nose and the esophagus. Fluid then is instilled into the tube, allowed to mix with stomach contents, and removed through suction or aspiration. Either procedure is most effective if accomplished within 4 hours for readily absorbed drugs (15).

The efficacy of ipecac treatment and lavage in removing gastric contents was compared in 20 patients, 12–20 months old, who had ingested salicylates (16). Each patient was lavaged with a small nasogastric tube and also given syrup of ipecac, and the amount of salicylate returned was measured. Approximately one-half of the patients were lavaged first, and the others were given syrup of ipecac first. Ipecac was superior to lavage in removing salicylate. In patients who had vomited with ipecac, little more salicylate was removed by subsequent lavage.

In another study, two adult patients who had ingested aspirin were lavaged first with 3 liters of normal saline through a small (20 French, or 6.7 mm) tube 10–15 minutes after ingestion and then given syrup of ipecac (17). Twenty-five tablets from one patient and 10–15 tablets from the other patient were included in the vomitus following ipecac administration. Lavage alone would have left a toxic dose of aspirin in the stomach.

It also was shown that, under optimal conditions and immediately after ingestion, dogs given sodium salicylate returned 38% of the ingested dose after lavage and 45% after ipecac-induced emesis (18). Of greater significance were the results under delayed conditions wherein the procedure was not instituted for 30 minutes with emesis or 60 minutes with lavage. The lavage was done at approximately the same time emesis occurred. Delayed emesis recovered 39% of the administered dose whereas delayed lavage recovered only 13% of the administered dose. In these studies, the lavage tube was considerably smaller than the 36–50 French (12.0–16.7 mm) orogastric tubes that are recommended for acute poisoning (19). The larger lavage tubes might return significantly more stomach contents than either the smaller tubes or ipecac alone. However, there are no data to support this hypothesis, and at present emesis is preferred over lavage unless induction of emesis is contraindicated.

Contraindications to Emetics

CNS Depression or Seizures An emetic is not likely to produce vomiting in patients who have significant CNS depression as evidenced by lethargy, loss of gag reflex, or unconsciousness. If vomiting is produced, the risk of aspiration of vomitus into the lungs is significant. Thus, emesis and home treatment are inappropriate when CNS depression is present. These patients must be treated in an emergency treatment facility.

Patients who are convulsing or who have ingested convulsants and are seizure prone may aspirate their vomitus if when given an emetic they have a seizure. Additionally, an emetic may produce seizures in susceptible patients or worsen an existing seizure.

Ingestion of Caustics Patients who have ingested a caustic substance should not be made to vomit. Caustic agents are strong acids and bases that can produce severe burns of the mucous membranes of the GI tract including the mouth and esophagus. If emesis is induced, these tissues are re-exposed to the caustic agent, and more damage may occur. In addition, if the esophagus is already damaged, the force of vomiting may cause esophageal or gastric perforation.

When ingestion of a caustic agent is suspected, the patient should immediately be given water or milk to drink (if the patient is conscious and able to drink) to dilute the caustic agents. Attempts to neutralize the caustic agent using an acid or base could generate heat and produce more serious injury and, therefore, must be avoided. Most patients who have ingested a caustic agent should be referred to a medical facility.

Antiemetic Drug Ingestion Emetics should be administered with caution in cases of undesired or excessive antiemetic drug ingestion. If an emetic is not given soon after an antiemetic has been ingested, a significant emetic failure rate may result. Although two studies suggest that this is not a problem clinically, emetics still must be used cautiously in these patients (20, 21). If an emetic is given in the hospital setting and vomiting does not occur, gastric lavage may be necessary to remove the initially ingested antiemetic substance.

Petroleum Distillate Ingestion Patients who have ingested petroleum distillates (such as kerosene, gasoline, and furniture polish) traditionally have not been given emetics. It was thought that induced vomiting increased the likelihood of aspiration of the petroleum distillate into the lungs, leading to alveolar irritation and pneumonitis. When small amounts of petroleum distillates (less than 30 ml or 1 ml/kg) have been ingested, emptying the stomach is unnecessary, and emetics should not be considered. When large amounts of a petroleum distillate capable of producing systemic toxicity have been taken, or when a potentially dangerous chemical, such as a pesticide, is dissolved in a petroleum distillate base, emptying the stomach may be necessary. The likelihood that 1 ml/kg or ounce of an absorbable petroleum distillate will produce systemic toxicity if ingested is unclear. Some of the CNS effects may be secondary to aspiration and not due to a direct effect of the petroleum distillate. Some suggest that it is safe and allow larger amounts (90–120 ml) to remain in the GI tract (22).

A retrospective study showed that of patients who had ingested petroleum distillates a lower percentage developed aspiration pneumonitis when vomiting was induced with ipecac than with either lavage or spontaneous vomiting (23). Other research has shown that aspiration pneumonitis is less likely to occur in ipecac-treated patients than in those who were lavaged (24). The pneumonitis that developed in this study was less severe in the ipecac-treated patients than in those who were lavaged (24). Based on these findings, it was suggested that ipecac be used instead of gastric lavage for alert patients who ingested an excessive quantity of petroleum distillate.

Syrup of Ipecac

Generally, syrup of ipecac is the emetic of choice. Syrup of ipecac is prepared from ipecac powder, a natural product derived from *Cephaelis ipecacuanha* or *acuminata*, and contains approximately 2.1 g of powdered ipecac/30 ml. Vomiting probably is produced by both a local irritant effect on the GI mucosa and a central medullary effect (stimulation of the CTZ) (25). The central effect is probably caused by emetine and cephaeline, two alkaloids present in ipecac.

When a patient asks to purchase syrup of ipecac, the pharmacist should determine whether it is to be used immediately to treat a poison ingestion or is being purchased to keep in the home in the event an ingestion occurs. If the purchase is for immediate use, the pharmacist should determine whether that use is appropriate and if the local poison center or other medical adviser has been contacted. If not, the pharmacist should contact the poison center to alert it of the problem and receive instructions on how to manage the ingestion so that he or she can instruct the purchaser.

If the purchase is for later use, the pharmacist should discuss poison prevention with the patient, distribute poison prevention materials, and provide the patient with the telephone number of the nearest poison center. Additionally, the patient should be advised that whenever possible in poisoning emergencies, syrup of ipecac should not be given without first consulting a pharmacist, physician, or poison center.

Toxicity   Toxicity following syrup of ipecac administration is rare. After therapeutic doses, diarrhea and slight CNS depression are common; mild GI upset may last for several hours following emesis. Clinical experience has shown that ingestion of 30 ml of syrup of ipecac (the largest amount available over the counter in a single unit of purchase) is safe in children over 1 year old. In larger doses, ipecac is cardiotoxic if absorbed and may cause bradycardia, atrial fibrillation, and hypotension (26).

Fluidextract of ipecac is 14 times stronger than syrup of ipecac and should no longer be found in any pharmacy. Severe toxicity and death have occurred when fluidextract of ipecac was given by mistake (27–30).

The death of a 14-month-old child following administration of less than 30 ml of ipecac syrup given to her for an ingestion of amaryllis leaves was not a direct result of the pharmacologic effects of ipecac but rather due to an anatomic defect (31).

Dosages   In children over 1 year of age, the recommended dose of syrup of ipecac is 15 ml (1 tbsp). Because children under 1 year may not have as well-developed a mechanism to prevent aspiration, ipecac should not be administered without medical supervision.

Ipecac does not work well if the stomach is nearly empty. Therefore, it is recommended that at least 3–4 glasses of water be given immediately after the ipecac to distend the stomach partially. Vomiting should occur in 15–20 minutes. If vomiting has not occurred in 20 minutes, another 15 ml of syrup of ipecac should be given. No additional doses should be administered once 30 ml has been given.

The initial dose of syrup of ipecac for adults is 15–30 ml. Generally, no more than a total of 30 ml should be given although some recommend a maximal dose of 60 ml in adults. One study suggests that the time to induce vomiting is longer when milk is given with the ipecac than when other fluids are used (32). Therefore, other fluids, such as water, should be used instead of milk.

The effect of other protein-containing substances that might be in the stomach when ipecac is given is not known. Syrup of ipecac is virtually 100% effective when 15 ml or more is given (33, 34). Whether the fluids are given before or after the ipecac or whether the fluids are tepid (40°C) or cold (10°C) does not affect the time for vomiting to occur (35, 36). Although no scientific evidence exists, patients who are ambulatory seem to vomit more quickly than those who are not. Therefore, children should be encouraged to play quietly rather than recline, and adults should be encouraged to move around. Stimulation of the posterior pharynx by inserting a finger into the throat also may help to initiate vomiting.

If the patient is to be brought to an emergency facility or physician's office, the patient should be made to vomit in a bucket or container so that the vomitus can be inspected for evidence of the poison. It is not necessary or advisable to wait for the patient to vomit before transporting; a bucket should be provided if emesis occurs en route to the hospital.

Drug Interactions   The only well-documented drug interaction with syrup of ipecac involves activated charcoal. Activated charcoal is used as an adsorbent in many poisoning cases. When it is administered with ipecac, the ipecac is adsorbed by the charcoal (37), and emesis is prevented. In addition, the adsorptive capacity of the charcoal is reduced. If both activated charcoal and ipecac are used, the activated charcoal must be given after successful vomiting has been induced by the ipecac.

Activated Charcoal

Activated charcoal is an effective adsorbent for most drugs and chemicals. It is most often administered as a water slurry (60–100 grams) in 250 ml of water in adults. Once the decision to use activated charcoal has been made and the proper dose determined, measuring the amount is difficult. To alleviate this problem, preweighed packages in the appropriate amount should be available in glass or polyethylene containers. The slurry can be prepared by adding water to the container and shaking it (38). Optimally, it should be given as soon as possible after ingestion; however, it has been shown to be effective even when delayed by several hours, especially in the absence of bowel sounds. Although not effective for all ingestions, activated charcoal can reduce absorption of the many common causes of poisonings such as analgesics (salicylates, acetaminophen, and propoxyphene), sedative-hypnotics, and tricyclic antidepressants (see Table 1). There is no systemic toxicity and no maximum dose limit. Contrary to popular belief, burnt toast is not a substitute for activated charcoal and is not indicated in the treatment of poisoning.

Previously, a "universal antidote" mixture of activated charcoal, magnesium oxide, and tannic acid was used. This combination is ineffective since the adsorptive capacity of the charcoal is diminished and may produce significant toxicity due to the tannic acid (39).

Following ingestion of activated charcoal, a saline cathartic such as magnesium sulfate may be adminis-

Table 1. Ability of activated charcoal to adsorb different compounds

Compounds adsorbed by activated charcoal

Acetaminophen	Hexachloro-	Phenol
Aconitine	phene	Phenolphthalein
Alcohol	Imipramine	Phenothiazines
Amphetamines	Iodine	Phosphorus
Antimony	Ipecac	Phenylpropanol-
Antipyrine	Isoniazid	amine
Atropine	Kerosene	Potassium
Arsenic	Malathion	permanganate
Barbiturates	Mefenamic acid	Primaquine
Camphor	Meprobamate	Probenecid
Cantharides	Mercuric	Propantheline
Chlordane	chloride	Propoxyphene
Chloroquine	Methyl salicylate	Quinacrine
Chlorpheniramine	Methylene blue	Quinidine
Cocaine	Morphine	Quinine
Colchicine	Muscarine	Salicylamide
2,4-Dichlorophen-	Narcotics	Salicylates
oxyacetic acid	Nicotine	Selenium
Digitalis	Nortriptyline	Silver
Digitoxin	Opium	Stramonium
Diphenylhydan-	Oxalates	Strychnine
toin	Paracetamol	Sulfonamides
Ergotamine	Parathion	Tricyclic
Ethclorvynol	Penicillin	antidepressants
Glutethimide		

Compounds with little or no adsorption

Alkali	DDT	*N*-Methyl
Boric acid	Ferrous sulfate	carbamate
Cyanide	Mineral acids	

Adapted with permission of the American College of Physicians from J. Grensher, H. C. Mofenson, A. L. Picchioni, and P. Fallon, *J. Am. Coll. Emerg. Phys., 8,* 261–263 (1979).

tered to speed elimination of the charcoal-drug complex and the adsorbed drug.

Other Methods to Induce Emesis

Vomiting may be induced in numerous ways. Syrup of ipecac is the only safe and effective nonprescription emetic. Home remedies other than ipecac are frequently ineffective and, in some cases, dangerous.

Mechanically induced vomiting is produced by giving the patient fluids and then manually stimulating the gag reflex at the back of the throat with either a blunt object or a finger. Care must be taken not to injure the patient during this procedure. The percentage of persons who vomit following this procedure has been shown to be low, and the mean volume of vomitus is small compared with that induced by syrup of ipecac (40). However, if an emergency exists and no appropriate emetic or medical care is available, it may be a worthwhile initial effort to induce vomiting by mechanical stimulation.

Salt water is an unpalatable, unreliable, and potentially dangerous emetic. Salt water may be quite toxic owing to sodium absorption, and in fact, fatalities have been produced in children and adults from the use of salt as an emetic (41–45). If vomiting is not produced, severe hypernatremia may result. It is estimated that one tablespoonful of salt contains about 250 mEq of sodium. If retained and absorbed, this amount would raise the serum sodium level by 25 mEq/liter in a 3-year-old child with an estimated total body water of 10 liters. Salt water should not be used under any circumstances (46).

Mustard water is an unreliable and unpalatable emetic and should not be routinely recommended.

Copper and zinc sulfate have been used as emetics and act by producing direct gastric irritation leading to reflex stimulation of the vomiting center. Copper sulfate is usually given in a dose of 150–250 mg dissolved in 30–60 ml water. In three children who vomited soon after the administration of copper sulfate as an emetic, only 54–67% of the dose was recovered in the vomitus (47). In the same study, all six children who had been given copper sulfate as an emetic had significant increases in serum copper levels (15–105 μg/100 ml). However, no evidence of copper intoxication, such as jaundice or oliguria, was noted. Copper sulfate administered to another patient with a three-fourths gastrectomy caused renal failure and death (48). Based on the available data, copper sulfate is an effective emetic, but concerns about copper absorption and its potential toxicity preclude routine recommendation of this form of induction of emesis (49).

Apomorphine produces rapid emesis; however, it is available only by prescription and must be given parenterally. Apomorphine may produce or worsen already existing CNS and respiratory depression. Naloxone can usually reverse these effects. In several cases, significant respiratory and/or CNS depression unresponsive to naloxone developed in patients who had been given apomorphine (50).

Antiemetics

Nausea and vomiting are symptoms common to many serious and minor disorders. The pharmacist should be very cautious about patient self-medication of these symptoms and should question the patient appropriately to be satisfied that referral is not indicated.

Evaluation

The following are some of the more important considerations to determine whether an antiemetic is indicated.

Age of Patient

Vomiting in newborns results from a number of serious abnormalities, including obstruction of the GI tract and disorders of neuromuscular control, and may quickly lead to acid-base disturbances and dehydration. Physician referral is recommended for further work-up of any vomiting in newborns. Nonprojectile vomiting, where milk appears to spill gently from the mouth, is common in infants. Often the causes are simple, such as overfeeding, feeding too quickly, ineffective burping, laying the infant down after feeding, and the immaturity of the esophageal sphincters. Forceful vomiting may be the result and characteristic of esophageal reflux. Such vomiting may be persistent and lead to failure to gain weight. These can be resolved without drug therapy and should be excluded as causes in any evaluation (51).

One of the more common causes of vomiting in children is acute gastroenteritis. Opinions vary on whether drug therapy should be directed at the symptom, vomiting, or at the primary condition; there are no acceptable data on the effects of nonprescription antiemetics on vomiting with gastroenteritis in children. Some sources question the safety of treating children with antiemetics in an acute, self-limiting disorder (52, 53). It has been suggested that vomiting in gastroenteritis is a body defense that sheds the pathogen and should not be suppressed. This theory awaits confirmation.

Nondrug remedies such as Coca-cola syrup and carbonated beverages have been used to control vomiting, apparently on an empirical basis. Vomiting may be produced by acidosis and dehydration secondary to severe diarrhea, and practitioners have noted that rehydration may control this vomiting (54).

Pregnancy and Menstrual Cycle

Nausea and vomiting may be one of the earliest symptoms of pregnancy. A woman who notes nausea and vomiting in the early part of the day and who has no other symptoms except a missed menstrual cycle and perhaps weight gain should be referred for a pregnancy test and follow-up. Even if the woman is known to be pregnant, it is important to exclude causes of vomiting other than pregnancy, such as urinary tract infections and appendicitis.

Treatment of morning sickness has been characterized as "therapeutic nihilism" since the thalidomide tragedy, and most physicians are reluctant to prescribe any drug for a pregnant woman. Commonly used, nonprescription antiemetics have not been evaluated for, nor are they promoted for, use in nausea and vomiting of pregnancy. Some practitioners have suggested trying small frequent meals to control morning sickness, although the benefits of this approach are not clear (7, 55). Others have suggested treating morning sickness with soda crackers and cola in the morning (56) and that they be given at room temperature after the fizz has been allowed to disperse. Allowing the fizz to disperse would decrease the likelihood of stomach distention and discomfort. One report indicates that the effect of cola drinks in delaying gastric emptying is dependent upon its content of carbohydrates and phosphoric acid. The study demonstrated that Tab, a noncarbohydrate cola drink, had a similar but lesser effect on gastric emptying (57). Nausea and vomiting also occur frequently in women during the third and fourth weeks of the menstrual cycle, possibly because of increased gonadotropin levels.

Due to the publicity surrounding Bendectin, a commonly prescribed antiemetic for the morning sickness of pregnancy, pharmacists are likely to be questioned by their pregnant patients regarding the teratogenic potential of prescription and nonprescription antinauseant medication. Bendectin (doxylamine succinate and pyridoxine hydrochloride) was suspected of being associated with a risk of congenital heart and limb defects in infants born to women who used the drug in early pregnancy (58). However, epidemiologic studies could not demonstrate sufficient evidence of a teratogenic effect which, if it exists, is extremely rare. The FDA has advised, however, that the drug be prescribed only for those patients, "who are unresponsive to conservative measures such as eating soda crackers or drinking hot or cold liquids . . . (or whose symptoms) interfere with normal eating habits or daily activities, and are sufficiently distressing to require drug intervention" (59, 60, 61). Of the nonprescription antiemetics, only the benzhydryl piperazine compounds have been suspected of having teratogenic potential, and these also were reviewed and cleared of suspicion.

Current Drug Use

Some drugs are known to cause nausea and vomiting as a side effect or as a toxic effect. For example, digitalis toxicity may be manifested as nausea and vomiting. One consequence of congestive heart failure is visceral congestion, which also can produce GI symptoms. Other drugs, such as tetracyclines, estrogens, and the opiate analgesics, frequently cause nausea and vomiting as side effects.

Symptoms Requiring Physician Referral

A patient who vomits forcefully several times per day for 2–3 days or who has blood in the vomitus should be referred to a physician for diagnosis.

Patients who complain of abdominal pain, vomiting, particularly projectile vomiting, and headache should be referred to a physician. Patients with vomiting and diarrhea of gastroenteritis in whom even a slight electrolyte imbalance may be critical, such as the newborn or very young child, should also be referred to a physician.

Vomiting has been described as being symptomatic of a form of anorexia nervosa, a psychological disorder in which patients attempt to lose weight by repeated vomiting and chronic use of purgatives and diuretics (62). Patients with such a history should be referred for medical and psychological management of the underlying problem.

Ingredients in Nonprescription Products

The available nonprescription antiemetic preparations have been evaluated and are promoted only for nausea and vomiting of motion sickness (antihistamines and carbohydrates) and nausea associated with overeating or "upset stomach" (bismuth compounds). In addition, bismuth compounds are said to be effective in the nausea and vomiting associated with gastroenteritis. Therefore, the pharmacologic properties of antiemetic agents pertinent only to relieving nausea and vomiting from these causes are discussed (Table 2).

Motion sickness is caused by a visual and vestibular imbalance. When these stimuli are not in accord, mo-

Table 2. FDA categorization of antiemetic single active ingredients

Active ingredient	Antiemetic category
Aminoacetic acid	II
Bismuth subsalicylate	III
Cyclizine hydrochloride	I
Dimenhydrinate	I
Diphenhydramine hydrochloride	III
Meclizine hydrochloride	I
Phenyl salicylate	II
Phosphorated carbohydrate	III
Scopolamine hydrochloride	III
Zinc phenolsulfonate	II

Reprinted from the *Federal Register*, *44*, 41068 (1979)

tion sickness may occur, particularly when the head rotates in two axes simultaneously. Motion sickness can often be prevented by taking an antiemetic 30–60 minutes before traveling (63). The primary agents used to prevent or control motion sickness are the parasympatholytics, antihistamines, and phenothiazines. These compounds have CNS activity; although the precise mechanism in preventing vomiting is unknown, it is assumed to relate to increased thresholds associated with afferent input to the chemoreceptor trigger zone. Most compounds studied have varying success rates in controlling nausea and vomiting, according to length of therapy, duration of pretreatment, duration and type of motion, and individual susceptibility to motion sickness. The ability of an agent to prevent motion sickness is not correlated with its potency as an antihistamine, anticholinergic, or phenothiazine tranquilizer (6, 64). The FDA advisory review panel has stated that the effectiveness of antiemetic agents for the treatment of nausea and vomiting not associated with motion sickness has not been determined and the only indication established at this time is for "prevention and treatment of nausea associated with motion sickness" (63).

Classic studies of the usefulness of antiemetics in motion sickness have identified scopolamine, particularly in conjunction with amphetamine, as being probably the most effective agent in preventing vomiting (65). However, these agents are available only by prescription and have produced significant side effects in therapeutic doses. Cyclizine, meclizine, and dimenhydrinate are nonprescription antiemetics generally recognized as safe and effective. Well-controlled double-blind clinical studies are needed to compare the antiemetic effect of scopolamine at the adult dose of 0.25 mg every 4–6 hours with that of placebo (5, 65).

The nonprescription antihistaminic preparations are all effective antiemetics under various conditions that induce motion sickness. There is little evidence of superiority of one agent over another in all cases.

In young children, motion sickness associated with car travel may be alleviated by placing the child in a car seat (66). The resulting elevation is sufficient to allow vision out the front window. Apparently, the elevation allows the child to focus on relatively still objects and may control the motion sickness (67).

Cyclizine and Meclizine

Cyclizine and meclizine are members of the benzhydryl piperazine group of antihistamine compounds. They are reported to depress labyrinth excitability and are safe and effective in the management of motion sickness (65, 68–70).

Doses of meclizine for adults are 25–50 mg once per day, administered orally 1 hour before departure and repeated every 24 hours. The drug has a relatively long duration of action, and studies have suggested that it provides 24-hour protection against motion sickness (71). Meclizine is not recommended for use in children under 12.

Adult doses of cyclizine are 50 mg up to 4 times/day (65). For children 6–12 years old, the dose is 25 mg up to 3 times/day. Cyclizine is not recommended for use in children under 6. To be effective in preventing motion sickness, the drug should be administered 30 minutes before departure.

Drowsiness with therapeutic doses can occur and is the most common unwanted effect of these agents. Patients should be cautioned not to drive a car or operate hazardous machinery while using meclizine or cyclizine. The effects are additive to those of other CNS depressants such as alcohol and tranquilizers. In large doses, these agents also produce anticholinergic effects, including blurred vision and dry mouth. It is apparent, however, that anticholinergic activity does not correlate with the efficacy of the antihistamine (cyclizine is a weak anticholinergic). The drugs should be used with caution in patients with asthma, narrow-angle glaucoma, obstructive disease of the GI or genitourinary tracts, or prostatic enlargement because of the potential exacerbation of symptoms.

In 1966, the FDA required that products containing meclizine and cyclizine carry a warning against their use by pregnant women. This warning was based on animal studies in several species that suggested that the drug may have teratogenic or embryolethal potential. Subsequent epidemiologic studies of many pregnant women have not shown an increase in embryo deaths or malformations in children of women who used these drugs during early pregnancy (72, 73). The warning against the use of these drugs in pregnant women is no longer required; however, these agents are not promoted for nonprescription use for morning sickness of pregnancy.

Dimenhydrinate

Dimenhydrinate is the 8-chlorotheophyllinate salt of the antihistamine diphenhydramine. Both dimenhydrinate and diphenhydramine hydrochloride are effective antiemetics for motion sickness, although their precise mechanism is unknown (69, 71, 74).

Usual doses for adults are 50–100 mg, 2–4 times/day administered 30–60 minutes before departure (51). The dose for children 2–5 years old is 12.5–25 mg up to 3 times/day.

Since drowsiness can occur at recommended doses, patients should be cautioned about driving a car or operating hazardous machinery (75). Alcohol may potentiate the drowsiness and CNS depression, and thus should be avoided. In doses of 50 mg, dimenhydrinate can cause anticholinergic side effects such as dry mouth (71); patients with narrow-angle glaucoma, prostatic hypertrophy, or asthma should be cautioned about exacerbation of their symptoms.

One individual was reported to have taken between 15 and 25 tablets of dimenhydrinate (50 mg), which caused delirium, visual and auditory hallucinations, pupil dilation, and dry mouth (76). In another case report, 10 50-mg tablets were ingested, which caused cholinergic hypofunction and toxic psychosis (77). Dimenhydrinate has been implicated in one case report of allergy associated with fixed-drug eruptions. The eruption appeared as "dusky red, later brownish plaques with well defined borders and edematous or bullous centers" (78).

Oral and facial dyskinesias were reported after chronic use of antihistamines, and dystonia was reported even with acute use (79, 80). A 4-year-old child manifested dystonic posture and torticollis 2 hours after taking 50 mg of diphenhydramine.

Although not documented clinically, it is possible that diphenhydramine salts mask the vestibular toxicity of aminoglycoside antibiotics (such as streptomycin and kanamycin) (81). A study of the control of vestibular toxic effects of streptomycin with dimenhydrinate suggests that the potential interaction warrants careful patient monitoring if both drugs are used (82).

Phosphorated Carbohydrate

Phosphorated carbohydrate solution is a mixture of levulose (fructose) and dextrose (glucose) with phosphoric acid added to adjust the pH to between 1.5 and 1.6. Studies evaluating its effectiveness in the vomiting of childhood, pregnancy, and motion sickness have been criticized as being poorly designed (83–87). The mechanism of action is suggested to be a delay in gastric emptying time because of the high osmotic pressure of the solution (87). However, there is no evidence that an increase in gastric emptying time affects nausea and vomiting, particularly if it is due to a disturbance in the semicircular canals.

The usual adult dose of the phosphorated carbohydrate is 15–30 ml (1–2 tbsp) at 15-minute intervals until vomiting ceases. Doses should be limited to 5/hour. The solution should not be diluted, and the patient should not consume other liquids for 15 minutes after taking a dose. If vomiting does not cease after five doses, a physician should be contacted.

According to the FDA advisory review panel on laxative, antidiarrheal, emetic, and antiemetic drug products, there is insufficient evidence available to establish the effectiveness of phosphorated carbohydrate as an antinauseant/antiemetic, and appropriate studies should be done to document effectiveness (86). Large doses of levulose may cause abdominal pain and diarrhea. Uric acid levels in the urine and serum were reported to have increased in healthy volunteers when levulose (500 mg/kg) was given orally (88). Practitioners should be aware of the high glucose content and associated problems in diabetics. In addition, the product contains fructose and should not be used by individuals with hereditary fructose intolerance.

Bismuth Compounds

The nonprescription bismuth preparations are promoted for the relief of symptoms of nausea and upper GI distress, particularly those related to the consumption of certain foods or excess quantities of food. The proposed mechanism of action is a coating effect of the bismuth preparation on the gastric mucosa, although this phenomenon has been questioned (86). There is no evidence that bismuth compounds affect gastric emptying time, tone of the stomach wall, or intragastric pressure to relieve symptoms induced by overeating. Unpublished data provided by the manufacturer suggest a consumer preference for this product in treating such self-defined symptoms as "indigestion," "gas," and "full stomach" (89). However, no convincing objective data show that bismuth compounds decrease nausea and vomiting due to overeating. One study of bismuth subsalicylate in dogs and humans found that bismuth subsalicylate given before or in connection with 7.5 ml of syrup of ipecac prevented subsequent vomiting (the effective dose of syrup of ipecac in humans is 15 ml) (90). The bismuth subsalicylate may have bound the ipecac, preventing its absorption and subsequent action. The use of low-dose ipecac to duplicate the conditions of a patient's "upset stomach" is highly questionable.

Bismuth subsalicylate also has been studied in the prevention and relief of abdominal cramps, nausea, vomiting, and diarrhea associated with gastroenteritis. In one study, bismuth subsalicylate, at a dose of 30–60 ml each ½ hour for 8 doses, decreased subjective complaints of nausea and abdominal cramping associated with enteric infections (excluding *Shigella*) acquired in Mexico (91). After 3.5 hours of therapy, 90% of subjects expressed relief of all symptoms compared with 70% of placebo-treated control subjects.

In a second study on the prevention of gastroenteritis in Mexico, bismuth subsalicylate in a dose of 60 ml, 4 times/day, appeared to decrease the incidence of gastroenteritis compared to placebo-treated control subjects (92). Adhering to such a regimen would require a traveler to pack 21 8-oz bottles of bismuth subsalicylate for a 3-week vacation in Mexico. However, once an individual became ill, he or she had the same amount of nausea and vomiting regardless of treatment.

Another study on laboratory-induced viral gastroenteritis found the only significant effect of bismuth subsalicylate in 39 ill volunteers was to decrease the duration of abdominal cramping (median of 2 hours in the treated group compared with 9 hours in the placebo control group) (93). There was no difference between the groups in the number of episodes of vomiting and diarrhea and no difference in the severity of illness. Dosage in this study was 30 ml/30 minutes for a total of 8 doses. Bismuth subsalicylate may decrease subjective complaints of abdominal cramping and nausea associated with certain types of gastroenteritis, although the patient's primary complaint is likely to be diarrhea. (See Chapter 5, *Antidiarrheal and Other Gastrointestinal Products*.)

Bismuth salts appear to be poorly absorbed from the GI tract. Several studies report the absence of detectable bismuth in the urine of human subjects given high doses or treated over a long period. Detectable but unpredictable blood levels of salicylate have been reported after the ingestion of 30–45 ml of bismuth subsalicylate (equivalent to ingesting 357.5–536.3 mg of salicylic acid). Blood levels ranged from barely detectable to 6.2 mg/100 ml (94). Patients who have salicylate allergies, such as asthmatics, should be cautioned about the salicylate content of these products. Nonacetylated salicylates have not been associated with precipitating asthmatic attacks (95).

The manufacturer's maximum recommended dose of bismuth subnitrate provides 5.6 g for adults and 0.475 g for children (3–6 years old) within 4 hours. There is a risk of methemoglobinemia in children under 2 years old due to absorption of nitrate and nitrite from bismuth subnitrate (94, 96). Isolated cases of eruption like those of pityriasis rosea due to bismuth injections have been reported, but no reaction to oral use of bismuth salts has been reported (97). A possible relationship between toxic encephalopathy and ingestion of insoluble bismuth salts has been reported (98). A series of 45 patients treated with bismuth subnitrate (4–20 g/day) for periods ranging from 4 weeks to 30 years developed acute encephalopathies. The toxic phenomenon does not appear to be directly proportional to bismuth consumption and may represent an idiosyncratic reaction. Epidemiologic findings suggest possible transformation of bismuth to a toxic form by certain bacteria in the bowel of affected individuals. Because of the restricted geographical pattern of the reactions that have been reported (primarily in France and Australia), the FDA does not intend to restrict the use of bismuth-containing compounds at this time. However, further study is necessary to determine the effectiveness of bismuth subsalicylate in reducing or controlling nausea and vomiting (99). Pharmacists should note that the patient's tongue, dentures, and/or stools may darken with use of bismuth compounds.

Summary

Emetics are useful in cases of oral poisoning to remove gastric contents and to prevent further absorption of the ingested agent. Syrup of ipecac is the most effective and safest nonprescription emetic for this purpose. It should be kept in all homes with young children and used with the guidance of a Poison Control Center or physician if an ingestion occurs.

Nonprescription antiemetics are useful in limited, patient-diagnosed situations, such as prevention of motion sickness. Antiemetics should always be used with caution because of the potential danger of masking the symptoms of organic disease. The pharmacist should ascertain the reason for purchasing a nonprescription antiemetic and suggest referral if necessary. Chronic unsupervised use of antiemetics, especially for an "upset stomach," should be discouraged, and the patient should be encouraged to seek additional medical help for continuous discomfort.

References

1. H. L. Borison and S. L. Wang, *Pharmacol. Rev.*, *5*, 193–230 (1953).
2. A. J. Cummins, *Am. J. Dig. Dis.*, *3*, 710–721 (1958).
3. T. R. Hendrix, in "Medical Physiology," 14th ed., Vol. 2, V. Mountcastle, Ed., C. V. Mosby, St. Louis, Mo., 1980, p. 1336.
4. "Harrison's Principles of Internal Medicine," 9th ed., G. W. Thorn, R. D. Adams, E. Braunwald, K. J. Isselbacher, and R. G. Petersdorf, Eds., McGraw-Hill, New York, N.Y., 1980, p. 194.
5. J. Kirsner, in "Pathologic Physiology: Mechanisms of Diseases," 5th ed., W. Sodeman and W. Sodeman, Jr., Eds., W. B. Saunders, Philadelphia, Pa., 1974, p. 711.
6. J. Brand and W. Perry, *Pharmacol. Rev.*, *18*, 895 (1966).
7. I. Gordon et al., in "Gastroenterologic Medicine," M. Paulson, Ed., Lea and Febiger, Philadelphia, Pa., 1969, pp. 468, 1233–1234.
8. "Williams Obstetrics," L. Hellman and J. Prichard, Eds., Meridith, New York, N.Y., 1971, pp. 343–344.
9. M. L. Soule et al., *Obstet. Gynecol.*, *55*, 696 (1980).
10. "Accident Facts," National Safety Council, 1980.
11. Statistics quoted by telephone, The National Poison Center Network, 1981.
12. R. Sobel, *Pediat. Clin. N. Amer.*, *17*, 653 (1970).
13. R. H. Dreisbach, "Handbook of Poisoning," 10th ed., Lange, Los Altos, Calif., 1980.
14. R. E. Gosselin, H. C. Hodge, R. P. Smith, and M. N. Gleason, "Clinical Toxicology of Commercial Products," 4th ed., Williams and Wilkins, Baltimore, Md., 1976.
15. R. H. Dreisbach, "Handbook of Poisoning," 10th ed., Lange, Los Altos, Calif., 1980, p. 20.
16. L. Boxer, F. P. Anderson, and D. S. Rowe, *J. Pediatr.*, *74*, 800 (1969).
17. L. Goldstein, *J. Am. Med. Assoc.*, *208*, 2162 (1969).
18. F. Arnold, Jr., J. B. Hodges, Jr., R. A. Barta, Jr., S. Spector, I. Sunshine, and R. Wedgewood, *Pediatrics*, *23*, 286 (1959).
19. B. Rumack, "Poisindex," Micromedex, Denver, Colo., 1981.
20. A. S. Manoguerra and E. P. Krenzelok, *Am. J. Hosp. Pharm.*, *35*, 1360 (1978).
21. M. E. Thoman and H. J. L. Verhulst, *J. Am. Med. Assoc.*, *196*, 433 (1966).
22. R. W. Moriarty, *Drug Ther.*, *9*, 135–139 (1979).
23. S. Molinas, National Clearinghouse for Poison Control Centers, U.S. Public Health Service, Washington, D.C., March-April 1966.
24. R. C. Ng, H. Darwish, and D. A. Stewart, *Can. Med. Assoc. J.*, *111*, 537 (1974).
25. "The Pharmacological Basis of Therapeutics," 6th ed., A. G. Gilman, L. S. Goodman, and A. Gilman, Eds., Macmillan, New York, N.Y., 1980, p. 1609.
26. J. McLeod, *N. Engl. J. Med.*, *268*, 146 (1963).
27. J. D. Speer, W. O. Robertson, and L. R. Schultz, *Lancet*, *1*, 475 (1963).
28. T. Bates and E. Grunwaldt, *Am. J. Dis. Child.*, *103*, 169 (1962).
29. R. Allport, *Am. J. Dis. Child.*, *98*, 786 (1959).
30. R. Smith and D. Smith, *N. Engl. J. Med.*, *265*, 23 (1964).
31. W. O. Robertson, *Vet. Human Toxicol.*, *21*, 87 (1979).
32. R. J. Varipapa and G. M. Oderda, *N. Engl. J. Med.*, *296*, 112 (1977).
33. W. Robertson, *Am. J. Dis. Child.*, *103*, 58 (1972).
34. W. MacLean, *J. Pediatr.*, *82*, 121 (1973).
35. D. B. Bukis, L. Kiwahana, and W. O. Robertson, *Vet. Human Toxicol.*, *20*, 90 (1978).
36. R. W. Spiegel, I. Abdouch, and D. Munn, *Clin. Toxicol.*, *14*, 281 (1979).
37. D. O. Cooney, *J. Pharm. Sci.*, *67*, 426 (1978).
38. J. Grensher, H. C. Mofenson, A. L. Picchioni, and P. Fallon, *J. Am. Coll. Emerg. Phys.*, *8*, 261–263 (1979).
39. "AMA Drug Evaluations," 4th ed., American Medical Association, Chicago, Ill., 1980, pp. 1438–1439.
40. I. A. Dabbous, A. B. Bergman, and W. O. Robertson, *J. Pediatr.*, *66*, 952 (1965).
41. J. Barer, L. L. Hill, R. M. Hill, and W. M. Martinez, *Am. J. Dis. Child.*, *125*, 889 (1973).
42. F. DeGenaro and W. Nyhan, *J. Pediatr.*, *78*, 1048 (1971).

43. D. Ward, *Br. Med. J.*, *2*, 432 (1963).
44. B. Lawrence and B. Hopkins, *Med. J. Aust.*, *1*, 1301 (1969).
45. W. Robertson, *J. Pediatr.*, *78*, 877 (1971).
46. *Federal Register*, *42*, 31803 (1977).
47. N. Holtzman and R. Haslam, *Pediatrics*, *42*, 189 (1976).
48. R. S. Stein, D. Jenkins, and M. E. Korns, *J. Am. Med. Assoc.*, *235*, 801 (1976).
49. W. D. Meester, *Vet. Human Toxicol.*, *22*, 225–234 (1980).
50. J. Schofferman, *J. Am. Coll. Emerg. Phys.*, *5*, 22 (1976).
51. A. Schaffer, *Surg. Clin. N. Am.*, *50*, 853 (1970).
52. O. Anderson, *Pediatrics*, *46*, 319 (1970).
53. M. Casteels-Van Dael *et al.*, *Arch. Dis. Child.*, *45*, 130 (1970).
54. H. Hirschhorn and W. B. Greenough, in "Davidson's Principles and Practices of Medicine," 19th ed., A. M. Harvey, Ed., Appleton-Century-Crofts, New York, N.Y., 1976, p. 1264.
55. *Medical Letter on Drugs and Therapeutics*, *16*, 46 (1974).
56. W. A. Check, *J. Am. Med. Assoc.*, *242*, 2518 (1979).
57. J. B. Houston and G. Levy, *J. Pharm. Sci.*, *64*, 1504–1507 (1975).
58. K. Rothman, *Am. J. Epidemiol.*, *109*, 433 (1979).
59. A. A. Mitchell, L. Rosenberg, S. Shapiro, and D. Slone, *J. Am. Med. Assoc.*, *245*, 2311–2314 (1981).
60. *FDA Drug Bulletin*, March (1981).
61. J. F. Cordero, G. P. Oakley, F. Greenberg, and L. M. James, *J. Am. Med. Assoc.*, *245*, 2307–2310 (1981).
62. P. J. Beumond, G. C. George, and D. E. Smart, *Psychol. Med.*, *6*, 617 (1976).
63. *Federal Register*, *44*, 41068 (1979).
64. H. I. Chinn and P. K. Smith, *Pharmacol. Rev.*, *7*, 53 (1955).
65. C. D. Wood and A. Graybiel, *Clin. Pharmacol. Ther.*, *11*, 621 (1970).
66. E. L. Schor, *N. Engl. J. Med.*, *301*, 1066 (1979).
67. W. M. Jay et al., *N. Engl. J. Med.*, *302*, 1091 (1980).
68. L. B. Gutner et al., *Arch. Otolaryngol.*, *59*, 503 (1954).
69. H. I. Chinn et al., (Army/Navy/Air Force Motion Sickness Team), *J. Am. Med. Assoc.*, *160*, 755 (1956).
70. R. Trumbull, H. I. Chinn, C. H. Maag, L. J. Milch, S. W. Handford, R. Seibert, P. Sterling, and P. K. Smith, *Clin. Pharmacol. Ther.*, *1*, 280 (1960).
71. H. I. Chinn, S. W. Handford, P. K. Smith, T. E. Cone, Jr., R. F. Redmond, J. V. Maloney, and C. M. Smythe, *J. Pharmacol. Ther.*, *108*, 69 (1953).
72. L. Milkovich and G. Vander Berg, *Am. J. Obstet. Gynecol.*, *125*, 244–248 (1976).
73. S. Shapiro et al., *Am. J. Obstet. Gynecol.*, *128*, 480–485 (1977).
74. S. W. Handford, T. E. Cone, Jr., H. I. Chinn, and P. K. Smith, *J. Pharmacol. Exp. Ther.*, *111*, 447 (1954).
75. C. D. Wood, R. E. Kennedy, A. Graybiel, R. Trumbull, and R. J. Wherry, *J. Am. Med. Assoc.*, *198*, 1155 (1966).
76. J. Brown and H. Sigmundson, *Can. Med. Assoc. J.*, *101*, 49 (1969).
77. S. A. Nigro, *J. Am. Med. Assoc.*, *203*, 301 (1968).
78. C. Stritzler and A. W. Kopf, *J. Invest. Dermatol.*, *34*, 319 (1960).
79. R. P. Granacher, *N. Engl. J. Med.*, *296*, 516 (1977).
80. R. Sorner, *N. Engl. J. Med.*, *296*, 633 (1977).
81. P. Hansten, "Drug Interactions," 4th ed., Lea and Febiger, Philadelphia, Pa., 1979, p. 131.
82. L. L. Titche and A. Nady, *Dis. Chest*, *20*, 324 (1951).
83. J. E. Bradley, L. Proutt, E. R. Shipley, and R. H. Oster, *J. Pediatr.*, *38*, 41 (1951).
84. A. B. Crunden, Jr., and W. A. Davis, *Am. J. Obstet. Gynecol.*, *65*, 311 (1953).
85. H. A. Agerty, *Adult Child*, *1*, 66 (1969).
86. *Federal Register*, *44*, 41065 (1979).
87. J. B. Houston and G. Levy, *J. Pharm. Sci.*, *64*, 1504 (1975).
88. J. Perkeentupa and K. Raivis, *Lancet*, *2*, 528 (1967).
89. Norwich Pharmaceutical Company, unpublished data, Communication with FDA Advisory Review OTC Panel on Laxative, Antidiarrheal, Emetic, and Antiemetic Products, 1974.
90. M. M. Goldenberg, L. J. Honkomp, and C. S. Davis, *J. Pharm. Sci.*, *65*, 1398 (1976).
91. H. L. DuPont, P. Sullivan, L. K. Pickering, G. Haynes, and P. B. Ackerman, *Gastroenterology*, *73*, 715 (1977).
92. H. L. DuPont et al., *J. Am. Med. Assoc.*, *243*, 237 (1980).
93. M. C. Steinhoff et al., *Gastroenterology*, *78*, 1495 (1980).
94. R. E. Gosselin, H. C. Hodge, R. P. Smith, and M. N. Goleason, in "Clinical Toxicology of Commercial Products, Acute Poisoning," 4th ed., Williams and Wilkins, Baltimore, Md., 1976, pp. 251, 295.
95. *Federal Register*, *42*, 35418 (1981).
96. "Accumulation of Nitrate," National Academy of Sciences, Washington, D.C., 1972, pp. 46–75.
97. W. L. Dobes and H. S. Alden, *South. Med. J.*, *42*, 572 (1949).
98. V. Supino-Viterbo, C. Sicard, M. Risvegliato, G. Rancurel, and A. Buge, *J. Neurol. Neurosurg. Psych.*, *40*, 748 (1977).
99. *Federal Register*, *44*, 41070 (1979).

Antiemetic Product Table

Product (Manufacturer)	Dosage Form	Active Ingredients	Other Ingredients
Bonine (Pfipharmecs)	chewable tablet	meclizine hydrochloride, 25 mg	
Dramamine (Searle)	tablet liquid	dimenhydrinate, 50 mg/tablet 3 mg/ml	sucrose, 54% (liquid) ethanol, 5% (liquid) cherry pit flavor, 0.2% (liquid)
Emetrol (Rorer)	liquid	invert sugar, 750 mg/ml phosphoric acid, 5 mg/ml	
Especol (Pfeiffer)	liquid	levulose (fructose), 330 mg/ml dextrose, 330 mg/ml phosphoric acid with controlled pH, 1.5–1.6	flavor
Marezine (Burroughs-Wellcome)	tablet	cyclizine hydrochloride, 50 mg	
Trav-Arex (Columbia Medical)	tablet	dimenhydrinate, 50 mg	

8

Ostomy Care Products

Michael L. Kleinberg and Melba C. Connors

Questions to Ask the Patient

What type of ostomy do you have? Where is it located?

How long have you had the ostomy?

Do you irrigate and/or use a bag?

What type of appliance are you using?

What is the stoma size?

Do you have problems with the skin surrounding the stoma?

Have you noticed any change in the contents of your fecal discharge or urinary output?

Are you experiencing any problems related to your ostomy such as diarrhea or gas?

Are you having any problems with odor or gas control?

Are you taking any medications?

An ostomy is the surgical formation of an opening, or outlet, through the abdominal wall for the purpose of eliminating waste. It is usually made by passing the colon, small intestine, or ureters through the abdominal wall. The opening of the ostomy is called the stoma. (The anatomy of the lower digestive tract is shown in Figure 1.) Major functions of the digestive system include digestion/absorption of food stuffs and water absorption. Digestion begins in the mouth and then continues in the stomach and small intestine; water absorption takes place in the large intestine. (See Chapter 3, *Antacid Products,* and Chapter 5, *Antidiarrheal and Other Gastrointestinal Products.*)

An understanding of the digestive process is important because ostomy surgery interrupts this process. The particular problems associated with each type of ostomy are directly related to the phase of digestion that is interrupted.

Ostomy surgery necessitates the use of an appliance designed to collect the waste material normally eliminated through the bowel or bladder. Approximately 90,000 ostomies are created annually in the United States, and more than 1 million patients have established stomas (1).

The idea of cutting into the abdominal cavity and creating an artificial opening is not new. This type of surgery was first suggested in 1710 by a French physician, Alexis Littre (2). Since that time, the technique of ostomy surgery has been refined greatly. The surgical creation of an ostomy is only the first step, however, in the rehabilitation of an ostomate (a person with an ostomy). Complete recovery depends on how well ostomy patients understand and adjust to their changed medical and physical circumstances.

Pharmacists involved in ostomy care must be familiar with the various types of ostomies and with the use and maintenance of the appliances for each type. They should also be prepared to provide patients with information on problems related to ostomy care such as skin care, diet, and drug therapy.

Because each ostomy patient is different, one patient may benefit from one type of appliance, while another may develop problems with it. The ostomy patient should be familiar with applying and fitting an appliance that affords maximum benefit. Proper patient counseling on diet, fluids, and medication is necessary to prevent complications.

Pharmacy involvement in ostomy care is important. The American Pharmaceutical Association identifies ostomy care as a clinical role for the pharmacist in direct patient care. The American Society of Hospital Pharmacists specifies experience in ostomy care in the new accreditation standards for residency training. Procurement and distribution of ostomy supplies and patient counseling are necessary services that can be provided by the pharmacist.

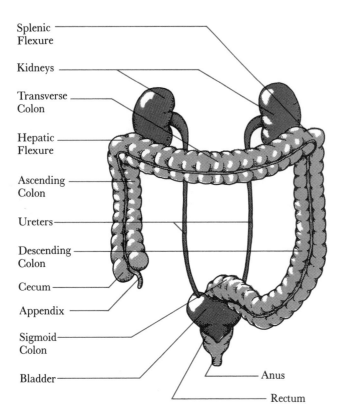

Splenic Flexure

Kidneys

Transverse Colon

Hepatic Flexure

Ascending Colon

Ureters

Descending Colon

Cecum

Appendix

Sigmoid Colon

Bladder

Anus

Rectum

Figure 1. Anatomy of the lower digestive and urinary tracts.

Types of Ostomies

Several types of ostomies are performed regularly. They include: ileostomy in which the entire colon and possibly part of the ileum is removed, colostomy (ascending, transverse, and descending or sigmoid) in which the colon is partially or entirely removed, and urostomy or urinary diversion in which the bladder may be removed. A discussion of each type follows. Special problems affecting patients often depend on the location of the ostomy. Skin irritation and electrolyte and fluid imbalance cause more problems in ostomates with a fluid or semisoft stoma discharge. This is a factor in ileostomies, ascending and transverse colostomies, and for those having a urinary diversion. Urostomates and ileostomates may also experience an increased incidence in kidney and gall bladder stone formation. Constipation may be a problem in patients with descending and sigmoid colostomies.

Ileostomy

An ileostomy is a surgically created opening between the ileum and abdominal wall, usually in cases of ulcerative colitis, Crohn's disease, trauma, familial polyposis, or necrotizing enterocolitis. The two most common disorders requiring ileostomy surgery, ulcerative colitis and granulomatous enterocolitis (Crohn's disease), are both considered inflammatory conditions affecting the intestines. Ulcerative colitis affects the large intestine and rectum. Its clinical course is often prolonged, with the patient experiencing remissions and exacerbations.

Crohn's disease may involve any part of the GI tract. As the disease progresses, the bowel wall thickens, causing the lumen to narrow. Obstruction may result, requiring surgery. Patients with these diseases may develop debilitating extraintestinal manifestations. In an acute episode, toxic megacolon and perforation are possible. These conditions require surgery. The entire colon is surgically removed or bypassed, and the ileum is brought to the surface of the abdomen (Figure 2A).

It should be mentioned that a total proctocolectomy, which results in an ileostomy, is considered a cure for the ulcerative colitis patient. Because of the possibility of recurrence, coupled with the total loss of large bowel function, the same surgical procedure is less often used in Crohn's disease.

The discharge from an ileostomy ranges from liquid to semisoft because it contains fluid that normally would be absorbed from the large bowel. For this reason, it is especially important for ileostomates to pay close attention to adequate fluid intake. Their bodies have lost the capacity to reabsorb water from the large bowel, and they must compensate for this water loss by maintaining an adequate intake.

Excoriation of the skin is a common problem for ileostomates. The continuous flow of liquid, semisoft discharge contains active pancreatic enzymes that irritate and digest unprotected skin. Diligent hygiene and special protective measures can help alleviate these problems. Patients with standard ileostomies are never continent. The flow is continuous, and an appliance must be worn at all times.

Researchers are working continually on ways to render the ileostomy continent. One procedure, developed by Dr. Nils Kock, of Sweden, may be an alternative for those who meet certain criteria (4). The surgeon creates a pouch internally, made from 35 cm of ileum. An intussusception of the bowel is used to create a "nipple" that renders the patient continent for stool and flatus. The distal limb of the ileum is brought to the abdomen. A flush stoma is made just above the hairline. The pouch is emptied by inserting a catheter through the nipple into the pouch. At first, the pouch holds approximately 75 ml. It stretches with use so that 6 months postoperatively it can hold 600–800 ml without discomfort or danger. At this time, the pouch needs to be drained only 3 or 4 times/day.

Since the diseases and conditions predisposing one to requiring ileostomy surgery are found primarily in persons 15–25 years old, the advantages of this operation are obvious. For those in the prime of their athletic, social, and sexual life, the absence of an external pouch allows a speedy adjustment and rehabilitation. Not everyone is a candidate for this surgery, however. Other factors taken into consideration are the patient's age (between 15 and 60 is felt to be ideal), intelligence, absence of Crohn's disease, motivation, other handicaps, and general health.

Colostomy

A colostomy is the creation of an artificial opening using part of the large intestine or colon. Major indications for performing a colostomy include obstruction of the

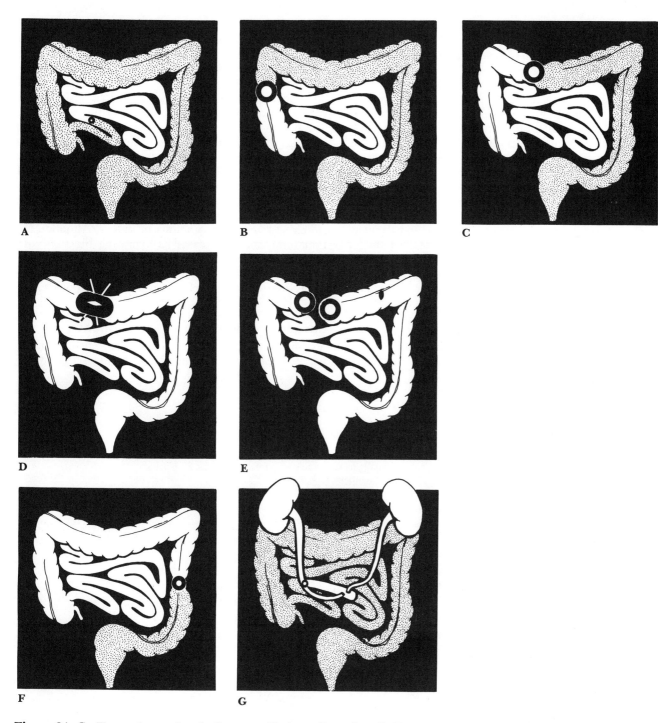

Figure 2A–G. Types of ostomies. **A**, Ileostomy. **B**, Ascending colon. **C**, Transverse colostomy. **D**, Loop ostomy. **E**, Double-barrel colostomy. **F**, Descending or sigmoid colostomy. **G**, Ileal conduit. Adapted from the "Hollister Ostomy Reference Chart," © Copyright 1978, 1979, 1980, Hollister, Incorporated (all rights reserved) and from J. R. Wuest, *J. Am. Pharm. Assoc., NS15*, 626 (1975).

colon or rectum, cancer of the colon or rectum, genetic malformation, diverticular disease, trauma, and loss of anal muscular control. There are three types of colostomies (Figure 3), each named for the portion of the bowel that is brought to the outside of the body to form the stoma: ascending colostomies; transverse colostomies (further subdivided into temporary loop ostomies, double-barrel colostomies, and permanent stoma colostomies); and descending and sigmoid colostomies.

When certain conditions are present in the lower bowel, it may be necessary to perform a temporary colostomy so that the lower bowel can heal. Healing of the bowel for the primary condition may take several weeks, months, or years. Eventually, the colon and rectum are reconnected, and bowel continuity is restored. A permanent colostomy is formed when the rectum is removed. A colostomy, permanent or temporary, may be made in any part of the colon.

The type of colostomy the surgeon will perform depends on the condition being treated. If the disease entity is cancer, the section of bowel may be resected without a colostomy. If the lesion is in the rectum, however, then the entire rectum is removed, resulting in a permanent colostomy. The most common disease that may result in a colostomy is diverticulitis. It presents as small "balloon-like" areas in the lining of the large intestine. Sometimes these areas become irritated and rupture resulting in peritonitis, which usually requires emergency surgery. To protect the perforated section and/or the suture line when this area is surgically removed, a temporary colostomy may be performed. This can be made at any point in the bowel above the lesion. The more proximal the colostomy, the more water and frequent the output will be. When the abscess is resolved and/or the suture line healed, a comparatively minor operation is performed to restore the continuity of the large intestine.

Ascending Colostomy

The ascending colostomy retains the ascending colon but removes or bypasses the rest of the large bowel. This ostomy appears on the right side of the abdomen (Fig-

ure 2B). Its discharge is semiliquid because the fluid has not been reabsorbed. The patient must wear an appliance continually.

Transverse Colostomy

This opening usually is created on the right side of the transverse colon (Figure 2C) in one of two ways. The first method entails lifting a loop of the transverse colon through the abdominal incision. A rod or bridge then is placed under the loop to give additional support (Figure 2D) and removed after a few days. The second method is to divide the bowel completely and have two openings (double-barrel colostomy) (Figure 2E). In this case, the proximal stoma discharges fecal material, and the distal stoma secretes small amounts of mucus. Although the remaining colon increases its hydrating function with time, the discharge generally stays semisoft. Generally, irrigation does not produce control in those with transverse colostomies; therefore, an appliance is worn continually.

Descending and Sigmoid Colostomies

These ostomies are on the left side of the abdomen (Figure 2F). They can be made as double-barrel or single-

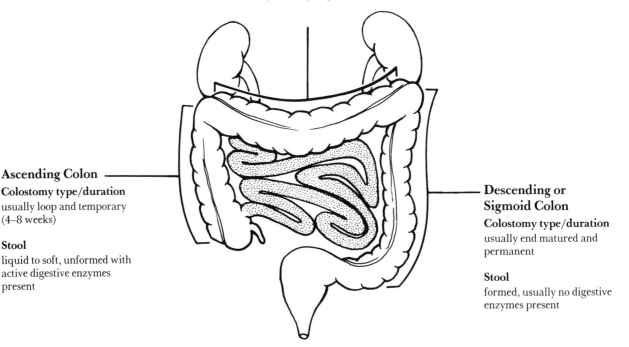

Transverse Colon

Colostomy type/duration
usually loop, or double-barrel and temporary (4–6 weeks)

Stool
soft, unformed, active digestive enzymes may be present

Ascending Colon

Colostomy type/duration
usually loop and temporary (4–8 weeks)

Stool
liquid to soft, unformed with active digestive enzymes present

Descending or Sigmoid Colon

Colostomy type/duration
usually end matured and permanent

Stool
formed, usually no digestive enzymes present

Figure 3. Colostomy care based on location and permanence. Copyright © 1977, American Journal of Nursing Company. Adapted with permission, from *American Journal of Nursing,* March, Vol. 77, No. 3, p. 443.

barrel openings. Because the fecal discharge is firm and often can be regulated by the patient, an appliance may not be needed. However, many patients prefer appliances to irrigation. Several factors that should be considered in connection with the decision to irrigate include (3)

- The capability of the patient to manage the irrigation procedure;
- The prognosis of the patient;
- The presence of stomal stenosis or peristomal hernia;
- The presence of radiation enteritis;
- Fear of the irrigation procedure.

Urinary Diversions

These diversions are performed as a result of bladder loss or dysfunction usually due to cancer, neurogenic bladder, or genetic malformation. An ileal or colon conduit is created by implanting the ureters into an isolated loop of bowel, the distal end of which is brought to the surface of the abdomen (Figure 2G). An appliance is worn continually. A ureterostomy involves detaching the ureters from the bladder and bringing them to the outside of the abdominal wall. This procedure is performed less frequently than the conduits because the ureters tend to stenose (narrow) unless they have been dilated permanently by previous disease.

Appliances and Accessories

The appliance is an extremely important aspect of the ostomate's well-being. The ostomate has lost a normal functioning body process; the appliance takes over that lost function and seemingly becomes a part of the body. The type of appliance depends on the type of surgery performed. Patients with regulated colostomies (irrigates routinely with no output from the stoma between irrigations) may wear closed-end appliances or security pouches. Those with unregulated colostomies and ileostomies usually wear open-end appliances to allow frequent emptying. The ideal appliance should be leakproof, comfortable, easily manipulated, odorproof, inconspicuous, inexpensive, and safe (5). Unfortunately, no one appliance meets all these criteria. Major manufacturers of ostomy products and accessories are listed in the appendix to this chapter.

Disposable Appliances

A disposable appliance consists simply of a plastic bag that can be attached to the skin and is intended for one-time use, after which it is discarded. It is usually transparent, so that a surgeon can examine the stoma without removing the appliance. Disposable (or postoperative) pouches are used in the hospital. If one has a slim flat abdomen and a well-constructed stoma, a temporary pouch can continue to be the appliance of choice after going home.

Reusable Appliances

An appliance consists of two main parts: a pouch that can be emptied and a faceplate that can be attached to the skin. These appliances are available in one piece (with the faceplate attached to the bag) or two pieces (with a removable faceplate). Reusable appliances have the advantages of strength, convexity, better adhesiveness, and lower cost. Disadvantages include the cleaning necessary to make it reusable. The two-piece appliance is more economical, because the pouch can be discarded as soon as it becomes stained or odorous, while the faceplate is retained. The one-piece appliance, however, is easier for some to use, because there are no parts to assemble.

The evolution of ostomy devices has led to the development of pouches that are lighter in weight and more comfortable to wear, easier to apply, more odorproof, and provide for increased wearing time. Some pouches now offer the potential advantage of using soft, nonocclusive adhesive, allowing the skin to breathe. The nonocclusive characteristic eliminates a potential source of skin irritation that can occur with conventional occlusive adhesives that seal the skin.

Reusable pouches may be drainable or nondrainable. The type of output from the stoma is usually a dominant factor in choosing a particular type. Because of the continuous liquid output, an ileostomy requires a drainable pouch, while colostomy pouches, for those controlled through irrigation, are nondrainable. There may be occasions, however, when a patient who usually used a nondrainable pouch will require a drainable device, as during a diarrhea episode. Even though ostomy appliances are categorized by the manufacturer according to the type of surgery performed, it is more useful to consider these appliances in terms of function rather than surgical procedure (6).

Accessories

Foam Pads

The foam pad is not an integral part of an appliance, but it can be very useful. Generally made of closed-pore nonabsorbent foam rubber, it is cemented between the faceplate of the appliance and the skin. The pad should be larger than the faceplate so that it covers the edge of the faceplate when one bends over. This prevents abrasion or ulceration of the skin above or below the faceplate.

Belts

Special belts attached to various appliances give additional support. Belts are made for specific appliances and generally are not interchangeable. Not all ostomates need to wear belts, but ileostomates and urostomates often do. Indications for use are a deeply convex flaceplate, poor wearing time, children, heavy perspiration, or personal preference. If it is worn too tight, "belt ulcers" may result. To be effective, the belt must be kept even with the belt hooks. If the belt slips up around the waist, it may cause poor adherence and possibly may cause a cut of the stoma.

Cement

The cement that holds the appliance to the skin usually is made of latex, a hydrocarbon solvent, and a protective additive such as zinc oxide. It is waterproof. However, the cement can be detrimental to the skin if it is not applied properly. It must be applied very thinly and allowed to dry before the appliance is applied. Many of these products are contact cements, and both surfaces (skin and appliance) must be glued. Sometimes a second coat is indicated for the faceplate, but the first coat should dry thoroughly before the second is applied. Allergy to the cement is rare.

Adhesive Disks

An alternative to cement is the double-faced adhesive disk. These seals are sized, so no cutting is necessary. For many ostomates, this is the preferred method of attaching the appliance to their skin since it is quick and easy. This technique may not be suitable for those with deep convex appliances, children, those with sensitivity to tape, or those who are prone to profuse perspiration. Tape sensitivity often may be handled by switching brands of tape. Another alternative is the use of Relia-Seal, which has a hypoallergenic pectin-based material on the side that touches the skin and an adhesive on the appliance side.

Skin Barriers

Skin barriers are intended to protect the skin immediately adjacent to the stoma and provide a barrier between the skin and the stoma discharge. Except for those with urinary diversions, a skin barrier should always be used with the appliance. Colly-Seel, karaya, Hollihesive, and Stomahesive are frequently used barriers. Colly-Seel contains very little karaya, being composed mainly of mono- and polysaccharides. Its composition is useful when used with liquid output such as urine. It is also used to correct peristomal hyperplasia. Karaya alone should not be used with urostomies because it tends to be broken down by the urine. Karaya rings are composed of karaya gum and glycerol, to make it soft, stretchable, and durable. These rings are available in different sizes so no cutting is necessary. They can fit irregularly shaped stomas, since they can be pulled into any shape desired.

Stomahesive

Stomahesive is composed of gelatin, pectin, carboxymethyl cellulose sodium, and polyisobutylene laminated between polyethylene film and an opaque paper backing. It is a versatile barrier because it has both wet and dry tack; it not only has good adherence to normal skin, but broken, weepy, and oozing skin, as well.

Stomahesive and Hollihesive are useful and effective skin barriers that provide protection against intestinal discharge. Both products may be described as a "blanket" or "wafer," which is worn next to the skin underneath the ostomy device. Each requires cutting a hole in the blanket to fit it snugly around the stoma.

Skin barrier products have been useful to prevent leakage around the stoma, thus reducing skin breakdown and increasing the wearing time of the device.

Skin barrier blankets or wafers are available with a flange incorporated into the outside surface, which allows the pouch to be attached directly to the skin barrier.

In addition to its major use in a wafer form, Stomahesive also is available as a powder and paste.

The wafer is used on a flat area of the skin and acts as a barrier against stoma discharge. The powder is used on weeping skin. Stomahesive powder incites granulation but does not sting on an open wound as do karaya products. It can be mixed with other substances, such as glycerol or water, and increases wearing time. The paste is used to seal around the stoma and to fill in creases in the skin. This will provide a flat surface for application of other skin barriers.

Karaya Gum

Karaya gum powder is made from the resin of the *Sterculia urens* tree found in India. It is used to absorb moisture on open, weepy skin. It also promotes granulation in open wounds, such as decubitus ulcers (7). It is inert and often is found in food products and many denture creams and pastes. It can be mixed with other substances, such as aluminum hydroxide gel or glycerol, for use in difficult bagging and/or excoriated skin situations. Karaya paste is useful for stoma care. A rim can be put around a stoma before the skin barrier is applied, leading to longer wearing time. It also can be used to fill in dips or scars.

Skin Protective Dressings

A waterproof dressing can be applied to the skin in a thin film, which might be described as a chemical bandage. After application, the product leaves a thin protective layer on the skin, that aids in the removal of adhesive tape and absorbs the stress normally applied to the top layers of the skin when the ostomy appliance is removed. Although these dressings promote skin protection, they do not replace skin barriers such as Stomahesive. When the skin is reddened, but unbroken, skin preparations give brief protection from the contact agent causing the redness. They also can help to "waterproof" tape around a draining wound. They come in varying forms: gel, bottle (with brush), spray can, roll on, and wipe-on packets.

Op Site, a versatile new product, comes in many different sizes, from one used for intravenous sites to a complete body wrap. It is a transparent, sterile material that is sticky on one side. It can be used as a dressing, as well as a second skin to which appliances can be affixed. It also can be used prophylactically to prevent skin irritation. It takes some dexterity to apply, however, and two persons may be needed to apply larger pieces. Tegaderm, like Op Site, has many advantages in addition to having easy application without aid.

Solvents

Solvents help to remove an appliance, to remove excess glue from the skin, and to clean the faceplate. Solvents are usually hydrocarbons. They should be used sparingly on the skin and washed off quickly since they can burn. Solvents should not be used on children. Additionally, solvents dry out and defat the skin, eventually leading to a longer wearing time of the appliance. Longer wearing time is important in terms of economy. Also, less frequent changes provide fewer opportunities for skin irritation.

Special Skin Care

Several companies manufacture products especially for the incontinent patient or others at high risk of excoriation. The products consist of a liquid cleaner that is gentle and renders output odorless, a cream that can be rubbed into the skin and to which the appliance will adhere, and an ointment that is not water soluble and gives high-grade protection to vulnerable areas where pouching is not appropriate.

Tape

Hypoallergenic tape provides appliance support. A strip may be applied across the top, bottom, and sides of the faceplate, with half on the faceplate and half on the skin.

Irrigating Sets

A patient having a colostomy distal to the splenic flexure, who gives no history of an irritable bowel, who is not a child nor has a disabling handicap, and who wants to maintain control without a pouch, is a candidate for irrigation. To be safe and effective, a colostomy irrigation set should be used, rather than a standard enema set. This set consists of a reservoir for the irrigating fluid, a tube, graduated clamp, soft catheter, and a dam (or cone) (Figure 4). Perforation of the bowel is a serious complication of irrigation. This hazard has been almost eliminated by the use of the cone-tip irrigator that can be inserted only one-half to one inch into the colostomy. Once in place, the cone provides an effective dam.

Although introducing water into the bowel stimulates peristalsis, control (meaning at least 24 hours without any output) is rarely achieved unless the colostomate instills and holds in a prescribed amount of water. The irrigating set also includes a sleeve that attaches to a faceplate which is held on to the patient by a belt. The distal end of the sleeve is inserted into the toilet. In this way, the returns go into the commode without any waste material to clean up in the bathroom after this procedure. Frequency of irrigation depends somewhat on the colostomate's normal bowel habits. The irrigation is not necessary for health. It is merely one method of management.

The only danger in this procedure is the risk of perforation. The well-lubricated catheter, used with a dam, needs only to be inserted to the point where the eye of the catheter is past the fascia (5–7.5 cm in the average person). As an alternative to the dam and catheter, a cone may be used. After control, patients may wear a piece of gauze over their stoma or wear a security pouch, or Stomacap, a small closed-end appliance that is attached to the body.

Deodorizers

Odor control is either local or systemic. Some agents are placed directly in the appliance to mask the odor of the fecal discharge. Liquid concentrates are available as companion products from most manufacturers of ostomy devices, which can be placed directly into the pouch to neutralize odor. Specially formulated bathroom sprays are also available. Ostomates sometimes place aspirin tablets in the pouch for odor control, but this practice should be discouraged, since aspirin may irritate the stoma. Chlorophyll, charcoal tablets, and bismuth subgallate and subcarbonate are taken orally.

The mechanism of action of bismuth subgallate is unknown but may involve inhibition of bacterial formation. The dose is 200 mg before each meal and at bedtime. (The instructions on the bottle are for diarrhea, not for a deodorant, which should be brought to the attention of the ostomate.) Bismuth subgallate also decreases peristaltic activity and causes the stool to turn a darker color. It also has been reported to cause side effects such as general malaise, lack of energy, and peculiar sensations in the fingers and toes, as well as memory loss. Fortunately, the side effects disappear when the medication is discontinued (8). A physician should be consulted before recommending these preparations.

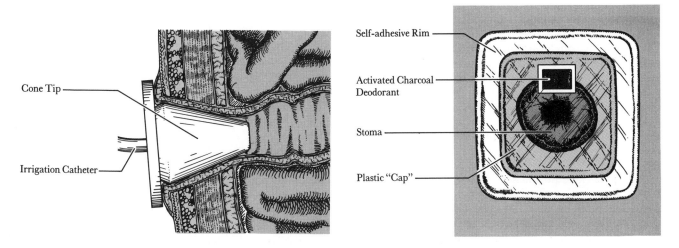

Figure 4. Colostomy irrigation set. A cone-tipped irrigator is preferred to a plain catheter to avoid possibility of false passage and bowel perforation. © Copyright 1978 CIBA-GEIGY Corporation. Adapted with permission from *Clinical Symposia*, illustrated by John A. Craig, M.D. All rights reserved.

In addition to local and systemic methods of odor control, other devices are available that fit directly on the pouch to filter and control gas and odors. One commercial device is a charcoal filter, which is placed on the pouch. Up-to-date pouches are also formulated with an odor-barrier film.

Fitting and Application

Measuring the stoma to determine the proper fit of an appliance is an important part of ostomy care. An appliance with an opening smaller than the stoma may cause abrasion of the stoma and poor wearing time. An appliance with an opening larger than necessary, even with a snug-fitting skin barrier, may allow skin excoriation and hyperplasia formation. Consideration in fitting the appliance includes body contour, stoma location, skin creases and scars, and the type of ostomy. Since faceplates can be obtained in different convexities, materials (flexible or rigid), and shapes (round or oval), one must be knowledgeable and experienced in selecting the appropriate combination for each individual's needs. The lack of uniformity in types of ostomies and ostomy equipment makes it difficult to give standard instructions for application. Some procedures for applying different types of appliances and accessories (Figure 5) are discussed (9, 10). An enterostomal therapist is an excellent resource to aid in the custom fitting of these appliances.

Disposable Adhesive Appliances
- Assemble the equipment.
- Remove the used appliance by gently peeling away the pouch from the skin. If necessary, solvent may be applied with a gauze pad or medicine dropper, one drop at a time, between the body and the bag. This should be followed quickly by nongreasy soap and water to remove the solvent and other residue. Rinse well and dry thoroughly.
- Measure the stoma (only when selecting an appliance, not routinely).
- Cut a hole in the skin barrier just the size of stoma. Cut a hole in the pouch ⅛ inch larger than stoma. (Some disposable pouches have precut, sized holes.)
- If a skin barrier is used, and in most cases it should be, place it snugly around the stoma.
- Peel the paper backing from the adhesive.
- Grasp both sides of the appliance and place the center opening over the stoma. Press gently around the stoma.
- Attach tail closure.
- Apply tape and/or belt, if desired.

Reusable Appliances
- Assemble the equipment.
- If a two-piece appliance is used, attach the pouch to the faceplate by stretching the opening in the pouch over the faceplate. Secure the attaching device around the pouch.
- Old cement should be removed from the faceplate by rubbing with a cotton ball or gauze pad dipped in solvent.

- Remove the used appliance by gently peeling away the pouch from the skin. Solvent may be applied as for a disposable appliance.
- Clean the skin with soap and water. Rinse and dry well.
- Apply one or two thin coats of cement to the clean faceplate, allowing each coat to dry thoroughly. An alternative is to apply a double-faced adhesive disk to the faceplate. If glue is used, apply a thin coat to the skin and allow to dry. For the majority of people who need a skin barrier, it should be applied snugly around the stoma.
- Grasp both sides of the appliance and place the center opening over the stoma. Press gently around the stoma.
- Clamp the bottom of the pouch.
- Apply tape and/or belt, if desired.

Relia-Seal
- Purchase the same size opening as in the faceplate.
- Peel the white paper covering from the pad and apply the Relia-Seal over the stoma.
- Peel the blue paper covering from the pad.
- Place the appliance over the Relia-Seal.

Stomahesive
- If stoma is small, it is not necessary to use entire sheet. Many times ¼ of a sheet is sufficient. This lessens the cost of changing the pouch, since 20 applications can be obtained from one box instead of five.
- Cut a hole in the wafer the same size as stoma.
- Peel the paper backing from the wafer and place this side on skin, fitting snugly around stoma.
- Attach the pouch in the manner described.

Hollihesive
- Measure the stoma with the enclosed cutting guide.
- Remove Hollihesive wafer from the envelope and remove the plastic cover from the wafer.
- Place the cutting guide over the backing paper on the reverse side and trace an outline of the circle onto the backing paper.
- Cut an opening in the wafer (wafer must fit snugly to provide adequate skin protection).
- Peel the remaining protective backing paper from wafer, and with the sticky side toward the skin, place the wafer over the stoma.
- Smooth the wafer against skin starting immediately below the stoma.
- Attach the pouch in the manner described.

Potential Complications

Ostomates may experience both psychologic and physical complications. The pharmacist should be prepared to handle these complications or refer the patient to an enterostomal therapist. A thorough explanation of the type of surgery to be performed, what to expect during the postsurgical recovery period, and an explanation of the appliances and supplies the patient will use often will alleviate the patient's anxiety.

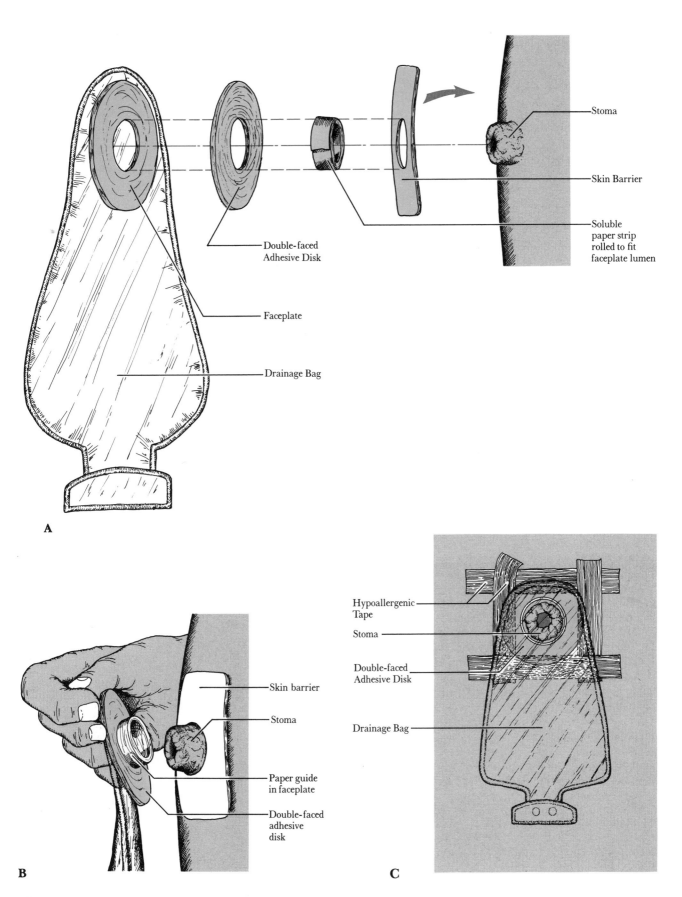

A

Double-faced
Adhesive Disk

Faceplate

Drainage Bag

Stoma

Skin Barrier

Soluble
paper strip
rolled to fit
faceplate lumen

B

Skin barrier

Stoma

Paper guide
in faceplate

Double-faced
adhesive
disk

C

Hypoallergenic
Tape

Stoma

Double-faced
Adhesive Disk

Drainage Bag

Figure 5A–C. Components of an ileostomy appliance. **A,** Drainable bag and skin barrier. **B,** After skin barrier is affixed to skin, the appliance is placed, using paper strip guide to align faceplate lumen over stoma. **C,** Hypoallergic type placed around faceplate in "picture frame" fashion.

Psychological Complications

Following ostomy surgery, depending on prior mental status and self-confidence, the patient may be psychologically depressed. There also may be the fear of not being able to engage in former work, participate in sports, perform sexually, or have children. The pharmacist should reassure the patient that the ability to carry out these activities or functions generally remains unchanged. However, the pharmacist should be aware that most males having a radical resection of the rectum or bladder are rendered organically impotent. Penile implants could enable a male to regain part or all of this function. If this is the patient's concern, a referral to his surgeon would be appropriate.

The United Ostomy Association, formed in 1962, is comprised of various ostomy organizations around the United States whose main purpose is to help ostomy patients by giving moral support and supplying information. The United Ostomy Association (2001 W. Beverly Boulevard, Los Angeles, California 90057) sponsors a yearly meeting and publishes a quarterly journal and other literature.

Enterostomal therapy is a comparatively new nursing specialty, in which registered nurses with postgraduate education from an accredited school for enterostomal therapy specialize in ostomy care. A listing of enterostomal therapists may be obtained from the Executive Secretary, International Association of Enterostomal Therapy, 505 N. Tustin, #219, Santa Ana, California 92704.

Physical Complications

Physical complications of ostomies include stenosis of the stoma, fistula formation, prolapse, retraction, and skin irritation. A continuing series of articles concerning physical problems, their assessment, and care are available (11).

Stenosis

Stenosis, or narrowing of the stoma, is caused by the formation of scar tissue. Excessive scar tissue usually is caused by improper surgical construction, postoperative ischemia, active disease, or alkaline stomatitis and/or dermatitis. Although dilation of the stoma often is advocated to prevent and/or palliate this problem, the only cure is revision of the stoma.

Fistula

The formation of an opening, or fistulous tract from inside the body to the skin, most often is a manifestation of inflammatory bowel disease. Other entities causing this complication are cancer, abscess formation, foreign body retention, radiation, tuberculosis, and trauma. Treatment includes hyperalimentation and/or surgery.

Prolapse

Prolapse, the abnormal extension of the bowel beyond the abdominal wall, frequently results from too large an opening in the abdominal wall. The danger of prolapse is the decrease in blood supply to the bowel outside the abdominal cavity. Treatment is surgical correction.

Retraction

Retraction is the recession of the stoma to a subnormal length caused by several factors, including active Crohn's disease. It also may damage the skin surface. Treatment is surgical correction.

Skin Irritation

Skin irritation can occur from a number of causes. The most common are: excoriation from the output, sensitivity to the product used, monilial infection, epithelial hyperplasia, alkaline dermatitis, infection, and Crohn's disease.

Output Excoriation   Excoriation, an abrasion of the epidermis by digestive enzymes from output, occurs when an improper pouch is worn, the lumen in the faceplate is too big, or the pouch has leaked without prompt replacement. This allows fecal or urinary output to come in contact with the skin. Fecal output may contain active pancreatic enzymes (especially in the case of an ileostomy) that digest the skin protein. The alkaline nature of the fecal output also is irritating to unprotected skin. Alkaline urine similarly is irritating and causes excoriation. These two conditions are treated differently. After diagnosis and treatment, a skin barrier and pouch may be applied. The pouch should be changed as infrequently as possible to lessen irritation, and treatment should be continued until the skin is clear.

Sensitivity   Preoperative patch testing of those who have a history of allergy, adhesive tape reaction, eczema, psoriasis, and those with very fair skin can help prevent skin irritation due to sensitivity to a product. Skin barriers can be used next to the skin instead of an adhesive disk or cement for adhering the appliance onto the skin. Op Site, covering the denuded area and 5 cm beyond, can relieve pain, promote healing, and provide a dry area for pouch application.

Monilial Infection   Yeast manifestation may be a problem in those wearing appliances continuously. An environment that is dark, warm, and moist provides an area for growth of *Candida* species. The primary symptom is itching. If the condition is diagnosed early, an application of nystatin powder is useful. If infection is allowed to continue unchecked, skin will become denuded, the faceplate will not stick, and additional skin irritation will result from the output. These preparations should be used every other day and for 1 week after skin has become clear.

One must determine whether the ostomate is taking antibiotics. Any antibiotic, but especially a broad-spectrum agent, changes the flora of the skin and the entrenched monilia become difficult to eradicate. Treatment for those on antibiotics should be given as outlined but continued for 1 month after the yeast is gone.

Hyperplasia   This overgrowth of hyperplastic skin occurs when the faceplate opening is too large. In the early stages, there is no pain, but later the affected skin cells multiply and cause agonizing pain. The condition resembles a mucosal malignancy. If it is detected early, the treatment is simple. A Colly-Seel is placed over this skin, fitting closely around the stoma. A faceplate that fits just ¹⁄₁₆ inch larger than the stoma is applied, and a snug belt is added. A mild case of hyperplasia generally resolves in 1 week. In severe cases, although treated the same, healing may take from 1 month to 6 weeks.

Alkaline Dermatitis Many patients with urinary diversions have problems with alkaline urine. Although normal urine is not particularly irritating on intact skin, urine that is alkaline may have gross effects on the stoma and skin. It is a major cause of frank blood in the pouch since the stoma is extremely friable.

The treatment is to acidify the urine. This can be done by avoiding alkaline ash foods, especially citrus fruits and juices which, although originally acidic, are excreted in alkaline form. Ascorbic acid or cranberry juice acidifies the urine.

The stoma and skin may be soaked with a 50% solution of white vinegar and water. The saturated cloth is renewed with new solution as often as necessary. This treatment must be repeated every 4 hours while awake. After the vinegar soaks, a heat lamp and hair dryer at the "cool" setting should be directed to the affected area for 20 minutes. The appliance then can be applied. If the manifestation is mild, this procedure can be conducted once every other day until the skin is clear.

Infection Ostomates are not affected more often with infection on the peristomal skin, or anywhere else, than nonostomates. A possible exception to this is those with Crohn's disease. When the infection occurs under the faceplate, however, it can be a problem. If the skin is indurated, swollen, and red, it may need incision and draining. At that time, a culture is taken and sent to the lab for culture and sensitivity. The appropriate antibiotic then can be prescribed topically and/or systemically. It may be a challenge to devise a way that contains the discharge, yet leaves the affected area accessible for treatment.

Excessive Sweating Sweating under the faceplate can cause poor wearing time, as well as monilial infection. Cement may be necessary to hold the appliance on, in addition to use of a belt. Discomfort from perspiration underneath the collection pouch can be alleviated by purchasing or making a cover or bib to keep the pouch material from touching the skin.

Importance of Diet

Diet plays an important role in management of the ostomy patient. Patients need to be counseled in proper diet since certain foods may cause irregularity and should be avoided, and other foods are necessary to maintain adequate nutritional balance.

The diet for an ostomate should be individualized. Some patients are placed on a low-residue diet (a diet low in fruits and vegetables) for the first few weeks following surgery to minimize waste discharge and intestinal obstruction. The low-residue diet includes (13) the following:

- **Meat**—bacon, liver, beef, chicken, and lamb;
- **Fish**—boiled or broiled;
- **Eggs**—boiled, scrambled, and poached;
- **Vegetables**—potato, plain rice;
- **Bread**—toast, white or rye; plain crackers;
- **Cereals**—Farina, Cream of Wheat, puffed rice or wheat, corn flakes, Rice Krispies, strained oatmeal, noodles, spaghetti without sauce;
- **Beverages**—decaffeinated coffee, tea, light cream, milk;
- **Soup**—without vegetables or spices;
- **Desserts**—custards, cornstarch puddings, junkets, gelatins, rice puddings, tapioca, simple cakes and cookies, plain ice cream, and sugar.

After this initial period, the ostomate may be allowed to eat all foods. It might be wise for the patient to try one different type of food at a time, enabling selective avoid-

Table 1. Drug effects on the ostomate

	Colostomate	Ileostomate	Urostomate
Dosage Forms			
Chewable tablets	1	1	1
Enteric-coated tablets	1	3	1
Sustained-release medication	1	3	1
Liquid medication	1	1	1
Gelatin capsules	1	1	1
Compounds			
Alcohol	1	1	1
Antibiotics (poorly absorbed)	1	2, 3	1, 2
Antidiarrheal agents	1, 2	1	1
Calcium-containing antacids	2	2	2
Corticosteroids	1	2	1
Diuretics	1	2	2
Magnesium-containing antacids	2	2	1
Opiates	1, 2	1	1
Salicylates	1	1	1
Salt substitutes	1	2	1
Stool softeners	1	2	1
Sulfa drugs	1	1	2
Vitamins	1	2	1

1, Probably no adverse effects; 2, may cause an increase in adverse effects, patient should be monitored; 3, may be ineffective, patient should be monitored.

ance of foods that produce unfavorable reactions. Problems associated with certain foods include (12)

- **Blockage**—This can be caused by high-fiber foods, seeds, corn, celery, popcorn, nuts, coleslaw, Chinese vegetables, coconut, grapefruit, raisins, dried fruit, or oranges.
- **Loose bowels**—This symptom may be caused by green beans, broccoli, spinach, prune juice, raw fruits, or beer.
- **Gas production**—This may be caused by foods from the cabbage family, onions, beans, cucumbers, radishes, or beer.
- **Odor-producing foods**—These foods include cheese, eggs, fish, beans, onions, vegetables of the cabbage family, some vitamins or medications, or asparagus. (Fecal odor may be reduced by consuming buttermilk or yogurt; urine odor responds to cranberry juice.)

Patients with a urinary ostomy, ileostomy, or ascending colostomy must include an adequate amount of fluid in their diets to prevent the precipitation of crystals or kidney stones in the urine. Absence of the large bowel may not allow normal absorption of water needed to maintain urinary volume. Additionally, to avoid potential intestinal blockage the ileostomate should chew all foods thoroughly. Good dental hygiene and regular dental visits are essential. Fibrous foods (popcorn, corn-on-the-cob, mushrooms, bran products, coconut, Chinese vegetables, raw celery and carrots, and nuts), especially when eaten outside of regular meal times, should be eaten in moderation.

Additional information on colostomy care is also important and it must be stressed that emotional and peer support are imperative for good patient compliance and management.

Use of Drugs

Because part or all of the colon is removed and intestinal transit time may be altered, the ostomate may have difficulty in taking prescription or nonprescription medication (Table 1).

Coated or sustained-release preparations may pass through the intestinal tract without being absorbed, and the patient may receive a subtherapeutic dose. The ostomate should look for any undissolved drug particles in the pouch. Liquid preparations or preparations crushed or chewed before swallowing are best. Patients should be cautioned about drugs that will discolor the urine or feces since ostomates may be more conscious of these discharges.

The ostomate also must be careful in taking antibiotics, diuretics, and laxatives. Antibiotics may alter the normal flora of the intestinal tract, causing diarrhea or

fungal infection of the skin surrounding the stoma. If diarrhea occurs, fluid and electrolyte intake should be increased. Antidiarrheal and antimotility drugs may affect ileal excreta (14). The physician may prescribe nystatin powder to treat fungal overgrowth.

Sulfa drugs should be used with caution. Crystallization in the kidney may be more prominent in patients having difficulty with fluid balance. To minimize this problem fluid intake should be increased and the urine should not be acidified. In patients with ileostomies whose fluid and electrolyte balance is more difficult to maintain, diuretics should be given with care since additional loss of fluid may cause dehydration (15). The ileostomate should be monitored for hyponatremia if salt substitutes are prescribed.

Laxatives may be used in colostomy patients, but only under close supervision. Ostomates tend to become obstructed, and the laxative's particular action may cause perforation. If the colostomate has constipation, a stool softener may be recommended. Antacids may also cause problems and should be taken with caution. Calcium-containing products may cause calcium stones in the urostomate; magnesium products may cause diarrhea in the ileostomate; and aluminum products may cause constipation in the colostomate.

Summary

With proper instructions and equipment, ostomates can lead normal, healthy lives. Pharmacists can help by giving patients the necessary information concerning treatment, ostomy supply service, and appropriate referrals to the enterostomal therapist.

References

1. J. R. Benfield, E. Fowler, and P. V. Barrett, *Arch. Surg.*, *107*, 62 (1973).
2. C. D. Cromar, *Dis. Colon Rectum*, *7*, 256 (1968).
3. R. Watt, *Am. J. Nurs.*, *77*, 442 (1977).
4. Z. Cohen and R. Stone, *Ostomy Manag.*, *2*, 4 (1980).
5. M. Sparberg, "Ileostomy Care," Charles C Thomas, Springfield, Ill., 1971, p. 18.
6. M. Gebhardt, S. Caiola, and F. Eckel, *Drug Intell. Clin. Pharm.*, *6*, 374 (1972).
7. G. Wallace and J. Hayter, *Am. J. Nurs.*, *74*, 1094 (1974).
8. D. Lowe, *Med. J. Aust.*, *2*, 664 (1974).
9. L. Gross, "Ileostomy: A Guide," United Ostomy Association, Inc., Los Angeles, Calif., 1974, p. 28.
10. N. N. Gill, J. Kerr, and R. B. Turnbull, "Instructions for the Care of the Ileostomy Stoma," Cleveland Clinic Foundation, Cleveland, Ohio, p. 3.
11. C. Travers, *J. Enterost. Ther.*, *7*, 8 (1980).
12. "Counseling for the Urostomate," E. R. Squibb and Sons, Princeton, N.J., 1979.
13. *U.S. Pharmacist*, *4*, 48 (1980).
14. P. Kramer, *Dig. Dis.*, *22*, 327 (1977).
15. N. D. Gallagher, D. D. Harrison, and A. P. Skyring, *Gut*, *3*, 219 (1962).

Appendix:
Major Manufacturers

- American Hospital Supply Corp.
1450 Waukegan Road
McGaw Park, Ill. 60085
Op Site.

- Atlantic Surgical Co., Inc.
1834 Landsdowne Avenue
Merrick, Long Island, N.Y. 11566
(516) 868-4545
Full line of appliances and auxiliary products.

- Blanchard Ostomy Products
2216 Chevy Oaks Circle
Glendale, Calif. 91206
(213) 242-6789
Appliances and karaya wafers.

- Byram Surgical, Inc.
2 Armonk Street
Bryan, Conn. 10573
(203) 531-6400
Appliances and supplies.

- Cipa
17 Fields Court
Brockton, Mass. 02401
Temporary pouches.

- Coloplast/Bard, Inc.
73 Central Avenue
Murray Hill, N.J. 07974
(201) 277-8000
Disposable pouches and auxiliary products.

- Richard Daniels
P.O. Box 2181
Dublin, Calif. 94556
Cellu-Rings.

- Davol, Inc.
Box D
Providence, R.I. 02901
(401) 463-7000
Irrigation equipment and Relia-Seal.

- The DePress Co.
130 Central Avenue
Holland, Minn. 49423
(616) 392-3145
Deodorant tablets.

- Diamond Shamrock Medical Products
6235 Packer Drive
P.O. Box 1101
Wausau, Wis. 45501
Full line of appliances and auxiliary supplies (including Crixilene).

- Duke Labs, Inc.
P.O. Box 529
South Norwalk, Conn. 06856
(203) 838-4737
Double-backed adhesive.

- Thomas Fazio Laboratories
P.O. Box 35
Assonet, Mass. 02702
(617) 823-0753
Appliances and supplies.

- Ferndale Labs and Surgical, Inc.
780 West Eight-Mile Road
Ferndale, Mich. 48220
(313) JO4-5780, LI8-0900
Deodorant tablets.

- Graham-Field Surgical Co., Inc.
3256 62nd Street
Woodside, N.Y. 11377
(212) 728-8770
Appliances and supplies.

- Foxy Enterprises
Plaza 16-E Lancaster Avenue
Ardmore, Pa. 19003
(215) 642-6207
Custom-made pouches.

- John F. Greer Co.
5335 College Avenue
P.O. Box 2898
Oakland, Calif. 94618
(415) 652-2213
Appliances and supplies.

- Gricks, Inc.
Hollis, N.Y. 11423
(212) 465-4440
Appliances and supplies.

- Hollister, Inc.
211 East Chicago Avenue
Chicago, Ill. 60611
(312) 642-2001
Disposable pouches and auxiliary products.
Hollihesive, Holliseal, and karaya paste.

- Imex Company
222 West 17th South
Salt Lake City, Utah 84115
(801) 486-1057
Disposable pouches.

- Johnson and Johnson Company
501 George Street
New Brunswick, N.J. 08903
(201) 524-0400
Paper tape.

- Eli Lilly and Co.
740 S. Alabama Street
Indianapolis, Ind. 46206
Oral deodorant (bismuth subcarbonate).

- Marlen Manufacturing and Development Co.
5150 Richmond Road
Bedford, Ohio 44146
(216) 292-7060
Full line of appliances and auxiliary products.

- Mason Laboratories
  P.O. Box 194
  Willow Grove, Pa. 19090
  (215) 659-1815, 659-1819
  Colly-Seel and Colly-Seel appliances.

- Medicon, Inc.
  Holbrook, Mass. 02343
  Karaya washers.

- The Medical Specialty Co., Inc.
  P.O. Box 3663, Dilweg Station
  Green Bay, Wis. 54303
  (414) 494-5082
  Appliances and supplies.

- Moran Medical Supplies
  P.O. Box 24, MIT Branch
  Cambridge, Mass. 02139
  (617) 862-7848
  Karaya washers.

- 3M Medical Products Division
  3M Center
  St. Paul, Minn. 55101
  (612) 733-1110
  Double-backed adhesive, adhesive foam pads,
  and micropore paper tape.
  Tegaderm

- Nu-Hope Labs., Inc.
  2900 Rowene Avenue
  Los Angeles, Calif. 90039
  (213) 666-5249
  Appliances and supplies.

- Osto Care Company
  P.O. Box 2131
  Sepulveda, Calif. 91343
  (213) 782-3100
  Carbo zinc stoma gaskets.

- The Parthenon Co., Inc.
  P.O. Box 11274
  Salt Lake City, Utah 84111
  (801) 355-7630
  Deodorant tablets, Devrom oral deodorant (bismuth
  subgallate), and Lite touch belts.

- The Perma-Type Co., Inc.
  P.O. Box 175
  Farmington, Conn. 06032
  (203) 677-7388
  Appliances and supplies.

- Perry Products
  3803 East Lake Street
  Minneapolis, Minn. 55406
  (612) 722-4783
  Nonadhesive appliances.

- Pettibone Labs., Inc.
  11 E. 44th Street
  New York, N.Y. 10017
  (212) 661-8117
  Ostobon deodorant.

- Requa Manufacturing Co., Inc.
  4510 Bullard Avenue
  Bronx, N.Y. 10470
  (212) FA5-8888
  Charcoal deodorant.

- Robinson Surgical Appliance Co.
  21 East Main Street
  Auburn, Wash. 98002
  (206) TE3-3161
  Appliances.

- H. W. Rutzen and Son
  345 West Irving Park Road
  Chicago, Ill. 60618
  Appliances.

- Rystan Company
  Dept. OR
  470 Mamaroneck Avenue
  White Plains, N.Y. 10605
  (914) 761-0044
  Derifil deodorant.

- E. R. Squibb and Sons, Inc.
  Hospital Division
  Princeton, N.J. 08540
  (609) 921-4000
  Kenalog spray, Mycostatin powder, Stomahesive,
  and disposable appliances.

- Sween Corporation
  Rapidan, Minn. 56079
  Skin care, deodorant, and cleansing supplies.

- Torbot Co.
  1185 Jefferson Boulevard
  Warwick, R.I. 02886
  (401) 739-2241
  Appliances and auxiliary supplies.

- United Surgical Corp.
  11775 Starkey Road
  Largo, Fla. 33540
  (813) 392-1261
  Full line of appliances and auxiliary supplies.

In addition to these products, the following general items are sold: mild detergents, available at grocery stores (Dreft, Lux, Vel, Joy); small (No. 20) and large (No. 4 or 5) binder clips available at stationery stores; G. E. Silicone Seal, available at hardware stores; girdles for men (Carter's "Trimmer," Arrow's "Mandate and Highrise," Jockey's "Vitalizer"); stretch girdles for women by Vassarette, Olga, Warner, Formfit, and Gossard; Tupperware; and "glucose" drinks (e.g., Gatorade, Olympade, Bulldog Punch, Sportade, Quick Kick).

Information taken from the *Ileostomy Guide,* United Ostomy Association, Los Angeles, Calif., 1974.

Ostomy Adhesive Disk Product Table

Product (Manufacturer)	Ingredients
A-D's (Gricks)	not stated
HolliHesive Skin Barrier (Hollister)	gelatin, pectin, carboxymethyl-cellulose sodium, polyisobutylene
HolliSeal Skin Barrier (Hollister)	gelatin, pectin, polyisobutylene
Pre-Cut Adhesive Supports (United)	rubber-based adhesive
Seal-Tite (United)	rubber-based adhesive
Universal Adhesive Gaskets (United)	rubber-based adhesive

Ostomy Cement Product Table

Product (Manufacturer)	Ingredients
Medical Adhesive (Hollister)	silicone base adhesive, hydrocarbon propellant
Mastisol (Ferndale)	gum mastic
Nu-Hope Adhesive (Nu-Hope)	natural rubber, hexane
Skin-Bond (United)	natural rubber, hexane
Skin-Bond (non-flammable) (United)	natural rubber, 1,1,1-trichloroethane
Skin-Hesive (United)	natural rubber, petroleum solvent

Ostomy Solvent Product Table

Product (Manufacturer)	Ingredients
Adhesive Remover (Hollister)	chloro-fluoro solvent, hydrocarbon propellant
Cleaning Solvent (Nu-Hope)	mineral spirits
Detachol (Ferndale)	paraffin hydrocarbons
HolliHesive Skin Barrier Remover (Hollister)	ethyl alcohol, organic solvents
StripEase (Medtech)	1,1,1-trichloroethane
Uni-Solve (United)	naphtha, 1,1,1-trichloroethane
Uni-Solve (nonflammable) (United)	1,1,1-trichloroethane
Universal Remover (Hollister)	organic solvents, silicone oil, ethyl alcohol

Ostomy Deodorizer Product Table

Product (Manufacturer)	Ingredients
Appliance	
Banish II (United)	zinc ricinoleate
Deo-Pel (Gricks)	not stated
Odo-Way (United)	chlorine-producing tablets
Oxychinol (Ferndale)	potassium oxyquinoline sulfate
QAD Tablets (Atlantic)	quaternary ammonium compound
Super Banish (United)	silver nitrate, ethylene thiourea
Uri-Kleen (United)	phosphoric acid
Internal	
Charcocaps (Requa)	activated charcoal, 260 mg
Derifil (Rystan)	chlorophyll, 100 mg

Ostomy Skin Protective Product Table

Product (Manufacturer)	Ingredients
Carbo Zinc (Nu-Hope)	karaya gum powder
Formula A Stretchable Karaya Washers and Sheets (United)	karaya gum powder, propylene glycol
Karaya gum (Various)	karaya gum powder
Nu-Cream (Nu-Hope)	vitamins A, B₆, D₂, E; *dl*-panthenol allantoin
Nu-Gard (Nu-Hope)	isopropyl alcohol, butyl ester of PVM/MA copolymer, dimethyl phthalate
Pro Cute (Ferndale)	stearic acid, cetyl alcohol, forlan-LM, ceraphyl 230, glycerin, triethanolamine, deltyl prime, P.V.P., sorbic acid, cetrimide, silicone, perfume and menthol
Relia-Seal (Davol)	not stated
Skin Gel (Hollister)	glycerin, allantoin, isopropyl alcohol, film formers, plasticizers
Skin-Prep (United)	poly MVE/MA *n*-butyl monoester
Sterile Wound Care Skin Barrier Blanket (Hollister)	gelatin, pectin, polyisobutylene
Stomahesive (Squibb)	not stated
Tincture of Benzoin (Various)	tincture of benzoin
Uni-Derm (United)	anhydrous lanolin, petrolatum, isopropyl palmitate
Uni-Salve (United)	petrolatum, casein

9 Cold and Allergy Products

Bobby G. Bryant and John F. Cormier

Questions to Ask the Patient

What symptoms do you have? Do you have a runny or stuffy nose, sore throat, cough, fever, earache? Do you have red, itchy eyes, sneezing, postnasal drip, or muscle aches?

How long have these symptoms been present?

Do you or members of your family have a history of allergies?

Do you have any respiratory disease (breathing problems) such as asthma or bronchitis?

Do you have diabetes, glaucoma, heart disease, thyroid problems, or high blood pressure? Are these conditions controlled?

What medicines are you taking? How long have you been taking them?

Which products have you used for your cold and allergy symptoms? Were they effective?

Does your job require you to remain alert to prevent an accident?

Although the common cold and allergic rhinitis are etiologically different, they present similar symptoms and respond to similar management approaches. This chapter provides the pharmacist with the information necessary to identify and distinguish between the common cold and allergic rhinitis, as well as other disorders that may mimic them, and to advise the patient on the proper use of cold and allergy products.

Types of Disorders

The common cold is a mixture of symptoms affecting the upper respiratory tract (Figure 1). It is also called a "cold," acute rhinitis, infectious rhinitis, coryza, or catarrh. The symptoms, which are usually acute and self-limiting, may be caused by one of many viruses. The main anatomical sites of infection may vary, and therefore a cold may present symptoms, individually or in combination, of the nose (rhinitis), throat (pharyngitis), larynx (laryngitis), or bronchi (bronchitis). The intensity of symptoms may vary from hour to hour. A reasonable approach is to treat the patient symptomatically, if necessary, with individual drugs (1).

Allergic rhinitis is the reaction of the nasal mucosa resulting from an antibody-mediated reaction to one or more inhaled antigens. It may be perennial because of the year-round presence of antigenic substances, or it may be seasonal and correspond with the periodic appearance of offending antigens. The most common type of allergic rhinitis is seasonal and is called hay fever or pollenosis.

Upper Respiratory Tract

The nose is a respiratory organ. As a passageway for airflow into and out of the lungs, it humidifies and warms inspired air and filters inhaled particles. Several anatomical features facilitate the performance of these functions. The nasal cavity is divided by a central septum and finger-like projections (turbinates) that extend into the cavity, increasing the nasal surface area (Figure 2).

The nasal passageway surface is coated with a continuous thin layer of mucus, a moderately viscous, mucoproteinaceous liquid secreted continuously by the mucous glands. Under normal conditions, foreign bodies such as dust, bacteria, powder, and oil droplets are trapped in the film and carried out of the nose into the nasopharynx. The turbinates facilitate this action by causing many eddies in the flowing air, forcing it to rebound in different directions before finally completing its passage through the nose. This rapid change in airflow enables air-suspended particles to precipitate against the nasal surfaces. High vascularity and resultant high-blood flow within the nasal mucosa help warm and humidify the inspired air.

Nerve control of the nasopharyngeal vascular bed is derived from both sympathetic and parasympathetic divisions of the autonomic nervous system. Stimulation of

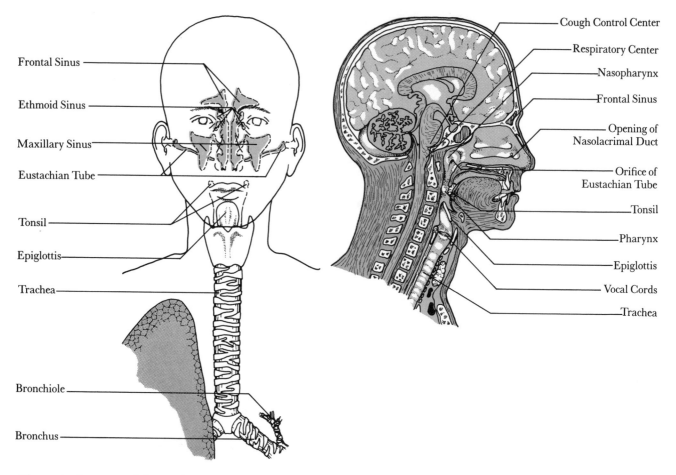

Figure 1. Anatomy of the respiratory passages.

the sympathetic fibers causes decreased activity of the mucous glands and vasoconstriction that reduces the size of the turbinates, widening the airway. Parasympathetic stimulation increases mucus production and narrows the airways by vasodilation and vascular engorgement of the mucosal tissue. Treatment may be directed toward eliciting a sympathetic response or blocking parasympathetic response.

The epithelium of the nasal passageways is ciliated. The constant beating of the cilia causes the mucus film to be moved continually toward the nasopharynx, carrying with it trapped particles to be expectorated or swallowed (2). Because this ciliary movement is one of the body's main defense mechanisms, care should be taken to avoid agents that impair this movement. Oils, especially mineral oil, and the overuse of topically applied decongestants may interfere with normal ciliary movement. Dust, fumes, smoke, and lack of humidity may also impair ciliary movement (3).

The mucous blanket is rich in lysozymes and contains glycoproteins and immunoglobulins (4). Lysozymes are an important defense against bacteria because they readily digest the lipid and carbohydrate cell wall of some bacteria and are responsible for the digestion of the cell wall of pollens and the subsequent release of antigenic substances. Mucous glycoproteins may inhibit some viruses temporarily by combining

with the virus protein coat. The union of inhibitor and virus is reversible; therefore, these inhibitors probably do no more than delay host cell invasion by virus particles. Immunoglobulins of low molecular weight, mainly IgA and IgG, also are contained in the mucus secretion. Although present in low concentrations, they may decrease the infectivity of certain viruses.

Viruses that attach to and invade respiratory tract host cells stimulate the infected cell to produce interferon. Interferon is active against not only the virus that caused its production but also against other unrelated viruses. It protects neighboring, noninfected cells against subsequent viral infection (5). Research is directed toward a better understanding of this substance as well as stimulating its endogenous development.

The cough reflex is an essential body defense mechanism by which the respiratory airways leading to the lungs are kept free of foreign matter. It occurs in health as well as disease and is frequently the symptom in various pathologic states. All areas of the respiratory tract (the trachea, larynx, bronchi, and terminal bronchioles), are sensitive to foreign matter and other causes of irritation such as irritant corrosive gases and infection. A cough may be caused by the stimulation of receptors (mechanoreceptors and chemoreceptors) located in the mucosa of the airways and lungs. Afferent impulses pass along nerve pathways to the cough center in the medulla, which coordinates efferent impulses to the diaphragm and intercostal and abdominal muscles. The cough response follows an automatic sequence of events leading to the rapid expulsion of air from the lungs designed to carry with it foreign bodies that have initiated the reflex. Localized bronchoconstriction also may play an important role in the stimulation of the cough reflex.

The sneeze reflex is very similar to the cough reflex, except that it is intended to clear the nasal passages instead of the lower respiratory tract. Irritation in the nasal passages initiates the sneeze reflex. The afferent impulses from the nose travel to the medulla, where the reflex is triggered. A series of reactions similar to those for the cough reflex takes place. In addition, the uvula is depressed, so that large amounts of air pass rapidly through the nose, as well as through the mouth, helping to clear the nasal passages of foreign matter (2).

The passageways of the trachea and lungs are lined with a ciliated, mucus-coated epithelium that aids in removing foreign matter. As in the nasal passageways, the cilia in the trachea and lungs also beat toward the pharynx, carrying mucus and trapped particles out of the respiratory tract.

The Common Cold

The common cold has been described as the most expensive single illness in the United States. In fact, more time is lost from work and school because of the common cold than because of all other diseases combined. The prevalence of common colds is approximately 15% of population/week during the winter months. Among the industrial employees in the United States, common colds account for one-half of all absences and one-quarter of the total time lost (6).

The American public buys approximately $500–700 million of nonprescription cough, cold, and allergy preparations each year, of which approximately 50% are purchased in pharmacies. Pharmacists should take advantage of these opportunities to interact with and assist the self-medicating patient in proper product selection and administration.

The common cold is spread directly from person to person with no intermediate source such as food, water, or animals. The only means by which spreading may be prevented is by isolating the infected individual. However, by the time a cold has been detected, the virus undoubtedly has already been transmitted to others through respiratory droplets (5).

There is an apparent relationship between the season of the year and the common cold. It is not known what the exact etiologic relationship is, but it is usual to observe three peak seasons of common colds per year. One of these occurs in the autumn, a few weeks after schools open; another occurs in midwinter; and a third occurs in the spring. These separate epidemics are associated with different viruses, each of which may have its own seasonal epidemiology. The U.S. Public Health Service studies show that during the winter quarter of the year, about 50% of the population experience a common cold; during the summer quarter, only about 20% are stricken with a cold (7).

The patient's age is related to the incidence of the common cold and to its complications. Children 1–5 years old are most susceptible, and each child averages 6–12 respiratory illnesses per year, most of which are common colds. Some practitioners feel that infants less than 6 months old are somewhat resistant to cold viruses, but this finding may be attributed to infants' relatively infrequent exposure to different environments. Individuals 25–30 years old average about six respiratory illnesses per year; older adults average two or three. Young children are more prone to complications of the

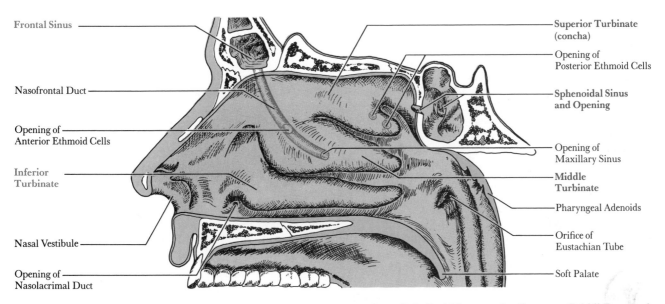

Frontal Sinus

Nasofrontal Duct

Opening of Anterior Ethmoid Cells

Inferior Turbinate

Nasal Vestibule

Opening of Nasolacrimal Duct

Superior Turbinate (concha)

Opening of Posterior Ethmoid Cells

Sphenoidal Sinus and Opening

Opening of Maxillary Sinus

Middle Turbinate

Pharyngeal Adenoids

Orifice of Eustachian Tube

Soft Palate

Figure 2. The nose and paranasal sinus. Reprinted with permission from "Medical Notes on the Common Cold," Burroughs Wellcome Co., Publication No. PI99-2, Research Triangle Park, NC., 1972.

common cold, such as middle ear inflammation (otitis media) and pneumonia, than older cold sufferers. However, many adults also suffer from these complications (4, 7).

Poor nutritional state, fatigue, and emotional disturbances are associated with greater susceptibility to infection as well as increased severity of infection and greater likelihood of complications (7). Body chills or wet feet in themselves do not induce the common cold. However, if the virus is a recent invader, the effects of exposure probably are contributory factors because such exposure is associated with a vasomotor effect that decreases the nasal mucosal temperature by several degrees. As a result of this temperature change, many people experience symptoms of nasal irritation such as sneezing and serous discharge. Changes in the nasal mucosa and a subsequent change in the character of the mucus may then facilitate viral invasion (7).

Allergic disorders involving the nasopharynx, such as hay fever, also seem to play a part in facilitating infection. The probable mechanism is the inflammatory changes occurring in the mucosa as a result of the antigen-antibody reaction, which may facilitate subsequent viral invasion.

Etiology

Viruses cause the common cold. More than 120 different viral strains that produce common cold symptoms in humans have been isolated (7). Known causative agents include the rhinoviruses (approximately 60 different serologic types), adenoviruses, coxsackieviruses, echoviruses, influenza viruses, and parainfluenza viruses. Of these, the rhinoviruses comprise the largest etiologic group, probably accounting for more than one-half of all common colds in adults (7). A significant number, 5–10%, of common colds are associated with more than one virus, and evidence of simultaneous infection with two viruses is not rare (4, 7).

Viruses differ from bacteria by their existence within the host cell, their chemical composition, their mode of replication, and their responsiveness to drug therapy (5). The process of a viral infection is divided into three states: entry into the host cell and nucleic acid release, genome replication and viral protein synthesis, and assembly of new virus particles and their release from the cell to infect additional host cells (8). There probably are several mechanisms by which the virus penetrates the host cell, but none is well defined. Once inside the host cell, the virus is attacked by host cell enzymes and possibly other substances, releasing the viral nucleic acid. In the second state of infection, the virus uses metabolic pathways of the host cell itself to duplicate the viral genome and synthesize viral proteins. Finally, these components are assembled into new, mature virus particles and are released by the host cell. The release may be rapid and may be accompanied by lysis and death of the host cell, although cell death may not always result. The new virus particles then infect adjacent cells by the same cycle.

When host cell injury or death occurs, the body's inflammatory defense mechanism is activated, causing pathologic changes and subsequent symptoms. These clinical manifestations of infection are not evident, however, until after extensive viral replication and inflammation have occurred.

Specific immunity against illness from reinfection with the same strain of virus is demonstrable in volunteers, and this clinical immunity is apparent for a period of about 2 years after infection. Reinfection, however, is not entirely prevented and usually results in a modified illness. The specificity of the antibody and its concentration at the infection site appear to be critical in the likelihood and extent of reinfection (4). These characteristics also underscore the difficulty of developing comprehensive vaccines to prevent the common cold.

Pathophysiology and Symptoms

Symptoms associated with the common cold are a manifestation of the pathologic changes (inflammation) that occur in the respiratory epithelium, secondary to viral invasion. The pathologic changes that make up the inflammatory response to one or more viruses are excess blood flow in the area (hyperemia), abnormal fluid accumulation in the intercellular spaces (edema), and profuse watery discharge from the nasal mucous membrane (rhinorrhea) (7).

The severity of the cellular damage (and hence the degree of inflammation and symptoms) is related to the type and virulence of the infecting virus and the extent of the infection. Various strains of influenza virus, for example, do a great deal more damage to the respiratory epithelium than those that cause the common cold. Therefore, "flu" symptoms are usually more severe than cold symptoms, and the predisposition to secondary bacterial complications is greater.

Although colds commonly involve the nasal structure, other sites along the respiratory tract may be affected. This condition is due to the predilection of certain viruses for pharyngeal, laryngeal, or bronchial cells and to the extension of the infectious process from the original invasion site (5).

Because the incubation period for these viral infections is relatively short (1–4 days), patients often report a rapid onset and progression of symptoms. Virus shedding usually begins 1–2 days before the onset of symptoms and is associated with epithelial sloughing and regeneration. A few days later, during the symptomatic phase, peak viral replication and host cell injury occur. With the intervention of body defenses, such as interferon, virus excretion ceases after several days, and symptoms decrease (4).

The clear, watery fluid that initially flows from the irritated nasal epithelium (nasal discharge or rhinorrhea) is the hallmark of the common cold. Although it is initially clear, it is followed shortly by a much thicker and tenacious mucoid and purulent secretion, largely composed of dead epithelial cells and white blood cells. The quantity of epithelial cells shed may be so high at times as to give the appearance of purulence. It is commonly assumed that these mucopurulent secretions are the result of secondary bacterial infection, but this is not always the case. Viruses may cause inflammatory reactions on their own, and the secretions occur even when there has been no change in the nasal bacterial flora.

Nasal congestion (swelling of the nasal turbinates) encroaches on the nasal lumen, which is also burdened with the increased secretions. Nasal discharge and congestion are the most commonly described discomforts associated with the common cold.

The combination of nasal irritation, discharge, and congestion (which cause further irritation) gives rise to sneezing. Sneezing is not as discomforting as the discharge and congestion and subsides when the infection and secretions clear.

Pharyngitis also may occur during a cold (4). This throat symptom is usually described as a "dryness" or "soreness" rather than actual pain such as that associated with bacterial pharyngitis or acute tonsillitis. Pharyngitis is attributed to edema of the pharyngeal mucosa, which activates sensory nerve fibers as the infection spreads to deeper tissue.

Pharyngitis is usually the result of the infectious process, and histamine release is not the target-offending agent. Most commonly, the symptom is soreness or dryness rather than actual pain, as in the more severe cell injury and inflammation of bacterial infections.

Environmental factors also may lead to pharyngitis. Overuse of tobacco products and ingestion of large amounts of concentrated, alcohol-containing beverages, or other irritating substances are factors associated with pharyngeal irritation and sore throat. Rarely, irritant gas inhalation also may be an etiologic factor.

Diseases in which pharyngitis may be a symptom include not only the common cold but also streptococcal infection of the throat, scarlet fever, tonsillitis, influenza, measles, and smallpox. It is important that the etiology be uncovered so that appropriate measures may be taken. An acute sore throat with a nonbacterial infection usually has a much slower onset than bacterial pharyngitis with milder constitutional symptoms, normal or slightly elevated temperature, and a dry, raspy, possibly tickling sensation in the throat when swallowing.

This irritation of the pharnyx ("tickling") also may cause a nonproductive cough. In addition, the cough may result from irritation of tracheal or bronchial mucous membranes due to the direct extension of the inflammation or from infectious material dripping from the nasopharynx (postnasal drip). At its onset the cough is usually dry and nonproductive. Later stages of the common cold are characterized by heavy bronchial congestion resulting from the cellular debris of local phagocytic activity added to the respiratory tract fluids in the bronchial and nasal passage secretions and draining into the lower respiratory tract. Ciliary activity may not be sufficient to remove these fluids, and coughing is necessary to clear the lower tract of accumulated phlegm.

Another possible manifestation of the common cold is laryngitis, which is associated with hoarseness or loss of voice. It also may be caused by the spread of infection, or it may be an irritation secondary to drainage from the nasopharynx.

A hot or warm sensation ("feverishness") is another fairly common complaint. In general, little or no fever is actually present. Finally, headache, which usually occurs in the early stages of the cold, may be caused by the infection and inflammation of the nasal passages and paranasal sinuses.

Complications

In an otherwise healthy individual the common cold is self-limiting; the course of symptoms is 5–7 days. It is not uncommon (but not inevitable) for complications to develop during or immediately following a common cold. The pharmacist should be familiar with possible complications, their causes, and how they are treated. Viral infection induces swelling and some exudation, but it causes no significant change in the bacterial flora of the nasopharynx. If the inflammatory changes are of sufficient magnitude, passages connecting the paranasal sinuses and middle ear become obstructed, and under these conditions, infection may occur from secondary bacterial growth. In addition, it has been reported that viral respiratory infections trigger a substantial proportion of wheezing attacks in young asthmatic children (9).

The most common bacterial complications are purulent sinusitis, otitis media, bacterial pneumonia, and tonsillitis (10). Young children are especially prone to otitis media and pneumonia. Children's eustachian tubes are short, relatively horizontal, and rather narrow. This configuration facilitates fluid accumulation in the middle ear as well as rapid blockage in response to only a slight degree of inflammation. A young child's bronchiolar passages also are smaller in diameter than those of older children and adults and become blocked more easily. The smaller passages and the child's lack of conscious effort to cough up accumulated fluids in the lower tract lead to stasis of the fluids, inflammation, and secondary bacterial infection.

These complications usually manifest themselves by worsening of local symptoms (earache, headache, or cough), development of a fever, and failure of the cold to improve in the expected time. Such manifestations in a person with a recent cold probably are caused by secondary bacterial invaders for which culture and sensitivity tests and appropriate prescribed antibiotic therapy are indicated.

Conditions Mimicking the Common Cold

Other infectious diseases present initial manifestations identical to those of the common cold (10). The pharmacist should be aware of these disorders because some of them have potentially serious implications for which a physician should be consulted. Using strictly palliative therapy in situations that may not be self-limiting has little effect on the underlying problem and may delay necessary treatment. A patient's "sore throat," alone or in conjunction with other symptoms, may be caused by bacteria, a virus, or another irritative process. For example, a sore throat in a child may be a bacterial pharyngitis due to beta-hemolytic *Streptococcus* species. If symptomatic therapy alone is recommended and the child is suffering from beta-hemolytic streptococcal pharyngitis, the possible sequela of rheumatic fever or glomerulonephritis may develop. Appropriate antibiotic therapy may help prevent these dangerous sequelae.

Table 1. Distinguishing bacterial from nonbacterial sore throats

	Bacterial sore throat	Nonbacterial sore throat
Onset	Rapid	Slower
Soreness	Marked	Seldom marked
Constitutional symptoms	Marked	Mild
Upper and lower respiratory symptoms	Present in 50% of cases	Usual
Lymph nodes	Large, tender	Slight enlargement, not tender

Adapted from V. Bulteau, *Med. J. Aust.*, 2, 1053 (1966).

Sore throat in children should be evaluated by a physician as soon as possible, and symptomatic therapy should be employed only to provide relief until a physician can be seen. Sore throat in an adult patient may be due to a variety of causes, some of which may be amenable to self-medication (Table 1).

Influenza   A viral respiratory tract infection that may mimic a cold is called influenza, or the flu. Flu is usually distinguishable from the common cold by its epidemic occurrence and by fever, dry cough, joint and muscle ache, and more significant general malaise. Although treatment is symptomatic, it usually is more vigorous than cold treatment, and complications, especially secondary bacterial infections, are more likely to develop. This outcome is especially true in elderly and debilitated patients, who should be referred to a physician when influenza is suspected.

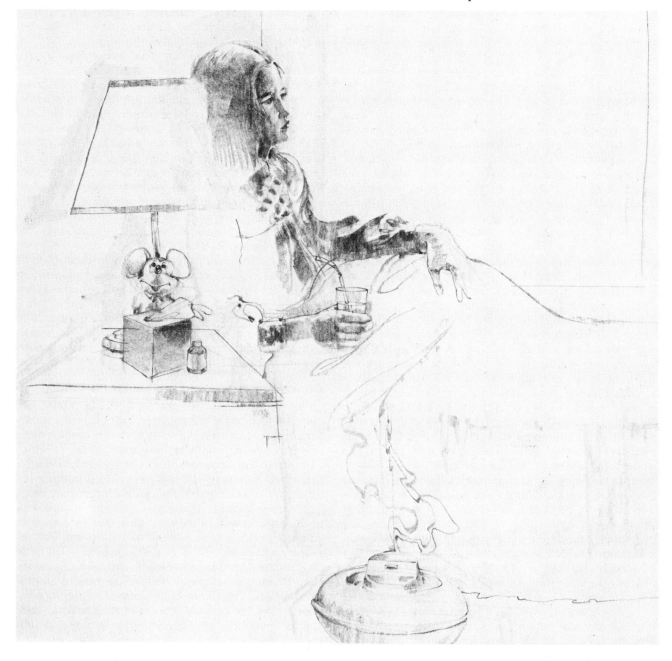

Measles The incidence of measles (rubeola) has been drastically reduced by immunization; when it does occur, it is associated with a prodrome that includes fever, rhinitis, dry cough, and conjunctivitis. Initially, it is difficult to distinguish from the common cold. However, in about 3 days, a red rash indicative of measles develops over the face, trunk, and extremities. The appearance of Koplik's spots is pathognomonic (characteristic) of measles. These spots usually appear 1–2 days before the rash as tiny "table salt crystals," usually on the mucous membranes of the cheek. Although treatment is symptomatic (along with patient isolation), a physician should be notified because secondary bacterial infections and postmeasles encephalitis may develop. Also, local public health regulations may require reporting measles.

German Measles Another viral disease in which fever, malaise, and rhinitis coincide with the eruption of a fine red rash is German measles (rubella). It is recommended that this disorder also be brought to a physician's attention because of possible complications. An important concern is the devastating effect that rubella may have on a fetus in utero. If a pregnant woman is exposed to a case of rubella (actual or suspected), she must be referred to a physician to determine her degree of immunity to the virus.

Allergy A history of allergy and a review of symptoms help differentiate allergic rhinitis from the common cold. Hay fever may be suspected in young children who suffer from repeated cold-like symptoms. Persistent symptoms of a cold are often the first clue to allergy rhinitis. Since a cold usually lasts only several days, a patient who presents with a stuffy nose for several weeks may have allergic rhinitis or some other form of noninfectious rhinitis.

Treatment

Self-medication of the common cold is intended to provide palliation of symptoms. There are no curative remedies, only drugs that bring temporary relief while the cold runs its course and the normal body defenses attempt to remove the viral invaders and repair the damage. In general, additional bed rest and prevention of chilling add to the patient's comfort. Adequate fluid intake is necessary to prevent dehydration and to decrease the viscosity of respiratory secretions. A well-balanced diet should be maintained.

Nasal Congestion and Discharge Treating nasal congestion is valuable in that it not only relieves the discomfort but also prevents excessive nose blowing, which may further irritate mucous membranes and the nostrils. Excessive nose blowing also may force infected fluids into nasal sinuses and the eustachian tubes, extending the infection and discomfort. Decongestants (sympathomimetic amines) applied as drops or spray to the nasal mucosa or administered systemically are effective vasoconstrictors that help decrease edema and swelling of the nasal mucosa. The watery nasal discharge found in the early stages of the common cold may be minimized by decongestant use.

Cough The first step in attempting to control a cough is to provide the respiratory tract with adequate fluids either by increasing oral fluid intake or by humidifying the inspired air. If the cough is dry, hyperactive, and annoying, a cough suppressant is indicated; an expectorant agent, by virtue of its action, theoretically would be useful in providing a demulcent effect, but none has been proven effective (1). These two agents are frequently found together in nonprescription products. If the cough is productive and frequency is tolerable, ensuring adequate fluid intake may be all that is needed. Regardless of the character of the cough (productive or nonproductive), if it is bothersome and not related to asthma, a cough suppressant may be beneficial. This is particularly true if the cough interferes with sleep. The tickling sensation in the pharynx that causes a cough may be treated initially with a demulcent, such as hard candy or cough drops, but if the cough becomes more intense, a cough suppressant may be recommended (1).

Dry or Sore Throat A sore throat in a child is difficult to evaluate and should not be self-medicated: The child should be seen by a physician.

Lozenges and gargles containing antiseptics and/or topical anesthetics are heavily promoted for treating sore throat. However, aside from a demulcent effect, the use of an antibacterial lozenge or gargle is irrational because the antibacterial ingredients are not effective against viruses.

If the throat is dry or raspy, hard, sour candy may be used to stimulate saliva flow, which acts as a demulcent. A frequently overlooked measure in soothing an inflamed throat is the regular use of a warm, normal saline gargle (2 tsp of salt/qt of water). If these measures do not provide adequate relief, lozenges or sprays containing a local anesthetic (phenol, hexylresorcinol, or benzocaine) may be used every 3–4 hours for temporary symptomatic relief.

Laryngitis Acute laryngitis presents a therapeutic problem—the only direct way to reach the inflamed laryngeal tissue is by inspired air. Lozenges and gargles do nothing to relieve hoarseness; their ingredients or the saliva that they stimulate do not reach this area. Water vapor inhalation (steam or cool mist) several times a day has proven beneficial in acute laryngitis. The value of adding any medications to steam has not been established. Inhaling irritants (smoking) should be avoided, and the voice should be rested as much as possible.

Feverishness and Headache Vague complaints of feverishness and headache, although not necessarily occurring together, may be treated with the same remedies. Aspirin or acetaminophen, in the proper dosage, is usually effective. In conjunction with fluids and rest, aspirin or acetaminophen are very useful because of their analgesic/antipyretic properties. Fever (orally measured temperature greater than 98.9–99.6° F) is seldom associated with the common cold, and the lasting benefit of the antipyretic property of aspirin or acetaminophen is doubtful. When a fever is present and persists for more than 24 hours in spite of treatment, a physician should be consulted. In the interim, aspirin or acetaminophen will provide temporary relief of fever symptoms. If fever persists in spite of these medical measures, the patient should be sponged or bathed in cool or tepid, not cold, water. The use of diluted isopropyl alcohol (50:50 in water) also has been recommended as adjunctive antipyretic therapy. In spite of this sponging solution's proven effectiveness, its use has been associated with two drawbacks (11). First, it has been found that there is significantly more discomfort associated with its use than with tepid water and second, coma following acute alcohol poisoning has been reported in patients sponged with isopropyl alcohol (11, 12). Therefore, the most rational approach to fever reduction in adults and children is aspirin or acetaminophen and/or tepid water sponging (13).

Physician-directed treatment is usually unnecessary unless there is concern that the patient has something other than a cold, the symptoms are severe, or secondary complications are present or suspected. Severely debilitated patients, however, should seek advice from their physician, as should patients with other chronic disorders (such as emphysema and cystic fibrosis) in which a respiratory infection may pose serious problems or the usual nonprescription remedies may be contraindicated.

Allergic Rhinitis

Etiology

Allergic rhinitis may begin at almost any age, although the incidence of first onset is greatest in children and young adults and decreases with age. Heredity seems to play a role. Allergic rhinitis itself is not genetically transmitted; however, the heightened predisposition to become sensitized following exposure to adequate concentrations of an allergen is transferred (14).

Pollens from plants that depend on the wind for cross-pollination and mold spores are the main agents responsible for seasonal allergic rhinitis. Ragweed pollen accounts for about 75% of seasonal rhinitis patients in the United States; grass pollens, 40%; and tree pollens, about 9%. Approximately 25% suffer from both grass and ragweed allergic rhinitis, and about 5% suffer from all three allergies (15).

The seasonal appearance of symptoms is a reflection of the pollen or spores in the air. Of the airborne mold spores, *Alternaria* and *Hormodendrum* species are the most common and also may cause seasonal allergic rhinitis (16). These spores are most prevalent from mid-March to late November. Tree pollination begins in late March and extends to early June. Grasses generally pollinate from mid-May to mid-July. Ragweed pollen has a long season, extending from early August to early October or to the first killing frost. The pollinating season is relatively constant from year to year for a particular plant in a given locale. Weather conditions such as temperature and rainfall influence the amount of pollen produced but not the actual onset or termination of a specific season (14). The appearance of seasonal allergic rhinitis symptoms is influenced by the patient's geographic location and specific hypersensitivities.

Perennial allergic rhinitis symptoms are usually caused by house dust, animal dander, and feathers. Occupational causes may include wheat flour, various grains, cotton and flax seeds, and enzymes used in detergents. The continued presence of the allergens results in patient symptoms that are persistent more or less year round. In addition, some patients may exhibit perennial allergic rhinitis symptoms with seasonal exacerbations.

Pathophysiology

Allergic rhinitis symptoms may be due to many different etiologic allergens. These allergens, which are primarily protein in nature, may, when deposited on the nasal mucosa, initiate an inflammatory response by the body and produce symptoms characteristic of allergic rhinitis.

The pathologic inflammatory process of seasonal allergic rhinitis develops within minutes after an allergen is deposited on the nasal mucous membrane of an allergy-prone individual. Pollen itself is not believed to be directly antigenic. However, the lysozyme component of nasal mucus may degrade the pollen cell wall to allow for the release of the proteinaceous contents. This released protein may be an antigen. The antigen stimulates lymphoid tissue in the respiratory tract to produce a specific type of immunoglobulin, IgE (reagin). These reaginic antibodies have a special affinity for circulating basophils and tissue mast cells. The cells pick up many IgE molecules on their surfaces and thus become sensitized. Subsequent exposure to the same antigen, by its deposition on nasal mucosa, causes an antigen-antibody reaction, which causes vasoactive chemical mediators to be released from these sensitized host cells. These mediators include histamine, slow-reacting substances of anaphylaxis, eosinophilic chemotactic factor, and possibly others.

The nasal mucosa is particularly vulnerable to this immediate type of allergic reaction because the allergen is deposited directly where it may act locally and because the mediators are very active vasodilators that are released in a highly vascularized area. The immediate effects are vasodilation, increased vascular permeability, and increased mucus secretion, all of which are responsible for the symptoms.

The longer the symptoms persist, from whatever cause, the more chronic and irreversible changes such as thickening of the mucosal epithelium, connective tissue proliferation, loss of epithelial cilia, and development of polyps of the nose or sinuses may be noted.

Symptoms

Major symptoms of allergic rhinitis are edema and symptoms resulting from the engorgement of the nasal mucosa—sneezing, rhinorrhea, nasal pruritus, and nasal congestion are the most common. Sudden sneezing attacks may consist of 10–20 sneezes in rapid succession (Table 2).

Rhinorrhea is typically a watery, thin discharge that may be quite profuse and continuous. Purulent discharge does not occur in uncomplicated allergic rhinitis; its presence indicates a secondary infection.

Table 2. Characteristics of the various types of rhinitis

Rhinitis	Allergic		Infectious	Nonallergic (vasomotor)
	Seasonal	Perennial		
Etiology	IgE-mediated immunologic reaction		Respiratory infection	Autonomic nervous system disorder
Seasonal pattern	Yes	Present year-round	Often worse in winter	Worse in changing seasons
Recurrences	Mild symptoms between attacks		Clears completely	Frequently continuous
Family history of allergy	Common	Common	Occasional	Occasional
Systemic symptoms	Rare	Rare	Common	Rare
Other allergic symptoms (asthma, eczema)	Common	Common	Occasional	Occasional
Pruritus	Yes	Yes	No	Mild or absent
Fever	No	No	Occasional	No
Conjunctivitis	Yes	Yes	No	No
Discharge	Water-like	Water-like	Mucopurulent	Water-like
Paroxysmal sneezing	Yes	Yes	No	Yes

The nasal congestion of allergic rhinitis is due to swollen turbinates. If the nasal obstruction is severe, it may cause headaches or earaches. With continuous, severe nasal congestion, loss of smell and taste may occur. Itching of the nose also may be a prominent feature, particularly in children, and causes frequent nose rubbing.

Conjunctival symptoms commonly associated with allergic rhinitis include itching and lacrimation. These symptoms are caused by the trapping of pollen grains in the conjunctival sac and subsequent antigen-antibody reaction as well as possible lacrimal duct congestion caused indirectly by the nasal congestion. Patients with severe eye symptoms often complain of photophobia and sore, tired eyes. Dark circles or greater than normal discolorations beneath the eyes are called "allergic shiners." This discoloration is more common in perennial rhinitis than in the seasonal variant.

A characteristic of seasonal allergic rhinitis is the periodicity of its appearance. Careful patient history indicates when the symptoms first began and the intervals at which they were exacerbated. With seasonal rhinitis the allergic reaction often begins with sneezing and progresses to rhinorrhea, then possibly to severe nasal obstruction, at which time sneezing may be absent and rhinorrhea minimal. Perennial rhinitis is more likely to begin with nasal obstruction and postnasal discharge than with sneezing and rhinorrhea (17).

The symptoms of allergic rhinitis may exhibit periodicity even within the season. Most patients tend to exhibit more intense symptoms in the morning and on windy days due to increased pollen in the air. Symptoms may diminish when it rains and the pollen is cleared from the air.

It is more difficult to associate perennial rhinitis than seasonal rhinitis with the environment; the patient history may be helpful in these cases. The most common perennial allergens are house dust and household pet dander with which the patient may be in contact during all seasons. Many patients with perennial allergic rhinitis have continuous symptoms because of the presence of dander or dust in their environment. However, other patients who have multiple overlapping allergies can be symptomatic each season for different reasons. The patient with mold, grass, ragweed, and house-dust allergies may be symptomatic all year.

Generally, allergic rhinitis tends to show increasingly severe symptoms for 2–3 years until a somewhat stabilized condition is reached. With seasonal allergic rhinitis, symptoms then tend to be exacerbated annually. There is no effective means of predicting whether symptoms will increase or decrease in severity. In fact, for reasons not well understood, hypersensitivity may disappear after several years. The pharmacist may differentiate seasonal allergic rhinitis from perennial allergic rhinitis by questioning the patient concerning the appearance and disappearance of symptoms. Important to the differentiation of seasonal allergic rhinitis from perennial allergic rhinitis is the presence of acute exacerbations. Patients with seasonal allergic rhinitis generally have a marked increase in symptoms corresponding to an increase in the amount of allergen in the air. The treatment is similar with both of these conditions.

Complications

Patients with allergic rhinitis may develop complications due to chronic nasal inflammation including recurrent otitis media with hearing loss, sinusitis, and loss of epithelial cilia. Hyposmia (decreased sense of smell acuity), nasal polyps, and vocal changes may complicate allergic rhinitis. The mechanism may be due to a chronic mucosal inflammation, which would explain why these complications are more often seen in patients with the perennial form (18). Complications of allergic rhinitis seem to be more prominent in children. Often a child develops a characteristic manner of rubbing the nose in an upwards direction with the palm of the hand to relieve itching and spread the nasal wall to produce better nasal ventilation. This persistent rubbing is called the allergic salute. Nasal allergy in children may also lead to bony structural changes in the palate and a depression of cheek bone prominence. The resultant crowding of incisor teeth is called the Gothic arch. Children with chronic, recurrent rhinitis may develop a hearing impairment due to the involvement of the eustachian tubes and middle ear.

Allergic rhinitis and asthmatic attacks often may be precipitated by the same agents. If allergic rhinitis symptoms are prolonged, a slight cough and a feeling of constriction in the chest or asthmatic wheezing may follow. These are dangerous signals—a warning of possible asthma onset. Because one-third or more of all patients with allergic rhinitis may develop asthma, these signs should be the basis for directing the patient to a physician for diagnosis and treatment (19).

Perennial allergic rhinitis is associated with chronic symptoms that may lead to anatomical changes within the nasal and sinus cavities. The resulting complications include loss of epithelial cilia and development of nasal polyps. Because the symptoms are chronic and complications may develop, all perennial allergic rhinitis sufferers should be under a physician's care.

Conditions Mimicking Allergic Rhinitis

It is also important for pharmacists to recognize common disease entities that may mimic signs or symptoms of allergic rhinitis. The main clinical entity in differential diagnosis of seasonal allergic rhinitis is infectious rhinitis. A mucopurulent discharge, the possibility of fever and other systemic symptoms, and the lack of pruritus often distinguish infectious from allergic rhinitis (Table 2). Chronic sinusitis, recurrent infectious rhinitis, abnormalities of nasal structures, such as septal deviations, and nonseasonal, nonallergic, noninfectious rhinitis of unknown etiology (vasomotor rhinitis) may be confused with perennial allergic rhinitis (10). A physician should be consulted to differentiate among these conditions.

Other conditions that may mimic allergic rhinitis symptoms are rhinitis medicamentosa (nasal congestion rebound from overuse of topical decongestants), reserpine rhinitis, foreign bodies in the nose, and cerebrospinal rhinorrhea. Rhinitis medicamentosa is a condition resulting from the overuse of topically applied vasoconstrictors. The pharmacist may identify this condition by questioning the patient about past use of nose drops or sprays for nasal congestion. Preparations containing reserpine or other antiadrenergic antihypertensives may cause marked nasal congestion. Often, this side effect is transient and subsides with continued antihypertensive administration. However, if it persists and is bothersome, topical decongestant treatment may be tried.

In rare instances the presence of a foreign body in the nose may be mistaken for chronic allergic rhinitis. Examination by a physician is necessary. Cerebrospinal rhinorrhea may follow a head injury; it is characterized by the discharge of a clear, watery fluid, usually from one nostril.

Treatment

Allergic rhinitis treatment involves

- Avoidance of allergens to prevent the immunologic response;
- Injection of allergen extracts to alter the immunologic response to the allergens (immunotherapy);
- Pharmacologic treatment to minimize or counteract the consequences of the immunologic response once it has occurred.

In most cases of allergic rhinitis, total avoidance of the allergen is difficult because airborne allergens are so widely distributed and, in most cases, patients are sensitive to more than one allergen. However, avoidance of certain situations (burning leaves, sleeping with bedroom windows open, and driving in the countryside when pollen counts are especially high) decreases exposure to environments or situations conducive to encountering potential allergens. The mechanical filters in most air conditioners help reduce the number of allergens if they are changed regularly (monthly), if doors and windows are kept closed, and if the air is recirculated. An electrostatic precipitator in conjunction with a central heating and air conditioning unit is even more effective in reducing house dust and other potential allergens. An effective environmental control for house-dust allergy is covering the bedding mattress (where the house dust mite lives) with a plastic cover and sealing the pillow in a plastic casing.

When brief exposure to an allergen is unavoidable, a proper face mask effectively filters the inhaled air. Such masks are sold by industrial or scientific supply firms as well as pharmacies for protection against noxious dust. The commonly used gauze masks are ineffective. The pharmacist should explain to the patient specific measures that decrease the likelihood of exposure to the offending allergen.

Immunotherapy (hyposensitization) attempts to raise a person's threshold for symptoms following exposure to the allergen. Although the mechanisms of immunotherapy are not understood completely, it is believed that blocking antibodies are produced when the patient is given a continuing series of allergen injections in specified incremental doses. A successful treatment regimen enables the patient to develop increased allergen tolerance. The indications for immunotherapy, a relatively long-term treatment modality, are relative rather than absolute. For example, if a patient's symptoms are mild and last only a few weeks, the patient may be well managed by symptomatic therapy alone. For those whose reaction to the allergens is much more severe or who cannot tolerate symptomatic treatment, immunotherapy may be considered.

Immunotherapy begins with the proper identification of the offending allergen, most commonly by skin tests measuring the patient's response to test allergens introduced intracutaneously. After the offending allergen is identified, an extract is injected in small amounts at frequent intervals. Studies indicate that in pollen allergy, 70–80% of the patients treated with immunotherapy experience beneficial results (14, 19, 20). However, most of the studies on the efficacy of immunotherapy relate to successes with ragweed and grass.

Immunotherapy does not cure the disease but reduces the number of symptoms, making it easier to control the allergy by symptomatic medication. Patients who experience allergic rhinitis symptoms throughout the year, whose allergic reactions tend to be severe, and who do not demonstrate a beneficial response from self-medication may be candidates for immunotherapy and should be advised by the pharmacist to seek the aid of a physician.

Pharmacologic Agents

The primary pharmacologic agents employed in treating these disorders are the antihistamines (H_1-blockers) and the alpha-adrenergic agonists (decongestants). Antihistamines are valuable because they competitively inhibit the effects of histamine released as a result of the antigen-antibody reaction. The alpha-adrenergic agonists, on the other hand, reverse the effects of histamine or viral inflammation by constricting dilated blood vessels, thereby diminishing nasal congestion.

Antihistamines

Histamine is a common biogenic amine found in every body tissue; most, however, is found in the mast cells. In these cells, histamine is localized and stored in granules and generally becomes active only when the cells are lysed. It may be released to exert its effects as a result of an antigen-antibody reaction (allergy) or physical damage (trauma or infection). Histamine has its most significant effects on the cardiovascular system, exocrine glands, and smooth muscles. Its major effects in the common cold and allergic rhinitis are profound vasodilation, increased capillary permeability, and edema. These effects are more pronounced in highly vascularized areas such as the nose.

Histamine is released in both the common cold and allergy, but the actual cause of its release and the amount released differ, and therefore the magnitude of its contribution to the symptoms is different. In allergy the antigen-antibody reaction leads to cellular damage of specific sensitized cells (mast cells) and consequent release of histamine that initiates the local inflammatory response. In colds, the local inflammatory response results from widespread cellular injury caused by virus particle invasion. Therefore, the vasodilation and resultant edema associated with a cold may be attributed not only to histamine release but also (and perhaps predominantly) to the body's inflammatory defense and the release of inflammatory mediators in addition to histamine.

Antihistamines are chemical agents that exert their effect in the body primarily by competitively blocking the actions of histamine at receptor sites (21, 22). They are classified as "pharmacologic antagonists" of histamine with a mechanism of action analogous to other pharmacologic antagonists such as antiadrenergics and anticholinergics. They do not prevent histamine release, and because they act by competitive inhibition, if the histamine concentration at the receptor site exceeds the drug concentration, histamine effects predominate. It has been observed that most antihistamines can be classified as either H_1-receptor blockers, which block the smooth muscle response, or H_2 receptor blockers, whose primary effect is blocking histaminic stimulation of gastric acid secretion (23). Those antihistamines that block the H_1 receptor are potentially useful in allergic rhinitis and to a lesser extent in cold treatment.

Although antihistaminic activity is the dominant effect of these agents, antihistamines are structurally similar to other pharmacologic classes of drugs (anticholinergic, local anesthetic, and ganglionic-blocking and adrenergic-blocking agents) and exert various combinations and degrees of side effects. In some cases, the side effects have been used to achieve a therapeutic goal (such as CNS depression for insomnia and local anesthetic effects for pruritus). However, these side effects, especially drowsiness, may be bothersome and potentially dangerous.

The most commonly used nonprescription antihistamines and their usual dosages are shown in Table 3. Brompheniramine maleate, chlorpheniramine maleate, doxylamine succinate, phenindamine tartrate, pheniramine maleate, promethazine maleate, pyrilamine maleate, and thonzylamine hydrochloride are recognized by the FDA advisory review panel on nonprescription cold, cough, allergy, bronchodilator, and antiasthmatic drug products as being safe for nonprescription use and effective in suppressing the symptoms of allergic rhinitis when taken in the dosage specified. Conclusive evidence is still lacking as to the safety and effectiveness of phenyltoloxamine citrate (1). Methapyrilene was removed from the market in 1979 because of reports of cancer in laboratory animals.

Antihistamines are most effective in controlling allergic rhinitis (1). They are rarely effective in vasomotor rhinitis.

Some regular antihistamine users may find that they do not obtain the same degree of relief after several weeks or months. One reason for this apparent decreased effectiveness is that some antihistamines are capable of hepatic enzyme induction, resulting in increased metabolism in the liver. Enzyme induction by antihistamines is a possible cause of diminished effectiveness of other drugs. However, the clinical significance of such interactions is undetermined. The various antihistamine classes differ in their capacity to induce hepatic enzymes. Some practitioners have found that if tolerance develops, some patients may benefit by switching to another antihistamine. Further studies are needed to evaluate the effectiveness of this technique.

Although antihistamines have no ability to prevent or abort the common cold, they are found in many cold remedies. A rationale for their inclusion in these products probably stems from their anticholinergic action, which decreases the amount of mucus secretion, relieving the rhinorrhea. Although some people experience a drying effect, the anticholinergic activity of the antihistamines is actually very weak, and this action may be insignificant at the dosage levels of the various nonprescription preparations.

Table 3. Antihistamine dosage

Drug (by chemical class)	Dosage (maximum dose/24 hours)		
	Adults	Children 6 to <12 years	Children 2 to <6 years
Ethanolamines			
Diphenhydramine hydrochloride[a]	25–50 mg every 4–6 hours (300 mg)	12.5–25 mg every 4–6 hours (150 mg)	6.25 mg every 4–6 hours (37.5 mg)
Doxylamine succinate	7.5–12.5 mg every 4–6 hours (75 mg)	3.75–6.24 mg every 4–6 hours (37.5 mg)	Professional labeling only: 1.9–3.125 mg every 4–6 hours (18.75 mg)
Phenyltoloxamine citrate	50 mg every 4–6 hours (300 mg)	Information inadequate to establish dosage	Information inadequate to establish dosage
Ethylenediamines			
Pyrilamine maleate	25–50 mg every 6–8 hours (200 mg)	12.5–25 mg every 6–8 hours (100 mg)	6.25–12.5 mg every 6–8 hours (50 mg)
Thonzylamine hydrochloride	50–100 mg every 4–6 hours (600 mg)	25–50 mg every 4–6 hours (300 mg)	12.5–25 mg every 4–6 hours (150 mg)
Alkylamines			
Pheniramine maleate	12.5–25 mg every 4–6 hours (150 mg)	6.25–12 mg every 4–6 hours (75 mg)	3.125–6.25 mg every 4–6 hours (37.5 mg)
Brompheniramine maleate	4 mg every 4–6 hours (24 mg)	2 mg every 4–6 hours (12 mg)	1 mg every 4–6 hours (6 mg)
Chlorpheniramine maleate	4 mg every 4–6 hours (24 mg)	2 mg every 4–6 hours (12 mg)	1 mg every 4–6 hours (6 mg)
Miscellaneous			
Phenindamine tartrate	25 mg every 4–6 hours (150 mg)	12.5 mg every 4–6 hours (75 mg)	6.25 mg every 4–6 hours (37.5 mg)

The FDA advisory review panel on nonprescription cold, cough, allergy, bronchodilator, and antiasthmatic products has recommended all of these ingredients as safe and effective (Category I) except phenyltoloxamine citrate, for which there is insufficient evidence (Category III).

[a]Diphenhydramine hydrochloride, as a single-entity product, is not available without a prescription as of January 1, 1982.

In general, antihistamines possess a high therapeutic index (toxic dose/therapeutic dose), and serious toxicities are seldom noted in adults. At recommended labeled doses, most nonprescription antihistamines also are safe for use in children. As with most drugs, however, accidental overdose in children may lead to profound symptoms, such as excitement, ataxia, incoordination, muscular twitching, generalized convulsions with pupillary dilation, and skin flushing. Treatment is symptomatic and usually requires supportive therapy with artificial respiration.

The major contraindication to antihistamine use, which is the agent's sedative property, is relative. Degrees of drowsiness associated with antihistamines vary, but none is entirely free of this side effect. The ethanolamines, such as diphenhydramine hydrochloride, have a pronounced tendency to induce sedation. The alkylamines (chlorpheniramine maleate) possess weak sedative properties, and the ethylenediamines (pyrilamine maleate) are approximately intermediate in their sedative properties (24). Although most individuals acquire a tolerance to this effect, the alkylamines probably are the most suitable agents for daytime use (24). In one study, persistent drowsiness was reported to be uncommon when therapy was initiated with a low dose of drug at bedtime, and the dose increased progressively over a 10-day period as tolerated (25). If a person's job or other activities require a high degree of mental alertness, any antihistamine must be used cautiously until its effect is determined by the individual. The effects of alcohol and other CNS depressants including hypnotics, sedatives, analgesics, and antianxiety agents may be enhanced by the antihistamines. If concurrent administration is necessary, caution must be exercised because of the increased possibility of drowsiness (24, 26). Patients should be warned of "hidden" sources of alcohol contained in some nonprescription medications.

A paradoxical effect frequently seen in children is CNS stimulation rather than depression, causing insomnia, nervousness, and irritability (phenindamine). For this reason, antihistamines must be used cautiously in children with convulsive disorders or hyperkinesis (1, 20). The anticholinergic properties of an antihistamine may predominate in some individuals. Antihistamines may cause dry mouth, blurred vision, urinary retention (in older males suffering from an enlarged prostate), and constipation as a result of their anticholinergic effects; these effects, however, are usually associated with high doses. Because of the potential drying effect on respiratory secretions and potential airway obstruction, some practitioners believe that antihistamines should not be given to asthmatics (27). The agents may be useful, however, in special situations where the physician may elect a trial course of antihistamine therapy in patients not adequately controlled with the usual antiasthmatic regimen (4). This may be particularly useful in patients with an allergic component to their asthma.

The cholinergic-blocking properties of the antihistamines may pose a problem for patients whose glaucoma is being controlled with an anticholinesterase. Such an effect is unpredictable; because of the potential consequences, a patient being treated for narrow-angle glaucoma probably should take antihistamines only under a physician's supervision. Ninety-five percent of all patients with glaucoma have the wide-angle type and antihistamines are not contraindicated in these patients.

The cholinergic-blocking effect of antihistamines has a quantitatively unpredictable additive effect with anticholinergic drugs. Although excessive cholinergic blockage effects are usually of minor clinical significance, effects such as urinary retention, constipation, and dry mouth may be bothersome (1).

Hypersensitivity reactions may develop with the antihistamines, but this effect is more common with topical application than with oral use (23). Antihistamine overdose may cause dermatitis, psychosis, convulsions, and facial dyskinesias (28, 29, 30, 31).

Topical Decongestants

Various sympathomimetic amines have been used to provide relief from the nasal stuffiness of colds and allergic rhinitis. These drugs, which differ primarily in their duration of action, are contained in many nonprescription products promoted for hay fever and colds. Nasal decongestants stimulate the alpha-adrenergic receptors of the vascular smooth muscle, constricting the dilated arteriolar network within the nasal mucosa and reducing blood flow in the engorged edematous nasal area. This constriction results in shrinkage of the engorged mucous membranes, which promotes drainage, improves nasal ventilation, and relieves the feeling of stuffiness.

The ideal topical decongestant agent should have a prompt and prolonged effect. It should not produce systemic side effects, irritation to the mucosa with resultant harmful effects on the cilia of the respiratory tract, or rebound congestion. An ideal topical sympathomimetic amine has not yet been found (32).

Intranasal application of commercially available decongestants provides prompt and dramatic decrease of nasal congestion. Shrinking of the mucous membrane not only makes breathing easier but also permits the sinus cavities to drain.

It is important that the patient follow the label directions regarding the frequency and duration of use. Topical application of these drugs is often followed by a rebound phenomenon (rhinitis medicamentosa) in which the nasal mucous membranes become even more congested and edematous as the drug's vasoconstrictor effect subsides. This secondary congestion is believed to result from ischemia caused by the drug's intensive local vasoconstriction and local irritation of the topically applied agent itself. If the use of a topical nasal decongestant is restricted to 3–4 days or less, rebound congestion is minimal; with chronic use and/or overuse of these agents, rebound nasal stuffiness may become quite pronounced. This phenomenon represents a vicious cycle because it leads to more frequent use of the agent that causes it. To determine the possible existence of this condition, the pharmacist should question a patient concerning prior use of nasal sprays, drops, or inhalants. If the pharmacist suspects that the patient is experiencing this rebound phenomenon, the patient should be referred to a physician. Topical decongestant therapy should be discontinued, and systemic decongestants and/or isotonic saline drops may be used.

The patient should be instructed on the proper administration of topical decongestants to obtain maximum relief without encountering side effects from the drug's systemic absorption. These products are available as drops or sprays. Nasal decongestant sprays are packaged in flexible plastic containers that produce a fine mist when squeezed. The patient should administer nasal sprays in the upright position, squeezing once into each nostril. The nose should be blown to remove mucus 3–5 minutes after spraying. If there is still congestion, another dose should be administered that should reach farther into the nasal cavities and to the surfaces of the turbinates.

Some persons may prefer to administer the decongestant solution with a nasal atomizer. Most commercial spray containers are designed to deliver the approximate dose with one squeeze; the atomizer, however, is not so calibrated. Also, using an atomizer may increase the possibility of contaminating the solution. If the patient prefers to use a nasal atomizer, instructions should be provided on the proper use of the particular atomizer, including the liquid level and proper placement within the nostril, and the hazards of misuse. The patient should be instructed to remove the solution and rinse the atomizer after use to guard against solution contamination. Naphazoline solutions should not be used in atomizers containing aluminum parts because drug degradation will result.

Nasal drops usually do not cover the entire nasal mucosa and may pass to the pharynx, where they may be swallowed. Although systemic absorption through the nasal mucosa is minimal because of the local vasoconstriction induced by the drug, if an excess amount drains through the nasal passage and is swallowed, absorption and systemic effects are then possible. The amount of medication swallowed may be minimized by proper administration.

To administer nasal drops, the patient should recline on a bed with the head tilted back over the edge or should recline on the side, holding the head lower than the shoulders. The drops should be placed in the lower nostril without touching the nasal surface with the dropper. After the drops have been instilled into each nostril, the patient should breathe through the mouth and remain in the reclining position for about 5 minutes. To ensure more uniform absorption of the medica-

Table 4. Topical nasal decongestant dosage

Drug and concentration	Dosage		
	Adults, drops or sprays	Children 6 to < 12 years drops or sprays	Children 2 to < 6 years[a]
Ephedrine, 0.5% (various salts)	2–3 (≥ 4 hours)	1–2 (≥ 4 hours)	—
Naphazoline hydrochloride, 0.05%	1–2 (≥ 6 hours)	Not recommended (refer to 0.025%)	—
0.25%	—	1–2 (≥ 6 hours)	—
Oxymetazoline hydrochloride, 0.05%	2–3 (morning and evening)	Same as for adults	Not recommended (refer to 0.025%)
0.025%	—	—	2–3 (morning and evening)
Phenylephrine hydrochloride, 0.5%	2–3 (≥ 4 hours)	Not recommended (refer to 0.25%)	Not recommended (refer to 0.125%)
0.25%	Same as 0.5%	2–3 (≥ 4 hours)	Not recommended (refer to 0.125%)
0.125%	—	—	2–3 drops (≥ 4 hours)
Xylometazoline hydrochloride, 0.1%	2–3 (8–10 hours)	Not recommended (refer to 0.05%)	Not recommended (refer to 0.05%)
0.05%	—	2–3 (8–10 hours)	2–3 (8–10 hours)

The FDA advisory review panel on cold, cough, allergy, bronchodilator, and antiasthmatic products has recommended these ingredients as safe and effective (Category I) at the dosages specified. Only drops should be used in children 2 to <6 years, since the spray is difficult to use in the small nostril. These products should not be used in patients with chronic rhinitis because of the risk of rhinitis medicamentosa.

[a]For children under 6 there is no recommended dosage of ephedrine, naphazoline, or oxymetazoline except under the advice and supervision of a physician.

tion, the head may be turned from side to side while the patient is reclining.

A topical decongestant in spray form is probably more convenient for adults and older children. Sprays also may afford better decongestion by reaching greater areas of the mucous membranes. Drops are the most effective means of administering a topical decongestant to children under 6 years old because of their smaller nostril openings.

Several agents are commonly used as topical nasal decongestants. The primary difference lies in their intensity and duration of action (Table 4).

Ephedrine

Ephedrine is the prototype of the topical sympathomimetic decongestant. Various ephedrine salts provide rapid nasal decongestion applied topically in 0.5–1.0% concentrations. Ephedrine's peak effects are achieved 1 hour after administration. The aqueous solution of topical ephedrine as drops or sprays is the only vehicle recommended by the FDA advisory review panel on nonprescription cold, cough, allergy, bronchodilator, and antiasthmatic drug products since oily solutions may lead to lipoid pneumonia (1). Products containing ephedrine should be shielded from direct light, since decomposition will be hastened by such exposure. Ephedrine in a concentration of 0.5% should be administered as 2 or 3 drops or sprays for adults or 1 or

2 drops or sprays for children 6–12 years old, not more frequently than every 4 hours. However, ephedrine is not recommended in children less than 6 years of age except under the advice and supervision of a physician (33).

Phenylephrine

Phenylephrine hydrochloride is one of the most effective nonprescription nasal decongestants (34). It is commonly applied as 2 or 3 drops or sprays of a 0.25–0.5% solution every 4 hours. The use of stronger solutions except under a physician's direction is hazardous. This agent may produce a marked irritation of the nasal mucosa in some individuals, in addition to the irritation already present from the pathologic condition of the allergic disorder or cold. If this reaction occurs, phenylephrine use should be stopped immediately.

Phenylephrine hydrochloride is also available as an aqueous jelly. A small amount of jelly is placed in each nostril and snuffed well back into the nasal passage. This dosage form is not convenient and is not widely used, and its effectiveness has not been established. Nasal decongestant jellies are used most commonly by otorhinolaryngologists for office examination or treatment. Theoretically, a more prolonged decongestant effect may be achieved with nasal jellies, which may have an emollient and protective action on the nasal mucosa, but these effects also have not been proven (35).

Naphazoline

Naphazoline hydrochloride is a more potent vasoconstrictor than phenylephrine hydrochloride. It produces CNS depression rather than stimulation when it is absorbed systemically. Because of its systemic effects, this agent is not recommended for use in children under 6 years old except on the advice and supervision of a physician (1). Naphazoline hydrochloride is commonly administered as 1 or 2 drops or sprays of a 0.05% solution every 6 hours. It may be irritating to the mucosa and may sting when administered; use should be discontinued if this adverse effect persists or worsens.

Oxymetazoline and Xylometazoline

Longer-acting topical nasal decongestants, such as oxymetazoline hydrochloride and xylometazoline hydrochloride, have a decongestant effect that may last 5–6 hours, with a gradual decline thereafter (1, 36, 37, 38). Because of their longer duration, these agents are easier to use; but, because they are used only twice per day, potential rebound congestion or rhinitis medicamentosa is not less likely to occur. Oxymetazoline may be administered as 2 or 3 drops or sprays in the morning and evening; xylometazoline may be administered in the same amount every 8–10 hours (1).

Levodesoxyephedrine and Propylhexedrine

These sympathomimetic amines are volatile and commonly used in inhalants. Both of these aromatic amines are classified as Category I when used as two inhalations in each nostril not more frequently than every 2 hours. While children 6 years and older may use the adult dose of propylhexidrine, the dose of levodesoxyephedrine should be halved to 1 inhalation not more frequently than every 2 hours. Neither of these products is promoted for use in children less than 6 years old.

The use of nasal inhalers is associated with potential problems, such as the inadvertent loss of the active agent when the cap is not properly replaced. Also, there may not be sufficient nasal airflow to distribute the agent throughout the nasal cavity. These agents have been implicated as being irritating to the nasal mucosa and as interfering with ciliary action, as have all effective topical nasal decongestants. As with other topical amines, overuse produces side effects of local irritation and rebound congestion.

Oral Decongestants

Administering sympathomimetic amines orally distributes the drug through the systemic circulation to the vascular bed of the nasal mucosa. The oral decongestant agents have the advantage of a longer duration of action in comparison with certain topically applied decongestants. However, they cause less intense vasoconstriction than the topically applied sprays or drops. Oral agents have not been associated with rebound congestion or rhinitis medicamentosa because of their lesser degree of vasoconstriction and the lack of local drug irritation (24).

These agents do not exert their action exclusively on the vasculature of the nasal mucosa; in doses large enough to bring about nasal decongestion they also affect other vascular beds (24). Although the vasoconstriction produced by oral decongestants usually does not increase blood pressure, individuals predisposed to hypertension may experience a change in blood pressure. These decongestants may cause cardiac stimulation and the development of arrhythmias in individuals so predisposed. In patients with glucose intolerance or Type I diabetics, sympathomimetic administration may be a problem because these drugs increase blood glucose levels. However, hyperglycemia is a beta$_2$-adrenergic effect and most oral decongestants (except ephedrine) have primarily alpha-adrenergic stimulating properties. Labeling instructions on products containing sympathomimetics should indicate that patients with hypertension, hyperthyroidism, diabetes mellitus, or ischemic heart disease should use these products only on the advice of a physician.

Sympathomimetic amines are contraindicated in patients receiving monoamine oxidase (MAO) inhibitor therapy for depression because a hypertensive crisis may result. They should be used cautiously in hypertensive patients stabilized with guanethidine (39). These warnings apply largely to the oral agents and are not likely to occur with topically applied drugs.

Table 5. Oral nasal decongestant dosage

| Drug | Dosage (maximum dose/24 hours) | | |
	Adults	Children 6 to <12 years	Children 2 to <6 years[a]
Phenylephrine	10 mg every 4 hours (60 mg)	5 mg every 4 hours (30 mg)	2.5 mg every 4 hours (15 mg)
Phenylpropanolamine	25 mg every 4 hours (150 mg)	12.5 mg every 4 hours (75 mg)	6.25 mg every 4 hours (37.5 mg)
Pseudoephedrine	60 mg every 6 hours (240 mg)	30 mg every 6 hours (120 mg)	15 mg every 6 hours (60 mg)

The FDA advisory review panel on nonprescription cold, cough, allergy, bronchodilator, and antiasthmatic products has recommended these ingredients as safe and effective (Category I) at the dosages specified.

[a]There is no recommended dosage for children under 2 years of age except under the advice and supervision of a physician.

Ephedrine, phenylpropanolamine hydrochloride, phenylephrine hydrochloride, and pseudoephedrine are oral sympathomimetic amines commonly incorporated into cold and allergy products (Table 5). According to classification by the FDA advisory review panel, only phenylpropanolamine, phenylephrine, and pseudoephedrine have been shown to be effective as oral decongestants (1).

Ephedrine

According to the FDA advisory review panel on cold, cough, allergy, bronchodilator, and antiasthmatic drug products, ephedrine is effective as a bronchodilator for asthma but has not been proven effective as a nasal decongestant (40). Orally, in doses of 12.5–25 mg every 4 hours for adults and children 12 years and over, ephedrine is effective as a bronchodilator for use in treating symptoms of asthma. The bronchodilator effects usually appear within 30 minutes to 1 hour following oral administration. Ephedrine has CNS stimulatory effects.

Phenylpropanolamine

Phenylpropanolamine hydrochloride resembles ephedrine in its action but is somewhat more active as a vasoconstrictor and less active as a CNS stimulant and bronchodilator. The peak effect occurs approximately 3 hours after administration.

Phenylephrine

Phenylephrine hydrochloride is rapidly hydrolyzed partially in the GI tract, and the amount delivered to the bloodstream by the oral route is hard to predict, but effectiveness as an oral decongestant has been demonstrated (1). Phenylephrine is a common ingredient of cold preparations but is usually present at inadequate dosage levels.

Pseudoephedrine

Pseudoephedrine is another effective vasoconstrictor. It has less vasopressor action than ephedrine and causes little CNS stimulation. The doses given in Table 5 reflect a recent relabeling requirement following an FDA decision that data do not support the advisory review panel's original recommendation for a 360-mg adult daily dose of pseudoephedrine. The FDA's latest labeling requirement sets the adult daily dose at 240 mg. The daily dose for children 6–12 years of age has been changed from 180 mg to 120 mg, and for children 2–6 years of age from 90 mg to 60 mg. The peak effect of a 60-mg dose occurs approximately 4 hours after administration. Since pseudoephedrine has a short duration of effect several companies have marketed slow-release formulations to maintain more constant relief from nasal airway obstruction. Patients who have nasal stuffiness interfering with night-time sleep may benefit from a slow-release pseudoephedrine formulation. However, most of the sustained-release products are prescription items.

Antitussives and Expectorants

The cough associated with the common cold may be either productive or nonproductive (dry cough). The productive cough is useful and essential if it helps to remove accumulated secretions and debris (phlegm) from the lower tract. Although a patient with "chest congestion" is expected to expectorate phlegm ("productive" cough) during coughing, this does not necessarily occur. It would be inappropriate, however, to describe the cough as "nonproductive" because this description usually is related to dry, noncongested coughing. For the sake of distinction in this section as well as rationale for product selection later, a cough will be classified in one of the following categories:

- **Congested/productive**—cough associated with chest congestion and the expectoration of phlegm;
- **Congested/nonproductive**—cough associated with chest congestion and scant expectoration of phlegm;
- **Dry/nonproductive**—cough not associated with chest congestion.

By referring to these categories the pharmacist will be able to determine when and which type of agent should be used. The first two categories could be undiagnosed symptoms of asthma since intermittent asthmatics may only develop symptoms during a viral respiratory infection.

Excessive coughing, particularly if it is dry and nonproductive, not only is discomforting but also tends to be self-perpetuating because the rapid air expulsion further irritates the tracheal and pharyngeal mucosa. The general types of antitussive agents available for self-medication are expectorants and cough suppressants. Table 6 indicates the sites at which the cough reflex may be blocked as well as the mechanism of the agents.

Expectorants

The use of expectorants in clinical practice is a controversial issue revolving around doubts of therapeutic efficacy. The controversy stems from the lack of objective

Table 6. Blockade of cough reflex

Site	Mechanism	Blocking agents
Sensory nerves	Reduction of primary irritation; inhibition of bronchoconstriction; inhibition of afferent impulses	Demulcents/expectorants; bronchodilators; local anesthetics
Cough center (medulla)	Depression	Opiate and nonopiate suppressants
Motor nerves	Inhibition of efferent impulses	Local anesthetics

Adapted from H. Salem and D. M. Aviado, *Drug Inform. J., 8,* 111 (1974).

experimental data showing that an expectorant decreases sputum viscosity or eases expectoration more than a placebo. In fact, in spite of the widespread use of guaifenesin, one study states that "from a scientific point of view [this drug] probably has no rational use in clinical medicine as an expectorant" (41). Other literature also questions the efficacy of expectorants, stating that "the use of expectorants is based primarily on tradition and the widespread subjective clinical impression that they are effective" (24). The apparent difficulty in accumulating objective evidence stems from two factors: insufficient evidence as to which physiochemical property of respiratory secretions correlates best with ease of expectoration, and lack of appropriate techniques and instrumentation (1). The FDA advisory review panel on nonprescription cold, cough, allergy, bronchodilator, and antiasthmatic drug products was unable to classify any claimed expectorant as Category I (generally recognized as safe and effective).

Fluid intake and maintaining adequate humidity of the inspired air are important to respiratory tract fluid mucus production and therefore are essential in cold therapy. These measures may be accomplished by increasing fluid intake (6–8 glasses/day) in patients who do not have fluid restrictions and by using a cool mist or hot steam vaporizer.

Subjective findings constitute the basis for continued expectorant use. In fact, according to the panel, "until such objective methods become available, the panel will consider well-controlled, double-blind subjective studies in the assessment of efficacy" (1). Table 7 lists the usual dose and dosage range of the most commonly used expectorants.

There are no apparent absolute contraindications to the use of orally administered expectorants. The toxicity associated with expectorant drugs varies among agents. In general, the most common adverse effect to anticipate is gastric upset.

Ammonium Chloride   Ammonium chloride is believed to increase the amount of respiratory tract fluid by reflex stimulation of bronchial mucous glands resulting from irritation of the gastric mucosa. In the presence of renal, hepatic, or chronic heart disease, doses of 5 g have caused severe poisoning (42). A relative contraindication exists when ammonium chloride is used in patients with hepatic, renal, or pulmonary insufficiency; doses larger than those recommended may predispose to metabolic acidosis. Because ammonium chloride acidifies the urine, it may affect the excretion of other drugs (39). This effect probably is not significant because the usual daily dosage range as a systemic acidifier is 4–12 g, which is greatly in excess of the safe range for nonprescription use (43).

Guaifenesin (Glyceryl Guaiacolate)   Guaifenesin, in the doses recommended for nonprescription use, also is thought to act by reflex gastric stimulation. In spite of its mechanism of action, its use at these doses is seldom associated with gastric upset and nausea. However, one controlled study has shown that guaifenesin neither increases the volume of sputum production nor

decreases viscosity (44). Another controlled study demonstrated that guaifenesin has no effect on bleeding time or platelet aggregation in patients (45).

Ipecac Syrup   Administration 3 or 4 times/day of 0.5–1.0 ml of ipecac syrup (see Table 8 for concentration) is believed to increase respiratory secretion flow by gastric irritation. Little is known regarding the toxicity associated with ipecac. The chief alkaloids, emetine and cephaeline, however, are very toxic. There is no information on the absorption of small oral doses from the GI tract or on the cumulative effects of repeated oral administration (1). For this reason the panel has recommended a 1-week time limit when ipecac preparations are used for self-medication. Ipecac is not recommended for use in children under 6 years of age.

Terpin Hydrate   This volatile oil derivative is believed to act by direct stimulation of lower respiratory tract secretory glands in the doses recommended for nonprescription use. Because of the elixir's high alcohol content, the potential for alcohol abuse should be recognized; however, misuse is associated far more frequently with terpin hydrate and codeine elixir. Terpin hydrate elixir is not recommended for use in children under 12 years old (1). Some GI distress, such as nausea and vomiting, has been noted in the recommended dosage.

Beechwood Creosote and Potassium Guaiacolsulfonate   The apparent usefulness of beechwood creosote and potassium guaiacolsulfonate as expectorants is due to the local irritating effects of guaiacol, the major constituent of the former and the active moiety of the latter. Guaiacol, like guaifenesin, apparently increases respiratory tract fluid by a gastric reflex action. It is believed that potassium guaiacolsulfonate is metabolized in vivo to liberate guaiacol but this has never been clearly established.

Although a dosage for beechwood creosote has been proposed, the panel was unable to establish a dosage for potassium guaiacolsulfonate (1, 43).

Other ingredients of unproven effectiveness in cold products associated with expectorant claims include

- Benzoin preparations;
- Camphor;
- Eucalyptus oil;
- Menthol;
- Peppermint oil;
- Pine tar;
- Sodium citrate;
- Tolu;
- Turpentine oil.

Antitussives

Antitussives (cough suppressants) are indicated when there is a need to reduce the frequency of a cough, especially when it is the dry/nonproductive type (24, 46). The mechanism by which the narcotic and nonnarcotic agents affect a cough's intensity and frequency depends on the principal site of action: CNS depression of the cough center in the medulla or suppression of the nerve receptors within the respiratory tract (1).

Table 7. Expectorant dosage

Drug	Dosage (maximum dose/24 hours)		
	Adults	Children 6 to <12 years	Children 2 to <6 years[a]
Ammonium chloride	300 mg every 2–4 hours	150 mg every 2–4 hours	75 mg every 2–4 hours
Beechwood creosote	250 mg every 4–6 hours (1,500 mg)	125 mg every 4–6 hours (750 mg)	62.5 mg every 4–6 hours (375 mg)
Guaifenesin	200–400 mg every 4 hours (240 mg)	100–200 mg every 4 hours (1,200 mg)	50–100 mg every 4 hours (600 mg)
Potassium guaiacolsulfonate	Not established	Not established	Not established
Syrup of ipecac	0.5–1.0 ml (of syrup containing not less than 123 mg and not more than 157 mg of total ether-soluble alkaloids of ipecac/100 ml) 3 or 4 times/day	0.25–0.5 ml (of syrup containing not less than 123 mg and not more than 157 mg of total ether-soluble alkaloids of ipecac/100 ml) 3 or 4 times/day	Not recommended
Terpin hydrate	200 mg every 4 hours (1,200 mg)	100 mg (of terpin hydrate alone or in a nonalcoholic mixture, not the elixir for children under 12) every 4 hours (600 mg)	50 mg (of terpin hydrate alone or in a nonalcoholic mixture, not the elixir for children under 12) every 4 hours (300 mg)

The FDA advisory review panel on nonprescription cold, cough, allergy, bronchodilator, and antiasthmatic products has concluded that the available data are insufficient to permit classification of these ingredients (Category III).

[a]There is no recommended dosage for children under 2 years of age except under the advice and supervision of a physician.

Codeine Codeine is the antitussive against which all other antitussives are compared (19). The FDA advisory review panel on cold, cough, allergy, bronchodilator, and antiasthmatic drug products has concluded that under usual conditions of therapeutic use, codeine has low-dependency liability (47). The average adult antitussive dose is 15 mg (with a range of 10–20 mg). At this dosage, codeine provides effective cough relief (see Table 8 for children's dosage). Stringent controls have been placed on codeine-containing nonprescription products as a result of their misuse. There is no danger of psychological and physical dependence when codeine is used in recommended amounts for short periods. On a weight basis, the respiratory depressant effect of codeine is about one-fourth that of morphine. Even when the dose is increased, commensurate increase in respiratory depression does not necessarily occur. In doses commonly used in nonprescription cough products, in an otherwise healthy person the effects on respiration are not apparent. Codeine is thought by some investigators to have a drying effect on the respiratory mucosa; this property would be detrimental in asthma and/or emphysema patients because of the increased viscosity of respiratory fluids and decreased cough reflex (32).

In clinical practice the adverse effects most commonly encountered with codeine include nausea, drowsiness, lightheadedness, and constipation, especially when recommended dosage levels are exceeded. Allergic reactions and pruritus also may occur but are not as common. These reactions may be more common in atopic or histamine-sensitive patients (48). In general, antitussive codeine doses are well tolerated. Codeine's CNS depressant effect is additive to that of other CNS depressants, and such agents should be used cautiously when given concurrently.

Codeine use is contraindicated in individuals with chronic pulmonary disease, where mucosal drying and slight respiratory depression, in addition to impairment of the clearing of the airway of secretions, may be additionally detrimental (1). Codeine should be avoided by patients who have experienced codeine-induced allergic manifestations (pruritus or rash). Codeine is safe and effective used as directed for cough.

Dextromethorphan Dextromethorphan is a methylated dextro-isomer of levorphanol, but, unlike its analgesic counterpart, it has no significant analgesic properties and does not depress respiration or predispose to addiction (46). Some investigators believe that dextromethorphan and codeine are equipotent; others give a slight edge to codeine (46). Unlike codeine, increasing the dose of dextromethorphan to 30 mg does not increase its antitussive effects (46).

Adverse effects produced by dextromethorphan hydrobromide at recommended nonprescription dosages are mild and infrequent. Drowsiness and GI upset are the most common complaints. Accidental poisonings in children have resulted in stuporousness and disturbances in gait, with rapid recovery after emesis (46). Larger doses in the abuse range have produced intoxication with bizarre behavior but no dependence (48).

Dextromethorphan hydrobromide at nonprescription dosages (Table 8) is a safe and effective antitussive for which there are no apparent contraindications unless, of course, the patient is hypersensitive to it (1).

Diphenhydramine Diphenhydramine hydrochloride, a potent antihistamine, is a safe and effective nonprescription antitussive, according to the FDA advisory review panel. However, the commissioner has disagreed with this recommendation and as of January 1, 1982, had not issued any decision on the question of exempting diphenhydramine from prescription requirement (49). In spite of this disagreement between the panel and the commissioner, on August 7, 1981, the FDA approved an NDA for Benylin Cough Syrup, containing 12.5 mg diphenhydramine hydrochloride/5 ml, which is available without a prescription. Although this concentration is identical to the prescription-only Benadryl Elixir, the cough syrup contains less alcohol (5% versus 14%), as well as several inactive ingredients such as the Category II expectorants, ammonium chloride and sodium citrate. At the present time, Benylin Cough Syrup is the only diphenhydramine-containing preparation available without a prescription.

Objective results of clinical studies indicate that diphenhydramine, in 25- and 50-mg doses, significantly reduced coughing in chronic cough patients. Diphenhydramine's antitussive effect is due to a central mechanism involving the medullary cough center. A peripheral action may also contribute to its effectiveness but further studies will be necessary to establish this point. (See Table 8 for dosage recommendations.)

The adverse effects associated with diphenhydramine hydrochloride are typical of other antihistamines. The most commonly encountered adverse effects are sedation and anticholinergic (atropine-like) effects. Because of these properties, diphenhydramine hydrochloride should not be taken by individuals in whom anticholinergics are contraindicated (those with narrow-angle glaucoma or prostatic hypertrophy) or in situations where mental alertness is required, such as driving a car.

Diphenhydramine should be used cautiously in individuals taking tranquilizers, sedatives, or hypnotics, because of its additive CNS depressant effect. Likewise, ingesting alcohol will have additive depressant effects, and caution must be exercised in taking diphenhydramine hydrochloride. Diphenhydramine hydrochloride should be used cautiously in patients taking other anticholinergic drugs because of additive effects (50). Diphenhydramine hydrochloride, like codeine and dextromethorphan hydrobromide, is a safe and effective antitussive but has a high likelihood of producing side effects, which must be kept in mind when recommending it.

Noscapine Noscapine is an opium alkaloid related to papaverine. Although it is used in only a few nonprescription preparations, its limited availability is not an indication of its effectiveness—it has been reported to reduce the frequency and severity of allergic cough (43, 46). Nevertheless, the FDA advisory review panel has suggested additional testing to establish its effectiveness (1). Noscapine's antitussive effectiveness is dose related, and although some investigators believe that it is equipotent on a weight basis to codeine, safe nonprescription adult dosages range from 15–30 mg every 4–6 hours, not to exceed 180 mg/day (Table 8).

Table 8. Antitussive dosage

| Drug | Dosage (maximum dose/24 hours) | | |
	Adults	Children 6 to <12 years	Children 2 to <6 years[a]
Codeine	10–20 mg every 4–6 hours (120 mg)	5–10 mg every 4–6 hours (60 mg)	2.5–5 mg every 4–6 hours (30 mg)
Dextromethorphan	10–20 mg every 4 hours or 30 mg every 6–8 hours (120 mg)	5–10 mg every 4 hours or 15 mg every 6–8 hours (60 mg)	2.5–5 mg every 4 hours or 7.5 mg every 6–8 hours (30 mg)
Diphenhydramine hydrochloride[b]	25 mg every 4 hours (150 mg)	12.5 mg every 4 hours (75 mg)	6.25 mg every 4 hours (37.5 mg)
Noscapine hydrochloride[c]	15–30 mg every 4–6 hours (180 mg)	7.5–15 mg every 4–6 hours (90 mg)	3.75–7.5 mg every 4–6 hours (45 mg)

The FDA advisory review panel on nonprescription cold, cough, allergy, bronchodilator, and antiasthmatic products has recommended all of these ingredients as safe and effective (Category I) except noscapine hydrochloride, for which there is insufficient evidence (Category III).

[a] There is no recommended dosage for children under 2 years of age except under the advice and supervision of a physician.
[b] Diphenhydramine, as a single-entity product, is not available without a prescription as of January 1, 1982.
[c] Category III, additional evidence of safety and effectiveness required.

In therapeutic doses, noscapine shows little or no effect on the CNS or respiratory system and has neither analgesic properties nor addictive liabilities. Constipation and other GI reactions have not been encountered to a significant degree. Noscapine is apparently safe at currently available nonprescription dosages, but effectiveness has yet to be proven.

The following ingredients may have antitussive properties but need to be tested for effectiveness.

- Beechwood creosote;
- Camphor (topical/inhalant);
- Caramiphen edisylate (ethanedisulfonate);
- Carbetapentane citrate;
- Cod liver oil;
- Elm bark;
- Ethylmorphine hydrochloride;
- Eucalyptol/eucalyptus oil (topical/inhalant);
- Horehound (horehound fluidextract);
- Menthol/peppermint oil (topical/inhalant);
- Thymol (topical/inhalant);
- Turpentine oil (spirits of turpentine) (topical/inhalant).

Oral Antibacterials and Anesthetics

A sore throat may indicate a more serious disease that demands medical attention (for example, streptococcal pharyngitis), and self-treatment may mask the symptoms. When the sore throat symptom is not related to environmental factors, to allergic rhinitis, or to a cold, a physician should be consulted. Failure to consult a physician may result in a worsening of the condition and development of complications. If the sore throat symptoms can be self-medicated, there are many products to choose from that are promoted for relief, but only those containing local anesthetics have any basis for effectiveness. Since most of these products are lozenges, sprays and mouthwashes, gargles, and throatwashes, effectiveness is limited to the mucous membranes of the oral tract which can be reached by the dosage form.

Antibacterial Agents

The primary purpose of a mouthwash is to cleanse and soothe. Most mouthwashes are promoted for bad breath with the suggestion that these products kill germs. The American Dental Association Council on Dental Therapeutics does not recognize substantial contributions to oral health from medicated mouthwashes (51). Much of the controversy surrounding the use of these products stems from the problems associated with substantiating germicidal or germistatic claims. There is no method that effectively compares the germicidal activity in the test tube with that in the oral cavity. There is also no adequate evidence that individuals benefit from a nonspecific change in the oral cavity flora; it is possible that alteration of the normal oral cavity flora actually may allow invasion by pathogenic organisms. In addition, most infectious sore throats are viral in origin, and using a lozenge or gargle promoted as an "antibacterial" does not influence the viral pharyngitis.

The antimicrobial substances in most commercial mouthwashes are phenols, alcohol, quaternary ammonium compounds, volatile oils, oxygenating agents, and iodine-containing preparations. These agents are believed to be of little value in treating sore throat symptoms.

Anesthetic Agents

A possible benefit of oral mouthwashes and gargles is derived from the anesthetic compounds they contain. These agents temporarily desensitize the sensory nerves in the pharyngeal mucosa, affording transient relief. The danger remains, however, in masking a symptom of a condition which may be harmful. Many commercially available lozenges also are promoted to treat sore throat symptoms. They usually contain an antibacterial agent in combination with a local anesthetic. The beneficial effect of this combination is probably caused by the anesthetic agent.

There is much controversy surrounding the effectiveness of the different anesthetic ingredients in lozenges and mouthwashes promoted for sore throats. The value and effectiveness of a local anesthetic agent usually are established by testing on human skin, oral mucosa, or tongue, not by pharyngeal tests. Consequently, patient satisfaction is probably the best indicator of these products' effectiveness until they meet the regulations being proposed by the FDA advisory review panel on nonprescription dentifrice and dental care drug products.

Benzocaine   Benzocaine is beneficial in diminishing sore throat symptoms in concentrations of 5–20%. Concentrations of less than 5% are not considered beneficial. There are currently no nonprescription preparations containing an effective benzocaine concentration.

Phenol and Phenol-Containing Salts   These agents are included in several nonprescription lozenges. They are effective in concentrations of 0.5–1.5%.

Benzyl Alcohol   Benzyl alcohol is an effective oral anesthetic agent used in concentrations of as much as 10%.

The pharmacist should recommend a product that contains an effective dose of a local anesthetic and a minimum of extraneous compounds, since their effectiveness or value is doubtful. Moreover, extraneous compounds may increase the risk of a hypersensitivity reaction. The pharmacist also should try to follow up on patient response to recommended agents for future suggestions as to alternative nonprescription therapy for pharyngeal soreness.

Anticholinergics

Some nonprescription cold remedies contain atropine or a mixture of belladonna alkaloids. The rationale for their inclusion is that their drying effect provides symptomatic relief from the "runny nose" associated with the cold and allergic rhinitis.

Although anticholinergics can dry excessive nasal secretions, the doses commonly found in nonprescription remedies (0.06–0.2 mg total alkaloids) have not been shown to accomplish this objective. To make up for this therapeutic shortcoming, these agents are usually found in products that also contain an antihistamine. The additive anticholinergic effect obtained from such a combination theoretically may help reduce secretions resulting from the common cold, but this claim remains to be proven for specific combinations. Such a combination exposes the patient to the antihistamine's unwanted sedative effects. It hardly seems rational to combine the therapeutic effect of one drug (in subtherapeutic amounts) with an unpredictable side effect of another in an attempt to achieve the effects obtainable with a larger (therapeutic) dose of the former.

Drug interactions involving anticholinergics are unlikely at the doses used in a cold or allergy remedy when no other ingredients are present that have anticholinergic effects. However, hypersensitivity to these relatively small amounts does occur. If a hypersensitive individual also suffers from narrow-angle glaucoma or enlarged prostate, a physician should be contacted before a preparation containing an anticholinergic is taken.

Pending further definitive dosage data, the anticholinergics available in nonprescription products should not be considered significant contributors to the relief of cold or allergy symptoms (1). Therefore their presence in a product should not be a criterion for product selection.

Antipyretics/Analgesics

In the common cold there is seldom an actual clinical fever. More often it is a feeling of warmth but with little or no temperature elevation. The usefulness of aspirin or acetaminophen lies in relieving the discomforts of generalized aches and pains or malaise associated with the viral infection. (See Chapter 11, *Internal Analgesic Products*.)

Ascorbic Acid (Vitamin C)

The claim that ascorbic acid is effective in preventing and treating the common cold is controversial. Linus Pauling, who popularized its use for the cold, recommends 1–5 g per day as a prophylactic measure and as much as 15 g per day to treat a cold (52). Many studies have been conducted, and although some have shown trends in favor of ascorbic acid's effectiveness, they have not shown the vitamin to be unequivocally effective in any dosage in either preventing colds or reducing their severity or duration (53, 54).

The potential for adverse effects associated with these large doses is also a debated issue. The most frequently noted adverse effect is diarrhea. Precipitation of urate, oxalate, or cystine stones in the urinary tract has been seen, although the potential for this problem increases with higher doses. The effects on the urinary excretion of other drugs also must be investigated because of ascorbic acid's ability to acidify the urine (55).

Urinary acidification increases the possibility of aminosalicylic acid crystalluria in patients receiving aminosalicylic acid in the free acid form. It also increases the excretion of drugs that are weak bases (e.g., amphetamines), reducing their effect, and increases renal tubular salicylate reabsorption, increasing serum salicylate concentrations. Ascorbic acid in doses large enough to acidify the urine (4–12 g/day) should not be given with aminosalicylic acid and should be used cautiously when salicylates are taken in large doses (3–5 g/day).

Ascorbic acid has been implicated in an interaction with warfarin in which the anticoagulant's hypoprothrombinemic effect was diminished (26, 39). Only isolated incidents were reported, however, and it is felt that the interaction either was dose dependent or occurred only in certain patients. Until further clarification is provided, practitioners should be aware of this possible interaction and inquire about ascorbic acid intake in patients who respond erratically to an anticoagulant. The possibility of an exaggerated hypoprothrombinemic response also must be kept in mind when these patients stop taking the vitamin.

Diabetic patients taking ascorbic acid and testing the urine by the glucose oxidase test may encounter false negative results; the copper reduction method may produce false positive results (39).

Adjunctive Therapy

Inhaling water vapor is an adjunctive therapeutic measure that provides a demulcent action on the respiratory mucosa and adds to and dilutes respiratory tract fluid, decreasing its viscosity (46). Humidifying the inspired air usually aids in relieving the cough and hoarseness associated with laryngitis. Humidification may be a prophylactic measure against upper respiratory infections when people are exposed to low relative humidities. This is usually the case during the winter months, when doors and windows are closed and the heat is on. With inspiration of dry air the mucus viscosity increases, and irritation of the respiratory mucosa may develop, creating a predisposition to viral or bacterial invasion. The relative humidity may be as low as 10% in the home on a cold day; 40–50% is necessary for comfort, and 60–80% is better for persons with respiratory problems. However, at this level, condensation on windows and walls is a limiting factor.

The oldest method of humidifying the air involves generating steam from a pot of boiling water or, more commonly, from an electric steam vaporizer. A newer method involves a cool mist vaporizer from which fine droplets of water are formed by pumping water through a fine screen. Therapeutically, the steam vaporizer does not seem to offer an advantage over the cool mist type. The cool mist vaporizers are safe in that they do not generate heat or hot water; however, they are noisier, and humidify somewhat more slowly than the steam vaporizers, they become quickly contaminated, and they may lower room temperature because the water particles absorb heat from the surrounding air, chilling the air and causing air saturation at a lower temperature. In one study, 24 hospitalized patients contracted systemic infections with *Acinetobacter calcoaceticus* during a 4-month period. Cold-air humidifiers at patients' bedsides were implicated as the source of infection in six. The outbreak was terminated with the removal of the humidifiers (56). It is important to follow the manufacturer's directions for cleaning the unit to avoid bacterial overgrowth (a problem not encountered with steam vaporizers). Steam vaporizers do not incur the hazards of contamination and do not lower room temperature.

If humidification is supplemented with a volatile substance (menthol or compound benzoin tincture), a steam vaporizer must be used. It has not been established whether these volatile substances are of therapeutic value, and therefore they may have no advantage over inhaling plain water vapor. In some cases they may even cause irritation of the respiratory tract and could be potentially dangerous if they reached high concentrations in a small enclosed room.

As an adjunctive measure, humidifying the inspired air is important. Either a steam-generated unit or a cool mist vaporizer may be used as prophylaxis and should be used at the cold's onset. It is also important to increase oral fluid intake to prevent dehydration during a cold.

Product Selection Guidelines

The effectiveness of many products available for self-medication of colds may be questionable, but they are generally safe when used as directed. Allergic rhinitis treatment provides comfort until the acute symptoms subside. Past experience may influence selection. Nevertheless, the pharmacist must be prepared to distinguish between the common cold and allergic rhinitis on the basis of symptoms, recognize complications that may arise or have arisen, and recommend the proper approaches for control of the symptoms (self-medication or consulting a physician), including drugs, adjunctive measures, and duration of treatment.

Patient Considerations

When symptoms usually associated with the common cold are present, recognizing the underlying disorder is not difficult. However, recognition of the allergic rhinitis condition is often more involved. In both conditions the pharmacist should conduct a brief but careful history of the present illness. This history should provide information useful in distinguishing one disorder from another and in identifying those disorders which should or should not be self-medicated. The following specific points should be investigated:

- Abruptness of onset;
- Symptomatology;
- Intensity;
- Duration;
- Recurrence.

Common cold onset generally is associated with a prodrome ("running nose" or dry throat); in fact, it is very common for people to predict that they are "coming down with a cold."

Early in a cold's development the symptoms are not very intense. As the infection runs its course, the symptoms may get worse, subject to patient variability and depending on the infecting organism. The intensity of symptoms in allergic rhinitis is based on the amount of allergen encountered and the degree of individual hypersensitivity. Generally, the symptoms are most intense following allergen exposure and subside over time unless additional exposures are encountered.

Duration of cold symptoms is a very important detail in deciding which course of action should be taken. Typically, the common cold lasts 4–7 days. If the problem persists beyond this time with no apparent improvement or if the cold symptoms tend to be recurrent, a physician should be consulted for an evaluation. Duration of allergic rhinitis symptoms is extremely variable, partially because of individual sensitivity to the allergen. If the patient has received no relief in 10 days of self-treatment, physician follow-up evaluation and proper management are indicated.

The recurrent nature of seasonal allergic rhinitis is a hallmark in differentiating this condition from other nonallergic respiratory conditions. The recurrence of symptoms often follows high pollen counts or patient activities that result in increased allergen exposure. If the symptomatology is present throughout the year or if it persists after the first killing frost, the condition may be perennial allergic rhinitis. Referral to a physician is desirable with perennial allergic rhinitis because of the prolonged duration of symptoms and the potential for developing complications.

Information on medications that have already been tried will aid the pharmacist not only in assessing the patient's current status but also in selecting a product. If, in the pharmacist's judgment, the measures were appropriate and were not effective, the patient should be encouraged to see a physician. If no medication was tried or if inadequate or inappropriate measures were taken, the pharmacist should recommend a more appropriate course of therapy. When a patient seeks the pharmacist's assistance in selecting a cold or allergy remedy, the pharmacist should question the individual as to the presence of other acute or chronic illnesses. This process may identify patients for whom certain preparations should be used cautiously, if at all.

Orally administered preparations containing sympathomimetics should be given only on the advice of a physician to patients with hyperthyroidism (the patient is already predisposed to tachycardia and arrhythmias), hypertension (especially moderate to severe, where additional peripheral vasoconstriction may cause significant blood pressure elevation), diabetes mellitus (especially in insulin-dependent diabetics and in cases where glycogenolysis may cause the diabetes to go out of control), and ischemic heart disease or angina (where an increase in heart rate may precipitate an acute angina attack and possibly a subsequent myocardial infarction). These concerns center primarily around the oral administration of sympathomimetic decongestants, where systemic effects are predictable. Judiciously administered decongestant drops, sprays, or inhalations provide a local intranasal action without significant concern of systemic absorption.

Theoretically, all of these effects may occur when the sympathomimetics reach the systemic circulation. In actual practice, however, the effect on a diabetic has not been a particular problem, except in an extremely unstable (brittle) diabetic. Should a diabetic patient take a liquid cough/cold preparation containing sugar? The syrup vehicle may contain as much as 85% (weight per volume) sucrose, and each gram of sucrose has about 4 cal (17 kcal/tsp). If 4 tsp (about 70 kcal) are taken in 1 day, the additional (nondietary) calories may be clinically significant in a brittle diabetic. Consequently, a sugar-free preparation is preferable. In a stable diabetic, however, these additional calories probably would be of little concern. (See Chapter 13, *Diabetes Care Products.*)

Another factor that pharmacists should take into consideration in dealing with a diabetic patient is the alcohol contained in the product. Alcohol, like sucrose, also will provide calories, more calories, in fact, than an equal weight of sucrose. Because most liquid cough remedies contain alcohol (1–25%, each gram providing about 7 kcal), it is clear that a brittle diabetic taking a "usual" dose might experience some difficulty with diabetes control.

Persons taking disulfiram also must be cautious of alcohol in cough syrups. The minimum amount necessary to trigger an adverse reaction has not been established.

The anticholinergic properties of antihistamines are usually not prominent in nonprescription preparations. However, the anticholinergic effects of atropine and other belladonna alkaloids in some allergy and cold remedies pose a potential problem. In cases of glaucoma or urinary retention secondary to prostatic hypertrophy, preparations containing anticholinergic agents and antihistamines, especially in combination, should be used only on a physician's advice.

The pharmacist should have a medication history to avoid possible drug interactions and to identify and avoid drug allergies or idiosyncrasies. In addition, a history of chronic topical nasal decongestant use may help identify rhinitis medicamentosa.

Product Considerations

In view of the number of cold and allergy products (single-entity and combinations) it is important that the pharmacist become familiar with a few preparations, especially those found safe and effective by FDA advisory review panels and those found empirically useful, and recommend these products preferentially. The pharmacist who recommends a nonprescription product needs to know what effect is sought, which drug entity will produce this effect, how much of the drug is necessary to produce this effect, and which nonprescription product satisfactorily meets these needs.

If only one effect is sought (nasal decongestion), a preparation with a single agent in a full therapeutic dose should be used. When more than one effect is desired, selection becomes more complex. Several single-entity products may be used, but this solution is not usually acceptable to the patient and a combination product will usually be preferable. The pharmacist should be selective in recommending a combination because many of these preparations are extreme examples of "shotgun therapy." One highly regarded medical text states that "the numerous compounded remedies, including those with vitamins, bioflavonoids, quinine, alkalinizers, multiple analgesics, antihistamines, decongestants, and tranquilizers, are developed for sales profit in a large market of uninformed and uncritical people" (4).

Combinations recommended by the FDA advisory review panels provide a reasonable basis for selection when directions for use are followed carefully.

The pharmacist should select a combination product containing the desired agents in full therapeutic doses, with as few additional ingredients as possible. This goal, however, seldom is achievable. The pharmacist must decide which effect is most important and select the combination on the basis of the agent that will produce this effect. For example, antihistamine efficacy in common cold treatment is doubtful, and this drawback is magnified by the subtherapeutic doses contained in some nonprescription remedies. An antihistamine-decongestant product therefore should be selected on the basis of the decongestant, with only secondary consideration being given to the antihistamine. Alternatively, the antihistamine is the important ingredient when selecting a product for allergic rhinitis.

There is no evidence that incorporating other ancillary agents or other ingredients of the same pharmacologic class in a subtherapeutic dose provides more relief or even as much relief as one agent in its full therapeutic dose. There is also no evidence that supports an increased efficacy when two or more antihistamines are combined within a product (57). The addition of a decongestant in sufficient dose to the antihistamine in the allergic rhinitis product is rational and may provide additional relief of symptoms.

Combination products containing analgesic/antipyretic agents generally should not be recommended. Their routine use carries the risk of masking a fever that may indicate a bacterial infection. Such agents should be administered separately and only when needed.

Similarly, preparations that do not disclose the amounts of ingredients on the package should not be recommended. It would be difficult for a pharmacist to justify recommending a product to ameliorate a symptom when there is no indication as to how much of the active ingredients the product contains.

In general, the use of timed-release preparations allows better patient compliance and increased patient convenience. However, some practitioners feel that these advantages may be outweighed by the fact that drug bioavailability in this dosage form may be neither uniform nor reliable. The pharmacist's recommendation of a timed-release preparation should be based on the presence of indicated agents in therapeutic doses and, in the pharmacist's experience, the product's success record.

There is much controversy concerning the advantages of oral nasal decongestants over the topical agents. Proponents of oral decongestants state that these agents can affect all respiratory membranes, that they are unaffected by the character of mucus, that they do not induce pathologic changes in the nasal mucosa, and that they relieve nasal obstruction without the additional irritation of locally applied medication.

There is also evidence to support the value of topically applied vasoconstrictors (58). Although nasal sprays and drops do not represent the ideal dosage form, they do provide rapid relief. Because the relief is so dramatic, the patient tends to overuse topical agents, risking drug-induced irritation of the nasal mucosa, alteration of the mucosal ciliary movement, and possibly rhinitis medicamentosa.

Combining topical therapy with oral decongestant therapy is also a controversial procedure. However, judicious use of an oral decongestant proven safe and effective along with a fast-acting topical agent presents a definite advantage. With this combination the patient experiences rapid relief from the topically applied decongestant and possibly a greater degree of relief through the systemic circulation from the oral agent if given in an adequate dose. Depending on the topical agent being used, a longer-lasting effect also is possible with this combined therapy.

Patient Consultation

In almost all cases of self-medication the pharmacist is the first and only knowledgeable professional contacted. If the pharmacist takes the time to identify the patient's problem and ensure proper product selection, advice regarding proper use also must be considered essential to fulfilling professional responsibility.

Patients cannot always be depended on to read and/or follow the package instructions. There is a tendency to believe in the philosophy that "if one is good, two are better." This is not always the case, however. Pharmacists should caution patients against increasing the dose and/or frequency of administration of any medication.

Even when antihistamines are taken in recommended amounts, they may cause transient drowsiness. Patients should be advised of this effect, especially if they are taking a prescription medication that also depresses the central nervous system. They should be advised as to the possible effects and should determine what effect the medication has on them before engaging in activities requiring mental alertness.

Nasal solutions may become contaminated. The pharmacist should recommend that the tip of the dropper or the spray applicator be rinsed in hot water after use, that only one person use the spray or drop applicator, and that the bottle or spray be discarded when the medication is no longer needed. Contamination of the nasal dropper also may be minimized by not touching the nose or the nasal surface with the dropper itself. In patients with allergic rhinitis, the presence of coughing, wheezing, tightness in chest (asthma), pain above the teeth, on the sides of the nose or around the eyes (sinusitis), and earache are all indications for medical advice. In addition, if nonprescription drugs are not markedly effective or if side effects are persistent even at reduced doses, the patient should consult a physician.

Nondrug measures (humidification, increased fluid intake, and local heat) may be recommended, and although these suggestions may not seem acceptable to the patient who desires a medication, they may be quite beneficial. The pharmacist's recommendation that the patient use humidification and/or increase fluid intake is in the patient's best interest. Normal saline gargles several times per day help relieve an inflamed throat, and the tepid water sponge bath with or without aspirin

or acetaminophen usually causes an elevated temperature to fall dramatically.

A cold usually lasts 7 days. The duration of therapy depends on which day in the course of the cold the medication is begun. If symptoms persist beyond the arbitrary, yet fairly reliable, 7-day limit in spite of adequate therapy, a physician should be consulted. If after 2–3 days of therapy the symptoms do not improve or become more intense, or if a fever, a very painful sore throat, or a cough productive of a mucopurulent sputum develops, the patient also should seek a physician's diagnosis.

It is important that the patient realize that a cold will resolve in spite of the medication and other measures recommended, that the medication is intended only to relieve discomfort, and that relief should occur in a week or less. The concern for duration of self-medication stems not only from the potential adverse effects of some medications but also from the minority of cold sufferers who may develop complications, such as secondary bacterial infections. If the pharmacist does not stipulate a time limit for therapy, patients may unknowingly continue self-medicating with little effect, prolonging their discomfort and delaying the time for a physician's diagnosis and appropriate treatment.

Product selection must be based not only on the presence of an effective agent in a therapeutic amount but also on underlying disorders that may be influenced adversely by the recommended therapy. Having chosen the product, the pharmacist must then ensure that the patient knows how to take the medication and what to expect from it with regard to symptomatic relief as well as adverse effects. The patient must be told for how long the medication should be taken. Realizing that questions may arise later, the pharmacist should encourage the patient to return or call back.

Summary

By evaluating the presenting symptoms the pharmacist usually can distinguish the common cold from disorders such as the flu or allergic rhinitis and offer proper suggestions for treatment. The pharmacist also can offer the allergic rhinitis sufferer medications to provide symptomatic relief. By conducting a careful history and recognizing the pertinent symptoms, a partial diminution of the symptoms may be achieved through advice and medication.

Recommendations for the common cold should be directed at relieving symptoms while those for allergic rhinitis should be directed at preventing symptoms. The pharmacist's endorsement of a shotgun remedy is irrational, since the intensity of symptoms will vary from hour to hour. Recommending a particular product is also irresponsible if the product contains agents in less than therapeutic amounts.

Common cold treatment objectives include reducing nasal secretions, opening congested nasal passages, reducing frequency of a cough, soothing a sore throat, overcoming the hoarseness of laryngitis, and relieving feverishness and headache. For allergic rhinitis the treatment is directed at blocking or competing with the effect of released histamine, relieving nasal congestion, and palliating secondary symptoms such as pharyngitis and headache. For nasal congestion, topically applied phenylephrine hydrochloride (0.25–0.5%) used every 4 hours if needed or oxymetazoline hydrochloride (0.05%) used twice per day if needed is very effective. To augment the effects of the topical decongestant, an oral nasal decongestant also may be recommended. Pseudoephedrine, 60 mg every 4 hours, or phenylpropanolamine, as much as 50 mg 3 times/day, is usually effective.

The very few oral nasal decongestants available as single-entity products should be recommended. Topically applied products should contain only the decongestant. For example, antihistamines add no beneficial effect to a topical decongestant preparation and may increase the likelihood of a hypersensitivity reaction. Oral antihistamines in combination with nasal decongestants may be indicated in allergic rhinitis.

The frequency of cough resulting from colds can usually be controlled by humidification of the inspired air (vaporizers), a demulcent/expectorant to the mucosa (hard candy or cough drop), and/or a cough suppressant (codeine or dextromethorphan). Humidification should be started early in the course of a cold and continued throughout. Products that contain a cough suppressant in combination with an expectorant should not be recommended. In the case of a dry cough, the dose of the cough suppressant is the criterion by which a product is selected. Productive coughs should not be treated with cough suppressants. Administration of 15 mg of codeine or dextromethorphan usually decreases the cough's frequency and intensity.

The dry, sore throat present in colds and to a lesser extent in allergic rhinitis may be relieved by dissolving a piece of hard candy in the mouth to stimulate saliva flow. Frequent warm normal saline gargles may relieve symptoms. Topical antibacterials for a viral infection or allergic rhinitis are unwarranted. Significant relief may be obtained from a lozenge or throat spray containing an anesthetic such as hexylresorcinol or phenol in sufficient concentration. A sore throat that is markedly sore and accompanied by swollen lymph nodes, fever, and constitutional symptoms may be caused by bacterial rather than viral infection. The patient should be directed to seek medical care for appropriate diagnostic tests and antimicrobial therapy. For nonbacterial pharyngitis, a sore throat product may be used for as long as the symptom persists.

Laryngitis may be managed by water vapor inhalation, by voice rest, and by avoiding inhaled irritants such as tobacco smoke. Dissolving lozenges in the mouth or gargling does little to reach the inflamed laryngeal tissues.

Relief from feverishness and headache may be provided by using an analgesic/antipyretic, either aspirin or acetaminophen. Products containing these agents in combination with several other ingredients are not recommended. Taking aspirin or acetaminophen regularly during the common cold or acute allergic rhinitis masks the possible development of a fever, which may indicate secondary bacterial infection. An antipyretic agent should be used to bring relief only as needed.

Antihistamines are effective in allergic rhinitis; their role in common cold treatment is at best only adjunctive by virtue of mild anticholinergic drying effects. Chlorpheniramine maleate, administered orally in doses of as much as 4 mg, is effective in the treatment of allergic rhinitis and only slightly sedative. There is marked individual variability to the different antihistamines. The pharmacist should be aware of this variability and should be prepared to suggest an alternative if relief is not obtained with the original agent. As with the nasal decongestants, most antihistamines are found in combination with other ingredients in commercial preparations and should not be recommended. The only rational combination for allergic rhinitis treatment is an oral antihistamine with an oral nasal decongestant. Other ingredients found in nonprescription products are of dubious efficacy.

The duration of therapy depends on when during the course of a cold the patient decides to start treatment. In any case, the patient should be able to stop treatment on the sixth or seventh day of the cold. Slight symptoms, such as cough, may persist for another day or so and, if necessary, should be treated.

The duration of treatment of allergic rhinitis should be limited to 3 days when topical nasal decongestants are used, in order to minimize the chances of rhinitis medicamentosa. Generally, oral decongestant therapy should be limited to 10 days. The patient's need of the oral agents for longer than 10 days may indicate the development of complications, and the patient should be referred to a physician. An antihistamine product may be used prophylactically in acute allergic rhinitis. The duration of antihistamine therapy should coincide with the appearance and disappearance of the particular allergen.

Patients who have a common cold or allergic rhinitis offer the pharmacist many opportunities to be involved. Although pharmacists often cannot counsel every cold and/or hay fever sufferer, they should be available on request and volunteer as other professional responsibilities permit.

References

1. *Federal Register, 41*, 38312 (1976).
2. A. C. Guyton, "Textbook of Medical Physiology," W. B. Saunders, Philadelphia, Pa., 1976, pp. 525–527.
3. I. Ziment, "Respiratory Pharmacology and Therapeutics," W. B. Saunders, Philadelphia, Pa., 1978, p. 44.
4. "Cecil-Loeb Textbook of Medicine," P. B. Beeson and W. McDermott, Eds., W. B. Saunders, Philadelphia, Pa., 1979, pp. 230–235.
5. A. G. Christie, "Infectious Disease—Epidemiology and Clinical Practice," Churchill Livingstone, New York, N.Y., 1974, pp. 316–318, 359–360, 363.
6. "Cecil's Textbook of Medicine," 15th ed., W. B. Saunders, Philadelphia, Pa., 1980, p. 231.
7. "Medical Notes on the Common Cold," Burroughs Wellcome, Research Triangle Park, N.C., 1972.
8. W. B. Pratt, "Fundamentals of Chemotherapy," Oxford University Press, New York, N.Y., 1972, p. 232.
9. *Journal of Pediatrics, 87*, 578–590 (1973).
10. "Current Medical Diagnosis and Treatment," M. A. Krupp and M. J. Chatton, Eds., Lange Medical, Los Altos, Calif., 1979, pp. 104–105.
11. R. W. Steele, P. T. Tanaka, R. P. Lara, and J. W. Bass, *J.*

Pediatr., 77, 824 (1970).

12. S. W. McFadden and J. E. Haddow, *Pediatrics, 43,* 622 (1969).
13. *Federal Register, 42,* 35346 (1977).
14. J. I. Tannenbaum, in "Allergic Diseases—Diagnosis and Management," R. Patterson, Ed., Lippincott, Philadelphia, Pa., 1972, pp. 161–195.
15. W. B. Sherman, "Hypersensitivity Mechanisms and Management," W. B. Saunders, Philadelphia, Pa., 1968.
16. J. M. O'Loughlin, *Drug Ther., 4,* 47 (April 1974).
17. P. M. Seebohm, *Postgrad. Med., 53,* 52 (1973).
18. J. A. Church, *Clin. Pediatr., 19,* 657 (1980).
19. L. Tuft, "Allergy Management in Clinical Practice," C. V. Mosby, St. Louis, Mo., 1973, pp. 185–238.
20. L. H. Criep, *J. Am. Med. Assoc., 166,* 572 (1965).
21. "Basic Pharmacology in Medicine," J. R. DiPalma, Ed., McGraw-Hill, New York, N.Y., 1976, pp. 280–290.
22. "International Encyclopedia of Pharmacology and Therapeutics," Vol. I, Section 74, M. Schachter, Ed., Pergamon, New York, N.Y., 1973, p. 127.
23. "The Pharmacological Basis of Therapeutics," A. G. Gilman, L. Goodman, and A. Gilman, Eds., Macmillan, New York, N.Y., 1980, pp. 610–614, 626–627.
24. "AMA Drug Evaluations," 4th ed., American Medical Association, Chicago, Ill., 1980, pp. 438, 441, 452, 453, 468, 474.
25. L. Schaaf, L. Hendeles, and M. Weinberger, *J. Allergy Clin. Immunol., 63,* 129 (1979).
26. "Evaluations of Drug Interactions," 2nd ed., American Pharmaceutical Association, Washington, D.C., 1976.
27. "Manual of Medical Therapeutics," 22nd ed., Little, Brown, Boston, Mass., 1977, p. 157.
28. B. J. Thack, T. N. Chase, and J. F. Basma, *N. Engl. J. Med., 293,* 486–487 (1975).
29. *American Journal of Hospital Pharmacy, 33,* 1200–1207 (1976).
30. *Medical Journal of Australia, 1,* 112–113 (1978).
31. *Drugs, 12,* 258–273 (1976).
32. "Drill's Pharmacology in Medicine," J. R. DiPalma, Ed., McGraw-Hill, New York, N.Y., 1971, p. 655.
33. *Federal Register, 41,* 38397 (1976).
34. D. M. Aviado, "Sympathomimetic Drugs," Charles C Thomas, Springfield, Ill., 1970, pp. 282, 288, 382.
35. E. W. Martin, "Techniques of Medication," Lippincott, Philadelphia, Pa., 1979, p. 91.
36. J. T. Connell, *Ann. Allergy, 27,* 541 (1969).
37. G. Aschan and B. Drettner, *Eye Ear Nose Throat Mon., 43,* 66 (1964).
38. *Federal Register, 41,* 38398 (1976).
39. P. D. Hansten, "Drug Interactions," Lea and Febiger, Philadelphia, Pa., 1979.
40. *Federal Register, 41,* 38370 (1976).
41. S. R. Hirsch, *Drug Ther., 5,* 179 (1975).
42. C. J. Polson and R. N. Tattersall, "Clinical Toxicology," Lippincott, Philadelphia, Pa., 1969, p. 92.
43. "The United States Dispensatory," 27th ed., A. Osol and R. Pratt, Eds., Lippincott, Philadelphia, Pa., 1973, pp. 354, 571, 794, 947.
44. *Chest, 63,* 9 (1973).
45. *Journal of Pediatrics, 89,* 653 (1976).
46. "Drugs of Choice, 1980/1981," W. Modell, Ed., C. V. Mosby, St. Louis, Mo., 1980, pp. 450–465.
47. *Federal Register, 41,* 38339 (1976).
48. Committee on Drugs, American Academy of Pediatrics, *Pediatrics, 62,* 118–122 (1978).
49. *Federal Register, 41,* 52536 (1976).
50. Parke, Davis, and Company, package literature.
51. "Accepted Dental Therapeutics," 38th ed., American Dental Association, Chicago, Ill., 1979.
52. L. Pauling, "Vitamin C and the Common Cold," Freeman, San Francisco, Calif., 1970.
53. *Medical Letter on Drugs and Therapeutics, 16,* 85 (1974).
54. J. L. Coulehan, *Postgrad. Med., 66,* 153–160 (1979).
55. *Medical Letter on Drugs and Therapeutics, 12,* 105 (1970).
56. P. W. Smith and R. M. Massanari, *J. Am. Med. Assoc., 237,* 795 (1977).
57. L. Hendeles, M. Weinberger, and L. Wong, *Am. J. Hosp. Pharm., 37,* 1496 (1980).
58. *Annals of Otology, Larngology, and Rhinology, 86,* 310–317 (1977).

Antitussive Product Table

Product[a] (Manufacturer)	Cough Suppressant	Expectorant	Sympatho-mimetics	Antihistamine	Other Ingredients
Actol Expectorant (Beecham Labs)	noscapine, 6 mg/ml	guaifenesin, 40 mg/ml			alcohol, 12.5% fruit flavoring
Alamine (North American)			phenylpropanolamine hydrochloride, 3.75 mg/ml	chlorpheniramine maleate, 0.4 mg/ml	alcohol, 5% green mint flavor
Alamine-C (North American)	codeine phosphate[b], 2 mg/ml		phenylpropanolamine hydrochloride, 3.75 mg/ml	chlorpheniramine maleate, 0.4 mg/ml	alcohol, 5% grape flavor
Alamine Expectorant (North American)	codeine phosphate[b], 2 mg/ml	guaifenesin, 20 mg/ml	phenylpropanolamine hydrochloride, 3.75 mg/ml		menthol, 0.2 mg/ml alcohol, 7.5% grape flavor
Alo-Tuss Tablets (North American)	dextromethorphan hydrobromide, 10 mg		phenylephrine hydrochloride, 5 mg	chlorpheniramine maleate, 2 mg	salicylamide, 2.27 mg phenacetin, 100 mg caffeine, 10 mg
Ambenyl-D (Marion)	dextromethorphan hydrobromide, 3 mg/ml	guaifenesin, 20 mg/ml	pseudoephedrine hydrochloride, 6 mg/ml		alcohol, 9.5% sucrose, 47%
Amonidrin Tablets (O'Neal, Jones & Feldman)		ammonium chloride, 200 mg guaifenesin, 100 mg			
Baby Cough Syrup (DeWitt)		ammonium chloride, 4.43 mg/ml			glycerin, 68.6 mg/ml licorice extract, 0.43 mg/ml
Bayer Cough Syrup for Children (Glenbrook)	dextromethorphan hydrobromide, 1.5 mg/ml		phenylpropanolamine hydrochloride, 1.8 mg/ml		alcohol, 5%
Benylin (Parke-Davis)	diphenhydramine hydrochloride, 2.5 mg/ml				alcohol, 5%
Benylin DM (Parke-Davis)	dextromethorphan hydrobromide, 2 mg/ml				alcohol, 5% ammonium chloride, 25 mg/ml sodium citrate, 10 mg/ml
Breacol (Glenbrook)	dextromethorphan hydrobromide, 2 mg/ml		phenylpropanolamine hydrochloride, 7.5 mg/ml	chlorpheniramine maleate, 0.8 mg/ml	alcohol, 10%
C3 Capsules (Menley & James)	dextromethorphan hydrobromide, 30 mg		phenylpropanolamine hydrochloride, 50 mg	chlorpheniramine maleate, 4 mg	
Cerose DM[c] (Ives)	dextromethorphan hydrobromide, 2 mg/ml	potassium guaiacolsulfonate, 17.2 mg/ml ipecac fluidextract, 0.034 mg/ml	phenylephrine hydrochloride, 1 mg/ml	phenindamine tartrate, 1 mg/ml	sodium citrate, 39 mg/ml citric acid, 13 mg/ml alcohol, 2.5%

Antitussive Product Table, continued

Product[a] (Manufacturer)	Cough Suppressant	Expectorant	Sympatho-mimetics	Antihistamine	Other Ingredients
Cetro-Cirose[c] (Ives)	codeine phosphate[b], 1 mg/ml	potassium guaiacolsulfonate, 17.2 mg/ml ipecac fluidextract, 0.034 mg/ml			sodium citrate, 39 mg/ml citric acid, 13 mg/ml alcohol, 1.5%
Cheracol (Upjohn)	codeine phosphate[b], 2 mg/ml	guaifenesin, 20 mg/ml			alcohol, 3%
Cheracol D (Upjohn)	dextromethorphan hydrobromide, 2 mg/ml	guaifenesin, 20 mg/ml			alcohol, 3%
Chlor-Trimeton Expectorant (Schering)		ammonium chloride, 20 mg/ml guaifenesin, 10 mg/ml	phenylephrine hydrochloride, 2 mg/ml	chlorpheniramine maleate, 0.4 mg/ml	sodium citrate, 10 mg/ml alcohol, 1%
Chlor-Trimeton Expectorant with Codeine (Schering)	codeine phosphate[b], 2 mg/ml	ammonium chloride, 20 mg/ml guaifenesin, 10 mg/ml	phenylephrine hydrochloride, 2 mg/ml	chlorpheniramine maleate, 0.4 mg/ml	sodium citrate, 10 mg/ml alcohol, 5.25%
Codimal DM[c] (Central)	dextromethorphan hydrobromide, 2 mg/ml	potassium guaiacolsulfonate, 16.66 mg/ml	phenylephrine hydrochloride, 1 mg/ml	pyrilamine maleate, 1.66 mg/ml	sodium citrate, 43.2 mg/ml citric acid, 10 mg/ml alcohol, 4%
Codimal Expectorant (Central)		potassium guaiacolsulfonate, 20 mg/ml	phenylpropanolamine hydrochloride, 5 mg/ml		sodium citrate, 43.2 mg/ml citric acid, 10 mg/ml
Codimal PH (Central)	codeine phosphate[b], 2 mg/ml	potassium guaiacolsulfonate, 16.66 mg/ml	phenylephrine hydrochloride, 1 mg/ml	pyrilamine maleate, 1.66 mg/ml	sodium citrate, 43.2 mg/ml citric acid, 10 mg/ml
Colrex[c] (Rowell)	dextromethorphan hydrobromide, 2 mg/ml		phenylephrine hydrochloride, 1 mg/ml	chlorpheniramine maleate, 0.4 mg/ml	cherry flavor alcohol, 4.5%
Colrex Expectorant[c] (Rowell)		guaifenesin, 20 mg/ml			alcohol, 4.7% butterscotch mint flavor
Conar[c] (Beecham Labs)	noscapine, 3 mg/ml		phenylephrine hydrochloride, 2 mg/ml		mint flavor
Conar Expectorant (Beecham Labs)	noscapine, 3 mg/ml	guaifenesin, 20 mg/ml	phenylephrine hydrochloride, 2 mg/ml		orange flavor
Conex (O'Neal, Jones & Feldman)		guaifenesin, 10 mg/ml	phenylpropanolamine hydrochloride, 2.5 mg/ml	chlorpheniramine maleate, 0.4 mg/ml	methylparaben, 0.13% propylparaben, 0.03%
Conex with Codeine (O'Neal, Jones & Feldman)	codeine phosphate[b], 2 mg/ml	guaifenesin, 10 mg/ml	phenylpropanolamine hydrochloride, 2.5 mg/ml	chlorpheniramine maleate, 0.4 mg/ml	methylparaben, 0.13% propylparaben, 0.03%

Antitussive Product Table, continued

Product[a] (Manufacturer)	Cough Suppressant	Expectorant	Sympatho mimetics	Antihistamine	Other Ingredients
Consotuss (Merrell-Dow)	dextromethorphan hydrobromide, 3 mg/ml			doxylamine succinate, 0.75 mg/ml	alcohol, 10%
Coricidin (Schering)	dextromethorphan hydrobromide, 2 mg/ml	guaifenesin, 20 mg/ml	phenylpropanolamine hydrochloride, 2.5 mg/ml		
Coryban-D[c] (Pfipharmecs)	dextromethorphan hydrobromide, 1.5 mg/ml	guaifenesin, 10 mg/ml	phenylephrine hydrochloride, 1 mg/ml		alcohol, 7.5% acetaminophen, 24 mg/ml
Coryzex Capsules (Vitarine)	dextromethorphan hydrobromide, 10 mg		phenylpropanolamine hydrochloride, 12.1 mg	chlorpheniramine maleate, 1 mg	citric acid, 4 mg
Cosanyl DM Improved Formula (Health Care Industries)	dextromethorphan hydrobromide, 3 mg/ml		*d*-pseudoephedrine hydrochloride, 6 mg/ml		alcohol, 6% peach flavor
Cosanyl Improved Formula (Health Care Industries)	codeine phosphate[b], 2 mg/ml		pseudoephedrine hydrochloride, 6 mg/ml		alcohol, 6% sucrose, 325 mg/ml
Cotussis (Merrell-Dow)	codeine phosphate[b], 2 mg/ml	terpin hydrate, 4 mg/ml			alcohol, 20%
DayCare Capsules (Vicks)	dextromethorphan hydrobromide, 10 mg		phenylpropanolamine hydrochloride, 12.5 mg		acetaminophen, 325 mg
DayCare Liquid (Vicks)	dextromethorphan hydrobromide, 0.67 mg/ml		phenylpropanolamine hydrochloride, 0.83 mg/ml		acetaminophen, 20 mg/ml
Dimacol Liquid and Capsules (Robins)	dextromethorphan hydrobromide, 3 mg/ml 15 mg/capsule	guaifenesin, 20 mg/ml 100 mg/capsule	pseudoephedrine hydrochloride, 6 mg/ml 30 mg/capsule		alcohol, 4.75% (liquid)
Dondril Anticough Tablets (Whitehall)	dextromethorphan hydrobromide, 10 mg		phenylephrine hydrochloride, 5 mg	chlorpheniramine maleate, 1 mg	
Dorcol Pediatric Cough Syrup (Dorsey)	dextromethorphan hydrobromide, 1.0 mg/ml	guaifenesin, 10 mg/ml	phenylpropanolamine hydrochloride, 1.25 mg/ml		alcohol, 5%
Dr. Drake's (Roberts)		ipecac fluidextract			alcohol, 2.25% castor oil glycerin benzoic acid camphor gum arabic anise oil
Dristan Cough Formula (Whitehall)	dextromethorphan hydrobromide, 1.5 mg/ml	guaifenesin, 6 mg/ml	phenylephrine hydrochloride, 1 mg/ml	chlorpheniramine maleate, 0.2 mg/ml	
Efricon (Lannett)	codeine phosphate[b], 2.19 mg/ml	ammonium chloride, 18 mg/ml potassium guaiacolsulfonate, 18 mg/ml	phenylephrine hydrochloride, 1 mg/ml	chlorpheniramine maleate, 0.4 mg/ml	sodium citrate, 12 mg/ml banana flavor

Antitussive Product Table, continued

Product[a] (Manufacturer)	Cough Suppressant	Expectorant	Sympatho-mimetics	Antihistamine	Other Ingredients
Endotussin-NN (Endo)	dextromethorphan hydrobromide, 2 mg/ml	ammonium chloride, 8 mg/ml		pyrilamine maleate, 1.5 mg/ml	alcohol, 4%
Endotussin-NN Pediatric (Endo)	dextromethorphan hydrobromide, 1 mg/ml	ammonium chloride, 12 mg/ml			alcohol, 4%
Fedahist Expectorant (Dooner/Rorer)		guaifenesin, 20 mg/ml	pseudoephedrine hydrochloride, 6 mg/ml	chlorpheniramine maleate, 0.4 mg/ml	
Fedahist Syrup and Tablets (Dooner/Rorer)			pseudoephedrine hydrochloride, 6 mg/ml, 60 mg/tablet	chlorpheniramine maleate, 0.4 mg/ml, 4 mg/tablet	
Formula 44 Cough Control Discs (Vicks)	dextromethorphan hydrobromide, 5 mg				benzocaine, 1.25 mg menthol anethole peppermint oil } 0.35%
Formula 44 Cough Mixture (Vicks)	dextromethorphan hydrobromide, 1.5 mg/ml			doxylamine succinate, 0.75 mg/ml	alcohol, 10% sodium citrate, 50 mg/ml
Formula 44-D (Vicks)	dextromethorphan hydrobromide, 2 mg/ml	guaifenesin, 10 mg/ml	phenylpropanolamine hydrochloride, 2.4 mg/ml		alcohol, 20%
2/G (Dow)		guaifenesin, 20 mg/ml			alcohol, 3.5% corn derivatives
2/G-DM (Dow)	dextromethorphan hydrobromide, 3 mg/ml	guaifenesin, 20 mg/ml			alcohol, 5% corn derivatives
GG-Cen Capsules and Syrup (Central Pharmacal)		guaifenesin, 200 mg/capsule 20 mg/ml			alcohol, 10% (syrup)
G G Tussin (Vitarine)		guaifenesin, 20 mg/ml			alcohol, 3.5%
G-Tussin DM (Columbia)	dextromethorphan hydrobromide, 3 mg/ml	guaifenesin, 20 mg/ml			alcohol, 1.4%
Halls (Warner-Lambert)	dextromethorphan hydrobromide, 1.5 mg/ml		phenylpropanolamine hydrochloride, 3.75 mg/ml		alcohol, 22% menthol eucalyptus oil glycerin
Histadyl EC (Lilly)	codeine phosphate[b], 2 mg/ml	ammonium chloride, 22 mg/ml	ephedrine hydrochloride, 1 mg/ml	chlorpheniramine maleate, 0.4 mg/ml	alcohol, 5% menthol, 0.13 mg/ml
Hytuss Tablets[c] (Hyrex)		guaifenesin, 100 mg			
Hytuss 2X Capsules (Hyrex)		guaifenesin, 200 mg			

Antitussive Product Table, continued

Product[a] (Manufacturer)	Cough Suppressant	Expectorant	Sympatho-mimetics	Antihistamine	Other Ingredients
Kiddies Pediatric (Vitarine)		potassium guaiacolsulfonate, 5.83 mg/ml ammonium chloride, 5.83 mg/ml			alcohol, 2% cocillana bark extract menthol, 0.02 mg/ml wild cherry flavor sucrose, 360 mg/ml
Kleer Chewable Tablets (Scrip)	dextromethorphan hydrobromide, 2.5 mg		phenylephrine hydrochloride, 5 mg	chlorpheniramine maleate, 2 mg	
Kolephrin GG/DM (Pfeiffer)	dextromethorphan hydrobromide, 3 mg/ml	guaifenesin, 30 mg/ml			sucrose, 226 mg/ml
Kolephrin Non-Narcotic (Pfeiffer)	dextromethorphan hydrobromide, 1.5 mg/ml		phenylephrine hydrochlorife, 1 mg/ml	pyrilamine maleate, 2 mg/ml	sodium salicylate, 65 mg/ml sucrose, 340 mg/ml
Kolephrin with Codeine (Pfeiffer)	codeine phosphate[b], 1.5 mg/ml		phenylephrine hydrochloride, 1 mg/ml	pyrilamine maleate, 2 mg/ml	sodium salicylate, 65 mg/ml sucrose, 340 mg/ml
Kophane Syrup (Pfeiffer)	dextromethorphan hydrobromide, 2 mg/ml	ammonium chloride, 18 mg/ml	phenylpropanolamine hydrochloride, 1 mg/ml	chlorpheniramine maleate, 0.1 mg/ml	sucrose, 340 mg/ml
Lanatuss[c] (Lannett)		guaifenesin, 20 mg/ml	phenylpropanolamine hydrochloride, 1 mg/ml	chlorpheniramine maleate, 0.4 mg/ml	sodium citrate, 39.4 mg/ml citric acid, 12 mg/ml
Mercodol with Decapryn (Merrell-Dow)	codeine phosphate[b], 2 mg/ml		phenylephrine hydrochloride, 1 mg/ml etafedrine hydrochloride, 2 mg/ml	doxylamine succinate, 1.2 mg/ml	alcohol, 5% sucrose, 600 mg/ml calories, 3/ml
Naldecon CX (Bristol)	codeine phosphate[b], 2 mg/ml	guaifenesin, 40 mg/ml	phenylpropanolamine hydrochloride, 3.6 mg/ml		
Naldecon DX (Bristol)	dextromethorphan hydrobromide, 1.5 mg/ml	guaifenesin, 20 mg/ml	phenylpropanolamine hydrochloride, 1.8 mg/ml		alcohol, 5%
Naldecon EX (Bristol)		guaifenesin, 30 mg/ml	phenylpropanolamine hydrochloride, 9 mg/ml		alcohol, 0.6%
Naldetuss (Bristol)	dextromethorphan hydrobromide, 3 mg/ml		phenylpropanolamine hydrochloride, 3.5 mg/ml	phenyltoloxamine citrate, 1.5 mg/ml	acetaminophen, 32.4 mg/ml sucrose, 620 mg/ml

Antitussive Product Table, continued

Product[a] (Manufacturer)	Cough Suppressant	Expectorant	Sympatho-mimetics	Antihistamine	Other Ingredients
N-N Cough Syrup (Vitarine)	dextromethorphan hydrobromide, 2 mg/ml	potassium guaiacolsulfonate, 13 mg/ml ammonium chloride, 13 mg/ml		chlorpheniramine maleate, 0.1 mg/ml	alcohol, 5% glycerin menthol sucrose, 360 mg/ml wild cherry flavor
Noratuss (North American)	codeine phosphate[b], 0.67 mg/ml	ammonium chloride, 6.48 mg/ml potassium guaiacolsulfonate, 1.08 mg/ml terpin hydrate, 1.08 mg/ml			cocillana extract, 0.89 mg/ml sodium benzoate, 0.1% cherry flavor
Nortussin (North American)		guaifenesin, 20 mg/ml			alcohol, 3.5% cherry flavor
Novahistine Cough Formula (Dow)	dextromethorphan hydrobromide, 5 mg/ml	guaifenesin, 20 mg/ml			alcohol, 7.5%
Novahistine Cough and Cold Formula (Dow)	dextromethorphan hydrobromide, 5 mg/ml		pseudoephedrine hydrochloride, 15 mg/ml	chlorpheniramine maleate, 1 mg/ml	alcohol, 5%
Novahistine DH (Dow)	codeine phosphate[b], 2 mg/ml		phenylpropanolamine hydrochloride, 3.75 mg/ml	chlorpheniramine maleate, 0.4 mg/ml	alcohol, 5% calories, 2.3/ml
Novahistine DMX (Dow)	dextromethorphan hydrobromide, 2 mg/ml	guaifenesin, 20 mg/ml	pseudoephedrine hydrochloride, 6 mg/ml		alcohol, 10% calories, 3.2/ml
Novahistine Expectorant (Dow)	codeine phosphate[b], 2 mg/ml	guaifenesin, 20 mg/ml	phenylpropanolamine hydrochloride, 3.75 mg/ml	chlorpheniramine maleate, 0.4 mg/ml	alcohol, 7.5%
Ornacol Capsules and Liquid (Menley & James)	dextromethorphan hydrobromide, 30 mg/capsule		phenylpropanolamine hydrochloride, 25 mg/capsule		
Orthoxicol (Upjohn)	dextromethorphan hydrobromide, 2 mg/ml		methoxyphenamine hydrochloride, 3.4 mg/ml		sucrose, 600 mg/ml calories, 3/ml
Pediaqull (Philips Roxane)		guaifenesin, 10 mg/ml	phenylephrine hydrochloride, 0.5 mg/ml		alcohol, 5% sorbitol, 15% corn syrup, 30% currant and caramel flavors
Pertussin 8-Hour Cough Formula (Chesebrough-Pond)	dextromethorphan hydrobromide, 1.5 mg/ml				alcohol, 9.5% sucrose, 385 mg/ml calories, 2.6/ml
Pertussin Cough Syrup for Children (Chesebrough-Pond)	dextromethorphan hydrobromide, 0.7 mg/ml	guaifenesin, 5 mg/ml			alcohol, 8.5%

Antitussive Product Table, continued

Product[a] (Manufacturer)	Cough Suppressant	Expectorant	Sympatho-mimetics	Antihistamine	Other Ingredients
Pinex Regular & Concentrate (Roberts)	dextromethorphan hydrobromide				alcohol, 3% (reg.) alcohol, 16% (conc.) honey glycerin sucrose
Prunicodeine[c] (Lilly)	codeine sulfate[b], 2 mg/ml	terpin hydrate, 5.83 mg/ml			alcohol, 25% wild cherry white pine sanguinaria
Quelidrine (Abbott)	dextromethorphan hydrobromide, 2 mg/ml	ammonium chloride, 8 mg/ml ipecac fluidextract, 0.001 ml/ml	ephedrine hydrochloride, 1 mg/ml phenylephrine hydrochloride, 1 mg/ml	chlorpheniramine maleate, 0.4 mg/ml	alcohol, 2%
Queltuss Tablets (O'Neal, Jones & Feldman)	dextromethorphan hydrobromide, 15 mg	guaifenesin, 100 mg			
Quiet-Nite (Rexall)	dextromethorphan hydrobromide, 0.5 mg/ml		ephedrine sulfate, 0.33 mg/ml	chlorpheniramine maleate, 0.06 mg/ml	acetaminophen, 20 mg/ml alcohol, 25%
Robitussin (Robins)		guaifenesin, 20 mg/ml			alcohol, 3.5%
Robitussin A-C (Robins)	codeine phosphate[b], 2 mg/ml	guaifenesin, 20 mg/ml			alcohol, 3.5%
Robitussin-CF (Robins)	codeine phosphate[b], 2 mg/ml	guaifenesin, 20 mg/ml	phenylpropanolamine hydrochloride, 2.5 mg/ml		alcohol, 1.4%
Robitussin DAC (Robins)	codeine phosphate[b], 2 mg/ml	guaifenesin, 20 mg/ml	pseudoephedrine hydrochloride, 6 mg/ml		alcohol, 1.4%
Robitussin-DM (Robins)	dextromethorphan hydrobromide, 3 mg/ml	guaifenesin, 20 mg/ml			alcohol, 1.4%
Robitussin-PE (Robins)		guaifenesin, 20 mg/ml	pseudoephedrine hydrochloride, 6 mg/ml		alcohol, 1.4% sucrose, 714 mg/ml
Romilar III (Block)	dextromethorphan hydrobromide, 1 mg/ml		phenylpropanolamine hydrochloride, 2.5 mg/ml		alcohol, 20% flavor
Romilar Capsules (Block)	dextromethorphan hydrobromide, 15 mg		phenylephrine hydrochloride, 5 mg	chlorpheniramine maleate, 1 mg	acetaminophen, 120 mg
Romilar CF (Block)	dextromethorphan hydrobromide, 3 mg/ml	ammonium chloride, 1%			alcohol, 20% flavor
Romilar Children's (Block)	dextromethorphan hydrobromide, 0.5 mg/ml				sodium citrate citric acid grape flavor

Antitussive Product Table, continued

Product[a] (Manufacturer)	Cough Suppressant	Expectorant	Sympatho-mimetics	Antihistamine	Other Ingredients
Ryna-C[c] (Wallace)	codeine phosphate[b], 2 mg/ml		pseudoephedrine hydrochloride, 6 mg/ml	chlorpheniramine maleate, 0.4 mg/ml	
Ryna-CX[c] (Wallace)	codeine phosphate[b], 2 mg/ml	guaifenesin, 20 mg/ml	pseudoephedrine hydrochloride, 6 mg/ml		
Silexin Cough Syrup and Tablets (Otis Clapp)	dextromethorphan hydrobromide	guaifenesin (syrup)			benzocaine (tablet)
Sorbutuss[c] (Dalin)	dextromethorphan hydrobromide, 2 mg/ml	guaifenesin, 20 mg/ml ipecac fluidextract, 0.0006 ml/ml			potassium citrate, 17 mg/ml citric acid, 7 mg/ml mint flavor glycerin-sorbitol vehicle
St. Joseph Cough Syrup for Children (Plough)	dextromethorphan hydrobromide, 1.5 mg/ml				alcohol, 0.38% sodium citrate menthol
Sudafed Cough Syrup (Burroughs Wellcome)	dextromethorphan hydrobromide, 2 mg/ml	guaifenesin, 20 mg/ml	pseudoephedrine hydrochloride, 6 mg/ml		alcohol, 2.4% sucrose, 640 mg/ml
Supercitin[c] (Vitarine)	dextromethorphan hydrobromide, 2 mg/ml			chlorpheniramine maleate, 0.2 mg/ml	acetaminophen, 12 mg/ml sorbitol
Toclonol Expectorant[c] (Cenci)	carbetapentane citrate, 1.5 mg/ml	terpin hydrate, 3.33 mg/ml			alcohol, 7.2% sodium citrate, 13.23 mg/ml citric acid, 1.33 mg/ml glycerin, 0.56 ml/ml menthol, 0.166 mg/ml
Tolu-Sed[c] (First Texas)	codeine phosphate[b], 2 mg/ml	guaifenesin, 20 mg/ml			alcohol, 10%
Tolu-Sed DM[c] (First Texas)	dextromethorphan hydrobromide, 2 mg/ml	guaifenesin, 20 mg/ml			alcohol, 10%
Tonecol (A.V.P.)	dextromethorphan hydrobromide, 2 mg/ml	guaifenesin, 5 mg/ml	phenylephrine hydrochloride, 1 mg/ml	chlorpheniramine maleate, 0.2 mg/ml	alcohol, 7% sodium citrate, 3 mg/ml cherry flavor
Triaminic Expectorant (Dorsey)		guaifenesin, 20 mg/ml	phenylpropanolamine hydrochloride, 2.5 mg/ml	pheniramine maleate, 1.25 mg/ml pyrilamine maleate, 1.25 mg/ml	alcohol, 5%
Triaminic Expectorant with Codeine (Dorsey)	codeine phosphate[b], 2 mmg/ml	guaifenesin, 20 mg/ml	phenylpropanolamine hydrochloride, 2.5 mg/ml	pheniramine maleate, 1.25 mg/ml pyrilamine maleate, 1.25 mg/ml	alcohol, 5%

Antitussive Product Table, continued

Product[a] (Manufacturer)	Cough Suppressant	Expectorant	Sympatho-mimetics	Antihistamine	Other Ingredients
Triaminicol (Dorsey)	dextromethorphan hydrobromide, 3 mg/ml	ammonium chloride, 18 mg/ml	phenylpropanolamine hydrochloride, 2.5 mg/ml	pheniramine maleate, 1.25 mg/ml pyrilamine maleate, 1.25 mg/ml	
Tricodene Forte (Pfeiffer)	dextromethorphan hydrobromide, 2 mg/ml		phenylpropanolamine hydrochloride, 2.5 mg/ml	chlorpheniramine maleate, 0.4 mg/ml	sucrose, 600 mg/ml
Tricodene #1 (Pfeiffer)	codeine phosphate[b], 1.6 mg/ml			pyrilamine maleate, 0.83 mg/ml	sucrose, 333 mg/ml
Tricodene #2 (Pfeiffer)	codeine phosphate[b], 1.1 mg/ml			pyrilamine maleate, 0.83 mg/ml	sucrose, 330 mg/ml
Tricodene Pediatric (Pfeiffer)	dextromethorphan hydrobromide; 2 mg/ml		phenylpropanolamine hydrochloride, 2.5 mg/ml		sucrose, 600 mg/ml
Tricodene Sugar Free Syrup[c] (Pfeiffer)	dextromethorphan hydrobromide, 2 mg/ml	ammonium chloride, 18 mg/ml		chlorpheniramine maleate, 0.1 mg/ml	
Trind-DM (Mead Johnson)	dextromethorphan hydrobromide, 1.5 mg/ml		phenylpropanolamine hydrochloride, 2.5 mg/ml	chlorpheniramine maleate, 0.4 mg/ml	alcohol, 5%
Tussagesic Suspension (Dorsey)	dextromethorphan hydrobromide, 3 mg/ml	terpin hydrate, 18 mg/ml	phenylpropanolamine hydrochloride, 2.5 mg/ml	pheniramine maleate, 1.25 mg/ml pyrilamine maleate, 1.25 mg/ml	acetaminophen, 24 mg/ml
Tussagesic Tablets (Dorsey)	dextromethorphan hydrobromide, 30 mg	terpin hydrate, 180 mg	phenylpropanolamine hydrochloride, 25 mg	pheniramine maleate, 12.5 mg pyrilamine maleate, 12.5 mg	acetaminophen, 325 mg
Tussar-2 (Armour)	codeine phosphate[b], 2 mg/ml carbetapentane citrate, 1.5 mg/ml	guaifenesin, 10 mg/ml		chlorpheniramine maleate, 0.4 mg/ml	alcohol, 5% sodium citrate, 26 mg/ml citric acid, 4 mg/ml methylparaben, 0.1%
Tussar DM (Armour)	dextromethorphan hydrobromide, 3 mg/ml		phenylephrine, 1 mg/ml	chlorpheniramine maleate, 0.4 mg/ml	methylparaben, 0.2%
Tussar-SF[c] (Armour)	codeine phosphate[b], 2 mg/ml carbetapentane citrate, 1.5 mg/ml	guaifenesin, 10 mg/ml		chlorpheniramine maleate, 0.4 mg/ml	alcohol, 12% sodium citrate, 26 mg/ml citric acid, 4 mg/ml methylparaben, 0.1%

Antitussive Product Table, continued

Product[a] (Manufacturer)	Cough Suppressant	Expectorant	Sympatho-mimetics	Antihistamine	Other Ingredients
Tusscapine Suspension and Tablets (Fisons)	noscapine, 3 mg/ml 15 mg/tablet				sucrose, 85 mg/ml sorbitol, 0.3 ml/ml glycerin, 0.03 ml/ml saccharin sodium, 1 mg/ml lime flavor (suspension) raspberry flavor (tablet)
Tussciden Expectorant (Cenci)		guaifenesin, 20 mg/ml			sucrose, 28%
Vicks Cough Syrup (Vicks)	dextromethorphan hydrobromide, 0.7 mg/ml	guaifenesin, 5 mg/ml			alcohol, 5% sodium citrate, 40 mg/ml
Vicks Cough Silencer Lozenges (Vicks)	dextromethorphan hydrobromide, 2.5 mg				benzocaine, 1 mg menthol anethole pepper-mint oil } 0.35%
Viromed Tablets (Whitehall)	dextromethorphan hydrobromide, 7.5 mg	guaifenesin, 50 mg	pseudoephedrine hydrochloride, 15 mg	chlorpheniramine maleate, 1 mg	aspirin, 325 mg
Viromed Liquid (Whitehall)	dextromethorphan hydrobromide, 0.67 mg/ml		pseudoephedrine hydrochloride, 1 mg/ml		alcohol, 16.63% acetaminophen, 21.67 mg/ml sodium citrate, 16.7 mg/ml

[a] Liquid unless specified otherwise.
[b] Schedule V drug: nonprescription sale forbidden in some states.
[c] Sugar free.

Lozenge Product Table

Product (Manufacturer)	Anesthetic	Antibacterial Agents	Other Ingredients
Cépacol (Merrell-Dow)		cetylpyridinium chloride, 1:1,500	benzyl alcohol, 0.3%, sucrose, 1 g
Cépacol Troches (Merrell-Dow)	benzocaine, 10 mg	cetylpyridinium chloride, 1:1,500	sucrose, 1 g
Cépastat[a] (Merrell-Dow)		phenol, 1.45%	menthol, 0.12% eucalyptus oil, 0.04% sorbitol
Cherry Chloraseptic (Eaton)		phenol, sodium phenolate (total phenol, 1.4%) (these ingredients are also anesthetic)	
Children's Cepastat[a] (Merrell-Dow)		phenol, 0.73%	menthol, 0.12% sorbitol mannitol

Lozenge Product Table, continued

Product (Manufacturer)	Anesthetic	Antibacterial Agents	Other Ingredients
Children's Chloraseptic (Norwich-Eaton)	benzocaine, 5 mg		
Children's Hold 4 Hour Cough Suppressant (Beecham Products)			dextromethorphan, 3.75 mg phenylpropanolamine, 6.25 mg
Chloraseptic Cough Control (Norwich-Eaton)		phenol sodium phenolate (total phenol, 32.5 mg) (these ingredients are also anesthetic)	dextromethorphan hydrobromide, 10 mg
Colrex Troches (Rowell)	benzocaine, 10 mg	cetylpyridinium chloride, 2.5 mg	black currant flavor sucrose, 3.74 g
Conex (O'Neal, Jones & Feldman)	benzocaine, 5 mg	cetylpyridinium chloride, 0.5 mg	methylparaben, 2 mg propylparaben, 0.5 mg sucrose, 738 mg
Hold (Beecham Products)	benzocaine		dextromethorphan hydrobromide
Hold 4 Hour Cough Suppressant (Beecham Products)	benzocaine, 3.75 mg		dextromethorphan hydrobromide, 7.5 mg
Isodettes Super (Norcliff Thayer)	benzocaine, 10 mg	cetalkonium chloride, 4 mg	
Meloids Pastilles (Cunningham)			licorice, 98 mg sugar, 48 mg capsicum, 2 mg menthol, 1.8 mg sucrose, 48 mg
Menthol Chloraseptic (Eaton)		phenol, sodium phenolate (total phenol, 1.4%) (these ingredients are also anesthetic)	
Mycinettes Sugar Free[a] (Pfeiffer)	benzocaine, 15 mg	cetylpyridinium chloride, 2.5 mg	
N'Ice Sugarless Cough Lozenges[a] (Beecham Products)			menthol, 6 mg sorbitol
Oracin (Vicks)	benzocaine, 6.25 mg		menthol, 0.08%
Oradex-C (Commerce)	benzocaine, 10 mg	cetylpyridinium chloride, 2.5 mg	
Robitussin-DM Cough Calmers (Robins)			dextromethorphan hydrobromide, 7.5 mg guaifenesin, 50 mg sucrose, 3.63 g
Semets (Beecham Labs)	benzocaine, 3 mg	cetylpyridinium chloride, 1:1,500	
Sepo (Otis Clapp)	benzocaine		
Spec-T Sore Throat Anesthetic (Squibb)	benzocaine, 10 mg		sucrose, 3.7 mg
Spec-T Sore Throat/Cough Supressant (Squibb)	benzocaine, 10 mg		dextromethorphan hydrobromide, 10 mg sucrose, 3.6 mg

Lozenge Product Table, continued

Product (Manufacturer)	Anesthetic	Antibacterial Agents	Other Ingredients
Spec-T Sore Throat/Cough Suppressant (Squibb)	benzocaine, 10 mg		phenylephrine hydrochloride, 5 mg phenylpropanolamine hydrochloride, 10.5 mg sucrose, 3.7 g
Sucrets (Beecham Products)		hexylresorcinol, 2.4 mg	
Sucrets Cough Control Formula (Beecham Products)	benzocaine, 3.75 mg		dextromethorphan hydrobromide, 7.5 mg
Sucrets Cold Decongestant Formula (Beecham Products)	benzocaine, 5 mg		phenylephrine hydrochloride, 5 mg phenylpropanolamine hydrochloride, 10 mg
Synthaloids (Buffington)	benzocaine	calcium-iodine complex	sucrose, 800 mg
Thantis (Hynson, Westcott & Dunning)		meralein sodium, 8.1 mg	salicyl alcohol, 64.8 mg sucrose, 660 mg
Throat Discs (Marion)			capsicum peppermint anise cubeb glycyrrhiza extract linseed
Trocaine (North American)	benzocaine, 10 mg	cetylpyridinium chloride, 2.5 mg	terpin hydrate, 15 mg
Trokettes (Vitarine)	benzocaine, 10 mg	cetylpyridinium chloride, 1:3,000 cetalkonium chloride, 1:3,000	orange flavor
Vicks Throat Lozenges (Vicks)	benzocaine, 5 mg	cetylpyridinium chloride, 1.66 mg	menthol camphor eucalyptus oil
Victors (Vicks)			menthol eucalyptus oil

[a] Sugar free

Cold and Allergy Product Table

Product (Manufacturer)	Dosage Form	Sympathomimetic Agents	Antihistamine	Analgesic	Other Ingredients
Alka-Seltzer Plus (Miles)	effervescent tablet	phenylpropanolamine bitartrate, 24.08 mg	chlorpheniramine maleate, 2.0 mg	aspirin, 324 mg	
Allerest (Pharmacraft)	time capsule	phenylpropanolamine hydrochloride, 50 mg	chlorpheniramine maleate, 4 mg		
Allerest Headache Strength (Pharmacraft)	tablet	phenylpropanolamine hydrochloride, 18.7 mg	chlorpheniramine maleate, 2 mg	acetaminophen, 325 mg	

Cold and Allergy Product Table, continued

Product (Manufacturer)	Dosage Form	Sympathomimetic Agents	Antihistamine	Analgesic	Other Ingredients
Allerest Regular and Children's (Pharmacraft)	tablet	phenylpropanolamine hydrochloride, 18.7 mg 9.4 mg (children's)	chlorpheniramine maleate, 2 mg 1 mg (children's)		
Allergesic (Vitarine)	tablet	phenylpropanolamine hydrochloride, 18.7 mg	chlorpheniramine maleate, 2 mg		sucrose, 64.8 mg
Anodynos Forte (Buffington)	tablet	phenylephrine hydrochloride, 10 mg	chlorpheniramine maleate, 2 mg	salicylamide acetaminophen	caffeine
Aspirin Free Dristan (Whitehall)	tablet	phenylephrine hydrochloride, 5 mg	chlorpheniramine maleate, 2 mg	acetaminophen	caffeine
Bayer Children's Cold Tablets (Glenbrook)	tablet	phenylpropanolamine hydrochloride, 3.125 mg		aspirin, 81 mg	
Cerose Compound Capsules (Ives)	capsule	phenylephrine hydrochloride, 10 mg	chlorpheniramine maleate, 4 mg	acetaminophen, 325 mg	
Chlor-Trimeton (Schering)	syrup tablet		chlorpheniramine maleate, 0.4 mg/ml 4 mg/tablet		
Chlor-Trimeton Decongestant (Schering)	tablet	pseudoephedrine sulfate, 60 mg	chlorpheniramine maleate, 4 mg		
Codimal (Central)	tablet capsule	pseudoephedrine hydrochloride, 30 mg	chlorpheniramine maleate, 2 mg	salicylamide, 150 mg acetaminophen, 150 mg	
Colrex (Rowell)	capsule	phenylephrine hydrochloride, 5 mg	chlorpheniramine maleate, 2 mg	acetaminophen, 325 mg	
Conex DA (O'Neal, Jones & Feldman)	tablet	phenylpropanolamine hydrochloride, 50 mg	phenyltoloxamine citrate, 50 mg		sucrose, 20 mg
Conex Plus (O'Neal, Jones & Feldman)	tablet	phenylpropanolamine hydrochloride, 25 mg	phenyltoloxamine citrate, 25 mg	acetaminophen, 250 mg	
Congespirin (Bristol-Myers)	chewable tablet	phenylephrine hydrochloride, 1.25 mg		aspirin, 81 mg	sucrose, 194.5 mg
Contac (Menley & James)	time capsule	phenylpropanolamine hydrochloride, 50 mg	chlorpheniramine maleate, 4 mg		
Contac Severe Cold Formula (Menley & James)	capsule	pseudoephedrine hydrochloride, 30 mg	chlorpheniramine maleate, 1 mg	acetaminophen, 500 mg	dextromethorphan hydrobromide, 15 mg
Coricidin (Schering)	tablet		chlorpheniramine maleate, 2 mg	aspirin, 325 mg	
Coricidin "D" (Schering)	tablet	phenylpropanolamine hydrochloride, 12.5 mg	chlorpheniramine maleate, 2 mg	aspirin, 325 mg	
Coricidin Demilets (Schering)	children's chewable tablet	phenylpropanolamine hydrochloride, 6.25 mg	chlorpheniramine maleate, 1 mg	aspirin, 80 mg	

Cold and Allergy Product Table, continued

Product (Manufacturer)	Dosage Form	Sympathomimetic Agents	Antihistamine	Analgesic	Other Ingredients
Coricidin Medilets (Schering)	children's chewable tablet		chlorpheniramine maleate, 1 mg	aspirin, 80 mg	
Coryban-D (Pfipharmecs)	capsule	phenylpropanolamine hydrochloride, 25 mg	chlorpheniramine maleate, 2 mg		caffeine, 30 mg
Co Tylenol (McNeil)	tablet capsule	pseudoephedrine hydrochloride, 30 mg	chlorpheniramine maleate, 2 mg	acetaminophen, 325 mg	dextromethorphan hydrobromide, 15 mg
Co Tylenol (McNeil)	liquid	pseudoephedrine hydrochloride, 2 mg/ml	chlorpheniramine maleate, 0.13 mg/ml	acetaminophen, 21.67 mg/ml	dextromethorphan hydrobromide, 1 mg/ml alcohol, 7.5%
Children's Co Tylenol Liquid Cold Formula (McNeil)	liquid	phenylpropanolamine hydrochloride, 1.25 mg/ml	chlorpheniramine maleate, 0.2 mg/ml	acetaminophen, 32 mg/ml	alcohol, 8.5%
Covanamine (Wallace)	liquid	phenylpropanolamine hydrochloride, 1.25 mg/ml phenylephrine hydrochloride, 0.75 mg/ml	pyrilamine maleate, 1.25 mg/ml chlorpheniramine maleate, 0.2 mg/ml		
Covangesic (Wallace)	tablet	phenylpropanolamine hydrochloride, 12.5 mg phenylephrine hydrochloride, 7.5 mg	pyrilamine maleate, 12.5 mg chlorpheniramine maleate, 2.0 mg	acetaminophen, 275 mg	
Dalca (B.F. Ascher)	tablet	phenylpropanolamine hydrochloride, 12.5 mg		magnesium salicylate, 325 mg	
Decapyryn (Merrell-Dow)	syrup		doxylamine succinate, 1.25 mg/ml		
Demazin (Schering)	syrup repetabs	phenylephrine hydrochloride, 0.5 mg/ml 20 mg/tablet	chlorpheniramine maleate, 0.2 mg/ml 4 mg/tablet		alcohol, 7.5% (syrup)
D-Feda (Dooner/Rorer)	time capsule	pseudoephedrine hydrochloride, 60 mg			
Dimetane Decongestant (Robins)	tablet liquid	phenylephrine hydrochloride, 10 mg (tablet) 1 mg/ml (liquid)	brompheniramine maleate, 4 mg (tablet) 0.4 mg/ml (liquid)		alcohol, 2.3% (liquid)
Dristan (Whitehall)	tablet	phenylephrine hydrochloride, 5 mg	chlorpheniramine maleate, 2 mg	aspirin, 325 mg	caffeine, 16.2 mg aluminum hydroxide magnesium carbonate
Dristan (Whitehall)	time capsule	phenylephrine hydrochloride, 20 mg	chlorpheniramine maleate, 4 mg		
Dristan-AF Tablets (Aspirin-Free) (Whitehall)	tablet	phenylephrine hydrochloride, 5 mg	chlorpheniramine maleate, 2 mg	acetaminophen, 325 mg	caffeine, 16.2 mg

Cold and Allergy Product Table, continued

Product (Manufacturer)	Dosage Form	Sympathomimetic Agents	Antihistamine	Analgesic	Other Ingredients
Dristan Capsules (Whitehall)	capsule	phenylpropanolamine hydrochloride, 12.5 mg	chlorpheniramine maleate, 2 mg	aspirin, 325 mg	caffeine, 16.2 mg
Duadacin (Hoechst-Roussel)	capsule	phenylephrine hydrochloride, 5 mg	pyrilamine resin adsorbate equiv. to pyrilamine maleate, 12.5 mg chlorpheniramine maleate, 1 mg	salicylamide, 200 mg acetaminophen, 120 mg	ascorbic acid, 50 mg caffeine, 30 mg
Duradyne-Forte (O'Neal, Jones & Feldman)	tablet	phenylephrine hydrochloride, 5 mg	chlorpheniramine maleate, 2 mg	salicylamide, 225 mg acetaminophen, 160 mg	caffeine, 30 mg sucrose, 44 mg
Emagrin Forte (Otis Clapp)	tablet	phenylephrine hydrochloride, 5 mg		acetaminophen	atropine sulfate, 0.06 mg caffeine
Endecon (Endo)	tablet	phenylpropanolamine hydrochloride, 25 mg		acetaminophen, 325 mg	
Euphenex (O'Neal, Jones & Feldman)	tablet		phenyltoloxamine citrate, 25 mg	acetaminophen, 300 mg	caffeine, 15 mg sucrose, 67 mg
Extendac (Vitarine)	extended-action capsule	phenylpropanolamine hydrochloride, 50 mg	pheniramine maleate, 12.5 mg chlorpheniramine maleate, 1 mg		belladonna alkaloids, 0.2 mg
Fedahist (Dooner/Rorer)	tablet syrup	pseudoephedrine hydrochloride, 60 mg/tablet 6 mg/ml	chlorpheniramine maleate, 4 mg/tablet 0.4 mg/ml		
Fedrazil (Burroughs Wellcome)	tablet	pseudoephedrine hydrochloride, 30 mg	chlorcyclizine hydrochloride, 25 mg		sucrose, 113 mg
Fendol (Buffington)	tablet	phenylephrine hydrochloride, 10 mg		salicylamide acetaminophen	caffeine atropine sulfate, 0.13 mg
Gonex (O'Neal, Jones & Feldman)	tablet	phenylpropanolamine hydrochloride, 25 mg phenylephrine hydrochloride, 2.5 mg	pyrilamine maleate, 12.5 mg chlorpheniramine maleate, 1 mg		
Headway (Vicks)	capsule tablet	phenylpropanolamine hydrochloride, 18.75 mg	chlorpheniramine maleate, 2 mg	acetaminophen, 325 mg	
Hista-Compound No. 5 (North American)	tablet		chlorpheniramine maleate, 2 mg	salicylamide, 175 mg acetaminophen, 150 mg	
Hot Lemon (Rexall)	tablet	phenylephrine hydrochloride, 10 mg	chlorpheniramine maleate, 2 mg	acetaminophen, 600 mg	ascorbic acid, 60 mg
Kiddisan (O'Neal, Jones & Feldman)	chewable tablet	phenylephrine hydrochloride, 1.25 mg	chlorpheniramine maleate, 0.5 mg	salicylamide, 80 mg	ascorbic acid, 30 mg

Cold and Allergy Product Table, continued

Product (Manufacturer)	Dosage Form	Sympathomimetic Agents	Antihistamine	Analgesic	Other Ingredients
Kolephrin (Pfeiffer)	capsule	phenylephrine hydrochloride, 10 mg	chlorpheniramine maleate, 2 mg	acetaminophen, 196 mg salicylamide, 130 mg	caffeine, 65 mg
Naldegesic (Bristol)	tablet	pseudoephedrine hydrochloride, 15 mg		acetaminophen, 325 mg	
Neorhiban (O'Neal, Jones & Feldman)	tablet	phenylpropanolamine hydrochloride, 12.5 mg	phenyltoloxamine citrate, 25 mg	acetaminophen, 195 mg	sucrose, 35 mg
Neo-Synephrine Day Relief (Winthrop)	time-release capsule	pseudoephedrine hydrochloride, 120 mg			
Nor-Lief (North American Pharmacal)	chewable tablet	phenylephrine hydrochloride, 5 mg	chlorpheniramine maleate, 0.5 mg		ascorbic acid, 15 mg
Novafed (Dow)	syrup	pseudoephedrine hydrochloride, 6 mg/ml			alcohol, 7.5%
Novafed A (Dow)	syrup	pseudoephedrine hydrochloride, 6 mg/ml	chlorpheniramine maleate, 0.4 mg/ml		alcohol, 5%
Novahistine Cold Tablets (Dow)	tablet	phenylpropanolamine hydrochloride, 18.75 mg	chlorpheniramine maleate, 2 mg		
Novahistine Elixir (Dow)	syrup	phenylpropanolamine hydrochloride, 3.75 mg/ml	chlorpheniramine maleate, 0.4 mg/ml		alcohol, 5%
Novahistine Fortis (Dow)	capsule	phenylephrine hydrochloride, 10 mg	chlorpheniramine maleate, 2 mg		
Novahistine Melet (Dow)	chewable tablet	phenylephrine hydrochloride, 10 mg	chlorpheniramine maleate, 2 mg		
Novahistine Sinus Tablets (Dow)	tablet	pseudoephedrine hydrochloride, 30 mg	chlorpheniramine maleate, 2 mg	acetaminophen, 325 mg	
NyQuil (Vicks)	liquid	ephedrine sulfate, 0.267 mg/ml	doxylamine succinate, 0.25 mg/ml	acetaminophen, 20 mg/ml	alcohol, 25% dextromethorphan hydrobromide, 0.5 mg/ml
Ornex (Menley & James)	capsule	phenylpropanolamine hydrochloride, 18 mg		acetaminophen, 325 mg	
Peletac (Vitarine)	time-release capsules	phenylpropanolamine hydrochloride, 50 mg	chlorpheniramine maleate, 4 mg		sucrose, 5 mg
Pfeiffer Allergy Tablets (Pfeiffer)	tablet		chlorpheniramine maleate, 4 mg		
Pyrroxate (Upjohn)	capsule	phenylpropanolamine hydrochloride, 25 mg	chlorpheniramine maleate, 4 mg	acetaminophen, 500 mg	
Ryna (Wallace)	liquid	pseudoephedrine hydrochloride, 6 mg/ml	chlorpheniramine maleate, 0.4 mg/ml		
Sinacon (Glaxo)	tablet	pseudoephedrine hydrochloride, 15 mg		acetaminophen, 325 mg	

Cold and Allergy Product Table, continued

Product (Manufacturer)	Dosage Form	Sympathomimetic Agents	Antihistamine	Analgesic	Other Ingredients
Sinapils (Pfeiffer)	tablet	phenylpropanolamine hydrochloride, 12.5 mg	chlorpheniramine maleate, 1.0 mg	acetaminophen, 325 mg	caffeine, 32.5 mg sucrose, 11.6 mg
Sinarest (Pharmacraft)	tablet	phenylpropanolamine hydrochloride, 18.7 mg	chlorpheniramine maleate, 2 mg	acetaminophen, 325 mg	
Sinarest Extra Strength (Pharmacraft)	tablet	phenylpropanolamine hydrochloride, 18.7 mg	chlorpheniramine maleate, 2 mg	acetaminophen, 500 mg	
Sine-Aid (McNeil)	tablet	phenylpropanolamine hydrochloride, 25 mg		acetaminophen, 325 mg	
Sine-Off (Menley & James)	tablet	phenylpropanolamine hydrochloride, 18.75 mg	chlorpheniramine maleate, 2 mg	aspirin, 325 mg	
Sine-Off Extra Strength (Menley & James)	capsule	phenylpropanolamine hydrochloride, 18.75 mg		acetaminophen, 500 mg	
Sine-Off Non-Aspirin Formula (Menley & James)	tablet	phenylpropanolamine hydrochloride, 18.75 mg	chlorpheniramine maleate, 2 mg	acetaminophen, 500 mg	
Sinulin (Carnrick)	tablet	phenylpropanolamine hydrochloride, 37.5 mg	chlorpheniramine maleate, 2 mg	acetaminophen, 325 mg salicylamide, 250 mg	homatropine methylbromide, 0.75 mg
Sinurex (Rexall)	tablet	phenylpropanolamine hydrochloride, 25 mg	phenyltoloxamine citrate, 22 mg	acetaminophen, 325 mg	
Sinustat (Vitarine)	tablet	phenylpropanolamine hydrochloride, 25 mg	phenyltoloxamine citrate, 22 mg	acetaminophen, 325 mg	sucrose, 9 mg
Sinutab (Warner-Lambert)	tablet	phenylpropanolamine hydrochloride, 25 mg	phenyltoloxamine citrate, 22 mg	acetaminophen, 325 mg	
Sinutab Extra Strength (Warner-Lambert)	tablet capsule	phenylpropanolamine hydrochloride, 25 mg/tablet, 18.75 mg/capsule	phenyltoloxamine citrate, 22 mg/tablet, chlorpheniramine maleate, 2 mg/capsule	acetaminophen, 500 mg	
Sinutab II (Warner-Lambert)	tablet	phenylpropanolamine hydrochloride, 25 mg		acetaminophen, 325 mg	
St. Joseph Cold Tablets for Children (Plough)	chewable tablet	phenylpropanolamine hydrochloride, 3.125 mg		aspirin, 81 mg	sucrose, 96.2 mg
Sudafed (Burroughs Wellcome)	tablet syrup	pseudoephedrine hydrochloride, 30 mg/ tablet, 6 mg/ml			sucrose, 76 mg/tablet, 700 mg/ml
Sudafed Plus (Burroughs Wellcome)	liquid tablets	pseudoephedrine hydrochloride, 6 mg/ml 60 mg/tablet	chlorpheniramine maleate, 0.4 mg/ml 4 mg/tablet		
Super Anahist (Warner-Lambert)	tablet	phenylpropanolamine hydrochloride, 25 mg		acetaminophen, 325 mg	

Cold and Allergy Product Table, continued

Product (Manufacturer)	Dosage Form	Sympathomimetic Agents	Antihistamine	Analgesic	Other Ingredients
Triaminic (Dorsey)	syrup	phenylpropanolamine hydrochloride, 2.5 mg/ml	pheniramine maleate, 1.25 mg/ml pyrilamine maleate, 1.25 mg/ml		
Triaminicin (Dorsey)	tablet	phenylpropanolamine hydrochloride, 25 mg	chlorpheniramine maleate, 2 mg	aspirin, 450 mg	caffeine, 30 mg
Triaminicin Allergy (Dorsey)	tablet	phenylpropanolamine hydrochloride, 37.5 mg	chlorpheniramine maleate, 4.0 mg		
Triaminicin Chewables (Dorsey)	chewable tablet	phenylpropanolamine hydrochloride, 6.25 mg	chlorpheniramine maleate, 0.5 mg		sucrose, 52.5 mg
Trind (Mead Johnson)	syrup	phenylpropanolamine, 2.5 mg/ml	chlorpheniramine maleate, 0.4 mg/ml		alcohol, 5%
Tri-Nefrin (Pfeiffer)	tablet	phenylpropanolamine, 25 mg	chlorpheniramine maleate, 4.0 mg		
Ursinus (Dorsey)	in-lay tablet	phenylpropanolamine hydrochloride, 25 mg	pheniramine maleate, 12.5 mg pyrilamine maleate, 12.5 mg	calcium carbaspirin (equiv. to 300 mg of aspirin)	
Valihist (Otis Clapp)	capsule	phenylephrine hydrochloride, 10 mg	chlorpheniramine maleate, 1 mg	acetaminophen	caffeine
VapoRub (Vicks)	ointment				camphor menthol turpentine spirits eucalyptus oil cedar leaf oil myristica oil thymol } 14%
VapoSteam (Vicks)	liquid (for vaporizers)				polyoxyethylene dodecanol, 1.8% eucalyptus oil camphor menthol } 12.4% tincture of benzoin, 5% alcohol, 55%
Vasominic TD (A.V.P.)	tablet	phenylpropanolamine hydrochloride, 50 mg	pheniramine maleate, 25 mg pyrilamine maleate, 25 mg		
Viro-med (Whitehall)	liquid tablet	pseudoephedrine hydrochloride, 1 mg/ml pseudoephedrine, 15 mg/tablet	chlorpheniramine maleate, 1 mg/tablet	acetaminophen, 20 mg/ml aspirin, 325 mg/tablet	alcohol, 16% dextromethorphan hydrobromide, 0.66 mg/ml guaifenesin, 50 mg/tablet
4-Way Cold Tablets (Bristol-Myers)	tablet	phenylephrine hydrochloride, 12.5 mg	chlorpheniramine maleate, 2.0 mg	aspirin, 324 mg	

Topical Decongestant Product Table

Product (Manufacturer)	Application Form	Sympathomimetic Agents	Preservative	Other
Afrin (Schering)	nasal spray nose drops	oxymetazoline hydrochloride, 0.05%	benzalkonium chloride, 0.2 mg/ml phenylmercuric acetate, 0.02 mg/ml	sorbitol, 57 mg/ml aminoacetic acid, 3.8 mg/ml sodium hydroxide
Afrin Pediatric (Schering)	nose drops	oxymetazoline hydrochloride, 0.25 mg/ml	benzalkonium chloride, 0.02 mg/ml phenylmercuric acetate, 0.02 mg/ml	aminoacetic acid, 3.8 mg/ml sorbitol, 57.1 mg/ml
Alconefrin (Alcon)	nose drops	phenylephrine hydrochloride		
Allerest (Pharmacraft)	nasal spray	phenylephrine hydrochloride, 0.5%	benzalkonium chloride	edetate disodium sodium bisulfite saline phosphate buffer
Ayr (B.F. Ascher & Co.)	nose drops		benzalkonium chloride edetic acid	sodium chloride, 0.65%
Ayr (B.F. Ascher & Co.)	nasal spray		benzalkonium chloride edetic acid	sodium chloride, 0.65%
Benzedrex (Menley & James)	inhaler	propylhexedrine, 250 mg		aromatics menthol
Cerose Compound Capsules (Ives)	capsules	phenylephrine hydrochloride, 10 mg	chlorpheniramine maleate, 4 mg	acetaminophen, 325 mg
Coricidin (Schering)	nasal spray	phenylephrine hydrochloride, 0.5%		
Dristan (Whitehall)	inhaler nasal spray	propylhexedrine (inhaler) phenylephrine hydrochloride, 0.5% (spray)	benzalkonium chloride, 0.02% (spray) thimerosal, 0.002% (spray)	pheniramine maleate, 0.2% (spray) menthol eucalyptol methyl salicylate
Dristan Long Lasting Nasal Mist (Whitehall)	nasal spray	xylometazoline hydrochloride, 0.1%	benzalkonium chloride, 0.02% thimerosal, 0.002%	
Dristan Long Lasting Menthol Nasal Mist (Whitehall)	nasal spray	xylometazoline hydrochloride, 0.1%	benzalkonium chloride, 0.02% thimerosal, 0.002%	menthol camphor eucalyptol
Dristan Menthol Nasal Mist (Whitehall)	nasal spray	phenylephrine hydrochloride, 0.5%	benzalkonium chloride, 0.02% thimerosal, 0.002%	pheniramine maleate, 0.2% camphor eucalyptol menthol
Duramist PM (Pfeiffer)	nasal spray	xylometazoline, 0.1% (w/v)	thimerosal, 0.002%	
Duration (Plough)	nasal spray nose drops	oxymetazoline hydrochloride, 0.05%	phenylmercuric acetate, 0.002%	
Duration Mentholated Vapor Spray (Plough)	nasal spray	oxymetazoline hydrochloride, 0.05%	phenylmercuric acetate, 0.002%	menthol camphor eucalyptol
Efedron Nasal Jelly (Hyrex)	jelly	ephedrine hydrochloride, 0.6%	chlorobutanol	cinnamon oil menthol sodium chloride, 0.85%

Topical Decongestant Product Table, continued

Product (Manufacturer)	Application Form	Sympathomimetic Agents	Preservative	Other
I-Sedrin Plain (Lilly)	nose drops	ephedrine, 1%	chlorobutanol, 0.5%	glucono delta lactone, 1.1%
Nasal Douche Powder (Alvin Last)	powder			sodium bicarbonate sodium chloride sodium borate menthol eucalyptol
Neo-Synephrine (Winthrop)	nasal spray nose drops nasal jelly	phenylephrine hydrochloride, 0.25 and 0.5% (spray) 0.125, 0.25, 0.5, and 1% (drops) 0.5% (jelly)	benzalkonium chloride, 0.02% (spray) 0.125% (drops) thimerosal, 0.001% methylparaben (drops) propylparaben (drops) sodium bisulfite (drops) phenylmercuric acetate (jelly)	
Neo-Synephrine Mentholated (Winthrop)	nasal spray	phenylephrine hydrochloride, 0.5%	benzalkonium chloride, 0.02% thimerosal, 0.001%	menthol
Neo-Synephrine II (Winthrop)	nasal spray nose drops	xylometazoline hydrochloride, 0.1% (spray) 0.1% and 0.05% (drops)	benzalkonium chloride, 0.02% thimerosal, 0.001%	
Neo-Synephrine 12 Hour (Winthrop)	nasal spray nose drops	oxymetazoline hydrochloride, 0.05% (spray) 0.05% (drops) 0.025% (children's drops)	benzalkonium chloride phenylmercuric acetate, 0.002%	
Neo-Synephrine 12 Vapor Nasal Spray (Winthrop)	nasal spray	oxymetazoline hydrochloride, 0.05%	benzalkonium chloride thimerosal	camphor eucalyptol menthol methyl salicylate
Newphrine (Vitarine)	nose drops	phenylephrine hydrochloride, 0.25%	methylparaben, 0.02% propylparaben, 0.01%	sodium bisulfite, 0.2%
NTZ (Winthrop)	nose drops nasal spray	phenylephrine hydrochloride, 0.5%	benzalkonium chloride, 1:5000	thenyldiamine hydrochloride, 0.1%
Privine (Ciba)	nose drops nasal spray	naphazoline hydrochloride, 0.05%	benzalkonium chloride, 1:5000	
Salinex (Fleming)	nasal mist		benzalkonium chloride, 0.01%	sodium chloride, 0.4% hydroxypropyl methylcellulose propylene glycol
Sinarest (Pharmacraft)	nasal spray	phenylephrine hydrochloride, 0.5%	benzalkonium chloride sodium bisulfite	
Sine-Off Once-A-Day (Menley & James)	nasal spray	xylometazoline hydrochloride, 0.1%	thimerosal, 0.001%	menthol eucalyptol camphor methyl salicylate
Sinex (Vicks)	nasal spray	phenylephrine hydrochloride, 0.50%	thimerosal, 0.001%	menthol eucalyptol camphor methyl salicylate
Sinex-L.A. (Vicks)	nasal spray	oxymetazoline, hydrochloride, 0.05%	thimerosal, 0.001%	

Topical Decongestant Product Table, continued

Product (Manufacturer)	Application Form	Sympathomimetic Agents	Preservative	Other
Sinutab (Warner-Lambert)	nasal spray	xylometazoline, 0.1%	benzalkonium chloride, 0.02%	
St. Joseph (Plough)	nasal spray nose drops	oxymetazoline hydrochloride, 0.025%	phenylmercuric acetate, 0.002%	
Super Anahist (Warner-Lambert)	nasal spray	phenylephrine hydrochloride, 0.25%	thimerosal, 0.002%	alcohol, 0.038% thonzonium bromide, 0.05%
Va-Tro-Nol (Vicks)	nose drops	ephedrine sulfate, 0.50%	thimerosal, 0.001%	menthol eucalyptol camphor methyl salicylate } 0.06%
Vicks (Vicks)	inhaler	levodesoxyephedrine, 50 mg		menthol camphor methyl salicylate bornyl acetate
4-Way (Bristol-Myers)	nasal spray	phenylephrine hydrochloride, 0.05% nephazoline hydrochloride, 0.05%		pyrilamine maleate, 0.2%

10 Asthma Products

J. Robert Powell and Lawrence J. Hak

Questions to Ask the Patient

Has a physician diagnosed your condition as asthma?

Are you under the care of a physician?

Do you have any other medical problems such as heart disease, seizures, high blood pressure, hyperthyroidism, or diabetes?

What medications are you taking?

Which asthma products have you used before? Were they effective?

Did they cause any problems (side effects)? If so, what were they?

Physiology of the Respiratory System

The respiratory system is a series of airways, starting with the nose and mouth and leading ultimately to air sacs. The mouth and nasal passages lead to the pharynx, which branches into the esophagus and the trachea. The trachea divides into two large bronchi that supply air to the lungs. Each bronchus progressively divides into smaller airways (bronchioles), leading through the alveolar ducts to the alveoli (1).

As an airway branches, the walls become progressively thinner; at the level of the alveoli, all that remains is a thin layer of cells surrounded by pulmonary capillaries. Respiration, which is an exchange of gases, occurs in the alveoli. Oxygen passes across the alveolar walls into the capillaries, and carbon dioxide diffuses in the opposite direction.

The lungs are essentially elastic air sacs suspended in the airtight thoracic cavity. The movable walls of this cavity are formed by the sternum, ribs, and diaphragm. As the thoracic cavity expands, the pressure within the cavity becomes less than the atmospheric pressure, air enters, and the lungs expand. This process is accomplished by means of two simultaneous mechanisms. The diaphragm, when relaxed, is a dome-shaped muscle that extends upward into the thoracic cavity. As the diaphragm contracts, it becomes flattened and moves downward into the abdomen, causing an increase in the longitudinal size of the thoracic cavity. The ribs are attached to the spinal vertebrae and join together at the sternum (breast bone). Contraction of the external intercostal muscles raises the ribs, causing an elevation and forward movement of the sternum and an increase in the diameter of the chest cavity. During inspiration, the diaphragm and the ribs move simultaneously, expanding the thoracic cavity, and the lungs fill with air.

During normal respiration, inhaled air is cleaned and humidified before it is delivered to the alveoli. The nasal cavities are lined with highly vascular mucous membranes and ciliated epithelial cells. As air passes over these areas, it is warmed, humidified, and filtered. Dust particles, bacteria, and other foreign matter are trapped in the mucus and propelled toward the pharynx by the movement of the nasal cilia. Humidification and filtration continue as air passes through the trachea, bronchi, and bronchioles, which also are lined by a ciliated mucous membrane. Trapped particles are moved upward by the wavelike movement of the cilia and are deposited in the oral cavity where they are either expelled or swallowed.

Bronchial smooth muscle tone is under neural and humoral control. Stimulation of beta₂-adrenergic receptors, which can be found in the bronchioles, causes bronchodilation. The parasympathetic system also controls bronchial smooth muscle by means of the vagus nerve. Stimulation of this system causes bronchoconstriction. Under normal circumstances these two mechanisms are balanced.

Origins of Asthma

Bronchial asthma is defined as "a disease characterized by an increased responsiveness of the trachea and bronchi to various stimuli and manifested by a widespread narrowing of the airways that changes in severity either spontaneously or as a result of therapy" (2).

The overall incidence of asthma in the United States is reported to be about 3% (3). However, the actual incidence may be much higher, since symptoms of the disease may occur intermittently and vary in severity (4).

About 50% of asthmatic patients develop the disease before the age of 10, and another 30% before age 30. However, asthma may develop even in later years. In children under the age of 10, the incidence of the disease is 50% higher in boys than in girls. In the 30-year age group, the incidence of asthma is equal in both sexes. Although it is a common childhood disease, asthma may go into permanent or temporary remission by adulthood. A long-term study of childhood asthma reported that at 20-years followup, 70% of the patients were symptom free (5). In the majority of individuals, if the disease has not resolved, it can be reasonably well controlled. In a series of 6,000 asthma patients, 15% required emergency medical care during the course of a year, and only 1.5% required hospitalization (4).

Patients are generally characterized as having either extrinsic (allergenic) or instrinsic (nonallergenic) asthma (Table 1). A personal history or family history of allergy, seasonal variation in symptoms, positive skin tests, and elevated circulating immunoglobulin E (IgE) levels are characteristics of extrinsic asthma. Patients with intrinsic asthma usually have a negative family history of allergy, negative skin tests, and normal levels of IgE but may develop nasal polyps and aspirin sensitivity (6–8). About 2–10% of asthmatic patients develop an acute asthma attack after taking as little as 300 mg of aspirin (9, 10). Many patients, however, present characteristics of both extrinsic and intrinsic asthma.

Asthma exacerbations are generally precipitated by respiratory tract infection, particularly viral infection; an allergic response to drugs; inhaled allergens such as pollen, dust, or mold; inhaled pollutants; exercise; or a psychophysiologic response to stress (11, 12) (Figure 1). Multiple factors may induce an exacerbation in a patient's symptoms. An allergic response is the major precipitating factor in about 25% of the asthmatic population, and respiratory infections are a major factor in about 40%.

Pathophysiology of Asthma

The mechanism by which asthma attacks occur continues to be major area of research, and has recently been reviewed (12). There is general agreement that the common finding in all patients with asthma is hyper-

irritability of the tracheobronchial tree. In patients with allergic asthma, an antigen sensitizes T-cell lymphocytes, which in turn stimulate B-cell lymphocytes to proliferate and produce IgE. The circulating IgE attaches to mast cells. On subsequent exposure to antigen these sensitized mast cells become activated and release chemical mediators of immediate hypersensitivity (histamine, slow-reacting substance of anaphylaxis, eosinophil chemotactic factor, prostaglandins, and others). These chemical mediators are capable of constricting bronchiolar smooth muscle, increasing vascular permeability, aggregating platelets, and stimulating an inflammatory reaction.

In patients who do not have an allergic component to their disease, an imbalance in autonomic nervous function may be involved. Neural control of the lungs is channeled through the parasympathetic fibers in the vagus nerve and sympathetic fibers that arise from ganglia in the thorax. Normal tone of the bronchiolar smooth muscle is maintained by the vagus. Direct stimulation of the vagus causes constriction of the trachea, bronchi, and large bronchioles as well as increased goblet cell secretion and dilated pulmonary vessels, resulting in bronchospasm and excess mucus production. There are also receptors in the larynx and lower airways. Activation of these receptors by excessive coughing, laughing, or inhalation of irritants, produces stimulation of cholinergic pathways, resulting in a cough reflex and bronchospasm. Bronchospasm is the constriction of smooth muscles that line the tracheobronchial tree, resulting in a decrease in airway caliber and air flow. All of these actions may be blocked by the administration of atropine. Beta$_2$-adrenergic stimulation opposes vagal effects and causes relaxation of the smooth muscle of the airways, constriction of pulmonary vessels, and inhibition of glandular secretions.

The activities of the mast cell and bronchiolar smooth muscle appear to be modulated by the intracellular concentration of the cyclic nucleotides 3':5' guanosine monophosphate (cyclic GMP) and 3':5' adenosine monophosphate (cyclic AMP). Cyclic GMP enhances the release of the chemical mediators from mast cells and promotes bronchoconstriction. Beta$_2$-adrenergic stimulation increases cyclic AMP and opposes the actions of the cholinergic system. Theophylline inhibits the enzyme phosphodiesterase, which inactivates cyclic AMP and cyclic GMP. Increasing cyclic AMP concentration by this effect is believed to be the major mechanism for the bronchodilatory effect of theophylline.

A relative decrease in beta$_2$-adrenergic activity has been proposed as a mechanism for bronchoconstriction (13, 14). In asthmatics, administration of a beta$_2$-blocking agent may precipitate an attack. In contrast, nonasthmatic patients whose beta-receptors have been completely blocked by drugs such as propranolol do not experience bronchospasm.

As mentioned earlier, the common finding in all patients with asthma is the hyperirritability of the tracheobronchial tree. The mechanism that causes this is unclear. There are individuals who are clearly allergic, while in others, several types of stimuli may evoke bronchoconstriction. Whatever the etiology, the hallmark of

Table 1. Clinical characteristics of asthma		
	Extrinsic, atopic	Intrinsic, nonatopic
Onset of symptoms	Childhood	Adults over age 35
Family history of allergy	Positive	Negative
Skin tests	Positive	Negative
IgE	Elevated	Normal
Aspirin sensitivity	Negative	Positive

the asthma attack is reversible airway obstruction, which may be caused by excessive smooth muscle contraction, mucosal edema and mucous plugs that block terminal bronchioles and decreased clearance of secretions.

Symptoms

Asthma characteristically occurs in episodes lasting from a few minutes to several days. Some individuals are often symptom-free between attacks, while others

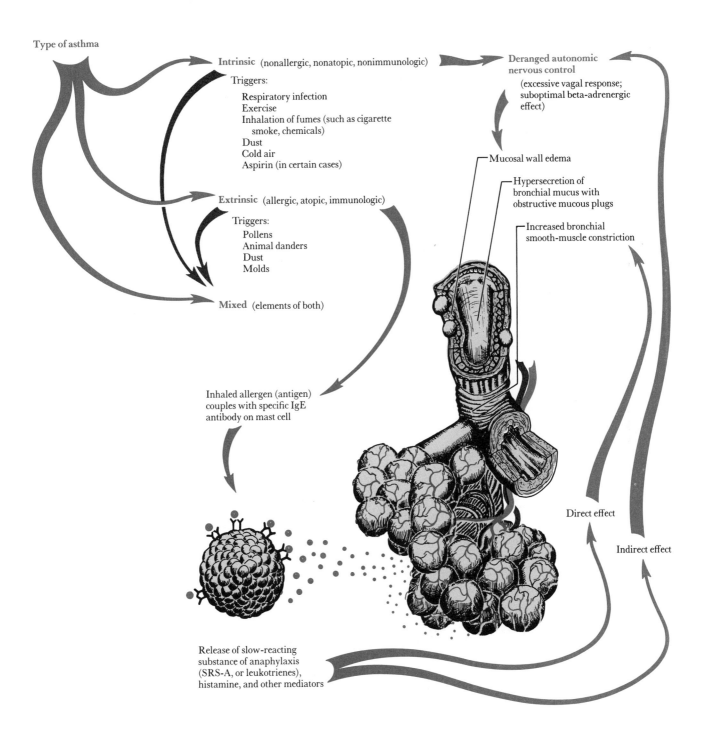

Figure 1. Mechanisms of asthma. Few patients have the pure form of any of these major clinical types of asthma, but most asthmatic patients can be classified as having predominantly extrinsic, intrinsic, or mixed disease. Adapted with permission from *Patient Care,* August 15, 1981, Copyright © 1981, Patient Care Communications, Inc., Darien, Ct. All rights reserved.

may have continuous mild wheezing for prolonged periods.

Attacks, which often occur in the middle of the night, usually begin with tightness in the chest. Coughing and wheezing may occur separately or together and may increase in severity over time. Dyspnea (difficult breathing) is severe, and expiration is more difficult than inspiration. As a result, in prolonged or severe attacks the lungs become overinflated, and there is audible wheezing and physical exhaustion. The sputum is viscid and difficult to expectorate.

Patient Assessment

In most cases, the patients themselves make the diagnosis of asthma after several episodes of intermittent shortness of breath and wheezing (3). Tightness in the chest and cough are frequently present and usually come and go with each attack. In some cases, however, chronic cough and shortness of breath may occur. Many patients have mild asthma that does not progress; in others, the condition may worsen and be accompanied by the following symptoms:

- Dyspnea and wheezing;
- Cough;
- Tachycardia;
- Retraction of the sternocleidomastoid muscle;
- Apprehension;
- Chest distention;
- Tenacious sputum;
- Flaring nostrils.

Sinus tachycardia with a pulse rate up to 120/min is a very common finding (15). Sternocleidomastoid muscle retraction is a consistent finding in patients with severely impaired pulmonary function (16).

The question as to whether the pharmacist should evaluate patients' symptoms and recommend a nonprescription agent for the treatment of asthma is difficult to answer, but the following should be considered. If the symptoms are new and the patient has not been diagnosed by a physician as having asthma, physician referral for evaluation is essential. Nonprescription medication for asthma relief should never be used unless a diagnosis of asthma has been established by a physician. Diagnosis is important to rule out other causes of pulmonary symptoms such as physical obstruction from a tumor, congestive heart failure, and chronic bronchitis. It is also important to establish a baseline for disease severity, explore the etiology of the patient's asthma so that the causative factor may be removed, and avoid nonprescription medications that may worsen other conditions.

For instance, if a patient with new pulmonary symptoms describes a history of hypertension or heart disease, physician referral is essential, since patients with congestive heart failure may awaken in the middle of the night with dyspnea and cough resulting from pulmonary edema. Shortness of breath and chest pain in women taking oral contraceptives may be signs of pulmonary emboli rather than asthma, and the patient should be referred to a physician.

People with chronic bronchitis and emphysema have symptoms similar to asthma. However, these symptoms are usually continuous, not episodic, and should not be treated with nonprescription drugs except under a physician's care.

If a diagnosis of asthma has been established previously, it is important to determine how severe the symptoms are and which self-treatment approaches have already been tried. In determining the severity of asthma symptoms, the patient may need immediate medical help if he or she is unable to complete a full sentence without stopping for shortness of breath, if discomfort persists while at rest after bronchodilator administration, or if the bronchodilator does not completely relieve the symptoms. If a bronchodilator (aerosol, oral, or both) is being used, but the dyspnea becomes worse, a severe attack may be imminent, and the patient should see a physician immediately. Patients with progressive dyspnea and wheezing, and who are dependent on nonprescription products may be in danger of acute pulmonary complications that may lead to hospitalization. In patients with intermittent asthma, or in those whose symptoms are relieved with therapy, evaluation of symptoms becomes more difficult. Significant airway obstruction may be present even when symptoms are absent. In this situation, spirometric measurements will most accurately reflect the status of airway function (16). In one group of patients who were symptomatic, the patients were more accurate in guessing the severity of their airway obstruction than were experienced physicians on the basis of a physical examination (17). However, in another group of asthmatics, 15% of patients were unable to sense significant airway obstruction (18).

Although it is clear that patients with mild, seasonal asthma are often relieved without medication, the difficulty is in distinguishing these patients from those with significant airway obstruction who may go on to develop a severe attack. From the available evidence it seems that this judgment can best be made by the objective measurement of pulmonary function. It therefore seems prudent that therapy of all patients with asthma should be determined on the basis of periodic pulmonary function tests.

Treatment

Drugs available without a prescription for the treatment of asthma are limited to the epinephrine aerosol, ephedrine as a single entity and in combination dosage forms, such as theophylline, ephedrine, phenobarbital, and theophylline only in combination dosage forms. Prescription drugs available for the treatment of chronic asthma include isoproterenol, metaproterenol, albuterol or isoetharine; terbutaline or metaproterenol tablets; single entity theophylline dosage forms; cromolyn; and aerosol or oral corticosteroids (Table 2).

General Pharmacology

Beta$_2$-adrenostimulant bronchodilators (isoproterenol and terbutaline) are associated with an increased intracellular cyclic AMP concentration (Figure 2). Anticho-

Table 2. Characteristics of bronchodilator drugs

Drug	Route of administration	Availability	Pharmacologic activity			Anticholinergic	Duration of action (hours)
			Sympathomimetic				
			Alpha	Beta$_1$	Beta$_2$		
Epinephrine	Inhalation	OTC	a	a	+++		1–2
	IM, SC	Rx	+++	+++	+++		variable, <8
Ephedrine	PO: syrup, capsules, combination tablets	OTC	+++	++	++		3–5
	IV, IM, SC	Rx					<6
Isoproterenol	Inhalation	Rx		a	+++		1–2
	IV, SL			+++	+++		<1
Isoetharine	Inhalation	Rx		a	+++		1–3
Metaproterenol	Inhalation	Rx		a	+++		1.5–3
	PO: tablets, syrup			++	+++		4
Terbutaline	Tablet	Rx		+	+++		4–8
	SC						1.5–4
Theophylline (Various salts)	PO: combination liquids and tablets	OTC		+[b]	+++[b]		4–12
	PO: single entity liquids and tablets sustained release	Rx		+[b]	+++[b]		
	PR, IV						
Atropine	IV, inhalation	Rx				+++	<1

+ Relative intensity of effect.
[a] Inhalation confers more beta$_2$ activity than systemic administration.
[b] Although theophylline is not a sympathomimetic drug, it has nearly identical effects.

linergic bronchodilators (atropine) inhibit the formation of cyclic GMP (19). Similarly, drugs with the opposite effects such as propranolol and bethanechol, can be expected to cause bronchospasm in patients with asthma. Other drugs that can induce bronchospasm are aspirin and other prostaglandin synthetase inhibitors, tartrazine dye in some patients, metoprolol, and phenylephrine.

For clinical purposes, it is more important to understand the pharmacologic effects of stimulating the different receptors (Table 3). The ideal drug for the treatment of bronchospasm would induce bronchodilation and stimulate mucociliary clearance. The only desirable property of alpha-adrenergic stimulation is the decongestant effect. The concomitant effects of bronchoconstriction, vasoconstriction, urinary retention, and mydriasis are clearly undesirable and are reflective of the clinical adverse effects of systemically administered epinephrine or ephedrine (Table 2). In some patients with bronchospasm and rhinorrhea (hay fever), it may be desirable to also have decongestant effects. However,

patients with bronchospasm and rhinorrhea who need a nasal decongestant may be treated more effectively with an alpha-adrenostimulant nasal spray and a bronchodilator that does not produce undesirable systemic alpha-adrenergic effects (such as beta-adrenostimulants, and theophylline). Care should be taken to avoid rhinitis medicamentosa due to long-term use of a nasal decongestant spray.

Beta$_1$-adrenostimulant activity (cardiac stimulation) is also not a desirable effect, whereas beta$_2$-adrenostimulant activity most closely approaches the ideal drug characteristics in the treatment of asthma. Isoproterenol has roughly equivalent beta$_1$ and beta$_2$ effects compared with the newer, relatively selective beta$_2$ drugs, including metaproterenol, terbutaline, and albuterol. Terbutaline, for example, induces bronchodilation and stimulates mucociliary clearance. However, up to 33% of patients on oral terbutaline may experience skeletal muscle tremor, which can be severe (20). The ultimate clinical benefit from using a systemic beta$_2$-adrenostimulant is unclear. Peripheral vasodilation from systemic

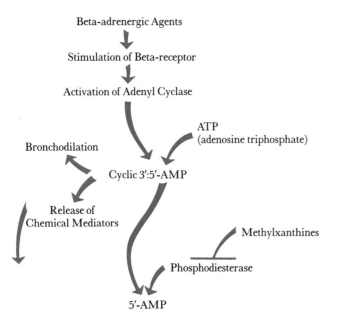

Figure 2. Beta-adrenergic agents.

beta₂-stimulation causes a decrease in blood pressure, producing a compensatory increase in heart rate to maintain cardiac output (21). An early study comparing the relative effects of graded intravenous doses of isoproterenol (beta₁, beta₂) with albuterol (beta₂) found albuterol produced less tachycardia at the same degree of bronchodilation. Isoproterenol produced a similar increase in both tachycardia and bronchodilation as the dose was increased (22). A study in patients with chronic obstructive pulmonary disease and pre-existing premature ventricular contractions found that terbutaline (beta₂) produced a greater increase in heart rate

and tended to produce a greater increase in premature ventricular contractions than theophylline or ephedrine at similar levels of bronchodilation (23). Hence, the newer beta₂-adrenostimulants should be regarded as "relatively selective" at best.

Anticholinergic drugs such as atropine are potent bronchodilators. However, when used systemically, the undesirable attendant pharmacologic effects (tachycardia, urinary retention, decreased mucociliary clearance, and mydriasis) limit the clinical utility. Parenteral administration or inhalation of atropine is occasionally used in hospitalized patients after all other drugs have failed to provide adequate relief.

Route of administration has a profound effect on the pulmonary selectivity of sympathomimetic and anticholinergic bronchodilators. At the same degree of bronchodilation, oral or intravenous terbutaline produces more tremor, hypotension, and tachycardia than does inhalation (21). The same is true for metaproterenol and epinephrine (24). When these drugs are inhaled, much less drug reaches the systemic circulation because the dose is smaller and there is drug metabolism in the lung. This phenomenon is analogous to the use of atropine ophthalmic drops to produce mydriasis. Local administration does not usually result in systemic effects at normal doses. It seems that the pattern of bronchodilation (large central bronchi versus small peripheral bronchioles), is similar by inhalation or systemic administration (24). Two significant advantages of the newer relatively selective beta₂-adrenostimulants (metaproterenol, terbutaline, and albuterol) are that they can be administered by mouth and their duration of action is longer.

Historically, there has been concern about patients becoming tachyphylactic or resistant to the bronchodilator effects of sympathomimetic bronchodilators. For an individual asthma patient who worsens, it would be difficult to determine if the drug has become ineffective due to tachyphylaxis or simply because the disease has worsened due to external or unidentified internal

Organ	Sympathomimetic			Anticholinergic
	Alpha	Beta₁	Beta₂	
Bronchopulmonary	Bronchoconstriction Decongestant		Bronchodilation Stimulate mucociliary clearance	Bronchodilation Inhibit mucociliary clearance
Heart		Increased heart rate, contractility, and automaticity		Increased heart rate and contractility
Peripheral blood vessels	Contraction		Dilation	
Urinary bladder	Difficulty in micturation			Difficulty in micturation
Eye	Mydriasis			Mydriasis Failure of accommodation
Skeletal muscle			Tremor	

Table 3. Clinical drug-induced effects on the various organs and tissues

causes. The best available evidence indicates that after treating patients with oral terbutaline for 1 year, resistance did not develop to the bronchodilation or cardiac stimulant effects of intravenous isoproterenol (25). However, there was a decrease in the tremorogenic effects within 1 month. Although biochemical tolerance has been reported, clinical resistance to sympathomimetic bronchodilators remains under investigation.

Ingredients in Nonprescription Products

Epinephrine

Epinephrine is useful for the treatment of periodic, chronic, and acute severe bronchospasm and also in prophylaxis against exercise-induced bronchospasm. For periodic or chronic asthma, epinephrine is administered by inhalation (metered aerosol or nebulized solution). Acute, severe asthma can be treated by subcutaneous or intramuscular injection. Although the various epinephrine products differ slightly in the drug dose delivered, there is no difference between inhalation epinephrine products purchased with or without a prescription.

Epinephrine has roughly equipotent alpha, beta$_1$, and beta$_2$-adrenostimulant effects, which are dose dependent. The effects of epinephrine are terminated by the drug being taken up by sympathetic nerve endings and by sympathetically innervated tissues (26). In the nerve ending, epinephrine is metabolized by monoamine oxidase and in the innervated tissues by catechol-o-methyltransferase. Epinephrine and isoproterenol are ineffective when taken by mouth since there is nearly complete metabolism by monoamine oxidase in the GI tract and the liver. Adverse effects of epinephrine (tachycardia, cardiac arrhythmias, hypertension, tremor, and anxiety) are almost always associated with the parenteral route of administration. These effects would not be expected by the inhalation route except in an extreme overdose situation.

The peak effect of both epinephrine and isoproterenol aerosol occurs within 5 minutes. The peak effect of metoproterenol occurs between 15 and 30 minutes after administration. The duration of bronchodilation from epinephrine and isoproterenol is about 1–2 hours compared with 3–4 hours for metaproterenol. Several of the investigational beta$_2$-adrenostimulant aerosols have a duration of action of 6 hours.

Probably the most significant problem associated with nonprescription epinephrine aerosols is that most patients do not administer the drug correctly. One study of hospitalized patients found that 47% did not use their aerosol correctly (27). The most commonly observed error was that the patient actuated the aerosol after the inspiration was complete. Even after the patients who used the aerosol incorrectly were taught the correct procedure, upon retesting at a later date, approximately two-thirds had reverted to their old incorrect techniques. These were patients who had serious diseases and would be expected to be under a physician's care.

Although directions for the correct technique of aerosol administration are printed and supplied with nonprescription epinephrine preparations, possibly more than 50% of patients may use these products in-

correctly. When a nonprescription epinephrine aerosol is purchased in a pharmacy, it is the professional responsibility of the pharmacist to instruct the patient on the correct administration technique. The correct procedure is to have the patient shake the aerosol and then insert the mouthpiece in the mouth and close the teeth and lips around the mouthpiece. An alternative method is for the patient to hold the mouthpiece at the level of the lips with the mouth open. The patient exhales completely and then as the patient begins a deep inspiration, the cannister is actuated. The inspiration continues to completion and the patient holds his or her breath for several seconds and then exhales. A second dose may be administered several minutes later as the first dose reaches the maximal effect. In this way, the second dose may reach deeper into the smaller bronchioles not reached by the first dose. The pharmacist should watch the patient use the device to ensure that the instructions have been understood. If an aerosol is not administered correctly, it may be worthless in relieving bronchospasm.

In the 1960's in Great Britain, there were reports of a rapidly increasing mortality in asthmatic patients, particularly in children 10–14 years old (28–30). It appeared that patients may have been overdosing themselves with preparations that delivered a larger dose than was available in the United States. This, combined with cardiac arrhythmias associated with Freon propellant exposure may have caused sudden death. Although this possibility cannot be discounted, it seems more likely that these patients may have avoided medical attention and aggressive treatment too long. Instead of pure bronchospasm, the patient may have had mucosal edema, increased mucous viscosity, and plugging of airways. Here lies the dilemma associated with the use of nonprescription drugs to treat bronchospasm from seasonal allergy, asthma, or chronic bronchitis. If the condition is self-limiting and does not become progressively worse, nonprescription bronchodilators may be effective, much like aspirin for relieving a simple headache. However, if the patient's condition worsens, competent medical care must be sought. To tread this fine line can be dangerous, and the patient and his or her family should know when to abandon self-treatment and immediately seek medical care.

The FDA advisory review panel on nonprescription cough, cold, allergy, bronchodilator, and antiasthmatic drug products recommended that inhalation of nonprescription epinephrine preparations be placed in Category I (safe and effective). Their recommendations for dosing and labeling are (31): In adults and children 4 years and above inhalation dosage is 1–3 inhalations of a 1% aqueous solution of L-epinephrine or the equivalent in a pressurized preparation not more often than every 3 hours, except under the advice and supervision of a physician. For children under 4 years, there is no recommended dosage except under the advice and supervision of a physician. Children and adolescents should not have unsupervised access to this inhaler. There is the possibility of abuse of this material and possible adverse effects on the heart if excessively used (32). These dosages should be safe and effective, however, it may be more efficacious in some patients to space two inhalations several minutes apart. The panel indicated that this preparation should not be taken at higher than recommended doses except under the advice and supervision of a physician since it may cause nervousness and rapid heart beat. If symptoms are not relieved within 20 minutes or become worse, the drug should be discontinued and a physician should be contacted immediately. Patients with heart disease or high blood pressure should avoid self-medication with epinephrine except under the advice and supervision of a physician. In addition, the drug is contraindicated in those taking a prescription antihypertensive or antidepressant drug containing monoamine oxidase inhibitors. The caution to seek medical attention if symptoms are not relieved or worsen within 20 minutes assumes that the patient would have taken 3 doses by that time. If the epinephrine is going to relieve bronchospasm, the effect should occur 5–10 minutes after the last inhalation. This may be life-saving advice for the pharmacist to give the patient. In the recommended dosage it is unlikely that epinephrine aerosol will worsen either cardiac disease or hypertension. However, some patients may have a tendency to overdose particularly when relief is not produced. It is similarly unlikely that aerosol epinephrine in the recommended dosage will produce drug interactions.

Ephedrine

As a bronchodilator, ephedrine is only useful for the treatment of mild to moderate seasonal or chronic asthma. Parenteral ephedrine is rarely, if ever, recommended as a bronchodilator. Although ephedrine sulfate is available on a nonprescription basis for use as a single entity in a 25 mg capsule and a syrup, by far the most abundantly available preparations are combination tablets, elixirs, and suspensions. Drugs combined with ephedrine in these dosage forms include theophylline, phenobarbital, guaifenesin, chlorobutanol, and pyrilamine. These combinations are discussed below.

Ephedrine has roughly equivalent alpha, beta$_1$, and beta$_2$ activity. The pharmacologic actions of ephedrine are produced by an indirect effect whereby ephedrine induces the release of norepinephrine from sympathetic nerve endings and by a less significant direct stimulation of adrenoceptors. Since ephedrine causes the release of norepinephrine, the administration of ephedrine to a patient who has been receiving a monoamine oxidase inhibitor, which decreases the degradation and increases the storage of norepinephrine, could result in severe hypertension. Although this is a potentially fatal interaction, there is very little clinical information available. Tricyclic antidepressants may partially block the action of ephedrine.

The major route of ephedrine elimination is as the unchanged drug in urine (33–35). Although the average elimination half-life is 6 hours, the half-life will be decreased by urinary acidification and increased by alkalinization. Metabolic routes of elimination include *N*-demethylation and oxidative deamination.

The peak bronchodilation effect occurs in 1 hour and lasts about 5 hours (36–38). There is far more dis-

cussion of ephedrine tachyphylaxis or tolerance than is evidenced as a significant problem in the literature (37–39).

The principal adverse effects of ephedrine are CNS stimulation, nausea, tremors, tachycardia, and urinary retention. Other than urinary retention, this similar pattern of adverse effects is produced by theophylline. Of all the bronchodilators, CNS stimulation is produced only by ephedrine and theophylline. Reports indicate that chronic ephedrine overdosage may result in either severe cardiac toxicity or psychosis (40, 41). The latter report indicated that ephedrine may be a potential drug of abuse, producing symptoms of schizophrenia similar to that found in amphetamine psychosis. Ephedrine, caffeine, and phenylpropanolamine are frequent ingredients of drugs manufactured to physically resemble amphetamine dosage (42).

With the development of new drugs over the last decade, ephedrine seems to have fallen into disfavor by many clinicians in the treatment of serious chronic or intermittent bronchospasm. It is difficult to determine from the available studies if ephedrine is clearly inferior to oral theophylline, oral metaproterenol, terbutaline, albuterol, or inhaled sympathomimetic drugs. A limitation in evaluating the literature is that the comparative efficacy studies have usually compared one dosage regimen of ephedrine with the other drug. These studies frequently find that ephedrine produces less or nearly equivalent bronchodilation and either a similar or greater frequency of adverse effects compared with terbutaline, carbuterol, or theophylline (38, 43, 44). Therefore, it seems that ephedrine is, at best, no more effective and not less toxic than other oral bronchodilators and, at worst, is less effective and more toxic.

The FDA advisory review panel on nonprescription cough, cold, allergy, bronchodilator, and antiasthmatic drug products recommended ephedrine preparations be considered safe and effective (Category I) as a bronchodilator in adult oral dosages of 12.5–25 mg given not more often than every 4 hours, not to exceed 150 mg in 24 hours.

The panel strongly recommended that ephedrine be available as scored tablets containing 12.5 mg and 25 mg ephedrine/tablet to permit flexibility in dosage (45). Additionally, the panel recommendations include ephedrine dosages in children 2–12 years old to the health professions, but not to the general public. In children 6–12 years old, oral dosage is 6.25–12.5 mg, no more than every 4 hours, and not to exceed 75 mg in 24 hours. In children 2–6 years, oral dosage is 0.3–0.5 mg/kg of body weight, no more than every 4 hours and not to exceed 2 mg/kg of body weight in 24 hours (45).

The panel warns that this product should not be given to children under 12 years of age except under the advice and supervision of a physician. Based on these recommendations, it is likely that the panel feels ephedrine would be unsafe but not ineffective for unsupervised use in children. For children under 2 years of age, there is no recommended dosage except under the advice and supervision of a physician. There is insufficient information as to the possible toxic effect of ephedrine in this age group.

Ephedrine is available as a base, as hydrochloride and sulfate salts, and as a racemic ephedrine hydrochloride. Dosage recommendations do not account for these differences. If symptoms are not relieved within 1 hour or become worse, the product should be discontinued and a physician should be consulted immediately. Adverse effects include nervousness, tremor, sleeplessness, nausea, and loss of appetite.

The FDA advisory review panel on nonprescription cough, cold, allergy, bronchodilator, and antiasthmatic drug products recommended that ephedrine not be taken by patients with heart disease, high blood pressure, thyroid disease, diabetes, or difficulty in urination due to enlargement of the prostate gland. Ephedrine should not be taken concurrently with antihypertensive or antidepressant drugs containing monoamine oxidase inhibitors. These warnings are reasonable and worthy of emphasis when advising a patient who is purchasing ephedrine, particularly for the first time. The panel's maximal dosage recommendation (150 mg/day) is approximately one-half of the current maximal ephedrine hydrochloride dosage, which is allowable with current Tedral labeling (288 mg/day). This ephedrine dosage, contained in some commercial products, is likely to produce adverse effects in many patients and could be dangerous. Usually nonprescription ephedrine will not be purchased as a single entity drug. The dosage form will usually contain theophylline and other drugs. The ephedrine dosage in these combinations is not different than for single-entity ephedrine dosage forms. The above warnings deserve even more emphasis for combination dosage forms since both ephedrine and theophylline cause nervousness, tremor, sleeplessness, nausea, and can be dangerous in selected patients with seizure disorders or cardiac arrhythmias. The panel did not address the relative safety of single-entity versus combination ephedrine dosage forms.

Theophylline

Theophylline is effective in the treatment of periodic, chronic, and acute, severe bronchospasm and in prophylaxis against exercise-induced bronchospasm. Although theophylline is not a sympathomimetic drug, the pharmacologic effects in patients are nearly identical to a beta-adrenostimulant. Several studies indicate 5–20 mg/liter is the therapeutic theophylline plasma concentration range (46–51). A plasma theophylline concentration above 20 mg/liter can cause nausea, vomiting, cardiac tachyarrhythmias, and seizures. Critical reviews of theophylline clinical pharmacology are available (52, 53). Although there is little information directly comparing the relative efficacy and adverse effects of theophylline and beta$_2$-adrenostimulants, cardiac adverse effects including tachycardia and arrhythmias, are uncommon within the therapeutic range (47, 50, 51). In a direct comparison of theophylline and terbutaline in patients with bronchoconstriction and premature ventricular contractions, at the same level of bronchodilation, theophylline produced both less tachycardia and fewer premature ventricular contractions (23). For these reasons, theophylline has been listed as a relatively selective beta$_2$-adrenostimulant in Table 3. Theo-

phylline is the only bronchodilator that increases gastric acidity (54). Patients with peptic ulcers or a hiatal hernia should be warned of this effect. Theophylline and ephedrine, the only oral nonprescription bronchodilators, are also the only bronchodilators that cause CNS stimulation.

Although single-entity theophylline oral dosage forms, available in solution and in tablets, have not been relegated to prescription-only availability by law, there is no nonprescription, single-entity theophylline oral dosage form available. Nonprescription theophylline dosage forms are only available in combination with ephedrine and other drugs. Prescription theophylline, or theophylline salts or complexes, are available in the following dosage forms: aqueous solution, elixir, uncoated tablet, enteric coated tablet, sustained-release tablets and capsules, suppository, retention enema, and in IV and IM injections. Aminophylline should not be given IM because it is painful and offers no advantage over other dosage forms. Nonprescription theophylline products contain anhydrous and hydrous theophylline and theophylline calcium salicylate. Prescription products contain these ingredients in addition to other salts (Table 4). None of these salts or complexes appear to offer any therapeutic advantage over pure theophylline.

The principal determinants of the theophylline plasma concentration for a given dosage regimen are the rate and extent of drug absorption (bioavailability) and drug clearance. Theophylline is rapidly and completely absorbed from uncoated tablets and oral solutions and may be complete with some sustained-release dosage forms (55–57). Food does not decrease the extent, but may decrease the rate of absorption (58). Theophylline absorption may be incomplete or erratic from enteric coated tablets, suppositories, and some sustained-release products (59–60). Suppositories are frequently expelled prior to the time required for complete absorption, about 6 hours. For most purposes, the only dosage forms that are necessary are uncoated tablets, oral solutions, sustained-release tablets or capsules, and IV injections. Oral solutions are principally useful in patients who cannot swallow tablets. Sustained-release preparations may decrease the required dosing frequency (from every 6 hours to every 8 or 12 hours), and will make the theophylline plasma concentration less variable. Pa-

Table 4. Theophylline content of various preparations	
	Theophylline (%)
Theophylline anhydrous	100
Theophylline hydrous	91
Aminophylline	80
Oxtriphylline	65
Theophylline calcium salicylate	48
Theophylline sodium glycinate	50
Theophylline monoethanolamine	75

tients with a high theophylline clearance and short elimination half-life will have a large difference between the maximal (peak) and minimal (trough) theophylline plasma concentration. For example, theophylline plasma levels may vary from greater than 20 mg/liter to less than 5 mg/liter at steady-state. Since both therapeutic and toxic effects of theophylline are correlated to the plasma drug concentration, it may be more desirable to decrease fluctuations in serum concentration while maintaining an acceptable dosing interval by using a sustained-release preparation. Unfortunately, children who have the shortest theophylline half-life and stand to gain the most from a sustained-release preparation, frequently have difficulty swallowing these large dosage forms.

Theophylline clearance is primarily determined by hepatic metabolism with less than 10% eliminated unchanged in the urine. Although the theophylline metabolite, 3-methylxanthine, is active as a phosphodiesterase inhibitor, the plasma levels are usually low compared with the parent drug. Theophylline clearance is increased by tobacco and marijuana smoking, charcoal-broiled beef, a high protein diet, (61–66), and phenobarbital. Theophylline clearance is decreased by hepatic failure, severe congestive heart failure, viral respiratory infections, vaccines, severe pulmonary obstruction, propranolol (should not be used in patients with bronchospasm), erythromycin, troleandomycin, and cimetidine (67–74). These factors can alter theophylline clearance by 50–75%. Compared with adults, children have a high clearance and premature infants have a low clearance (75, 76). There is no conclusive evidence that elderly patients have altered clearance (69). Theophylline clearance tends to be dynamic as changes occur in the severity of the above diseases, as interacting drugs are added or discontinued, as smoking status changes, as diet changes, and as the patient ages (77, 62). There is an indication that theophylline clearance is dose-dependent. However, this phenomenon has not been completely elucidated, and the clinical importance remains uncertain (78).

Dosing theophylline can be complex if the effects of the various factors that alter theophylline clearance are taken into consideration. Since these factors may alter theophylline clearance 2–3 fold, and the factors are variable, a fixed theophylline dose for all patients (as is the case with nonprescription dosage recommendations) may not be safe or effective. Furthermore, the safest method of chronic theophylline dosing will utilize theophylline plasma concentration determinations. Although it is unlikely that many patients taking a nonprescription theophylline product will have severe cardiac, hepatic, or pulmonary failure, it is likely that some patients may smoke, experience a viral respiratory infection, alter their diet, or may be prescribed erythromycin or cimetidine.

The FDA advisory review panel on nonprescription cough, cold, allergy, bronchodilator, and antiasthmatic drug products recommended theophylline be regarded as safe and effective (Category I) bronchodilator in adult oral dosages of 100–200 mg, based on the anhydrous theophylline equivalent, taken every 6 hours not to exceed 800 mg in 24 hours. It is not recommended in children under 12 except under the advice and supervision of a physician, since excessive use may cause toxic effects and even death. The panel recommended that scored compressed tablets in dosage units of 50 mg, 100 mg, and 200 mg of anhydrous theophylline equivalent be made available for nonprescription use (84). However, the FDA did not agree with the Category I classification by the panel (nor the recommendation that theophylline be available as a single-entity nonprescription drug).

The recommended dosage of this drug should not be exceeded except under the advice and supervision of a physician, and it should not be taken if nausea, vomiting, or restlessness occur. If asthmatic symptoms are not relieved within 1 hour or become worse, a physician should be contacted immediately. The drug is contraindicated in patients already taking a drug or suppository containing any form of theophylline, except under the supervision of a physician.

The panel recommended that labeling provided to health professionals (but not to the general public) may contain the following additional dosage information: In children 2 to under 12 years old, oral dosage based on the anhydrous theophylline equivalent, is 3.33 mg/kg of body weight 3 times/day every 8 hours, not to exceed 10 mg/kg in 24 hours (79).

As with ephedrine, the panel seemed to recognize that unsupervised use of theophylline in children may be unsafe. The dosing recommendations for Tedral (130 mg theophylline, 24 mg ephedrine hydrochloride, 8 mg phenobarbital) are: adults, 1 or 2 tablets every 4 hours; children over 60 lb, one-half the adult dose. At the maximal Tedral recommended dosage an adult could receive 1,560 mg theophylline/day. If it is assumed that theophylline is completely absorbed and theophylline clearance is 40.9 ml/hr/kg for a 70 kg adult, for a nonsmoker who is not seriously ill and has no other factor affecting theophylline clearance, the mean expected theophylline plasma concentration would be 22.7 mg/liter (95% confidence interval 10–51 mg/liter) (69). Using a similar projection for a 60-lb child who takes one Tedral tablet every 4 hours using a mean clearance of 87 ml/hr/kg (75), the expected mean theophylline plasma concentration would be 13.7 mg/liter (range 5.4–38.4 mg/liter).

The panel's recommendations are reasonable and certainly safer than the current labeling of nonprescription theophylline products. The fact that theophylline toxicity has not been commonly reported from nonprescription products is probably due to patients taking less than the maximal dosage recommendations and the possibility that patients who do become sick from an overdose, recognize this and either discontinue the drug or decrease the dosage. The manufacturers dosage recommendations as currently written may be a public health hazard.

Combination Products

The major ingredients in bronchodilator combination products are theophylline and ephedrine. Both drugs have individually been demonstrated to be effective bronchodilators. However, for the combination to offer an advantage over a single drug, it seems reasonable that either a greater degree of bronchodilation should be achieved with theophylline and ephedrine than with either drug alone or that at the same degree of bronchodilation, the combination should produce fewer adverse effects than with either drug alone.

To determine the maximal degree of bronchodilation from two single drugs and the combination, a study would need to increase the dose of each bronchodilator alone to the dose above which bronchodilation does not increase. Then, either the alternate drug could be added to determine if further bronchodilation could be achieved or a dose-response curve could be constructed with a fixed combination to maximal bronchodilation. Based on the studies reviewed, these criteria have not been met (24, 80–84). Most investigators have studied the bronchodilating effects of a single dose or multiple dosing regimen for theophylline, ephedrine, and the combination of theophylline and ephedrine in the same doses as when administered alone. In general, investigators find that the combination produces more bronchodilation than either single drug. Unfortunately, this does not exclude the possibility that the same degree of bronchodilation achieved with the combination could also be achieved by increasing the dose of either single

drug. The doses chosen for theophylline in these studies often do not achieve theophylline plasma concentrations within the therapeutic range.

Similarly, there is no evidence to indicate that at the same degree of bronchodilation, the combination of theophylline and ephedrine is less toxic than either single drug. To the contrary, the incidence of adverse effects seems to be higher (24, 63). This is not surprising since the adverse effect patterns for theophylline and ephedrine are similar, e.g., nausea, agitation, and tachycardia. It would seem more rational to combine theophylline with an oral beta$_2$-adrenostimulant for which the adverse effect patterns are somewhat different (85). Even more advantageous might be the combination of theophylline with a beta$_2$-adrenostimulant aerosol.

Hence, the fixed combination of theophylline and ephedrine may offer no advantage over either single drug and may be more toxic.

Phenobarbital was originally added to the theophylline-ephedrine combination to offset the CNS stimulant properties of the bronchodilators. One study supported by the manufacturer of Tedral found this proposed effect of phenobarbital could not be detected. If used in the maximal dosage, Tedral would supply an adult with 96 mg phenobarbital/day. Theoretically, since phenobarbital is completely absorbed, a 70 kg adult with an average clearance of 3.0 ml/hr/kg, would be estimated to have a steady-state phenobarbital plasma level of 19 mg/liter (range 15–27 mg/liter with the anticonvulsant therapeutic range being 10–30 mg/liter) (86, 90). Since it appears that phenobarbital offers no therapeutic advantage and may induce the metabolism of other drugs, therapy may be unnecessarily complicated.

Other Agents

Antihistamines   Some combination asthma products have contained antihistamines to antagonize histamine effects. However, they have no effect on bradykinin and slow-reacting substance of anaphylaxis and thus are ineffective as therapeutic agents for asthma. Antihistamines have anticholinergic activity causing watery secretions in the bronchi to be reduced and resulting in the formation of thicker mucus that is more difficult to expectorate. It is unlikely that this would be a significant problem in ambulatory patients taking recommended antihistamine doses.

Expectorants   Many asthma products contain expectorants, especially guaifenesin and potassium iodide. These agents are probably no more effective as expectorants than adequate hydration of the patient. Therefore their use in asthma is questionable. Because of the concern for iodide toxicity the FDA advisory review panel on cough and cold drug products recommended that iodide-containing products (expectorants) be restricted to prescription status.

Antitussives   Antitussives, such as codeine and dextromethorphan hydrobromide, are used occasionally in asthma products. Coughing is the major mechanism for removing bronchial secretions and mucus plugs. There-

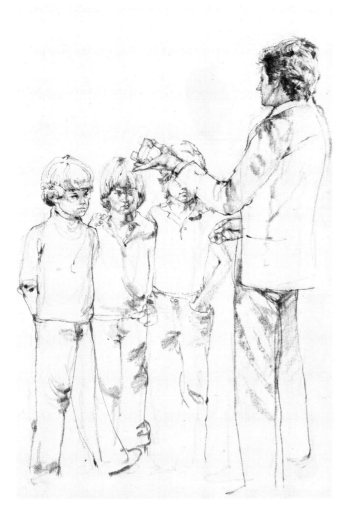

fore antitussives generally should not be used for asthma, since the cough usually has a useful effect.

Product Selection Guidelines

Before recommending a nonprescription product for asthma it is important that the pharmacist have a good understanding of the patient's condition. A complete patient profile alerts the pharmacist to conditions such as heart disease, diabetes, hypertension, aspirin sensitivity, and prescription medications being taken that can duplicate or interact with nonprescription products. It also may provide an indication concerning the patient's compliance with drug regimens. Regular dosing with oral agents to maintain therapeutic drug blood levels is necessary to prevent asthma symptoms. Patients who consistently forget to take oral medications may do better by treating symptoms as they occur with an aerosolized product.

It must also be remembered that the patient is usually the best judge of whether a particular agent is effective or not. After recommending an agent, the pharmacist should alert the patient to discontinue the product and seek medical assistance if symptoms are not relieved within 1 hour or become worse. Nothing is gained by continuing ineffective therapy. When nonprescription medications do not provide sufficient relief, physician referral is the necessary next step.

Education in asthma medication use is as important as drug choice. Improper use of aerosol agents may decrease effectiveness and increase side effects. If headache, nervousness, or palpitations occur, the medication should be discontinued. The mouthpiece should be washed daily with warm water to prevent clogging, and it should always be kept free of particles. Gargling after each use prevents dry mouth and throat irritation.

Patients with aspirin sensitivity should be cautioned that some asthma combination drug preparations contain aspirin. However, the FDA panel has recommended that no aspirin be included in products used for asthma (87). If nausea, vomiting, or restlessness occurs after taking nonprescription xanthine preparations, the dosage should be reduced. If an adverse effect occurs while taking theophylline, the drug should be stopped and medical attention sought to establish a safe and effective dose. Excessive use of coffee or medications, or foods containing methylxanthines (caffeine, theobromine, or theophylline) should be avoided because they increase the risk of apparent theophylline toxicity. When stressful situations, such as exercise, are unavoidable, prophylactic use of an aerosol prior to exposure may prevent an asthmatic attack.

Summary

It seems that the most commonly available oral nonprescription bronchodilator preparation, which contains a fixed dose of theophylline, ephedrine, and phenobarbital is less rational and, perhaps, less safe than many prescription bronchodilators.

There is no evidence to indicate that expectorant (guaifenesin) or antihistamine drugs contained in oral nonprescription bronchodilator combinations are beneficial (89, 90).

Mild seasonal or intermittent bronchospasm is usually self-limiting and may only produce discomfort. A patient who experiences seasonal asthma may feel comfortable with self-treatment, but unfortunately it is difficult to distinguish those patients who will worsen and those who will remain stable or improve. Although nonprescription epinephrine aerosol seems safe, there is no evidence that oral ephedrine or theophylline-ephedrine combination products are safer than prescription-only bronchodilators. Theophylline-ephedrine combinations at their current labeled dosages are probably not as safe as prescription aerosol bronchodilators or cromolyn. Perhaps combination products should be re-evaluated for nonprescription availability, particularly at current dosage labeling.

The FDA advisory review panel on nonprescription cough, cold, allergy, bronchodilator, and antiasthmatic drug products recommended that bronchodilators are generally safe and effective for nonprescription use at recommended dosages in relieving the shortness of breath caused by bronchospasm. However, the panel emphasized that these preparations should not be used unless a diagnosis of asthma and a dosage schedule of nonprescription medicine has been established by a physician. In addition, patients with asthma may also require prescription drugs that may have serious dangers and side effects, requiring continued medical supervision (91).

Availability of nonprescription bronchodilators outside of pharmacies should also be a matter of concern. Who instructs patients purchasing an epinephrine aerosol in a grocery or department store on the correct manner of drug administration? Who warns patients in these environments about adverse effects and dosing or checks on other drugs the patient is taking? Weight-reducing preparations sold in health food stores commonly contain ephedrine, caffeine, and phenylpropanolamine. These drugs are also purchased for their stimulant properties by drug abusers. In these situations, the nonprescription availability of these drugs may not have a beneficial effect on the public health. There are inconsistencies among the availability of these nonprescription drugs, the labeled doses, and the current standards for appropriate asthma therapy.

References

1. P. M. Penna, *J. Am. Pharm. Assoc., NS13,* 690, (1973).
2. American Thoracic Society, *Am. Rev. Resp. Dis., 85,* 762 (1962).
3. "Prevalence of Selected Chronic Respiratory Conditions in the United States—1970," Vital and Health Statistics, Series 10, No. 84, DHEW Publication No. (HRA) 74–1511, National Center for Health Statistics, Health Resources Administration, Rockville, Md., September 1973.
4. M. H. Williams, *Sem. Resp. Med., 1,* 283–286 (1980).
5. F. M. Rackemann and M. C. Edwards, *N. Engl. J. Med., 246,* 815 (1952).
6. A. L. Sheffer and M. D. Valentine, *Med. Clin. North Am., 53,* 239 (1969).
7. R. P. McCombs, *N. Engl. J. Med., 286,* 1186 (1972).
8. D. A. Mathison, D. D. Stevenson, E. M. Tan, and J. H. Vaughan, *J. Am. Med. Assoc., 244,* 1134 (1973).
9. R. F. Lockey, D. L. Rucknagel, and N. E. Vanselow, *Ann. Intern. Med., 78,* 57 (1973).

10. R. D. Snyder and G. L. Siegel, *Ann. Allergy, 25,* 377 (1967).
11. D. D. Stevenson, D. A. Mathison, E. M. Tan, and J. H. Vaughan, *Arch. Intern. Med., 135,* 777 (1975).
12. E. R. McFadden, *Sem. Resp. Med., 1,* 287 (1980).
13. A. Szentivanji, *J. Allergy, 42,* 203 (1968).
14. A. Szentivanji, *Ann. Allergy, 24,* 253 (1966).
15. A. S. Rebuck and J. Read, *Am. J. Med., 51,* 788 (1971).
16. E. R. McFadden, Jr., R. Kiser, and W. J. Degroot, *N. Engl. J. Med., 288,* 221 (1973).
17. C. S. Shim and M. H. Williams, *Am. J. Med., 68,* 11 (1980).
18. A. R. Rubinfeld and M. C. F. Pain, *Lancet, 1,* 882 (1976).
19. N. Svedmyr and B. G. Simonson, *Pharmac. Ther. B., 3,* 397 (1978).
20. H. Formgren, *Scand. J. Resp. Dis., 56,* 321 (1975).
21. G. Thiringer and N. Svedmyr, *Scand. J. Resp. Dis., 101,* (95) (1977).
22. J. W. Paterson, R. J. Courtnay Evans, and J. F. Prime, *Br. J. Dis. Chest, 65,* 21 (1971).
23. A. S. Banner, E. V. Sunderrajan, M. K. Agarwal, and W. W. Addington, *Arch. Intern. Med., 139,* 434 (1979).
24. C. Shim and M. H. Williams, Jr., *Ann. Intern. Med., 93,* 428 (1980).
25. S. Larsson, N. Svedmyr, and G. Thiringer, *J. Allergy Clin. Immunol., 59,* 93 (1977).
26. L. L. Iversen, *Br. J. Pharmacol., 41,* 571 (1971).
27. C. Shim and M. H. Williams, Jr., *Am. J. Med., 69,* 891 (1980).
28. J. M. Smith, *Lancet, 1,* 1042 (1966).
29. M. J. Greenberg and A. Pines, *Br. Med. J., 1,* 563 (1967).
30. P. D. Stolley, *Am. Rev. Resp. Dis., 105,* 883 (1972).
31. "Bronchial Asthma, Mechanisms and Therapeutics," E. B. Weiss and M. S. Segal, Eds., Little, Brown, Boston, Mass., 1976.
32. *Federal Register, 41,* 38372 (1976).
33. G. R. Wilkinson and A. H. Beckett, *J. Pharmacol. Exp. Ther., 162,* 139 (1968).
34. P S. Sever, L. G. Dring, and R. T. Williams, *Eur. J. Clin. Pharmacol., 9,* 193 (1975).
35. M. E. Pisckup, C. S. May, R. Ssendagire, and J. W. Paterson, *Br. J. Clin. Pharmacol., 3,* 123 (1976).
36. E. Bresnick, J. F. Beaky, L. Levinson, and M. S. Segal, *J. Clin. Invest., 28,* 1182 (1949).
37. D. G. Tinkelman and S. E. Avner, *J. Am. Med. Assoc., 237,* 553 (1977).
38. T. D. James and H. A. Lyons, *J. Am. Med. Assoc, 241,* 704 (1979).
39. C. S. May, M. E. Pisckup, and J. W. Patterson, *Br. J. Clin. Pharmacol., 2,* 533 (1975).
40. W. V. Mieghem, E. Stevens, and J. Cosemans, *Br. Med. J., 1,* 816 (1978).
41. M. G. Roxanas and J. Spaulding, *Med. J. Aust., 2,* 639 (1977).
42. U.S. Drug Enforcement Administration, *Microgram, 13,* 143 (1980).
43. D. P. Taskin, R. Meth, D. H. Simmons, and Y. E. Lee, *Chest, 68,* 155 (1975).
44. M. M. Weinberger and E. A. Bronsky, *J. Pediatr., 84,* 421 (1974).
45. *Federal Register, 41,* 38370 (1976).
46. R. Maselli, G. Casal, and E. F. Ellis, *J. Pediatr., 76,* 777 (1970).
47. J. W. Jenne, E. Wyze, F. S. Rood, and F. M. MacDonald, *J. Clin. Pharmacol. Ther., 13,* 349 (1972).
48. P. A. Mitenko and R. I. Ogilvie, *N. Engl. J. Med., 289,* 600 (1973).
49. J. Pollack, F. Dieckel, D. Cooper, and M. M. Weinberger, *Pediatrics, 60,* 840 (1977).
50. L. Hendeles, L. Bighley, R. H. Richardson, C. D. Hepler, and J. Carmichael, *Drug Intell. Clin. Pharm., 11,* 12 (1977).
51. M. H. Jacobs, R. M. Senior, and G. Kessler, *J. Am. Med. Assoc., 235,* 1983 (1976).
52. R. I. Ogilvie, *Clin. Pharmacokinet., 3,* 267 (1978).
53. J. R. Powell and J. E. Jackson, in "Applied Pharmacokinetics," W. E. Evans, J. Schentag, and W. Jusko, Eds., Applied Therapeutics, San Francisco, Calif., 1981, pp. 139–166.
54. L. J. Foster, W. L. Trudeau, and A. L. Goldman, *J. Am. Med. Assoc., 241,* 2613 (1979).
55. R. A. Upton, L. Sansom, T. Quentert, J. R. Powell, J. F. Thiercelin, V. P. Shah, P. E. Coates, and S. Riefehman, *J. Pharmacokinet. Biopharm., 8,* 229 (1980).
56. R. A. Upton, J. F. Thiercelin, T. Quentert, L. Sansom, J. R. Powell, P. E. Coates, and S. Reigelman, *J. Pharmacokinet. Biopharm., 8,* 131 (1980).
57. M. Fixley, D. D. Shen, and D. L. Azarnoff, *Am. Rev. Resp. Dis., 115,* 955 (1977).
58. P G. Welling, L. L. Lyons, W. A. Craig, and G. A. Trochta, *J. Clin. Pharmacol. Ther., 17,* 475 (1975).
59. R. A. Upton, J. R. Powell, T. Quentert, J. F. Thiercelin, L. Sansom, P. E. Coates, and S. Riegelman, *J. Pharmacokinet. Biopharm., 8,* 151 (1980).
60. J. F. Thiercelin, L. Sansom, J. R. Powell, and S. Riegelman, *Proceedings of the First European Congress of Biopharmaceutics and Pharmacokinetics,* Clermont, France, in press.
61. J. W. Jenne, H. Nagasawa, R. McHugh, F. MacDonald, and E. Wyse, *Life Sci., 17,* 195 (1975).
62. J. R. Powell, J. F. Thiercelin, S. Vozeh, L. Sansom, and S. Riegelman, *Am. Rev. Resp. Dis., 116,* 17 (1977).
63. W. J. Jusko, J. J. Schentagg, J. H. Clark, M. Gardner, and A. M. Turchak, *J. Clin. Pharmacol. Ther., 24,* 406 (1978).
64. A. Kappas. A. P. Alvares, K. E. Anderson, E. J. Pantuck, C. B. Pantuck, R. Chang, and A. H. Conney, *J. Clin. Pharmacol. Ther., 23,* 445 (1978).
65. A. Kappas, K. E. Anderson, A. H. Conney, and A. P. Conney, and A. P. Alvares, *J. Clin. Pharmacol. Ther., 20,* 643 (1977).
66. R. A. Landay, M. A. Gonzalez, and J. C. Taylor, *J. Allergy Clin. Immunol, 62,* 27 (1978).
67. K. M. Piafsky, D. S. Sitar, R. E. Ragno, and R. I. Ogilvic, *N. Engl. J. Med., 296,* 1495 (1977).
68. A. Mangione, T. E. Imhoff, R. V. Lee, L. Y. Shum, and W. J. Jusko, *Chest, 73,* 616 (1978).
69. J. R. Powell, S. Vozeh, P. Hopewell, J. Costello, L. B. Sheiner, and S. Riegelman, *Am. Rev. Resp. Dis., 118,* 229 (1978).
70. K. W. Renton, *Lancet, 2,* 160 (1978).
71. K. W. Renton, J. D. Gray, and R. I. Hall, *J. Can. Med. Assoc., 123,* 288 (1980).
72. K. Conrad and D. Myman, *J. Clin. Pharmacol. Ther., 28,* 463 (1980).
73. B. J. M. Zarowitz, S. J. Szefler, and G. M. Lasezkay, *J. Clin. Pharmacol. Ther., 29,* 601 (1981).
74. J. E. Jackson, J. R. Powell, M. Wandell, J. Bentley, and R. Dorr, *Am. Rev. Resp. Dis., 123,* 615 (1981).
75. E. F. Ellis, R. Koysooko, and G. Levy, *Pediatrics, 58,* 542 (1976).
76. J. V. Aranda, D. S. Sitar, W. D. Parsons, P. M. Loughnan, and A. H. Niems, *N. Engl. J. Med., 295,* 413 (1976).
77. S. Vozeh, J. R. Powell, S. Riegelman, J. F. Costello, L. B. Sheiner, and P. C. Hopewell, *J. Am. Med. Assoc., 240,* 1882 (1978).
78. L. J. Lesko, *Clin. Pharmacokinet., 4,* 449 (1979).
79. *Federal Register, 41,* 38373 (1976).
80. B. G. Simonsson and N. Svedmyr, *Pharmac. Ther. B., 3,* 239 (1977).
81. M. M. Weinberger, E. Bronsky, G. Bensch, G. Bock, and J. Yecies, *J. Clin. Pharmacol. Ther., 17,* 585 (1975).
82. J. A. Sims, G. A. do Pico, and C. E. Reed, *J. Allergy Clin. Immunol., 62,* 15 (1978).
83. W. F. Taylor, S. C. Siegal, R. J. Busser, J. Strick, and E. M. Heimlick, *Ann. Allergy, 26,* 523 (1968).
84. J. A. Sims and C. E. Reed, *J. Allergy Clin. Immunol., 55,* 95 (1975).
85. J. D. Wolfe, D. P. Taskin, B. Calvarese, and M. Simmons, *N. Engl. J. Med., 298,* 363 (1978).
86. E. A. Nelson, J. R. Powell, K. Conrad, K. Likes, J. Byers, S. Baker, and D. Perrier, *J. Clin. Pharmacol. Ther., 29,* 273 (1981).
87. *Federal Register, 41,* 38326 (1976).
88. P. G. Welling, L. E. Schmitz, J. R. Wills, and R. K. Bush, *Internat. J. Pharmaceutics, 4,* 135 (1979).
89. S. R. Hirsh, P. F. Viernes, and R. C. Korey, *Chest, 63,* 9 (1973).
90. J. D. Leopold, J. P. R. Hartley, and A. P. Smith, *Br. J. Clin. Pharmacol., 8,* 249 (1979).
91. *Federal Register, 41,* 38370 (1976).

Asthma Product Table

Product (Manufacturer)	Dosage Form	Ephedrine	Epinephrine	Theophylline	Other Ingredients
Amodrine (Searle)	tablet	25 mg (as racemic hydrochloride)			aminophylline, 100 mg phenobarbital, 8 mg
AsthmaHaler (Norcliff Thayer)	oral inhalant		7 mg/ml (as bitartrate)		propellant 12, 114, 11
AsthmaNefrin (Norcliff Thayer)	inhalant solution		2.25% (epinephrine base as racemic hydrochloride)		chlorobutanol, 0.5%
Breatheasy (Pascal)	inhalant		2.2% (as hydrochloride)		benzyl alcohol, 1% isotonic salts, 0.5%
Bronitin (Whitehall)	tablet	24 mg		130 mg	guaifenesin, 100 mg pyrilamine maleate, 16 mg
Bronitin Mist (Whitehall)	inhalant		7.0 mg/ml (as bitartrate)		freon propellant
Bronkaid (Winthrop)	tablet	24 mg (as sulfate)		100 mg (anhydrous)	guaifenesin, 100 mg magnesium trisilicate, 74.52 mg
Bronkaid Mist (Winthrop)	inhalant		0.5%		ascorbic acid, 0.07% alcohol, 34% hydrochloric and nitric acid buffers
Bronkotabs (Breon)	tablet	24 mg (as sulfate)		100 mg	guaifenesin, 100 mg phenobarbital, 8 mg
Phedral (North American)	tablet	24.3 mg		129.6 mg	phenobarbital, 8.1 mg
Primatene M (Whitehall)	tablet	24 mg (as hydrochloride)		130 mg	pyrilamine maleate, 16 mg
Primatene Mist (Whitehall)	inhalant		5.5 mg/ml		alcohol, 34% freon propellant
Primatene P (Whitehall)	tablet	24 mg (as hydrochloride)		130 mg	phenobarbital, 8 mg
Tedral (Parke-Davis)	tablet elixir suspension	24 mg/tablet 1.2 mg/ml (elixir) 2.4 mg/ml (suspension) (all as hydrochloride)		130 mg/tablet (anhydrous) 6.5 mg/ml (elixir) 13 mg/ml (suspension)	phenobarbital, 8 mg/tablet 0.4 mg/ml (elixir) 0.8 mg/ml (suspension)
Thalfed (Beecham Labs)	tablet	25 mg (as hydrochloride)		120 mg (hydrous)	phenobarbital, 8 mg
Vaponefrin Solution (Fisons)	inhalant		2.25% (epinephrine base as racemic hydrochloride)		chlorobutanol, 0.5%
Verquad (Knoll)	tablet suspension	24 mg/tablet 2.4 mg/ml (both as hydrochloride)		130 mg/tablet 13 mg/ml (both as calcium salicylate)	guaifenesin, 100 mg/tablet or 10 mg/ml phenobarbital, 8 mg/tablet or 0.8 mg/ml

11 Internal Analgesic Products

W. Kent Van Tyle

Questions to Ask the Patient

Where is the pain? Is it in one place or does it spread to other parts of the body?

What type of pain do you have? Is it sharp, dull, aching, knife-like, etc.?

Does the pain occur at any particular time of the day? Does anything make it worse or better?

Do you have any other symptoms that you feel might be associated with the pain you have or any idea as to the reason for the pain (physical injury)?

What pain reliever has worked for you before?

What have you already taken? How much and for how long?

Does aspirin upset your stomach?

Have you ever had an allergic reaction to aspirin?

Do you now have or have you ever had asthma, allergies, or ulcers?

Are you now taking medication for gout, arthritis, or diabetes?

Are you now taking medication that thins your blood?

Have you ever had any problem with your blood being slow to clot?

(If appropriate) How high is your fever, and how long have you had a fever?

Internal analgesics are used to relieve pain. Certain compounds in this group also possess pharmacologic activities that make them valuable for reducing elevated body temperature and for ameliorating various inflammatory conditions.

Even though pain is a common experience, it is not a simple condition to define. Pain is a sensation, but it is also an interpretation of that sensation that can be influenced by many factors. Fatigue, anxiety, fear, and the anticipation of more pain all affect the perception of and reaction to pain. Studies show that various personality types may experience pain differently; the introverted personality has a lower pain threshold than the extrovert (1). In addition, the perception of pain may be modified significantly by suggestion. Studies indicate that approximately 35% of patients suffering pain from a variety of causes report their pain as being "satisfactorily relieved" by placebo (2).

Etiology

Pain is usually a protective mechanism, occurring when tissue is damaged or when cells are altered by pain stimuli that threaten to produce tissue damage. Pain resulting from a functional disturbance or pathology is called "organic" pain. In contrast, "psychogenic" pain is a symptom of an underlying emotional disturbance and is not a consequence of organic pathology.

Origin and Perception of Pain

Pain is categorized, according to its origin, as either somatic or visceral. Somatic pain arises from the musculoskeletal system or skin; visceral pain originates from the organs or viscera of the thorax and abdomen.

Free nerve endings serve as pain receptors to initiate nerve impulses which travel through specialized pain fibers through the spinal cord and/or brain stem to specific receiving areas of the brain. These receptors are found throughout the superficial skin layers and in certain deeper tissues such as membranous bone covering, arterial walls, muscles, tendons, joint surfaces, and membranes lining the skull. Pain-evoking stimuli have in common the ability to injure cells and to release proteolytic enzymes and polypeptides that stimulate nerve endings and initiate the pain impulse (3). Prostaglandins appear to sensitize nerve endings to polypeptide-induced stimulation (4).

Pain fibers enter the dorsal roots of the spinal cord and interconnect with other nerve cells that cross to the opposite side of the cord and ascend to the brain. A pain impulse terminates in the thalamus, where the conscious perception of pain appears to be localized, or in well-defined areas of the cerebral cortex, where recognition and interpretation of the nature and location of the pain impulse occur.

Pain initiation, transmission, and perception are essentially the same for both visceral and somatic pain. One important distinction, however, is that highly localized visceral damage rarely causes severe pain. Diffuse stimulation of nerve endings throughout an organ is required to produce significant visceral pain. Conditions producing visceral pain include ischemia of organ tissue, chemical destruction of visceral tissue, spasm of visceral smooth muscle, and physical distention of an organ or stretching of its associated mesentery (3).

In evaluating the etiology and therapy of pain, it is important to recognize the potential for referred pain. Referred pain is perceived as coming from a part of the body other than that part actually initiating the pain signal. Unlike somatic pain, visceral pain cannot be localized by the brain as coming from a specific organ. Instead, most visceral pain is interpreted by the brain as coming from various skin or muscle segments (it is "referred" to various body surface areas) (Table 1). When a pharmacist is advising the patient as to the need of or potential benefit to be derived from nonprescription analgesic products, an appreciation for the sites of referred visceral pain is invaluable. Failure to recognize the possibility of referred visceral pain could mean that a serious visceral pathology might go undiagnosed and untreated while ineffective self-medication with nonprescription anagesics is attempted. Consequently, effective medical treatment may be dangerously delayed.

Pain Responsive to Nonprescription Analgesics

The analgesic products available for self-medication are more effective in treating musculoskeletal (somatic) pain than visceral pain (5). Nonprescription analgesic therapy is used most frequently for headache or for pain associated with peripheral nerves (neuralgia), muscles (myalgia), or joints (arthralgia).

Headache

The most common form of pain is headache. Estimates are that each week, 15% of the population experiences headache pain (6). Headache may be classified as either intracranial or extracranial, depending on the area of initiation of the pain (7).

Intracranial headache results from inflammation or traction of sensitive, primarily vascular, intracranial structures. Its etiology includes tumor, abscess, hematoma, or infection. Intracranial headache is an uncommon situation, but because of the potential seriousness of its underlying causes it requires immediate medical attention.

Because headache may be a symptom of a serious underlying pathology, the pharmacist should evaluate the potential for intracranial headache and should be prepared to recommend medical attention when appropriate. Intracranial headache produced by tumor or meningeal traction is "deep, aching, steady, dull, and

seldom rhythmic or throbbing (8)." The pain may be continuous, is generally more intense in the morning, and may be associated with nausea and vomiting. Pain location cannot be used to differentiate headache of intracranial origin. Concomitant disturbances in sensory function such as blurred vision, dizziness, or hearing loss or changes in personality, behavior, speech patterns, or memory are signals to seek immediate medical attention.

Table 1. Body surface areas associated with referred visceral pain

Origin of visceral pain	Localization of pain on body surface
Appendix	Around umbilicus localizing in right lower quadrant of abdomen
Bladder	Lower abdomen directly over bladder
Esophagus	Pharynx, lower neck, arms, midline chest region
Gallbladder	Upper central portion of abdomen; lower right shoulder
Heart	Base of neck, shoulders, and upper chest; down arms (left side involvement more frequent than right)
Kidney and ureters	Regions of lower back over site of affected organ; anterior abdominal wall below and to the side of umbilicus
Stomach	Anterior surface of chest or upper abdomen
Uterus	Lower abdomen

Adapted from A. C. Guyton, "Textbook of Medical Physiology," 6th ed., W. B. Saunders, Philadelphia, Pa., 1981, pp. 618–620 and L. Zetzel, in "Textbook of Medicine," Vol. 1, 13th ed., P. B. Beeson and W. McDermott, Eds., W. B. Saunders, Philadelphia, Pa., 1971, p. 1327.

The more common headache forms are extracranial and of diverse etiology. Migraine headache is characterized by intense throbbing, hemicranial pain lasting from several hours to 2 days. The pain often is preceded by visual disturbances; numbness and tingling in the lips, face, or hands; and dizziness and confusion. As the pain increases in intensity, it is often accompanied by nausea and vomiting (3, 8, 9). A hereditary association is seen in 60–80% of patients with migraine; there is a 3:1 female predominance; and stress, hormonal changes, dietary chemicals, and other environmental factors can trigger an attack (10–12). Abnormalities in platelet aggregation resulting in increased plasma serotonin levels are seen in patients with migraine. Increased platelet aggregation occurs during the preheadache phase and parallels increased plasma serotonin levels (13–15). Preheadache vasoconstriction occurs in migraine possibly in response to the increased plasma serotonin levels and is followed by both intracranial and extracranial vasodilation (16). Because of the resulting vascular tone loss, the arteries begin to pulsate with the rising and falling intravascular pressure, and intense pain results from the distention and traction of the affected arteries (12, 16). Preliminary research suggests that drugs, such as aspirin, that inhibit platelet aggregation and the associated serotonin release may be of prophylactic value in reducing the frequency of migraine attacks (17, 18).

The "tension" headache is the result of spasms of the somatic musculature of the neck and scalp. Symptoms include a feeling of tightness or pressure at the base of the head or in the muscles of the back of the neck. Pain with a tension headache is often located in the forehead or at the base of the skull and is usually bilateral.

The sinus headache may be distinguished from headache of other etiology because its location is restricted to the frontal areas of the head and behind or around the eyes. Sinus headaches often recur and subside at the same time each day, and the pain often is intensified by bending over. Sinus pain may be present upon awakening and may subside after a few hours with facilitated sinus drainage. Accompanying symptoms include rhinorrhea, nasal congestion, and a feeling of sinus pressure. The underlying cause is irritation and edema of the nasal and sinus mucous membranes with resultant pressure placed on sinus walls. Infection or allergy is the usual cause, and short-term decongestant therapy often is helpful in facilitating sinus drainage and reducing intrasinus pressure. (See Chapter 9, *Cold and Allergy Products.*)

In addition to being a symptom of sinus headache, pain around or behind the eyes may be caused by uncorrected visual problems associated with difficulty in focusing on near or far objects. An attempt to gain clear vision by tonic ciliary muscle contractions may result in extraocular muscle spasm and referred retro-orbital pain. If retro-orbital headache recurs persistently, referral for ophthalmologic examination is indicated. Recurrent facial or mandibular pain may indicate the need for professional dental examination and treatment.

Neuralgia

Pain generated along the course of a sensory nerve is called neuralgia. The trigeminal nerve frequently is affected, and trigeminal neuralgia is characterized by sharp, stabbing pain in the face or jaw region occurring in brief, agonizing episodes. The cause of trigeminal neuralgia is unknown, but it apparently is not the result of organic damage to the nerve (19, 20). Because of the intense pain of trigeminal neuralgia, therapy with drugs more potent than those available in nonprescription medications may be required.

Dull, aching facial pain localized in the trigeminal nerve area may occur in association with or during recovery from an upper respiratory tract infection. Although the pain often is described as "neuralgia," the exact etiology usually is unknown. Nevertheless, nonprescription analgesics frequently are helpful in alleviating this type of facial pain.

Myalgia

Pain from skeletal muscle (myalgia) is common. The most frequent cause is strenuous exertion of an unconditioned body. However, prolonged tonic contraction produced by tension or by maintaining a certain body position for extended periods also may produce muscle pain (7). Myalgia usually responds well to nonprescription analgesics and adjunctive treatment with rubefacients, counterirritants, and heat. (See Chapter 27, *External Analgesic Products.*)

Arthralgia

The most frequent cause of joint pain is inflammation of the synovial membrane (arthritis) or the associated bursae (bursitis). Joints that require free movement between two bones are constructed to maintain the articulating ends of the bones bathed in a lubricating synovial fluid. The two opposing bone ends are held in position by tough, fibrous tissue that forms an enclosure around the bone ends. The inner lining of this fibrous enclosure is the synovial membrane, which produces the lubricating synovial fluid (21). Bursae are sac-like structures that contain fluid formed at sites of joint friction (where a tendon passes over a bone).

Rheumatoid arthritis is a chronic inflammation of synovial membranes, often occurring at multiple sites and having a predilection for smaller joints such as those of the hands, fingers, wrists, feet, and toes. Symptoms include joint stiffness, especially after arising in the morning, pain with joint motion, and swelling and tenderness of affected joints. Studies indicate that approximately 2.5–3% of the adult population has this condition, the highest incidence occurring in people over 40 (22). Although the cause of rheumatoid arthritis is obscure, hereditary factors have been demonstrated, and an immunologic mechanism has been proposed.

Because of the slow, subtle nature of the onset of rheumatoid arthritis, many people attempt self-medication in the initial stages on the premise that advancing age inevitably brings aches and pains. As the disease progresses, it is a common practice to increase the dosage of nonprescription analgesics voluntarily to maintain relief from arthritic pain. The pharmacist should caution the patient about the potential for chronic toxicity, drug interactions, or other adverse effects and should be on guard for symptoms that indicate overmedication or progression of the disease. Also, because rheumatoid arthritis is a progressive, degenerative disease, medical attention must be encouraged to institute physical therapy and exercise in order that the maximum possible mobility of affected joints is maintained.

Bursitis

This condition may be caused by trauma, gout, infection, or rheumatoid arthritis. Although the most common site of bursa inflammation is the shoulder, the knee (housemaid's knee), and the elbow (tennis elbow) also may be affected. Common symptoms include pain and limited motion of the affected joint. Depending upon the severity, the pain usually will respond to nonprescription analgesic therapy. Limiting motion of the affected joint often hastens recovery (23, 24).

Mechanisms of Normal Thermoregulation and Fever

In a normothermic individual, the internal body temperature is maintained within 1°F of its normal mean temperature by a complex thermoregulatory system. Although the normal mean body temperature is 98.6°F (37°C) measured orally, normal body temperature may range from approximately 97°F (36.1°C) to more than 99°F (37.2°C). When measured rectally, these normal values are 1°F higher (22).

To maintain a constant body temperature, the thermoregulatory system must balance heat production with heat loss. Thermoregulation is accomplished by keeping the temperature control center in the hypothalamus continually apprised of body temperature. Temperature-sensitive neurons located in the hypothalamus and skin relay body temperature information to the hypothalamus. Responding to this information, the hypothalamus initiates responses either to conserve heat and to increase heat production or to increase heat loss.

The skin is the primary site of heat loss from the body. Heat is carried by the blood from internal structures to the body surface where it is lost to the surroundings by radiation, conduction, and evaporation. The heat loss rate from the skin is related directly to the cutaneous blood flow rate, which in turn is a reflection of the degree of tone in the cutaneous vasculature. Consequently, the hypothalamic thermoregulatory center can change the rate of heat loss by altering vasoconstriction in the cutaneous vasculature. It also facilitates cooling by stimulating sweating, which increases the evaporative heat loss rate from the skin. Heat production can be enhanced by hormonally mediated increases in cellular metabolism and by increased muscle tone and shivering.

Fever, or the elevation of body temperature above normal, may occur as the result of infection by various organisms including both gram-negative and gram-positive bacteria, viruses, fungi, yeasts, and protozoa (25). Other causes of fever include drugs, dehydration, tissue damage, antigen-antibody reactions, and malignancies. Pyrogens, or fever-producing substances, are categorized as either exogenous or endogenous. Exogenous pyrogens (those not produced by the body) include the endotoxins produced by gram-negative bacteria. Endogenous pyrogens are small proteins produced and released within the body by liver and spleen cells, monocytes, eosinophils, and neutrophils (26). Pyrogen release occurs as a consequence of the phagocytosis of an infectious agent or in response to stimulation by bacterial endotoxin or antigen-antibody complexes (25–28). The production and release of endogenous pyrogen constitute the common pathway of fever production by all pyrogens.

Experimental evidence in animals strongly suggests that prostaglandins of the E series are produced in response to circulating endogenous pyrogen and that the E prostaglandins act on the anterior hypothalamus to elevate the set point above its normal level, thereby producing fever. Endogenous pyrogen increases the concentration of E prostaglandins in cerebrospinal fluid, and drugs that inhibit the synthesis of E prostaglandins in response to endogenous pyrogen have antipyretic activity (29–36). In response to E prostaglandins and changes in monoamine concentration, the hypothalamus directs the re-establishment of body temperature to correspond to the new elevated set point (26, 27). Within hours the body temperature reaches this new set point, and a febrile condition results. During the period of upward temperature readjustment, symptoms of chills and shivering are experienced, even though the body temperature is elevated above normal. These are manifestations of peripheral heat conservation and production mechanisms, such as peripheral vasoconstriction and increased skeletal muscle tone, which produces shivering.

Fever produces a clouding of intellectual function, disorientation, and possibly delirium. Headache is common in a febrile individual and is thought to be the result of dilation and stretching of the larger arteries at the base of the brain. Tachycardia often occurs concomitantly with fever and is usually of little concern unless there is a history of impaired cardiovascular function (37).

Fever itself does not require therapy unless there is a possibility of CNS damage, cardiovascular insufficiency, or significant discomfort to the patient. Temperatures as high as 105°F (40.6°C) usually are tolerated by adults. However, children are more prone to convulsions with temperatures in this range. When body temperature rises above 106°F (41.1°C), tissue damage begins. The brain is acutely sensitive to temperatures in this range because damaged brain tissue does not regenerate. Body temperatures above 110°F (43.3°C) are fatal within hours (38).

Treatment

On the basis of careful patient history evaluation, the pharmacist should decide whether the pain or fever can be self-medicated or if physician referral is necessary. If the condition is amenable to self-medication with a nonprescription analgesic/antipyretic, the pharmacist should recommend an appropriate product.

Salicylates

By virtue of their historical significance, extent of use, and spectrum of pharmacologic activity, the salicylates represent the prototype of non-narcotic analgesics. They produce their pharmacologic effects primarily through the production of salicylate ion in the body. Several forms of salicylate are available.

The salicylates have analgesic, antipyretic, and anti-inflammatory activity and are most effective in treating mild to moderate pain of the dull, aching type that originates in somatic structures. In doses of 325–650 mg, "controlled experiments have repeatedly shown aspirin to be superior to placebo in pathologic pain of a wide variety of etiologies" (39). Salicylates produce analgesia both centrally, by acting on hypothalamic structures, and peripherally, by inhibiting pain impulse production in pain receptors (5, 40). Certain prostaglandins sensitize peripheral pain receptors, making them more sensitive to chemical or mechanical initiation of pain impulses (4, 41). Salicylates inhibit prostaglandin synthesis and desensitize pain receptors to the initiation of pain impulses by decreasing prostaglandin production at inflammation and trauma sites (42).

Salicylate therapy for fever reduction is initiated most frequently in children because of their propensity for fever-induced convulsions. Salicylates effectively reduce elevated body temperature by causing the hypothalamic thermoregulatory center to re-establish a normal set point. Heat production is not inhibited, but rather, heat loss is augmented by increased cutaneous blood flow and sweating induced by the reset thermoregulatory center. Salicylates exert their antipyretic effect by inhibiting prostaglandin production in the hypothalamus (5, 43, 44).

The adult oral aspirin dosage considered to be safe for self-medication by the FDA advisory review panel on nonprescription internal analgesic and antirheumatic drug products is 352–360 mg every 4 hours while symptoms persist, not to exceed 4 g in 24 hours. On the basis of pharmacokinetic considerations, the panel recommends that the maximum single dose be 975 mg (45). This dose is to be administered only once as a single dosage or as the initial (loading) dosage in a multiple-dose regimen. These dose recommendations apply to aspirin use either as an analgesic or as an antipyretic. The panel recommendations for pediatric aspirin dosage are summarized in Table 2.

Although the efficacy of salicylates in treating inflammatory conditions such as rheumatic fever and rheumatoid arthritis is well established, the mechanism by which these beneficial effects are produced is not. Studies show that the anti-inflammatory effect of salicylates is the result of their inhibition of prostaglandin synthesis (42, 46). Prostaglandins of the E type are formed at inflammation sites where they produce vasodilation and potentiate plasma exudate formation produced by other mediators such as histamine and bradykinin (47, 48). Research in animals shows a correlation between potentiation of plasma exudate formation and the vasodilator activity of prostaglandins and suggests that prostaglandins probably do not increase vascular permeability and plasma exudate formation directly in inflammation (49). Therefore at least part of the anti-inflammatory effect of salicylates is attributable to decreased prostaglandin synthesis at inflammation sites, with a resultant decrease in vasodilation and plasma exudate formation.

Aspirin doses in the range of 4–6 g/day often are effective in relieving symptomatic pain associated with rheumatoid arthritis. Proposed nonprescription labeling regulations for aspirin direct the patient not to exceed 4 g in a 24-hour period. Consequently, self-medication with aspirin for arthritis may be inadequate therapy because the aspirin dose required for efficacy is often greater than that deemed safe for self-medication (50). Furthermore, some patients may require higher aspirin doses to attain adequate salicylate serum levels for optimal anti-inflammatory effects. The dose required may vary from 4–10 g/day (51).

Contraindications to Salicylate Use

Impaired Platelet Aggregation and Hypoprothrombinemia Aspirin may comprise hemostasis by inhibiting platelet aggregation and by reducing plasma prothrombin levels. In a normal individual, a single 650-mg (10 g) dose of aspirin approximately doubles the mean bleeding time for 4–7 days (5, 52). This increase in bleeding time is due primarily to inhibited platelet aggregation and not to hypoprothrombinemia. Decreased platelet aggregation is the result of an irreversible aspirin-induced inhibition of prostaglandin synthesis in the platelet (53–55). Salicylate doses of more than 6 g/day are required to reduce plasma prothrombin levels, and the minimal prolongation of prothrombin time that occurs with these doses is rarely clinically significant (5, 52). Salicylates reduce plasma prothrombin levels by interfering with the use of vitamin K for prothrombin synthesis (56).

Platelet aggregation is an important hemostatic mechanism, especially in capillaries and other small blood vessels. When small vessel damage occurs, platelets adhere to exposed collagen fibers and aggregate to form a plug. A fibrin network forms, and a clot develops to stop bleeding from the damaged vessel. Platelet aggregation is an extremely important mechanism for controlling the oozing type of capillary bleeding. Aspirin may potentiate capillary bleeding from the GI tract, post-tonsillectomy tonsillar bed, and tooth sockets following dental extractions (57–59). Consequently, aspirin therapy should be discontinued at least 1 week before surgery, and aspirin should be used to relieve the

Table 2. Recommended pediatric single dosage schedule for aspirin and acetaminophen

Age of child (years)	Number of 80-mg pediatric dosage units to be taken every 4 hours[a]	Dosage (mg) every 4 hours	Maximum total 24-hour dosage (mg)
Under 2[b]			
2 to under 4	2	160	800
4 to under 6	3	240	1,200
6 to under 9	4	320	1,600
9 to under 11	5	400	2,000
11 to under 12	6	480	2,400

Adapted from the Report of the Advisory Review Panel on OTC Internal Analgesic and Antirheumatic Drug Products, *Federal Register*, 42(131), 35368 and 35445–50 (1977).

[a]Not to exceed five single dosages in 24 hours. No child should be given a nonprescription analgesic for more than 5 days or a nonprescription antipyretic for more than 3 days except under the advice and supervision of a physician.

[b]There is no recommended dosage except under the advice and supervision of a physician.

pain of tonsillectomy or dental extraction only under the advice and supervision of a physician or dentist. Additionally, the FDA advisory review panel on nonprescription internal analgesic and antirheumatic drug products recommends the following warning on all oral aspirin products to be chewed (chewable tablets or gums): "Do not take this product for at least 7 days after tonsillectomy or oral surgery except under the advice and supervision of a physician" (60).

Many patients are under the false impression that if there is "tooth" or "throat" pain, local placement of aspirin is more beneficial. Pharmacists should be aware of the potential dangers of gum ulceration with this practice and advise their patients appropriately.

Apirin use should be avoided by individuals with hypoprothrombinemia, vitamin K deficiency, hemophilia or history of other clotting disorders, and by those with a history of peptic ulcer or GI bleeding. In contrast to aspirin, acetaminophen does not affect platelet aggregation or bleeding time (52, 57). A recent study demonstrated that in both normal patients and hemophiliacs a 6-week course of acetaminophen (1,950 mg/day) had no effect on bleeding time or platelet aggregation (61). Therefore acetaminophen may be a useful analgesic in patients where concern about hemostasis contraindicates aspirin use.

Impaired Uric Acid Elimination   Salicylates affect uric acid secretion and reabsorption by the renal tubules. The result is dependent on the dose of salicylate administered. In low doses of 1–2 g/day, salicylates inhibit tubular uric acid secretion without affecting reabsorption. Consequently, low salicylate doses 1–2 g/day reduce urate excretion by the kidney, elevate plasma urate levels, and may precipitate an acute gout attack. Moderate doses (2–3 g/day) usually have no effect on uric acid secretion and high doses (>5 g/day) may increase uric acid excretion, resulting in decreased plasma urate levels. However, effective uricosuric doses of salicylates are poorly tolerated, making aspirin a poor choice as a uricosuric agent (5). For this reason, self-medication with salicylates by individuals with a history of gout should be discouraged.

GI Irritation and Bleeding   Dyspepsia with heartburn, epigastric distress, and nausea or vomiting occur in approximately 5% of patients taking aspirin (62). More common than dyspepsia is mild GI bleeding following aspirin ingestion in 40–70% of patients. The GI blood loss usually is in the range of 2–6 ml/day, but as much as 10 ml/day has been reported with normal analgesic doses (63, 64). GI blood loss usually is not clinically significant, but prolonged aspirin use may result in continued blood loss and a persistent iron-deficient anemia (65, 66). Gastroscopic examination in salicylate-treated patients often reveals ulcerative and hemorrhagic lesions of the gastric mucosa, although lesions are not always visible in those experiencing blood loss (5, 6, 67). A reappraisal of the evidence suggests that the incidence of aspirin-induced mucosal damage has been overestimated (68). Occult blood tests of stool are frequently false-positive in patients taking aspirin. Aspirin use should be discontinued 3 days before such tests.

Massive GI bleeding characterized by the vomiting of blood (hematemesis) or the presence of large amounts of digested blood in the stools (melena) has been linked to aspirin ingestion. Approximately 30–40% of hospital admissions for hematemesis and/or melena are attributable to prior salicylate use (69–71). Individuals who take aspirin at least 4 days per week during a 12-week period have a significantly greater likelihood of suffering major GI bleeding than the less frequent user or nonuser of aspirin. The incidence rate of hospital admissions for major upper GI bleeding attributable to regular aspirin use is estimated to be about 15/100,000/year (72). Aspirin is contraindicated in individuals having a history of peptic ulcer disease or GI bleeding because it may activate latent ulcers or aggravate existing ones. In addition, ingesting alcohol with aspirin appears to increase the incidence of GI bleeding, and patients taking aspirin daily should be advised of the potential hazards of alcohol ingestion (73, 74).

Aspirin Hypersensitivity   In predisposed individuals, aspirin may produce a hypersensitivity reaction characterized by any of the following symptoms: shortness of breath, skin rash and edema, hives (urticaria), severe asthma attack, anaphylaxis with laryngeal edema, bronchoconstriction, and shock. Aspirin hypersensitivity occurs most frequently in persons having a history of asthma or chronic urticaria. Up to 20% of such persons may exhibit aspirin hypersensitivity (75–78). In contrast, the incidence of aspirin hypersensitivity in the general population is estimated to be 0.3% (79).

There are two major types of aspirin hypersensitivity, which differ in mechanism, type of response, and cross-sensitivities (80). One type usually exhibits shortness of breath or asthma-like symptoms in response to aspirin. Evidence suggests that asthma-like symptoms are related to prostaglandin synthesis inhibition by aspirin, and cross-sensitivity has been demonstrated with other prostaglandin synthesis inhibitors including flufenamic acid, ibuprofen, indomethacin, mefenamic acid, and phenylbutazone (81–83). Acetaminophen does not usually show cross-sensitivity in this group (81).

The second aspirin-hypersensitive group exhibits skin reactions such as edema, rash, or hives. The mechanism for this reaction is unknown, and this group may be more susceptible to cross-sensitivity with acetaminophen but the frequency is still low (84). Acetaminophen cross-sensitivity has been estimated at 5–6% in persons intolerant to aspirin (85).

A history of asthma, chronic urticaria, or aspirin hypersensitivity contraindicates aspirin use for self-medication. In addition, a history of asthma-like reactions to the prostaglandin synthesis inhibitors also contraindicates self-medication with aspirin. Limited studies on cross-sensitivity suggest that in persons exhibiting asthma-like symptoms with aspirin, acetaminophen may be an acceptable analgesic/antipyretic drug. Finally, persons with known aspirin hypersensitivity should be cautioned about using other nonprescription medications that may contain aspirin or salicylates.

Drug Interactions Uricosuric agents such as probenecid and sulfinpyrazone are effective in treating gout because they block the tubular reabsorption of uric acid. Salicylates inhibit the uricosuric effects of both drugs by blocking this inhibitory effect on uric acid reabsorption (86, 87). Consequently, the concurrent administration of salicylates with either probenecid or sulfinpyrazone should be avoided because of the possibility of precipitating acute gouty attacks, hyperuricemia, or urate stone formation. Occasionally, salicylate doses of 650 mg or less, which do not produce serum salicylate levels above 5 mg/100 ml, do not appear to significantly affect probenecid uricosuria (88).

Because of their effects on hemostasis and GI mucosa, salicylates have the potential for producing hemorrhaging if administered with oral anticoagulants. The effect of oral anticoagulants on bleeding time may be enhanced by the salicylates, and the severity of salicylate-induced GI bleeding may be augmented as a result of hemostasis impairment by anticoagulant drugs (89). It is advised that the concurrent administration of salicylates and oral anticoagulants be avoided. For analgesic/antipyretic activity, acetaminophen is recommended for self-medication in patients receiving oral anticoagulant therapy (90).

Lowering of blood glucose levels by the sulfonylurea oral hypoglycemics may be enhanced when a salicylate is administered concurrently. Salicylates displace tolbutamide and chlorpropamide from plasma protein binding sites and have intrinsic hypoglycemic activity when taken by diabetics (5, 91). Controlled clinical studies documenting the significance of this interaction are lacking. However, in view of existing evidence, it is advisable to monitor closely diabetics who are receiving both salicylates and a sulfonylurea hypoglycemic agent, especially when the drug is started or doses are changed. In recommending a nonprescription analgesic for concurrent administration, the pharmacist should take into consideration that acetaminophen seems to have less potential for interaction than the salicylates.

All anti-inflammatory drugs, both steroidal and nonsteroidal, used to treat arthritis and other inflammatory diseases are potentially ulcerogenic. Because of possible enhanced GI erosion when these agents are used in combination with a salicylate, it is recommended that persons taking prescription anti-inflammatory drugs should not self-medicate concurrently with salicylates (92). There is no clinical evidence to suggest additive or synergistic anti-inflammatory activity with the concurrent administration of nonsteroidal

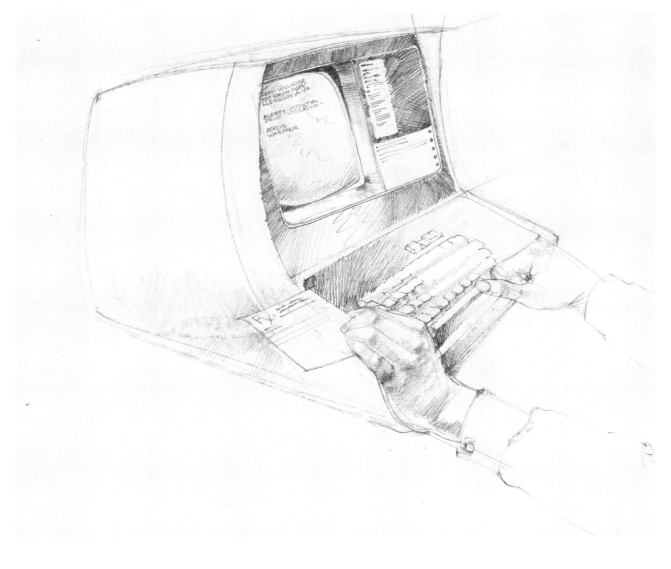

anti-inflammatory agents and salicylates. In this regard, the ulcerogenic potential with salicylates would make acetaminophen a more appropriate choice of therapy (93).

Salicylate Toxicity   Mild salicylate toxicity may occur in adults after repeated administration of large doses or in young children as a result of therapeutic overdosage. Symptoms consist of dizziness, ringing in the ears (tinnitus), difficulty in hearing, nausea, vomiting, diarrhea, mental confusion, and lassitude (5). Skin eruptions may appear if salicylates are continued for a week or longer, and more pronounced CNS symptoms may develop, such as incoherent speech, delirium, or hallucinations.

The mean lethal aspirin dose in adults is between 20 and 30 g, and the toxic dose for children is 150 mg/kg (94–96). Symptoms of salicylate poisoning include those cited for mild toxicity and hyperventilation, dimness of vision, mental confusion, delirium, hallucinations, convulsions, and coma. Acid-base disturbances are prominent and range from respiratory alkalosis to metabolic acidosis. Initially, salicylate effects on the respiratory center in the medulla produce hyperventilation and respiratory alkalosis. In severely intoxicated adults and in most children under 5, respiratory alkalosis rapidly changes to metabolic acidosis (5, 95, 96).

Salicylate poisoning affects other physiologic functions. The metabolic rate is increased, resulting in increased heat production and fever. Children are more prone than adults to develop high fever in salicylate poisoning (95, 96). Hypoglycemia results from increased tissue glucose use and may be especially serious in children (5). Bleeding may occur from the GI tract due to erosion of the mucosal lining, or hemorrhaging from other sites may occur as a consequence of salicylate inhibition of platelet aggregation (94, 96).

Emergency management of aspirin poisoning is designed to delay drug absorption and to remove it from the stomach. If the person is conscious and able to swallow, one or two glasses of milk should be given to dilute the drug, delay gastric emptying, and slow absorption. However, the volume of liquid given to children should not exceed 50 ml/10 kg (97).

Because of the rapid absorption of salicylates from the GI tract, emptying the stomach at home or enroute to an emergency medical facility is advised. Vomiting should be induced even if the patient has vomited spontaneously. An emetic dose of 1 tbsp (15 ml) of syrup of ipecac followed by ingestion of 8 oz of water should be given and the patient ambulated to favor emesis. If emesis does not occur in 30 minutes, the process should be repeated with the same ipecac dose. For children under 1 year of age, emesis should be induced only under medical supervision. Administering liquids or ipecac to a person who is convulsing or to one who is not completely conscious is absolutely contraindicated (94, 96, 97). It should also be noted that any patient suspected of taking a CNS depressant agent should not be given an emetic. Since it takes several minutes for the emetic to act, aspiration pneumonia may occur if the patient becomes obtunded prior to emesis.

Activated charcoal slurry (50 g in 400 ml of water) may be given orally and is very effective in delaying salicylate absorption from the stomach. When syrup of ipecac is used, emesis must occur before giving activated charcoal since ipecac will be absorbed on the charcoal, reducing the effectiveness of both (97). (See Chapter 7, *Emetic and Antiemetic Products*.)

Biopharmaceutics of Aspirin-Containing Products
The rate-limiting step for achieving therapeutic blood levels with solid dosage forms of aspirin is dissolution in the GI fluids rather than absorption from the gut (98). Factors affecting the dissolution rate include the degree of GI motility, the gastric fluid pH, gastric fluid volume, and the diffusion layer pH (the region of high salicylate concentration surrounding the dissolving aspirin particles). Aspirin's dissolution rate is increased by raising the volume and pH of the surrounding medium (99). Including alkaline buffering agents in the table formulation produces an elevated pH in the diffusion layer, increasing the aspirin dissolution rate. If formulated properly, buffered aspirin has significantly greater dissolution and absorption rates than nonbuffered aspirin (45, 100–102). However, there is no evidence from controlled clinical studies that buffered aspirin provides a more rapid onset or greater degree of pain relief than nonbuffered aspirin (100, 102).

The degree of salicylate-induced gastric irritation and erosion is a function of the salicylate concentration and the duration of exposure at the gastric mucosal surface. Although aspirin solutions also may produce GI erosion, undissolved apsirin particles are thought to be primarily responsible for gastric mucosal damage because they produce high salicylate concentrations at mucosal surfaces in the region of their diffusion layer (103). Buffered aspirin tablets produce less GI bleeding than nonbuffered tablets, presumably because they dissolve more rapidly, reducing the exposure time of the gastric mucosa to the offending aspirin particles (100, 104). Aspirin dissolution is favored when tablets are taken with a full glass (8 oz) of fluid.

Aspirin is absorbed more rapidly in solution than from either buffered or nonbuffered tablets because the dissolution factor is eliminated (101). Highly buffered aspirin solutions having a neutralizing capacity of at least 20 mEq of hydrochloric acid significantly decrease the amount of gastric bleeding (105, 106). However, the effervescent-type buffered aspirin solutions achieve their buffering action at the expense of a high sodium content. For this reason their use by patients whose sodium intake is restricted should be avoided. In addition, there is no valid evidence that highly buffered aspirin solutions produce more rapid or effective analgesia than either plain or buffered aspirin tablets (100).

Enteric-coated aspirin is specially formulated to prevent tablet dissolution until it reaches the more alkaline pH of the small intestine, preventing the gastric distress associated with dissolution in the stomach. However, aspirin absorption from enteric-coated tablets may be highly erratic. Tablets sometimes dissolve prematurely in the stomach and sometimes they do not dissolve at all (107). The variable aspirin absorption from enteric-coated tablets also is caused by differences in the tablets' gastric retention time (108, 109). However, enteric coating may reduce the likelihood of gastric and duodenal mucosal injury (110, 111). Studies indicate that current formulations of enteric-coated aspirin produce serum salicylate levels not significantly different from regular aspirin (112).

Timed-release aspirin is a formulation using encapsulation techniques attempting to prolong the product's duration of action. Such products are not useful for rapid pain relief because their absorption is delayed. However, the prolonged absorption may make timed-release aspirin useful as a bedtime medication. One study showed that 6–8 hours after ingestion of a single 1,300-mg aspirin dose the total serum salicylate concentration is significantly higher with the timed-release product tested than with regular tableted aspirin (113). Timed-release aspirin has been implicated in hemorrhagic gastritis and an increased incidence of deafness, but definitive clinical studies are not available (114–116).

Other Aspirin and Salicylate Dosage Forms

Carbaspirin calcium is a complex of urea and calcium acetylsalicylate that is hydrolyzed in the GI tract to aspirin, calcium, and urea (117). Although it may be absorbed more rapidly, there is no evidence that it offers a clinically significant advantage over aspirin in the rate at which analgesia is achieved (118). Because it is a larger molecule than aspirin, 414 mg is required to produce the same pharmacologic effect as 325 mg of aspirin. The recommended adult dose is 414–828 mg every 4 hours while symptoms persist, not to exceed 4,968 mg/24 hours (119).

Choline salicylate is the only liquid salicylate preparation available. It is absorbed from the stomach more rapidly than aspirin in tablet form, but this property has little clinical significance (119). Evidence suggests that choline salicylate is less potent than aspirin as an analgesic/antipyretic; however, it may produce less GI bleeding and distress (39, 118, 119). A dose of 435 mg of choline salicylate is equivalent to 325 mg of sodium salicylate. The recommended adult dose is 435–870 mg every 4 hours, not to exceed 5,220 mg/24 hours (119). The liquid form is often useful for arthritic patients who have difficulty swallowing tablets.

Magnesium salicylate is equivalent to sodium salicylate in analgesic/antipyretic potency. Claims remain to be proven that it might be indicated when aspirin cannot be tolerated (119). In addition, the possibility of systemic magnesium toxicity exists in persons with renal insufficiency who take maximum daily doses of magnesium salicylate. The recommended adult dose is 325–650 mg every 4 hours, not to exceed 4 g/24 hours (119). The FDA, however, is considering revision of the recommended adult dose for magnesium salicylate. Magnesium salicylate is available as the tetrahydrate such that the salicylate content of approximately 375 mg of magnesium salicylate tetrahydrate is equivalent to 325 mg of sodium salicylate.

Sodium salicylate produces blood salicylate levels as high as equimolar doses of aspirin; however, it is probably less effective than aspirin as an analgesic/antipyretic (120). The sodium content of the maximum daily sodium salicylate dose (25 mEq) is sufficient to contraindicate its use in persons on sodium-restricted diets. The recommended adult dose of sodium salicylate is 325–650 mg every 4 hours, not to exceed 4 g in 24 hours (119).

Aspirin and Pregnancy

Evidence from studies in laboratory animals and from retrospective studies in humans suggests that aspirin use during the latter months of pregnancy has adverse effects on both the mother and the fetus. The administration of 200 mg/kg/day of aspirin to rats during the last 6 days of pregnancy produced a prolongation of labor, a prolongation of parturition time, and increased in-utero fetal death (121).

A 20-year retrospective study of 103 women who took aspirin doses greater than 3,250 mg/day during the last 6 months of pregnancy suggests that aspirin has detrimental effects during pregnancy. In comparison with control groups of women, those using aspirin had significantly longer gestation periods, longer labor periods, and greater blood loss at delivery. These effects on pregnancy may be related to the inhibition of prostaglandin synthesis, platelet aggregation, and prothrombin synthesis by aspirin (122).

Studies of 144 women who used nonprescription analgesic preparations containing aspirin during pregnancy reached similar conclusions (123, 124). The major effects reported for regular aspirin use during pregnancy included an increased frequency of anemia during pregnancy, a prolonged gestation period, an increased incidence of complicated deliveries, a high incidence of antepartum and postpartum hemorrhage, increased perinatal mortality, and decreased neonate birth weight.

Interpretation of these results is complicated, however, by a higher incidence of smoking in the aspirin-using group and by the fact that the nonprescription analgesic products used by these women were combinations of either aspirin, salicylamide, and caffeine or aspirin, phenacetin, and caffeine. Smoking in itself has been established to have numerous detrimental effects on pregnancy including lower birth weight of the neonate, increased perinatal mortality, and increased spontaneous abortion (125). Another study of 1,515 mother-child pairs exposed to aspirin for at least 8 days/month during at least 6 months of the pregnancy found "no evidence that aspirin as used by pregnant women in the United States is related to perinatal mortality or low birth weight" (126). It is possible therefore that the differences in perinatal mortality and birth weight reported in the Australian studies are due to confounding factors such as smoking rather than totally to aspirin use (123, 124).

In attempting to reconcile the Australian (123, 124) and Boston Collaborative Drug Surveillance Program reports, the amount and frequency of aspirin use also must be considered (126). In the Australian study the group of women showing the greatest incidence of detrimental aspirin effect on pregnancy admitted taking nonprescription analgesic preparations every day during the pregnancy. This dosage represented a higher frequency of aspirin use than that evaluated in the Boston study.

Aspirin readily traverses the placenta and often is found in higher concentration in the blood of the neonate than in that of the mother (124, 127, 128). Normal analgesic aspirin doses taken by the mother before delivery may decrease platelet aggregation in the neonate (129) and possibly produce clinical bleeding (130). As a consequence of these observations, the FDA advisory review panel on nonprescription internal analgesic and antirheumatic drug products has recommended that aspirin-containing products not be used during the last 3 months of pregnancy except under the advice and supervision of a physician (60).

Aspirin and Antiplatelet Therapy

The use of aspirin under medical supervision for the prophylaxis or therapy of platelet-mediated thromboembolic or atherosclerotic disease has aroused considerable interest. When blood vessel damage occurs, platelets aggregate and adhere to collagen and other components of the damaged vessel wall, release granular contents including ADP, aggregate, and release thromboxane A_2, a highly unstable intermediate produced by prostaglandin biosynthetic pathways. Its release promotes further platelet aggregation, and it is a potent vasoconstrictor. The vessel wall also produces an unstable intermediate in prostaglandin synthesis called prostacyclin, a powerful vasodilator which inhibits both platelet adherence to the vessel wall and platelet aggregation. Prostacyclin seems to control homeostasis by limiting thrombus formation at sites of vessel wall damage. Its antiaggregatory effect counters the proaggregatory effect of platelet thromboxane A_2 (131, 132).

Aspirin irreversibly inhibits prostaglandin-dependent platelet aggregation and thromboxane A_2 synthesis by acetylating and inhibiting the prostaglandin synthetase (cyclo-oxygenase) enzyme in platelets (133). Aspirin destroys the ability of circulating platelets to synthesize prostaglandins and thromboxane A_2 for the entire life of the platelet, decreasing its ability to aggregate. Aspirin also acetylates vascular cyclo-oxygenase and inhibits the synthesis of prostacyclin in blood vessels, thereby allowing platelets to aggregate, a potentially detrimental, prothrombotic event. However, with appropriate aspirin dosage, selective inhibition of thromboxane A_2 production may potentially be achieved with minimal inhibition of prostacyclin (134, 135), allowing platelet aggregation to be controlled. Dosage requirements for this selective inhibition have yet to be determined adequately but may be as low as 40 mg (136, 137).

Preliminary clinical observations suggested that antiplatelet therapy might be effective in preventing transient ischemic attack (TIA) and stroke. A TIA is a sudden interruption of the blood flow to a portion of the brain or retina resulting in symptoms of neurologic deficit lasting for from a few seconds to 24 hours. Emboli consisting of platelet-fibrin masses or debris from atherosclerotic lesions are the most common cause

(138). The risk of stroke in a patient who has had a TIA is approximately 5–6% a year with the greatest risk in the first 3 months following the first attack (138).

The Canadian Cooperative Study found that a dose of 1,300 mg of aspirin/day produced a 48% decrease in the incidence of stroke and death in men who had had a TIA within 3 months of entering the study. However, no significant benefit of aspirin was found in women (139). A similar study in the United States also employing 1,300 mg/day demonstrated a reduction in TIA's by aspirin during the first 6 months following entry into the study, but no difference between the responses of men and women was demonstrated (140).

Numerous observations suggest a link between platelet-induced thromboembolism and myocardial infarction. In animal models of myocardial ischemia, aggregated platelets have been found in the coronary vessels, which may produce occlusion and myocardial injury (144). Patients dying suddenly with coronary atherosclerosis but no infarction often show platelet aggregates in the myocardial microcirculation (142). Several clinical studies have shown that patients with coronary artery disease have increased platelet aggregation and decreased platelet survival (143). The rationale for the use of antiplatelet drugs in patients with ischemic heart disease is to prevent the formation of a platelet-fibrin thrombus and its subsequent embolization in the coronary microcirculation.

Two studies have attempted to evaluate whether or not aspirin is effective in preventing reinfarction in men and women who have had at least one recently documented myocardial infarction. In the Medical Research Council study, 1,682 patients who had had a confirmed myocardial infarct were given 300 mg of aspirin 3 times/day for 1 year (144). There was a 17% reduction in mortality in the aspirin-treated group; however, this reduction was not statistically significant. The aspirin-treated group did have a statistically significant reduction in the incidence of nonfatal myocardial infarction.

The Aspirin Myocardial Infarction Study randomized 4,524 postinfarction patients into an aspirin-treated group receiving 1.0 g/day and a placebo-treated group (145, 146). After 3 years, death rates were not significantly different in the aspirin and placebo groups. However, there was a statistically significant reduction in the rate of recurrent, nonfatal myocardial infarctions and strokes in the aspirin-treated group. Both of these studies have been criticized on the basis that more patients in the aspirin group had congestive heart failure on entry into the study.

In summary, these studies suggest that the incidence of nonfatal myocardial reinfarction is reduced in postmyocardial infarction patients receiving aspirin. However, the reduction in mortality in these patients attributable to aspirin was not statistically significant.

Salicylamide

Although it is structurally similar to salicylates, salicylamide is not hydrolyzed to salicylic acid in the body, and its pharmacologic activity resides in the salicylamide molecule itself (147). Salicylamide's unusual pharmacokinetic character complicates interpretation of its efficacy and formulation factors. Oral salicylamide doses below 600 mg are almost completely metabolized to inactive metabolites during transit through the GI mucosa and hepatic circulation before ever reaching the systemic circulation. Consequently, "breakthrough doses" greater than 300–600 mg are required to saturate the intestinal and hepatic enzyme systems and to achieve effective systemic concentrations (148, 149).

Salicylamide has been shown to have greater analgesic effects in animals than aspirin (150, 151); however, studies in humans with pathologic pain have shown that salicylamide has no superiority over aspirin in doses below 600 mg and is indistinguishable from placebo (39, 150). Salicylamide has been proven consistently inferior to aspirin as an antipyretic in both animal and human studies and is estimated to be about half as potent as aspirin as an antipyretic (39, 45, 152, 153). Persons allergic to aspirin usually have no cross-sensitivity to salicylamide, and salicylamide does not increase prothrombin time (148, 154). The FDA advisory review panel on nonprescription internal analgesic and antirheumatic drug products concluded that salicylamide is probably ineffective in the recommended adult doses of 300–600 mg every 4 hours when used as a single analgesic or antipyretic agent and that there is insufficient evidence of efficacy when salicylamide is used as an adjuvant in combination with other analgesic-antipyretic ingredients. Higher doses (1,000 mg every 4 hours not to exceed 6,000 mg/24 hours) may be effective; however, there is insufficient evidence supporting the safety of salicylamide. There is no recommended dosage for children under 12 years except under the advice and supervision of a physician (148).

Para-aminophenols

Analgesic compounds in this class include acetaminophen and phenacetin. These compounds are analgesic-antipyretic and are effective in treating mild to moderate pain such as headache, neuralgia, and pain of musculoskeletal origin (39, 155). Although phenacetin is considered to be an effective analgesic-antipyretic, there are serious questions concerning its safety and abuse potential. The FDA advisory review panel on nonprescription internal analgesic and antirheumatic drug products has recommended that phenacetin be removed from all nonprescription products. The majority of a phenacetin dose is biotransformed to acetaminophen, which is thought to be primarily responsible for the analgesic-antipyretic activity (156). However, phenacetin also has been shown to have intrinsic analgesic-antipyretic activity in laboratory animals (156, 157). The mechanism and site of analgesic action of these compounds have not been definitely established (5).

Dosage Considerations

Studies document the analgesic efficacy of phenacetin and acetaminophen in doses of 325–650 mg (158–161). The recommended adult dose of acetaminophen is 325–650 mg every 4 hours, not to exceed a total of 3.9 g in 24 hours. Table 2 gives the recommended acetaminophen

pediatric dosage. Although comparative analgesic effectiveness is difficult to establish because of the nature of existing clinical testing procedures, acetaminophen and phenacetin are similar in potency to aspirin as analgesics and antipyretics (39). However, a single 1,000-mg acetaminophen dose is less effective than 600 mg of aspirin in relieving pain associated with rheumatoid arthritis when it is given as an analgesic supplement to regular anti-inflammatory drug therapy (162).

Both phenacetin and acetaminophen are effective antipyretic agents, and both reduce fever by acting on the hypothalamic thermoregulatory center to increase body heat dissipation. Acetaminophen reduces fever by inhibiting the action of endogenous pyrogen on the hypothalamus, through inhibition of prostaglandin synthesis (43, 163, 164). In febrile individuals, both compounds begin to reduce body temperature about 30 minutes after administration and produce their peak effect in 2–4 hours (158). Clinical studies indicate that acetaminophen and aspirin are equally effective as antipyretics (165–167).

Although there are reports of minimal anti-inflammatory activity with acetaminophen, the *p*-aminophenols have no therapeutic use as anti-inflammatory drugs (5, 39, 155, 168).

Toxicity of Para-aminophenols Although methemoglobin production contributes to phenacetin toxicity in acute overdose, therapeutic phenacetin doses in the 1–2 g/day range cause only minimal methemoglobinemia, which is usually of no clinical significance (5). Phenacetin-induced hemolytic anemia has been associated most frequently with chronic drug ingestion; however, clinically significant hemolysis may occur with the administration of a single dose of phenacetin. Phenacetin produces hemolytic anemia in an individual deficient in glucose 6-phosphate dehydrogenase or in an immunologically sensitive individual (169). In addition glucose 6-phosphate dehydrogenase deficiency is a genetically transferable enzyme deficiency that predisposes a person to acute, drug-induced hemolytic episodes. This deficiency occurs rarely in Americans of West European genetic origin but is common in some Mediterranean people and has an incidence of about 13% in American Negroes (170). In contrast, acetaminophen rarely produces hemolytic anemia and produces almost no methemoglobin formation (120, 171, 172).

Because it lacks many undesirable effects produced by aspirin, acetaminophen is gaining favor in the United States as the "common household analgesic" (5, 173). However, there is also growing concern that increasing household availability and the public's lack of recognition of acetaminophen toxicity will produce a new health hazard (174–177). Acute acetaminophen poisoning may produce fatal hepatic necrosis (178–180). Chronic excessive use of acetaminophen (> 5 g/day) for several weeks can produce hepatotoxicity, which is potentiated by chronic alcohol consumption (181, 182, 183).

In adults, symptoms of acute toxicity may occur following the ingestion of 10–15 g of acetaminophen (5, 184, 185). A single oral ingestion of 15–25 g is seriously

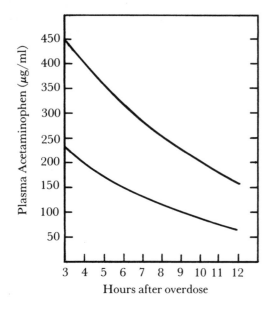

Figure 1. Nomogram for relation of acetaminophen levels to potential hepatotoxicity.

hepatotoxic and potentially fatal (186–188). However, estimates of the ingested acetaminophen dose are not reliable predictors of potential hepatotoxicity. Plasma acetaminophen levels should be determined following ingestion of a potentially toxic amount, and nomograms (Figure 1) have been established to relate plasma acetaminophen levels to the likelihood of hepatotoxicity (189, 190). The plasma acetaminophen half-life is prolonged in cases of hepatotoxicity and is a valuable predictor of hepatic necrosis. If the plasma acetaminophen half-life exceeds 4 hours, hepatic necrosis is likely to occur (191).

The progression of symptoms with acute acetaminophen poisoning include: vomiting within a few hours; anorexia, nausea, and stomach pain within 24 hours; evidence of hepatotoxity in 2–4 days with jaundice; and death at any time in 2–7 days (5, 184). In addition, kidney damage, disturbances in clotting mechanisms, metabolic acidosis, hypoglycemia, and myocardial necrosis may occur (5, 175, 176). A latent period with no visible symptoms follows the initial symptoms. This can be deceptive to both the patient and physician. In nonfatal cases, the hepatic damage is usually reversible (192). Emergency first-aid treatment of acetaminophen poisoning should include emesis with syrup of ipecac (192). Activated charcoal will reduce acetaminophen absorption significantly but is most effective if given immediately after emesis within the first 30 minutes following acetaminophen ingestion (193). Activated charcoal should not be employed if oral administration of acetylcysteine is anticipated since the charcoal may prevent adequate absorption of the antidote (194, 195). The dose and contraindication considerations for syrup of ipecac and activated charcoal previously discussed for salicylate poisoning also apply to acetaminophen overdose. (See Chapter 7, *Emetic and Antiemetic Products.*)

The oral administration of a solution of acetylcysteine (Mucomyst) has been reported to be effective without significant toxicity in preventing the hepatic necrosis of acetaminophen poisoning and is being evaluated for this purpose (196, 197). The initial dose of acetylcysteine should be given within 12 hours of overdose. The dose of acetylcysteine recommended for acetaminophen poisoning includes a loading dose of 140 mg/kg, followed in 4 hours with a maintenance dosage regimen of 70 mg/kg every 4 hours for 17 doses. Dilute with a soft drink or unsweetened grapefruit juice to 5% (198). Evidence suggests that IV administration of acetylcysteine is superior (199).

Analgesic Renal Toxicity

Reports first appeared in the 1950's linking chronic analgesic use to renal papillary necrosis and interstitial nephritis (200–203). The syndrome is characterized by asymptomatic sloughing of renal papillary tissue, sometimes with the elimination of "brown lumps" of necrotic tissue in the urine. Tissue necrosis may be accompanied by oliguria, nausea and vomiting, massive diuresis, or hematuria. Anemia may be present as the syndrome progresses, and final stages include renal insufficiency, hypertension, and death (204).

Analgesic nephropathy has been linked most consistently to the use of phenacetin-containing analgesic combination products. Current opinion suggests that aspirin alone is not an initiator of nephropathy but that it may worsen or perpetuate the progression of papillary necrosis and renal dysfunction (205–211). Aspirin-induced inhibition of prostaglandin synthesis has been suggested to contribute to the nephrotoxicity of aspirin-phenacetin combinations by causing ischemic changes in the ascending loop of Henle which predisposes the tissue to phenacetin-induced necrosis (212, 213).

In the United States, phenacetin-containing products are involved in almost all reported cases of analgesic-induced kidney disease (212). Numerous epidemiologic studies suggest temporal and dose relationships between phenacetin ingestion and renal dysfunction, and follow-up studies in countries after complete removal of phenacetin from nonprescription use support the causality assumption (214–220). Prolonged use of phenacetin-containing analgesics also has been associated with cancer of the renal pelvis and urinary bladder (221–225). Phenacetin has been used chronically for its stimulant and euphoric effects rather than for its analgesic/antipyretic action. The potential for abuse of this compound and the incidence of toxicity associated with it have prompted the FDA advisory review panel to recommend removing phenacetin from nonprescription drug products.

Product Selection Guidelines

In evaluating the relative merits of nonprescription internal analgesic products, the choices are aspirin or acetaminophen and the formulation of the product. Aspirin is the most frequently used nonprescription analgesic except when specifically contraindicated because of its effects on hemostasis or GI erosion or in case of hypersensitivity or drug interaction. Buffered aspirin and choline salicylate have the advantage of producing less GI distress. Highly buffered aspirin solutions produce less GI erosion, but they contain large amounts of sodium and should not be used by individuals on low-sodium diets. Enteric-coated aspirin products may reduce the likelihood of GI erosion but have a longer onset of action due to their delayed and possibly incomplete absorption. The delayed onset of such products precludes their use in acute pain when prompt relief is desired.

In many cases, acetaminophen is the drug of choice. It is less likely to trigger asthma-like symptoms in asthmatics, but hypersensitivity reactions to the drug have been reported (226). Because acetaminophen does not cause gastric mucosal erosion and does not affect platelet function, it may be recommended for individuals with a history of peptic ulcer disease (227). Although acetaminophen in a dose of 650 mg 4 times/day for a 2-week period significantly increased prothrombin time, two 650-mg doses 4 hours apart did not (228, 229). In addition, a 6-week course of acetaminophen (1,950 mg/day) does not affect bleeding time or platelet aggregation (61). Consequently, the intermittent use of acetaminophen by individuals receiving oral anticoagulant therapy should present no serious interaction. Because of its lack of anti-inflammatory activity, acetaminophen is not an acceptable substitute for aspirin in treating rheumatoid arthritis and similar inflammatory conditions. Acetaminophen is usually not as effective as aspirin if there is an inflammatory component to the pain, such as a sprain. Acetaminophen is the nonprescription analgesic of choice for patients taking uricosuric drugs because it does not antagonize the uricosuric effect (226). In addition, acetaminophen's stability in solution provides a convenient and palatable pediatric dosage form.

The rationale for including caffeine in many analgesic combinations remains obscure. "There is some inconclusive evidence to suggest that caffeine may exert additional analgesia when used in combination with other analgesics" (45). An evaluation of analgesic combinations in treating cancer pain showed that 65 mg of caffeine did not increase significantly the analgesic efficacy of 650 mg of aspirin (230).

Claims promoting "extra-strength pain relievers" require clarification. Such products are usually combinations of several analgesic ingredients and may include acetaminophen, salicylamide, and aspirin. Because the total analgesic ingredients may be more than 325 mg, the implication in these products' promotional materials is that they are "stronger" and hence more effective. These claims only confuse the consumer because combinations have not been proven more effective than the sum of their individual ingredients. In most controlled clinical trials, pain relief provided by analgesic combinations has not been superior to that of aspirin alone (5).

Summary

The appropriate choice of an analgesic/antipyretic agent involves a consideration of both patient and drug factors (Table 3). In determining the drug of choice for recommendation, the pharmacist must consider the following factors: the condition being treated; the nature and origin of the pain or fever; accompanying symptoms; a history of asthma, urticaria or other allergic disease, hypersensitivity reactions, peptic ulcer, or clotting disorders; and the concomitant use of other medication. In addition, product selection must include evaluation of the product's proven efficacy for the condition being treated, formulation factors that may give the patient more prompt relief or fewer side effects, and the potential for adverse effects from the product ingredients.

Table 3. Factors influencing the choice of analgesic agents

Patient	Drug
Condition being treated	**Efficacy of drug**
Type of pain	Analgesic potency
Accompanying symptoms	Antipyretic potency
	Anti-inflammatory potency
Frequency of dose and duration of treatment	Onset and duration of effect formulation factors
Patient profile	**Untoward effects of drug**
Age of patient	General acute and chronic toxicity
Drug allergy or idiosyncrasies	Allergenic potential and cross-sensitivity with other drugs
Pathologic conditions or susceptibility to untoward effects	Relative tendency to produce untoward effects
Concomitant use of other drugs, therapeutic diets or diagnostic procedures	Potential to modify pharmacologic activities of other drugs or endogenous compounds

References

1. D. R. Haslam, *Br. J. Psychol., 58,* 139 (1967).
2. H. K. Beecher, in "Nonspecific Factors in Drug Therapy," K. Rickels, Ed., Charles C Thomas, Springfield, Ill., 1968, p. 27.
3. A. C. Guyton, "Textbook of Medical Physiology," 6th ed., W. B. Saunders, Philadelphia, Pa., 1981, pp. 611–625.
4. S. H. Ferriera, M. Nakamura, and M. S. A. Castro, *Prostaglandins 16,* 31 (1978).
5. "The Pharmacological Basis of Therapeutics," 6th ed., A. G. Gilman, L. S. Goodman, and A. Gilman, Eds., Macmillan, New York, N.Y., 1980, pp. 682–705.
6. M. L. Tainter and A. J. Ferris, "Aspirin in Modern Therapy," Sterling Drug, New York, N.Y., 1969, p. 43.
7. H. G. Wolff, "Headache and Other Head Pain," 2nd ed., Oxford University Press, New York, N.Y., 1963.
8. "Textbook of Medicine," 15th ed., P. B. Beeson, W. McDermott, and J. B. Wyngaarden, Eds., W. B. Saunders, Philadelphia, Pa., 1979, pp. 728–733.
9. "Harrison's Principles of Internal Medicine," 9th ed., G. W. Thorn, R. D. Adams, E. Braunwald, K. J. Isselbacher, and R. G. Petersdorf, Eds., McGraw-Hill, New York, N.Y., 1980, pp. 21–22.

10. J. R. Saper, *J. Am. Med. Assoc., 239,* 2380, 2480 (1978).
11. V. S. Caviness, Jr., and P. O'Brien, *N. Engl. J. Med., 302,* 446 (1980).
12. R. J. Scheite and J. R. Hills, *Am. J. Hosp. Pharm. 37,* 365 (1980).
13. S. V. Deshmukh and J. S. Meyer, *Stroke, 7,* 11 (1976).
14. J. R. Couch, *Neurology, 26,* 348 (1976).
15. S. V. Deshmukh and J. S. Meyer, *Headache, 17,* 101 (1977).
16. J. Edmeads, *Headache, 17,* 148 (1977).
17. D. J. Dalessio, *J. Am. Med. Assoc., 239,* 52 (1978).
18. B. P. O'Neill and J. D. Mann, *Lancet, 2,* 1179 (1978).
19. "Textbook of Medicine," 15th ed., P. B. Beeson, W. McDermott, and J. B. Wyngaarden, Eds., W. B. Saunders, Philadelphia, Pa., 1979, p. 727.
20. "The Merck Manual," 13th ed., Merck, Rahway, N.J., 1977, p. 1464.
21. W. S. Gilmer, Jr., in "Concepts of Disease," J. B. Brunson and E. A. Gall, Eds., Macmillan, New York, N.Y., 1971, p. 746.
22. "Textbook of Medicine," 15th ed., P. B. Beeson, W. McDermott, and J. B. Wyngaarden, Eds., W. B. Saunders, Philadelphia, Pa., 1979, p. 186.
23. "The Merck Manual," 13th ed., Merck, Rahway, N.J., 1977, p. 1357.
24. "Textbook of Medicine,' 15th ed., P. B. Beeson, W. McDermott, and J. B. Wyngaarden, Eds., W. B. Saunders, Philadelphia, Pa., 1979, p. 205.
25. A. S. Milton, *J. Pharm. Pharmacol., 28,* 393 (1976).
26. C. A. Dinarello and S. M. Wolff, *N. Engl. J. Med., 298,* 607 (1978).
27. H. A. Bernheim, L. H. Block, and E. Atkins, *Ann. Intern. Med., 91,* 261 (1979).
28. L. Weinstein and M. N. Swartz, in "Pathologic Physiology—Mechanisms of Disease," 5th ed., W. A. Sodeman, Jr., and W. A. Sodeman, Eds., W. B. Saunders, Philadelphia, Pa., 1974, pp. 473–488.
29. W. Feldberg and K. P. Gupta, *J. Physiol. (London), 228,* 41 (1973).
30. W. Feldberg, K. P. Gupta, A. S. Milton, and S. Wendlandt, *J. Physiol. (London), 234,* 279 (1973).
31. W. Feldberg and P. N. Saxena, *J. Physiol. (London), 217,* 547 (1971).
32. W. Feldberg and P. N. Saxena, *J. Physiol. (London), 219,* 739 (1971).
33. C. A. Harvey and A. S. Milton, *J. Physiol. (London), 250,* 18P (1975).
34. C. A. Harvey, A. S. Milton, and D. W. Straughan, *J. Physiol. (London), 248,* 26P (1975).
35. A. S. Milton and S. Wendlandt, *J. Physiol. (London), 207,* 76P (1970).
36. A. S. Milton, *J. Pharm. Pharmacol., 28,* 393 (1976).
37. F. Allison, Jr., in "Concepts of Disease," J. G. Brunson and E. A. Gall, Eds., Macmillan, New York, N.Y., 1971, p. 443.
38. A. C. Guyton, "Textbook of Medical Physiology," 6th ed., W. B. Saunders, Philadelphia, Pa., 1981, pp. 886–898.
39. W. T. Beaver, *Am. J. Med. Sci., 250,* 577 (1965).
40. R. K. Lim, F. Guzman, D. W. Rodgers, K. Goto, C. Braun, G. D. Dickerson, and R. J. Engle, *Arch. Int. Pharmacodyn. Ther., 152,* 25 (1964).
41. S. H. Ferreira, *Nature New Biol., 240,* 200 (1972).
42. J. R. Vane, *Nature New Biol., 231,* 232 (1971).
43. R. J. Flower, *Am. Heart J., 86,* 844 (1973).
44. M. Perlow, C. A. Dinarello, and S. M. Wolff, *J. Infect. Dis., 132,* 157 (1975).
45. *Federal Register, 42,* 35360–63 (1977).
46. S. H. Ferreira and J. R. Vane, *Annu. Rev. Pharmacol., 14,* 57 (1974).
47. A. Willis, *J. Pharm. Pharmacol., 21,* 126 (1969).
48. T. J. Williams and M. J. Peck, *Nature, 270,* 530 (1977).
49. T. J. Williams, *Br. J. Pharmacol., 56,* 341P (1976).
50. *Federal Register, 42,* 35453–61 (1977).
51. E. Mongan, P. Kelly, K. Nies, W. W. Porter, and H. E. Paulus, *J. Am. Med. Assoc., 226,* 142 (1973).
52. J. H. Weiss, in "Aspirin, Platelets and Stroke," W. S. Fields and W. K. Hass, Eds., W. H. Green, St. Louis, Mo., 1971, p. 51.
53. H. J. Weiss and L. M. Aledort, *Lancet, 2,* 495 (1967).
54. J. B. Smith and A. L. Willis, *Nature, 231,* 235 (1971).
55. H. J. Weiss, *Am. Heart J., 92,* 86 (1976).
56. K. P. Link, R. S. Overman, W. R. Sullivan, C. F. Huebner, and L. D. Scheel, *J. Biol. Chem., 147,* 463 (1943).
57. C. Pochedly and G. Ente, *Pediatr. Clin. N. Am., 19,* 1104 (1972).
58. S. H. Reuter and W. W. Montgomery, *Arch. Otolaryngol., 80,* 214 (1964).
59. *Federal Register, 42,* 35385 (1977).
60. *Federal Register, 42,* 35412 (1977).
61. C. H. Mielke, D. Heiden, A. F. Britten, J. Ramos, and P. Flavell, *J. Am. Med. Assoc., 235,* 613 (1976).
62. A. Muir, in "Salicylates–An International Symposium," A. St. J. Dixon, B. K. Martin, M. J. H. Smith, and P. H. N. Wood, Eds., J. & A. Churchill, London, England, 1963, p. 230.
63. L. T. Stubbe, *Br. Med. J., 2,* 1062 (1958).
64. M. I. Grossman, K. K. Matsumoto, and R. J. Lichter, *Gastroenterology, 40,* 383 (1961).
65. W. H. J. Summerskill and A. S. Alvarez, *Lancet, 2,* 925 (1958).
66. H. Heggarty, *Br. Med. J., 1,* 491 (1974).
67. H. E. Paulus and M. W. Whitehouse, *Annu. Rev. Pharmacol., 13,* 107 (1973).
68. W. D. W. Rees and L. A. Turnberg, *Lancet, 2,* 410 (1980).
69. A. Muir and I. A. Cossar, *Br. Med. J., 2,* 7 (1955).
70. H. F. Lange, *Gastroenterology, 33,* 778 (1957).
71. A. S. Alvarez and W. H. J. Summerskill, *Lancet, 2,* 920 (1958).
72. M. Levy, *N. Engl. J. Med., 290,* 1158 (1974).
73. K. Goulston and A. R. Cooke, *Br. Med. J., 4,* 664 (1968).
74. C. D. Needham, J. Kyle, P. F. Jones, S. J. Johnson, and D. F. Kerridge, *Gut, 12,* 819 (1971).
75. G. A. Settipane and F. H. Chafee, *J. Allergy Clin. Immunol., 53,* 200 (1974).
76. B. Giraldo, M. N. Blumenthal, and W. W. Spink, *Ann. Intern. Med., 71,* 479 (1969).
77. B. T. Fein, *J. Allergy, 29,* 598 (1971).
78. M. Moore-Robinson and R. P. Warin, *Br. Med. J., 4,* 262 (1967).
79. R. A. Settipane, H. P. Constantine, and G. A. Settipane, *Allergy, 35,* 149 (1980).
80. *Federal Register, 42,* 35397–99 (1977).
81. A. Szczeklik, R. J. Gryglewski, and G. Czerniawska-Mysik, *Br. Med. J., 1,* 67 (1975).
82. A. Szczeklik and G. Czerniawska-Mysik, *Lancet, 1,* 488 (1976).
83. A. Szczeklik, R. J. Gryglewski, G. Czerniawska-Mysik, and A. Zmuda, *J. Allergy Clin. Immunol., 58,* 10 (1976).
84. J. A. M. Phills, L. Perelmutter, and A. Liakopoulou, *J. Allergy Clin. Immunol., 49,* 97 (1972).
85. G. A. Settipane, *Arch. Intern. Med., 111,* 328 (1981).
86. T. F. Yu, P. G. Dayton, and A. B. Gutman, *J. Clin. Invest., 42,* 1330 (1963).
87. "Evaluations of Drug Interactions," 2nd ed., American Pharmaceutical Association, Washington, D.C., 1976, p. 226.
88. P. D. Hansten, "Drug Interactions," 4th ed., Lea and Febiger, Philadelphia, Pa., 1979, p. 255.
89. "Evaluations of Drug Interactions," 2nd ed., American Pharmaceutical Association, Washington, D.C., 1976, p. 270.
90. "Evaluations of Drug Interactions," 2nd ed., American Pharmaceutical Association, Washington, D.C., 1976, p. 263.
91. H. Wishinsky, E. J. Glasser, and S. Perkal, *Diabetes, 11,* (suppl.) 18 (1962).
92. *Federal Register, 42,* 35453 (1971).
93. D. R. Millet, *Drug Intell. Clin. Pharm. 7,* 1513 (1981).
94. R. E. Gosselin, H. C. Hodge, R. P. Smith, and M. N. Gleason, "Clinical Toxicology of Commercial Products," 3rd ed., Williams and Wilkins, Baltimore, Md., 1969, pp. 209–214.
95. A. R. Temple, *Pediatrics, 62* (suppl.), 873 (1978).
96. H. B. Andrews, *Am. Fam. Physician, 8,* 102 (1973).
97. H. R. Dreisbach, "Handbook of Poisoning: Diagnosis and Treatment," 10th ed., Lange Medical, Los Altos, Calif., 1980, pp. 17–25, 289–295.
98. G. Levy and J. R. Leonards, in "The Salicylates—A Critical

Bibliographic Review," M. J. H. Smith and P. K. Smith, Eds., Interscience, New York, N.Y., 1966, pp. 5–47.

99. G. Levy, in "Salicylates–An International Symposium," A. St. J. Dixon, B. K. Martin, M. J. H. Smith, and P. H. N. Wood, Eds., J. & A. Churchill, London, England, 1963, pp. 9–16.

100. *Medical Letter on Drugs and Therapeutics, 16,* 57 (1974).

101. J. R. Leonards, *Clin. Pharmacol. Ther., 4,* 476 (1963).

102. *Federal Register, 42,* 35378 (1977).

103. K. W. Anderson, in "Salicylates–An International Symposium," A. St. J. Dixon, B. K. Martin, M. J. H. Smith, and P. H. N. Wood, Eds., J. & A. Churchill, London, England, 1963, pp. 217–223.

104. J. R. Leonards and G. Levy, *Arch. Intern. Med., 129,* 457 (1972).

105. J. R. Leonards and G. Levy, *Clin. Pharmacol. Ther., 10,* 571 (1969).

106. P. H. Wood, E. A. Harvey-Smith, and A. S. Dixon, *Br. Med. J., 1,* 669 (1962).

107. L. Stubbe, J. H. Pietersen, and C. van Heulen, *Br. Med. J., 1,* 675 (1962).

108. E. Nelson, *Clin. Pharmacol. Ther., 4,* 283 (1963).

109. J. R. Leonards and G. Levy, *J. Am. Med. Assoc., 193,* 99 (1965).

110. F. L. Lanza, G. L. Royer, and R. S. Nelson, *N. Engl. J. Med., 303,* 136 (1980).

111. G. R. Silvoso, K. J. Ivey, J. H. Butt et al., *Ann. Intern. Med., 91,* 517 (1979).

112. J. J. Oroczo-Alcala and J. Baum, *Arthritis Rheum., 22,* 1034 (1979).

113. L. E. Hollister, *Clin. Pharmacol. Ther., 13,* 1 (1972).

114. J. R. Hoon, *J. Am. Med. Assoc., 229,* 841 (1974).

115. R. R. Miller, *J. Clin. Pharmacol., 18,* 468 (1978).

116. R. John, *J. Am. Med. Assoc., 230,* 823 (1974).

117. "The Merck Index," 9th ed., Merck, Rahway, N.J., 1976, p. 209.

118. "Drugs of Choice—1980/1981," W. Modell, Ed., C. V. Mosby, St. Louis, Mo., 1980, p. 205.

119. *Federal Register, 42,* 35417–21 (1977).

120. "AMA Drug Evaluations," 4th ed., Publishing Sciences Group, Littleton, Mass., 1980, p. 77.

121. H. Tuchmann-Duplessis, D. Hiss, G. Mottot, and I. Rosner, *Toxicology, 3,* 207 (1975).

122. R. B. Lewis and J. D. Schulman, *Lancet, 2,* 1159 (1973).

123. E. Collins and G. Turner, *Lancet, 2,* 335 (1975).

124. G. Turner and E. Collins, *Lancet, 2,* 338 (1975).

125. J. E. Fielding, *N. Engl. J. Med., 298,* 337 (1978).

126. S. Shapiro, R. R. Monson, D. W. Kaufman, V. Siskin, O. P. Heinonin, and D. Slone, *Lancet, 1,* 1375 (1976).

127. G. Levy and L. K. Garrettson, *Pediatrics, 53,* 201 (1974).

128. P. A. Palmisano and G. Cassady, *J. Am. Med. Assoc., 209,* 556 (1969).

129. W. A. Bleyer and R. T. Breckenridge, *J. Am. Med. Assoc., 213,* 2049 (1970).

130. R. R. Haslam, H. Ekert, and G. L. Gillam, *J. Pediatr., 84,* 556 (1974).

131. S. Moncada and J. R. Vane, *Pharmacol. Rev., 30,* 293 (1979).

132. J. F. Mustard, R. L. Kinlough-Rathbone, and M. A. Packham, *Annu. Rev. Med., 31,* 89 (1980).

133. G. J. Roth, N. Stanford, and P. W. Majerus, *Proc. Nat. Acad. Sci., 72,* 3073 (1975).

134. G. Masotti, G. Galanti, L. Poggesi, R. Abbate, and G. G. Neri Serneri, *Lancet, 2,* 1213 (1979).

135. E. F. Ellis, K. F. Wright, P. S. Jones, P. W. Richardson, and C. K. Ellis, *J. Cardiovas. Pharmacol., 2,* 387 (1980).

136. E. M. G. Hoogendijk and J. W. Tencate, *Lancet, 1,* 372 (1980).

137. S. P. Hanley, J. Bevan, S. R. Cockbill, and S. Heptinstall, *Lancet, 1,* 969 (1981).

138. H. J. M. Barnett, *Med. Clin. N. Am., 63,* 649 (1979).

139. Canadian Cooperative Study Group, *N. Engl. J. Med., 299,* 53 (1978).

140. W. S. Fields, N. A. Lemak, and R. F. Frankowski, *Stroke, 8,* 301 (1977).

141. H. Vik-Mo, *Scand. J. Haematol., 19,* 68 (1977).

142. J. W. Haerem, *Artheroscelrosis, 15,* 199 (1972).

143. P. P. Steele, H. S. Weily, H. Davies et al., *Circulation, 48,* 1194 (1972).

144. P. C. Elwood and P. M. Sweetnam, *Lancet, 2,* 1313 (1979).

145. Aspirin Myocardial Infarction Study Research Group, *J. Am. Med. Assoc., 243,* 661 (1980).

146. R. J. Jones, *J. Am. Med. Assoc., 244,* 667 (1980).

147. D. C. Brodie and I. J. Szekely, *J. Am. Pharm. Assoc. Sci. Ed., 40,* 414 (1951).

148. *Federal Register, 42,* 35439–42 (1977).

149. L. Fleckenstein, J. M. Mazzullo, G. R. Mundy, R. A. Horvitz, and L. Lasagna, *Clin. Pharmacol. Ther., 17,* 233 (1975).

150. E. R. Hart, *J. Pharmacol. Exp. Ther., 89,* 205 (1947).

151. E. M. Bavin, F. J. Macrae, D. E. Seymour, and P. D. Waterhouse, *J. Pharm. Pharmacol., 4,* 872 (1952).

152. A. J. Vignec and M. Gasparik, *J. Am. Med. Assoc., 167,* 1821 (1958).

153. M. P. Borovsky, *Am. J. Dis. Child., 100,* 23 (1960).

154. A. J. Quick, *J. Pharmacol. Exp. Ther., 128,* 95 (1960).

155. L. O. Randall, in "Physiological Pharmacology," Vol. 1, W. S. Root and F. G. Hofmann, Eds., Academic, New York, N.Y., 1963, pp. 356–369.

156. B. B. Brodie and J. Axelrod, *J. Pharmacol. Exp. Ther., 97,* 58 (1949).

157. A. H. Conney, M. Sansur, F. Soroko, R. Koster, and J. J. Burns, *J. Pharmacol. Exp. Ther., 151,* 133 (1966).

158. P. K. Smith, "Acetophenetidin–A Critical Bibliographic Review," Interscience, New York, N.Y., 1958.

159. F. B. Flinn and B. B. Brodie, *J. Pharmacol. Exp. Ther., 94,* 76 (1948).

160. S. L. Wallenstein and R. W. Houde, *Fed. Proc., 13,* 414 (1954).

161. D. R. L. Newton and J. M. Tanner, *Br. Med. J., 2,* 1096 (1956).

162. E. C. Huskisson, *Br. Med. J., 4,* 196 (1974).

163. W. G. Clark and S. G. Moyer, *J. Pharmacol. Exp. Ther., 181,* 183 (1972).

164. R. J. Flower and J. R. Vane, *Nature, 240,* 410 (1972).

165. A. N. Eden, *Am. J. Dis. Child., 114,* 284 (1967).

166. S. J. Jaffe, *Arch. Intern. Med., 141,* 286 (1981).

167. L. Tarlin, P. Landrigan, R. Babineau, and J. J. Alpert, *Am. J. Dis. Child., 124,* 880 (1972).

168. J. Hajnal, J. Sharp, and A. J. Popert, *Ann. Rheum. Dis., 18,* 189 (1959).

169. M. Swanson, *Drug Intell. Clin. Pharm., 7,* 6 (1973).

170. P. A. Parks and J. Banks, *Ann. N.Y. Acad. Sci., 123,* 198 (1965).

171. L. O. Boreus and F. Sandberg, *Acta Physiol. Scand., 28,* 261 (1953).

172. E. Manor, A. Marmor, S. Kaufman, and H. Leiba, *J. Am. Med. Assoc., 236,* 2777 (1976).

173. E. E. Czapek, *J. Am. Med. Assoc., 235,* 636 (1976).

174. J. R. DiPalma, *Am. Fam. Physician, 13,* 142 (1976).

175. E. Sutton and L. F. Soyka, *Clin. Pediatr. (Philadelphia), 12,* 692 (1973).

176. H. Matthew, *Clin. Toxicol., 6,* 9 (1973).

177. R. Goulding, *Pediatrics, 52,* 883 (1973).

178. D. G. Davidson and W. N. Eastham, *Br. Med. J., 2,* 497 (1966).

179. P. G. Rose, *Br. Med. J., 1,* 381 (1969).

180. R. Clark, V. Borirakchanyavat, A. R. Davidson, R. P. H. Thompson, B. Widdop, R. Goulding, and R. Williams, *Lancet, 1,* 66 (1973).

181. J. D. Barker, D. J. De Carle, and S. Anuras, *Ann. Intern. Med., 87,* 299 (1977).

182. L. Harvey, L. B. Seeff, and H. J. Zimmerman, *Ann. Intern. Med., 92,* 511 (1980).

183. C. J. McClain, J. P. Kromhout, F. J. Peterson, and J. L. Holtzman, *J. Am. Med. Assoc., 244,* 251 (1980).

184. A. T. Proud and W. N. Wright, *Br. Med. J., 3,* 557 (1970).

185. M. Black, *Gastroenterology, 78,* 382 (1980).

186. J. Koch-Weser, *N. Engl. J. Med., 295,* 1297 (1976).

187. J. Ambre and M. Alexander, *J. Am. Med. Assoc., 238,* 500 (1977).

188. B. McJunkin, K. W. Barwick, W. C. Little, and J. B. Winfield, *J. Am. Med. Assoc., 236,* 1874 (1976).

189. B. Rumack and H. Matthew, *Pediatrics, 55,* 871 (1975).

190. L. F. Prescott, G. R. Sutherland, J. Park, I. J. Smith, and A. T. Proudfoot, *Lancet, 2,* 109 (1976).
191. L. F. Prescott, P. Roscoe, N. Wright, and S. S. Brown, *Lancet, 1,* 519 (1971).
192. E. P. Krenzelok, L. Best, and A. S. Manoguerra, *Am. J. Hosp. Pharm., 34,* 391 (1977).
193. G. Levy and J. B. Houston, *Pediatrics, 58,* 432 (1976).
194. B. H. Rumack and R. S. Peterson, *Pediatrics, 62* (suppl), 898–903 (1978).
195. A. S. Manoguerra, *Clin. Toxicol., 14,* 151–155 (1979).
196. R. G. Peterson and B. H. Rumack, *J. Am. Med. Assoc., 237,* 2406 (1977).
197. B. H. Rumack and R. G. Peterson, *Pediatrics, 62* (suppl.), 898 (1978).
198. R. D. Scalley and C. S. Conner, *Am. J. Hosp. Pharm., 35,* 964 (1978).
199. L. F. Prescott, *Arch. Intern. Med., 141,* 386 (1981).
200. O. Spuhler and H. N. Zollinger, *Z. Klin. Med., 151,* 1 (1953).
201. L. F. Prescott, *J. Pharm. Pharmacol., 18,* 331 (1966).
202. J. H. Shelley, *Clin. Pharmacol. Ther., 8,* 427 (1967).
203. M. H. Gault, T. C. Rudwal, W. D. Engles, and J. B. Dossetor, *Ann. Intern. Med., 68,* 906 (1968).
204. B. Koch, A. H. Irvine, J. R. McIver, and E. Liepa, *Can. Med. Assoc. J., 98,* 9 (1968).
205. L. F. Prescott, *Scott. Med. J., 14,* 82 (1969).
206. P. Kincaid-Smith, B. M. Saker, I. F. McKenzie, and K. Muriden, *Med. J. Aust., 1,* 203 (1968).
207. M. A. McIver and J. B. Hobbs, *Med. J. Aust., 1,* 197 (1975).
208. U. C. Dubach, B. Rosner, A. Muller, P. S. Levy, H. R. Baumeler, A. Peier, and T. Ehrensperger, *Lancet, 1,* 539 (1975).
209. R. D. Emkey and J. Mills, *J. Rheumatol., 1,* 126 (1974).
210. A. F. Macklon, A. W. Craft, M. Thompson, and D. N. S. Kerr, *Br. Med. J., 1,* 597 (1974).
211. R. J. Bulger, L. A. Healey, and P. Polinsky, *Ann. Rheum. Dis., 27,* 339 (1968).
212. *Federal Register, 42,* 35424–30 (1977).
213. R. S. Hanra and P. Kincaid-Smith, *Br. Med. J., 3,* 559 (1970).
214. K. Grimlund, *Acta Med. Scand., 174,* 3 (1963).
215. A. F. Burry, P. DeJersey et al., *Med. J. Aust., 1,* 873 (1966).
216. N. R. Eade and L. Lasagna, *J. Pharmacol. Exp. Ther., 155,* 301 (1967).
217. V. Bengtsson, *Acta Med. Scand., 388,* 5 (1962).
218. H. H. Pearson, *Med. J. Aust., 2,* 308 (1967).
219. D. Bell, D. N. S. Kerr, J. Swinney, and W. K. Yeates, *Br. Med. J., 3,* 378 (1969).
220. D. R. Wilson, *Can. Med. Assoc. J., 107,* 752 (1972).
221. N. Hultengren, C. Lagergren, and A. Ljungqvist, *Acta Chir. Scand., 130,* 314 (1965).
222. U. Bengtsson, L. Angevall, H. Ekman, and L. Lehman, *Scand. J. Urol. Nephrol., 2,* 145 (1968).
223. G. Hoybye and O. E. Nielson, *Scand. J. Urol. Nephrol, 5,* 190 (1971).
224. R. A. Mannion and D. Susmano, *J. Urol., 106,* 692 (1971).
225. T. A. Gonwa, W. T. Corbett, H. M. Schey et al., *Ann. Intern. Med., 93,* 249 (1980).
226. *Medical Letter on Drugs and Therapeutics, 13,* 74 (1971).
227. C. H. Mielke, Jr., and A. F. Britten, *N. Engl. J. Med., 282,* 1270 (1970).
228. A. M. Antlitz, J. A. Mead, Jr., and M. A. Tolentino, *Curr. Ther. Res., 10,* 501 (1968).
229. A. M. Antlitz and L. F. Awalt, *Curr. Ther. Res., 11,* 360 (1969).
230. C. G. Moertel, D. L. Ahmann, W. F. Taylor, and N. Schwartau, *J. Am. Med. Assoc., 229,* 55 (1974).

Internal Analgesic Product Table

Product[a] (Manufacturer)	Aspirin	Salicyl- amide	Acetami- nophen	Caffeine	Sodium	Other Ingredients
Acephen Suppositories (G & W Laboratories)			120 mg 650 mg		NS[b]	hydrogenated vegetable oil, polysorbate 80
Actamin (Buffington)			325 mg 500 mg		free	
Alka-Seltzer Efferves- cent Pain Reliever and Antacid (Miles)	324 mg				24 mEq	sodium bicarbonate, 1.904 g citric acid, 1.0 g;
Allerest Headache Strength (Pharmacraft)			325 mg		NS[b]	chlorpheniramine maleate, 2 mg phenylpropanolamine hydrochloride, 18.7 mg
Amphenol (O'Neal, Jones & Feldman)			325 mg		free	
Anacin (Whitehall)	400 mg			32.5 mg	NS[b]	
Anacin Tablets and Capsules, Maximum Strength (Whitehall)	500 mg			32 mg	0.006 mEq (tablet)	
Anodynos (Buffington)	NS[b]	NS[b]	NS[b]	NS[b]	free	
Arthralgen (Robins)		250 mg	250 mg		<0.04 mEq	
Arthritis Pain Formula (Whitehall)	486 mg (micro- nized)				NS[b]	aluminum hydroxide magnesium hydroxide
Arthritis Strength Bufferin (Bristol-Myers)	486 mg				NS[b]	magnesium carbonate, 145.8 mg aluminum glycinate, 72.9 mg
Arthropan Liquid (Purdue Frederick)					NS[b]	choline salicylate, 174 mg/ml (equivalent to 130 mg of aspirin)
A.S.A. Compound Capsules (Lilly)	227 mg			32.5 mg	<0.04 mEq	phenacetin, 160 mg
A.S.A. Enseals (Lilly)	325 and 650 mg				<0.04 mEq	enteric coating
Ascriptin (Rorer)	325 mg				NS[b]	magnesium hydroxide, 75 mg aluminum hydroxide gel, dried, 75 mg
Ascriptin A/D (Rorer)	325 mg				NS[b]	magnesium hydroxide, 150 mg aluminum hydroxide gel, dried, 150 mg

Internal Analgesic Product Table, continued

Product[a] (Manufacturer)	Aspirin	Salicyl-amide	Acetami-nophen	Caffeine	Sodium	Other Ingredients
Aspercin (Otis Clapp)	325 mg 500 mg (Extra)				free	
Aspergum (Plough) (chewing gum)	228 mg				0.003 mEq	
Aspirin Free Anacin-3 (Whitehall)			500 mg	32 mg	0.004 mEq	
Aspirin Suppositories (G & W Laboratories)	125 mg 300 mg 600 mg				NS[b]	hydrogenated vegetable oil
Bancap Capsule (O'Neal, Jones & Feldman)		200 mg	300 mg		free	
Banesin (O'Neal, Jones & Feldman)		200 mg	300 mg		free	
Bayer Aspirin (Glenbrook)	325 mg				3.2 mEq	
Bayer Children's Aspirin (Glenbrook)	81 mg				0.004 mEq	
Bayer Timed-Release Aspirin (Glenbrook)	650 mg				free	
BC Tablet and Powder (Block)	325 mg/tablet 650 mg (powder)		95 mg/tablet 195 mg (powder)		0.7 mEq 1.4 mEq	
Bromo-Seltzer (Warner-Lambert) (granules)			325 mg/capful		33 mEq/ capful	sodium bicarbonate and citric acid to yield 2.85 g of sodium citrate/capful
Buffaprin (Buffington)	325 mg 500 mg				free	magnesium oxide
Bufferin (Bristol-Myers)	324 mg				NS[b]	magnesium carbonate, 97.2 mg aluminum glycinate, 48.6 mg
Buffinol (Otis Clapp)	325 mg 500 mg (Extra)				free	magnesium oxide
Cama (Dorsey) (in-lay tablet)	600 mg				NS[b]	magnesium hydroxide, 150 mg aluminum hydroxide gel, dried, 150 mg
Capron Capsules (Vitarine)	227 mg		227mg	32 mg	free	
Congespirin Chewable (Bristol-Myers)	81 mg				NS[b]b	phenylephrine hydrochloride, 1.25 mg

Internal Analgesic Product Table, continued

Product[a] (Manufacturer)	Aspirin	Salicyl- amide	Acetami- nophen	Caffeine	Sodium	Other Ingredients
Cope (Glenbrook)	421.2 mg			32 mg	free	magnesium hydroxide, 50 mg aluminum hydroxide, 25 mg
Cystex (Cooper Vision)		65 mg			0.6 mEq	methenamine, 162 mg sodium salicylate, 97 mg benzoic acid 32 mg
Datril (Bristol-Myers)			325 mg		NS[b]	
Datril 500 (Bristol-Myers)			500 mg		NS[b]	
DeWitt Pills (DeWitt)		108.2 mg		6.5 mg	NS[b]	potassium nitrate, 56.4 mg uva ursi extract 32.4 mg buchu leaves, 7.8 mg
Doan's Pills (Jeffrey Martin)				32 mg	NS[b]	magnesium salicylate, 325 mg
Dolcin (Dolcin Corp.)	240.5 mg				NS[b]	calcium succinate monohydrate, 182 mg
Dularin Syrup (Dooner/Rorer)			24 mg/ml		free	
Duradyne (O'Neal, Jones & Feldman)	230 mg		30 mg	15 mg	NS[b]	phenacetin, 150 mg
Duragesic (Glaxo)	325 mg				NS[b]	salicylsalicylic acid, 162.5 mg
Ecotrin (Menley & James)	325 mg				0.001 mEq	enteric coating
Emagrin (Otis Clapp)	NS[b]	NS[b]		NS[b]	free	
Empirin (Burroughs Wellcome)	325 mg				free	
Excedrin (Bristol-Myers)	250 mg		250 mg	65 mg	NS[b]	
Excedrin P.M. (Bristol-Myers)	250 mg		250 mg		NS[b]	pyrilamine maleate, 25 mg
Febrinol (Vitarine)			325 mg		free	
Goody's Extra Strength Tablets (Goody's)	260 mg		130 mg	16.25 mg	NS[b]	

Internal Analgesic Product Table, continued

Product[a] (Manufacturer)	Aspirin	Salicyl- amide	Acetami- nophen	Caffeine	Sodium	Other Ingredients
Goody's Headache Powder (Goody's)	520 mg		260 mg	32.5 mg	35.3 mEq	
Liquiprin Solution (Norcliff Thayer)			48 mg/ml		<0.03 mEq/ml	
Meadache (Organon)		150 mg	150 mg	32 mg	free	phenyltoloxamine dihydrogen citrate, 44 mg
Measurin (Breon) (timed-release)	650 mg				NS[b]	
Mobigesic (B. F. Ascher)					NS[b]	magnesium salicylate, 300 mg
Momentum (Whitehall)	162.5 mg				0.0003 mEq	salicylsalicylic acid, 325 mg phenyltoloxamine citrate, 12.5 mg
Neocylate (Central Pharmacal)					free	potassium salicylate, 280 mg aminobenzoic acid, 250 mg
Nilain (A.V.P.)	325 mg		162.5 mg	32.5 mg	free	
Nilprin 7½ (A.V.P.)			486 mg		free	
Pabirin (Dorsey)	300 mg				0.04 mEq	aminobenzoic acid, 300 mg aluminum hydroxide gel, dried, 100 mg
PAC (Upjohn)	228 mg			32 mg	0.043 mEq	phenacetin, 163 mg
Panodynes Analgesic (Keystone)	260 mg	64.8 mg	64.8 mg	16.2 mg	free	
Percogesic (Endo)			325 mg			phenyltoloxamine citrate, 30 mg
Persistin (Fisons)	160 mg				NS[b]	salicylsalicylic acid, 485 mg
Rid-A-Pain (Pfeiffer)		97.2 mg	226.8 mg	32.4 mg	NS[b]	phenyltoloxamine citrate, 30 mg
S-A-C (Lannett)		230 mg	150 mg	30 mg		
Sal-Fayne Capsules (Cooper Vision)	227 mg			32.4 mg	NS[b]	phenacetin, 162 mg
Sinarest (Pharmacraft)			325 mg 500 mg (extra strength)		NS[b]	phenylpropanolamine hydrochloride, 18.7 mg chlorpheniramine maleate, 2 mg
Sine-Aid (McNeil)			325 mg		<0.09 mEq	phenylpropanolamine hydrochloride, 25 mg

Internal Analgesic Product Table, continued

Product[a] (Manufacturer)	Aspirin	Salicyl-amide	Acetami-nophen	Caffeine	Sodium	Other Ingredients
SK-APAP Tablets and Elixir (Smith Kline & French)			325 mg/tablet 24 mg/ml		0.004 mEq/ tablet 0.1 mEq/ml	alcohol, 8% (elixir)
Stanback Tablets and Powder (Stanback)	325 mg/tab-let 650 mg (powder)	200 mg (pow-der)		15 mg (powder)	0.003 mEq (powder)	
St. Joseph Aspirin (Plough)	325 mg				free	
St. Joseph Aspirin for Children Chewable Tablets (Plough)	81 mg				free	
Tempra Syrup and Drops (Mead Johnson)			24 mg/ml (syrup) 100 mg/ml (drops)		0.03 mEq/ ml (syrup) 0.08 mEq/ ml (drops)	alcohol, 10%
Tenol (North American)			325 mg		NS[b]	
Trigesic (Squibb)	230 mg		125 mg	30 mg	free	
Tylenol Extra Strength Tablets, Capsules, Liquid (McNeil)			500 mg/tablet, capsule 33.3 mg/ml		<0.04 mEq/ tablet, cap-sule 0.02 mEq/ ml	alcohol, 8.5%
Tylenol Tablets, Chewable Tablets, Drops, and Elixir (McNeil)			325 mg/tablet, capsules 80 mg/chewable tablet 100 mg/ml (drops) 32 mg/ml (elixir)		<0.04 mEq/ tablet, capsule, chewable tablet, ml (drops) 0.02 mEq/ ml (elixir)	alcohol, 7% (drops and elixir)
Uracel S (North American)					NS[b]	sodium salicylate, 324 mg
Valadol Tablets and Liquid (Squibb)			325 mg/tablet 24 mg/ml		0.05 mEq/ ml (liquid)	alcohol, 9% (liquid)
Valorin (Otis Clapp)			325 mg 500 mg		free	
Vanquish Caplet (Glenbrook)	227 mg		194 mg	33 mg	free	magnesium hydroxide, 50 mg aluminum hydroxide gel, dried, 25 mg

[a] Tablet unless specified otherwise.
[b] Quantity not specified.

12 Nutritional Supplement, Mineral, and Vitamin Products

Marianne Ivey and Gary Elmer

Questions to Ask the Patient

What are your age and weight?

Do you participate regularly in sports or do you have a job requiring physical activity?

Do you have any chronic illnesses (diabetes, ulcer, ulcerative colitis, or epilepsy)?

Do you donate blood? How often?

Are you currently taking any medicines (prescription or nonprescription)?

Are you menstruating now? Are you pregnant? Do you take oral contraceptives (birth control pills)?

How much alcohol do you drink in a day?

Do you eat meats, vegetables, dairy products, and grain products every day? Are you dieting or are you on a restricted diet?

Why do you feel you need a nutritional supplement/vitamin/mineral?

What are your symptoms? Have they appeared suddenly or gradually?

Are you taking any nutritional supplements, vitamins, or minerals now?

Do you smoke or are you around smokers daily?

American consumers are convinced that they need more and better nutrients than their diets provide, and accordingly spend about $3 billion a year on vitamin and nutritional products (1, 2). The health science professions frequently have associated good health with good nutrition. Actually, there is much to learn about adequate nutrition, and much that has been learned has not been communicated effectively to the public. In many cases, the average American diet does not need supplementation (3). Exceptions are described in the subsequent sections. Misconceptions about the value of supplementation were shown in a survey in which 75% of those interviewed believed that supplemental vitamins furnish energy (4).

Marketing practices may further confuse the issue. The label "organic" is misleading because all foods are organic. "Organically grown" foods are those that are grown without the use of agricultural chemicals and are processed without chemicals or additives. However, no laws exist that enforce the label, "organically grown," to comply with the definition. There is no evidence that organically grown food is more nutritious than foods grown using chemical fertilizers (5).

Frequently, "natural" vitamins are supplemented with the synthetic vitamin. For example, the amount of ascorbic acid acquired from rose hips (the fleshy fruit of a rose) is relatively small, and synthetic ascorbic acid is added to prevent an unreasonable tablet size (6). However, this addition is not indicated on the label, and the price of such products often is considerably higher than for the synthetic, equally effective vitamin.

The pharmacist as a public adviser should be aware that one of the greatest dangers of food fads is that they are sometimes used in place of sound medical care. The false hope of superior health or freedom from disease may attract individuals with cancer, heart disease, arthritis, or other serious illnesses, and the pharmacist should be aware of the limited therapeutic value, if any, of these fads.

In 1979 the FDA advisory review panel on nonprescription vitamin and mineral drug products released its report, which contained recommendations to the FDA. The panel designated the differences between a dietary supplement and a nonprescription drug. Accordingly, a dietary supplement of a vitamin or mineral is defined as a food intended to supplement a diet by increasing the total dietary intake of one or more essential vitamins or minerals. In contrast, a product containing a vitamin or mineral is a nonprescription drug when that vitamin or mineral is used to prevent imminent development of a disease or for treatment of a vitamin- or mineral-deficiency disease. Vitamins and minerals marketed for supplementing a diet are proposed to be regulated as "foods for special dietary use" and are distinguished from nonprescription drugs. A vitamin or mineral product would require a prescription when the vitamin or mineral is used in such doses or in combinations that require regular monitoring by a physician.

A nonprescription drug would be considered safe, effective, and appropriately labeled when there is identification of a disease or condition in a target population for which the nonprescription ingredient would be useful in treatment or prevention and when the instructions accompanying the drug are true, clear, and not misleading. The FDA recommends that terms such as "stress," "super potency," and "geriatric" in the brand name are inappropriate (7).

The FDA has issued bans against several claims and statements regarding foods and food supplements. Claims cannot be made that foods or diet supplements alone can prevent, cure, or treat illness or that ingredients such as rutin, inositol, bioflavonoids, and amino-benzoic acid have nutritional value. Another FDA rule requires that all nutrients (caloric, protein, carbohydrate, and fat) as well as the percentage of the U.S. recommended daily dietary allowance of vitamins and minerals be listed on the container of all food shipped interstate.

From 1973 to 1978, certain high-potency preparations of vitamins A and D (more than 10,000 IU of A and 400 IU of D) were restricted by the FDA to sale as prescription drugs. These regulations, after protracted litigation, were declared invalid and the regulations revoked as of March 14, 1978 (8). Unfortunately, there are now no restrictions whatsoever on the availability of even toxic potencies of these or any other vitamin.

Optimum Nutrition

Guidelines for optimum nutrition are provided by two organizations—the Food and Nutrition Board of the National Academy of Sciences-National Research Council and by the Food and Drug Administration. The former provides Recommended Dietary Allowance

Table 1. Recommended daily dietary allowances, revised 1980 Food and Nutrition Board, National Academy of Sciences-National Research Council[a]

Age, years, and sex group	Weight kg	Weight lb	Height cm	Height in	Protein (g)	Fat-soluble vitamins Vitamin A (μg RE[b])	Vitamin D (μg[c])	Vitamin E (mg α-TE[d])	Ascorbic Acid (mg)	Thiamine (mg)
Infants										
0.0–0.5	6	13	60	24	kg × 2.2	420	10	3	35	0.3
0.5–1.0	9	20	71	28	kg × 2.0	400	10	4	35	0.5
Children										
1–3	13	29	90	35	23	400	10	5	45	0.7
4–6	20	44	112	44	30	500	10	6	45	0.9
7–10	28	62	132	52	34	700	10	7	45	1.2
Males										
11–14	45	99	157	62	45	1,000	10	8	50	1.4
15–18	66	145	176	69	56	1,000	10	10	60	1.4
19–22	70	154	177	70	56	1,000	7.5	10	60	1.5
23–50	70	154	178	70	56	1,000	5	10	60	1.4
51+	70	154	178	70	56	1,000	5	10	60	1.2
Females										
11–14	46	101	157	62	46	800	10	8	50	1.1
15–18	55	120	163	64	46	800	10	8	60	1.1
19–22	55	120	163	64	44	800	7.5	8	60	1.1
23–50	55	120	163	64	44	800	5	8	60	1.0
51+	55	120	163	64	44	800	5	8	60	1.0
Pregnancy						+30	+200	+5	+2	+20	+0.4
Lactation						+20	+400	+5	+3	+40	+0.5

[a] The allowances are intended to provide for individual variations among most normal persons as they live in the United States under usual environmental stresses. Diets should be based on a variety of common foods to provide other nutrients for which human requirements have been less well defined.
[b] Retinol equivalents: 1 retinol equivalent = 1 μg retinol or 6 μg beta-carotene.
[c] As cholecalciferol: 10 μg cholecalciferol = 400 IU vitamin D.
[d] Alpha-tocopherol equivalents: 1 mg *d*-alpha-tocopherol = 1 α TE.
[e] Niacin equivalents: 1 mg niacin or 60 mg dietary tryptophan.
[f] The folacin allowances refer to dietary sources as determined by *Lactobacillus casei* assay after treatment with enzymes ("conjugases") to

Values (RDA) for essential nutrients based on sex, age, weight, and height (Table 1). Even though the RDA values are periodically updated, based on current information, they are only estimates of the amounts that will meet the needs of the majority of individuals in a population. They are set sufficiently high to compensate for individual variations due to minor illness and stress in normal individuals. In the most recent Food and Nutrition Board recommendations, an "estimated safe and adequate daily dietary intake" of other nutrients for which human requirements are not quantitatively known has been promulgated (Table 2). These data should be used merely as guidelines for nutritional assessment.

The FDA publishes a less comprehensive set of RDA values to be used for labeling purposes. These are known as the "U.S. Recommended Daily Allowance" (U.S. RDA) and are formulated under advisement from the National Research Council-National Academy of Sciences (Table 3). The pharmacist will find U.S. RDA values to be the most useful for patient discussions, because all vitamin and mineral product potencies are ex-pressed as percent of the adult U.S. RDA values. The reader will note that the U.S. RDA values are often higher than RDA values. This chapter uses U.S. RDA values for purpose of general discussion.

Nutritional Supplements

Often, patients requesting a nutritional supplement self-diagnose their condition. By careful evaluation the pharmacist can estimate the patient's nutritional status. If the evidence indicates the presence of a nutritional deficiency or any serious illness, the pharmacist should refer the patient to a physician for further diagnosis and treatment. Patients purchasing a nonprescription dietary supplement should be instructed as to its use, storage, and possible side effects.

Determining Nutritional Status

The assessment of nutritional status is very difficult. Clinical impressions about nutrition are often erroneous because the stages between the well-nourished and the poorly nourished states are not well defined. Only

Water-soluble vitamins					Minerals					
Riboflavin (mg)	Niacin (mg NE[e])	Pyridox-ine (mg)	Folacin[f] (μg)	Vitamin B$_{12}$[g] (μg)	Calcium (mg)	Phosphorus (mg)	Magne-sium (mg)	Iron (mg)	Zinc (mg)	Iodine (μg)
0.4	6	0.3	30	0.5	360	240	50	10	3	40
0.6	8	0.6	45	1.5	540	360	70	15	5	50
0.8	9	0.9	100	2.0	800	800	150	15	10	70
1.0	11	1.3	200	2.5	800	800	200	10	10	90
1.4	16	1.6	300	3.0	800	800	250	10	10	120
1.6	18	1.8	400	3.0	1,200	1,200	350	18	15	150
1.7	18	2.0	400	3.0	1,200	1,200	400	18	15	150
1.7	19	2.2	400	3.0	800	800	350	10	15	150
1.6	18	2.2	400	3.0	800	800	350	10	15	150
1.4	16	2.2	400	3.0	800	800	350	10	15	150
1.3	15	1.8	400	3.0	1,200	1,200	300	18	15	150
1.3	14	2.0	400	3.0	1,200	1,200	300	18	15	150
1.3	14	2.0	400	3.0	800	800	300	18	15	150
1.2	13	2.0	400	3.0	800	800	300	18	15	150
1.2	13	2.0	400	3.0	800	800	300	10	15	150
+0.3	+2	+0.6	+400	+1.0	+400	+400	+150	10[h]	+5	+25
+0.5	+5	+0.5	+100	+1.0	+400	+400	+150	10[h]	+10	+50

make polyglutamyl forms of the vitamin available to the test organism.
[g] The RDA for vitamin B$_{12}$ in infants is based on average concentration of the vitamin in human milk. The allowances after weaning are based on energy intake (as recommended by the American Academy of Pediatrics) and consideration of other factors, such as intestinal absorption.
[h] The increased requirement during pregnancy cannot be met by the iron content of habitual American diets or by the existing iron stores of many women; therefore, the use of 30–60 mg supplemental iron is recommended. Iron needs during lactation are not substantially different from those of nonpregnant women, but continued supplementation of the mother for 2–3 months after parturition is advisable in order to replenish stores depleted by pregnancy.

Table 2. Estimated safe and adequate daily dietary intakes of additional selected vitamins and minerals[a]

Age group, Years	Vitamins			Trace elements[b]				
	Vitamin K (µg)	Biotin (µg)	Pantothenic acid (mg)	Copper (mg)	Manganese (mg)	Fluoride (mg)	Chromium (mg)	Selenium (mg)
Infants								
0.0–0.5	12	35	2	0.5–0.7	0.5–0.7	0.1–0.5	0.01–0.04	0.01–0.04
0.5–1.0	10–20	50	3	0.7–1.0	0.7–1.0	0.2–1.0	0.02–0.06	0.02–.06
Children and adolescents								
1–3	15–30	65	3	1.0–1.5	1.0–1.5	0.5–1.5	0.02–0.08	0.02–0.08
4–6	20–40	85	3–4	1.5–2.0	1.5–2.0	1.0–2.5	0.03–0.12	0.03–0.12
7–10	30–60	120	4–5	2.0–2.5	2.0–3.0	1.5–2.5	0.05–0.2	0.05–0.2
11+	50–100	100–120	4–7	2.0–3.0	2.5–5.01	1.5–2.5	0.05–0.2	0.05–0.2
Adults	70–140	100–200	4–7	2.0–3.0	2.5–5.0	1.5–4.0	0.05–0.2	0.05–0.2

[a]From the Recommended Dietary Allowances, Revised 1980, Food and Nutrition Board of the National Academy of Sciences of the National Research Council. Because there is less information on which to base allowances, these figures are provided here in the form of ranges of recommended intakes.
[b]Since the toxic levels for many trace elements may be only several times usual intakes, the upper levels for the trace elements given in this table should not be habitually exceeded.

when emaciation from disease, economics, or climatic conditions are obvious are clinical impressions reliable.

There are guidelines, however, by which the pharmacist can gain a more objective impression of a patient's nutritional status. Knowing the population groups that are most often poorly nourished, exercising good observation skills, and knowing what questions may yield helpful information are valuable indicators. Frequently undernourished groups in the United States include infants, preschool children, lactating or pregnant women, the elderly, alcoholics, and the impoverished.

In addition, other populations at risk are people on restricted diets, persons with intestinal disease leading to malabsorption of nutrients, people who neglect their nutritional needs, people taking certain drugs that may affect absorption or nutrient interaction, and women of child-bearing age who have regular blood loss. Epidemiologic surveys have shown that school children, factory workers, businesspersons, and farmers are less likely to be poorly nourished.

The pharmacist should observe the patient's physical condition to help guide in diet supplementation. The texture, amount, and appearance of the hair may suggest nutritional status. The eyes, particularly the conjunctiva, may indicate vitamin A and iron deficiencies, and the mouth may show stomatitis, glossitis, or hypertrophic or pale gums. The number and general condition of the teeth may reflect the patient's choice of food. Visible goiter, skin color and texture, obesity or thinness relative to bone structure, and the presence of edema also may be indications of malnutrition. The edematous patient often looks well nourished but in fact may be severely protein malnourished. This is a common problem in the hospital, particularly among surgical patients or patients with edema due to liver, renal, or heart disease.

The more specific the information from the patient, the more helpful the pharmacist can be in determining the need for nutritional supplementation. Questions regarding foods generally not included in the diet may give the pharmacist more information. Previous treatment for similar symptoms also may be important.

Although nutritional deficiencies may lead to disease, disease may lead to nutritional deficiencies. It is the pharmacist's responsibility to refer patients with a suspected serious illness to a physician for a definitive assessment. Guidelines for the clinical appraisal of nutritional status include evaluation of medical and dietary history; growth, development, and fitness; signs consistent with deficiencies; and biochemical assessment. Rarely in the United States would the pharmacist ever encounter patients with severe deficiencies resulting in diseases such as scurvy (ascorbic acid deficiency), pellagra (niacin deficiency), or kwashiorkor (protein deficiency). Instead, milder forms of malnutrition are more frequently seen, often involving simultaneous deficiencies of more than one nutrient.

Protein and Calorie (Energy) Deficiency

In developing nations, protein-calorie malnutrition is fairly common. In the United States it is quite uncommon, except as a consequence of certain diseases; in fact, an excess intake of protein and energy is more common. The U.S. RDA for protein is 45 g for adults, and for energy it is 1,600–3,100 cal. In most cases, excess protein intake (to as much as 300 g) does not lead to disease conditions. Excess caloric intake, however, leads to obesity, with resulting increased risk for coronary, vascular, and other diseases.

Protein-calorie malnutrition can be caused by a food supply shortage or by inadequate information and understanding of nutrition or disease. Kwashiorkor is a protein deficiency; marasmus is caused by the inade-

Molybdenum (mg)	Electrolytes		
	Sodium (mg)	Potassium (mg)	Chloride (mg)
0.03–0.06	115–350	350–925	275–700
0.04–0.08	250–750	425–1,275	400–1,200
0.05–0.1	325–975	550–1,650	500–1,500
0.06–0.15	450–1,350	775–2,325	700–2,100
0.1–0.3	600–1,800	1,000–3,000	925–2,775
0.15–0.5	900–2,700	1,525–4,575	1,400–4,200
0.15–0.5	1,100–3,300	1,875–5,625	1,700–5,100

trauma, or radiation; severe burns; jaw fractures; neoplastic diseases; and renal disease. Protein and calorie intake in some very active people, such as athletes, dancers, and manual laborers, may not be adequate to meet their needs. However, in the United States, high activity levels are not very common for much of the population.

Several products are available for use as dietary supplements or tube feedings (oral, nasogastric, jejunostomy, or gastrostomy tubes). The pharmacist's role regarding these products may be more as a consultant to other health professionals and less as a primary therapist for the self-treating patient. The pharmacist should first establish why the patient believes a dietary supplement, vitamin-mineral supplement, tonic, or health food is needed. For weight loss or failure to gain weight in a highly active, otherwise healthy individual, a product with a high protein and calorie concentration may be recommended. Patients with a history of weight loss without apparent cause should be referred to a physician. The concern is the possibility of conditions such as diabetes or cancer for which expedient referral to a qualified practitioner or diagnostic clinic may be crucial.

Types of Formulas

Supplemental formula products are used as dietary adjuncts to a regular diet; they should not be used as the sole dietary product because they are not nutritionally complete. Some (Mull-Soy and Nutramigen) are milk free and can be used by individuals who have milk al-

quacy of calories and protein. In the United States, protein-calorie malnutrition is more commonly caused by conditions such as Crohn's disease; malabsorption syndromes; short bowel syndromes caused by surgery,

Table 3. U.S. Recommended Daily Allowances (U.S. RDA) for labeling purposes

	Unit	Infants	Children under 4 years of age	Adults and children 4 or more years of age	Pregnant and lactating women
Vitamin A	IU	1,500	2,500	5,000	8,000
Vitamin D	IU	400	400	400	400
Vitamin E	IU	5	10	30	30
Ascorbic acid	mg	35	40	60	60
Folacin	mg	0.1	0.2	0.4	0.8
Thiamine	mg	0.5	0.7	1.5	1.7
Riboflavin	mg	0.6	0.8	1.7	2.0
Niacin	mg	8	9	20	20
Pyridoxine	mg	0.4	0.7	2	2.5
Cyanocobalamin	μg	2	3	6	8
Biotin	mg	0.05	0.15	0.30	0.3
Pantothenic acid	mg	3	5	10	10
Calcium	g	0.6	0.8	1.0	1.3
Phosphorus	g	0.5	0.8	1.0	1.3
Iodine	μg	45	70	150	150
Iron	mg	15	10	18	18
Magnesium	mg	70	200	400	450
Manganese[a]	mg	0.5	1.0	4.0	4.0
Copper	mg	0.6	1.0	2.0	2.0
Zinc	mg	5	8	15	15
Protein	g		20(28)[b]	45(65)[b]	

[a]Proposed U.S. RDA.
[b]Values in parentheses are U.S. RDAs when protein efficiency ratio (PER) is less than that of casein; the other values are used when PER is equal to or greater than that of casein. No claim may be made for a protein with a PER equal to or less than 20% that of casein.

lergy disease as well as patients with lactose malabsorption resulting in distention and diarrhea. (See Chapter 14, *Infant Formula Products.*) One product (Controlyte) is restricted in its protein content and in electrolytes. It is appropriate for people with acute or chronic renal failure, where the diet must be carefully controlled. Many supplementary formula products may be combined with special recipes to make preparations such as desserts, malts, and shakes that still maintain the controlled intake.

Complete formulas can be used orally or as tube feedings, and they may be used as the sole dietary intake if the patient's electrolytes are monitored (9). They also may be used as supplementation to a regular diet. The complete formulas contain various ingredients that make them appropriate for special needs. Several (Instant Breakfast, Sustacal, and Meritene) are milk based; others (Compleat-B and Gerber Meat Base Formula) have a mixed food base. A third type provides a synthetic source of protein and carbohydrate. This type supplies the protein in the form of crystalline amino acids or protein hydrolysate, the carbohydrate in the form of oligosaccharides or disaccharides and the vitamins and minerals as the individual chemicals. These are chemically defined diets known as "elemental diets," and examples include Vivonex and Jejunal. Some other complete products (Precision LR, Flexical, and Portagen) are only partly chemically defined.

Nearly all chemically defined (elemental) diets have a very low fat content and contain electrolytes, minerals, trace elements, and water-soluble and fat-soluble vitamins. All the chemically based products require little or no digestion, are absorbed by a small part of the intestine, and have a low residue. The low residue reduces the number and volume of the stools, making these products appropriate for patients with ileostomies or colostomies who wish also to decrease fecal output. The low-residue products also may be appropriate for patients with brain damage from strokes, congenital defects or retardation, or for elderly persons with stool incontinence. Because of the ease of absorption and low fecal residues they are often used in postoperative care, in GI diseases, and in neoplastic disease where tissue breakdown is extensive.

Formulation and Dosage

Supplementary and complete formulas are available in several forms. Some are powders that must be diluted with water or milk, some are liquids that must be diluted further, and some are ready-to-use liquids. The extent of dilution is based on the amount of nutrients needed and the amount that can be tolerated. Most often, adults will not tolerate preparations of more than 25% weight/volume (w/v), which generally delivers 1.0 cal/ml, and infants, 12% w/v, which generally delivers 0.5 cal/ml. (Infants should be started on a concentration of 7–7.5% w/v, increasing to 12% over 4–5 days.) For children over 10 months, 15% w/v may be initiated, with gradual increases to 25%. Higher concentrations may cause osmotic diarrhea because of the sugar.

If the preparations are taken orally, 100–150 ml should be ingested at one time. Over the course of a day,

2,000 ml (about 2 qt) of most preparations provides about 2,000 cal. If the product is tube fed, 40–60 ml/hour may be given initially. The container should be kept cold to prevent bacterial growth, and all prepared products remaining after 24 hours should be discarded. The tubing should be rinsed 3 times/day with sterile water. If diarrhea, nausea, or distention occurs, the diet should be withheld for 24 hours, then gradually resumed. In elderly or unconscious patients or patients who recently have had surgery, elevating the head of the bed is advisable during administration of the preparation to avoid aspiration.

Cautions

Pharmacists should take care not to store products as they come from the manufacturer in areas with temperatures higher than 75° F (23.8° C) and should check expiration dates before dispensing.

Because all formulas are excellent media for bacterial growth, they should be prepared each day and refrigerated until used. If they become bacterially contaminated, they may cause diarrhea. Diarrhea also may occur from the osmotic carbohydrate load, especially simple sugars, or from fat intolerance. However, some elemental diets are fat free.

Patients must be monitored to detect biochemical abnormalities of electrolyte values and to ensure adequate nutrition and hydration. Urine and blood glucose concentrations should be measured; diabetics may require increased insulin doses. Edema may be precipitated or aggravated in patients with protein-calorie malnutrition or cardiac, renal, or hepatic disease because of the relatively high sodium content of the chemically defined diets. It has been emphasized that some commercially available nutritional products (Ensure and Ensure Plus) are a source of vitamin K supplementation, which may interfere with oral anticoagulant therapy (10). Frequently, hospital dieticians prepare formulas so that the electrolytes may be tailored to the individual patient.

Minerals

Trace mineral nutrition research has received considerable attention in recent years. Deficiency states and biologic functions are being defined in animal systems providing data that is assumed to apply generally to humans.

Unlike vitamins, the mineral content of plants varies according to the composition of the soil in which the plant is grown. This in turn affects the mineral content of the grazing domestic livestock. Mineral intake varies considerably from region to region, although the use of foods delivered from other locations tend to minimize intake variations. Marginal deficiencies of minerals have been reported only in certain segments of the population, although the increasing use of highly refined foods, which are low in minerals, contributes to the problem.

Optimal mineral intake values for humans are still imprecise. The U.S. RDA values for calcium, phosphorus, iodine, iron, magnesium, copper, manganese, and zinc are available (Table 3). However, only estimated ranges thought to be safe and adequate are published for chromium, selenium, fluoride, and molybdenum (Table 2). These ranges are based on the content of the "average" diet. Similarly, the possible adverse effects of long-term ingestion of high-dose mineral supplements are unknown. Pharmacists should encourage the consumer to achieve balanced mineral intake through attention to a proper diet, if possible, rather than the use of mineral supplements.

Iron

Iron deficiency anemia is still a widespread problem. Although it causes few deaths, it contributes to the poor health and suboptimal performance of many people. Furthermore, less severe iron deficiencies (those not resulting in frank anemia but rather more subtle clinical manifestations) may be quite common. Iron plays an important role in oxygen and electron transport. In the body it is either functional or stored. Functional iron is found in hemoglobin, myoglobin, heme enzymes, and cofactor and transport iron. Although functional in nature, the hemoglobin of the red blood cells also represents the major body store of iron containing 60–70% of total body iron. The rest is stored in the form of ferritin and hemosiderin. Ferritin is a micelle of ferric hydroxyphosphate surrounded by 24 identical protein units (11). Hemosiderin consists of aggregated ferritin molecules and additional components (12). The storage sites of ferritin and hemosiderin are the liver, spleen, and bone marrow.

Normally, adult males have about 50 mg of iron/kg; females have about 35 mg/kg (13). Hemoglobin is about 0.34% iron. The normal hemoglobin level in adult males is about 14–17 g/100 ml of blood and in adult females, it is 12–14 g/100 ml. The U.S. RDA for iron is 15 mg for infants, 10 mg for children under 4 years of age, and 18 mg for all adults.

Dietary iron is available in two forms. Heme iron is found in red meats and liver and is reasonably well absorbed (30–40%). Nonheme iron, the second form, constitutes most of the dietary iron and is poorly absorbed (about 5%). Published values for the iron content of foods and nutritional supplements are misleading in that under normal conditions only about 10% (total of heme plus nonheme iron) is absorbable. However, in the presence of an iron-deficient state, up to 20% may be absorbed.

Ingested iron, mostly in the form of ferric hydroxide, is solubilized in gastric juice and then reduced to the ferrous form. It is then chelated to substances such as ascorbic acid, sugars, and amino acids. These chelates have a low molecular weight and can be solubilized and absorbed before they reach the alkaline medium of the distal portion of the small intestine where precipitation occurs. Some of the transferrin iron is stored in the spleen, liver, and bone marrow. Iron is utilized in all cells of the body; however, most is incorporated into the hemoglobin of red blood cells. Iron is lost from the body by the sloughing of skin cells and GI mucosal cells in the urine, sweat, and feces; by hemorrhagic loss; and by menstruation.

Etiology of Iron Deficiency

Iron deficiency results from inadequate diet, malabsorption, pregnancy and lactation, or blood loss. Because the amount of normal excretion of iron through the urine, feces, and skin is very small, iron deficiency caused by poor diet or malabsorption may develop very slowly and manifest itself only after several years. The differential diagnosis of iron deficiency in an adult male or postmenopausal female should rule out iron deficiency due to blood loss. Blood loss occurs with conditions such as hiatus hernia, peptic ulcers, esophageal varices, diverticulitis, intestinal parasites (especially hookworm), regional enteritis, ulcerative colitis, and cancer. The pharmacist should be aware that anemia may be an indication of a more serious illness.

Blood loss may also occur from drug ingestion. Many drugs directly irritate the gastric mucosa or have an indirect effect on the GI tract. These drugs include the salicylates, analgesic/anti-inflammatory drugs such as indomethacin, phenylbutazone, reserpine, steroids, and most drugs used in the treatment of neoplasms, such as fluorouracil, mithramycin, and dactinomycin.

Menstrual blood losses may cause iron deficiency. Normally, the blood lost during a menstrual period is 60–80 ml; in 95% of women, this represents about 1.4 mg or less of iron lost (14). The iron loss due to menses, in addition to that normally lost by excretion and skin shedding, indicates a total daily requirement of absorbed iron of 0.7–2.3 mg. Although average U.S. diets contain about 5–7 mg of iron/1,000 cal, only 10% of iron in food is absorbed. Therefore, women on restricted diets may need supplemental iron. Some women who consider their menses normal, actually lose between 100 and 200 ml of blood/period. To make up this loss would require as much as 40 mg/day of iron in the diet, assuming about 10% of food iron is absorbed. Clearly, for these women supplemental iron is desirable. Formulation of a convenient diet to provide the excess iron demand during pregnancy would be difficult and supplements are therefore recommended as a component of prenatal care.

Another source of blood loss is through donation of blood. A donation is usually about 500 ml of blood. If the hemoglobin is normal, about 250 mg of iron is lost. This is not a significant problem in a healthy, well-nourished adult with adequate iron stores; however some blood donors, especially multiple or frequent donors, may benefit from short-term iron replacement following blood donation.

Iron deficiency may be caused by not eating enough animal protein and cereal food made with iron-fortified flour. Clay eating (geophagia) interferes with iron absorption by the chelation or precipitation of iron in the gut (14, 15). Achlorhydria and partial or total gastrectomy cause decreased iron absorption.

Evaluation

Early symptoms of iron deficiency frequently are vague and are related to other disease states. Easy fatigability, weakness, and lassitude cannot be related easily to iron deficiency. Often, patients without obvious symptoms have iron deficiency anemia, discovered during a routine medical examination. Other symptoms of anemia include pallor, dyspnea on exertion, palpitation, and a feeling of exhaustion. Coldness and numbness of extremities may be reported.

The pharmacist may ascertain the cause of the patient's disease by consulting the medication record. The patient might have been treated for ulcers or hemorrhoids, conditions that could cause blood loss. Checking the medication record for previous use of drugs such as phenylbutazone, reserpine, or warfarin might yield another reason for blood loss. Medications, such as aspirin, that may cause blood loss are bought without a prescription and often are not included on a medication record. In these cases the pharmacist must question the patient. A patient who indicates blood loss should be referred to a physician immediately. Abnormal blood loss may be indicated by any of the following symptoms:

- Vomiting blood ("coffee ground" vomitus);
- Bright red blood in the stool or black, tarry stools;
- Large clots or an abnormally large flow (200 ml or more) during the menstrual period;
- Cloudy or pink/red appearance of the urine (ruling out dyes in drugs that may cause urine discoloration).

Blood loss, particularly through the stool, is not always obvious to the patient. Before suggesting self-treatment, the pharmacist must consider the patient's medication history and overall appearance.

Other questions may be asked for indications of iron deficiency:

- Do you eat balanced meals on a regular basis?
- Do you have cravings for clay or ice (16)?
- Have you given blood recently?

The pharmacist should ascertain the chronicity of the patient's problem and whether medical care has been sought. Depending on the answers, the pharmacist might suggest iron supplementation with self-monitoring to check for improvement. It is well to remember, however, that the presence of anemia in patients other than those pregnant, lactating, menstruating, or on a restricted diet may be a symptom of a more serious disorder, and these individuals should be encouraged to seek medical diagnosis.

Treatment

If iron supplementation can be suggested safely, the pharmacist must determine which iron product is best. The choice of an iron preparation should be based on how well it is absorbed, how well it is tolerated in therapeutic doses, and price. Because ferrous salts are more soluble than ferric salts, it seems reasonable to choose an iron product of the ferrous group. Ferrous sulfate has been the standard against which other salts of iron—ferrous succinate, ferrous lactate, ferrous fumarate, ferrous glycine sulfate, ferrous glutamate, and ferrous gluconate—have been compared. All are absorbed about as well as ferrous sulfate. Ferrous citrate, ferrous tartrate, ferrous pyrophosphate, and some ferric salts are not absorbed as well (17).

Ferrous salts have been given in combination with ascorbic acid. At a ratio of 200 mg of ascorbic acid to 30 mg of elemental iron the increased amount of iron absorbed validated this practice (17). Some investigators believe that the cost of the iron-ascorbic acid combinations does not warrant its use for the moderate increase in iron absorption. As an economy measure, ascorbic acid tablets in relatively large doses may be given concurrently with an iron supplement. This type of therapy is probably more appropriate for people who have difficulty in absorbing adequate quantities of iron (infants and young children with severe anemia) (18).

In a 320-mg hydrated ferrous sulfate tablet, 20% (about 60 mg) is elemental iron. In patients with iron deficiencies, 20% of the elemental iron may be absorbed. If three 320-mg tablets/day are taken, 36 mg of iron may be absorbed. Between 36 and 48 mg of iron is enough to support maximum incorporation into red blood cells (0.3 g of hemoglobin/100 ml of blood) and replace iron stores.

Enteric-coated or delayed-release iron preparations are not pharmacologically advantageous. Because progressively less iron is absorbed as it moves from the duodenum to the ileum, the overall iron absorption is decreased by delaying the time of release (19). These products generally are more expensive than other iron preparations but do cause fewer symptoms of gastric irritation.

All iron products tend to irritate the GI mucosa. The symptoms are nausea, abdominal pain, and diarrhea. These symptoms may be decreased by decreasing the dosage or by giving iron with meals. Although giving iron with food is less irritating, food decreases the amount of iron absorbed by 40–50% (17). Periodically, physicians recommend iron with instructions for between-meal dosing. It is advantageous for absorption if the patient is able to tolerate the iron taken in this manner. If nausea or diarrhea is a problem, the pharmacist should be consulted; it usually is better to suggest taking the iron with food or decreasing the number of tablets than for the patient to decide to stop taking the supplement entirely.

Constipation, a frequent side effect of iron therapy, has prompted the formulation of medications that contain iron and a stool softener. However, not all patients become constipated with iron therapy.

Another observation with iron therapy is that stools become black and tarry. Usually, this effect is caused by unabsorbed iron, but it also may be caused by occult blood. Black tarry stools may indicate a serious GI problem; referral is indicated if an underlying GI condition is suspected or if there is a history of ulcerogenic (aspirin) or antiprothrombinemic (warfarin) use. If the stools do not darken during iron therapy, it may be that the iron tablet did not disintegrate.

Iron is chelated by many substances. Its interaction with antacids is therapeutically significant (20). The mechanism is probably related to the relative alkalinization of the stomach contents. Therefore, the chelate of iron with the antacid (magnesium trisilicate) is even more insoluble in the alkaline medium. Iron appears to chelate with several of the tetracyclines, resulting in decreased tetracycline and iron absorption (21). If simultaneous administration of the iron salt and tetracycline is necessary, patients should receive tetracycline 3 hours after or 2 hours before iron administration (22).

The manufacturers of allopurinol recommend that iron and allopurinol not be given together. In animals, allopurinol may increase hepatic uptake of iron; however, this effect has not been shown in humans.

Iron deficiency anemia is diagnosed by a physician or in a diagnostic clinic, on the basis of tests such as hemoglobin, hematocrit, serum iron, and iron-binding capacity. To monitor the effect of iron therapy, the pharmacist and physician may inquire about the patient's own perception of well-being. The physician generally uses the hemoglobin to measure the effect of iron therapy. The pharmacist might remind the patient who has a prescription for iron to have a blood test to check for the appropriate response in 1–2 months. Usually, hemoglobin and iron stores are corrected within 2–6 months, provided there is no ongoing bleeding and the diet is adequate.

Most healthy individuals who self-medicate, including menstruating females, will absorb adequate iron from 1 tablet/day of 300–325 mg of ferrous sulfate. However, the usual dose for iron deficiency is 2–4 tablets/day. One to two months of therapy is probably reasonable for self-medication with iron. If the patient has no response after this period, a physician should be consulted.

Iron Toxicity

Accidental poisoning with iron occurs most frequently in children. The sugar-coated, brown iron tablets look like chocolate and attract children. An accidental overdose could also occur from overingestion of chewable multivitamins containing iron. A 50% mortality has been associated with some series of cases but more recent experience suggests that a considerably lower mortality can be anticipated (23, 24). As few as 15 tablets of 300 mg of ferrous sulfate have been lethal, but the ingestion of as many as 70 tablets has been followed by recovery. Outcome depends upon speed of appropriate treatment.

The symptoms of acute iron poisoning are reflected by several organ systems. Because iron salts in large doses are corrosive to the gastric mucosa, pain, vomiting (the vomitus may contain blood and particles of the iron tablets), and diarrhea occur (ribbons of mucosa may be seen in the watery diarrhea) (25). These symptoms may lead to electrolyte imbalances and shock. In later phases of what may seem like recovery, pneumonitis (if the vomitus is aspirated) and acidosis may occur, and cardiovascular collapse may ensue. Autopsies frequently show liver damage, and there may be pyloric stenosis. Renal damage usually does not occur.

The treatment for iron toxicity may begin at home by immediately giving milk, eggs, or sodium bicarbonate solution to precipitate and bind iron. Vomiting should be induced on the way to the hospital. This can be accomplished with syrup of ipecac or by stroking the pharynx with a blunt object such as a spoon handle. Toxic ingestions of iron may be very dangerous and should immediately be referred to a poison control center or an emergency facility.

A more insidious kind of iron toxicity may occur during prolonged therapy with iron. In the treatment of refractory anemia, oral iron may be excessively absorbed, leading to iron overload. Alcoholic patients can also become overloaded with iron since wine contains iron, and alcohol increases ferric iron absorption. Patients with chronic liver disease and chronic pancreatic disease absorb more iron than normal from the gut. Iron overload also may occur if individuals who do not require iron supplementation take it for prolonged periods. Multivitamins with iron may be unknowingly abused in this manner by patients. The pharmacist should be aware of this possibility and should discourage the use of iron if no evidence indicates its need.

Calcium

Calcium is a major component of bones and teeth. It is necessary for the clotting of blood; the integrity of many cells, especially those of the neuromuscular system; and cardiac function. The present U.S. RDA of calcium for adults is 1 g, 600 mg for infants, and 800 mg for children under 4. During pregnancy and lactation 1.3 g/day is recommended.

The small intestine controls the amount of calcium absorbed. Patients taking relatively low amounts of calcium absorb proportionately more, and some taking large amounts excrete more as a fecal calcium. Calcium requirements also appear to increase as the consumption of protein increases (26, 27).

Decreased calcium levels may have profound and diverse consequences including convulsions, tetany, behavioral and personality disorders, mental and growth retardation, and bone deformities, the most common being rickets in children and osteomalacia in adults. Common causes of hypocalcemia and associated skeletal disorders are malabsorption syndromes, hypoparathyroidism, vitamin D deficiency, renal failure with resulting impairment in activation of vitamin D, long-term anticonvulsant therapy (increased metabolic inactivation of vitamin D), and decreased dietary intake of calcium, particularly during periods of growth, pregnancy, and lacatation, and in the elderly.

Serum levels may also be lowered by various medications. Corticosteroids inhibit calcium absorption in the gut. Several other drugs also lower calcium serum levels through various mechanisms and include phosphates, calcitonin, sodium sulfate, furosemide, mithramycin, anticonvulsants, magnesium, cholestyramine, and estrogen. Although furosemide lowers serum calcium, other diuretics increase serum calcium levels.

Therapy of calcium deficiencies hinges on the etiology of the disorder. Rich dietary sources of this element include milk and other dairy products. Dietary factors that increase calcium absorption include certain amino acids such as lysine, arginine, vitamin D, and lactose. Foods with high phosphate content (unpolished rice, hexaphosphoinositol in bran, or wheat meal), and foods high in oxalate content (cocoa, soy beans, kale, and spinach) decrease the efficiency of intestinal absorption of calcium (28).

The most common calcium salts available without a prescription are calcium carbonate, calcium gluconate, calcium lactate, and calcium phosphate. Treatment consists of 1–2 g of the salt or its equivalent daily with careful patient monitoring. Serum calcium should be maintained between 9 and 11 mg/100 ml of blood. Urine calcium is not an accurate reflection of serum calcium levels. One study supports the widely held view that calcium-rich foods and calcium supplements improve bone density in elderly patients with osteoporosis (29).

Calcium can be toxic. Large amounts taken as dietary supplementation or as antacids can lead to high levels of calcium in the urine and renal stones. The latter may result in renal damage. Hypercalcemia, with associated anorexia, nausea, vomiting, constipation, and polyurea, is also possible, particularly in patients taking high-dose vitamin D preparations.

Phosphorus

Phosphorus is essential for most metabolic processes. As phosphate, it serves as an integral structural component of the bone matrix (as calcium phosphate) and as a functional component of phospholipids, carbohydrates, nucleoproteins, and high-energy nucleotides. Accordingly, plasma phosphate levels are under tight biologic control involving the parathyroid hormone, calcitonin, and vitamin D.

There is a reciprocal relationship between calcium and phosphorus. Both minerals are regulated partially by parathyroid hormone. Secretion of parathyroid hormone stimulates an increase in calcium levels through increased bone resorption, gut absorption, and reabsorption in renal tubules. Parathyroid hormone causes a decrease in resorption of phosphate by the kidney tubules. Thus, when serum calcium is high, serum phosphate is generally low and the reverse is also true.

Phosphorus deficiencies are relatively uncommon. However, in patients with diabetic ketoacidosis, phosphorus deficiency can result from increased tissue catabolism, impaired glucose utilization and cellular phosphorus uptake, and increased renal excretion of phosphorus due to metablic acidosis (30).

Chronic use of antacids can also result in a deficiency due to formation of insoluble and poorly absorbed dietary phosphates. Symptoms include weakness, anorexia, bone demineralization, and hypocalcemia.

The opposite situation, hyperphosphatemia, along with hypocalcemia, and mild hypermagnesemia are usually present in acute renal failure. Hyperphosphatemia results from decreased renal phosphorus elimination in the face of continued release of phosphorus from the tissues (31).

The U.S. RDA values are identical to those of calcium except that infants are estimated to require 500 mg/day. Dietary sources of phosphorus are diverse because of the importance of this element in all living systems. Rich sources include seeds, nuts, eggs, meats, fish, and dairy products. Sodium and potassium phosphate salts are available without a prescription for those requiring supplements. In addition to being used to alleviate the deficiency state, phosphates have been employed to increase tissue calcium uptake in osteomalacia and to decrease serum calcium levels in hypercalcemia.

Iodine

Iodine is required to synthesize thyroxine and triiodothyronine, and in its absence, thyroid hypertrophy ensues. This results in the classical goiter that used to be prevalent in the midwest, where soils are iodide poor. The supplementation of iodized table salt with 0.01% potassium iodide has essentially eliminated goiter as a health problem in the United States.

Some concern exists that the iodine content of typical diets in the United States is too high. Surveys have revealed that the average iodine intake is 3–15 times the U.S. RDA of 0.15 mg for adults (32). No overt adverse effects have been found; however, these findings suggest that consumption of iodine supplements is unwarranted for most individuals. The U.S. RDA's are 0.045 mg for infants, 0.07 mg for children, and 0.15 mg for adults.

Magnesium

Magnesium, the fourth most abundant cation in the body, is required for bone structure, and is essential for the functioning of a number of critical enzymes including enzymes involved with ATP-dependent phosphorylation, protein synthesis, and carbohydrate metabolism. Magnesium tends to mimic calcium in terms of effects on the CNS and skeletal muscle. In fact, the normal response of the parathyroid glands to hypocalcemia is blunted by magnesium deficiency. One cannot correct tetany due to lack of calcium with calcium unless the magnesium deficiency is also corrected. Magnesium deficiency causes apathy, depression, increased CNS stimulation, delirium, and convulsions. Although muscle excitability is increased in hypomagnesemia, excess magnesium has a direct depressive effect on skeletal muscle. Advantage is taken of this activity in the use of magnesium sulfate to block the seizures of eclampsia.

Magnesium deficiencies are rarely noted in the normal adult population. Special situations, however, predispose toward suboptimal levels of magnesium (and other elements). Deficiencies have been observed in individuals with alcoholism, diabetes, chronic diarrhea, renal tubular damage, and with long-term intravenous feedings without magnesium supplementation. Hypermagnesemia is characterized by muscle weakness, CNS depression, hypotension, and confusion and can occur with overzealous use of magnesium sulfate (Epsom salts) as a cathartic or even magnesium-containing antacids in patients with severe renal failure.

The U.S. RDA values for magnesium are 400 mg for adults, 200 mg for children, and 70 mg for infants. An additional 50 mg is suggested during pregnancy and lactation.

Trace Elements

Trace elements, present in minute quantities in plant and animal tissues, are considered essential for physiologic processes. The RDA's for zinc and iodine are established. The requirements for the other trace elements are not accurately known. Based on the amount in the average diet, a range of intake values for these elements thought to be safe and adequate has been published by the Food and Nutrition Board, National Academy of Sciences (Table 2).

Zinc

Zinc is an essential constituent of a large number of metaloenzymes. Deficiencies adversely affect DNA, RNA, carbohydrate, and protein metabolism. In humans, zinc deficiencies have long been known to result in an impairment in healing, in taste and smell acuity, and in growth. In the Middle East, the use of unleavened whole-grain breads, rich in phytic acid (which binds zinc), has been associated with dwarfism and hypogonadism. This condition is relieved by supplemental zinc. Although zinc deficiencies are not widespread in the United States, marginally low values have been noted in certain population groups and have been associated with growth retardation in children and slow wound healing in adults (33, 34, 35). High-fiber diets rich in phytate, in addition to malabsorption syndromes, infection, myocardial infarction, major surgery, liver cirrhosis, pregnancy, and lactation, predispose an individual to a suboptimal zinc status.

Several studies (35–37) have demonstrated that oral zinc sulfate supplementation (200 mg, 3 times/day) hastened healing in zinc-deficient patients; zinc did not appear to be of benefit in those who had adequate zinc stores. The addition of zinc to the diets of patients with impaired wound healing who seem to be zinc deficient on the basis of a lowered serum zinc concentration seems to be indicated. However, the addition of extra zinc to the diets of patients who have normal serum zinc concentrations is not warranted on the basis of present evidence (38).

Zinc supplementation may be necessary in patients with large abdominal fluid losses because of surgical drains, ileostomies, vomiting, or diarrhea. Zinc deficiency may lead to a decrease in nitrogen retention (39). Patients with large GI losses of zinc were found to have significantly lower insulin and higher glucose levels (and lower lactate and pyruvate levels) than patients with normal GI loss (37).

Cirrhotic patients have been reported to have abnormal dark adaptation that does not respond to supplemental vitamin A (40). One study investigated the role that zinc deficiency may play in causing abnormal dark adaptation in cirrhotic patients. Administration of oral zinc corrected the abnormal adaptation (41). The study findings indicate that the improvement in dark adaptation by zinc may be due to enhanced activity of previously depressed retinol dehydrogenase.

Zinc is not without toxicity, although the emetic effect that occurs after consumption of large amounts of zinc serves to minimize the problems of accidental overdoses (36). Other reported signs of zinc toxicity in humans, in addition to vomiting, include dehydration, muscle incoordination, dizziness, and abdominal pain (36).

The adult U.S. RDA is 15 mg. The value for infants is 5 mg and for children is 8 mg. Typical Western diets supply 10–15 mg of zinc on a daily basis.

Copper

A major role for copper in iron metabolism has been elucidated and one of the prominent features of a copper deficiency is impaired iron absorption. This is most likely due to loss of activity of the copper metaloenzymes, ferroxidase, and ceruloplasmin with resulting hypochromic anemia (39). Other copper-containing enzymes are cytochrome-C oxidase, dopamine beta-hydroxylase, superoxide dismutase, tyrosinase, and lysyl oxidase. The latter enzyme is involved in crosslinking of collagen and elastin. In copper-deficient animals, bone cortices are fragile and thin due to failure of collagen crosslinking; angiorrhexis or spontaneous rupture of major vessels is also observed.

Copper is essential for structure and function of the CNS perhaps because of its involvement in the cytochromes, myelination, and dopamine beta-hydroxylase.

Copper deficiencies have been mostly observed in small premature infants where hepatic copper stores are low, in severely malnourished infants fed milk-based, low-copper diets, and in patients receiving total parenteral nutrition with inadequate copper (42).

Wilson's disease is an inborn error of metabolism with failure to eliminate copper resulting in CNS and kidney and liver damage. Acute copper toxicity symptoms include nausea, vomiting, diarrhea, hemolysis, convulsions, and GI bleeding.

The adult U.S. RDA is 2 mg. The value for children is 1 mg and for infants is 0.6 mg.

Manganese

Manganese is required for synthesis of the mucopolysaccharides of cartilage, for glucose utilization, for steroid biosynthesis, and for the activity of pyruvate carboxylase. Psychiatric abnormalities and neurologic disorders have been reported in occupational exposure to manganese oxide. This mineral can therefore be considered potentially toxic at high levels. Although manganese deficiencies have been experimentally produced in animals, they have never been detected in humans. The U.S. RDA value for adults is 4 mg, for children is 1 mg, and for infants is 0.5 mg.

Fluorine

Fluorine is present in the soil and water, but the content varies widely from region to region. Although it is essential for growth of animals, no deficiency state has been found in humans. The pharmacist's interest in this element relates to its demonstrated efficacy in helping to prevent dental caries. Most municipal water supplies are brought to 1 ppm of fluoride, a level that has been shown to be safe and to reduce caries in children by about 50%. (See Chapter 23, *Oral Health Products*.) Fluoride supplements should be routinely administered to children who consume water low in fluoride ion. The safe and adequate estimated range for children is 0.5–2.5 mg.

Excess fluoride can lead to toxicity, which can be either chronic or acute. Chronic toxicity is manifest as changes in the structure of bones and teeth. Bones become more dense, causing, in its most severe form, a disabling disease. The enamel of teeth acquires a mottled appearance consisting of white, patchy plaques, occurring with pitting brown stains. Prolonged ingestion of water containing more than 2 ppm has resulted in a significant incidence of mottling. Acute toxicity can be life threatening. The GI and central nervous systems are affected. Symptoms include salivation, abdominal pain, nausea, vomiting, and diarrhea. Because of the calcium-binding effect of fluoride, symptoms of calcium deficiency, including tetany, are seen. The patient may show mental irritability. Eventually, respiratory and cardiac failure may occur. The dose causing acute toxicity in adults is 5 g. Death has occurred after as little as 2 g but much larger doses have been treated successfully. In children, as little as 0.5 g of sodium fluoride may be fatal. Treatment includes precipitation of the fluoride by using gastric lavage with 0.15% calcium hydroxide solution, intravenous glucose and saline for hydration, and calcium to prevent tetany (43).

Chromium

The only defined function for chromium is as a component of glucose tolerance factor, a dietary organic chromium complex that appears to facilitate glucose utilization. In genetically diabetic mice, glucose tolerance factor administration (but not chromium itself) normalizes blood glucose levels (44). In humans, experimental administration of Brewer's yeast, a rich source of the as yet undefined glucose tolerance factor, has resulted in significant improvement of glucose utilization and a decrease in insulin requirements in some diabetics (45). More effort is warranted to define the therapeutic utility of chromium in diabetics.

One patient, receiving total intravenous feeding, developed a chromium deficiency that led to glucose intolerance and neuropathy. These symptoms were reversed after chromium supplementation (46).

The richest source of glucose tolerance factor chromium is Brewer's yeast. Smaller but significant amounts are present in liver, fish, whole grains, and milk. There is concern that the increasing consumption of refined foodstuffs will eventually lead to a marginal chromium deficiency in the population. Chromium intake in the United States is low (about 0.05 mg/day) compared with other countries (Egypt, 0.129 mg/day) but adverse effects have yet to be established. The estimated safe and adequate dietary intake for adults has been set at 0.05–0.20 mg/day. Chromium has a relatively high margin of safety.

Selenium

Selenium has been identified as an essential trace element in humans (47, 48). Selenium deficiencies are not common in the general population. Selenium deficiency has been reported in patients on long-term parenteral nutrition and in a child ingesting an inadequate diet (49, 50, 51). Selenium deficiencies are endemic in certain regions of China (52). The above deficiencies are characterized by cardiomyopathy. Selenium deficiency has also been reported in patients with alcoholic cirrhosis, probably due to insufficient diet or altered metabolism of selenium involving increased urinary or fecal output and resultant loss of the element (53). There appears to be an association between selenium deficiency and protein malnutrition disease (kwashiorkor) and multiple sclerosis (54, 55). Epidemiologic studies suggest that cancer and heart disease are most common in areas of low ambient selenium availability (56). A sta-

tistically significant inverse relationship was found between blood selenium levels in adult males and the total cancer mortality in 10 U.S. cities (57, 58). In the United States, the mortality in women with breast cancer is lower in areas in which grain and forage crops are high in selenium (59). In 110 cancer patients, lower serum selenium levels were usually associated with distant metastasis, multiple primary tumors, multiple recurrences, and a short survival time (60). As selenium levels reached or exceeded the mean value for the carcinoma group, the tumor was usually confined to the region of origin, distant metastasis occurred less frequently, and multiple primary lesions and recurrences seldom appeared. These findings warrant further investigation.

Excess selenium does not produce the same signs in humans as those observed in animals. However, excess selenium does produce growth retardation, muscular weakness, infertility, focal hepatic necrosis, dysphagia, dysphonia, bronchopneumonia, and respiratory failure (61, 62). Selenium has been implicated in four cases of amyotrophic lateral sclerosis in west central South Dakota, where naturally occurring intoxication is endemic in livestock (63).

Other Trace Elements

Molybdenum   Xanthine oxidase is a molybdenum-containing enzyme but no deficiency state has been observed in humans.

Cobalt   Cobalt is a component of vitamin B_{12}, but ingested cyanocobalamin is metabolized in vivo to form the B_{12} coenzymes. No deficiency state exists.

Silicon, Tin, Nickel, and Vanadium   Deficiency states involving these elements have been produced in animals only under stringent experimental conditions. They are presumed essential for humans but are obtained in small but adequate amounts in the diet.

Vitamins

Vitamins may be defined as chemically unrelated organic substances that are essential in small amounts for the maintenance of normal metabolic functions but are not synthesized within the body and, therefore, must be furnished from exogenous sources (64). Amino acids, proteins, fats, carbohydrates, and minerals are excluded from this definition (65). Vitamins generally are supplied adequately through most diets, and vitamin deficiencies that are diagnosed early usually can be corrected easily by administering large doses of the missing vitamin. The pharmacist should be aware of physical, environmental, or social conditions (such as vegetarian diets) that may be conducive to inadequate vitamin intake.

Fat-Soluble Vitamins

Vitamins A, D, E, and K are fat soluble and are absorbed in association with lipids; and therefore conditions that impair fat absorption, such as biliary cirrhosis, cholecystitis, and sprue, can lead to a deficiency of the fat-soluble vitamins. Similarly, drugs that affect lipid absorption, such as cholestyramine (binds bile acids thereby hindering lipid emulsification) and mineral oil (increases fecal elimination of lipids), may precipitate a deficiency of one or more fat-soluble vitamins.

Vitamin A

Vitamin A is needed to prevent night blindness and xerosis (drying) of the conjunctiva, the early symptoms of vitamin A deficiency. Drying of the epithelium on other sites of the body, nerve lesions, and increased pressure in the cerebrospinal fluid also may occur. Pregnant women must have an adequate vitamin A intake to avoid malformation of the fetus. Preformed vitamin A (retinol) can be obtained from animals, and carotenoids (provitamin A), of which the most active is beta-carotene, can be found in plants.

The term *vitamin A* designates several biologically active compounds. Vitamin A (retinol) and A_2 (3-dehydroretinol) are alcohols. Retinol is the major naturally occurring form. Because vitamin A and carotenoids are fat soluble, they are found mainly in fatty foods. Good sources are fish, butter, cream, eggs, milk, and organ meats. Four ounces of liver contain 37,000 units of vitamin A, a week's supply for the average adult. Carotenoids are the yellow-orange pigments of carrots, squash, and pumpkin, and they are also present in many dark, leafy vegetables. Deficiencies of vitamin A rarely occur in well-nourished populations, and when they do occur, they develop slowly since the body stores fat-soluble vitamins. Serum levels usually remain normal until the liver reserve becomes very small.

There are several etiologies of vitamin A deficiency. Before 1968, there was an epidemic of vitamin A deficiency in Brazil due to the provision of skim milk to Brazilian children without a supplementary vitamin A capsule. The skim milk was the dietary staple.

Diseases such as cancer, tuberculosis, pneumonia, chronic nephritis, urinary tract infections, and prostatic diseases may cause excessive excretion of vitamin A (66). Conditions in which there is fat malabsorption, such as GI diseases of sprue, obstructive jaundice, cystic fibrosis, and cirrhosis of the liver, may impair vitamin A absorption. Neomycin or cholestyramine may cause significant malabsorption of vitamin A and other fat-soluble vitamins and precipitate deficiencies upon long-term use. In the United States, vitamin A deficiency occurs more frequently because of diseases of fat malabsorption than because of malnutrition.

Vitamin A deficiency is a leading cause of childhood blindness worldwide. One of the earliest symptoms of the deficiency is night blindness, due to a failure of the retina to obtain adequate supplies of retinol for the formation of rhodopsin. If the lesion is not reversed, it may rapidly be followed by structural changes in the retina and xerosis (drying) of the conjunctiva. Bitot spots (small patches of bubbles that resemble tiny drops of meringue) may appear. The conjunctiva may look dry and opaque, and photophobia may occur. If the deficiency continues, xerosis of the cornea appears, followed by corneal distortion. The loss of continuity of the surface epithelium, with the formation of noninflammatory

ulcer and infiltration of the stoma, can lead to softening of the cornea, perforation prolapse of the iris, and permanent loss of vision (67).

Other features of vitamin A deficiency may be complicated by concurrent deficiencies of other nutrients. Notable, however, is the drying and hyperkeratinization of the skin, which predisposes patients to infections. The integrity of epithelial tissues depends on vitamin A activity.

The RDA values published by the Food and Nutrition Board, National Academy of Sciences, expresses potency in terms of a retinol equivalent (RE). This value compares activity of all carotenoids and other retinol derivatives to retinol. The U.S. RDA still retains the international unit (IU) as a measure of potency. The U.S. RDA for adults is 5,000 IU, which is equivalent to 1,000 RE. This is increased to 8,000 IU for pregnant and lactating women and decreased to 1,500 IU for infants and 2,500 IU for children. If the pharmacist establishes that the patient has poor dietary habits (alcoholism, anorexia, or an inadequate diet), a nonprescription multiple vitamin that contains the U.S. RDA of vitamin A should be recommended. Patients with corneal lesions due to hypovitaminosis A are treated with 50,000–200,000 IU/day of a water-dispersible, vitamin A preparation. In children under 5 years of age, 50,000 IU's have been reported to be effective (68). High-dose vitamin A therapy should only be undertaken with close medical supervision.

Vitamin A is appreciably stored and high doses can lead to a toxic syndrome known as hypervitaminosis A. The incidence of hypervitaminosis A is increasing because of publicity regarding the potential application of vitamin A in cancer. Toxicity in the form of bulging fontanel or hydrocephalus has occurred in infants given doses 10 times the RDA for several weeks (68). Fatigue, malaise, and lethargy are also common signs. Abdominal upset, bone and joint pain, throbbing headaches, insomnia, restlessness, night sweats, loss of body hair, brittle nails, exophthalmus, rough and scaly skin, peripheral edema, and mouth fissures may also occur. Severe constipation, menstrual irregularity, and emotional lability have been reported in some cases (69, 70). A single dose (2,000,000 IU or 400,000 RE) may precipitate acute toxicity 4–8 hours after ingestion. Headache is a predominant symptom, but it may be accompanied by diplopia, nausea, vomiting, vertigo, hypercalcemia, or drowsiness (71). Treatment consists of discontinuing vitamin A supplementation. The prognosis is good. Because of the dangers of high-dose vitamin A therapy, the FDA had ruled that products containing more than 10,000 IU of vitamin A/dose could not be sold without a prescription; however, this ruling has been reversed in a court decision. Carotene is not toxic because the rate of conversion of carotene to vitamin A is slow.

One of the most promising developments in vitamin research has been the discovery that vitamin A analogs show potential in the prevention and treatment of certain cancers and in the treatment of certain skin disorders. It has been long known that vitamin A deficiency in animals leads to hyperkeratosis and metaplasia (preneoplastic conditions) of epithelial tissues. Systemic administration of high doses of vitamin A can retard the development of these preneoplastic lesions (72, 73). Simultaneous administration of vitamin A with a carcinogen has been shown to block or delay carcinogenesis in laboratory animals (74). The disadvantage of this approach, which has direct significance to the pharmacist, is that the doses of vitamin A required to demonstrate antitumor or chemoprevention effects are sufficient to cause toxicity.

Recent research has been directed toward the development of analogs of retinoic acid with the goal of improving the therapeutic index of vitamin A. Although retinoic acid has activity in promoting normal epithelial differentiation, it is not stored and does not share other activities of retinol such as effects on vision and fertility. 13-*cis*-retinoic acid and certain other aromatic retinoic acid derivatives show particular promise (75–77) and have therapeutic and preventive activity against several experimental animal tumors. Dietary surveys have shown a lower incidence of lung cancer in smokers whose diet was high in vitamin A (78, 79).

The application of retinoids in cancer therapy is still under investigation. Meanwhile, pharmacists should stay abreast of developments so that consumer questions can be answered as accurately as possible. It behooves everyone to attempt to consume a diet that will provide the U.S. RDA for each vitamin. Those who have an elevated cancer risk (including smokers, familial polyposis patients, and individuals whose occupations expose them to carcinogens) may do well to pay particular attention to their intake of vitamin A. The pharmacist, however, should emphasize the dangers of megadose vitamin A therapy.

Experimental results also show promise for systemic retinoids in the treatment of acne, psoriasis, and other skin conditions characterized by hyperkeratosis (80–82). Topical retinoic acid is currently being used in the treatment of acne vulgaris, and therapy has proved to be quite successful. (See Chapter 29, *Acne Products*.)

Vitamin D

Vitamin D is a collective name for several structurally similar chemicals and their metabolites—ergocalciferol (vitamin D_2), derived from ergosterol, cholecalciferol (vitamin D_3), derived from cholesterol, and dihydrotachysterol, a synthetic reduction product of tachysterol. Cholecalciferol (vitamin D_3) is the natural form of vitamin D. It is synthesized in the skin from endogenous or dietary cholesterol on exposure to ultraviolet irradiation (sunlight). Ergocalciferol, which differs structurally only slightly from cholecalciferol, is of dietary importance. This is sometimes called synthetic vitamin D, a misnomer, because it is obtained by ultraviolet irradiation of ergosterol, a steroid found in plants and some fungi. Ergocalciferol and cholecalciferol are equipotent.

Studies have demonstrated that vitamin D requires activation involving both the liver and kidney. One metabolite, 25-hydroxycholecalciferol, is formed by the liver and is in turn hydroxylated to its most active form, 1,25-dihydroxycholecalciferol (83). These findings explain the observation Sof hypocalcemia in patients with renal failure and the failure of some of these patients to respond to even massive doses of vitamin D_3 (lowered kidney hydroxylation activity). Administration of 1,25-dihydroxycholecalciferol (available as calcitriol) to these patients has proved to be successful (84).

Vitamin D is needed to stimulate calcium absorption from the small intestine and to mobilize bone calcium. It is closely involved with parathyroid hormone, phosphate, and calcitonin in the hemostasis of serum calcium.

Vitamin D has properties of both hormones and vitamins. If there is sufficient exposure to sunlight, sterol in the skin is irradiated, and vitamin D is synthesized. If sun exposure is not sufficient, it is necessary to obtain preformed vitamin D from the diet.

The signs and symptoms of vitamin D deficiency diseases are reflected as calcium abnormalities, specifically, those involved with the formation of bone. As serum calcium and inorganic phosphate decrease, compensatory mechanisms attempt to increase the calcium. Parathyroid hormone secretion increases, possibly leading to secondary hyperparathyroidism. If physiologic mechanisms fail to make the appropriate adjustments in levels of calcium and phosphorus, demineralization of bone will ensue to maintain essential plasma calcium levels. During growth, demineralization leads to rickets; in adults it may lead to severe osteomalacia. Rickets is a failure of bone matrix mineralization. The epiphyseal plate may widen owing to failure of calcification combined with weight load on the softened structures. As a result, rickets is manifested by soft bones and deformed joints. The diagnosis is made radiologically by observing the bone deformities. The lack of adequate calcium in muscle tissue results in tetany.

Milk and milk products are the major sources of preformed vitamin D in the United States because milk is routinely supplemented with 400 IU/qt. Eggs are also a good source, and since the vitamin is stored in the liver, animal livers are rich in this vitamin. Because ultraviolet light is filtered out by water, fish synthesize their own vitamin D and are also a rich source of the vitamin.

Although the incidence of rickets in the United States is still low, the increasing popularity of vegetarian diets has led to rickets in children who abstain from milk and infants breast fed by mothers who did not drink milk or take prenatal vitamins (85, 86).

Vitamin D deficiencies caused by renal disease, malabsorption syndromes, short bowel syndromes, hypoparathyroidism, and familial hypophosphatemia are relatively common. The clinical significance of the decreased vitamin D levels noted in patients on long-term anticonvulsant drugs is still an important clinical question (87). Some clinicians recommend giving vitamin D 50,000 IU/day until serum calcium is normal and then giving 800–2,000 IU/day prophylactically to adult patients who are on continuous anticonvulsant therapy (88).

Large doses of vitamin D are prescribed for rickets (1,000–4,000 IU) (89). For adults with osteomalacia due to renal disease, 0.25–1.0 μg of calcitriol is often prescribed. Dihydrotachysterol, a synthetic analog that does not require kidney activation, may also be used.

The monitoring procedure for therapy, regardless of the particular vitamin D entity used, is extremely important. Urine and blood calcium levels must be checked to avoid hypercalcemia resulting from bone turnover and intestinal absorption. Because phosphate binds with calcium and may be deposited in soft tissue such as brain, eyes, heart, and kidney, phosphate in the serum also should be regulated. However, in vitamin D intoxication, the serum phosphate will usually be normal or slightly elevated.

Concurrent drug therapy must be monitored closely. Phosphate in chronically used drugs such as certain laxatives may lower the calcium level and contribute to a vitamin D deficiency. Patients who have vitamin D deficiency caused by renal problems should use caution in taking antacids. The pharmacist should point out to patients with renal problems that antacids should be chosen for the specific ingredients they contain; aluminum antacids may be chosen because they bind phosphates, and magnesium antacids avoided because of their toxicity in renal disease. A calcium antacid may be used to help increase serum calcium levels.

Vitamin D is toxic when taken in large doses for long periods. Adults should be limited to 400 IU/day as a general rule. Doses of 50,000–100,000 IU/day (1,250–2,500 μg cholecalciferol) are dangerous to adults and children. In infants, as little as 1,800 units/day may inhibit growth (89). Doses of 1,380–2,370 IU have not been shown to be detrimental to children, but doses exceeding 400 IU (25 μg cholecalciferol) are not advisable (90, 91).

The symptoms of hypervitaminosis D are anorexia, nausea, weakness, weight loss, polyuria, constipation, vague aches, stiffness, soft tissue calcification, nephrocalcinosis, hypertension, anemia, hypercalcemia, acidosis, and irreversible renal failure. The pharmacist should check the medication profile for a possible cause of the problem. For example, if a patient complained of bone pain and stiffness and the medication record showed therapy with vitamin D, the pharmacist might suspect hypervitaminosis. If a recent blood test has not been taken to measure serum calcium, a physician should be consulted.

Most persons obtain the U.S. RDA of vitamin D in dietary sources and by exposure to sunlight. If a patient asks for a vitamin D supplement and the pharmacist determines that the need is based on poor dietary intake or indoor confinement, a multiple-vitamin supplement may be recommended. Patients who request therapeutic doses of vitamin D should be referred to a physician if the pharmacist ascertains that a need exists. Liquid preparations that contain vitamin D should be measured carefully, particularly when given to infants. Patients using prescription vitamin D products should be encouraged to see a physician regularly.

Vitamin D is included in most multivitamin preparations and is available alone in various strengths for purchase by consumers. The FDA had placed all products containing more than 400 IU (10 μg cholecalciferol) on prescription-only status because of the potential for hypervitaminosis D, but this ruling has been reversed by court action. Two active metabolites, 25-hydroxycholecalciferol (Calciferol) and 1,25-dihydroxycholecalciferol [calcitriol (Rocaltrol)] are available by prescription for use in patients with hypocalcemia associated with renal failure. The former compound has the advantage of having a longer half-life but is less potent. Dihydrotachysterol, a vitamin D analog, available on prescription, is also useful in renal failure because it does not require metabolic activation.

Vitamin E

Vitamin E refers to a series of eight cyclic compounds, each containing a C-16 isopreneoid side chain. Alpha-tocopherol is the most active in the series and the one used to calculate the vitamin E content of foodstuffs. Plant oils contain considerable amounts of gamma-tocopherol, and although less than 10% as potent as alpha 1-tocopherol, it may contribute as much as 20% of ingested vitamin E activity. The Food and Nutrition Board of the National Academy of Sciences lists RDA values for vitamin E potency in terms of tocopherol equivalents (TE). One TE is equal to 1 mg of *d*-alpha-tocopherol, which is equivalent to about 1.5 IU. In addition, the U.S. RDA values are still expressed in terms of IU.

In spite of the seeming lack of a defined deficiency state in adults, vitamin E has received considerable interest in recent years through claims of its therapeutic efficacy for a variety of disorders. A deficiency syndrome involving premature infants fed a vitamin E depleted formula was noted in the late 1960's. Symptoms found were edema, hemolytic anemia, reticulocytosis, and thrombocytoses, which cleared upon supplementation with the vitamin (92). Earlier studies on adults revealed that chronic ingestion of a vitamin E–depleted diet resulted only in an increased propensity for hydrogen peroxide–induced erythrocyte hemolysis in vitro (93). Evidence for deposition of ceroid (age) pigments, creatininuria, altered erythropoiesis, and occurrence of a myopathy was found in a group of patients with vitamin E deficiency secondary to steatorrhea (94). In contrast to humans, most animals develop a characteristic and severe deficiency state. Just why humans are not so adversely affected by vitamin E depletion is unknown. It must be recognized that some of the claims for megavitamin use of vitamin E stem from deficiency symptoms noted in animals (muscular dystrophy, coronary diseases, sterility). The rationale for this type of vitamin E use is tenuous at best.

The biochemical function of this vitamin is still unresolved. Most investigators now believe that vitamin E serves in concert with selenium as a cellular antioxidant, protecting vital membranes from peroxidative damage. It may also have a more specific coenzyme role in heme biosynthesis, steroid metabolism, and collagen formation, but much remains to be learned relative to its molecular function.

It is unlikely that pharmacists will ever see a nutritional vitamin E deficiency in infants now that infant formulas are supplemented with the vitamin. Much interest centers on the pharmacologic activity of megadoses of the vitamin. Although most claims for the vitamin are unfounded, pharmacists are urged to keep an open mind on the therapeutic applications of vitamin E. Vitamin E does appear to have some utility for certain circulatory conditions and remains inadequately tested for other pathologies. Studies in Canada and Sweden showed a significant improvement in walking distance and in leg arterial flow in patients with intermittent claudication (95, 96). The treatments required at least 400 mg/day for at least 3 months. These studies have inexplicably attracted little interest in the United States. Relief of a related circulatory problem, nocturnal leg cramps, has also been reported using vitamin E (97).

There have also been claims that vitamin E is useful in coronary diseases, particularly angina (98). Numerous conflicting reports have been published on the value of tocopherols in this disease. Two recent, randomized double-blind studies, however, failed to find any significant benefit of vitamin E in the treatment of angina (99, 100). Careful studies have also failed to show that this vitamin is useful in improving athletic and sexual performance (101, 102, 103).

Other popular claims of the beneficial effects of vitamin E therapy have not been adequately investigated. Vitamin E appears to be essentially nontoxic, although the hazards of long-term therapy are unknown. One study failed to demonstrate any adverse effects in 28 volunteers ingesting 100–800 IU/day (67–536 alpha-tocopherol equivalents) for an average of 3 years (104). Nevertheless, the enhancement of warfarin anticoagulation has been reported and the pharmacist should caution patients taking anticoagulants to avoid vitamin E megadoses (105).

High doses of vitamin E have been reported to be of benefit in reducing the cardiotoxicity of doxorubicin, in treatment of glutathione peroxidase deficiency (a selenium enzyme) and in hemolysis associated with glucose-6-phosphate dehydrogenase deficiency (106, 107, 108). These uses rely on the physiologic antioxidant properties of this compound and represent a rational therapeutic use of the vitamin. Medical supervision of this therapy is essential. The use of endogenous vitamin E to relieve fibrocystic breast disease has been reported, although a final account of this research has yet to be published (109).

The U.S. RDA for vitamin E is 30 IU for adults, 10 IU for children, and 5 IU for infants. Requirements vary in proportion to the amount of polyunsaturated fatty acids in the diet. Although the polyunsaturated fatty acid content of the U.S. diet has increased in recent years, the plant oils responsible for the increase are rich in tocopherol. However, the exact requirement is a controversial issue. The Food and Nutrition Board has lowered its RDA value to 8–10 TE for adults (equivalent to about 12–15 IU). This change reflects the actual amount of vitamin E in the diet, which is approximately 12–15 IU for adults. It has been theorized that with the increasing oxidant insult in the environment in the form of atmospheric pollutants, the intake should be increased. However, the lack of evidence of deficiency at the present intake supports the lowering of the RDA from 30 to 12–15 IU. Until more information is available, intake at the higher end of the RDA range seems appropriate.

Foods rich in vitamin E activity include margarines (made from plant oils), green vegetables, and whole grains. Refining of grains to produce white flour removes most of the vitamin, and bleaching further depletes it. Meats, fruits, and milk contain very little vitamin E.

If vitamin E has been prescribed, iron should not be taken at the same time. Studies with supplementation of infant formulas containing iron and vitamin E show that blood tocopherol levels do not increase (110).

Vitamin K

Vitamin K is a fat-soluble vitamin found commonly in green leafy vegetables and a smaller amount in dairy products and fruits. A major amount of vitamin K required by humans is produced in the intestines by microbes.

There are only a small number of nonprescription products available containing vitamin K. There are no official RDA values for vitamin K, although the National Research Council indicated that a daily intake of 70–140 μg for adults is considered safe and effective (Table 2). Normal U.S. mixed diets contain 300–500 μg of vitamin K daily, so there is a low incidence of deficiency in healthy individuals. Since the absorption of vitamin K requires bile in the small intestine, anything that interferes with bile production or secretion may cause a deficiency, for instance, malabsorption syndromes and bowel resections. Liver disease may also cause vitamin K deficiency symptoms, since hepatic production of prothrombin clotting factor is decreased.

In addition to agents that interfere with all oil-soluble vitamins, such as cholestyramine resins and mineral oil, the oral anticoagulants are antagonists of vitamin K. Although antibiotics may potentially initiate a vitamin K deficiency by decreasing gut flora synthesis of the vitamin, this interaction is usually not seen if dietary intake is normal.

Vitamin K deficiencies are almost always associated with severe pathologic conditions in which the patient is receiving intensive medical care. Hemorrhage is the most common deficiency symptom. For minor bleeding, 1–5 mg of vitamin K is given, and for major hemorrhage, 20 mg. The cause of the deficiency will determine whether the oral route of administration is adequate. Vitamin K (phytonadione) is routinely given to neonates in doses of 1 mg to prevent hemorrhaging. This is necessary because placental transport of vitamin K is low and the neonate has yet to acquire a vitamin K–producing intestinal microflora.

Water-Soluble Vitamins

Ascorbic Acid (Vitamin C)

As a nutrient, ascorbic acid is necessary to prevent scurvy. Only humans and a few other species must consume ascorbic acid because it is not produced by the body. Today, scurvy is rare in the United States and develops only when psychiatric illness, alcoholism, age, GI disease, food fads, poverty, or ignorance cause inadequate nutritional consumption. Infants who are fed artificial formulas without vitamin supplements also may develop scurvy. In adults, scurvy occurs 3–5 months after all ascorbic acid consumption is stopped.

Ascorbic acid is necessary for biosynthesis of hydroxyproline, a precursor of collagen, osteoid, and dentin. A deficiency causes impairment of wound healing and reopening of old wounds. Early manifestations include anorexia, weakness, neurasthenia, and joint and muscle aches. Another early sign is prominent hair follicles on the thighs and buttocks due to plugging with keratin. The hair is coiled in the hair follicle and resembles a corkscrew, or it may be fragmented after it erupts. Bleeding abnormalities, such as hemorrhaging in the skin, muscles, joints, GI mucosa, and major organs, also occur. The gingiva become swollen, hemorrhagic, infected, and possibly necrotic; if left untreated, the teeth will fall out. Death may occur suddenly in untreated scurvy. In infants, ascorbic acid deficiency may cause retarded growth and development, skin and gum hemorrhaging, impaired bone development, and anemia.

Rarely are pharmacists confronted with overt symptoms of ascorbic acid deficiency. Only 10 mg/day of ascorbic acid prevents scurvy and a normal diet containing fresh fruits and vegetables contains many times more than this. The most common early symptom of a deficiency is prominent hair follicles. Rough skin probably will be a problem, most often in winter, when fresh fruits and vegetables are not as plentiful. The pharmacist should ask about the sites of the roughness and the appearance of the hairs. If there are no indications of a deficiency, the pharmacist should determine if more serious, hemorrhagic signs and symptoms exist, such as easy bruising, spontaneous petechiae or purpura (blood spots just under the skin). In the absence of these disorders, a multiple-vitamin product may be recommended. Most of these products contain 40 mg or more of ascorbic acid/dose. If the patient is already taking a daily vitamin supplement, additional ascorbic acid probably is not helpful. If hemorrhagic signs are present, the pharmacist should refer the patient to a physician because many serious diseases cause similar problems.

In patients with severe vitamin C deficiency, 300 mg of ascorbic acid/day for 5 days is recommended to build up the body store, followed by a daily dietary allowance of 45–65 mg, or a supplement in addition to diet. Infants who do not have ascorbic acid supplements in their formula should receive 35–50 mg/day; those who are breast fed by well-nourished mothers will receive a sufficient amount.

Ascorbic acid has been used for some time in the prevention and amelioration of the common cold (111, 112). Ascorbic acid advocates' claims are primarily based on personal experience and on the results of early trials of ascorbic acid for the common cold (113–115) that have been criticized on the basis of scope and experimental design (116). The claims have not been completely substantiated by the more than 10 randomized, double-blinded clinical trials conducted since 1970 (117–120). The results appear to depend on age, sex, and perhaps subjective factors. Positive findings could not be repeated in subsequent trials by the same investigator (117, 118). At best, megadoses resulted in only a small reduction in severity of cold symptoms. No consistent decrease in the incidence of colds in subjects taking prophylactic megadoses was found. One study found both natural and synthetic orange juice (the latter supplemented with ascorbic acid) containing 80 mg of ascorbic acid had the same effect (14–21% total reduction in symptoms) on the common cold as has been reported using megadoses (1–10 g) (121).

One valuable finding from these trials (which now involve over 7,000 human subjects) has been the seeming lack of toxicity of ascorbic acid. Megadoses of ascorbic acid, however, may be harmful in certain circumstances, and it is incumbent upon the pharmacist to estimate the risk/benefit ratio when advising patients on this vitamin. There have been isolated reports of toxicity including increased risk of oxalate urinary tract stone formation, possible ascorbate-mediated destruction of dietary vitamin B_{12}, an interaction of ascorbate and warfarin, and rebound scurvy upon sudden withdrawal of ascorbate. This latter phenomenon has been detected in infants whose mothers were taking megadoses during pregnancy.

Urine glucose tests are affected by large quantities of ascorbic acid in the urine. The TesTape and Clinistix tests may give false-negative readings while Benedict's solution and Clinitest tablets may give false-positive readings (122, 123). The pharmacist should instruct the patient on the procedure to modify the technique and minimize the interaction between tape tests and ascorbate. TesTape can be dipped in urine and the color inspection made at the moving front of the liquid since different diffusion rates allow the glucose to be chromatographically separated from the ascorbic acid.

Ascorbic acid (0.5–2 g/4 hours) has been used to acidify the urine in patients taking methenamine compounds for urinary tract infections. The lower pH of the urine facilitates hydrolysis of methenamine to the antibacterial product, formaldehyde. A drug interaction may result from use of high doses of ascorbic acid. When the urine is acidified, acidic drugs are reabsorbed more readily from the tubules resulting in higher blood levels (124). Basic drugs, such as tricyclic antidepressants and amphetamines, may be excreted more rapidly from acidified urine and their effect reduced by ascorbic acid therapy (125–127).

Additionally, crystalluria may be potentially caused by simultaneous administration of sulfonamides and ascorbic acid due to decreased solubility in the acidified urine. The clinical significance of ascorbic acid effects on the solubility and elimination of acidic and basic drugs is open to question because the decrease in urine pH has been shown to be less than 0.25 units (128, 129). Nevertheless, patients should be monitored if they are on acidic or basic medications and they initiate megadose ascorbic acid therapy.

Several other uses of ascorbic acid are worthy of mention. Marginal ascorbic acid deficiencies have been reported in institutionalized elderly patients and some studies have shown that ascorbic acid supplementation in these patients resulted in measurable improvement in general health and well-being (130). Lower-than-normal levels of ascorbic acid (and several other vitamins) have been noted in smokers and in women taking oral contraceptives. There is no evidence of scurvy in these individuals, but the pharmacist may reasonably suggest a multivitamin supplement for these patients. Ascorbic acid can also be used to increase iron absorption by virtue of its ability to form a soluble iron-chelate and by inhibiting the oxidation of Fe^{+2} to Fe^{+3}.

As discussed previously, ascorbic acid is necessary for collagen synthesis and has been used to promote healing following surgery, trauma, and fractures. Although there is not universal agreement on the value of this approach, recent studies indicate it may be beneficial. For example, decreased recovery time from cold sores, an increased healing rate of pressure sores, and a decreased incidence of rectal polyps have been reported following administration of gram quantities of ascorbic acid (131–134). These findings await confirmation by others, but at present there is evidence of the efficacy of ascorbic acid in the promotion of healing of certain lesions.

Conflicting data exist concerning the ability of ascorbic acid to lower cholesterol levels in nonascorbic, hypercholesterolemic patients (135, 136). Similarly, some studies reported prolonged survival of terminal cancer patients administered ascorbic acid megadoses, and others were unable to demonstrate an effect (137, 138). The usefulness of ascorbic acid in cancer and hypercholesterolemia remains unclear at this point.

The pharmacist is urged to weigh the relative risks and benefits of ascorbic acid therapy. Short-term use to promote healing, for example, or for serious disorders such as rectal polyps, may warrant a trial of ascorbic acid. The expense and potential risks of long-term ingestion of large quantities of ascorbate may be questionable for a seemingly minor beneficial effect on the common cold, a self-limiting condition.

The U.S. RDA of ascorbic acid for adults is 60 mg, for children is 40 mg, and for infants is 35 mg. Ascorbic acid tablets should be stored in a sealed container and kept away from heat and moisture to maintain potency.

Ascorbic acid tablets and liquid concentrations are available in many sizes as ascorbic acid and sodium ascorbate. Sodium ascorbate is the soluble salt for parenteral use.

Thiamine Hydrochloride (Vitamin B₁)

Thiamine is necessary for several critical functions in carbohydrate metabolism, and the amount of vitamin required increases with increased caloric consumption. Additionally, thiamine is essential in neurologic function; however, this mechanism is not completely understood. A thiamine deficiency can be diagnosed on the basis of impaired carbohydrate utilization with a resulting build-up of pyruvic acid or more commonly by analyzing the activity of erythrocyte transketolase, a thiamine-dependent enzyme.

The most familiar natural thiamine source is the hull of rice grains. Other good sources are pork, beef, fresh peas, and beans. It was in animals and humans whose diets consisted largely of polished rice that thiamine-deficiency disease (beriberi) was first observed. Today, beriberi caused by nutritional deficiency rarely occurs in the Western world, unless it is precipitated by economic or medical conditions.

Symptoms of thiamine deficiency are evident 12–14 days after thiamine intake is stopped. The abnormalities center in the cardiovascular and neurologic systems. The deficiency causes cardiac failure possibly accompanied by edema, tachycardia on only minimal exertion, enlarged heart, and electrocardiographic abnormalities. The patient may have pain in the precordial or epigastric area. The neuromuscular symptoms are paresthesia of the extremities of maximal use, weakness, and atrophy.

Individuals subsisting on a diet of 0.2–0.3 mg of thiamine/1,000 calories (slightly less than the thiamine requirement), may gradually become depleted and develop peripheral neuropathy. If the patient has been subsisting on substantially less than 0.2 mg of thiamine/1,000 calories, deficiency will be more severe. In addition to neurologic manifestations, cardiovascular symptoms will be more apparent (139).

Beriberi may develop in infants whose mothers are on a polished rice diet in regions where thiamine hydrochloride supplements are not used. The symptoms of infantile beriberi also are neurologic. Aphonia, or silent crying, may occur, and the signs of meningitis may be mimicked. Death will ensue if treatment is not initiated with thiamine.

The dosage of thiamine for the treatment of the symptoms of heart failure caused by this deficiency is 5–10 mg 3 times/daily. At this dose the failure is rapidly corrected, but the neurologic signs correct much more slowly. The dosage of thiamine for neurologic deficits is between 30 and 100 mg given parenterally for several days or until an oral diet can be started.

The alcoholic represents a special population in which thiamine deficiency is common. The diet of the alcoholic is often nutritionally imbalanced, and alcohol may impair thiamine transport across the intestine (140, 141). A more severe metabolic condition due to a thiamine deficit (Wernicke-Korsakoff syndrome) may also be seen in alcoholics (142). This syndrome may also occur in other patients who have been vomiting for extended periods or who are given glucose solutions without supplemental thiamine.

The neurologic signs (Wernicke's encephalopathy) are particularly evident. Nystagmus occurs when the patient is asked to gaze up and down along a vertical plane or from side to side along a horizontal plane. Death is common if treatment is withheld. Damage to the cerebral cortex may occur in patients who survive, and it can lead to Korsakoff's psychosis. The symptoms of the psychosis are impaired retentive memory and cognitive function; the patient commonly confabulates when given a piece of information or when asked a question.

Wernicke-Korsakoff syndrome has a high morbidity and some mortality. Irreversible neurologic damage may ensue if left untreated, necessitating institutionalization of the patient. Fortification of alcoholic beverages with thiamine has been suggested as a means of preventing this disorder (143). Thiamine is commonly given to patients who are admitted for alcohol detoxification and treatment. A thiamine-containing vitamin supplement is often prescribed for the alcoholic patient.

Several genetic diseases respond to administration of thiamine. These fall in the category of "vitamin-responsive inborn errors of metabolism" and generally are attributable to a defect in the binding of enzyme and cofactor. Large doses of vitamin (5–100 mg in the case of thiamine) saturate the enzyme and usually obviate the pathology. Examples of thiamine-responsive inborn errors are lactic acidosis (defective pyruvate carboxylase), branched-chain aminoacidopathy (defective branched-chain amino acid decarboxylase), and the Wernicke-Korsakoff syndrome (defective transketolase) (144–146). These diseases are relatively rare and constitute a rational but uncommon use for megadose thiamine.

The use of thiamine as a mosquito repellent remains controversial. Some sportspersons claim that a dose of 100 mg 3 times/day for 3 days before and during an outing will largely prevent mosquito bites, but published studies do not substantiate these claims (147, 148).

Thiamine is considered to be nontoxic when administered orally. Excess vitamin is rapidly eliminated in the urine. A few reports of itching, tingling, pain, and rare anaphylactic reactions have been noted upon parenteral thiamine administration.

The U.S. RDA for adults is 1.5 mg, for children under 4 years of age, 0.7 mg, and for infants, 0.5 mg. The requirement is increased to 1.7 mg during pregnancy and lactation.

Thiamine is available as an elixir, an injectable solution, and a tablet. If it is mixed in a solution, the solution should be acidic because thiamine is labile at an alkaline pH.

Riboflavin (Vitamin B₂)

Riboblavin is a constituent of two coenzymes (FAD and FMN) and is involved in numerous oxidation and reduction reactions. Riboflavin-dependent enzymes are called flavoproteins because the riboflavin is intimately associated with the enzyme. There are at least 40 flavoproteins in the body, including the cytochrome P-450 reductase enzyme involved in drug metabolism. Cellular growth cannot occur without riboflavin.

The U.S. RDA for riboflavin is 1.7 mg for adults and children over 4 years of age. Intake should increase to 2.0 mg during pregnancy and lactation. It seems that the need for riboflavin increases during periods of increased cell growth, such as during pregnancy and wound healing. Surveys have revealed lower than anticipated riboflavin levels in women taking oral contraceptives although the pathologic consequences are unknown as yet (149). Levels of pyridoxine, folic acid, and ascorbic acid are also somewhat lower in oral contraceptive users. Marginal riboflavin deficiencies have also been detected in inner-city youths, vegetarians, and alcoholics (150, 151, 152). It usually accompanies other vitamin deficiencies attributable to an inadequate diet. Milk is a common source of dietary riboflavin and low-riboflavin levels in some urban teenagers have been correlated with low-milk consumption (150). The same may be true for strict vegetarians (vegans). Other rich dietary sources are eggs, meat, fish, liver, and whole grains.

Because of the importance of riboflavin in metabolism, it is surprising that the deficiency state is not more severe. Initial symptoms are mainly cheilosis, angular stomatitis, glossitis, corneal vascularization, and a dermatitis evident in the genital region and over the joints. Symptoms of later stages of the deficiency are seborrheic dermatitis of the face and a generalized dermatitis over the rest of the body. Photophobia may occur, and the eyes may itch and burn. The symptoms of riboflavin deficiency may be indicative of other very serious conditions, such as blood dyscrasia.

A complete dietary history should be obtained from the patient. In some cases, a therapeutic trial 10 mg/day of riboflavin may be carried out before diagnosis is made. The therapeutic dose is 10 mg orally. Larger doses are not harmful but provide no additional benefit. The patient should be monitored to assess improvement of symptoms.

Riboflavin is not very soluble. If oral absorption is a problem, 25 mg of the soluble riboflavin salt may be given intramuscularly. Riboflavin is also given intravenously as a component of injectable multivitamins, but the dosage is relatively low (about 10 mg/dose). Intravenous doses of 50 mg of riboflavin can decrease pulse rates in adults. Excess riboflavin is excreted in the urine and has a yellow fluorescense.

In addition to treating a deficiency state, riboflavin has been used following eye surgery to prevent vascularization of the cornea. However, the efficacy of this approach is not well documented.

Niacin (Nicotinic Acid)

Niacin and niacinamide are constituents of the coenzymes nicotinamide adenine dinucleotide (NAD) and nicotinamide adenine dinucleotide phosphate (NADP). The coenzymes are electron transfer agents (they accept or donate hydrogen in the respiratory mechanism of all body cells). Niacin is unusual as a vitamin because humans can synthesize it from dietary tryptophan. Most individuals receive about half of their niacin requirement from tryptophan-containing proteins and the rest as preformed niacin or niacinamide. Both niacin and niacinamide are effective in treating the niacin deficiency state (pellagra). Niacin, in high doses, will lower triglycerides and cholesterol and will produce cutaneous vasodilation. Niacinamide, however, does not produce the flushing associated with high doses of niacin nor does it have an effect on plasma lipids.

The U.S. RDA for all adults and children over 4 years of age is 20 mg. Foods rich in niacin include lean meats, liver, kidney, fish, whole grains, legumes (peas and beans), and green vegetables.

Niacin requirements are increased under the following conditions:

- During periods of substantially increased caloric expenditure;
- During acute illness and convalescence after severe injury, infection, or burns;
- When the caloric intake of the diet is increased substantially;
- If the patient has a low tryptophan intake (low-protein diet or high intake of corn as a staple in the diet).

Pellagra is rare, occurring most frequently in alcoholics, the elderly, and individuals on bizarre diets. It also occurs in areas where much corn is eaten because the niacin in corn is bound to indigestible constituents, making it unavailable. The main body systems affected are the nervous system, the skin, and the GI tract. Symptoms affecting the nervous system are peripheral neuropathy, myelopathy, and encephalopathy. Mania may occur, and seizures and coma precede death. Before the cause was discovered, many psychiatric admissions were due to the symptoms of niacin deficiency. There is a characteristic rash in niacin-deficient patients. Skin over the face and on pressure points may be thickened and hyperpigmented, or may appear as a severe burn and become secondarily infected. The entire GI tract is affected, including angular fissures around the mouth, atrophy of the epithelium and a beefy-red color of the tongue, and hypertrophy of the papillae. Inflammation of the small intestine may be associated with episodes of occult bleeding and/or diarrhea. A summary of the symptoms of niacin deficiency in the various systems is called the "three D's"—diarrhea, dementia, and dermatitis.

The diagnosis is clear if all systems are affected. However, if the skin is unaffected, the diagnosis is much more difficult. A complete dietary history with subsequent calculation of the consumption of niacin may point to the disease. Treatment involves the ingestion of 300–500 mg of niacinamide daily in divided doses. Because other nutritional deficiences may be present, treatment may include the other B vitamins, vitamin A, and iron.

Niacin has been used in daily doses of 100 mg to 3 g for hyperlipidemias and hypercholesterolemia. This modality has been carefully evaluated by the Coronary Drug Project and found to be ineffective in terms of increasing the survival time of patients with prior myocardial infarctions (153). The adverse reactions experienced by the volunteers were significant and included GI irritation, elevated serum enzymes, and increased arrhythmia. Niacinamide does not have an effect on plasma lipids. Niacin is also used for patients with peripheral vascular disease, but there has been no agreement on the value of this approach. Dosages suggested by the manufacturer for these conditions are 150 mg/day in divided doses. Niacin and niacinamide, in doses of 3 g or more/day, have been used in megavitamin therapy for schizophrenia. Controlled studies do not show significantly different results when compared with placebo (154–156).

High dosages of niacin cause significant and potentially life-threatening side effects. Because of the effects on the GI tract, high doses of niacin are contraindicated in patients with gastritis or peptic ulcer. Niacin can release histamine, and its use in patients with asthma should be undertaken carefully. It also can impair liver function, causing cholestatic jaundice, and can disturb glucose tolerance and cause hyperuricemia. If niacin and niacinamide are used in high doses, laboratory parameters, suggested by the potential side effects, should be followed.

Niacin and niacinamide are available as tablets and capsules of many strengths, as injectable solutions, and as elixirs (50 mg/5 ml). Doses of niacin in supplemental products usually are 10–20 mg (prenatal multivitamins contain 20 mg of niacin).

Pyridoxine Hydrochloride (Vitamin B₆)

Pyridoxine hydrochloride, pyridoxal hydrochloride, and pyridoxamine are all equally effective in nutrition. Pyridoxine hydrochloride is the form most frequently used in vitamin formulations.

The U.S. RDA is 2 mg for adults and children 4 or more years of age, and 0.7 mg for children under 4 years of age, and 0.4 mg for infants. The adult requirement should be increased to 2.5 mg during pregnancy and lactation. Foods rich in pyridoxine hydrochloride are meats, cereals, lentils, nuts, and some fruits and vegetables such as bananas, avocados, and potatoes. Cooking destroys some of the vitamin. The average U.S. diet provides the U.S. RDA; certain restricted diets and haphazard diets do not. Artificial infant formulas are required to contain pyridoxine hydrochloride.

The symptoms of vitamin B₆ deficiency in infants are convulsive disorders and irritability. Treatment with pyridoxine hydrochloride (2 mg/daily for infants) brings the encephalogram back to normal. Symptoms in adults whose diets are deficient in pyridoxine hydrochloride or who have been given a pyridoxine hydrochloride antagonist are indistinguishable from those of niacin and riboflavin deficiencies. They include pellagra-like dermatitis, scaliness around the nose, mouth, and eyes, oral lesions, peripheral neuropathy, and dulling of mentation. Other conditions or circumstances may also be related to pyridoxine hydrochloride requirements. Treatment of sideroblastic anemia requires 50–200 mg/daily of pyridoxine hydrochloride to aid in the production of hemoglobin and erythrocytes. Because these amounts are more than physiologic requirements, the anemia is not a nutritional deficiency.

Several drugs affect pyridoxine hydrochloride utilization. Isoniazid and cycloserine (antitubercular drugs) seem to antagonize pyridoxine hydrochloride (157). Hydralazine appears to have this effect as well (158). Perioral numbness resulting from peripheral neuropathy is a clinical manifestation of this antagonism, occurring most frequently in patients with poor diets. Psychotic behavior or seizures, both produced by cycloserine, may sometimes be prevented with increased pyridoxine hydrochloride intake. To overcome the antagonism, 50 mg/day of pyridoxine hydrochloride with isoniazid and as much as 200 mg/day with cycloserine should be used. Another recommended dosage is 10 mg pyridoxine/100 mg isoniazid (158). Penicillamine may bind with pyridoxine hydrochloride, causing pyridoxine hydrochloride–responsive neurotoxicity.

Pyridoxine is intimately involved in all amino acid metabolism, particularly tryptophan metabolism. Low pyridoxine levels result in the appearance of excess xanthurenic acid, a tryptophan metabolite, in the urine. Pyridoxine status can be assessed by quantitation of urinary xanthurenic acid following administration of a loading dose of tryptophan. Estrogens seem to significantly increase xanthurenic acid production, and women taking oral contraceptives show laboratory signs of a pyridoxine deficiency (160–162). Supplementation

(2–40 mg) with pyridoxine returns the tryptophan metabolic pattern to normal. The pathologic consequences of these events are not known although a depressive syndrome occasionally experienced by women on oral contraceptives has responded to pyridoxine supplementation (20–100 mg) in those women who showed signs of a marginal deficiency (160, 163, 164). Levels of other vitamins are marginally lower in some oral contraceptive users. Multivitamin supplements may be worth considering for women taking oral contraceptives.

At least five pyridoxine-dependent inborn errors of metabolism have been shown to respond to large doses of pyridoxine (165, 166). Pyridoxine (100 mg 3 times/day) for at least 11 weeks has also been reported to relieve paresthesia and pain in the hands in patients with carpal tunnel syndrome (167).

Pyridoxine hydrochloride acts as an antagonist of the therapeutic action of levodopa, a drug used in treating parkinsonism, because it facilitates the transformation of levodopa to dopamine before the former can cross into the CNS central nervous system. The pharmacist should inform patients taking levodopa of the interaction and should advise these patients to avoid supplemental pyridoxine hydrochloride. However, it may be useful in the treatment of patients who have overdosed on levodopa. A vitamin product that does not contain pyridoxine hydrochloride has been formulated for parkinsonian patients taking levodopa. A combination product containing carbidopa and levodopa, a peripherally acting dopa decarboxylase inhibitor, is not affected by the concurrent administration of pyridoxine hydrochloride.

Pyridoxine is generally considered to be nontoxic although high doses (200–600 mg) have been shown to inhibit prolactin (168, 169). Prenatal vitamins contain 1–10 mg and would therefore not appear to have a significant toxic effect. Large doses of pyridoxine also increase the activity of plasma aminotransferase enzymes, the consequences of which are unknown.

Pyridoxine hydrochloride is available as a tablet in varying strengths and as an injectable solution (50 mg/ml and 100 mg/ml).

Vitamin B$_{12}$ (Cyanocobalamin)

Vitamin B$_{12}$ participates in methylation reactions and hence cell division, usually in concert with folic acid. Vitamin B$_{12}$ is necessary for recycling of folate and therefore a folate deficiency is observed as a feature of a vitamin B$_{12}$ deficiency. It is also necessary for metabolism of lipids, for maintenance of sulfhydryl groups in the reduced state, and in the formation of myelin.

Cyanocobalamin, the common pharmaceutical form of the vitamin, is chemically stable and is generated as part of the isolation scheme for vitamin B$_{12}$ from natural sources. In vivo, the cyanide moiety is metabolically removed to form the active coenzyme forms of the vitamin (methyl cobalamin and 5-deoxyadenosylcobalamin). The term *vitamin B$_{12}$* refers to all cobalamins that have vitamin activity in humans.

The U.S. RDA for vitamin B$_{12}$ is 2 μg for infants, 3 μg for children under 4 years of age, and 6 μg for adults and for children over 4 years of age. Requirements during pregnancy and lactation increase to 8 μg because of the need for vitamin B$_{12}$ participation in generation of new cells and in production of milk. Vitamin B$_{12}$ is produced almost exclusively by microorganisms, hence its presence in animal protein. It may also be found in small amount in the root nodules of legumes, again due to the presence of microorganisms.

In healthy individuals who have not restricted their diets, adequate vitamin B$_{12}$ levels are maintained by the body. Vitamin B$_{12}$ deficiency may be caused by inadequate ingestion, absorption, or utilization, or an increased requirement or excretion of this vitamin (170). Because vitamin B$_{12}$ is well conserved by the body through enterohepatic cycling, it requires years for the deficiency to develop. In patients whose deficiency is related to malabsorption (ileal diseases or resection), the reabsorption phase of the enterohepatic cycle is affected, and the deficiency may occur much earlier. Some people lack the glycoprotein (intrinsic factor) necessary for the absorption of vitamin B$_{12}$, resulting in pernicious anemia. Because of the lack of vitamin B$_{12}$ in vegetables, vegetarians who consume absolutely no animal products are at risk for developing a deficiency (171). Several cases of a vitamin B$_{12}$ deficiency have been reported in infants breast fed by vegetarian mothers (172, 173). Strict vegetarians should consider taking vitamin B$_{12}$ supplements or adjust their diet to consume vitamin B$_{12}$-containing fermented foods, such as soy sauce and meso.

Since vitamin B$_{12}$ is important for recycling folate to be used in cell production, the symptoms of a deficiency are manifested in organ systems with rapidly duplicating cells. Thus, an effect on the hematopoietic system results in anemia. The GI tract is also affected, with glossitis and epithelial changes occurring along the entire tract. Because of the importance of vitamin B$_{12}$ in the maintenance of myelin, deficiency states cause many neurologic symptoms, such as paresthesia (manifested as tingling and numbness in the hands and feet), progressing to unsteadiness, poor muscular coordination, mental slowness, confusion, agitation, optic atrophy, hallucinations, and overt psychosis. Surgical removal of portions of the stomach and small intestine often result in vitamin B$_{12}$ deficiency. Regional enteritis, tropical sprue, idiopathic steatorrhea, and celiac disease impair the absorption of vitamin B$_{12}$.

Certain drugs may cause poor absorption of vitamin B$_{12}$. Neomycin reduces the absorption, and the absorption is further decreased if colchicine is also a part of therapy (174, 175).

In the past, treatment of vitamin B$_{12}$ deficiency involved the administration of crude liver extracts orally and parenterally. Crystalline vitamin B$_{12}$ is now readily available; the preferred route is the parenteral form of the vitamin. Treatment of pernicious anemia or permanent gastric or ileal damage with injectable vitamin B$_{12}$ is lifelong.

Vitamin B$_{12}$ is available in tablet and injectable dosage forms. Oral forms can be used if the deficiency is nutritionally based; intramuscular or subcutaneous administration is necessary for deficiencies caused by malabsorption. Hydroxocobalamin is a longer-acting form equal in hematopoietic effect to cyanocobalamin. Because it is more extensively bound to blood proteins, it remains in the body for a longer period. Vitamin B_{12} has no therapuetic value beyond that of correcting vitamin B_{12} deficiencies. A deficiency can be corrected with 3 μg of oral vitamin B_{12} daily for adults or a minimum of 100 μg given parenterally each month. Doses larger than needed do not cause toxicity because excretion through the urine and bile occurs once tissue and plasma binding sites are saturated.

Patients should be cautioned by the pharmacist that an accurate diagnosis of the causes of a suspected anemia is essential for effective treatment. For example, folic acid deficiency anemia should be treated with folic acid, pernicious anemia with vitamin B_{12}, and iron deficiency anemia with iron. The use of shotgun antianemia preparations containing multiple hematinic factors should be discouraged.

Folic Acid

Folic acid is pteroylglutamic acid, the pharmaceutical form of the vitamin. In foods, folate exists as reduced pteroylpolyglutamates, which are readily cleaved by in-

testinal conjugases to the monoglutamic acid derivatives. The term *folacin* refers to all folic acid derivatives with vitamin activity, and the vitamin content of foods is calculated after hydrolysis of polyglutamates to the monoglutamic acid derivatives. In its function in the body, folic acid is closely related to vitamin B_{12}. Folates are reduced in vivo to tetrahydrofolic acid (THFA) through a complex process involving dihydrofolate reductase. Tetrahydrofolic acid is involved in the transfer of one carbon unit in the biosynthesis of purine, pyrimidine, serine, methionine, and choline. Several methylated folate intermediates exist and are interconvertible. Vitamin B_{12} is necessary for regeneration of tetrahydrofolic acid and completion of the folate cycle. Thus a folate deficiency can occur as a consequence of a vitamin B_{12} deficiency.

The U.S. RDA's for folic acid are 0.1 mg for infants, 0.2 mg for children under 4 years of age, 0.4 mg for adults and children 4 or more years of age, and 0.8 mg during pregnancy and lactation.

The folate content of food is subject to destruction depending on how it is processed. Canning, long expo-

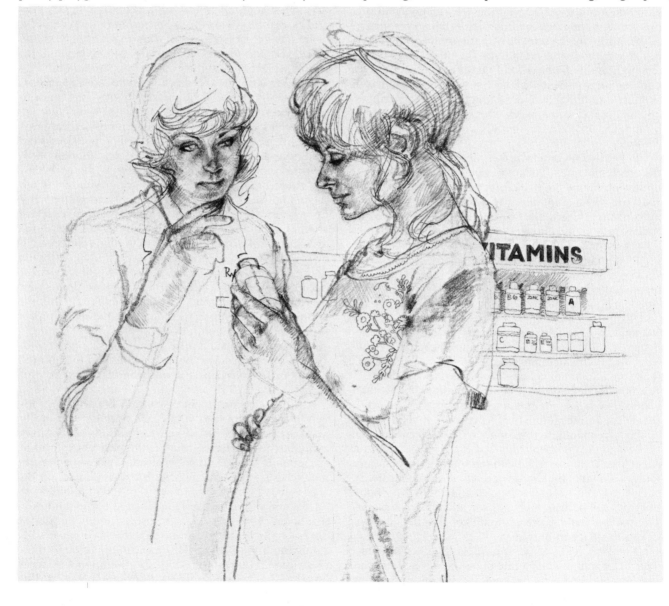

sure to heat, and extensive refining may destroy 50–100% of the folates. Generally, foods richest in folates are fresh green vegetables. Yeast and liver, and other organ meats, also contain folates.

The requirements for folic acid are related to metabolic rate and cell turnover. Thus, increased amounts of folic acid are needed during pregnancy (especially with twin or multiple fetuses); during infections; in hemolytic anemias and blood loss where red blood cell production must be increased to replenish blood supply; in infancy; and in cases of increased metabolic rates such as in hyperthyroidism. Rheumatoid arthritis, perhaps because of the proliferation of synovial membranes or the possible salicylate-induced folate loss, also increases folate requirements. Certain hematopoietic malignancies also cause an increased need for folic acid.

Folate deficiency may occur readily, particularly if fresh vegetables and fruits are not eaten. The symptoms of deficiency are much the same as those of vitamin B_{12} deficiency—sore mouth, diarrhea, and CNS symptoms such as irritability and forgetfulness. The most common feature of folic acid deficiency is megaloblastic anemia.

The causes of folic acid deficiency are similar to those of B vitamin deficiencies (poor diet and alcoholism). The diet should include foods that need little cooking because folates are heat labile. Conditions that cause rapid cell turnover may induce potentially life-threatening folic acid deficiency.

Several drugs taken chronically may increase the need for folic acid. Phenytoin and possibly other related anticonvulsants may cause an inhibition of folic acid absorption, leading to megaloblastic anemia (175). This problem is complicated further by the fact that folic acid supplementation may decrease serum phenytoin levels, decreasing seizure control (176). The pharmacist should keep this in mind, when dispensing folic acid to patients whose medication record indicates concurrent phenytoin use. The pharmacist should ask whether seizure activity is controlled. Another possible drug interaction occurs with oral contraceptive drugs, which may cause folic acid deficiencies (177). This effect is extremely rare and probably is not a significant side effect (178–180). Trimethoprim may act as a weak folic acid antagonist in humans. Megaloblastic anemia may be precipitated in patients who had a relatively low folate level at the onset of trimethoprim therapy; folate deficiency, however, is not a problem experienced by most patients using trimethoprim. Pyrimethamine, which is related to trimethoprim, in large doses may induce megaloblastic anemia. Folic acid may be administered to reverse the anemia because the mechanism of pyrimethamine's folic acid antagonism is inhibition of active tetrahydrofolate production (181). Methotrexate also causes folic acid antagonism; this effect is utilized in treatment of neoplastic diseases, and the toxicity produced in normal cells is controlled by the administration of folic acid in a procedure called leucovorin rescue.

Because vitamin B_{12} is essential for metabolism of folates, a megaloblastic anemia responsive to folate administration is a feature of pernicious anemia. Folic acid given without vitamin B_{12} to patients with pernicious anemia will correct the anemia but will have no effect on the more insidious damage to the nervous system. The symptoms of the damage include lack of coordination, impaired sense of position, and a spectrum of mental disturbances. Because of the potential for folic acid to mask the signs of pernicious anemia, products containing greater than 0.8 mg/dose are available only by prescription (182). The inclusion of vitamin B_{12} in oral preparations will not be helpful if the patient has a malabsorption syndrome; parenteral therapy is generally required.

The dose of folic acid for correction of a deficiency is usually 100 μg. If the deficiency occurs with conditions that may increase the folate requirement or suppress red blood cell formation (pregnancy, hypermetabolic states, alcoholism, or hemolytic anemia), the dose is 0.5–1 mg. Doses larger than 1 mg are not necessary, except in some life-threatening hematologic diseases. Maintenance therapy for deficiencies may be stopped after 1–4 months if the diet contains at least one fresh fruit or vegetable daily (183). For chronic malabsorption diseases, folic acid treatment may be lifelong and parenteral doses are usually needed. Folic acid toxicity is nearly nonexistent because of its water solubility and rapid excretion—15 mg can be given daily without toxic effect.

Pharmacists should refer for medical consultation all patients with suspected anemias.

Pantothenic Acid

Panthothenic acid is a precursor to coenzyme A, a product active in many biologic reactions in the body. It is contained in many foods, and deficiency states are rare except under experimental conditions. The U.S. RDA for pantothenic acid is 3 mg for infants, 5 mg for children under 4 years of age, and 10 mg for all adults and children 4 or more years of age. The Food and Nutrition Board of the National Academy of Sciences, does not list an RDA value for this vitamin but estimates a safe and adequate intake to be 2–3 mg for infants, and 4–7 mg for adults.

Pantothenic acid deficiency is very hard to detect. In malabsorption syndromes, it is difficult to separate pantothenic acid deficiency symptoms from many other ones. Pantothenic acid has been withheld experimentally, and the resulting symptoms are abdominal pain, vomiting, and cramps. Later, muscle tenderness, weakness, paresthesia, and insomnia occur. Administration of pharmacologic doses of pantothenic acid reverse these symptoms.

Pantothenic acid is not known to have any therapeutic use. It has gained some notoriety in recent years as an "antistress" formula and to prevent gray hair. These claims are not supported by experimental evidence. It frequently is incorporated into oral multiple-vitamin preparations. As much as 20 g has been administered, and the toxicity, which is minimal, appears as diarrhea (184).

Biotin

Although biotin is known to be necessary for carboxylation reactions in the body, knowledge as to the nutritional requirements for this member of the B-complex is imprecise. Biotin is widely distributed in animal tissue and appears necessary for the metabolism of certain amino acids. In rats, biotin also seems necessary for the appropriate utilization of glucose, and some of its effects are similar to those of insulin. In humans, biotin is synthesized by gut flora. Biotin deficiency in humans can be caused by the ingestion of a large number of egg whites, which contain avidin, a protein that binds biotin, preventing its absorption. Avidin causes a dermatitis, a grayish color of the skin, anorexia, anemia, hypercholesterolemia, and lassitude (185). Biotin deficiency symptoms have also been noted in patients on total parenteral nutrition without biotin supplements. In pregnant women, blood biotin levels decrease as gestation progresses.

In rats, a combination of oxytetracycline and succinylsulfathiazole inhibited the intestinal synthesis of biotin. A similar effect might be expected in humans after using gut-sterilizing antibiotics, but it has not been reported. The Food and Nutrition Board of the National Academy of Sciences does not list an RDA value for biotin, although 65–100 mg/day is listed as being safe and effective for adults (Table 2). The U.S. RDA values are 0.05 mg for infants, 0.15 mg for children under 4 years of age, and 0.30 mg for all adults and children 4 or more years of age.

Biotin has been incorporated into several multiple-vitamin preparations. It has been used therapeutically in infants and children to treat seborrheic dermatitis and propionic acidemia. There was slight improvement in muscle tone with oral doses (5–10 mg for 5 days) (186).

Bioflavonoids

The term *bioflavonoids* has been used to designate flavones and flavonols. Bioflavonoids were called vitamin P (for permeability), but this designation is no longer used because no vitamin activity has been documented. This group of agents includes rutin and hesperidin, which have stimulated controversy in the medical literature. The controversy stems from their proposed use in the treatment of vascular bleeding disorders such as vascular purpura, retinal hemorrhages, cerebrovascular accidents, and lymphedema (187, 188). Deficiency states have not been induced or discovered in humans or animals.

Choline

Choline is a precursor in the biosynthesis of acetylcholine and is an important donator of methyl groups used in the biochemical formation of other substances in vivo. It can be biosynthesized in humans by donation of methyl groups from methionine to ethanolamine. It is a component of phosphatidyl choline, commonly known as lecithin, and several other phospholipids. Choline and inositol are considered as lipotropic agents (agents involved in mobilization of lipids). They have been used in the treatment of fatty liver and disturbed fat metabolism, but their efficacy has not been established.

No choline deficiency disease in humans has been reported. Rats, hamsters, dogs, chickens, and pigs develop choline deficiency diseases including fatty liver,

cirrhosis, anemia, renal lesions, and hypertension. These findings have been the basis for treating alcoholics with choline, although the literature reports no therapeutic value. Although choline is found in egg yolks, cereal, fish, and meat, it is also synthesized in the body; therefore, it is doubtful that it is a vitamin. Choline is available as a tablet and powder and in combination with other nutritional ingredients.

Inositol

Inositol is a hexitol found in large amounts in muscle and brain tissues. It is widely distributed in nature and is synthesized in the body. In cell culture, inositol seems to be necessary for amino acid transport and for the movement of potassium and sodium. It is approximately one-third as effective as glucose in correcting diabetic ketosis. Inositol is available as a tablet or powder, but its value in human nutrition has not been documented. Like choline, it is considered a lipotropic agent but of unproven therapeutic value.

Vitamin F (Essential Fatty Acids)

Linoleic and linolenic acids are essential in human nutrition but do not meet the definition of a vitamin because they are required in large amounts (macronutrients). The Western diet, with its heavy use of polyunsaturated fats and oils, provides ample quantities of the essential fatty acids.

Vitamin B_{15} (Pangamic Acid)

Pangamic acid has no nutritional or therapeutic value.

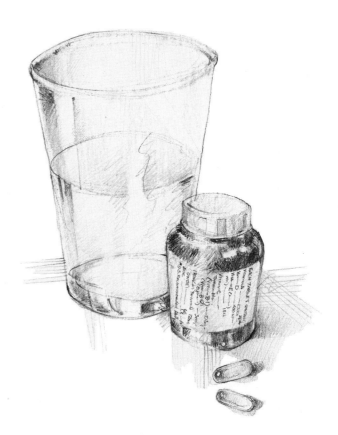

Vitamin B₁₇ (Laetrile)

Laetrile has no proven nutritional or therapeutic value.

Multivitamins

There is considerable controversy as to the need for multivitamin supplements in Western populations. Most health authorities would agree that attention to a balanced diet and adequate caloric intake obviates the necessity for supplemental vitamins for most individuals. There are certain segments of the population, however, that are known to be at risk for at least marginal vitamin deficiencies unless special attention is paid to diet or vitamin supplements are used. Multivitamin supplements may possibly be indicated in the following situations:

- **Iatrogenic situations**—oral contraceptive and estrogen users, patients on prolonged broad-spectrum antibiotics, patients receiving isoniazid, or patients on prolonged total parenteral nutrition;
- **Inadequate dietary intake conditions**—such as alcoholics, the impoverished, and the aged;
- **Increased metabolic requirements**—pregnancy, lactation, infants, severe injury, trauma, major surgery, or severe infection;
- **Patients with poor absorption**—due to such conditions as prolonged diarrhea, severe GI disorders and malignancy, sprue, obstructive jaundice, cystic fibrosis, or old age.

The pharmacist should be available to counsel patients on appropriate multivitamin selection. In general, a "supplemental" multivitamin preparation that would supply close to 100% of the U.S. RDA for each vitamin will meet the needs of most patients requiring or desiring supplements. The need for expensive high-potency, therapeutic vitamins is rare.

Patient Information

The following information may be helpful to your patients (189):

- Read the labels on all vitamin or vitamin and mineral preparations before you take them. Compare the contents and the amounts of vitamins and minerals with the RDA's.
- Take vitamins or vitamin and mineral supplements with meals. Iron supplements may cause less stomach upset if taken with meals.
- Do not take large doses of vitamins or minerals; large doses may be dangerous. It is best not to exceed the RDA. Follow label directions.
- Do not self-medicate a vitamin deficiency. If you feel that you are deficient, consult your physician or pharmacist.
- For proper nutrition, eat foods from the five basic food groups (meats, vegetables, fruits, dairy products, and grains). Vitamin supplements are not a substitute for a well-balanced diet.
- Liquid vitamin and mineral supplements may be mixed with food (fruit juice, milk, baby formula, or cereal).

- Iron supplements or vitamins with iron may make your stool turn black.
- Some vitamin supplements have a special coating and should be swallowed whole. Ask your physician or pharmacist if your medicine must be swallowed whole.
- Vitamin and combination vitamin and mineral supplements, like any medicine, should be stored out of the reach of children. This is especially important if there is iron in the product.
- Children's vitamins are not candy. Children should be taught that they are drugs and cannot be taken indiscriminately.

Summary

By being familiar with recommended dietary daily allowances of the various vitamins and minerals and knowing which natural sources provide these RDA's, the pharmacist can supply a valuable patient service. In addition, the pharmacist should be able to recognize symptoms of vitamin and mineral deficiencies; prompt physician referral often is crucial in these cases. A patient's cultural or socioeconomic background and physical condition are guidelines in helping the pharmacist determine nutritional status. Pregnant and lactating women require more nutrients than other normal healthy adults.

Supplementary formula products should be used as adjuncts to a regular diet and not as a substitute for food. Although dietary products can be obtained without a prescription, they are complex agents with specific indications. Medical assessment must precede their use. The pharmacist should review dilution, preparation technique, storage, and administration of these products with the patient and should offer to discuss with the patient unusual effects, such as diarrhea, that may be caused by the formulas. An antidiarrheal may be indicated or merely a change in administration or storage procedures. The pharmacist should not be reluctant to consult a dietician or physician (especially a gastroenterologist, oncologist, or surgeon, who often deal with nutrition problems) concerning nutritional supplementation and should refer patients when necessary.

As the pharmacist is well aware, there is a tendency for the health authorities and the public to become polarized over the vitamin issue. Some argue that vitamin supplements are unnecessary and that megavitamin therapy is dangerous. Others claim that everyone would benefit from supplements and megavitamins are the answer to most health problems. The truth probably lies somewhere in between the two extremes. Some segments of the population (geriatrics, alcoholics, patients with chronic diseases or recent trauma, and pregnant and lactating women) may benefit from supplemental multivitamins. Most others, provided that a balanced and varied diet is consumed, do not need supplements. There are specific situations where high doses of specific vitamins have been reported to be of therapeutic benefit, but for the most part the exaggerated claims of the megavitamin enthusiasts have not been confirmed. Furthermore, prolonged ingestions of vitamins at therapeutic levels have not been tested for safety and some vitamins, such as vitamins A and D and niacin, are known to be toxic in high doses. There is yet much to learn concerning the efficacy and safety of vitamin and vitamin analogs in therapy. The consumer should be cautioned against initiating self-medication with vitamin remedies. The chronic ingestion of large doses of any drug, including vitamins, for relief of a relatively mild and self-limiting condition such as the common cold is to be discouraged.

References

1. *Drug Topics, 125,* 45–47, 50 (1981).
2. *Drug Merchandising, 62,* 23–26 (1981).
3. D. Coldsmith, *Mod. Med., 43,* 121 (1975).
4. "A Study of Health Practices and Opinions," Final Report, Conducted for FDA, HEW Contract No. FDA 66–193, June 1972, and FDA Talk Paper, Oct. 6, 1972.
5. *Nutrition Reviews Supplement, 32,* 53 (1974).
6. A. Kamil, *J. Nutr., 4,* 92, (1972).
7. *Federal Register, 44,* 16132 (1979).
8. *Federal Register, 43,* 10551–52 (1978).
9. R. M. Kark, *J. Am. Diet. Assoc., 64,* 476 (1974).
10. R. O'Reilly and D. Rytand, *N. Engl. J. Med., 303,* 160 (1980).
11. R. R. Crichton, *N. Engl. J. Med., 284,* 1413 (1971).
12. T. H. Bothwell and C. A. Finch, "Iron Metabolism," Little, Brown, Boston, Mass., 1962.
13. Committee on Iron Deficiency, *J. Am. Med. Assoc., 203,* 407 (1968).
14. L. Hallberg, H. G. Harwerth, and A. Vannatti, "Iron Deficiency Pathogenesis, Clinical Aspects, Therapy," Academic, New York, N.Y., 1970, p. 169.
15. V. Minnich, A. Okcuoglu, Y. Tarcon, A. Arcasoy, S. Cin, O. Yorukoglu, F. Renda, and B. Demirag, *Am. J. Clin. Nutr., 21,* 78 (1968).
16. W. H. Crosby, *J. Am. Med. Assoc., 235,* 2765 (1976).
17. H. Brise and L. Hallberg, *Acta Med. Scand. Suppl., 376,* 23 (1962).
18. "Evaluations of Drug Interactions," 2nd ed., American Pharmaceutical Association, Washington, D.C., 1976, p. 74.
19. *Medical Letter on Drugs and Therapeutics, 20,* 46 (1978).
20. G. J. L. Hall and A. E. Davis, *Med. J. Aust., 2,* 95 (1969).
21. P. J. Neuvonen, G. Gothoni, R. Hackman, and K. Bjorksten, *Br. Med. J., 4,* 532 (1970).
22. "Evaluations of Drug Interactions," 2nd ed., American Pharmaceutical Association, Washington, D.C., 1976, p. 231.
23. H. W. Cann and H. L. Verhulst, *Am. J. Dis. Child., 99,* 688 (1980).
24. *Journal of Pediatrics, 77,* 117 (1970).
25. M. N. Gleason, R. Gosselin, H. Hodge, and R. Smith, "Clinical Toxicology of Commercial Products," 3rd ed., Williams and Wilkins, Baltimore, Md., 1969, p. 108.
26. S. Margen and D. H. Calloway, *Fed. Proc., 26,* 629 (1967).
27. R. M. Walker and H. M. Linkswiler, *J. Nutr., 102,* 1297 (1972).
28. "Modern Nutrition in Health and Disease," 6th ed., Lea and Febiger, Philadelphia, Pa., 1980, p. 300.
29. C. J. Lee, G. S. Lawler, and G. H. Johnson, *Am. J. Clin. Nutr., 34,* 819–823 (1981).
30. R. Kreisberg, *Ann. Intern. Med., 88,* 681 (1978).
31. "Harrison's Principles of Internal Medicine," 9th ed., G. W. Thorn, R. D. Adams, E. Braunwald, K. J. Isselbacher, and R. G. Petersdorf, Eds., McGraw-Hill, New York, N.Y., 1980, p. 1296.
32. J. A. T. Pennington, "Total Diet Study—Results and Plans for Selected Minerals in Foods," *FDA By-Lines, 10,* 179 (1980).
33. K. M. Hambridge, C. Hambridge, M. Jacobs, and J. Baum, *Pediatr. Res., 6,* 868 (1972).
34. T. Hallbröök and E. L. Lanner, *Lancet, 2,* 780 (1972).
35. K. Haeger and E. Lanner, *J. Vas. Dis., 3,* 77 (1974).
36. A. S. Prasad, in "Trace Elements in Human Health and Disease," A. S. Prasad and D. Oberleas, Eds., Academic, New York, N.Y., 1976, p. 15.
37. S. L. Wolman, G. H. Anderson, E. B. Marliss, and K. N. Jeejeebhoy, *Gastroenterology, 76,* 458 (1979).
38. K. Hambridge and B. Nichols, "Zinc and Copper in Clinical Medicine," S.P. Medical, New York, N.Y., 1978, p. 22.
39. G. R. Lee, D. M. Williams, and G. E. Cartwright, in "Trace Elements in Human Health and Disease," Vol. I, A. S. Prasad and D. Oberleas, Eds., Academic, New York, N.Y., 1976, pp. 373–90.
40. A. J. Patek and C. Haig, *J. Clin. Invest., 18,* 609 (1939).
41. I. Morrison, R. Russell, E. Carney, and E. Oaks, *Am. J. Clin. Nutr., 31,* 276 (1978).
42. M. F. Ivey, W. Mueller, M. Riella, and B. Scribner, *Am. J. Hosp. Pharm., 32,* 1032 (1975).
43. "The Pharmacological Basis of Therapeutics," 6th ed., A. G. Gilman, L. S. Goodman, and A. Gilman, Eds., Macmillan, New York, N.Y., 1980, p. 1546.
44. R. J. Doisy, M. S. Jastreski, and F. L. Greenstein, *Excerpta Med. Found. Int. Cong. Ser., 280,* 155 (1973).
45. R. J. Doisy, H. P. Streeten, J. M. Freiberg, and A. J. Schneiden, in "Trace Elements in Human Health and Disease," Vol. 2, A. S. Prasad and D. Oberleas, Eds., Academic Press, New York, N.Y., 1976, p. 84.
46. K. N. Jeejeebhoy, R. C. Chu, E. B. Marliss, G. R. Greenberg, and A. Bruce Robertson, *Am. J. Clin. Nutr., 30,* 531 (1977).
47. H. A. Schroeder, D. V. Frost, and J. J. Balassa, *J. Chron. Dis., 23,* 227 (1970).
48. H. A. Schroeder and A. D. Nason, *Clin. Chem., 17,* 461 (1971).
49. R. A. Johnson, S. S. Baker, J. T. Fallon, E. P. Maynard, J. N. Raskin, Z. Wen, K. Ge, and H. J. Cohen, *N. Engl. J. Med., 304,* 1210–1211 (1981).
50. W. W. King, L. Michael, W. C. Wood, R. A. Malt, and S. S. Baker, *N. Engl. J. Med., 304,* 1305 (1981).
51. P. J. Collipp and S. Y. Chen, *N. Engl. J. Med., 304,* 1309 (1981).
52. *Lancet, 2,* 889–890 (1979).
53. J. Aaseth, Y. Thomassen, J. Alexander, and G. Norhem, *N. Engl. J. Med., 303,* 944 (1980).
54. K. Schwartz, *Fed. Proc., 20,* Part 1, 665 (1961).
55. J. Wilstrom, T. Westermarck, and J. Palo, *Acta Neurol. Scand., 54,* 287 (1976).
56. D. V. Frost and D. Ingvoldstad, *Chem. Scr., A8,* 96 (1975).
57. R. J. Shamberger and D. V. Frost, *Can. Med. Assoc. J., 100,* 682 (1969).
58. G. N. Schrauzer, D. A. White, and C. J. Schneider, *Bioinorg. Chem., 7,* 23 (1977).
59. G. N. Schrauzer and D. Ishmael, *Ann. Clin. Lab. Sci., 4,* 441 (1974).
60. W. L. Broghamer, K. P. McConnell, and A. L. Blotcky, *Cancer, 37,* 1384 (1976).
61. R. S. Shakman, *Arch. Environ. Health, 28,* 105 (1974).
62. A. W. Kilness and F. H. Hochberg, *J. Am. Med. Assoc., 237,* 2843 (1977).
63. W. Mertz, *J. Am. Diet Assoc., 64,* 163 (1974).
64. *Federal Register, 44,* 16139 (1979).
65. *Journal of the American Medical Association, 233,* 550 (1975).
66. T. Moore, "Vitamin A," Elsevier, Amsterdam, Netherlands, 1957, p. 355.
67. "Modern Nutrition in Health and Disease," 6th ed., R. Goodhart and M. Shils, Eds., Lea and Febiger, 1980, p. 153.
68. A. Pirie and P. Ambunataham, *Am. J. Clin. Nutr., 34,* 34–40 (1981).
69. K. J. Hofman, F. J. Milne, and C. Schmidt, *S. Afr. Med., 54,* 579–580 (1978).
70. "Modern Nutrition in Health and Disease," 6th ed., R. S. Goodhart and M. E. Shils, Eds., Lea and Febiger, Philadelphia, Pa., 1980, p. 154.
71. K. J. Hofman, F. J. Milne, and C. Schmidt, *S. Afr. Med. J., 54,* 579 (1978).
72. U. Saffiotti, R. Montesano, and A. R. Sallakumar, *Cancer, 20,* 857 (1967).
73. E. W. Chu and R. A. Malmgren, *Cancer Res., 25,* 884 (1965).
74. M. B. Sporn, N. M. Dunlop, and D. L. Newton, *Fed. Proc., 35,* 1332 (1976).
75. H. Mayer, W. Bollag, R. Hanni, and R. Ruegg, *Experientia,*

340, 1105 (1978).

76. P. M. Newberne and V. Suphakarm, *Cancer*, *40*, 2553 (1977).
77. C. J. Grubbs, R. C. Moon, M. B. Sporn, and D. L. Newton, *Cancer Res.*, *37*, 599 (1977).
78. E. Bjilke, *Int. J. Cancer*, *15*, 561 (1975).
79. C. Mettlin, S. Graham, and M. Swanson, *J. Nat. Cancer Inst.*, *62*, 1435 (1979).
80. G. L. Peck, T. G. Olson, F. W. Yoder, J. S. Strauss, D. T. Downing, M. Pandya, D. Butkus, and J. Arnaud-Battandier, *N. Engl. J. Med.*, *300*, 329 (1979).
81. G. Heidbreder and E. Christophers, *Arch. Dermatol. Res.*, *264*, 331 (1979).
82. R. P. Haydey, M. F. Reed, L. M. Denbow, and J. F. Shupack, *N. Engl. J. Med.*, *303*, 560 (1980).
83. H. K. Schnoes and H. F. DeLuca, *Fed. Proc.*, *39*, 2723 (1980).
84. A. S. Brickman, J. W. Coburn, S. G. Massey, and A. W. Norman, *Ann. Intern. Med.*, *80*, 161 (1974).
85. S. Bachrack, J. Fisher, and J. S. Parks, *Pediatrics*, *64*, 871 (1979).
86. J. T. Dwyer, *Am. J. Dis. Child.*, *133*, 134 (1979).
87. S. Livingstone, W. Berman, and F. F. Pauli, *J. Am. Med. Assoc.*, *224*, 1634 (1973).
88. "The Medical Manual of Therapeutics," 22nd ed., N. V. Costrini and W. M. Thomas, Eds., Little, Brown, Boston, Mass., 1977, p. 308.
89. "The Pharmacological Basis of Therapeutics," 6th ed., A. G. Gilman, L. S. Goodman, A. Gilman, Eds., Macmillan, New York, N.Y., 1980, pp. 1544–1545.
90. S. Fomon, M. Youroszar, and L. Thomas, *J. Nutr.*, *89*, 345 (1966).
91. D. Fraser and R. Slater, *Pediatr. Clin. North Am.*, *5*, 417 (1958).
92. J. H. Ritchie, M. B. Fish, V. McMasters, and M. Grossman, *N. Engl. J. Med.*, *279*, 1185 (1968).
93. M. K. Horwitt, B. Century, and A. A. Zeman, *Am. J. Clin. Nutr.*, *12*, 99 (1963).
94. H. J. Binder, D. C. Herting, V. Hurst, S. C. Finch, and H. M. Spiro, *N. Engl. J. Med.*, *273*, 1289 (1965).
95. K. Haeger, *Am. J. Clin. Nutr.*, *27*, 1179 (1974).
96. H. T. G. Williams, D. Fenna, and R. A. MacBeth, *Surg. Gynecol. Obstet.*, *132*, 662 (1971).
97. S. Ayres and R. Mihan, *South. Med. J.*, *67*, 1308 (1974).
98. W. E. Shute, "Vitamin E for Ailing and Healthy Hearts," Pyramid, New York, N.Y., 1972.
99. T. W. Anderson and D. B. Reid, *Am. J. Clin. Nutr.*, *27*, 1174 (1974).
100. R. E. Gillilan and B. Modell, *Am. Heart J.*, *93*, 444 (1977).
101. I. M. Sharman, M. G. Down, and N. G. Norgan, *J. Sports Med.*, *16*, 215 (1976).
102. I. M. Sharman, M. G. Down, and R. N. Sen, *Br. J. Nutr.*, *26*, 265 (1971).
103. E. Herold et al., *Arch. Sex. Behav.*, *8*, 397 (1979).
104. P. M. Farrel and J. G. Bieri, *Am. J. Clin. Nutr.*, *28*, 181 (1975).
105. J. J. Shrogie, *J. Am. Med. Assoc.*, *232*, 19 (1975).
106. P. Sonneveld, *Cancer Treat. Rep.*, *62*, 1033 (1978).
107. L. A. Boxer, J. M. Oliver, S. P. Spielberg, J. M. Allen, and J. D. Schulman, *N. Engl. J. Med.*, *301*, 901 (1979).
108. L. Corash, S. P. Spielberg, C. Bartsocas, F. Boxer, R. Steinburg, M. Sheetz, M. I. Egan, J. Schlessleman, and J. D. Schulman, *N. Engl. J. Med.*, *303*, 416 (1980).
109. *Journal of the American Medical Association*, *244*, 1077 (1980).
110. L. A. Barness, F. A. Oski, M. Williams. G. Marrow, and S. Arnaud, *Am. J. Clin. Nutr.*, *21*, 40 (1968).
111. L. Pauling, "Vitamin C and the Common Cold," W. H. Freeman, San Francisco, Calif., 1970.
112. L. Pauling, "Vitamin C, the Common Cold and the Flu," W. H. Freeman, San Francisco, Calif., 1976.
113. G. Ritzel, *Helv. Med. Acta*, *28*, 63 (1961).
114. D. W. Cowen, H. S. Diehl, and A. B. Baker, *J. Am. Med. Assoc.*, *120*, 1267 (1942).
115. W. L. Franz, G. W. Sands, and H. F. Heyl, *J. Am. Med. Assoc.*, *162*, 1224 (1956).
116. M. H. M. Dykes and P. Meier, *J. Am. Med. Assoc.*, *231*, 1073 (1975).
117. T. W. Anderson, D. B. W. Reid, and G. H. Beaton, *Can. Med. Assoc. J.*, *107*, 503 (1972).
118. T. W. Anderson, G. Suranyi, and G. H. Beaton, *Can. Med. Assoc. J.*, *111*, 31 (1974).
119. J. C. Miller, W. E. Nance, J. A. Norton, R. L. Wolen, R. G. Griffith, and R. J. Rose, *J. Am. Med. Assoc.*, *237*, 248 (1977).
120. H. A. Pitt and A. M. Costrini, *J. Am. Med. Assoc.*, *241*, 908 (1979).
121. I. M. Baird, R. E. Hughes, H. F. Wilson, J. E. W. Davies, and A. N. Howard, *Am. J. Clin. Nutr.*, *32*, 1686 (1979).
122. J. Feldman, W. N. Kelley, and H. E. Lebovitz, *Diabetes*, *19*, 337 (1970).
123. J. Mayson, J. S. Schumaker, and R. M. Nakumura, *Am. J. Clin. Pathol.*, *58*, 297 (1972).
124. G. Levy and J. Leonards, *J. Am. Med. Assoc.*, *217*, 81 (1971).
125. F. Sioquist, *Clin. Pharmacol. Ther.*, *10*, 826 (1969).
126. L. Gram, B. Kofod, J. Christiansen, and O. J. Rafaelson, *Clin. Pharmacol. Ther.*, *12*, 239 (1971).
127. M. Rowland, *J. Pharm. Sci.*, *58*, 508 (1969).
128. M. C. Nakata, L. Shimp, T. Lampman, and D. C. McLeod, *Am. J. Hosp. Pharm.*, *34*, 1234 (1977).
129. D. V. Naccarto, *J. Am. Geriatr. Soc.*, *27*, 34 (1979).
130. C. J. Schorah, D. F. Scott, A. Newill, and D. B. Morgan, *Lancet*, *1*, 403 (1979).
131. G. T. Terezhalmy, J. Butcher, S. Rimmer, B. Day, and I. W. Dymock, *Oral Surg.*, *45*, 56 (1978).
132. T. V. Taylor, J. Butcher, S. Rimmer, B. Day, and I. W. Dymock, *Lancet*, *2*, 544 (1974).
133. J. J. DeCosse, *Surgery*, *78*, 608 (1975).
134. J. J. DeCosse, R. E. Condon, and M. B. Adams, *Cancer*, *40*, 2549 (1977).
135. C. R. Spittle, *Lancet*, *2*, 1280 (1971).
136. R. E. Hughes, *Proc. Roy. Soc. Med.*, *70*, 86 (1977).
137. E. Cameron and L. Pauling, *Proc. Natl. Acad. Sci.*, *U.S.A.*, *73*, 3685 (1976).
138. E. T. Creagan, C. G. Moertel, J. R. O'Fallon, A. J. Schutt, A. J. O'Connell, J. M. Rubin, and S. J. Frytak, *N. Engl. J. Med.*, *301*, 687 (1979).
139. "Modern Nutrition in Health and Disease," 9th ed., R. Goodhart and M. Shils, Eds., Lea and Febiger, Philadelphia, Pa., 1980, p. 686.
140. A. M. Hoyumpa, K. J. Breen, J. Schenker, and F. A. Wilson, *J. Lab. Clin. Med.*, *86*, 803 (1975).
141. A. M. Hoyumpa, H. M. Middleton, F. A. Wilson, and S. Schenker, *Gastroenterology*, *68*, 1218 (1975).
142. M. Victor, *Contemp. Neurol. Ser.*, *7*, 1–206 (1971).
143. B. S. Centerwald and M. H. Criqui, *N. Engl. J. Med.*, *299*, 285 (1978).
144. S. H. Mudd, *Fed. Proc.*, *30*, 970 (1971).
145. C. R. Scriver, *Metabolism*, *22*, 1319 (1973).
146. J. P. Blass and G. F. Gilson, *N. Engl. J. Med.*, *247*, 1367 (1977).
147. W. G. Strauss, H. I. Maiboch, and A. A. Khan, *Am. J. Trop. Med. Hyg.*, *17*, 411 (1968).
148. C. N. Smith, *Public Entomol. Soc. Am.*, *7*, 99 (1970).
149. L. J. Neuman, R. Lopez, H. S. Cole, M. C. Boria, and J. M. Cooperman, *Am. J. Clin. Nutr.*, *31*, 247 (1978).
150. R. Lopez, J. V. Schwartz, and J. V. Cooperman, *Am. J. Clin. Nutr.*, *33*, 1283 (1980).
151. J. G. Bergan and P. T. Brown, *Am. J. Diet. Assoc.*, *76*, 151 (1980).
152. R. S. Rivlin, *Nutr. Rev.*, *37*, 241 (1979).
153. The Coronary Drug Research Group, *J. Am. Med. Assoc.*, *231*, 360 (1975).
154. T. A. Ban and H. E. Lehman, *Can. J. Psychiatry*, *15*, 499 (1970).
155. J. F. Vallely, J. D. Lovegrove, and G. E. Hobbs, *Can. J. Psychiatry*, *16*, 433 (1971).
156. T. A. Ban and H. E. Lehman, *Can. J. Psychiatry*, *20*, 103 (1975).
157. "Evaluations of Drug Interactions," 2nd ed., American Pharmaceutical Association, 1976, p. 118.
158. N. H. Raskin, *N. Engl. J. Med.*, *273*, 1182 (1965).
159. "Applied Therapeutics for Clinical Pharmacists," 2nd ed., Applied Therapeutics, San Francisco, Calif., 1978, p. 337.
160. M. Baumblatt and F. Winston, *Lancet*, *1*, 832 (1970).
161. A. Lubby, P. Davis, M. Murphy, M. Gordon, M. Brin, and

H. Spiegel, *Lancet,* 2, 1083 (1970).

162. A. Lubby, P. Davis, M. Murphy, M. Gordon, M. Brin, and H. Spiegel, *Am. J. Clin. Nutr.,* 24, 684 (1971).

163. P. W. Adams, D. P. Rose, J. Folkard, V. Wynn, M. Seed, and R. Strong, *Lancet,* 1, 897 (1973).

164. P. W. Adams, V. Wynn, M. Seed, and J. Folkard, *Lancet,* 2, 516 (1974).

165. S. H. Mudd, *Fed. Proc.,* 30, 970 (1971).

166. C. R. Scrivor, *Metabolism,* 22, 1319 (1973).

167. J. M. Ellis, J. Azuma, T. Watanabe, K. Folkers, J. R. Lowell, G. A. Hurst, C. H. Ahn, E. H. Shiford, and R. F. Ulrich, *Res. Commun. Chem. Pathol. Pharmacol.,* 17, 165 (1977).

168. L. B. Greentree, *N. Engl. J. Med.,* 300, 141 (1979).

169. M. D. Foulkas, *Br. J. Obstet. Gynaecol.,* 80, 718 (1973).

170. "Modern Nutrition in Health and Disease," 6th ed., R. S. Goodhart and M. E. Shils, Eds., Lea and Febiger, Philadelphia, Pa., 1980, p. 235.

171. J. D. Hines, *Am. J. Clin. Nutr.,* 19, 260 (1966).

172. M. C. Higginbottom, L. Sweetman, and W. L. Nuhar, *N. Engl. J. Med.,* 299, 317 (1978).

173. J. Trader, B. Reibman, and D. Turkewitz, *N. Engl. J. Med.,* 299, 1319 (1978).

174. W. Faloon and R. Chodos, *Gastroenterology,* 56, 1251 (1969).

175. C. Gerson, *Gastroenterology,* 63, 246 (1972).

176. H. Kutt, J. Kaynes, and F. McDowell, *Arch. Neurol. (Chicago),* 14, 489 (1966).

177. T. Necheles and L. Snyder, *N. Engl. J. Med.,* 282, 858 (1970).

178. N. Elgee, *Ann. Intern. Med.,* 72, 409 (1970).

179. R. Swerdloff, W. Odell, G. Bray, R. Fiser, A. Wolfsen, D. Fisher, and M. Sperling, *West. J. Med.,* 122, 22 (1975).

180. A. Bingel and P. Benoit, *J. Pharm. Sci.,* 62, 179 (1973).

181. "The Pharmacological Basis of Therapeutics," 5th ed., L. S. Goodman and A. Gilman, Eds., Macmillan, New York, N.Y., 1975, p. 1058.

182. *Federal Register,* 41, 46172 (1976).

183. "Modern Nutrition in Health and Disease," 6th ed., R. S. Goodhart and M. E. Shils, Eds., Lea and Febiger, Philadelphia, Pa., 1980, p. 254.

184. "Modern Nutrition in Health and Disease," 6th ed., R. Goodhart and M. Shils, Eds., Lea and Febiger, Philadelphia, Pa., 1980, p. 214.

185. V. Sydenstricker, S. Singal, A. Briggs, and H. Isbell, *J. Am. Med. Assoc.,* 118, 1199 (1942).

186. N. Barnes, D. Hull, L. Balgobin, and D. Gompertz, *Lancet,* 2, 244 (1970).

187. E. Foldi-Borcsok and M. Foldi, *Am. J. Clin. Nutr.,* 26, 185 (1973).

188. R. Eastham, T. Perham, and P. Pocock, *Br. Med. J.,* 4, 491 (1972).

189. D. L. Smith, "Medication Guide for Patient Counseling," Lea and Febiger, Philadelphia, Pa., 1977, pp. 413–414.

Food Supplement Product Table

Product (Manufacturer)	Dosage Form[a]	Calories	Protein (g)	Carbo-hydrate (g)	Fat (g)	Vitamins, Minerals	Indicated Use
Amin-Aid (McGaw)	powder	665	6.6	124.3	15.7		nitrogen-restricted diets
Amin-Aid Instant Pudding (McGaw)	powder	695	6.6	131.7	15.7		nitrogen-restricted diets
Casec (Mead Johnson)	powder, 1 tbsp	17	4.0	trace	0.1	various[b,c]	sodium restriction cholesterol restriction
Citrotein (Doyle)	powder, 33.4 g	127	7.67	23.3	0.33	various[b,c] sodium, 5.7 mEq	supplementary nourishment
Compleat-B (Doyle)	liquid, 250 ml/ bottle	267	10.7	32	10.7	various[b,c] sodium, 22.46 mEq/bottle	tube feeding
	400 ml/ can	400	10.7	32	10.7	various[b,c]	
Compleat-Modified Formula (Doyle)	liquid, 250 ml	267	10.7	35.3	9.2	various[b,c]	tube feeding
Controlyte (Doyle)	powder, 100 g	504	0.04	72	24	sodium, 0.22 mEq potassium, 4 mg calcium, 2 mg phosphorus, 8 mg chloride, 5 mg	protein restriction electrolyte restriction high-calorie dietary supplement
Ensure (Ross)	liquid, 240 ml	250	8.8	34.3	8.8	various[b,c]	full liquid diet liquid supplement tube feeding
Ensure Plus (Ross)	liquid, 240 ml	355	13.0	47.3	12.6	various[b,c] 100% U.S. RDA/2,000 cal	high-calorie liquid food
Flexical (Mead Johnson)	powder	250	5.6	38.1	8.5	various[b,c] 100% U.S. RDA/3,000 cal	supplementary nourishment tube feeding
Gevral Protein (Lederle)	powder, 26 g	95.3	15.6	7.05	<0.52	various[b,c]	supplementary nourishment
Heatrol (Otis Clapp)	tablet					sodium, 10.8 mEq potassium, 21 mg calcium, 12 mg magnesium, 2.5 mg phosphate, 20 mg chloride, 420 mg	electrolyte replenishment for perspiration losses

Food Supplement Product Table, continued

Product (Manufacturer)	Dosage Form[a]	Calories	Protein (g)	Carbo-hydrate (g)	Fat (g)	Vitamins, Minerals	Indicated Use
Hepatic-Aid (McGaw)	powder	560	14.5	98.1	12.3		nutritional deficiencies resulting from chronic liver failure
Hepatic-Aid Instant Pudding (McGaw)	powder	585	14.5	104.5	12.3		nutritional deficiencies resulting from chronic liver failure
Instant Breakfast (various)	powder, 3.66 g	130	8.0	23	1.0	various[b,c]	supplementary nourishment
Isocal (Mead Johnson)	liquid, 240 ml	250	8.1	31.2	10.5	various[b,c]	supplementary nourishment tube feeding
Meritene (Doyle)	powder, 32.4 g	277	18	31	9	various[b,c] sodium, 10.9 mEq (powder) 10.9 mEq (liquid)	supplementary nourishment tube feeding
	liquid, 10 fl. oz./ can	300	18	34.5	10		
	8 fl. oz./ can	240	14.4	27.6	8		
Nutrament (Drackett)	liquid, 12 oz./ can	360	16	52	10	various[b,c]	supplementary nourishment
Osmolite (Ross)	liquid, 8 fl. oz.	250	8.8	34.3	9.1	various[b,c]	tube feeding
Polycose (Ross)	liquid, 120 ml	2 cal/ml		50/100 ml			carbohydrate calories
Precision High Nitrogen Diet (Doyle)	powder, 83 g	300	12.5	62	0.36	various[b,c] sodium, 12.2 mEq	low residue high protein requirement oral tube feeding
Precision Isotonic Diet (Doyle)	powder, 58.4 g	250	7.5	37.5	7.8	various[b,c] sodium, 8.7 mEq	food intolerance tube feeding supplementary nourishment
Precision LR Diet (Doyle)	powder, 85 g	317	7.5	71	0.45	various[b,c] sodium, 8.7 mEq	low residue supplementary nourishment tube feeding
Prototabs (North American)	tablet		0.25[d]				amino acid deficiency
Scott's Emulsion (Beecham Products)	liquid					cod liver oil vitamin A, 5,000 units vitamin D, 400 units	tonic food supplement
Sustacal (Mead Johnson)	liquid, 360 ml	360	21.7	49.6	8.3	various[b,c]	supplementary nourishment tube feeding

Food Supplement Product Table, continued

Product (Manufacturer)	Dosage Form[a]	Calories	Protein (g)	Carbo-hydrate (g)	Fat (g)	Vitamins, Minerals	Indicated Use
Sustagen (Mead Johnson)	powder, 100 g	390	23.5	66.5	3.5	various[b,c]	supplementary nourishment tube feeding
Very High Nitrogen (Ross)	powder	300	12.5	56.5	3.25	various[b,c]	tube feeding
Vivonex Standard (Norwich-Eaton)	powder, 80 g	300	6.2[d]	69.2	0.435	various[b,c]	maintenance elemental diet tube feeding
Vivonex High Nitrogen (Norwich-Eaton)	powder, 80 g	300	13.3[a]	63.0	0.261	various[b,c]	anabolic elemental diet tube feeding

[a] One serving. Powder must be added to liquid as package directs.

[b] Includes vitamins A, D, E, ascorbic acid, thiamine, riboflavin, niacin, pyridoxine hydrochloride, cyanocobalamin, and/or various other substances having vitamin activity.

[c] Includes iron, calcium, phosphorus, iodine, magnesium, copper, zinc, potassium, sodium, manganese, chromium, selenium and molybdenum.

Iron Product Table

Product (Manufacturer)	Iron	Vitamins	Other Ingredients
Chel-Iron Liquid and Tablets (Kinney)	ferrocholinate, 83.4 mg/ml 330 mg/tablet		
Chel-Iron Pediatric Drops (Kinney)	ferrocholinate, 208 mg/ml		
C-Ron (Rowell)	ferrous fumarate, 200 mg	ascorbic acid, 100 mg	
C-Ron Forte (Rowell)	ferrous fumarate, 200 mg	ascorbic acid, 600 mg	
C-Ron Freckles (Rowell)	ferrous fumarate, 100 mg (elemental iron, 33 mg)	ascorbic acid, 50 mg	
Cytoferin (Ayerst)	ferrous sulfate, 200 mg (elemental iron, 64 mg)	ascorbic acid, 150 mg	
Dical-D with Iron Capsules (Abbott)	10 mg (as ferric pyrophosphate)	ergocalciferol, 133 IU	dibasic calcium phosphate, 500 mg
Femiron (J. B. Williams)	ferrous fumarate, 20 mg		
Feosol Spansules and Tablets (Menley & James Labs)	ferrous sulfate, 250 mg/spansule 325 mg/tablet		
Feostat Drops, Chewable Tablets and Suspension (O'Neal, Jones & Feldman)	ferrous fumarate, 45 mg/0.6 ml (drops), 100 mg/tablet 100 mg/5 cc (suspension)		

Iron Product Table, continued

Product (Manufacturer)	Iron	Vitamins	Other Ingredients
Ferancee (Stuart)	elemental, 67 mg (as ferrous fumarate)	sodium ascorbate, 114 mg ascorbic acid, 49 mg	sodium, 0.52 mEq
Ferancee-HP (Stuart)	elemental, 110 mg (as ferrous fumarate, 330 mg)	sodium ascorbate, 281 mg ascorbic acid, 350 mg	sodium, 1.56 mEq
Fergon Capsules and Tablets (Breon)	ferrous gluconate, 435 mg/capsule 320 mg/tablet		
Fergon c̄ C Caplets (Breon)	ferrous gluconate, 450 mg	ascorbic acid, 200 mg	
Fer-In-Sol Drops, Syrup, and Capsules (Mead Johnson)	ferrous sulfate, 125 mg/ml (drops) 30 mg/ml (syrup) 190 mg/capsule		
Fermalox Tablets (Rorer)	ferrous sulfate, 200 mg		magnesium hydroxide, 100 mg aluminum hydroxide gel, dried, 100 mg
Fero-Grad-500 Tablets (Abbott)	105 mg (as ferrous sulfate)	sodium ascorbate, 500 mg	
Fero-Gradumet Tablets (Abbott)	105 mg (as ferrous sulfate)		
Ferrobid (Glaxco)	ferrous fumarate, 225 mg	ascorbic acid, 100 mg	copper sulfate, 8 mg
Ferro-Sequels (Lederle)	ferrous fumarate, 150 mg		docusate sodium, 100 mg
Ferrous Sulfate Tablets (Upjohn)	ferrous sulfate, 325 mg		
Fumaral Elixir and Spancaps (North American)	ferrous sulfate, 32.5 mg/ml ferrous fumarate, 330 mg/ capsule	ascorbic acid, 200 mg/ capsule	alcohol, 5% (elixir)
Hytinic Capsules and Elixir (Hyrex)	elemental, 150 mg/capsule 20 mg/ml (as polysaccharide– iron complex)		sodium, 0.2 mEq (capsules) 0.13 mEq/ml (elixir)
Iron and Vitamin C (Squibb)	50 mg (as ferrous fumarate)	sodium ascorbate, 25 mg	
Ironized Yeast (Glenbrook)	ferrous sulfate, 56.9 mg	thiamine, 0.33 mg	
Laud-Iron (Amfre-Grant)	ferrous fumarate, 324 mg/tablet 20 mg/ml		
Laud-Iron Plus Chewing Tablets (Amfre-Grant)	ferrous fumarate, 100 mg	cyanocobalamin, 5 μg	
Mol-Iron Chronsule Capsules (Schering)	ferrous sulfate, 390 mg		
Mol-Iron Liquid and Tablets (Schering)	ferrous sulfate, 48.7 mg/ml 195 mg/tablet		alcohol, 4.75% (liquid)
Mol-Iron with Vitamin C (Schering)	ferrous sulfate, 195 mg	ascorbic acid, 75 mg	

Iron Product Table, continued

Product (Manufacturer)	Iron	Vitamins	Other Ingredients
Mol-Iron with Vitamin C Chronsule Capsules (Schering)	ferrous sulfate, 390 mg	ascorbic acid, 150 mg	
Niferex Elixir, Capsules, and Tablets (Central Pharmacal)	elemental, 20 mg/ml 150 mg/capsule 50 mg/tablet (as polysaccharide–iron complex)		alcohol, 10% (elixir) sodium, 0.2 mEq (capsule) 0.07 mEq (tablet) 0.13 mEq/ml (elixir)
Niferex with Vitamin C Tablets (Central Pharmacal)	elemental, 50 mg (as polysaccharide–iron complex)	sodium ascorbate, 168.75 mg ascorbic acid, 100 mg	sodium, 0.07 mEq
Simron Capsules (Merrell-Dow)	elemental, 10 mg (as ferrous gluconate)		polysorbate 20, 400 mg
Toleron Suspension and Tablets (Wallace)	ferrous fumarate, 20 mg/ml 200 mg/tablet		
Tri-Tinic Capsules (North American)	ferrous fumarate, 110 mg	ascorbic acid, 75 mg folic acid, 0.5 mg cyanocobalamin, 7.5 μg	liver–stomach concentrate, 240 mg
Vitron-C (Fisons)	ferrous fumarate, 200 mg	ascorbic acid, 125 mg	

Multiple Vitamin Product Table

Product (Manufacturer)	Vitamin A (IU)	Vitamin D (IU)	Vitamin E (IU)	Ascorbic Acid (C) (mg)	Thiamine (B₁) (mg)	Riboflavin (B₉) (mg)	Niacin (mg)
Abdec Baby Drops[a] (Parke-Davis)	5,000	400		50	1.0[c]	1.2	10[d]
Abdec Kapseal (Parke-Davis)	10,000[q]	400	5	75	5.0[f]	3.0	25[d]
Abdol c̄ Minerals (Parke-Davis)	5,000[b]	400		50	2.5[f]	2.5	20[d]
Abron (O'Neal, Jones & Feldman)	8,000	400	30	100	3	3	20
Allbee-T (Robins)				500	15.5[f]	10.0	100[d]
Allbee with C (Robins)				300	15.0[f]	10.0	50[d]
Allbee C-800 (Robins)			45	800	15	17	100[d]
Allbee C-800 plus Iron (Robins)			45	800	15	17	100[d]
Aqua-A (Anabolic)	25,000[b]						
Aquasol E Capsules, Drops (USV)			100, 400 (capsules) 50[a] (drops)				
AVP Natal (A.V.P.)	5,000			100			
B6-Plus (Anabolic)					10[a]	2.4	20
B 12-Plus (Anabolic)							
B-C-Bid Capsules (Geriatric Pharm.)				300	15.0[f]	10.0	50[d]
B-Complex Capsules (North American)					1.5[c]	2.0	10[d]
B Complex Tablets (Squibb)					0.7	0.7	9
Becomco (O'Neal, Jones & Feldman)					2.25	2.6	30
Belfer (O'Neal, Jones & Feldman)				50	2	2	
Beminal 500 (Ayerst)				500	25.0	12.5	100.0[d]
Beminal Forte with Vitamin C (Ayerst)				250	25.0	12.5	50.0[d]
Beta-Vite Liquid[n] (North American)					10.0[c]		
Beta-Vite w/Iron Liquid[n] (North American)					10.0[c]		
Bewon Elixir[n] (Wyeth)					0.25[c]		
Brewers Yeast (North American)					0.06	0.02	0.15
Bugs Bunny (Miles)	2,500	400	15	60	1.05	1.2	13.5
Bugs Bunny Plus Iron (Miles)	2,500	400	15	60	1.05	1.2	13.5
Bugs Bunny with Extra C (Miles)	2,500	400	15	250	1.05	1.2	13.5
Calcium, Phosphate, and Vitamin D (Squibb)		180					
Calciwafers (Nion)				66.7			
Cal-M (Anabolic)		400			45[f]		90
Cal-Prenal (North American)	4,000[q]	400		50	2.0[c]	2.0	10[d]

Pyridoxine Hydrochloride (B6)(mg)	Cyanocobalamin (B12)(µg)	Folic Acid (µg)	Pantothenic Acid (µg)	Iron (mg)	Calcium (mg)	Phosphorus (mg)	Magnesium (mg)	Other Ingredients
1.0			5.0[e]					
1.5	2.0[g]		10.0[h]					
0.5	1.0[g]	100	2.5[i]	15[j]	44[k]	34[k]	1.0[j]	potassium, 5.0 mg[j] manganese, 1.0 mg[j] zinc, 0.5 mg[j] others[z]
4	12	400		60	260		100	iodine, 150 µg
10.0	5.0		23.0					desiccated liver, 150 mg
5.0			10.0[i]					
25	12		25[i]					
25	12	400	25[i]					
10.0				66[m]				purified veal bone ash, 500 mg
50							50[u]	potassium citrate, 50 mg
	250							
5.0	5.0							
0.1			1.0[i]					dried yeast, 100 mg desiccated liver, 70 mg
0.9	2.0							
3				27				sucrose, 7 g
2	10			94				sucrose, 60 mg
10.0	5.0				20.0			saccharin, 0.15 mg
3.0	2.5				10.0			
	25.0							
	25.0			75[o]				
0.007			0.05					
1.05	4.5	300						
1.05	4.5	300		15				
1.05	4.5	300						
					255	156		
					171.1[k] 35.3[p]	136.7[k]		
45					250			
1.0	2.0[r]	100		50[m]	230			iodine, 150 µg[l]

Multiple Vitamin Product Table, continued

Product (Manufacturer)	Vitamin A (IU)	Vitamin D (IU)	Vitamin E (IU)	Ascorbic Acid (C) (mg)	Thiamine (B₁) (mg)	Riboflavin (B₉) (mg)	Niacin (mg)
C-B Bone Capsules (USV)				250	25.0[f]	10.0	74[d]
Cebefortis (Upjohn)				150	5.0[f]	5.0	50[d]
Cebetinic (Upjohn)				25	2.0[f]	2.0	10[d]
Cecon Solution[a] (Abbott)				60			
Centrum (Lederle)	5,000	400	30	90	2.25	2.6	20[d]
Cetane (timed release) (O'Neal, Jones & Feldman)				500			
Cevi-Bid (Geriatric Pharm.)				500			
Ce-Vi-Sol Drops[a] (Mead Johnson)				35			
Cherri-B Liquid[a] (North American)					1.5[c]	0.3	6[d]
Chew-E (North American)			200				
Chew-Vite (North American)	5,000	400		50	3.0	2.5	20[d]
Clusivol 130 (Ayerst)	10,000	400	0.5	150.0	10.0[f]	5.0	50.0[d]
Clusivol Syrup (Ayerst)	25,000	400		15.0	1.0	1.0	5.0[d]
Cod Liver Oil Concentrate Capsules (Schering)	10,000	400					
Cod Liver Oil Concentrate Tablets (Schering)	4,000	200					
Cod Liver Oil Tablets with Vitamin C (Schering)	4,000	200		50			
Dayalets (Abbott)	5,000	400	30	60	1.5[c]	1.7	20[d]
Dayalets plus Iron (Abbott)	5,000	400	30	60	1.5[c]	1.7	20[d]
De-Cal (North American)		125					
Di-Calcium Phosphate Capsules (North American)		333					
Dical-D (Abbott)		133					
Dical-D with Vitamin C Capsules (Abbott)		133		15			
Drisdol Drops (Winthrop)		200					
Duo-CVP Capsules (USV)							
Dura-C 500 Graduals (Amfre-Grant)				500			
E-Ferol Succinate (O'Neal, Jones & Feldman)			200, 400				
Engran-HP (Squibb)	8,000	400	30	60	1.7	2.0	20

Pyridoxine Hydrochloride (B₆)(mg)	Cyanocobalamin (B₁₂)(μg)	Folic Acid (μg)	Pantothenic Acid (μg)	Iron (mg)	Calcium (mg)	Phosphorus (mg)	Magnesium (mg)	Other Ingredients
1.5	5.0		8.0					choline, 25 mg
1.0	2.0		10.0[i]					
0.5	5.0			38[p]				
3	9	400	10	27	162	125	100	biotin, 45 μg iodine, 150 μg copper, 3 mg zinc, 22.5 mg manganese, 7.5 mg potassium, 7.5 mg
								alcohol, 5%
0.09			0.12[h]					
1.0	1.0[r]							
0.5	2.5			15.0[j]	120.0[t]		3.0[j]	
0.6	2.0		3.0[h]				0.03	manganese, 0.5 mg zinc, 0.5 mg saccharin, 3.8 mg
2.0	6.0	400						
2.0	6.0	400		18				
					250			
					75[k] 14[p]	58[k]		
					120[k] 295[k]	90[k] 228[k]		dibasic calcium phosphate, 500 mg
					120[k]	90[k]		dibasic calcium phosphate, 500 mg
								citrus bioflavonoid compound, 200 mg
2.5	8.0	800		18	650		100	iodine, 150 μg

Multiple Vitamin Product Table, continued

Product (Manufacturer)	Vitamin A (IU)	Vitamin D (IU)	Vitamin E (IU)	Ascorbic Acid (C) (mg)	Thiamine (B_1) (mg)	Riboflavin (B_9) (mg)	Niacin (mg)
Epsilan-M (Warren-Teed)			100				
Feminins (Mead Johnson)	5,000	400	10	200	1.5[c]	3.0	15
Femiron with Vitamins (J. B. Williams)	5,000	400		60	1.5	1.7	20[d]
Feostim (O'Neal, Jones & Feldman)				20	3	1	
Ferritrinsic (Upjohn)				50	2.0[f]	2.0	10[d]
Filibon Tablets (Lederle)	5,000[q]	400	30	60[i]	1.5	1.7	20[d]
Flintstones (Miles)	2,500	400	15	60	1.05	1.2	13.5
Flintstones with Extra C (Miles)	2,500	400	15	250	1.05	1.2	13.5
Flintstones Plus Iron (Miles)	2,500	400	15	60	1.05	1.2	13.5
Folbesyn (Lederle)				180	10.0	5.0	50.0[d]
Ganatrex[a] (Merrell Dow)	5,000[b]	400	30	60	1.5[c]	1.7	20[d]
Geralix Liquid[y] (North American)					3.3[c]	1.7	
Geriamic (North American)				75	15.0[c]	5.0	30[d]
Gerilets (Abbott)	5,000	400	45	90[e]	2.25[f]	2.6	30[d]
Geriplex (Parke-Davis)	5,000[q]		5	50[e]	5.0[f]	5.0	15[d]
Geriplex-FS Kapseals (Parke-Davis)	5,000[q]		5	50[e]	5.0[f]	5.0	15[d]
Geriplex-FS Liquid[x] (Parke-Davis)					1.2[c]	1.7[k]	15[d]
Geritinic (Geriatric Pharm.)	5,000	400		60	3.0[f]	3.0	10[d]
Geritonic Liquid (Geriatric Pharm.)					1	1	10[d]
Geritol Junior Liquid[n] (J. B. Williams)	8,000[b]	400			5.0	5.0	100[d]
Geritol Junior Tablets (J. B. Williams)	5,000	100		30	2.5	2.5	20[d]
Geritol Liquid[n] (J. B. Williams)					5.0	5.0	100[d]
Geritol Tablets (J. B. Williams)				75	5.0	5.0	30[d]

Pyridoxine Hydrochloride (B₆)(mg)	Cyanocobalamin (B₁₂)(μg)	Folic Acid (μg)	Pantothenic Acid (μg)	Iron (mg)	Calcium (mg)	Phosphorus (mg)	Magnesium (mg)	Other Ingredients
25	10.0	100	10.0	18				zinc, 10.0 mg
2.0	5.0	100	10.0[i]	20[m]				
	5			20[m]				
		33		60[j]				intrinase, 1/3 NF XI unit desiccated liver, 100 mg
2	6	400		18[m]	125[t]		100[u]	iodine, 150 μg others[z]
1.05	4.5	300						
1.05	4.5	300						
1.05	4.5	300		15				
3.0	9.0	400						
2.0	6.0							alcohol, 15% invert sugar
0.7					33[w]		0.33	alcohol, 15% choline bitartrate, 100 mg inositol, 100 mg others[z]
0.5	3.0		2.0[i]	50				brewer's yeast, 50 mg choline bitartrate, 25 mg methionine, 25 mg inositol, 20 mg
3.0	9.0	400	15	27				biotin, 0.45 mg
	2.0[g]			30[j]	59[k]	46[k]		aspergillus oryzae enzymes, 162.5 mg choline dihydrogen citrate, 20 mg others[z]
	2.0[g]			30[j]	59[k]	46[k]		aspergillus oryzae enzymes, 162.5 mg docusate sodium, 100 mg others[z]
1.0	5.0[g]			15[v]				poloxamer 188, 200 mg alcohol, 18%
0.1	5.0		1.0[i]	195				inositol, 20 mg yeast concentrate, 22.4 mg potassium, 30 mg[q] choline bitartrate, 30 mg others[z]
0.1	3			35[v]	10	8	1[j]	manganese, 0.5 mg alcohol, 20%
1.0	3.0		4.0[h]	100[v]				
1.0	2.5		2.0[i]	25[j]				
1.0	3.0		4.0[h]	100[v]				methionine, 75 mg/oz. choline bitartrate, 100 mg
0.5	3.0		2.0[i]	50[j]				

Multiple Vitamin Product Table, continued

Product (Manufacturer)	Vitamin A (IU)	Vitamin D (IU)	Vitamin E (IU)	Ascorbic Acid (C) (mg)	Thiamine (B$_1$) (mg)	Riboflavin (B$_9$) (mg)	Niacin (mg)
Gerix Elixir[x] (Abbott)					6.0[c]	6.0	100[d]
Gerizyme[y] (Upjohn)					3.3[c]	3.3	33.3[d]
Gest (O'Neal, Jones & Feldman)	4,000	200		30	1.7	2	
Gevrabon[x] (Lederle)					5.0	2.5	50[d]
Gevral (Lederle)	5,000[q]		30	60	1.5[f]	1.7	20[d]
Gevral Protein (Lederle)	2,167[b]	217	4.3	22	2.2	2.2	6.5[d]
Gevral T Capsules (Lederle)	5,000[q]	400	45	90	2.25	2.6	30[d]
Gevrite (Lederle)	5,000[b]			60	1.5	1.7	20[d]
Golden Bounty B Complex with Vitamin C (Squibb)				100	4.0	4.8	4.67
Hi-Bee W/C Capsules (North American)				300	15.0[f]	10.0	50[d]
Hi-Bee Plus (North American)				300	20		100[d]
Iberet (Abbott)				150[e]	6.0[f]	6.0	30[d]
Iberet-500 (Abbott)				500[e]	6.0[f]	6.0	30[d]
Iberet Oral Solution[n] (Abbott)				37.5	1.5[c]	1.5	7.5[d]
Iberet-500 Oral Solution[n] (Abbott)				125	1.5[c]	1.5	7.5[d]
Iberol (Abbott)				75[e]	3.0[f]	3.0	15[d]
Incremin with Iron Syrup[n] (Lederle)					10.0[c]		
K-Forte Potassium Supplement with Vitamin C Chewable (O'Connor)				10 25			
Lederplex Capsules (Lederle)					2.0	2.0	10[d]

Pyridoxine Hydrochloride (B6)(mg)	Cyanocobalamin (B12)(µg)	Folic Acid (µg)	Pantothenic Acid (µg)	Iron (mg)	Calcium (mg)	Phosphorus (mg)	Magnesium (mg)	Other Ingredients
1.64	6.0			15				
1.0	3.3		3.3[h]	5[p]	100[w]		3.5[j]	inositol, 100 mg potassium, 10.0 mg[j] alcohol, 18% others[z]
				18	130			
1.0	1.0		10.0	15			2.0	manganese, 2 mg alcohol, 18% zinc, 2 mg inositol, 100 mg choline, 100 mg iodine, 100 µg[l] others[z]
2.0	6	400		18[m]	162[k]	125[k]	100[u]	iodine, 150 µg
0.22	0.87		2.2[i]	4.3[m]	359	52.8[k]	0.4	choline, 21 mg inositol, 22 mg lysine monohydrate, 1.1 g iodine, 40 µg[l] copper, 400 µg[u] zinc, 220 µg[u] manganese, 400 µg[u] potassium, 13 mg
3.0	9.0	400		27[m]	162[k]	125[k]	100[u]	potassium, 5.0 mg[j] zinc, 22.5 mg iodine, 225 µg[l] copper, 1.5 mg others[z]
2.0				18[m]	230[t]			
	25.0[r]							
5.0			10.0[i]					
5			20[i]				70	zinc sulfate, 80 mg
5.0	25.0		10.0[i]	105				
5.0	25.0		10.0[i]	105				
1.25	6.25		2.5[h]	26.25				
1.25	6.25		2.5[h]	26.25				
1.5	12.5		3.0[i]	105				
5.0	25.0			30[o]				sorbitol, 3.5 g lysine monohydrochloride, 300 mg
								potassium, 39 mg[p] (also citrate and chloride, 1 mEq) 99 mg[p] (2.5 mEq)
0.2	1.0	3.0[i]						liver fraction and desiccated liver, 340 mg choline, 20 mg inositol, 10 mg

Multiple Vitamin Product Table, continued

Product (Manufacturer)	Vitamin A (IU)	Vitamin D (IU)	Vitamin E (IU)	Ascorbic Acid (C) (mg)	Thiamine (B$_1$) (mg)	Riboflavin (B$_9$) (mg)	Niacin (mg)
Lederplex Liquid[n] (Lederle)					2.5	2.5	12.5[d]
Lederplex Tablets (Lederle)					2.0	2.0	10[d]
Lipoflavonoid Capsules (Cooper Vision Pharmaceuticals)				100	0.33[c]	0.33	3.33[d]
Lipotriad Capsules (Cooper Vision Pharmaceuticals)					0.33[c]	0.33	3.33[d]
Lipotriad Liquid[n] (Cooper Vision Pharmaceuticals)					1.0[c]	1.0	10[d]
Livitamin Capsules (Beecham Labs)				100	3.0[f]	3.0	10[d]
Livitamin Chewable (Beecham Labs)				100[j]	3.0[f]	3.0	10[d]
Livitamin Liquid[y] (Beecham Labs)					3.0[c]	3.0	10[d]
Lufa Capsules (USV)			4		2.0[f]	2.0	5.0[d]
Methischol Capsules (USV)					3.0[f]	3.0	10[d]
Mucoplex (ICN)						1.5	
Multicebrin (Lilly)	10,000	400	6.6	75	3[c]	3	25
Multiple Vitamins (North American)	5,000	400		50	3.0[f]	2.5	20[d]
Multiple Vitamins with Iron (North American)	5,000	400		50	2.0[f]	2.5	20[d]
Multivitamins (Rowell)	5,000	400	10	50	2.5[f]	2.5	20[d]
Myadec (Parke-Davis)	10,000	400	30	250	10.0[f]	10.0	100[d]
Natabec (Parke-Davis)	4,000[q]	400		50	3.0[f]	2.0	10[d]
Natalins Tablets (Mead Johnson)	8,000	400	30	90	1.7	2.0	20
Neo-Calglucon[n] (Dorsey)							
Norlac (Rowell)	8,000	400	30	90	2	2	20
Nutra-Cal (Anabolic)	1,250[b]	100	3	7.5			

Pyridoxine Hydrochloride (B$_6$)(mg)	Cyanocobalamin (B$_{12}$) (μg)	Folic Acid (μg)	Pantothenic Acid (μg)	Iron (mg)	Calcium (mg)	Phosphorus (mg)	Magnesium (mg)	Other Ingredients
0.25	6.25		2.5[h]					liver fraction and desiccated liver, 590 mg; choline, 25 mg; inositol, 5 mg
0.1	1.0		3.0[i]					liver fraction and desiccated liver, 250 mg; choline, 50 mg; inositol, 25 mg
0.33	1.67		0.33[i]					choline bitartrate, 233 mg; lemon-bioflavonoid complex, 100 mg
0.33	1.67		0.33[i]					choline bitartrate, 233.3 mg
1.0	5.0		1.0[i]					sugar free
3.0	5.0		2.0[i]	33[m]				desiccated liver, 150 mg; copper, 0.66 mg[j]
3.0	3.0	5.0		2.0[i]	17[m]			copper, 0.33 mg[u]
3.0	5.0		2.0[h]	36				liver fraction 1, 500 mg; copper, 0.66 mg[j]
2.0	1.0		1.0[h]					unsaturated fatty acids, 423 mg; choline bitartrate, 233 mg; desiccated liver, 87 mg; methionine, 66 mg; inositol, 40 mg
2.0	2.0[r]		2.0[h]					choline bitartrate, 240 mg; methionine, 110 mg; inositol, 83 mg; others[z]
	5.0							liver fraction A, 375 mg; liver fraction 2, 375 mg
1.2	3							
1.0	1.0		1.0[i]					
1.0	1.0		1.0	15[m]				
0.5	2.0		5[i]					
5.0	6.0	400	20	20[m]			100[u]	copper, 2.0 mg[j]; zinc, 20 mg[j]; manganese, 1.25 mg[j]; iodine, 150 μg[l]
3.0	5.0			150[j]	600[t]			
4.0	8.0	800		45	200		100	iodine, 150 μg
					115			calcium glubionate, 1.8 g; benzoic acid, 5 mg
4	8	400		60	200		100	iodine, 150 μg; copper, 2 mg; zinc, 15 mg
					185	125	62	iodine, 0.025 mg

Multiple Vitamin Product Table, continued

Product (Manufacturer)	Vitamin A (IU)	Vitamin D (IU)	Vitamin E (IU)	Ascorbic Acid (C) (mg)	Thiamine (B_1) (mg)	Riboflavin (B_9) (mg)	Niacin (mg)
Nutriganic (Commerce)	10,000	400	12.5	150	25	25	50[d]
Obron-6 (Pfipharmecs)	5,000	400		50	3.0	2.0	20
One-A-Day (Miles)	5,000	400	15	60	1.5	1.7	20
One-A-Day Core C 500 (Miles)	5,000	400	15	500	1.5	1.7	20
One-A-Day Plus Iron (Miles)	5,000	400	15	60	1.5	1.7	20
One-A-Day Vitamins Plus Minerals (Miles)	5,000	400	15	50	1.5	1.7	20
Optilets-500 (Abbott)	10,000	400	30	500[e]	15.0[f]	10.0	100[d]
Optilets-M-500 (Abbott)	10,000	400	30	500[e]	15.0[f]	10.0	100[d]
Orexin Softabs (Stuart)					10.0[f]		
Os-Cal (Marion)		125					
Os-Cal 500 (Marion)		125					
Os-Cal Plus (Marion)	1,666	125		33	0.5	0.66	3.33[d]
Os-Cal Forte (Marion)	1,668	125	0.8	50	1.7	1.7	15[d]
Paladac[n] (Parke-Davis)	5,000[b]	400		50	3.0[c]	3.0[k]	20[d]
Paladac c̄ Minerals (Parke-Davis)	4,000[q]	400	10	50[e]	3.0[f]	3.0	20[d]
Panuitex (O'Neal, Jones & Feldman)	6,000	400		100	1.5	2.5	15[d]
Peritinic (Lederle)				200	7.5	7.5	30[d]
Poly-Vi-Sol Chewable (Mead Johnson)	2,500	400	15	60	1.05	1.2	13.5
Poly-Vi-Sol with Iron Chewable (Mead Johnson)	2,500	400	15	60	1.05	1.2	13.5
Poly-Vi-Sol Drops[a] (Mead Johnson)	1,500	400	5	35	0.5	0.6	8
Poly-Vi-Sol with Iron Drops[a] (Mead Johnson)	1,500	400	5	35	0.5	0.6	8

Pyridoxine Hydrochloride (B$_6$)(mg)	Cyanocobalamin (B$_{12}$)(µg)	Folic Acid (µg)	Pantothenic Acid (µg)	Iron (mg)	Calcium (mg)	Phosphorus (mg)	Magnesium (mg)	Other Ingredients
15	50		12.5[i]	50[p]	53.5	24.3	7.2[p]	inositol, 250 mg; choline bitartrate, 150 mg; betaine hydrochloride, 25 mg; para-aminobenzoic acid, 15 mg; glutamic acid, 25 mg; rutin, 5 mg; citrus bioflavonoids, 15 mg; biotin, 1 µg; liver, 50 mg; bone meal, 162 mg; cooper gluconate, 7.2 mg; zinc gluconate, 2.2 mg; potassium iodide, 0.1 mg
8.2	2.0		0.92	33	243		1	potassium, 1.7 mg; zinc, 0.4 mg; manganese, 0.33 mg (sugar free)
2.0	6.0	400						
2[i]	6	400						
2.0	6.0	400		18				
2.0	6.0	400	10.0	18	100	100	100	zinc, 15 mg; copper, 2.0 mg; iodine, 150 µg
5.0	12.0		20.0[i]					
5.0	12.0		20.0[i]	20			80	copper, 2.0 mg; zinc, 1.5 mg; manganese, 1 mg; iodine, 150 µg
5.0	25.0							
					250			
					500			
0.5	0.03			16.6	250			zinc, 0.75 mg; manganese, 0.76 mg; copper, 0.036 mg; iodine, 0.036 mg
2	1.6			5	250		1.6	zinc, 0.5 mg; manganese, 0.3 mg; copper 0.3 mg; iodine, 0.05 mg
1.0	5.0[g]		5.0[e]					
1.0	5.0[g]		5.0[i]	5[k]	23[k]	17[k]	1.0[u]	potassium, 2.5 mg[j]; iodine, 50 µg[l]
3	2		5[i]	48[m]	250[t]			sucrose, 70 mg
7.5	50.0	50	15.0	100[m]				docusate sodium, 100 mg
1.05	4.5	300						
1.05	4.5	300		12				
0.4								
0.4				10				

Multiple Vitamin Product Table, continued

Product (Manufacturer)	Vitamin A (IU)	Vitamin D (IU)	Vitamin E (IU)	Ascorbic Acid (C) (mg)	Thiamine (B₁) (mg)	Riboflavin (B₉) (mg)	Niacin (mg)
Probec-T (Stuart)				600[e]	15.0[f]	10.0	100[d]
Roeribec (Pfipharmecs)				500	10.0	10.0	100[d]
Rogenic (O'Neal, Jones & Feldman)				100			
Selenace (Anabolic)	10,000		200	250			
Simron Plus (Merrell-Dow)				50			
Spancap C Capsules (North American)				500			
S.S.S. Tonic[y] (S.S.S.)					1.7	0.8	6.6[d]
S.S.S. Tablets (S.S.S.)				75	5	2.4	30
Stresscaps Capsules (Lederle)				300	10.0	10.0	100[d]
Stresstabs 600 (Lederle)			30	600	15.0	15.0	100[d]
Stresstabs 600 with Iron (Lederle)			30	600	15	15	100[d]
Stresstabs 600 with Zinc (Lederle)			45	600	20	10	100[d]
Stuart Formula (Stuart)	5,000[b]	400	15	60	1.5[f]	1.7	20[d]
Stuart Hematinic Liquid[n] (Stuart)					1.7[c]	1.7	10[d]
Stuartinic (Stuart)				300 225[e]	6.0[f]	6.0	20[d]
Stuart Prenatal (Stuart)	8,000[q]	400	30	60	1.7[f]	2.0	20[d]
Sugar Calcicaps (Nion)		133					
Super D Cod Liver Oil[n] (Upjohn)	4,000	400					
Super D Perles[n] (Upjohn)	10,000	400					
Super Plenamins (Rexall)	8,000	400	1.8	56	2.3[c]	2.35	18
Surbex (Abbott)					6.0[f]	6.0	30[d]
Surbex-T (Abbott)				500[e]	15.0[f]	10.0	100[d]
Surbex with C (Abbott)				250[e]	6.0[f]	6.0	30[d]
Surbex 750 with Iron (Abbott)			30	750[c]	15[f]	15	100[d]
Surbex 750 with Zinc (Abbott)			30	750[c]	15[f]	15	100[d]
Tega-C Caps (Ortega)				500			
Tega-C Syrup[n] (Ortega)				500			
Tega-E Caps (Ortega)			400 1,000				
Thera-Combex H-P Kapseals (Parke-Davis)				500	25.0[f]	15.0	100[d]
Theragran (Squibb)	10,000	400	15	200	10.3	10.0	100[d]
Theragran Liquid[n] (Squibb)	10,000	400		200	10.0	10.0	100[d]
Theragran-M (Squibb)	10,000	400	15	200	10.0	10.0	100[d]

Pyridoxine Hydrochloride (B_6)(mg)	Cyanocobalamin (B_{12}) (μg)	Folic Acid (μg)	Pantothenic Acid (μg)	Iron (mg)	Calcium (mg)	Phosphorus (mg)	Magnesium (mg)	Other Ingredients
5.0	5.0		20.0[l]					
8.2	4.0		18.0[i]					(sugar free)
6	25			60				desiccated liver
								selenium (yeast), 50 μg
1.0	3.33	100		10[p]				polysorbate 20, 400 mg
	0.2			33[v]				
0.5	1.5			50	2			copper, 1 mg
2.0	4.0		20.0[i]					
5.0	12.0		20.0[l]					
25	12	400	20[i]	27[m]				copper, 3 mg
10	25	400	25[m]	115[m]				zinc, 23.9 mg[j] docusate sodium, 50 mg
2.0	6.0	400		18	160	125	100	iodine, 150 μg
0.5			1.43[h]	22[p]				liver fraction 1, 54.0 mg
1.0	25.0		10.0[i]	100[m]				
4.0	8.0	800		60[m]	200[j]		100[u]	iodine, 150 μg[l]
					334	41.7		
1.0	1.5							
2.5	5.0		10.0[i]					
5.0	10.0		20.0[i]					
2.5	5.0		10.0[i]					
25	12	400	20	27				
20	12	400	20					zinc, 22.5 mg
10.0	5.0[g]		18.4[h]					
4.1	5.0		21.4[i]					
4.1	5.0		18.4[h]					
4.1	5.0		20.0[i]	12			65	copper, 2.0 mg zinc, 1.5 mg manganese, 1.0 mg iodine, 150 μg

Multiple Vitamin Product Table, continued

Product (Manufacturer)	Vitamin A (IU)	Vitamin D (IU)	Vitamin E (IU)	Ascorbic Acid (C) (mg)	Thiamine (B_1) (mg)	Riboflavin (B_9) (mg)	Niacin (mg)
Theragran-Z (Squibb)	10,000	400	15	200	10.3	10	100
Therapeutic Vitamins (North American)	1,000[b]	400	15	200	10.0[f]	10.0	100[d]
Thera-Spancap (North American)	10,000	400		150	6.0[f]	6.0	60[d]
Thex Forte (Medtech)				500	25	15	100[d]
Tonebec (A.V.P.)				300	15.0[f]	10.0	5[d]
Tri-B-Plex (Anabolic)					50	20	100[d]
Tri-Vi-Sol Chewable (Mead Johnson)	2,500	400		60			
Tri-Vi-Sol Drops (Mead Johnson)	1,500	400		35			
Tri-Vi-Sol with Iron Drops (Mead Johnson)	1,500	400		35			
Unicap (Upjohn)	5,000	400	15	60	1.5[c]	1.7	20
Unicap Chewable (Upjohn)	5,000	400	15	60	1.5[f]	1.7	20[d]
Unicap T (Upjohn)	5,000	400	15	300	10.0[f]	10.0	100[d]
Verazinc (O'Neal, Jones & Feldman)							
Vi-Aqua (USV)	5,000	400	1.0	50.0	5.0	5.0	20[d]
Vicon Iron (Glaxo)			30	300	2.0[f]	2.0	20[d]
Vicon-C (Glaxo)				300	20.0[f]	10.0	100[d]
Vicon Plus (Glaxo)	4,000[q]		50	150	10.0[f]	5.0	25[d]
Vigran (Squibb)	5,000	400	30	60	1.5	1.7	20
Vigran Chewable (Squibb)	2,500	400	10	40	0.7	0.8	9
Vigran plus Iron (Squibb)	5,000	400	30	60	1.5	1.7	20
Vio-Bec (Rowell)				500	25.0[f]	25.0	100[d]
Vio-Geric (Rowell)	5,000	400	30	60	5	5	20
Vi-Penta Infant Drops[a] (Roche)	5,000	400	2	50			
Vi-Penta Multivitamin Drops[a] (Roche)	5,000[b]	400	2	50	1.0[c]	1.0	10[d]
Vitagett (North American)	5,000[b]	400	3	50	3.0[f]	2.5	20[d]
Vita-Kaps Tablets (Abbott)	5,000	400		50[e]	3.0[f]	2.5	20[d]
Vita-Kaps-M Tablets (Abbott)	5,000	400		50[e]	3.0[f]	2.5	20[d]

Pyridoxine Hydrochloride (B_6)(mg)	Cyanocobalamin (B_{12})(μg)	Folic Acid (μg)	Pantothenic Acid (μg)	Iron (mg)	Calcium (mg)	Phosphorus (mg)	Magnesium (mg)	Other Ingredients
4.1	5.0		18.4	12				iodine, 150 μg copper, 2 mg zinc, 22.5 mg manganese, 1 mg
5.0	5.0[r]		20.0[i]					
6.0	6.0[r]		6.0[i]					
5			10[i]					
5.0			10.0[i]					
25	12.5	200	50[i]					biotin, 300 μg
				10				
2.0	6.0	400						
2.0	6.0	400						
6.0	18.0	400	10.0[i]	18.0				potassium, 5.0 mg[j] copper, 2.0 mg[j] manganese, 1.0 mg[j] iodine, 150 μg[l] zinc, 15.0 mg
								zinc sulfate, 220 μg
0.5	1.0		5.0[h]					
5.0			10[i]	30[m]			35[u]	zinc, 10 mg[j]
5.0			20.0[i]				70[j]	zinc, 80 mg[j]
2.0			10.0[i]				70[j]	zinc, 80 mg[j] manganese chloride, 4 mg
2.0	6.0	400						
0.7	3.0	200						
2.0	6.0	400		27				
25.0			40.0[i]					
2.4	6	400		18	220	125	100	iodine, 150 μg copper, 2 mg zinc, 15 mg
1.0			10.0[h]					biotin, 30 μg
1.5	2.5		5.0[i]	13[j]	215[k]	166[k]	7.5[j]	potassium, 5.0 mg[j] manganese, 1.5 mg[j] zinc, 1.4 mg[j]
1.0	3.0							
1.0	3.0			10				zinc, 7.5 mg copper, 1.0 mg manganese, 1.0 mg iodine, 150 μg

Multiple Vitamin Product Table, continued

Product (Manufacturer)	Vitamin A (IU)	Vitamin D (IU)	Vitamin E (IU)	Ascorbic Acid (C) (mg)	Thiamine (B_1) (mg)	Riboflavin (B_9) (mg)	Niacin (mg)
Vitamin-Mineral Capsules (North American)	5,000[b]	400		50[e]	3.0[f]	2.5	20[d]
Viterra (Pfipharmecs)	5,000	400	3.7	50	3.0	3.0	25
Viterra High Potency (Pfipharmecs)	10,000	400	5	150	10.0	10.0	100
Vi-Zac (Glaxo)	5,000		50	500			
VM Preparation[x] (Roberts)					3.0[c]	2.0	20[d]
Z-Bec (Robins)			45	600	15	10.2	100
Zinkaps (Ortega)							
Zymacap Capsules (Upjohn)	5,000	400	15	90	2.25	2.6	30[d]
Zymalixir Syrup[n] (Upjohn)					1.0[c]	1.0	8.0[d]
Zymasyrup[n] (Upjohn)	5,000	400		60	1.0[c]	1.0	10[d]

Vitamin formulations change frequently; therefore, the product label should be consulted before dispensing.
[a] Quantities given are per 0.6 ml.
[b] Palmitate.
[c] Hydrochloride.
[d] Niacinamide.
[e] Sodium salt.
[f] Mononitrate.
[g] Crystalline.

[h] Panthenol.
[i] Calcium salt.
[j] Sulfate.
[k] Phosphate.
[l] Potassium iodide.
[m] Fumarate.
[n] Quantities given are per 5 ml.
[o] Pyrophosphate.
[p] Gluconate.
[q] Acetate.

[r] Concentrate.
[s] Ferrocholinate.
[t] Carbonate.
[u] Oxide.
[v] Ammonium citrate.
[w] Glycerophosphate.
[x] Quantities given are per 30 ml.
[y] Quantities given are per 15 ml.
[z] Also contains other vitamins and/or minerals.

Pyridoxine Hydrochloride (B₆)(mg)	Cyanoco-balamin (B₁₂)(μg)	Folic Acid (μg)	Panto-thenic Acid (μg)	Iron (mg)	Calcium (mg)	Phospho-rus (mg)	Magne-sium (mg)	Other Ingredients
1.0	2.0		2.0[i]	13[j]	46[k]	35[k]	1.0[j]	potassium, 5.0 mg[j] manganese, 1.5 mg[j] zinc, 1.4 mg[j]
0.82	2.0		4.6	10	140	70	5.0	zinc, 1.2 mg copper, 1.0 mg manganese, 1.0 mg iodine, 150 μg (sugar free)
1.6	5.0		4.6	10	50		5.0	zinc, 1.2 mg copper, 1.0 mg manganese, 1.0 mg iodine, 150 μg (sugar free)
								zinc, 80 mg[j]
				50	94	94		manganese, 2 mg
10.0	6.0		25.0					zinc, 22.5 mg
								zinc, 25 mg[j]; 110 mg[j]; and 220 mg[j]
3.0	9.0	400	15.0					
0.5	2.0			15[p]				liver concentrate, 65 mg alcohol, 1.5%
0.5	3.0		3.0[h]					alcohol, 2%

13 Diabetes Care Products

R. Keith Campbell

Questions to Ask the Patient

Is there a history of diabetes in your family?

When were you last tested for diabetes? What were the results of those tests?

How long have you had diabetes?

How do you feel about having diabetes? Do members of your family understand the condition and the factors that affect control?

Do you belong to the local diabetes association?

How long has it been since you discussed your diabetes treatment program with your physician?

Do you use insulin?

If you use insulin, where do you inject it? How much do you inject? Do you rotate the sites of injection? How many times a day?

What drugs have been prescribed for you? Are you taking anything for diabetes?

Are you taking any other medicines, such as pain killers or cough medicines?

Are you allergic to sulfa drugs? Are you allergic to beef or pork insulin?

Explain how you test your urine using TesTape, Clinitest tablets, or Diastix.

Do you test your urine for glucose at home? Does any other person help you in testing your urine?

Do you test your blood glucose? Are you familiar with the strips you can use to test your blood glucose at home?

What kind of diet has your physician prescribed?

Do you have a regular schedule for exercise?

Do you use any of the current popular ''fad'' diets?

How much alcohol (including wine and beer) do you drink in a week?

What do you think has affected the control of your diabetes? Are you eating differently? Are you exercising more or less? Have you had any infections? Is there anything that is emotionally upsetting you?

Diabetes mellitus is a disease that requires a total health team effort if it is to be managed successfully. The physician must diagnose the condition accurately, classify the type of diabetes properly, and motivate the patient to learn to control and monitor the condition. The dietician explains the importance of diet control and the food exchange system. The nurse helps the patient to develop a positive attitude, learn how to perform laboratory tests, monitor control, inject insulin, and keep records of the factors that affect diabetic control. The pharmacist's easy access to the patient offers a unique opportunity to help the patient maintain a proper therapeutic regimen. The pharmacist can answer patient questions about the disease, urine and blood testing, drug therapy, diet, and proper foot care. In addition, the pharmacist can stress the importance of complying with the physician's, nurse's, and dietician's instructions, and monitor the control of diabetic patients, particularly in relation to the use of drugs (1, 2).

Approximately 5 million diabetics are being treated in the United States, and another 2 million have undiagnosed diabetes (mild symptoms or asymptomatic). Another 5 million will develop diabetes sometime during their lives. The prevalence of diabetes is approximately 5% of the population. Roughly 25% of the population (50 million people) either have diabetes, will develop diabetes, or have a relative with diabetes. It is the third leading cause of death and is responsible for approximately 5% of hospital admissions (3).

The incidence of diabetes is increasing at a 6% annual rate (4). Diabetes kills nearly 40,000 people each year in the United States, and about 300,000 more die of its complications (5). It is now the number one cause of new blindness in the United States; more than one-half of the heart attacks that occur are related to diabetes; five of every six amputations due to gangrene are a result of diabetes; diabetic kidney disease is common and often fatal; neurologic complications are remarkably frequent; and complications of pregnancy due to diabetes are well recognized. Coronary artery disease is seven times more prevalent in diabetic women than in normal women (6). Women are 50% more likely to have diabetes than men; nonwhites are 20% more likely to have it than whites; low-income people (with incomes under $5,000/year) are three times more likely to have it than middle- and upper-income people; and the chance of developing it doubles with every 20% of excess weight and decade of life (3).

This increase in the number of diabetics identified is due to a sharp increase in the geriatric population, who are more prone to develop the disease; more sophisticated methods of screening and diagnosis; and third-generation diabetics who never would have been born without the discovery of insulin (6).

It is estimated that in 1979 diabetics generated total costs of $15.7 billion (7). The "average" diabetic generated costs of $2,421 during 1979. Economic costs are 13% higher for insulin-dependent diabetics than for "average" diabetics (7). Unfortunately, the diabetic is sometimes neglected by manufacturers of pharmaceuticals, health and beauty aids, food, drinks, and candy. Diabetics are offered a bewildering selection of products that are improperly formulated or poorly labeled to be safe to use (5). The pharmacist has an excellent opportunity to help these patients by reiterating instructions and warning signs and by assessing patient ability to carry out self-help measures. The pharmacist also can serve as a consultant to both physician and patient concerning the disease and the drugs and devices used in its treatment (8).

Classification of Diabetes

Diabetes mellitus is a difficult condition to define because it is really a variety of conditions that have hyperglycemia as the common physiologic problem that needs to be brought under control. Diabetes mellitus is defined as chronic hyperglycemia. This is the common denominator for the several types and is responsible for the symptoms and complications of the disease. There is decreased utilization and increased production of glucose due to an absolute or relative deficiency of insulin, high amounts of glucagon, high amounts of insulin-antagonizing substances, such as growth hormone, sympa-

Table 1. New classification of diabetes and glucose intolerance	
New names	**Old names**
Clinical categories	
Type I: Insulin-dependent diabetes mellitus (IDDM)	Juvenile diabetes
	Juvenile-onset diabetes
	Ketosis-prone diabetes
	Growth-onset diabetes
	Brittle diabetes
Type II: Noninsulin-dependent diabetes mellitus (NIDDM)	Adult-onset diabetes
	Maturity-onset diabetes
Type a: nonobese	Ketosis-resistant diabetes
Type b: obese	Stable diabetes
	Maturity-onset diabetes of youth
Diabetes mellitus associated with other conditions or syndromes	Secondary diabetes (drug-induced diabetes; impaired glucose tolerance due to other hormonal irregularities)
Impaired glucose tolerance (IGT)	Asymptomatic diabetes
	Chemical diabetes
	Subclinical diabetes
	Borderline diabetes
	Latent diabetes
Gestational diabetes	Gestational diabetes
Statistical risk	
Previous abnormality of glucose tolerance	Latent diabetes
	Prediabetes
Potential abnormality of glucose tolerance	Potential diabetes
	Prediabetes

Reprinted with permission from *Diabetes, 28* (12), 1039 (1979).

thomimetic amines, and corticosteroids (9), or decreased insulin receptors on cell membranes. Insulin deficiency is associated with the utilization of protein and fat stores for energy. Diabetes mellitus may progress from nearly normal metabolism to a totally deficient state (10).

The several types of diabetes have different etiologies, clinical courses, and methods of treatment. Properly classifying a diabetic into one of several categories in which hyperglycemia is a clinical finding is critical in developing a treatment protocol to bring the patient under control. Diabetics may be classified in several ways: according to the degree of glucose tolerance, age, and other data, such as genetic or acquired background, age of onset (juvenile or adult), body weight, degree of hyperglycemia or glucosuria or both, susceptibility to ketoacidosis, insulin dependency, degree of severity and stability, treatment priorities, and the presence or absence of large and small blood vessel lesions (1, 11–15).

A classification of diabetes and other categories of glucose intolerance based on contemporary knowledge of this heterogeneous syndrome is now being used to ensure consistency in treatment (16). Table 1 summarizes the new classification system and compares it with the old methods. Table 2 shows a classification according to the distinguishing features of the two major clinical types of diabetes.

A clinical classification of diabetes that is useful to physicians and pharmacists in developing treatment protocols also is shown in Table 2 (17). This method uses specific radioimmunoassay techniques for measuring circulating insulin levels and divides diabetics into two subgroups.

Insulinopenic (Type I) diabetes, a severe form, occurs most often in juveniles but may also appear occasionally in nonobese elderly adults. Insulinotardic diabetes, a milder form of the insulinopenic condition, occurs predominantly in nonobese adults. About 10% of the diabetics in the United States are classified as insulinopenic and 15% are insulinotardic (17).

The remaining 75% are insulinoplethoric (Type II) diabetics. This mild, nonketotic condition is usually seen in frankly obese women, 40–65 years old, and occasionally in children. The obesity is a result of excessive caloric intake, possibly facilitated by hunger resulting from mild postprandial hypoglycemia after excess insulin release.

Table 2. Distinguishing features of two major types of diabetes mellitus

	Insulin-dependent Type I (IDDM)	Noninsulin-dependent Type II (NIDDM)
Age of onset	Usually, but not always, during childhood or puberty	Frequently over 35
Type of onset	Abrupt	Usually gradual
Prevalence	0.5%	2–4%
Incidence	<10%	>75%
Family history of diabetes	Infrequently positive	Commonly positive
Primary cause	Pancreatic beta cell deficiency	End organ (insulin receptors) unresponsiveness to insulin action
Nutritional status at time of onset	Usually undernourished	Obesity usually present
Postglucose plasma or serum insulin[a], μU/ml	Absent	>100 at 2 hours
Symptoms	Polydipsia, polyphagia, and polyuria	Maybe none
Hepatomegaly	Rather common	Uncommon
Stability	Blood sugar fluctuates widely in response to small changes in insulin dose, exercise, and infection	Blood sugar fluctuations are less marked
Possible etiologic factors include:		
Inheritance	Associated with specific HLA tissue types, but only 40–50% concordance in twins	95–100% concordance in twins, but not associated with specific HLA tissue types
Autoimmune disease	50–80% circulating islet cell antibodies	Negative; <10% circulating islet cell antibodies
Viral infections	Coxsackie, mumps, influenza	No evidence
Proneness to ketosis	Frequent, especially if treatment program is insufficient in food and/or insulin	Uncommon except in the presence of unusual stress or moderate to severe sepsis

Table 2. continued

	Insulin-dependent Type I (IDDM)	Noninsulin-dependent Type II (NIDDM)
Insulin defect	Defect in secretion; secretion is impaired early in disease; secretion may be totally absent late in disease	Insulin deficiency present in some patients; others are insulin resistant Insulin deficiency—in most patients, there is failure of insulin secretion to keep pace with inordinate demands engendered by the obese state; this defect may appear initially as a failure to respond to glucose alone, suggesting an impairment in the glucoreceptor of the pancreatic beta cell Insulin resistance—in some patients, there is a defect in tissue responsiveness to insulin and evidence of hyperinsulinemia, in such patients, insulin resistance may be mediated by decreased number of insulin receptors in target cells
Plasma insulin (endogenous)	Negligible to zero	Plasma insulin response may be either, adequate but delayed so that postprandial hypoglycemia may be present when diabetes is discovered or diminished but not absent
Vascular complications of diabetes and degenerative changes	Infrequent until diabetes has been present for ~5 years	Frequent
Usual causes of death	Degenerative complications in target organs, e.g., renal failure due to diabetic nephropathy	Accelerated atherosclerosis, e.g., myocardial infarction; to lesser extent, microangiopathic changes in target tissues, e.g., renal failure
Diet	Mandatory in all patients	If diet is utilized fully, hypoglycemic therapy may not be needed
Insulin	Necessary for all patients	Necessary for 20–30% of patients
Oral agents	Rarely efficacious	Often efficacious

[a]Normal response is between 50 and 135 μU/ml at 60 minutes and less than 100 μU/ml at 120 minutes after 100 g of oral glucose.

Etiology

The most common factors predisposing to the development of diabetes are heredity, obesity, age, stress, hormonal imbalance, vasculitis of the vessels supplying the beta-cells of the pancreas, and viruses affecting the autoimmune responses of the body (1, 18).

Type I diabetes due to a defect in pancreatic beta-cell function may have many causes. Genetic defects in production of certain macromolecules may interfere with proper insulin synthesis, packaging, or release, or the beta-cells may not recognize glucose signals or replicate normally (19). Extrinsic factors that affect beta-cell function include damage caused by viruses such as mumps or Coxsackie B_4, by destructive cytotoxins and antibodies released by sensitized lymphocytes, or by autodigestion in the course of an inflammatory disorder involving the adjacent exocrine pancreas.

An underlying genetic defect in beta-cell replication or function may predispose the patient to development of beta-cell failure after viral infection. Cells have many different antigen types. Specific histocompatibility locus antigen (HLA) genes may increase susceptibility to a diabetogenic virus, or certain immune-response genes may predispose patients to a destructive autoimmune response against their own islet cells. In the severe form of Type I diabetes, circulating islet-cell antibodies have been detected in as many as 80% of the cases tested in the first few weeks of the diabetes onset (19). The HLA linkage and islet-cell antibodies are not features of insulinoplethoric diabetes (19). In insulinotardic patients, as in severe Type I diabetics, the patient may inherit a response to a viral infection that causes a beta-cell defect as a consequence of viral stress.

In Type II diabetics who have excess insulin and are always obese, hyperinsulinism and insulin resistance may be correlated with a decrease in insulin receptors (20). Moreover, studies have shown that the tissues of insulin-resistant, obese patients exhibit reduced insulin binding. The reduced number of insulin receptors is the basic, and often reversible, defect in insulin-resistant patients (20).

Normal Carbohydrate Metabolism

The important carbohydrate metabolism sites sensitive to insulin are the liver, where glycogen is formed, stored, and broken down; skeletal muscle, where glucose is oxidized to produce energy; and adipose tissue, where glucose may be converted to fatty acids, glyceryl phosphate, and triglycerides. Some important effects of insulin on carbohydrate metabolism in these tissues are increased glucose uptake by the tissues, increased glucose oxidation by all pathways, increased energy production from glucose, increased muscle and liver glycogen levels, decreased hepatic glucose output, increased synthesis of fatty acids and triglycerides, decreased lipolysis, decreased production of ketone bodies, and enhanced incorporation of amino acids into proteins.

In the normal patient, insulin—in concert with glucagon, somatostatin, growth hormone, corticosteroids, epinephrine, and other chemicals—maintains the blood glucose between 40 and 160 mg/100 ml (mg %) at all times. In reference to all hormones and other chemicals that affect insulin and carbohydrate metabolism, if any are increased or decreased (as by drug therapy), they can cause a normal person to become diabetic or a diabetic to lose control.

Diabetic Carbohydrate Metabolism

Insulin-Dependent (Type I) Diabetics

With an understanding of carbohydrate metabolism in the nondiabetic, it is relatively easy to imagine what occurs in a Type I diabetic unable to utilize glucose in muscle and adipose tissue. When a meal is ingested, blood glucose levels increase. With no insulin available to facilitate glucose transport into the fat or muscle tissue, hyperglycemia results. In an attempt to provide glucose to the glucose-deficient tissue, amino acids are converted into glucose by gluconeogenesis, and liver glycogen is converted to glucose by glucogenolysis. However, without insulin, the tissues cannot utilize this glucose either and the hyperglycemia becomes even more pronounced.

The blood glucose level at which glucose first appears in the urine is clinically referred to as the renal threshold for glucose. Normally, glucose does not spill into the urine until the venous blood glucose reaches 180 mg/100 ml. In diabetic patients, the threshold level for glucose may increase to 250 mg/100 ml. The threshold level will also increase with advancing age.

The increased osmotic load in the kidney draws body water with it and is responsible for the excretion of large amounts of urine (polyuria) and the loss of fluid. The resulting water loss causes a compensatory increase in thirst (polydipsia) and may cause significant hypovolemia, electrolyte loss, and cellular dehydration. This diuresis can lead to dry skin and eventually dehydra-

tion. Since fats rather than carbohydrates are being metabolized, weight loss occurs over a period of time. The tissue cells, being "hungry" for carbohydrates, signal the person to eat (polyphagia), and eating continues to increase the blood glucose level.

Figure 1 shows the clinical manifestations that result in an untreated insulinopenic diabetic. Note the signs of insulin deficiency that result in abnormal urine and blood values. A properly trained diabetic patient can test for these abnormalities in the urine and blood to monitor how well the diabetes is being controlled.

Insulin also has a direct inhibitory effect on the enzyme lipoprotein lipase, which mobilizes body fat (lipolysis). Hormones such as glucocorticoids and epinephrine enhance lipolysis. When there is a shortage of insulin, lipase activity is enhanced, and fat is mobilized by conversion to free fatty acids which circulate through the blood. The ketone bodies that result from the breakdown of free fatty acids eventually lead to acidosis because the ketone bodies are naturally acidic. This acidosis can lead to deep and labored breathing, sometimes called "air hunger" or Kussmaul breathing. The breath will have a fruity acetone odor. Ketones can also depress the CNS, resulting in coma and death if insulin is not administered.

Noninsulin-Dependent (Type II) Diabetics

Whereas Type I diabetes typically has a rapid onset with the usual signs of polyuria, polyphagia, polydipsia, weakness, weight loss, and dry skin, Type II diabetes frequently is unaccompanied by any symptoms (21). Type II diabetes (Figure 2) is discovered most often when glucose is found in the urine or when elevated blood glucose is found on a routine examination. Careful study of this older, obese group of diabetics reveals glucosuria, proteinuria, postprandial hyperglycemia, microaneurysms, and even retinal exudates.

The most interesting abnormal finding in obese Type II diabetics is that they have normal or even greater than normal blood insulin levels. Glucose is transported into muscle and fat cells and, therefore, these patients are not ketosis prone and seldom develop ketoacidosis. However, because of their high blood glucose levels, they may develop nonketotic hyperglycemic coma. Increased obesity in these patients may cause hyperinsulinemia, resulting in fewer insulin receptors and thus producing the clinical finding of hyperglycemia. Weight reduction to an ideal body weight allows the blood glucose levels of most Type II patients to return to normal (21).

Consequences of Diabetic Disease

Diabetics frequently develop kidney failure (nephropathy), lesions of the eye (retinopathy), and atrophy of the peripheral nerves (neuropathy). Generally, these processes occur because the walls of the capillaries that supply these areas with blood and nutrients thicken. The molecular mechanisms leading to these late complications of diabetes have not been established conclusively (22, 23).

Over the years there has been considerable debate on whether the lesions that develop within the diabetic's

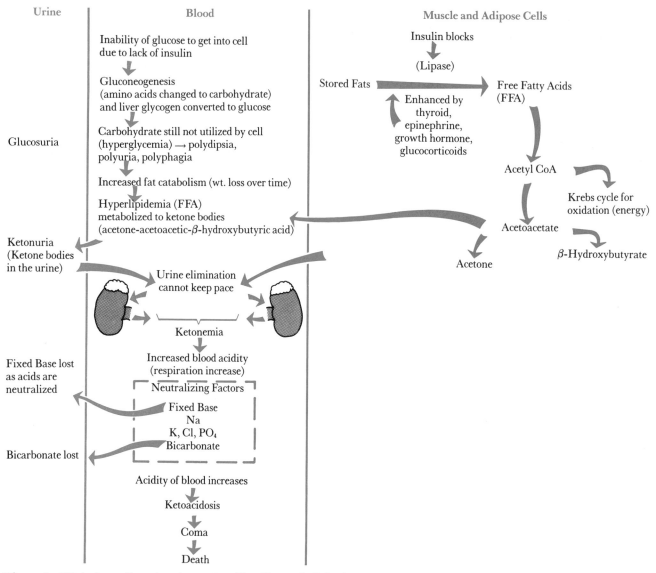

Figure 1. Clinical manifestations in untreated insulinopenic diabetics.

retina, kidneys, nerves, and vascular system are due to a disorder in the structure and function of blood vessels or whether they are a consequence of prolonged hyperglycemia caused by inadequate metabolic control (22, 24). Today few physicians believe that microvascular complications occur independently of hyperglycemia and insulin deficiency and that control of metabolic events is not a factor in their progress. There is substantial evidence that supports the concept that the microvascular complications of diabetes are decreased by reduction of blood glucose concentrations (22, 23). Because of these findings, there is a renewed emphasis on strict, but reasonable, control to prevent severe diabetic complications.

Disturbances in polyol and glycoprotein metabolism have been implicated in diabetic neuropathy (23). During periods of hyperglycemia, neuronal intracellular glucose concentrations rise because nerve tissue does not require insulin for glucose uptake. Aldose reductase and sorbitol dehydrogenase are two enzymes utilized in non-insulin-dependent pathway of metabolizing glucose

that produces abnormally high amounts of fructose and sorbitol. These enzymes normally involved in glucose metabolism became saturated with glucose, and other metabolic pathways, such as the polyol pathway, metabolize the excess glucose, thus increasing sorbitol levels.

Both sorbitol and fructose have been found in increased amounts in the nerves of hyperglycemic diabetic animals. The accumulation of these polyols could produce osmotic injury to the nerve with myoinositol depletion. It has been demonstrated that either elimination of hyperglycemia by insulin or exogenous repletion of myoinositol prevents the development of diabetic neuropathy in experimental diabetic animals. In addition, it was clinically demonstrated that when acutely elevated blood glucose levels in diabetics are normalized, symptoms of neuropathy may be more severe and then disappear (22, 23).

The basic morphologic lesion of diabetic micro-angiopathy is widespread thickening of capillary basement membranes. The direct cause of this thickening is unknown; however, since basement membranes are composed of collagen-like glycoproteins whose synthesis is controlled by both post-transcriptional and genetic factors, environmental influences could be important. Increased capillary permeability, which occurs early in human diabetes, may be normalized by control of hyperglycemia and may worsen with deterioration of control. Other abnormalities of glycoprotein metabolism have been found in both Type I and Type II diabetics. These findings include increased levels of a minor hemoglobin component, hemoglobin A_1c, which now is used clinically to monitor diabetes control (23). Hemoglobin A_1c levels reflect mean blood glucose concentration over a period of weeks and are sensitive in assessing cumulative control of hyperglycemia (25). Capillary basement membrane thickening may represent only one facet of a generalized abnormality in glycoprotein metabolism due to hyperglycemia or other sequelae of insulin deficiency or absence.

Atherosclerotic lesions in the diabetic appear to be the same as those in the nondiabetic, but they develop earlier, occur more often, and generally are more severe. It has been suggested that lower than normal levels of plasma high-density lipoproteins may be contributory factors. Atherosclerotic lesions produce symptoms in various areas. Peripheral lesions may cause intermittent claudication, gangrene, and impotence. Widespread disease of small vessels is common. Coronary heart disease and stroke may complicate the disease. Cardiomyopathy and silent myocardial infarction may also occur in diabetics (26). Hyperglycemia may impair the phagocytic activity of the body's white blood cells. Most chronic adverse conditions in the diabetic can be traced to an inadequate blood supply to the area. Besides the vascular and nerve changes that can take place in diabetics with prolonged hyperglycemia, diabetics frequently experience difficulty in eradicating bacterial infections (27).

Type I and Type II diabetics also suffer from occlusive vascular changes in the lower extremities as a result of both atherosclerosis and damage to smaller arteries (microangiopathies). After age 40, the incidence of gangrene in the feet is 50 times greater in diabetics than in nondiabetics (27).

In insulinotardic diabetics, hyperglycemia results after food ingestion. As with Type II diabetics, prolonged hyperglycemia may result in serious complications. However, in insulinotardic diabetics, the beta-cells eventually respond and release insulin. Consequently, the symptoms that bring the insulinotardic patient to the physician often are those of hypoglycemia (fatigue, weakness, nervousness, anxiety, trembling, headache, sweating, hunger, dizziness, nausea, visual disturbances, tingling of the tongue or lips, unsteadiness, drowsiness, and mental confusion).

Screening for Diabetes

The pharmacist's role in promoting and supporting diabetes detection programs cannot be overstressed. During the screening program, as well as at other times, the pharmacist should be able to answer any questions that the diabetic patient may have. In a 3-week period, the pharmacist may see up to 70% of the community residents; this contact provides an excellent opportunity to screen patients for diabetes. Possible diabetics can then be referred to physicians for a complete physical examination, history, and laboratory analysis (28).

If all pharmacists set aside 1 day each month to screen patients for diabetes, they would have a substantial impact on detecting the more than 2 million undiagnosed diabetics in the United States. The actual screening itself is quite simple. Dextrostix, alcohol swabs, lancets, literature, and an analyzing machine to test Dextrostix color changes (Dextrometer) are all that is needed. Pharmacists interested in diabetes-screening programs or in diabetic patient education can find assistance from the sources listed in Appendix 1, "Information for Pharmacists."

One screening program involves taking a blood sample from the subject's finger or earlobe. The blood is then analyzed instrumentally, using a blood glucose analyzer. In some states, only licensed medical technicians, registered nurses, or physicians may withdraw blood from patients legally. Contact with a volunteer nurses' association may be of value in launching a screening program (28).

Several criteria can be used by the pharmacist to select patients for a screening program. Patients with all types of cardiac problems, including high blood pres-

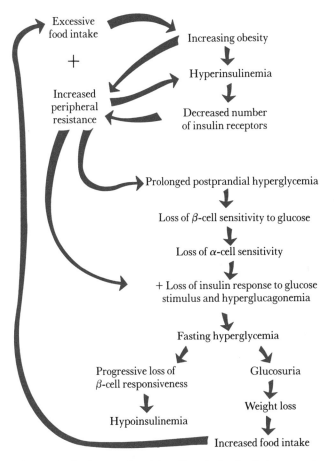

Figure 2. Pathogenesis of insulinoplethoric diabetes mellitus.

sure, stroke, congestive heart failure, and angina, have a higher incidence of diabetes. Diabetes is also more common in patients who have suffered from hyperthyroidism, Addison's disease, and Cushing's syndrome. At least 75% of all diabetics have relatives with diabetes. Approximately 80% of diabetics in the 40–65-year-old age group are overweight (29).

Symptoms

The pharmacist should obtain a careful patient history before attempting an evaluation. In addition to the more common symptoms of diabetes (polydipsia, polyphagia, and polyuria), there are several other symptoms that the pharmacist should be aware of in detecting potential diabetics; these symptoms follow. Pharmacists who detect these medical problems should refer the patient to a physician who specializes in treating diabetes.

Weight Loss

Weight loss when eating regular meals is a sign of diabetes. Other conditions that cause this phenomenon are hyperthyroidism, cancer, anorexia nervosa, and other chronic diseases.

Recurrent Monilial Infections

This condition is common in diabetics, especially fungal infections of the vulva and anus in women. Chronic skin infections, carbuncles, furuncles, and eczema are also more common in diabetics.

Gout

The percentage of patients with gout who have diabetes (5–10%) is higher than the norm. Thus, patients with gout are at higher risk and should be screened for diabetes.

Prolonged Wound Healing

Minor cuts and scratches take at least twice as long to heal in a diabetic.

Visual Disturbances

These may be the only symptoms the diabetic experiences early in the disease; patients who wear glasses may notice that increasingly stronger lenses are required at relatively short time intervals. Ophthalmologists detect a large number of diabetic patients (27). Cataracts and open-angle glaucoma in older diabetics are common. Research suggests that an increased level of sorbitol may result in the frequency of cataracts seen in diabetic patients. Sorbitol is the intermediate in the metabolism of glucose to fructose by the polyol pathway. Sorbitol poorly diffuses out of the cell and accumulates in certain tissues when hyperglycemia is present. This fact and reduced nucleotide and ketone levels contribute to the pathologic changes in diabetes mellitus. Cataract formation occurs due to the high sugar alcohol concentration in the lens, which causes an influx of water and eventual disruption of lens fiber membranes.

Psychologic Changes

Some of the first symptoms of hypoglycemia affecting the nervous system are irritability, nervousness, and anxiety. Generalized fatigue and depression occur more often in diabetics. Frequent emotional flare-ups may signal that the body's biochemistry is not normal, possibly because of diabetes.

Laboratory Diagnosis

If a patient has glucose in the urine or higher than normal glucose in the blood or presents with one or more of the symptoms of diabetes, the physician should administer an oral glucose tolerance test or other appropriate screening test. Patients with borderline oral glucose tolerance tests should be rechecked periodically, especially when they become symptomatic.

Other tests used as diagnostic or screening tests for diabetes include the fasting blood sugar, the 2-hour postprandial blood glucose test, and the hemoglobin A_1c.

Nondiabetic causes of glucose intolerance include liver disease, prolonged physical inactivity, acute stress, fever, trauma, surgery, heart attack, starvation, hypokalemia, renal disease, and endocrine diseases. A positive test for glucose in the urine is not necessarily diagnostic for diabetes, but it is an indication for more definitive testing. Glucosuria is symptomatic of many other conditions such as pregnancy or impaired renal function. Glucosuria generally occurs when the blood glucose level is 180 mg/100 ml or greater and rarely occurs when it is less than 130 mg/100 ml (31). The renal threshold for glucose increases with age, so that older diabetics may not demonstrate glucosuria despite a high blood glucose level.

Treatment

The objectives of diabetic control in order of importance are relief of diabetic symptoms, avoidance of hypoglycemic reactions, maintenance of optimal weight, maintenance of blood glucose between 80 and 130 mg/100 ml before meals and between 130 and 230 mg/100 ml after meals, production of little or no glucosuria, and the prevention of ketoacidosis (32). These objectives can be met only through the combined efforts of the physician, nurse, dietician, pharmacist, and patient. Sulfonylureas, insulin, and diet are used to control the condition, and nonprescription products formulated especially for use by the diabetic patient are helpful. Diet, exercise, and insulin must be delicately balanced in Type I patients and calories restricted in Type II patients. Multiple injections or the use of an insulin infusion pump improve control with fewer complications. Strict control of blood glucose levels may delay the late complications of diabetes (33–38).

Diabetic Medicines

The medicines used to treat diabetes can be categorized into two broad areas: oral hypoglycemic agents and insulin. The use of oral hypoglycemic agents has been controversial from the standpoint of effectiveness and long-term side effects. However, when used properly, they are both safe and effective. Pharmacists should monitor patients using oral hypoglycemic agents for reactions with products that can cause either hypoglycemia or hyperglycemia, which may affect diabetic con-

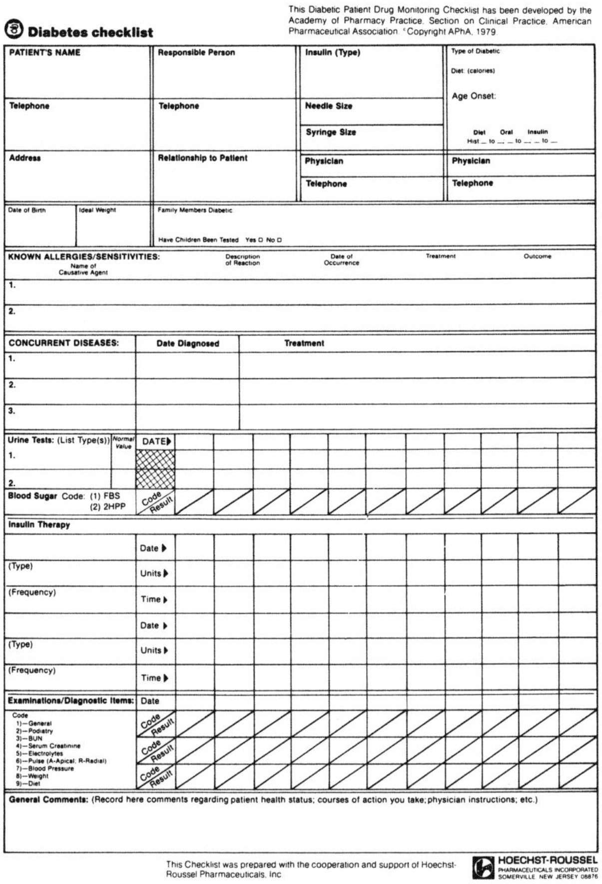
Diabetes checklist

This Diabetic Patient Drug Monitoring Checklist has been developed by the Academy of Pharmacy Practice, Section on Clinical Practice, American Pharmaceutical Association. ©Copyright APhA, 1979

PATIENT'S NAME	Responsible Person	Insulin (Type)	Type of Diabetic / Diet (calories) / Age Onset:
Telephone	Telephone	Needle Size / Syringe Size	Diet Oral Insulin Hist _ to _ to _ to _
Address	Relationship to Patient	Physician / Telephone	Physician / Telephone
Date of Birth / Ideal Weight	Family Members Diabetic / Have Children Been Tested Yes □ No □		

KNOWN ALLERGIES/SENSITIVITIES: Name of Causative Agent / Description of Reaction / Date of Occurrence / Treatment / Outcome
1.
2.

CONCURRENT DISEASES: / Date Diagnosed / Treatment
1.
2.
3.

Urine Tests: (List Type(s)) / Normal Value / DATE
1.
2.
Blood Sugar Code: (1) FBS (2) 2HPP / Code / Result

Insulin Therapy
(Type) (Frequency) Date / Units / Time
(Type) (Frequency) Date / Units / Time

Examinations/Diagnostic Items: Date
Code
1)—General
2)—Podiatry
3)—BUN
4)—Serum Creatinine
5)—Electrolytes
6)—Pulse (A-Apical, R-Radial)
7)—Blood Pressure
8)—Weight
9)—Diet
Code / Result

General Comments: (Record here comments regarding patient health status; courses of action you take; physician instructions; etc.)

This Checklist was prepared with the cooperation and support of Hoechst-Roussel Pharmaceuticals, Inc.
HOECHST-ROUSSEL PHARMACEUTICALS INCORPORATED SOMERVILLE, NEW JERSEY 08876

Figure 3. Diabetic patient drug monitoring checklist.

trol. A diabetic patient drug monitoring checklist (Figure 3) can be used by the pharmacist to monitor all aspects of a diabetic patient's treatment.

Although insulin must be prescribed initially by a physician, pharmacists frequently are the health care professionals consulted concerning problems. Therefore, pharmacists should be familiar with the various strengths and sources of insulin and with different onsets and durations of action.

Oral Hypoglycemic Agents

Although this chapter deals with nonprescription products used in diabetes, the pharmacist's understanding of the proper use of sulfonylureas is necessary.

Sulfonylureas stimulate insulin secretion by the pancreas and possibly increase the number of insulin receptors. The four products used in the United States are summarized in Table 3, plus glyburide, which will soon be available. The differences in metabolism of each sulfonylurea account for clinical differences with reference to the onset and duration of action.

The most common side effect with the sulfonylureas is hypoglycemia. Frequent "drug-drug" interactions resulting in enhanced hypoglycemia occur with alcohol, anabolic steroids, chloramphenicol, dicumarol, monoamine oxidase inhibitors, phenylbutazone, propranolol, salicylates, and sulfonamides (31). Drugs that may interfere with diabetes control by causing hyperglycemia include asparaginase, clonidine, corticosteroids, dextrothyroxine, diazoxide, ethacrynic acid, furosemide, glucagon, levodopa, lithium, niacin (high doses), oral contraceptives, phenytoin, probenecid, sympathomimetic amines, thiazide diuretics, and tricyclic antidepressants (16, 31).

Chlorpropamide is the most potent sulfonylurea in use in the United States. It can cause an increased sensitivity to circulating levels of antidiuretic hormone in approximately 4% of patients (39, 40). The chlorpropamide-induced inappropriate antidiuretic hormone activity is reversible. Improvement occurs within a week after the medication is discontinued. In insulinotardic and insulinoplethoric diabetics, diet is the main method of treatment, and sulfonylureas should be used only when diet fails. The physician should determine what constitutes dietary failure.

Conditions in which oral antidiabetic agents are usually contraindicated include acidosis, severe infections accompanying diabetic onset, major surgery (during and after), sulfa sensitivity, and pregnancy.

Pharmacists dispensing sulfonylureas should explain to the patient that the medication is used to treat diabetes and that it is important to take the medication regularly, exactly as prescribed by the physician. If the patient develops adverse drug reactions to the sulfonylureas, such as sore throat, fever, mouth sores, or dark-colored urine, the physician should be contacted. The pharmacist should advise the patient to use alcoholic beverages and drugs containing salicylates cautiously and stress the necessity of using the product in conjunction with the prescribed diet (41, 42). Pharmacists should be aware that approximately 40% of noninsulin-dependent diabetics do not achieve satisfactory control with oral agents. Secondary failures occur in patients who initially respond to oral agents but subsequently fail to be adequately controlled. The secondary failure rate ranges from 3% to 30%. This failure rate tends to increase year after year for patients experiencing initial satisfactory control. The continuous satisfactory control rate is approximately 20–30% (43).

The University Group Diabetes Program (UGDP) cooperative study concluded that tolbutamide was no more effective than diet alone in the treatment of diabetes. Those patients treated with tolbutamide had a significantly higher rate of cardiac deaths than control subjects. The validity of the study has been extensively questioned. Despite the reported findings, many physicians continue to advocate the use of the oral sulfonylureas for selected noninsulin-dependent diabetics. Sulfonylureas also are possible teratogens; they should not be used early in pregnancy and are absolutely contraindicated late in gestation, since they may cause prolonged and severe hypoglycemia (42).

Insulin

Type I diabetics who have absolute insulin deficiency must be treated with exogenous insulin. Generally, persons who require insulin initially tend to be younger than 30, lean, prone to developing ketoacidosis, and markedly hyperglycemic, even in the fasting state (21). Insulin is also indicated for adult-onset diabetics with

Table 3. Basic biopharmaceutics and pharmacokinetics of the oral hypoglycemics

	Recommended dose (g)	Maximum dose (g)	Half-life (hours)	Onset (hours)	Duration (hours)	Metabolism and excretion	Comments
Tolbutamide (Orinase)	0.5–3.0 divided doses	2–3	5.6	1	6–12	Totally metabolized to inactive form; inactive metabolite excreted in kidney	Generally first drug of choice; most benign; least potent; short half-life; especially useful in kidney disease
Acetohexamide (Dymelor)	0.25–1.5 single or divided doses	1.5	5	1	10–14	Metabolite's activity equal to or greater than parent compound; metabolite excreted by kidney	Essentially no advantage over tolbutamide, although a few patients who fail on tolbutamide are controlled; significant uricosuric effects
Tolazamide (Tolinase)	0.1–1.0 single or divided doses	0.75–1.0	7	4–6	10–14	Absorbed slowly; metabolite active but less potent than parent compound; excreted by kidney	Essentially no advantage over tolbutamide; said to be equipotent with less severe side effects
Chlorpropamide (Diabinese)	0.1–0.5 single dose	0.5	35	1	72	Previously thought not to be metabolized but recently found that metabolism may be quite extensive; significant percentage excreted unchanged	Most potent in use; caution in elderly patients and those with kidney disease; disulfiram-like reactions may occur with alcohol
Glyburide[a] (Diabeta, Micronase)	0.005–0.01 single or divided doses	0.02	Biphasic 3.2 + 10	1.5	24	50% absorbed; completely metabolized in liver to nonactive derivatives; excreted in urine and bile 1:1	50–200 times more potent than other agents; good for kidney-diseased patients; no disulfiram reaction; low toxicity

[a]Approval by FDA expected soon.

insulinopenia who do not respond to diet therapy, either alone or combined with oral hypoglycemic drugs (19). Insulin therapy is necessary in some Type II diabetic patients who are subjected to stresses such as infections, pregnancy, and surgery. Occasionally in Type II diabetics, doses of 10–20 units of intermediate-acting insulins are needed to bring hyperglycemia under control. Thus, all classes of diabetics should be trained to inject themselves with insulin.

Diabetic children should begin giving themselves their own injections at around 8–9, although parents should administer one or two injections each week to stay in practice and should inject in areas difficult for the child to reach (44, 45). By combining the appropriate modification of diet, exercise, and variable mixtures of short- and longer-acting insulins, it has been possible to achieve acceptable control of blood glucose (19).

Use in Ketoacidosis   Diabetic ketoacidosis constitutes an acute medical emergency, necessitating immediate diagnosis and therapy. It accounts for less than 1% of the deaths occurring in the diabetic population; however, the mortality associated with these acute episodes is 5–15%, indicating the need for strict attention to detail and management (46). The physician can diagnose diabetic ketoacidosis rapidly by assessing urinary glucose and ketones, arterial blood pH and blood gases, and serum ketone and glucose values.

Shock and cerebral edema are among the complications encountered in diabetic ketoacidosis. Shock generally develops as a consequence of life-threatening stress such as sepsis, myocardial infarction, or acute pancreatitis (46). Treatment is directed at plasma volume expansion and correction of acidosis and hypotension. Low-dose intravenous insulin regimens are recommended to treat diabetic ketoacidosis and nonketotic hyperosmolar coma. Regular insulin is the only insulin useful in treating ketoacidosis (24).

Insulin Preparations The insulins are divided into three groups, according to their duration of action. Short-acting insulins include semilente and regular insulin. Intermediate-acting insulins include NPH, lente, and globin zinc insulin. The long-acting insulins include protamine zinc and ultralente insulin. Lente insulin is a combination of 70% ultralente and 30% semilente insulin. The NPH insulin is a combination of two parts regular insulin and one part protamine zinc insulin.

In March 1980 the Food and Drug Administration decertified U-80 insulin, leaving two strengths of insulin available for diabetic patients: U-40 and U-100. Some patients who use small insulin doses still prefer U-40 insulin, but manufacturers, the FDA, and the American Diabetes Association with the support of the American Pharmaceutical Association are attempting to convert all patients to U-100 insulins. Standardizing the strengths should help to eliminate errors resulting from the use of incorrectly calibrated syringes and to reduce confusion in mixing insulins. Insulin vials and syringes are color coded to lessen these errors and to aid in identification. The U-40 insulin vials (40 units/ml) and the syringes designed to be used with U-40 insulins are color coded red; U-100 insulin vials and syringes are color coded orange with black lettering.

Methods to increase the duration of action of regular insulin include the addition of zinc, protein molecules, and acetate buffers. Globin, NPH, and protamine zinc are examples of insulins in which zinc and proteins have been added. The lente insulins result in longer- or shorter-acting types of insulin when the amounts of acetate buffer and zinc added to the insulin are varied.

All insulins except globin have a neutral pH; globin insulin has an acid pH. All regular insulins are at a normal pH of 7.4. Regular and globin insulins are clear solutions, but all other available insulins are cloudy suspensions.

Clinical Considerations in Insulin Use The animal from which the insulin is derived can influence its effect on blood glucose control and insulin resistance and sensitivity (47). Most commercially available insulins are derived from a mixture of beef and pork, although pure pork or pure beef insulin is available. High purification of pork insulin is clinically important in reducing insulin dose, lipoatrophy (subcutaneous concavities caused by a wasting of the lipid tissue), and insulin-binding capacity of serum. About 80% of the patients with persistent local allergy to mixed beef-pork insulin improve if treated with pure pork insulin (9). Beef insulin has greater antigenicity because it differs from human insulin by three amino acids; pork differs by only one amino acid (9). Biosynthetic human insulin has been developed by the Eli Lilly Company and is now being tested. It should be less antigenic than other sources of insulin.

Another factor that affects insulin use in diabetic patients is purity. New analytical techniques using chromatography and electrophoresis to separate and isolate proteins have made purer forms of insulin readily available. The average content of certain minor components of insulin, such as proinsulin, desamido insulin, arginine insulin, esterified insulin, and glucagon has been decreased, resulting in fewer insulin sensitivity reactions. The new forms of insulin often are referred to as "single-peak" insulins because their spectrophotometric curves show lower amounts of noninsulin protein material and increased amounts of insulin. The purity of insulins has been improved from 92% to approximately 98% (21). It is possible to purify insulin to the "monocomponent" insulin (99% pure) level, but a preparation of this purity is seldom required.

In 1980, Novo and Nordisk Laboratories, two foreign manufacturers of insulin, as well as Eli Lilly and Company, introduced the more purified forms of insulin in the United States. The purity of these new insulins is based on the amount of proinsulin. The newer insulins have less than 10 ppm of proinsulin. One study showed that this purified type of insulin produces less antigenicty and, in the average patient, allows a 15% decrease in dose (48). E. R. Squibb & Sons, Inc., purchases its insulin from Novo Laboratories and has primarily purified insulins available.

Diabetic patients who demonstrate a sensitivity to insulin usually develop redness at the injection site. When a diabetic initially begins taking insulin, these reactions are quite common and may occur over several weeks before gradually subsiding. If the reactions continue, however, they may be treated with an antihistamine such as diphenhydramine.

Insulin resistance, a state requiring more than 200 units/day of insulin for more than 2 days in the absence of ketoacidosis or acute infection, occurs only in about 0.001% of diabetic patients. These patients almost invariably have high titers of insulin-neutralizing antibodies. Glucocorticoids are indicated (60–80 mg/day prednisone) (49). Purified pork insulin (Iletin II) is also recommended.

Another factor that can affect the clinical use of insulin preparations is how they are administered parenterally (50). Insulin injection by the intramuscular route provides faster insulin absorption with a concomitant greater drop in plasma glucose than does injection by the subcutaneous route. Intravenous insulin produces the highest pharmacologic level of insulin in the least time.

Insulin absorption is affected by exercise. Leg exercise accelerates insulin absorption from the leg. Arm or abdominal injection avoids the acceleration during leg exercise and reduces exercise-induced hypoglycemia (51). Thus, a diabetic whose day includes a hard game of tennis might do well to inject that day's insulin into the abdomen rather than into the arm or leg (52, 53). If more than 60 units of insulin are injected at one site, there is potential for erratic absorption. Thus, patients receiving large doses of insulin should either split the doses and inject in two different sites or should be monitored closely (54).

Another complication of insulin therapy is insulin lipodystrophy. Lipodystrophy occurs in two forms: lipoatrophy (the breakdown of subcutaneous fatty tissue, leaving hollowed areas under the skin) and lipohypertrophy (the hyperdevelopment of fatty tissue, causing bulges under the skin) (55). Lipodystrophic changes usually are unattractive and may be difficult for the patient to accept. Lipoatrophy improves in the majority of patients when purified pork insulin is substituted for less purified forms (56, 57). Lipohypertrophy is generally seen in patients who use the same sites for repeated insulin injection. However, it may decrease insulin absorption from the affected site. This condition provides one of the main reasons for educating patients to rotate their injection sites.

Mixing and Storage   Neutral regular insulin may be mixed with NPH or lente insulin in any proportion desired. The NPH-regular combination and the lente mixed with regular are stable for only 5 minutes (54). Regular insulin may be added to protamine zinc insulin. However, because of the excess protamine in protamine zinc insulin, mixtures in a ratio of less than 1:1 have the same activity as protamine zinc insulin alone. As the proportion of regular to protamine zinc insulin approaches 2:1, a time-activity curve approximating that of NPH insulin is obtained. When the ratio exceeds 2:1 (that is, when the amount of regular insulin is increased further), the time-activity of the mixture approaches that of a regular NPH combination.

Regular and protamine zinc insulin should be mixed just before injection. Semilente, ultralente, and lente insulins may be combined in any ratio desired at any time. Because of excess globin molecules in globin insulin, mixing with regular insulin produces globin insulin and therefore has no advantage.

Regular insulin may be mixed in any proportion with normal saline for use in an infusion pump, but the combination should be used within 2–3 hours after mixing, since pH changes and dilution of buffer may affect stability. Regular insulin may be mixed with Lilly's Insulin Diluting Fluid in any proportion and will be stable indefinitely. Diabetic patients using insulin infusion pumps may use either normal saline or Lilly's Insulin Diluting Fluid to dilute the insulin used in the pump. However, the mixture is more stable using the insulin diluting fluid than with normal saline.

As the purity of insulins has improved, the problem of stability in mixing insulins has decreased. However, two mixtures of insulin requiring special attention are the combination of regular insulin with lente insulin and regular insulin with NPH. In general, these insulins should be used within 5 minutes after mixing to ensure the proper effect (54).

Because insulin is a heat-labile protein, care must be exercised in storing all preparations so that potency and maximum stability will be maintained. Insulin's potency is not significantly decreased if stored at temperatures of 68–75° F. Color changes may be associated with a denaturation of protein and should be interpreted as evidence of potency loss. At 100° F all insulins lose a significant amount of potency within 1–2 months. Patients may keep vials of insulin currently in use out of the refrigerator. Insulin should be stored in a cool area, away from radiators or sunny windows. When traveling in warm climates, insulin should either be kept in a cooler or packed between several layers of clothing in a suitcase (58). With regular insulin, loss of potency begins after 18 months if the insulin is kept at room temperature. With regular insulin there is an increase in the rate of potency loss as the temperature increases. The lente forms of insulin retain their potency when stored at room temperature for 24 months, but signs of loss of potency such as discoloration and clumping may occur after 30 months. With NPH and protamine zinc insulin, loss of potency does not occur at room temperature for up to 36 months. Thus, insulins are stable unrefrigerated for long periods. However, the pharmacist should advise patients to keep extra bottles of insulin in the refrigerator and keep the bottle in current use at room temperature.

Higher temperatures may cause the suspensions of insulin (NPH, protamine zinc, and lente) to clump. Potency is not necessarily lost, but there is a problem in drawing up the correct dose when clumping has occurred. Freezing also may cause clumping but does not necessarily affect potency (24). Injection of insulin at room temperature is recommended because refrigerator-temperature insulin produces more pain.

Adverse Reactions   The major complication of insulin therapy is hypoglycemia. Factors predisposing the patient to insulin reactions include insufficient food intake (skipping meals, vomiting, or diarrhea), excessive exercise, inaccurate measurement of insulin, concomitant intake of hypoglycemic drugs, or termination of the diabetogenic conditions. Symptoms include a parasympathetic response (nausea, hunger, or flatulence), diminished cerebral function (confusion, agitation, lethargy, or personality changes), sympathetic responses (tachycardia, sweating, or tremor), coma, and convulsions. Ataxia and blurred vision are common (59). In elderly patients with decreased nerve function, diabetes with advanced neuropathy, or patients receiving beta-blockers, the symptoms of hypoglycemia are sometimes lacking, and the reaction may go undetected and untreated. All manifestations of hypoglycemia are relieved rapidly by glucose administration.

Because of the potential danger of insulin reactions, the diabetic patient should always carry packets of table sugar or a candy roll for use at the onset of hypoglycemic symptoms. Patients may also drink orange juice or any sugar-containing beverage or food. An ampule of glucagon (1 mg) should be provided to every insulin-dependent diabetic to be injected by family or friends in case of unconsciousness. Pharmacists should be familiar with the mixing technique for glucagon and be able to instruct patients. Glucagon should be reconstituted with the accompanying solvent, and 0.5–1.0 mg should be administered in the same manner as insulin. Normally, the patient will regain consciousness within 5–10 minutes and be able to swallow some sweetened water. If there is no response after 5–10 minutes, a second injection may be given. If the response is still insufficient, more intensive treatment is indicated. The patient should be taken to an emergency room or physician immediately (60).

If a hypoglycemic person is mistakenly thought to be hyperglycemic and given insulin, severe hypoglycemia and subsequent brain damage may result. When there is doubt whether a diabetic is hypoglycemic or hyperglycemic, sugar should be given initially until the condition can be evaluated accurately.

Nondrug Therapy

One objective in maintaining diabetic control is maintaining normal weight. The pharmacist should stress the importance of proper exercise and diet.

Exercise

Although exercise is nearly always recommended by physicians as part of the treatment of diabetes, it is seldom prescribed. Physicians should prescribe an individualized daily exercise schedule for diabetic patients. Exercise lowers blood glucose by allowing glucose to penetrate the muscle cell and be metabolized without the assistance of insulin. Glucose may be utilized to varying degrees without insulin in all types of cells (17).

Exercise also improves circulatory function, an important factor in diabetic management; helps maintain normal body weight; and aids breathing, digestion, and metabolism. An exercise log may help the patient maintain a regular daily schedule. Patients who monitor their own blood glucose become motivated to exercise because they easily see the beneficial effects of exercise on maintaining good blood glucose control.

Diet

Diet is the most critical treatment in Type II diabetics and, in combination with exercise and insulin, is a necessary treatment for Type I diabetics (61). However, diet therapy failure occurs often and creates feelings of frustration, pessimism, failure, and anger, which in turn result in poorly informed and inadequately motivated patients (62). This is an area where the pharmacist can have strong impact by providing patient education on proper diet and nutrition.

Factors in Dietary Control Successful diet programs require behavior modification on the part of the patient. Patients should be encouraged to join groups such as Weight Watchers and to keep a diet log similar to the exercise log. They should record (for 4–10 days) each time they eat, how much they eat, and why they eat, whether food ingestion was due to social pressure, loneliness, depression, nervousness, or the time of day, or whether the patient truly needed nourishment. By having patients use smaller plates, take only one helping of food, and try to be conscious of why they eat, it is possible to change their dietary behavior (63). In addition, diet support groups can be of help in modifying behavior.

One reason for diet therapy failure in diabetics is that physicians or dieticians prescribe changes in diet without first adjusting the dose of insulin or oral agents. The first step in diet therapy should be to prescribe an exercise program, lower the medication dose, and put the patient on a diet containing fewer calories.

Insulin overtreatment is probably one of the most common causes of inadequate diabetic control and weight gain (64). In one group of diabetic patients, 75% needed a reduction in insulin dose of at least 10%; 35% of the overtreated patients had large appetites, and 30% had hepatomegaly and headaches (64). Diabetic patients should be educated to determine whether or not they have involved themselves in a vicious cycle of taking too much insulin and then consuming food up to that level of insulin.

The pharmacist has a supportive role to play in diet therapy. Pharmacists need to encourage diabetic patients to follow the prescribed diet and should discourage prolonged fasting or using fad diets to lose weight. Patients should obtain dietician or physician approval for any change in dietary habits. The pharmacist should caution diabetic patients that "dietetic" labeling of products does not mean "diabetic." Patients should be encouraged to read the labels of all foods marked "dietetic" because the foods may not be sugarless or even intended for diabetics. Some dietetic foods actually have more calories than regular food.

Artificial Sweeteners In general, there are two ways in which food may be adapted or prepared for the diabetic: by restricting the sugar content and by restricting both the sugar content and caloric value (65). In preparing special foods, sucrose is omitted, and other sweetening agents may be substituted. The safety of some of these substitutes often has been questioned. Saccharin, which is 400 times as sweet as sucrose, is the most common sucrose substitute in the United States. Because it has been implicated in causing malignant tumors in rats, the FDA requires a warning on all products containing saccharin. The FDA also requires all retail establishments selling saccharin-containing products to display a warning statement concerning saccharin. Cyclamates are used as a sugar substitute in other countries and eventually may be permitted back on U.S. markets, since little evidence of harm to humans has been documented (65).

Sorbitol is a glucose alcohol that is 60% as sweet as sugar. It is absorbed slowly from the gut with little effect on the blood glucose levels. Sorbitol is without side effects unless large quantities are taken, when osmotic effects may cause diarrhea and abdominal discomfort. However, it is converted to glucose and metabolized, and its energy value as calories must be counted for patients in whom weight control is necessary. Sorbitol is one of the end products of the polyol pathway of glucose metabolism that results in some of the late complications of diabetes. However, the amount in foods is not considered to be a risk factor to diabetics unless very large amounts are consumed.

Fructose is another sucrose substitute that is an end product of glucose metabolism by insulin-independent pathways and thus has a potential for adding to the late complications of diabetes (65). The American Diabetes Association warns diabetic patients that fructose has the same caloric content as table sugar (66). Diabetics planning to use fructose as a substitute sweetener should first consult with their physician (66). A summary statement by the American Diabetes Association on the use of fructose, sorbitol, and xylitol as sugar substitutes concludes: "The day-long quantitative reduction of hyperglycemia that may result from substantial substitution of these sweeteners for glucose and sucrose in the diabetic diet, and the long-term effectiveness and safety when they are ingested in substantial quantities and mixed meals, has not been established" (66).

The G. D. Searle Company has been given approval to manufacture aspartame. Aspartame is a combination of two naturally occurring amino acids. The agent is 200 times sweeter than sugar and yields only one-tenth of a calorie/tsp.

Dietary Cautions The aim of dietary treatment in diabetes is to control weight and blood glucose levels and to prevent the development and progression of vascular complications. Because about 75% of the deaths among diabetics are due to cardiovascular disease, compared with 50% of deaths in the general population, diabetics should avoid dietary factors, such as animal fats, which have been shown to result in cardiovascular disease (67). The American Diabetes Association has recommended a diet that contains 50% carbohydrates, 20% protein, and no more than 35% fat. Cholesterol is also restricted to less than 300 mg/day. Simple and refined sugars should be avoided in all diabetics because of the stress put on the patient (19). Complex carbohydrates are recommended since they are slowly broken down to simple carbohydrates and require smaller quantities of insulin. Simple carbohydrates produce a rapid increase in blood glucose and stress on the pancreas.

Many diabetic patients believe that since diabetes results in increased blood glucose levels, carbohydrates in general should be avoided. One long-term clinical trial showed that an increased proportion of dietary carbohydrate (bread, potatoes, or rice and not simple sugars) does not cause deterioration of diabetic control, provided that the total calories are limited to maintain or achieve ideal body weight (19). Diabetic patients who follow their diet therapy are able to keep their serum triglyceride and serum cholesterol levels within a normal range (19). Restriction of saturated fats and avoidance of pie, sugar, syrups, candy, alcoholic beverages, sweetened soft drinks, and cake are advised for all diabetics.

Diabetic patients who use a well-planned diet do not require vitamin supplements on a routine basis. However, supplemental vitamins and minerals may be useful in cases of imbalanced diets, malnutrition, illness, or surgery.

Patients taking vitamin supplements that contain high amounts of ascorbic acid should keep in mind that these vitamins may affect urine test values (false-positive results with Clinitest and false-negative results with glucose oxidase stick tests).

A high-fiber diet is valuable in the diabetic patient. Adequate dietary roughage reduces intraluminal pressure in the bowel and decreases the absorption rate of saccharides (61). When guar and pectin, components of dietary fiber, were added to a carbohydrate meal, the postprandial rise of blood glucose was delayed significantly (68). Fiber does not have miraculous weight-controlling properties. It simply makes it easier for a person to take in fewer calories without feeling hungry. Patients changing to a high-fiber diet should be warned to do it gradually. A sudden large increase may cause temporary flatulence and bloating (69).

Alcohol In general, alcohol use is discouraged in diabetic patients. However, diabetics should be assessed individually to determine if the advantages of alcohol, such as reducing emotional tension, relieving anxiety, and stimulating appetite, outweigh its potential effect on blood glucose control (67).

Either hyperglycemia or hypoglycemia may develop in diabetics who ingest alcohol. Hypoglycemia is the most common effect. The hypoglycemic effect of alcohol is believed to be due to either increased early endogenous insulin response to glucose or to inhibition of hepatic gluconeogenesis. Relatively small quantities of alcohol (48 ml of 100 proof) may cause this effect. If a diabetic patient is fasting and consumes alcohol, hypoglycemia may be severe. If a diabetic has adequate amounts of glucose in the blood, then alcohol has a less clinically significant effect (70).

The additive hypoglycemic effects of alcohol with insulin have produced severe hypoglycemia resulting in coma, brain damage, and even death. Diabetic patients who are well fed and drinking alcoholic beverages with a high level of carbohydrates eventually develop hyperglycemia.

Tolbutamide and chlorpropamide have been reported to interact with alcohol resulting in a "disulfiram-like" reaction (71).

It has been recommended that diabetics avoid alcoholic beverages, if possible, including alcohol-containing drug products (72). However, avoidance is not always possible or desired, and more individualized guidelines should be established.

Alcohol consumed in moderate quantities may have beneficial effects (70). Diabetics who wish to drink should use small quantities of dry wines. Some diabetologists advocate the use of small amounts of dry wine for their diabetic patients. Dry wine has been considered by many as part of the therapy in diabetes (73). Alcohol is one of the most readily oxidizable food substances known and, unlike sugar, can be metabolized readily without insulin participation. After the ingestion of sweet wine, blood glucose levels may rise.

Several studies have shown that diabetics who are on a diabetic diet alone or taking insulin or a sulfonylurea can consume up to 2 ounces (60 ml) of dry wine without any significant alteration in the blood glucose values (70, 73). The data available concerning diabetics drinking strong forms of alcohol, such as distilled liquors (gin), are different. If strong alcohol is drunk in excess, ketosis may arise, but there is little evidence to demonstrate concern over consumption of moderate amounts of hard liquor.

A typical 4-oz serving of dry table wine contains 90–100 calories with a sugar content generally averaging 400 mg. Rosé wines tend to be sweeter; a 4-oz serving contains about 1.3 g of sugar. Champagne contains about 1.4 g of sugar. The sweeter white wines may contain as much as 5 g glucose/4-oz serving. The caloric intake for fortified wines is about twice as much as for an equal volume of dry wine, and the sugar content may be as high as 6 g/2-oz serving of sweet sherries, ports, and muscatels. Four ounces of dry wine could be consumed with the evening meal without difficulty as long as calorie and carbohydrate adjustments were made for the wine (73).

Preventing Complications

The complications of diabetes include microangiopathy, macroangiopathy, dermopathy, retinopathy, neuropathy, and nephropathy, and a decreased ability to overcome infections. The prevention of complications through good diabetic control is the ultimate goal. Diabetic patients must be careful in using products that influence their diabetes. For instance, the ingestion of large quantities of aspirin or even ascorbic acid may influence urine tests and affect diabetic control. Nasal sprays, asthma, allergy and hay fever medications, decongestants, and cold and cough preparations that can contain sympathomimetic amines should also be used with caution, especially in poorly controlled diabetic patients. Diabetics should avoid medications containing either sugar or alcohol. Antihistamines or other products that produce drowsiness may result in skipped insulin doses.

Specific measures to prevent problems that require special attention in diabetic patients include general hygiene, foot care (see Chapter 33, *Foot Care Products*), dental care (see Chapter 23, *Oral Health Products*), and prevention of hypoglycemic episodes.

General Hygiene

Diabetic patients are more susceptible to bacterial infection and particularly to monilial infection than the general population (74). The most easily infected part of the body is the skin. Infections in diabetic patients with vascular disease or hyperglycemia heal slowly. Minor cuts and scratches should be cleansed thoroughly with soap and water. Any diabetic with a serious cut, burn, or puncture should see his or her physician immediately.

Monilial infections of the vagina and anus are much more common in patients with glycosuria. The first order of treatment of monilial infections in diabetic patients is to eliminate glycosuria. A product found useful in treating pruritus ani contains three parts Amphogel, one part kaolin powder, and one part Unibase. Application of this mixture to the anal area reduces itching and irritation. Daily bathing with thorough drying is also recommended for diabetic patients. Diabetics should use mild soaps and avoid all harsh chemicals including caustic powders, iodine preparations, and any other product that may produce or exacerbate vascular or neurologic complications.

Foot Care

Gangrene has been reported to be 50 times more frequent in diabetics over 40 years of age than in nondiabetics of the same age (75). Before the advent of antibiotics, amputation of the leg was performed in 9 of 10 diabetic patients undergoing surgery for gangrene of the foot. Even with the discovery of antibiotics, approximately 50% of major leg amputations are performed on diabetic patients (75). Diabetics are predisposed to infection because of vascular changes, as well as neuropathy in the lower extremities. If feet are exposed to minor trauma or infection, the thick-walled vessels become obliterated more easily, and gangrene may occur (75). (See *Plate 1-1.*)

Control of diabetes is the first step in foot care. To prevent foot problems, diabetic patients must be educated to care properly for their feet. Other measures in addition to the procedures described in Chapter 33, *Foot Care Products,* include the following:

- Rub dry feet thoroughly with either vegetable oil, lanolin, or an appropriate commercial product to keep them soft and prevent dryness. (If feet become too soft and tender, they should be rubbed with alcohol once a week) (19). Feet that are too soft and overly moist are more susceptible to skin infections such as athlete's foot; excessively dry skin may crack and fissure allowing infection to enter.
- Avoid bruises, cuts, and skin irritations, and avoid burning or freezing the skin of the feet.
- Avoid going barefooted;
- Toenails should be cut or filed straight across, never shorter than the underlying soft tissue of the toe; never cut the corner of the nails.
- Never cut corns or calluses.
- Prevent callus formation under the ball of the foot by exercise, finishing each step on the toes and not on the ball of the foot; wear shoes that fit well and do not have excessively high heels.
- Avoid corn medications, all of which contain keratolytic agents.
- Never apply heat of any kind to the feet (60).
- Do not sit with crossed legs, since this posture constricts the circulation and promotes nerve pressure.
- Never assume that sensation or circulation is normal in the feet.
- Select a podiatrist familiar with diabetic foot problems.

Some diabetologists believe that circulation may be improved by the use of contrast baths. With the contrast bath, a bath thermometer and two pails are required. One pail is filled with water at 105° F and the other with water at 50° F (use a thermometer). The feet and legs are immersed alternately for 4 minutes in the warm water and 1 minute in the cold water, and this process is repeated five times; however, the feet should not be soaked for long periods (60).

Patients with any type of foot problem should see a physician or podiatrist immediately. All diabetic patients should examine their feet daily for cuts, scratches, and changes in color (29, 76). It is also recommended that diabetic patients abstain from the use of tobacco, which can cause vasoconstriction in the extremities and is an important risk factor in the development of coronary artery disease.

Dental Care

Hidden abscesses of the teeth are common in hyperglycemic patients. Diabetic patients should have their teeth checked at least 2 times/year. Diabetic patients should brush and floss their teeth at least 2 times/day, and the gums should be massaged with a brush or fingers. At the first sign of abnormal condition of the gums, the patient should consult a dentist since uncontrolled diabetes seems to accentuate periodontal disease. Diabetic patients should inform their dentists that they are diabetic.

Product Selection Guidelines

Pharmacists should be able to advise the diabetic patient on purchasing the proper equipment. Injection aids are available for patients with handicaps such as impaired vision (77). Patients who travel should take special precautions. An identification tag should be worn and sufficient insulin and syringes should be available when traveling.

Urine testing is important in controlling diabetes. The pharmacist should be able to explain the use of urine testing kits (glucose oxidase methods versus Clinitest) to diabetic patients, as well as the need to keep accurate records. The pharmacist should also be able to discuss concurrent drug interferences with each urine testing method. In addition, the pharmacist should be aware of any effects other nonprescription products may have on diabetic patients. Because these patients are more subject to certain types of infections (monilial infections), the pharmacist should recommend that appropriate products be kept handy and that strict hygiene measures be followed.

Syringes and Needles

Pharmacists have a responsibility to ensure that the diabetic patient is purchasing the proper type of insulin and the proper insulin syringe corresponding to the strength of insulin used. Problems with insulin dosage occur when patients use the wrong syringe with their insulin. Insulin is administered in units and not in milliliters; therefore, syringes are calibrated in units (28). The calibration of the syringe should correspond to the concentration of the insulin used (U-40 syringes should be used only with U-40 insulin).

Two types of syringes are available: glass (reusable) and plastic (disposable). Both short and long syringes are available; the long type resembles the tuberculin syringe and holds 1 ml of insulin. The long syringe is preferred most often. Automatic injectors are available but these take only the short-type syringe. Although some centers recommend the automatic injector for use with children, many believe that children should be taught to inject themselves.

The advantages of disposable syringes and needles include assured sterility, ease of penetration due to 25% less angle in the cut, side bevels, thinner metal, and silicone coating. However, they are more expensive than the glass syringes. Reusing disposable syringes should be discouraged because of the possibility of infection and the potential for dulling the needle. However, one study showed that plastic disposable syringes can be reused for at least 3 days with safety and patient satisfaction (78).

Some disposable syringes (Becton-Dickinson's Plastipak and Sherwood's Monoject) contain less "dead space," which can be an important factor in diabetes control. Dead space volume is defined as the volume of insulin contained in the hub of the syringe, the hub of the needle, and the shaft of the needle (79). This volume becomes a potential source of error when two different fluids are drawn, measured, and mixed in the same syringe, and it also wastes insulin.

The amount of dead space volume of various U-100 insulin syringes from various manufacturers was significant in all but the Becton-Dickinson Plastipak insulin syringe and needle (79). In another study, dead space in some commercially available disposable insulin syringes caused substantial differences in the actual mixed dose delivered (80). Errors of up to 60% in the amount of intermediate-acting insulin were found.

New disposable syringes with a capacity of 0.5 ml may be used with U-100 insulin only. Patients who inject 50 units or less of U-100 insulin/dose may use these syringes, with the advantage that the syringe is graduated in 1-unit increments, allowing more accurate measurement of the dose. Other syringes, both glass and disposable, are graduated in 2-unit increments. The least accurate type uses 5-unit increments.

Insulin Infusion Pumps

The use of portable, battery-driven infusion pumps for the administration of insulin to diabetic patients has gained much support. When insulin infusion pumps are used by patients in conjunction with home monitoring of blood glucose, the diabetic patient can maintain blood glucose that approximate normal levels. Many diabetologists and diabetic patients support the idea that close monitoring of blood glucose will help prevent the late complications of diabetes mellitus. One of the few methods available to diabetic patients to achieve this objective is through the use of insulin infusion pumps and through self-monitoring of blood glucose (38).

There are several products being promoted to ambulatory diabetic patients. The first is the Auto-Syringe, model AS*6C. It weighs 9.5 oz and is small in size. It is battery operated and uses a 3-ml disposable syringe. Its adjustable control allows for the infusion of a preprogrammed, constant-rate (basal) amount throughout the day. A manually actuated, push-button feature facilitates the administration of a pulse dose of insulin before meals (bolus) to accommodate postprandial hyperglycemia. The device is available from Auto-Syringe, Inc., Hooksett, N.H., and requires a physician's order.

Another model is the Mill Hill Infuser Insulin Pump and is available from Harvard Apparatus, South

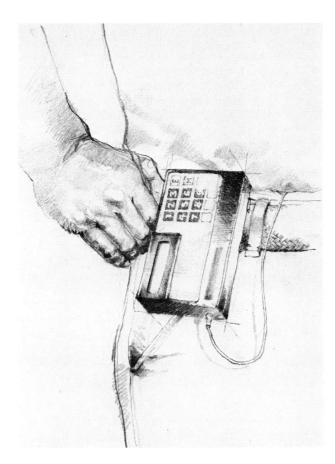

Natick, Mass. It is slightly larger than the Auto-Syringe and uses a 6-ml syringe. It also is lightweight and battery operated but is less versatile than the other two models. The latest insulin infusion pump is the CPI/LILLY Model 9100. It is manufactured by an Eli Lilly–owned company, Cardiac Pacemakers, Inc., St. Paul, Minn. It has the advantage of using regular insulin without dilution. The patient thus injects a significantly smaller volume of fluid subcutaneously. It also helps the patient think in terms of units of insulin rather than a percent of volume of the syringe, as is the case with the other two models. It can be programmed to give a supplemental dose during the middle of the night and also has several unique safety and alarm features. The pumps are connected to the patient through a catheter and a 27-gauge needle that is inserted subcutaneously in the abdomen. The injection sites are changed every 2–3 days. Patients need to be thoroughly educated with reference to the dilution of insulin and the proper use of the infusion pump.

The insulin infusion market is changing rapidly. The sizes of pumps are getting smaller, and the features of the pumps are improving in alarm systems and simplicity of use. Not all diabetic patients are candidates for insulin pump therapy.

Candidates for insulin pump therapy include

- Pregnant diabetics;
- Diabetics with complications;
- Diabetics with a renal transplant;
- Brittle (difficult to control) diabetics;
- Motivated Type I diabetics.

(At present, Type II and diabetic children are not encouraged to use an insulin pump.)

The objectives of insulin pump therapy include

- Normalization of blood glucose values (700–140 mg/deciliter);
- Maintenance of blood glucose values under 200 mg/deciliter;
- Normalization of glycosylated hemoglobin values;
- Prevention or reversal of diabetic complications;
- Maintenance of daily activities;
- Increased lifestyle flexibility (pump patients can more easily adjust to eating, sleeping, and exercise schedules);
- Avoidance of weight gain by maintenance of a well-planned diabetic diet;
- Avoidance of infection and complications with pump procedures;
- Achievement of a sense of well being.

Patients selected for insulin pump therapy must be willing and highly motivated, capable of being educated, responsible for keeping records and following specific procedures, willing to perform and log blood tests daily, and willing to be hospitalized for 1–2 days if necessary.

A Mizzy Syrijet Mark IV needleless insulin jet injector has been developed by Mizzy, Inc., Clifton Forge, Va. This well-designed device allows patients to inject insulin subcutaneously 4 to 6 times/day in response to blood glucose levels, allowing maintenance of these levels within normal limits (81). The Syrijet is relatively easy to use and maintain and provides the patient with a means of administering multiple injections of insulin in a relatively painless manner with less scarring at the injection site. Two other needleless injectors include GT Injector, American Medical Products, Greensburg, Pa., and MediJector, De Rata Corp., Minneapolis.

The role of these open-looped systems in delivering insulin to the diabetic patient will be significant in the next few years. Closed-loop systems are also being studied and are in the investigational stage of development. Unlike the open-loop systems, these closed-loop systems can monitor serum glucose levels and deliver programmed amounts of insulin in response to a particular amount of serum glucose. Such systems include implantable devices and the artificial pancreas. Pharmacists should review the literature closely to remain current with the new products available.

Techniques and Methods

Mixing Insulins

It is important that the patient understand how to mix insulin properly within the syringe. The technique generally recommended is as follows:

- Observing aseptic technique, inject a volume of air equal to the dose into the first vial of intermediate- or long-acting insulin. Withdraw the needle without withdrawing the dose.
- In the usual manner, take the second vial of regular or short-acting insulin; inject air and withdraw the proper dose of insulin.

- Invert the first vial of intermediate- or long-acting insulin several times. Withdraw the dose of this insulin into the syringe containing the regular insulin; remove the syringe from the vial.
- Holding the syringe with needle upright, draw an air bubble into the syringe, invert the syringe, and roll the bubble through to mix.
- Expel the air bubble and administer the insulin to the patient in the usual manner.
- Some insulins may also be premixed in a bottle in the proper short-, intermediate-, and long-acting proportions.

Sterilization Methods

Glass syringes and needles can be sterilized by storing them in alcohol or by boiling them in distilled water before each use. Even if the syringe is kept in alcohol, it should be boiled at least once a week. A product available for sterilizing glass syringes, Ster-Inge, is portable, safe, reusable every 90 minutes, and provides the patient with a sterile syringe and needle for each injection. One-half cup of fresh, distilled water should be used each time a syringe and needle are sterilized. If tap water is used for sterilization, the syringe may become caked on the inside with hard water deposits. These deposits can be removed by soaking the syringe in vinegar. Removal of the deposits is necessary since they may interfere with complete sterilization of the syringe. Additionally, particles may be injected into the body with the insulin. Heavily chlorinated water or chemical solutions for the sterilization of syringes should be avoided.

When boiling is inconvenient, the syringe and the needle may be sterilized by immersion in 70% ethyl alcohol or 91% isopropyl alcohol for at least 5 minutes. No other kind of alcohol should be used. The syringe then must be dried thoroughly by pumping the plunger in and out several times. If large quantities of isopropyl alcohol are introduced into a vial of insulin, the preparation turns cloudy. In addition, introduction of alcohol under the skin, even in minimal amounts, may lead to considerable irritation. Isopropyl alcohol is preferred because there is less corrosion and because it is not denatured, does not counteract insulin, and contains less water that can cause hydrolysis of insulin (82). Pharmacists should encourage their patients to use the plastic disposable syringes and discontinue use of the glass syringes.

Injection Technique

Pharmacists should make sure that their diabetic patients know the correct manner of drawing insulin into a syringe. The following procedure is recommended:

- Wash the hands with soap and water.
- Make sure that the proper equipment is used—correct insulin in the correct strength from the animal source normally used.
- Roll the insulin bottle between the hands, inverting to ensure mixing. To avoid generating air bubbles in the insulin, do not shake the bottle.
- Wipe off the top of the bottle with a piece of cotton moistened with alcohol.

- Remove the clean syringe from storage. Touch only the handle of the plunger or the barrel of the syringe. Avoid touching the hub of the needle.
- If necessary, remove any excess water or alcohol from the syringe by pushing the plunger back and forth a few times. If any liquid is left in the syringe, it will cause an error in measuring the insulin. For disposable syringes, this step is unnecessary.
- Pull the plunger backward to the prescribed number of units on the barrel.
- Put the needle through the rubber cap on the bottle and force the air into the bottle by pushing the plunger down.
- Turn the bottle upside down and pull the plunger back slowly to the prescribed number of units. If air bubbles appear in the barrel, hold the bottle up straight and force the air back into the bottle by pushing the plunger. It may be necessary to tap the barrel of the syringe briskly with the fingers to remove some of the air bubbles.
- When the correct number of units of insulin (without air bubbles) has been measured, pull the bottle away from the needle.
- Lay the syringe on a flat surface such as a table or shelf with the needle over the edge to avoid contamination.
- Check the record to see where insulin was injected the previous day. Injection sites should be rotated.
- Clean the injection site with a cotton ball moistened with alcohol, or use an alcohol swab.
- Pinch a fold of skin with one hand. With the other hand, hold the syringe like a pencil and push the needle quickly through the fold of skin at a 45–90° angle, depending on the degree of obesity. Before injecting the insulin, draw back slightly on the plunger (aspirate) to be sure a blood vessel has not been hit. If blood appears in the syringe barrel, withdraw the needle and repeat the injection in another spot.

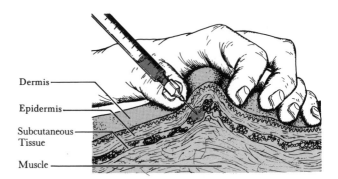

Dermis

Epidermis

Subcutaneous Tissue

Muscle

Figure 4. Correct method of insulin injection. Avoid areas already fibrotic or atrophic. Prevent fibrosis or atrophy by injection in one site at no less than 10 day intervals. Properly injected insulin leaves only the needle puncture dot to show the injection site. Several techniques are good; the one illustrated serves well because the needle penetrates the skin at its thinnest area (dimple) and must enter the subcutaneous space. The needle angle should be 60° or more.

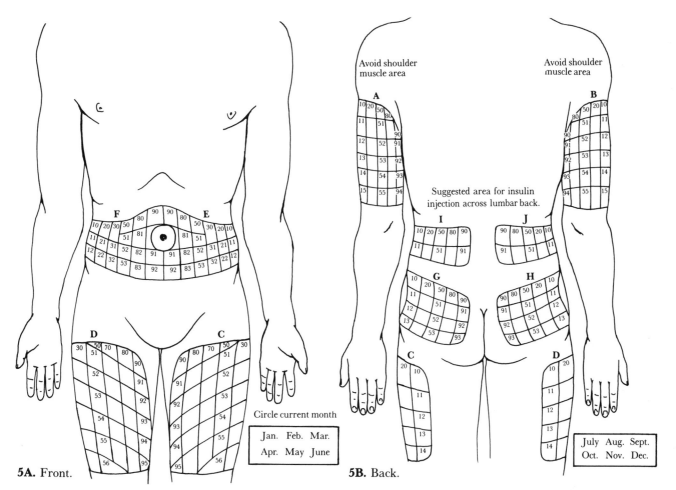

5A. Front.   **5B.** Back.

Figure 5A and B. Record of insulin injection sites. This body map is designed to systematically record insulin injection sites. The diagram is for both hospital and home use: The numbers printed in the squares are mainly for hospital recording of insulin injection sites on each patient's chart. The numbers may be used at home, but a simpler method of recording would be to write the date of each injection in the corresponding square on the map at the time of injection. With continued use, this diagram will facilitate the rotation of insulin injection sites over the entire body and thereby avoid injection too often in a single location. "The Body Map," adapted with permission from the Baptist Hospitals Foundation, Birmingham, Ala.

- Inject the insulin by pressing the plunger in as far as it will go.
- Withdraw the needle quickly and press on the injection site with the cotton ball moistened with alcohol.
- Record the injection site.
- Discard the syringe and needle, if disposable, by breaking the needle to prevent reuse.

Patients should be taught that insulin is to be injected deep into subcutaneous tissue. Properly injected insulin leaves only the needle puncture dot to show the injection site. The technique for injection may need to be altered with each individual, depending on the amount of subcutaneous fat present. For many, a 60° angle or more with the skin stretched will accomplish the deep subcutaneous injection needed (Figure 4). For a thin person, a 45° angle with the skin pinched up may be best to avoid penetrating the muscle. The purpose of pinching is to lift the fat off the muscle. Fibrosis and atrophy can be prevented by injection in the same site at no less than 14-day intervals.

The needle sizes recommended for diabetic patients for subcutaneous injection are in the 25–28 gauge and

⅜–⅝-inch range. Once patients use the 27 or 27½–28 gauge needle, it is difficult to get them to return to the 25 or 26-gauge needles due to less pain at the injection site.

Pharmacists should stress to their diabetic patients the importance of rotating injection sites. Injection sites include the arms, thighs, hips, and abdomen (Figures 5 A and B). Rotation entails moving in a straight line, giving each injection approximately 1 inch (2.5 cm) apart. For example, the patient starts on the right arm and gives four injections, moving in a straight line, and then finishes the line by moving to the left arm; the patient proceeds to the right leg, then the left leg, left abdomen, right abdomen, right hip, and left hip. Then the patient returns to the beginning, dropping down approximately 1 inch below the original line.

If insulin leaks through the puncture in the skin, the needle should be inserted at a right angle to the skin, and a longer needle should be used. It should be stressed to patients that proper rotation helps to avoid local irritation, tissue reaction, and lipodystrophy.

Injection aids are available for visually impaired diabetic patients (77). For blind persons, special aids may be used, or disposable syringes may be filled and stored by a sighted person. Additional information can be obtained from the New York Association for the Blind and the American Foundation for the Blind.

Cautions in Traveling

Diabetic patients traveling abroad should take their own syringes since there is no uniformity of syringes in foreign countries. For instance, it may be difficult to find a U-100 syringe. They also should bring additional insulin to ensure that they have insulin derived from the same protein source. Traveling diabetics should control their diets carefully and also carry candy or sugar to combat possible hypoglycemic attacks.

All diabetics, but especially traveling diabetics, should carry a card or wear an identification bracelet that shows that they are not intoxicated in the event that a hypoglycemic or hyperglycemic attack occurs. Diabetics changing time zones should plan their diet, exercise, and insulin adjustments carefully. It is wise for diabetic patients to carry some insulin and syringes with them rather than placing all of it in their luggage. Not only is this good practice in case luggage is lost, but keeping insulin on the person also avoids exposing it to extreme temperature changes (83).

The sale of syringes in various states differs. In some states, there are no regulations governing the sale of insulin syringes. In others, the sale of syringes must be made by a pharmacist. Certain states require a prescription for the purchase of syringes and needles. The patient should be aware that procedures may be different and take the appropriate precautions.

Blood and Urine Testing and Record Keeping

The pharmacist's role in emphasizing the importance of urine and blood glucose testing and keeping records of urine and blood glucose levels, medication, dose, diet, and exercise is significant in improving the patient's diabetic control (84). The pharmacist should assist the patient in selecting and using urine and blood testing equipment. In addition, the pharmacist should make available samples of testing products in the pharmacy's diabetic center so that the patients may practice technique and demonstrate their ability to properly test their urine or blood for glucose and ketones. Pharmacists should also encourage diabetic patients to bring in their blood or urine test, weight, and medication use records to check how well the patient's diabetes is being controlled.

Proper urine or blood testing for glucose and acetone, as well as adequate records of daily control, is essential for diabetic patients. Pharmacists should monitor patients' drug therapy for drugs that interfere with either the copper reduction or glucose oxidase methods of testing for glucose in the urine.

Factors in Selection

Proper blood and urine testing is especially important to the diabetic patient who is using insulin and must adjust the daily insulin dose according to test results (85). Several studies have shown that most diabetic patients do not perform urinary glucose tests properly (86-88) and, therefore, care should be used in adjusting the insulin dose based on patient tests of urine glucose. Periodic plasma glucose measurements with Dextrostix or Chemstrips bG are recommended to confirm impressions obtained from urine tests (79).

One study demonstrated that the unpredictability of Clinitest in the critically ill is due not only to error, but also to a changing rate of renal glucose reabsorption (89). It was concluded that blood glucose values are essential to rational dosing of insulin in the critically ill patient. A diabetic patient's control may be vastly improved by self blood glucose determinations using the available home blood glucose tests.

In ambulatory diabetic patients who have a relatively normal renal threshold for glucose (160–200 mg/100 ml), the testing of urine glucose is a valuable means of determining diabetic control. The renal glucose threshold varies dramatically from individual to individual. In older patients, the renal glucose threshold increases. Conditions other than diabetes that may cause glucosuria are pheochromocytoma, acute pancreatitis, ingestion of very large amounts of glucose and other reducing sugars (fructose, lactose, and galactose), acromegaly, and Cushing's syndrome. Other factors that may cause unreliable urine glucose determinations include residual urine (prostrate hypertrophy) and neurogenic bladder, which is a complication of diabetes that prevents the collecting of urine specimens at the correct time.

Numerous factors need to be considered in selecting a product to test the urine or blood of a diabetic patient.

Diabetic Category   Type II diabetics who are being treated with diet, or diet and sulfonylureas, need test their urine only 1 time/day approximately 2 hours after the main meal. Type II diabetics also are not as concerned with the quantitative amount of glucose in their urine and therefore can use glucose oxidase tests such as TesTape or Clinistix. Labile Type I diabetics receiving exogenous insulin should test their urine 3–4 times/day, using quantitative or semiquantitative methods such as Clinitest or Diastix. All unstable, pregnant diabetics and those showing signs of long-term complications should test their blood glucose 7 times/day.

Patient Ability and Motivation   Patients unable to perform the more complex tests should be tested with simple tests, even though they are not as quantitative. Willingness of the patient to learn and perform the more complicated test (the more complex drop method of Clinitest versus the strip method of TesTape or Diastix) also should be taken into account. Willingness is also a factor in selection of home blood glucose tests.

Physical Handicaps   Patients with poor vision, which is common in diabetics, may be unable to see the Clinitest drops and therefore would have difficulty performing the test. Special kits are available for visually impaired diabetics. Patients with trembling hands cannot perform the Clinitest test correctly (84). Not only is there a problem in the accuracy of the test results with these patients but the tablets contain sodium hydroxide, and the test solution could be caustic if it were accidentally splashed on the skin.

Patients who are ketosis prone should be educated not only to test their urine for glucose but also to test their blood. Patients who show positive results for glucose in urine and blood tests should also test their urine for ketones. All diabetic patients should periodically test their urine for protein as a warning of nephropathy. Protein in the urine can be tested easily by using Uristix, Labstix, Albustix, or Combistix.

Blood Glucose Tests

The ability to achieve and maintain normal blood glucose levels helps to prevent or delay the complications of diabetes, particularly retinopathy and nephropathy, and is the major objective of home blood glucose monitoring (90). The speculations concerning the benefits of tight control are supported by researchers with patients utilizing daily home blood glucose monitoring (90–93).

Evaluations of patients who monitor their own blood glucose have shown (94, 95):

- Patients were motivated to maintain their blood glucose within normal range by the frequent checking of blood glucose at home. Consequently, they became eager to regulate their daily lives. This positive attitude was observed in all cases.
- The method encouraged patients to become more involved in dietary control.
- Since blood glucose and urine glucose were checked simultaneously, the relationship between the two became obvious. The renal threshold for blood glucose could be demonstrated.
- Because the patient checked blood glucose daily instead of occasionally, more information on diabetic control became available, which facilitated proper insulin dosage. Adjustment of insulin dosage could be made with confidence.
- The metabolic disorder could be normalized quickly.

Even though a few diabetics are not candidates for home blood glucose monitoring, others enthusiastically follow protocol if sophisticated, intelligent training is provided. Eventually, most diabetics will test their blood glucose levels. The following types of diabetic patients should be strongly encouraged to self-test their blood glucose: patients with abnormal or unstable renal threshold; patients with renal failure; unstable, insulin-dependent diabetics; patients with impaired color vision; patients who have difficulty recognizing true hypoglycemia; and pregnant diabetics (95).

Calibrated Blood Glucose Tests   The ability to determine blood glucose levels using home glucose tests is rapidly changing the methods patients use to monitor the control of their diabetes. At the present time, there are three completely calibrated systems available to monitor blood glucose in the United States:

- The Dextrometer and Glucometer, manufactured by the Ames Division of Miles Laboratories, are about the size of a large pocket calculator. The components used with these Ames products include Dextrostix Reagent Strips, Dextro-Chek Standard Solution, Dextro-Chek Control Solution, Glucometer Calibration Chips, and Dextro-Log Glucose Test Record.
- The Stat-Tek is made by Bio-Dynamics and is slightly larger than a tape recorder. The components are Stat-Tek Glucose Strips, an ampul of glucose control, an ampul file, and a dial meter disk.

Both instruments work in a similar way. Drops of blood cover the reagent area of a reagent strip, which is then inserted into a slot in the instrument. Readings on the Glucometer and Dextrometer are displayed by a direct digital readout lighted number. On the Stat-Tek, readings are shown on a dial meter disk. Both instruments have power cords that plug into wall sockets; however, the Ames meter has an accessory rechargeable battery pack. The Glucometer and Dextrometer have a slightly wider measurement range, 0–399 mg/100 ml versus 50–350 mg/100 ml for Stat-Tek. Dextrostix can be read both by meter and visually by comparing the reacted strip to a color chart on the bottle label. For accurate performance, both reflectance colorimeters should be calibrated frequently (95). The Glucometer has the advantage of being battery operated, smaller, easily calibrated, and less expensive. It also has a timing mechanism that indicates when 60 seconds has elapsed.

The Stat-Tek twin-beam electronic photometer is manufactured in Europe under the name Reflomat. It is important to note that Stat-Tek does not work with the Ames Dextrostix, and the Ames Dextrometer and Glucometer do not work with the Stat-Tek strips. Both products can be ordered through surgical supply houses or through the local representatives for Ames or Bio-Dynamics. When the equipment is used according to instructions, the accuracy of Stat-Tek, Dextrometer, and Glucometer is stated to be approximately plus or minus 10% (95).

Visual Blood Glucose Tests   There are two methods available on the market to monitor blood glucose by visual estimation. Dextrostix, which is used with a Glucometer and Dextrometer, can be read visually. Blood placed on the strip induces alpha-color change which is compared with a color chart on the side of the bottle. Visual estimation of blood glucose without the Dextrometer is possible, although less accurate.

Chemstrip bG has been developed by Bio-Dynamics exclusively for visual estimation of blood glucose; it is not intended to be used with the Stat-Tek photometer. It has two reagent test areas.

Both Chemstrip bG and Dextrostix use one large drop of capillary blood. This is wiped off the Chemstrip with a cotton ball and washed off the Dextrostix with water after 60 seconds. The colors on the strip are matched against the color scale on the bottle. The test strips have expiration dates, and outdated strips should not be used since they do not give accurate results. Both test strips should be stored at temperatures under 86° F. They should not be refrigerated or allowed to freeze. Bottle caps should be replaced immediately and tightly after removing a reagent strip to keep the strips free of moisture. Visidex, a visually read blood glucose strip, will be available from Ames.

In addition to these test devices, patients also should purchase alcohol swabs, blood lancets, and other accessory items. Devices to help patients obtain a drop of blood include Autolet and Autoclix. Cost may be a factor for some patients. Most insurance companies, under the provisions of major medical plans, will reimburse patients for the cost of home glucose monitoring devices (96). Pharmacists can become distributors for the blood testing devices by contacting the manufacturers and receiving special training.

Urine Glucose Tests

There are two methods of testing for glucose in the urine: copper reduction tests (Clinitest) and glucose oxidase tests (Clinistix, TesTape, Diastix). In the copper reduction tests, cupric sulfate (blue) in the presence of glucose yields cuprous oxide (green to orange). Copper reduction tests are not specific for glucose and may detect the presence of other reducing substances in the urine. Care must be exercised when using the copper reduction test materials. As mentioned earlier, the tab-

Table 4. Comparison of urine glucose tests

Product	Old "plus" value	Glucose concentration	
		Percent	mg/dl
Glucose oxidase method[a]			
TesTape	0	Negative	Negative
(Lilly)	+	1/10	100
	++	1/4	250
	+++	1/2	500
	++++	2 or greater	2,000 or greater
		Negative	Negative
Diastix strips		1/10	Trace
(Ames)	+	1/4	250
	++	1/2	500
	+++	1	1,000
	++++	2 or greater	2,000 or greater
Copper reduction method[b]			
Clinitest tablets: 5-drop		Negative	Negative
method		1/4	Trace
(Ames)	+	1/2	500
	++	3/4	750
	+++	1	1,000
	++++	2	2,000
Clinitest tablets: 2-drop		Negative	Negative
method		Trace	Trace
(Ames)	"Plus" system	1/2	500
	never used	1	1,000
		2	2,000
		3	3,000
		5	5,000

Adapted with permission from "Facts and Comparisons," Erwin K. Kastrup, Ed., Facts and Comparisons, Inc., St. Louis, Mo., 1980 (December).

[a]More sensitive than copper reduction tests, specific for glucose.

[b]Not specific for glucose, may include other reducing substances.

Urine glucose tests now yield quantitative results:

Urine glucose testing is an established method of monitoring patient response to drug or dietary therapy in diabetes mellitus. Semiquantitative testing for urine glucose by diabetic patients has been simplified by the availability of various in vitro rapid testing products designed for in-home use. These include the dip-and-read reagent strips or tape (glucose oxidase method) and reagent tablets (copper reduction method).

In the past, results of these tests have been reported using a "plus" system. Color changes developing after a specified reaction period are compared to color blocks on a standardized color chart provided with the test product. Each color block is assigned a "plus" value ranging from 11 to 41 corresponding to a percent concentration of glucose in the urine. The "plus" system has created confusion in evaluation of test results because of the lack of uniformity among products in terms of the "plus" value assigned to a given concentration (in mg/dl) of urine glucose.

At the recommendation of the American Diabetes Association the old "plus" reporting system is being deleted from all products of the Ames Company used for in vitro urine glucose testing in the home. Color blocks for these Ames products are now being assigned percent (%) values. Since percentage values always indicate the same level of glycosuria regardless of the test product being used, reporting test results in percent will be more meaningful and less confusing to the practitioner.

The change of this system will require some initial patient education. The information in Table 4 has been provided to aid the practitioner in this effort. The table shows the correlation between "plus" values and urine glucose percentage for those products most often used for semiquantitative determination of reducing sugars in the urine.

lets and solution are very caustic and handling or splashing should be avoided. The tablets can be very dangerous if accidentally ingested and must be kept out of the reach of children.

A second method is based on the enzyme glucose oxidase. Glucose in the urine in the presence of glucose oxidase yields gluconic acid and peroxide (H_2O_2), which, in the presence of *o*-tolidine, results in a color change and is the basis of glucose oxidase tests.

Pharmacists should explain to patients that the results of the various urine glucose tests are not interchangeable. Therefore, it is important that the patient understand which testing method the physician referred to when recommending a sliding scale for adjusting insulin dose. For example, a +1 with the Clinitest represents 0.005% glucose, whereas with Diastix it represents 0.0025% glucose, and with TesTape it represents 0.001% glucose. Table 4 shows comparative readings for various urine glucose tests (97).

Patients who are taking drugs that can interfere with urine glucose testing methods should be instructed to test their urine using both the copper reduction method and glucose oxidase method (Tables 5, 6, 7, 8). If the test results differ, there is a strong possibility that a drug is interfering with the test results.

Tests for Urinary Ketones

Since the ketones in the blood overflow into the urine, urinary ketone levels can be tested to detect whether or not ketoacidosis is occurring. All diabetic patients should be counseled on the proper testing for ketones in the urine. The basis for the test is that sodium nitroprusside alkali in the presence of acetone or acetoacetic acid turns lavender. The detection levels, moisture resistance, and quantitation of some ketone tests have been improved over what has been previously available.

Acetest reagent tablets are specific for acetoacetic acid and acetone. Acetest will not react with beta-hydroxybutyric acid. It also will detect as little as 5 mg of acetoacetic acid/100 ml in urine. In serum plasma or whole blood, Acetest will detect 10 mg of acetoacetic acid/100 ml.

Ketostix will detect 5–10 mg of acetoacetic acid/100 ml of urine. The test is easier than Acetest to perform and no dropper is required (98). The new improved Ketostix only tests for acetoacetic acid and thus shows a false-negative result if the patient produces acetone or beta-hydroxybutyric acid. It is also difficult to find a substance at home to test the reliability of the Ketostix. Acetest can be tested for reliability by using nail polish remover that contains acetone.

Tests for Other Chemicals

Several products are available that test urine for pH, protein, glucose, acetone, bilirubin, blood, and/or urobilinogen. These multiple tests are not used often by patients and are more commonly used in physicians' offices, but patients may be instructed to use one of these reagents to test for various chemicals in the urine that may indicate the degree of diabetic control. Fresh urine is required in all of the tests. Urine may be refrigerated for a short time (up to 4 hours before testing) but the actual test must be run with the specimen at room temperature.

Table 5. Substances interfering with glucose oxidase tests

False positive

Chloride	Hydrogen peroxide
Glucose hypochlorite	Peroxide

False negative

Alcaptonuria	5-Hydroxyindole acetic acid
Ascorbic acid	
Aspirin	5-Hydroxytryptamine
Bilirubin	5-Hydroxytryptophan
Catalase	L-Dopamine
Catechols	Levodopa
Cysteine	Meralluride injection
3,4-Dihydroxyphenyl-acetic acid	Methyldopa (Aldomet)
	Sodium bisulfate
Epinephrine	Sodium fluoride
Ferrous sulfate (Feosol)	Tetracycline (Tetracyn, Achromycin) with vitamin C
Gentisic acid	
Glutathione	
Homogentisic acid	Uric acid

From *Contemporary Pharmacy Practice, 3*, 224–225 (1980).

Table 6. Minimal concentrations of chemicals that produce false glucose oxidase reactions

Chemical	Concentration in urine (mg/ml)	False positive or false negative
Homogentisic acid	0.05	False negative
L-Dopamine	0.6	False negative
Levodopa	2.5	False negative
Methyldopa	5.0	False negative
5-Hydroxytryptophan	1.0	False negative
5-Hydroxytryptamine	1.0	False negative
Cysteine	9.0	False negative
Glutathione	9.0	False negative
Sodium bisulfate	5.0	False negative
Glucuronic acid conjugates	20	False negative
Glucose hypochlorite		False positive
Chlorine		False positive
Peroxide		False positive
Hydrogen peroxide		False positive
Ascorbic acid	0.08	False negative
Gentisic acid	0.05	False negative
5-Hydroxyindole acetic acid	0.25	False negative

From *Contemporary Pharmacy Practice, 3*, 224–225 (1980).

Identification Tags

All diabetics should wear an identification bracelet, necklace, tag, or card. This identification may be life-

Table 7. Substances interfering with copper-reduction tests that give false-positive results

False positive

Abscorbic acid	Levodopa
Cephaloridine	Metaxalone (Skelaxin)
Cephalothin	metabolite
Dilute urine	Methyldopa
Gentisic acid (aspirin)	Penicillin
Glucuronic acid conjugates	Probenecid (Benemide)
	Reducing sugars
Homogentisic acid	Salicylates
Isoniazid	Streptomycin
Lactose in pregnant women	

From *Contemporary Pharmacy Practice, 3,* 224–225 (1980).

Table 8. Minimal concentrations of chemicals that produce false copper reduction reactions

Chemical	Concentration in urine (mg/ml)	False negative or false positive
Isoniazid	5	False positive
Streptomycin	5	False positive
Cephaloridine	5	False positive
Cephalothin	5	False positive
Fructose	10	False positive
Galactose	10	False positive
Lactose	10	False positive
Maltose	10	False positive
Penicillin	10,000 U/ml	False positive

From *Contemporary Pharmacy Practice, 3,* 224–225 (1980).

saving if hypoglycemia or ketoacidosis occurs. If a diabetic patient becomes unconscious through an accident or hypoglycemic or hyperglycemic coma, medications regularly taken by the patient may be missed. A hypoglycemic (insulin) reaction may be confused with drunkenness; there have been reports of diabetic patients being jailed rather than given medical care (74).

A tag that can be seen easily on any patient should indicate that the patient is diabetic and receiving medication. A diabetic identification card should include the patient's name, address, and telephone number, the amount and type of medication used, the patient's physician, and how the physician can be contacted.

Diabetic patients should be encouraged to inform friends, teachers, and others of their condition. Some patients are embarrassed that they have the condition and need special coaxing to overcome this problem. Diabetic patients should also carry a candy roll or quick energy source such as glucose. The MedicAlert Identification bracelet may be obtained from MedicAlert Foundation, P.O. Box 1009, Turlock, Calif. 95380.

Nonprescription Products Affecting Diabetes

Reading the label on all food and drug products is essential to maintaining diabetic control. Patients should develop this habit early to avoid potential adverse effects.

Sugar-Containing Products

A list of sugar-free pharmaceutical preparations is useful so that the pharmacist may suggest a suitable sugar-free product for diabetic patients; see Appendix 2, "Sugar-Free" Preparations by Therapeutic Category. For instance, cough preparations that contain simple syrup could have a clinically significant effect on a brittle insulinopenic diabetic. However, the amount of extra sugar ingested to relieve a cough would not be significant in most well-controlled diabetics. To put this into perspective, the difference between a large and small orange could include more sugar than would be found in 2 tsp of most cough syrups. Although sugar-containing medicinals may affect control in some diabetics, those who are properly educated to monitor their condition should have no clinically significant problems.

Alba Foods is promoting to diabetics a number of its nonfat, dry milk products with no sugar added. These products are low in calories (60–80 calories/serving) and low in fat. By making adjustments in their exchange diets, diabetics are provided an opportunity to consume a low-fat, low-calorie milkshake or hot chocolate-type drink.

Diabetics should read labels carefully to ensure that the dietetic product will fit into their diet plan. Many dietetic products cost much more than the nondietetic counterparts and actually have as many, if not more, calories.

Sympathomimetic Amines

Ephedrine, pseudoephedrine, phenylpropanolamine, phenylephrine, and epinephrine increase blood glucose and cause increased blood pressure by vasoconstriction. These substances should be used cautiously in diabetic patients. Sympathomimetic amines do not have as potent an effect on blood glucose as does epinephrine, which can stimulate glycogenolysis. Hyperglycemia, acetonuria, and glycosuria have been reported in three nondiabetic children who received therapeutic oral doses of phenylephrine (99–101). The major problem would occur in unstable Type I diabetics; the effect should not be significant in most Type II diabetics.

Salicylates

Aspirin products do not bear a warning statement for diabetic patients. However, aspirin in diabetics may cause hypoglycemia, possibly by stimulation of general cellular metabolism. In Type I diabetics, the degree of hypoglycemia resulting from large doses of aspirin (5–6 g) could stimulate a hypoglycemic reaction (27). However, the clinical significance of aspirin is questionable if a diabetic patient is monitoring diabetes control. In addition, aspirin may cause misleading results in urine tests for glucose, but it is a dose-related phenomena. False-negative glucose oxidase readings have been associated with doses of aspirin of approximately 2.5 g. False-positive glucosuria by the copper reduction method can also occur with similar doses of aspirin.

Diabetic Patient Monitoring

The therapeutic goal of diabetes therapy (insulin, diet, exercise, or drug) is to control the patient's blood glucose. Diabetic patients vary considerably in their responses to therapy and in their adherence to prescribed instructions. The pharmacist can play a key role in assisting the patient to adhere to the prescribed regimen.

A two-page diabetic patient monitoring checklist has been developed by the APhA Academy of Pharmacy Practice Section on Clinical Practice to help the pharmacist perform the monitoring function (Figure 4). The checklist is a patient profile, especially designed to record data necessary to effectively monitor the drug therapy of the diabetic patient. Use of the checklist enables the pharmacist to gather pertinent information about the patient, such as blood and urine glucose test results and blood pressure readings; prescribed therapy (special diet and therapy for concurrent diseases); and the patient's drug therapy, including a special section for recording insulin type(s), dosage, and dosage changes. The checklist may be used as the sole patient profile, or it may be used in conjunction with existing profiles.

The checklist, available in pads of 50 from the American Pharmaceutical Association, also includes an instruction booklet containing specific instructions and suggestions for use, a completed sample checklist, and a suggested transmittal form for obtaining blood glucose data from the patient's physician. The transmittal form, which can be reproduced easily on a 5″ × 8″ card, is given to the patient; the patient asks the physician to complete the form during a regular office visit and then returns it to the pharmacist.

Patient Education

Patient education is the key to success in controlling the diabetic patient. Some diabetologists insist that the patient know as much about diabetes from the practical management aspect as the physician (102).

Behavioral and Psychosocial Issues in Diabetes

To be successful in the treatment program of diabetics, each health team member must be sensitive to the emotional problems encountered by diabetics.

Anxiety and depression are major emotions experienced by diabetic patients. This can be partially overcome by empathetic teachers in a well-planned educational program. After being exposed to the many aspects of diabetic education, the patient may feel confused and anxious. Imagine experiencing in a several-hour or even several-day program a learning process that includes the following: the causes and complications of diabetes, food types, diet exchanges, urine testing, blood testing, effects of exercise, insulin mixing and injection, rotation of injection sites, foot care, treatment of insulin reactions, travel tips, what to do during sick days, and miscellaneous products. There may be a high level of anxiety with reference to understanding the treatment aspects of diabetes and the day-to-day regimen that must be followed to keep diabetes under control.

Many diabetics live with fear because of the grave implications of the disease. Fear of an early death, the thought of suffering from diabetic complications, and the embarrassment of strange behavior or possibly convulsions during an insulin reaction may strongly affect behavior and decrease good diabetic control. For instance, patients who have suffered a serious insulin reaction often keep their blood glucose high to avoid a repeat episode Some diabetics try to "beat the odds" or "live each day to the fullest" and don't fully comply with the treatment regimen. Some patients may overindulge themselves and rationalize that having a chocolate shake, for example, will not cause a medical emergency, pain, or any other acute symptom. However, bad habits such as overeating are easily formed and difficult to break, leading to poor diabetic control. Often, diabetics feel guilty when they are noncompliant with the prescribed treatment protocol. However, the treatment protocol is stringent and can cause frustration; there is seldom positive feedback as to whether the diabetic is following the proper procedures to maintain control and avoid complications. Blood glucose self-monitoring is one of the most significant advances in diabetes care in the past 40 years. With proper patient education, blood glucose self-testing allows the diabetic to tightly monitor his or her own blood glucose and regulate diet, exercise, and medicines.

Living with the fear of complications, in addition to the daily demands of a rigorous medical regimen, is very stressful, not only for the diabetic but for the entire family. Many diabetics are subject to powerful, unpredictable mood and behavioral changes due to metabolic imbalance (103). Moreover, chronic, nonmetabolic stresses associated with the disease include the need for diet management, rigid meal schedules, blood testing, various daily therapeutic decisions, insulin injections if required, and alterations in lifestyle. These stresses frequently result in significant emotional disequilibrium and occasionally in clinical psychiatric disorders. Impaired self-esteem is common (103). Denial, anxiety, hostility, and depression also occur and may impair interpersonal relationships at various levels.

Despite continuing gains in understanding this disease, the present state of knowledge remains insufficient to prevent the disease, cure it, or provide diabetic patients with optimally effective treatment. The search for a means of prevention and a cure continues. However, there is a need to focus energies on easing the emotional burdens and improving the quality of life for diabetics and their families.

There is still hope: hope for a cure; for a better way to control blood glucose; for a food that tastes great and is noncaloric; for an artificial sweetener that is safe; and for a health team that understands the varied emotional states of the diabetic patient and cares enough to provide honest, helpful, and informed information.

Education, periodic re-education, and support systems from friends and family members are essential in fighting the burdens accompanying diabetes. Since diabetes is a particularly difficult disease for children and adolescents, it is especially important that positive steps be taken to help these persons understand their emotions. Diabetes is the only disease in which the patient and the parents are expected to make independent therapeutic decisions based on daily clinical observation. Although this day-to-day control of the disease is dependent upon the efforts of the patient and family members, it has been repeatedly demonstrated that an understanding of the disease and mastery of the necessary skills required are inadequate in a large proportion of diabetics and their families (103). Although improved understanding leads to improved care and outcome, there is a lack of accessible and well-designed education programs. At every age, these issues affect not only the patient but also family, friends, teachers, employers, and the entire community of the diabetic. Clearly the emotional, social, economic, and public health problems of diabetes are enormous. The role of the pharmacist in helping to overcome some of these problems is significant.

Diabetics live with their disease 24 hours a day, so it is essential that they understand the condition and know when they are in trouble and need to call for help. Every diabetic patient should know the following:

- What diabetes is and why treatment is necessary;
- How to select the proper foods at each meal;
- How to test urine for sugar and acetone;
- How to test blood for glucose;
- How to administer insulin;
- The symptoms of uncontrolled diabetes and ketosis;
- The symptoms of hypoglycemia;
- The emergency treatment of hypoglycemia;
- When to return for follow-up;
- How to contact the attending physician, pharmacist, or emergency department;
- Precautionary measures while traveling;
- How to modify treatment for exercise or illness;
- How to care for the feet;
- The dosage and time of administration of oral agents, if appropriate.

A team approach to patient education is essential. The physician explains the disease and the treatment objectives to the patient. The dietician emphasizes the importance and methods of reaching and maintaining an ideal body weight. The nurse usually trains the patient in using syringes and needles, mixing insulins, and injecting insulin subcutaneously; the nurse also gives advice on proper personal hygiene, foot care, urine testing techniques, and record keeping.

Pharmacists have a special role in patient education concerning mixing, storing, and injecting insulin. They also should be able to answer questions about blood and urine testing, record keeping, foot care, diet, treatment of cuts and scratches, the use of antihistamines and decongestants, products safe to use in weight control, and the alcohol and sugar content of both prescription and nonprescription drugs.

The pharmacist's role in patient education is significant. The challenge of understanding diabetic products and teaching patients how to use them properly has many benefits. Diabetic patient education methods have been summarized in some excellent articles available from major manufacturers (46, 61, 104–111). Additional diabetes information sources for pharmacists and their patients are listed in Appendix 1. With the aid of this information, pharmacists should be prepared to discuss with patients any of the following topics:

- The relationship among diet, exercise, and insulin;
- The strength, dose, times of administration, and types of insulin;
- The correct use of insulin syringes, needles, and dead space;
- Diabetic diet and the prescribed caloric level;
- Injection sites and proper site rotation;
- Syringe preparation technique (insulin withdrawal and mixture);
- Oral hypoglycemic agents (dosage and times of administration);
- The availability and use of insulin infusion devices;
- Blood and urine testing methods and techniques;
- Urine testing times (Type I versus Type II diabetics);
- Proper interpretation of testing results and record keeping;
- Symptoms of hypoglycemic versus hyperglycemic reactions;
- Appropriate treatment for hypoglycemic and hyperglycemic reactions;
- Proper identification, including diabetic information card and MedicAlert emblems;
- Skin and foot care, and personal hygiene.

Pharmacists interested in giving special care to diabetic patients can use a number of educational techniques.

Diabetic Care Center

To emphasize to diabetic patients that the pharmacist is truly concerned and interested in serving their needs, a clearly identified section may be established in the pharmacy. The center should include a complete line of diabetic products: sugar-free food and drink products, nonprescription products safe for use by diabetics (sugar-free cough syrup), booklets about diabetes, and diabetic services available. An area also may be set up in which patients can practice testing their urine or blood and using syringes properly.

Diabetic Detection Programs

Free diabetes testing kits may be distributed to pharmacy patients. The American Diabetes Association may be helpful in providing information on how to set up a detection program. It is a good idea to establish 1–2 days each month when patients can be tested for diabetes in the pharmacy.

Diabetic "Hotline"

Pharmacists who are knowledgeable about diabetes may advise patients with questions concerning diabetes and diabetic products to call them for information.

Communication

Team effort and coordination are vital in patient education, and communication must be part of that effort. Pharmacists concerned about diabetes control should become involved in their local diabetes association or local Juvenile Diabetes Foundation. In addition, they should become familiar with community internal medicine specialists who treat diabetes and should develop a working relationship with them.

A system for communicating with diabetic patients may be developed. Using a diabetic patient drug monitoring checklist or merely a series of questions allows the pharmacist to show concern for the patient and gather information helpful in monitoring the condition.

Summary

Diabetes control requires team effort on the part of the physician, dietician, nurse, pharmacist, and patient. The pharmacist may play an important role by monitoring patient therapy and being informed about all aspects of the disease. Patient consultation should reinforce the patient's understanding of diabetes and should emphasize the importance of controlling blood glucose levels, urine tesing, and accurate record keeping.

Concerned pharmacists may join their local diabetes associations and consult recent literature to keep their knowledge up to date. Products for diabetics including both nonprescription medicines and food and beverage preparations may be displayed in the pharmacy's diabetic center along with diabetic patient information.

The pharmacist should be able to explain to the patient the purpose and methods of mixing, storing, and injecting insulins properly. The necessity of regular, scheduled exercise and a balanced, nutritious diet in combination with prescribed medicine should be made clear to the patient. Only by educating patients about diabetes is it possible to bring the disease under control.

References

1. R. A. Kerr, *New Environ. Pharm., 3*(2), 9 (1976).
2. A. R. Van Son, *Wellcome Trends Hosp. Pharm., 5*(3), 1 (1977).
3. "1976 Fact Sheet," Juvenile Diabetes Foundation, New York, N.Y., 1976.
4. "1977 Fact Sheet," Juvenile Diabetes Foundation, New York, N.Y., 1977.
5. *American Druggist, 176*(3), 54 (1977).
6. M. Ellenberg, *Pharm. Times, 40*(6), 56 (1974).
7. W. G. Platt and S. G. Sudovar, "The Social and Economic Costs of Diabetes: An Estimate for 1979, A Summary," Pracon, Inc., Washington, D.C., 1979, pp. 3–4.
8. M. A. Kimble, *J. Am. Pharm. Assoc., NS14,* 80 (1974).
9. P. G. Sesin, *Apothecary, 89*(5), 22 (1977).
10. E. Cerasi and R. Luft, "Pathophysiology of Diabetes Mellitus: Diagnosis and Treatment," Vol. 3, American Diabetes Association, New York, N.Y., 1971, p. 37.
11. K. E. Sussman, in "The Older Diabetic Patient," Upjohn, Kalamazoo, Mich., 1973, p. 20.
12. W. B. Spaulding, W. O. Spitzer, and P. W. Truscott, *Can. Med. Assoc. J., 89,* 329 (1963).
13. M. Fabrykant and B. I. Ashe, *J. Am. Geriatr. Soc., 11,* 68 (1963).
14. G. J. Hamwi, S. S. Fajans, G. F. Cahill, Jr., W. V. Greenberg, R. C. Hardin, E. A. Haunz, D. M. Kipnis, R. H. Unger, and K. M. West, *Diabetes, 16,* 540 (1967).
15. N. Baumslag, R. E. Yoadaiken, and J. C. Varady, *Diabetes, 19,* 664 (1970).
16. National Diabetes Data Group, *Diabetes, 28*(12), 1039 (1979).
17. P. H. Forsham, in "Diabetes Rounds," Medcom, New York, N.Y., 1973, p. 8.
18. J. Palmer, "Diabetes Update," Vol. 1, Diabetes Education Center, Deaconess Hospital, Spokane, Wash., 1977, p. 1.
19. J. H. Karam, in "Current Medical Diagnosis and Treatment," M. A. Krupp and M. J. Chatton, Eds., Lange Medical, Los Altos, Calif., 1980, p. 749.
20. K. D. Hepp, *Diabetologia, 13,* 177 (1977).
21. T. G. Skillman and M. Tzagournis, "Diabetes Mellitus," Upjohn, 1977, pp. 3, 14.
22. J. E. Gerich, *Am. Fam. Physician, 16,* 85 (1977).
23. J. Skyler, *Diabetes Care, 2*(6), 499 (1979).
24. "Diabetes Mellitus," 8th ed., S. O. Waife, Ed., Lilly Research Laboratories, Indianapolis, Ind., 1980, p. 1, 169.
25. C. R. Shulman, "The New Diabetic," American Family Physician—Monograph (April 1979).
26. Daniel W. Foster, in "Harrison's Principles of Internal Medicine," 9th ed., K. J. Isselbacher, R. D. Adams, E. Braunwald, R. G. Petersdorf, and J. D. Wilson, Eds., McGraw-Hill, New York, N.Y., 1980, pp. 1741–1754.
27. T. A. Gossell and R. J. Wuest, "Diabetes Mellitus, Part 1," Chain Store Age Continuing Education Program, New York, N.Y., 1977, p. 93.
28. "A Pharmacist's Guide to Diabetes Mellitus," School of Pharmacy, University of California, San Francisco, Calif., 1977, p. 52.
29. O. C. Olson, "Instruction Book for Diabetic Patients," 9th ed., Diabetes Education Center, Deaconess Hospital, Spokane, Wash., 1977, pp. ii–iii.
30. M. J. C. Crabbe et al., *Lancet, 2,* 1268–1270 (1980).
31. M. A. Kimble, in "Applied Therapeutics for Clinical Pharmacists," 2nd ed., L. Y. Young and M. A. Kimble, Eds., Applied Therapeutics, Inc., San Francisco, Calif., 1978, pp. 451–490.
32. "Monograph: 2, Diabetes, J. M. Moss, D. E. DeLawter, and C. R. Meloni, Pfizer Laboratories, New York, N.Y., 1974, p. 24.
33. R. Engerman, J. Bloodsworth, and S. Nelson, *Diabetes, 26,* 760 (1977).
34. D. Job, E. Eschwege, C. Guyot-Argenton, J. P. Aubry, and E. Tchobroutsky, *Diabetes, 25,* 463 (1976).
35. P. H. Forsham, in "Diabetes Mellitus," M. Ellenberg and A. Rifkin, Eds., McGraw-Hill, New York, N.Y., 1971, p. 697.
36. G. D. Molnar, *Mayo Clinic Proc., 47,* 709 (1972).
37. B. I. Chazon, *Diabetologia, 6,* 565 (1970).
38. A. Schiffrin, E. Colle, and M. Belmonte, *Diabetes Care, 3*(6), 643 (1980).
39. D. Fine and H. Shedrovilsky, *Ann. Intern. Med., 72,* 83 (1970).
40. P. N. Weismann, L. Shenkman, and R. I. Gregerman, *N. Engl. J. Med., 284,* 65 (1971).
41. D. L. Smith, "Medication Guide for Patient Counseling," Lea and Febiger, Philadelphia, Pa., 1977, p. 396.
42. R. K. Maudlin and L. Y. Young, "Drug Consultation Guide," Drug Intelligence Publications, Inc., Hamilton, Ill., 1976.
43. S. W. Shen and R. Bressler, *N. Engl. J. Med., 296,* 787–793 (1977).
44. D. G. Eastman, R. A. Guthrie, J. W. Hare, A. Krosnick, J. J. Kristan, C. R. Shuman, and K. E. Sussman, *Patient Care, 19*(9), 12 (1975).
45. D. W. Guthrie, *Am. J. Nurs., 77*(2), 48, 54 (1977).
46. P. Felig, *Postgrad. Med., 59,* 109 (1976).
47. T. Deckert, O. O. Anderson, and J. E. Poulsen, *Diabetologia, 10,* 703 (1974).
48. P. Daggert, B. E. Mustaffa, and J. Nabarro, *Practitioner, 218,* 563 (1977).
49. *American Journal of Hospital Pharmacy, 37,* 1105 (1980).
50. S. M. O. Guerra and A. E. Kitabchi, *J. Clin. Endocrinol. Metabl., 42,* 868 (1976).
51. V. Koivisto and P. Felig, *N. Engl. J. Med., 298,* 79 (1978).
52. *Medical World News, 18*(14), 15 (1977).
53. *Annals of Internal Medicine, 92,* 59 (1980).
54. J. Galloway, personal communication of unpublished research

on insulin mixtures and insulin absorption, Eli Lilly and Company, Indianapolis, Ind., December 15, 1980.

55. "Joslin Diabetes Manual," 11th ed., L. P. Krall, Ed., Lea and Febiger, Philadelphia, Pa., 1978, p. 657.

56. B. M. Watson and J. S. Calder, *Diabetes, 20,* 628 (1971).

57. D. K. Yue and J. R. Turtle, *Diabetes, 26,* 341 (1977).

58. M. A. Koda-Kimbler, "Applied Therapeutics for Clinical Pharmacists," 2nd. ed., Applied Therapeutics, San Francisco, 1978, pp. 448–493.

59. K. E. Sussman, J. R. Crout, and A. Marble, *Diabetes, 12,* 38 (1963).

60. "Joslin Diabetes Manual," 11th ed., L. P. Krall, Ed., Lea and Febiger, Philadelphia, Pa., 1978, pp. 97, 152, 184–186.

61. A. Bloom, *Clin. Endocrinol. Metab., 6,* 499 (1977).

62. J. K. Davidson, *Postgrad. Med., 59,* 114 (1976).

63. L. Howard, *Am. Fam. Physician, 12,* 152 (1975).

64. *Diabetes Outlook, 11*(6), 2 (1976).

65. J. M. Court, *Med. J. Aust., 1,* 841 (1976).

66. J. M. Olefsky and P. Crapo, *Diabetes Care, 3*(2), 390 (1980).

67. "Diabetes and Cardiovascular Disease," Publication No. (NIH)77-1212, Department of Health, Education, and Welfare, 1977, p. 8.

68. D. J. A. Jenkins, D. V. Goff, A. R. Leeds, K. G. M. M. Alberti, T. M. S. Wolever, M. A. Gassull, and T. D. R. Hockaday, *Lancet, 2,* 172 (1976).

69. H. R. Murdock, *Geriatrics, 27*(7), 93 (1972).

70. J. McDonald, *Diabetes Care, 3*(5), 629 (1980).

71. "Evaluations of Drug Interactions," 2nd ed., American Pharmaceutical Association, Washington, D.C., 1976, p. 240.

72. G. E. Dukes, J. G. Kuhn, and R. P. Evens, *Am. Fam. Physician, 16*(3), 97 (1977).

73. S. Dippe, in "Important Data on Diabetes," Northern California Diabetes Association and Geigy Pharmaceuticals, San Francisco, Calif., 1970, p. 23.

74. P. P. Lamy and M. E. Kittler, *J. Am. Pharm. Assoc., NS10,* 610 (1970).

75. M. C. Robson and L. E. Edstron, *Surg. Clin. North Am., 57,* 1089 (1977).

76. M. Kahan and Y. J. Chafiian, *Hosp. Med., 8*(2), 15 (1972).

77. R. K. Campbell, *American Pharmacy, NS21*(1), 30 (1981).

78. M. Crouch, A. Jones, E. Kleinbeck, E. Reece, A. Bessman, *Diabetes Care, 2*(5), 418 (1979).

79. M. Kochwar and L. K. Fry, *Drug Intell. Clin. Pharm., 8,* 33 (1974).

80. R. Rosoff, *Acad. Gen. Pract., 10*(7), 3 (1975).

81. T. S. Danowski and J. H. Sunder, *Diabetes Care, 1*(1), 27 (1978).

82. J. C. Scheller and M. D. Ormsby, *Hosp. Pharm., 6*(7), 7 (1971).

83. O. Aagenes and H. K. Akerblom, *Acta Paediatr. Belg., 30,* 126 (1977).

84. C. J. Nelson, *Drug Intell. Clin. Pharm., 8,* 422 (1974).

85. S. R. Abel and R. W. Bennett, *Apothecary, 89*(3), 12 (1977).

86. J. M. Feldman and F. L. Leborwitz, *Diabetes, 22,* 115 (1977).

87. G. M. Shenfield and J. M. Steel, *Practitioner, 218,* 147 (1977).

88. J. I. Malone, A. L. Rosenbloom, A. Grgic, and F. T. Weber, *Am. J. Dis. Child., 130,* 1324 (1976).

89. D. Smith and D. Angaran, "Urine glucose estimation of blood glucose in the critically ill," paper presented at the American Society of Hospital Pharmacists Midyear Meeting, Atlanta, Ga., December 1977.

90. T. S. Danowski, O. Ohler, and E. R. Fisher, *Diabetes Care, 3*(1), 94 (1980).

91. R. L. Engerman, M. D. Paris, and J. M. B. Bloodworth, "Retinopathy in Experimental Diabetes: Its Relevance to Diabetes in Man," Proceedings of the VII Congress of the International Diabetes Federation, Excerpta Medica International Congress Series, *231,* 261 (1970).

92. D. Job, B. Eschwege, C. Guyot et al., *Diabetes, 24*(Suppl 2), 397 (1975).

93. M. S. Maur, J. Barbosa, R. R. Vernier, G. Tchobroutsky, C. Kjellstrand, T. Buselmeier, R. Simmons, J. Najarian, F. Goetz, *N. Engl. J. Med., 295,* 916 (1976).

94. Y. Ikeda, *Diabetologia, 15,* 91 (1978).

95. C. Christiansen and M. Sachse, *The Diabetes Educator, 6*(3), 13 (1980).

96. R. K. Campbell, "Current Concepts in the Treatment of Diabetes Mellitus," a continuing education program sponsored by the Washington State University College of Pharmacy and published by The Ames Company, Elkhart, Ind., 1980, p. 23.

97. P. A. Lawrence, *Am. Diabetes Assoc. Forecast, 25*(2), 1, 12 (1972).

98. K. F. A. Soliman, D. Davis, and P. Wallace, *Contemp. Pharm. Prac., 3,* 215–227 (1980).

99. L. Baker et al., *Am. J. Dis. Child., 3,* 59 (1966).

100. S. Inoue, *J. Allergy, 40,* 337 (1967).

101. D. Porte Jr., *Arch. Int. Med., 123,* 253 (1969).

102. M. Ellenberg, *N.Y. State J. Med., 77,* 62 (1977).

103. B. Hamburg, L. Lipsett, A. Drash, and G. Inoff, "Behavioral and Psychosocial Issues in Diabetes: Summary of Proceedings of the National Conference," *Diabetes Care, 3*(2), 379–381 (1980).

104. C. A. Sczupak and W. F. Conrad, *Am. J. Hosp. Pharm., 34,* 1238 (1977).

105. K. W. Schilling, *Am. J. Hosp. Pharm., 34,* 1242 (1977).

106. R. D. Scalley, K. Fiegen, and E. Kearney, *Am. J. Hosp. Pharm., 34,* 1245 (1977).

107. E. W. Buruchien, *Drug Topics, 120*(21), 31 (1976).

108. L. A. Gieselman, "The Development and Evaluation of an Individualized Diabetic Education Program," 2nd Annual University of Nebraska Hospital Pharmacy Resident Seminar, 1975, p. 1.

109. D. W. Guthrie, *Am. J. Nurs., 77*(2), 48 (1977).

110. A. H. Dube, *N.Y. State J. Med., 69,* 1169 (1969).

111. B. J. Dye, C. A. Blainey, P. L. Byre, and J. P. Palmer, *J. Fam. Pract., 5,* 341 (1977).

Appendix 1
Diabetes Information Sources

Information for Pharmacists

- Alba Foods
  c/o Weldon Farm Products, Incorporated
  24 W. 57th Street
  New York, N.Y. 10019
  "The Alba Story: An Information Guide for Health Professionals."

- The Ames Company
  Division of Miles Laboratories, Incorporated
  P.O. Box 70
  Elkhart, Ind. 46514
  "Current Concepts in the Treatment of Diabetes Mellitus," R. K. Campbell, 1980.

- Becton, Dickinson, and Company
  Rutherford, N.J. 07070
  "Getting Started: Audiovisual Instructional Diabetes Education Program," a slide/cassette presentation covering the drawing and injection of insulin, site selection and rotation, and mixing of insulins, 1980.

- California Syllabus
  1494 MacArthur
  Oakland, Calif. 94602
  "A Pharmacist's Guide to Diabetes Mellitus," University of California at San Francisco School of Pharmacy, 1977.

- Diabetes Education Center
  4959 Excelsior Boulevard
  Minneapolis, Minn. 55416
  "Diabetes Manual," 1980.
  "The First International Workshop on Diabetes in Camping."
  "Fast Food Exchange List," 1978.
  Several cookbooks for diabetics, 1971–1978.

- Eli Lilly and Company
  Lilly Research Laboratories
  Indianapolis, Ind. 46206
  "Diabetes Mellitus," 8th ed., S. O. Waife, Ed., 1980.
  "Insulin: Its Source and Action," M. Kory, 1964.
  "The New Lilly Insulins: Questions and Answers for Pharmacists," 1980.
  "Continual Improvements in Manufacturing Techniques Have Led to Improved Diabetic Therapy," 1980.
  "Diabetes Therapy, Parts 1 and 2," a continuing education program for pharmacists, R. H. Raash, June 1981.

- National Diabetes Information Clearinghouse
  805 15th Street, N.W., Suite 500
  Washington, D.C. 20005
  "Teaching Guides for Diabetes Education Programs: Selected Annotations," June 1979.
  "Educational Materials for and About Young People with Diabetes: Selected Annotations," NIH Publication No. 80-1871.

- Novo Laboratories
  "Diabetic Ketoacidosis: Practical Guidelines for Patient Management," K. E. Alberti and J. S. Skyler, April 1981.

- Pfizer Laboratories
  Division of Pfizer Incorporated
  235 E. 42nd Street
  New York, N.Y. 10017
  "Diabetes Mellitus Reference Book," P. Felig and R. Sherwin, 1980.
  "Diabetes Outlook—Newest Developments in Diagnosis and Management," published 10 times yearly for Pfizer Laboratories by Science and Medicine Publishing Company, 515 Madison Avenue, New York, N.Y. 10022.

- Smith, Kline & French Laboratories
  Philadelphia, Pa. 19101
  "Low-Dose Insulin Therapy in Diabetic Ketoacidosis," in *Therapeutics Drug Monographs for the Pharmacist,* Biomedical Information Corporation, 919 Third Avenue, New York, N.Y. 10022, 1977.

- The Upjohn Company
  Kalamazoo, Mich. 49001
  "The Child with Diabetes Mellitus," R. L. Jackson and R. A. Guthrie, September 1975.
  "On Spontaneous Hypoglycemia," J. W. Conn and S. Pek, 1970.
  "Diabetes Mellitus," T. G. Skillman and M. Tzagournis, 1979.
  "Factors That Have Been Observed to Affect Blood Glucose Levels," March 1970.

Information for Patients

- American Diabetes Association, Incorporated
  600 Fifth Avenue
  New York, N.Y. 10020
  "What You Need to Know About Diabetes," 1976.
  "Some Facts About Diabetes," 1978.
  "Career Choices for Diabetics," 1979.
  "Employment Opportunities and Protections for Diabetics," 1979.
  "Anger—A Message to the Adolescent with Diabetes," 1979.
  "What Is the American Diabetes Association?" 1978.
  "Present Status of the Oral Drugs," 1979.
  "What the Teacher Should Know About the Student with Diabetes Mellitus," 1979.
  "Helping Your Child With Diabetes," 1978.
  "Diabetes Mellitus," 4th ed., Sussman and Metz, 1975.

- American Pharmaceutical Association
  2215 Constitution Avenue, N.W.
  Washington, D.C. 20037
  "The Diabetic Patient Drug Monitoring Checklist," 1979.
  "Eye Care for the Diabetic Patient," R. K. Campbell, 1980.
  "Diabetic Self-Monitoring Checklist," R. K. Campbell, 1982.

- The Ames Company
  Division of Miles Laboratories, Incorporated
  P.O. Box 70
  Elkhart, Ind. 46514
  "Mr. Hypo Is My Friend: A Handbook for the Young Diabetic," 1975.
  "Care of the Child with Diabetes: A Guidebook for Parents and Teachers of Diabetics," 1977.
  "Home Urine Testing for the Diabetic," P. Sylbert, 1976.
  "Plain Talk for Parents of Diabetic Children: A Guide-

book for Parents of Diabetics," 1978.
"Straight Talk About Diabetes: A Guidebook for the Teenagers and Young Adult Diabetic," 1977.
"Toward Good Control: Guidebook for Diabetics," 1977.
"Shopping List for Diabetic Patients," 1978.
"Take Charge of Your Diabetes," C. M. Peterson, 1981.

● Baptist Hospitals' Foundation of Birmingham, Incorporated
3201 Fourth Avenue S.
Birmingham, Ala. 35222
"Body Map for Diabetics—To Record the Systematic Rotation of Insulin Injection Sites," 1974.

● Becton, Dickinson, and Company
Rutherford, N.J. 07070
Diabetes I.D. Card
Insulin Reaction Wallet Card
"The Importance of Proper Dosage Accuracy for the Diabetic," 1977.
"An Illustrated Guide to Proper Diet Control for the Diabetic," 1977.
"Drawing and Injecting Insulin," 1980.
"Site Selection and Rotation," 1980.
"Mixing Insulins," 1980.
"Managing Diabetes at Home," 1980.
"Footnotes for Better Diabetes Care," 1980.
"Dining Out Made Simple," 1980.
"Exercise and Its Benefits," 1980.
"Answers to Questions About Sick Days," 1980.
"Fast Food Guide," 1980.
"Getting Started at Home," 1980.

● California Canners & Growers Cookbook Department
3100 Ferry Bldg.
San Francisco, Calif. 94106
"Diet Delight Cookbook for Diabetic Children," 3rd ed., J Jones.

● Geigy Pharmaceuticals
Division of Ciba-Geigy Corporation
Ardsley, N.Y. 10502
"Living with Diabetes," 1972.
"Urine Test Record," 1972.
"Daily Food Care Checklist," 1972.

● Health Education
Metropolitan Medical Center
900 S. Eighth Street
Minneapolis, Minn. 55404
"A Survival Kit for Diabetics: Healthy Living, Healthy Eating and a Healthy Future," A. K. J. Skaalure and S. Weinzierl.
"Diabetes: Healthy Living, Healthy Eating and a Healthy Future," video/cassette programs, 1980.

● The Juvenile Diabetes Foundation
23 E. 26th Street
New York, N.Y. 10010
"What You Should Know About Juvenile Diabetes," plus numerous other brochures on subjects relevant to Type I diabetics.
"Having Children—A Guide for the Diabetic Woman," R. Hausknecht.

● Eli Lilly and Company
Lilly Research Laboratories
Indianapolis, Ind. 46206

"What Is Diabetes?" 1976.
"A Guide for the Diabetic," 1975.
"The Progress of Insulin," 1977.
"Tony and Mark Score a Winning Run Over Diabetes," 1977.
"TesTape for Fast, Accurate Determination of Glucose in Urine," 1975.
"Complete Diet Plan Packet with Sample Diets for Diabetics," 1979.

● Medidisc Corporation
P.O. Box 14306
N. Palm Beach, Fla. 33408
"Electameal Medidisc: A Meal Planning Chart for Diabetics," 1976.

● Monoject, Division of Sherwood Medical
Dept. T.I., 1831 Olive Street
St. Louis, Mo. 63103
"How to Take Insulin," in English, Spanish, or French.
"Insulin Injection Site Selectors."
"Professional Outline: Diabetes and Pregnancy," Garvey.
"Aids for People with Diabetes Catalog."
"The Baby Team," Coustan and Garvey, 1979.

● Pfizer Laboratories
Division of Pfizer Incorporated
235 E. 42nd Street
New York, N.Y. 10017
"Home Self Management Center Program on Diabetes: You Are in Control," 1978.
"You're Not A Diabetic, Are You?" 1975.
"Understanding Your Diabetes," 1981.

● The Radwyn
Suite E-15
Bryn Mawr, Pa. 19010
"Insulin Injection Simplified Site Selector," A. Fischer, 1977.

● E. R. Squibb and Sons, Incorporated
Princeton, N.J. 08540
"Don't Be Afraid of Diabetes: A Handbook for Diabetics," 1977.
"Vacationing with Diabetes, Not From Diabetes," S. Mirsky, 1978.

● The Upjohn Company
Kalamazoo, Mich. 49001
"You and Diabetes," January 1979.
"Urine Test Record," July 1971.
"Calorie Control for You," 1972.

● USP Convention Incorporated
12601 Twinbrook Parkway
Rockville, Md. 20852
"A Guide to the Use of Oral Antidiabetic Medicines," 1980.
"A Guide to the Use of Insulin," 1980.
"A Guide to the Use of Glucagon," 1980.

Miscellaneous

The pharmacist should contact the local diabetes association for brochures to provide to diabetics.
● "Juvenile Diabetes—Adjustment and Emotional Problems," New Jersey State Department of Health, Diabetic Control Program, P.O. Box 1540, Trenton, N.J. 08625. Single copies free.

- "How to Live with Diabetes," H. Dolger, Upjohn (available only through bookstores).
- "Joslin Diabetes Manual," 11th ed., L. P. Krall, Ed.; available from Lea & Febiger, Philadelphia, Pa., 1978.

New information is constantly being published to help the diabetic patient maintain control. Pharmacists should ask the representatives of major pharmaceutical companies about what information is available for them and their diabetic patients.

Appendix 2: "Sugar-Free" Preparations by Therapeutic Category

Drugs containing sugar or other agents that have caloric value have the potential to interfere with the control of blood glucose in diabetic patients. The rule of thumb for diabetics is to avoid medicinal agents containing sugar. Pharmacists should note, however, in monitoring diabetic patients that the amount of sugar or calories in a single dose of any product is not likely to cause an acute problem in most diabetic patients, depending on the type of diabetes and the methods used by the patient to control the condition. Diabetics who are ill should be trained to monitor their blood glucose levels carefully. For example, if a drug that contains ingredients producing calories is prescribed to treat an infection, a patient who is closely monitoring blood glucose levels can detect an increase and make adjustments in diet and drug therapy to counteract the calories produced by ingesting the drug.

In addition, pharmacists should note that the sweetening agent in most of the products listed is saccharin. Proposed regulations by the FDA limiting or banning the use of saccharin could greatly change the list of sugar-free medicines. Since the list could change frequently, the pharmacist should check the label for sugar content of each drug prescribed for a diabetic. The pharmacist should also check for sugar substitutes such as sorbitol, fructose, and alcohol, which can provide calories.

The following list of sugar-free preparations can be used to assist the pharmacist and physician in selecting products that are free of sucrose in a given therapeutic class. **Sugar-free products have caloric value and should not be confused with low-calorie items.**

Systemic Alkalinizers
Polycitra-LC, Willen
Bicitra, Willen

Amino Acids
Lipomul Oral, Upjohn
L-Lysine, Nature's Bounty
Lycolan Elixir, Lannett
L-Tryptophan, Freeda Pharm.
L-Tryptophan, Nature's Bounty
L-Tryptophan, O.L.C. Labs
L-Tryptophan, Orlove's Lincoln Crawford Pharm. Labs
PDP Liquid Protein, Wesley Pharm.

Analeptics
Cenalene, Central
Coramine, Ciba

Analgesics
Acetaminophen Elixir, Beecham Labs, Lannett
Aminodyne, Bowman

Conex Liquid, O'Neal, Jones & Feldman
Conex Codeine Liquid, O'Neal, Jones & Feldman
Covangesic, Mallinckrodt
Donalex Elixir, Lannett
Elixir Aminodyne, Bowman
Paregoric USP, Abbott
SK-APAP Elixir, SKF Labs
Tylaprin Elixir, Cenci
Tylenol Drops, McNeil

Antacids and Combinations
AlternaGEL, Stuart
Aludrox, Wyeth
Amitone, Norcliff Thayer
Camalox Suspension, Rorer
Creamalin, Winthrop
Delcid, Merrell
Di-Gel Liquid (mint, lemon, and orange flavored), Plough
Estomul-M Liquid, Riker
Eugel Tabs, Reid Provident
Gaviscon Liquid, Marion
Gelusil Liquid-Flavor Pack, Warner-Chilcott
Gelusil II, Warner-Chilcott
Gelusil M Liquid, Warner-Chilcott
Kolantyl Gel, Merrell
Maalox Suspension, Rorer
Maalox Plus Suspension, Rorer
Maalox Therapeutic Concentrate, Rorer
Magnatril Suspension, Lannett
Magnesia and Alumina Oral Suspension USP, Abbott, Philips Roxane
Milk of Bismuth, Parke-Davis
Milk of Magnesia USP, Bowman
Mylanta Liquid, Stuart
Mylanta II Liquid, Stuart
Pepto-Bismol, Norwich
Riopan Plus, Ayerst
Riopan Suspension, Ayerst
Silain-Gel Liquid, Robins
Titralac Liquid, Riker
Trisogel, Lilly
WinGel, Winthrop

Antiasthmatics
Aerolate, Fleming
Alevaire, Breon
Alupent Syrup, Boehringer Ingelheim
Bronkometer, Breon
Bronkosol, Breon
Droxine S. F., Sherry Kershman
Elixir Adolphyllin, Bowman
Elixicon Suspension, Cooper
Ephed-Organidin Elixir, Wallace
Isuprel Mistometer, Breon
Isuprel Solutions, Breon
Lanophyllin Elixir, Lannett
Lixaminol AT Elixir, Ferndale
Lixaminol Elixir, Ferndale
Lufyllin Elixir, Mallinckrodt
Mucomyst-10%, Mead Johnson
Mucomyst-20%, Mead Johnson
Mini-Lix Elixir, Ferndale
Metaprel Syrup, Dorsey
Mudrane GG Elixir, Poythress
Neothylline Elixir, Lemmon
Neothylline GG, Lemmon
Organidin Solution, Wallace
Somophyllin Oral Liquid, Fisons

Synophylate, Central
Tedral Elixir, Warner-Chilcott
Tedral Pediatric Suspension, Warner-Chilcott
Theoloxir, Panray
Theo-Organadin Elixir, Wallace
Theophyl-225 Elixir, Knoll
Theophylline Elixir, Philips Roxane

Antidepressants

Sinequan Oral Concentrate, Pfizer

Antidiarrheals

ColyMycin Pediatric Suspension, Warner-Chilcott
Corrective Mixture, Beecham Labs
Corrective Mixture with Paregoric, Beecham Labs
Devrom, Parthenon
Infantol Pink, First Texas
Infantol White, First Texas
Kao-Con, Upjohn
Kaolin Mixture with Pectin NF, Abbott
Kaolin-Pectin Suspension, Philips Roxane
Kaopectate, Upjohn
Kaopectate Concentrate, Upjohn
Konsyl Powder, Burton-Parsons
Lomotil Liquid, Searle
Lomoxate, Cord
Opecto Elixir, Bowman
Paregoric, Parke-Davis
Paregoric USP, Lannett, Philips Roxane
Parepectolin, Rorer
Pargel, Parke-Davis (discontinued but available)
Pektamalt, Warren-Teed
Pepto Bismol, Norwich-Eaton
Quintess, Lilly

Antiepileptics

Mysoline Suspension, Ayerst
Paradoine Solution, Abbott

Antiflatulents

Di-Gel Liquid (mint, lemon, and orange flavored), Plough
Mylicon Drops, Stuart
Riopan-Plus, Ayerst

Antihistamines/Decongestants

A.R.M. Tabs, Menley James
Ciramine, Zemmer
Covanamine, Mallinckrodt
Covangesic Liquid, Mallinckrodt
Dimetapp Elixir, Robins
Histatapp Elixir, Upsher-Smith
Histosal Tabs, Ferndale
Nasal Decongestant Elixir, Bowman
Phenergan Syrup, Wyeth
Phenergan Fortis Syrup, Wyeth
Ryna Liquid, Mallinckrodt
Sine-Off AF Extra Strength Tabs, Menley James
SK-Diphenhydramine, SKF Labs
Veltap Elixir, Lannett

Anti-infectives

Declomycin Syrup, Lederle
Furadantin Oral Suspension, Norwich-Eaton
Furadantin Sodium Sterile, Norwich-Eaton
Furoxone Liquid, Norwich-Eaton
Mandelamine Suspension Forte, Warner-Chilcott
Minocin Syrup, Lederle
Mycifradin Sulfate Oral Solution, Upjohn

NegGram Suspension, Winthrop
Nydrazid Syrup, Squibb
Proklar Suspension, O'Neal, Jones & Feldman
Robitet Syrup, Robins
Rondomycin Syrup, Wallace
Sulfaloid Suspension, O'Neal, Jones & Feldman
Terramycin Syrup, Pfizer
Tetracyn Syrup, Pfipharmecs
Vibramycin Syrup, Pfizer

Antiparkinsonism Agents

Artane Elixir, Lederle

Antipsychotics

Loxitane Oral Concentrate, Lederle

Antispasmodics

Antrocol Elixir, Poythress
Pamine PB Drops, Upjohn

Cough Medicines

Brown Mixture, Bowman
Brown Mixture, N.F., Lannett
Cerose, Ives Labs
Cerose-DM Expectorant, Ives Lab
Cetro-Cerose, Ives Labs
Clistin Expectorant, McNeil
Codimal DM, Central
Colrex Syrup, Rowell
Colrex Compound Elixir, Rowell
Colrex Expectorant, Rowell
Conar Liquid, Beecham Labs
Conex Liquid, O'Neal, Jones & Feldman
Contac Jr., Menley James
Coryban-D Cough Syrup, Pfipharmecs
Dilocol, Bell
Elixir Terpin Hydrate and Codeine (various
  manufacturers)
Ephed-Organidin, Wallace
Hycomine Syrup, Endo
Lanatuss, Lannett
Omni-Tuss, Pennwalt
Ornacol Liquid, SKF Labs
Potassium Iodide Liquid, Philips Roxane
Promex, Lemmon
Prunicodeine, Lilly
Queltuss, O'Neal, Jones & Feldman
Robitussin-CF Liquid, Robins
Ryna-C, Mallinckrodt
Ryna-CS Liquid, Mallinckrodt
S-T Expectorant SF & D-F, Scot-Tussin
S-T Forte, Sugar-Free, Scot-Tussin
Scot-Tussin Sugar-Free, Scot-Tussin
Sorbutuss, Dalin
Syrup Bowtussin, Bowman
Tolu-Sed, First Texas
Tolu-Sed DM, First Texas
Tricodene "NN," Pfeiffer
Tussar SF, Armour
Tussionex, Pennwalt
Tussi-Organidin Elixir, Wallace
Tussirex Sugar-Free, Scot-Tussin
Tuss-Ornade, SKF Labs

Dental/Oral Preparations

Baby Oragel, Commerce
Cepacol Mouthwash, Merrell
Cepastat Mouthwash/Gargle, Merrell

Chloraseptic Mouthwash and Gargle, Norwich-Eaton
Fluorigard Mouthrinse, Colgate-Palmolive
Luride Drops, Hoyt
Oracin, Squibb
Phos-Flur Rinse-Supplement, Hoyt
Point Two Mouthrinse, Hoyt
Thera-Flur Gel-Drops, Hoyt

Diagnostic Agents

Gastrografin, Squibb

Dietary Substitutes

Co-Salt, Norcliff Thayer
Sweeta Liquid, Squibb

Hematinics

Amicar Syrups, Lederle
Chel-Iron Drops, Kinney
Chel-Iron Liquid, Kinney
Ferrolip Syrup, Flint
Gerivites Tabs, Nature's Bounty
Hytinic, Hyrex Pharm
Iberet Liquid, Abbott
Iberet-500 Liquid, Abbott
Incremin with Iron Syrup, Lederle
Niferex, Central
Nu-Iron, Mayrand
Pedicran with Iron Liquid, Scherer
Secran/Fe Elixir, Scherer
Toleron Suspension, Mallinckrodt
Vita-Plus H Half Strength Sugar-Free, Scot-Tussin
Vita-Plus H Liquid, Scot-Tussin
Vita-Plus H Sugar-Free, Scot-Tussin

Laxatives

Aromatic Cascara Fluidextract USP, Abbott, Lannett,
  Parke-Davis, Philips Roxane
Castor Oil (flavored), Philips Roxane
Castor Oil USP, Lannett, Philips Roxane
Castor Oil, Squibb
Colace, Liquid 1%, Mead Johnson
Cologel, Lilly
Doxinate Solution 5%, Hoechst-Roussel
Evac-Q-Mag, Magnesium Citrate Solution NF,
  Warren-Teed
Haley's MO, Winthrop
Hypaque oral powder (radiopaque), Winthrop
Kondremul, Fisons
Kondremul with Cascara, Fisons
Kondremul with Phenolphthalein, Fisons
Konsyl, Burton Parsons
Milk of Magnesia, Lilly, Parke-Davis, Squibb
Milk of Magnesia-Cascara Suspension, Philips Roxane
Milk of Magnesia-Mineral Oil Emulsion, Philips Roxane
Milk of Magnesia-Mineral Oil Emulsion (flavored),
  Philips Roxane
Milk of Magnesia USP, Lannett, Philips Roxane
Mineral Oil, Squibb
Mineral Oil USP, Abbott, Philips Roxane
Mint-O-Mag, Squibb
Neoloid, Lederle
Peri-Colace, Mead Johnson
Phospho-Soda, Fleet
Sodium Phosphate and Biphosphate Oral Solution USP,
  Philips Roxane

Potassium Products

Cena-K, Century
Elixir Potassium Gluconate, Bowman
Kaochlor S-F 10% Liquid, Warren-Teed
Kaochlor-Eff, Warren-Teed
Kaon-Cl 20% Liquid, Warren-Teed
Kaon Elixir (grape and lemon-lime flavor), Warren-Teed
Kay Ciel Elixir, Cooper
Kay Ciel Powder, Cooper
Kaylixir, Lannett
KEFF, Lemmon
KLOR-CON Liquid 20%, Upsher-Smith
KLOR-10% Liquid, Upsher-Smith
KLOR-CON Powder, Upsher-Smith
Kloride Elixir, Federal
Klorvess Effervescent Tabs, Dorsey
Klorvess Granules, Dorsey
Kolyum Liquid, Pennwalt
Liquid Potassium Triplex, Lilly
Pan-Kloride Elixir, Panray
Potasalan Elixir, Lannett
Potassium Chloride (10% and 20%), Cenci, Lederle
Potassium Chloride Liquid 10%, Abbott
Potassium Chloride, 10% Solution, Bowman
Potassium Chloride Oral Solution USP (5%, 10%, and 20%),
  Philips Roxane
Potassium Chloride Powder, Philips Roxane
Potassium Gluconate, Lederle
Potassium Gluconate Elixir NF, Philips Roxane
Potassium Triplex, Lilly
Rum-K, Fleming

Sedatives/Tranquilizers

Amytal Elixir, Lilly
Butabarbital Sodium Elixir, Lannett
Butazem Elixir, Zemmer
Butisol Sodium Elixir, McNeil
Haldol Concentrate, McNeil
Hyonatol-B Elixir, Bowman
Infadorm Drops, Reid Provident
Lithonate-S, Rowell
Loxitane Oral Concentrate, Lederle
Mellaril Concentrate, Sandoz
Permitil, Squibb
Serentil Concentrate, Boehringer Ingelheim
Thorazine Concentrate, SKF Labs
Triclos, Merrell
Vesprin High Potency Suspension, Squibb
Vistaril Oral Suspension, Pfizer

Vitamin Preparations/Nutritionals

Ad-Cebrin with Fluoride Drops, Lilly
Arcobee with C Capsules, Nature's Bounty
B & C Liquid, Nature's Bounty
C-B Time Liquid, Arco
Cecon, Abbott
Ce-Vi-Sol Drops, Mead Johnson
Cod Liver Oil, Squibb
Cod Liver Oil (mint-flavored), Squibb
Combinate 28 in 1 Tablets, Spencer-Mead
Flura-Drops, Kirkman
Flura-Loz, Kirkman
Formula-75 Tablets, Hudson
Hycal, Beecham Labs
Incremin with Iron Syrup Vitamins B-1, B-6, B-12
Iradicav SnF₂, Johnson & Johnson
Iron, B Complex, & Vitamin C Liquid, Abbott
Kari-Rinse, Lorvic

Lanoplex Elixir, Lannett
Lipotriad, Cooper
Liqui-Cee, Arnar-Stone
Luride, Hoyt
Luride Lozi-Tabs, Hoyt
Luride-SF Lozi-Tabs, Hoyt
Lycolan Elixir, Lannett
Mega-B Tablets, Arco
Megadose Tablets, Arco
M.V.I., USV Pharm
Neutra-Phos, Willen
Neutra-Phos K, Willen
Novacebrin Drops, Lilly
Novacebrin with Fluoride Drops, Lilly
Obron-6 Tablets, Pfipharmecs
Osteon-D Tablets, Pasadena
Pediaflor, Ross
Phos-Flur, Hoyt
Point Two, Hoyt
Poly-Vi-Flor Drops, Mead Johnson
Poly-Vi-Flor/Iron Drops, Mead Johnson
Poly-Vi-Sol Drops, Mead Johnson

Poly-Vi-Sol/Iron Drops, Mead Johnson
Relevite Improved Tablets, Scott-Alison
RoeriBeC Tablets, Pfipharmecs
Super D Cod Liver Oil, Upjohn
Thera-Flur, Hoyt
Thera-Flur-N, Hoyt
Theragran Liquid, Squibb
Theravim Tablets, Hudson
Tri-Vi-Flor Drops, Mead Johnson
Tri-Vi-Sol Drops, Mead Johnson
Tri-Vi-Sol/Iron Drops, Mead Johnson
Vi-Daylin Drops, Ross
Vi-Daylin ADC Drops, Ross
Vi-Daylin ADC/Fluoride Drops, Ross
Vi-Daylin ADC Plus Iron Drops, Ross
Vi-Daylin/Fluoride Drops, Ross
Vi-Daylin Plus Iron Drops, Ross
Vi-Penta Infant Drops, Roche
Vi-Penta F Infant Drops, Roche
Vi-Penta Multivitamin Drops, Roche
Vi-Penta F Multivitamin Drops, Roche
Viterra High Potency Tablets, Pfipharmecs

Insulin Preparations Product Table

Product[a] (Manufacturer)	Species[b] Source	Onset[c] (hours)	Peak[c] (hours)	Dura-tion[c] (hours)	pH	Buffer	Preserv-ative	Purity[d] ppm of Proinsulin	Stability[e] at Room Temp. (months)	Zinc Content (mg/ 100 U)	Protein (mg/ 100 U)
Rapid Acting[e]											
Actrapid Regular Insulin (Novo)	P	0.5	2.5–5	8	7.4	acetate	phenol	<10	10–18	none	none
Beef Regular Iletin II (Lilly)	B	0.5–1	2–4	5–7	7.4	neutral	phenol	<10	10–18	0.01–0.04	none
Insulin Quick Velosulin (Nordisk)	P	0.5	1–3	8	7.4	sodium phos-phate, 2.4 mg/ ml	*m*-cresol	<10	10–18	none	none
Regular Iletin I (Lilly)	B,P	0.5–1	2–4	5–7	7.4	neutral	phenol	<50	10–18	0.01–0.04	none
Pork Regular Iletin II (Lilly)	P	0.5	2–4	5–7	7.4	neutral	phenol	<10	10–18	0.01–0.04	none
Regular Insulin (Squibb)	P	0.5–1	2–3	6	7.4	none	phenol	<25	10–18	0.01–0.04	none
Regular Purified Insulin (Squibb)	P	0.5–1	2–3	6	7.4	none	phenol	<10	10–18	0.01–0.04	none
Semilente Iletin I (Lilly)	B,P	1	4–6	12–14	7.4	acetate	methyl-paraben	<50	24	0.12–0.25	none
Semilente Insulin (Squibb)	B	1	4–6	12–14	7.4	acetate	methyl-paraben	<25	24	0.12–0.25	none
Semitard Insulin Zinc Suspension (Novo)	P	1.5	5–10	16	7.4	acetate	methyl-paraben	<10	10–18	0.15	none
Sterile Diluting Fluid for Neutral Regular Insulin Injection (Lilly)					neutral	10% hydro-chloric acid and/ or 10% sodium hydrox-ide	phenol		10–18		
Intermediate											
Beef Lente Iletin II[f] (Lilly)	B	1–3	6–12	24–28	7.4	acetate	methyl-paraben	<10	24–30	0.12–0.25	none
Beef NPH Iletin II[g] (Lilly)	B	3–4	6–12	24–28	7.4	phos-phate	phenol, *m*-cresol	<10	36	0.01–0.04	prota-mine, 0.5

Insulin Preparations Product Table, continued

Product[a] (Manufacturer)	Species[b] Source	Onset[c] (hours)	Peak[c] (hours)	Duration[c] (hours)	pH	Buffer	Preservative	Purity[d] ppm of Proinsulin	Stability[e] at Room Temp. (months)	Zinc Content (mg/ 100 U)	Protein (mg/ 100 U)
Insulatard NPH (Nordisk)	P	1.5	4–12	24	7.4	phosphate	*m*-cresol, phenol	<10	20+	0.25	protamine, 0.5
Lentard Insulin Zinc Suspension (Novo)	B,P	2.5	7–15	24	7.4	acetate	methylparaben	<10	24+	0.15	none
Lente Iletin I[f] (Lilly)	B,P	1–3	6–12	24–28	7.4	acetate	methylparaben	<50	18–20	0.2–0.25	none
Lente Iletin II (Lilly)	P	1–3	6–12	24–28	7.4	acetate	methylparaben	<10	24+	0.12–0.25	none
Lente Insulin[f] (Squibb)	B	1–2	8–12	24–28	7.4	acetate	methylparaben	<25	24–30	0.12–0.25	none
Lente Purified Insulin (Squibb)	B	1–2	8–12	24–28	7.4	acetate	methylparaben	<10	24–30	0.12–0.25	none
Mixtard, NPH + Regular Insulin (Nordisk)	P	0.5	4–8	24	7.4	phosphate	*m*-cresol, phenol	<10	24+	0.25	protamine, 0.2
Monotard Pork Insulin Zinc Suspension (Novo)	P	2.5	7–15	22	7.4	acetate	methylparaben	<10	24+	0.15	none
NPH Iletin[g] (Lilly)	B,P	3–4	6–12	24–28	7.4	phosphate	phenol, *m*-cresol	<50	36	0.01–0.04	protamine, 0.5
NPH Iletin II (Lilly)	P	3–4	6–12	24–28	7.4	phosphate	phenol, *m*-cresol	<10	36	0.01–0.04	protamine, 0.5
NPH (Isophane) Insulin[g] (Squibb)	B	1–1.5	8–12	24–28	7.4	phosphate	phenol, *m*-cresol	<25	36	0.25–0.35	protamine 0.5
NPH Purified Insulin (Squibb)	B	1–1.5	8–12	24–28	7.4	phosphate	phenol, *m*-cresol	<10	36	0.25–0.35	protamine, 0.5
Protaphane (NPH) Insulin (Novo)	P	1–1.5	8–12	24–28	7.4	phosphate	phenol, *m*-cresol	<10	36	0.25–0.35	protamine, 0.5
Sterile Diluting Fluid for Dilution of NPH Iletin (Lilly)					neutral	10% hydrochloric acid and/ or 10% sodium hydroxide	phenol, *m*-cresol		36		

Insulin Preparations Product Table, continued

Product[a] (Manufacturer)	Species[b] Source	Onset[c] (hours)	Peak[c] (hours)	Duration[c] (hours)	pH	Buffer	Preservative	Purity[d] ppm of Proinsulin	Stability[e] at Room Temp. (months)	Zinc Content (mg/ 100 U)	Protein (mg/ 100 U)
Long-Acting											
Beef Protamine[h] **Zinc Iletin II** (Lilly)	B	4–6	14–24	36+	7.4	phosphate	phenol	<10	36	0.2–0.25	protamine, 1.25
Protamine Zinc Iletin[h] (Lilly)	B,P	4–6	14–24	36+	7.4	phosphate	phenol	<50	36	0.2–0.25	protamine, 1.25
Protamine Zinc Iletin II (Lilly)	P	4–6	12–24	36+	7.4	phosphate	phenol	<10	36	0.2–0.25	protamine, 1.25
Protamine Zinc Insulin[h] (Squibb)	B	4–8	14–20	36	7.4	phosphate	phenol	<25	36	0.2–0.25	protamine, 1.25
Ultralente Iletin I (Lilly)	B,P	4–6	18–24	36+	7.4	acetate	methylparaben	<50	24–30	0.2–0.25	none
Ultralente Insulin (Squibb)	B	4–6	18	36	7.4	acetate	methylparaben	<25	24–30	0.2–0.25	none
Ultratard Zinc (Novo)	B	4	10–30	36	7.4	acetate	methylparaben	<10	24+	0.15	none

Miscellaneous	Description
Glucagon for Injection (Lilly)	Used parenterally (subcutaneously, intramuscularly, or intravenously) for treatment of hypoglycemia. Stable in solution up to 3 months. Stimulates the conversion of liver glycogen to glucose. Intravenous glucose is drug of choice in hypoglycemia if available. To use, lyophilized glucagon is dissolved using accompanying solution and then injected.
Glutose (Reactose)	(Paddock Laboratories, 2744–46 Lyndale Ave. South, Minneapolis, MN 55408.) Oral glucose solution used to treat insulin reaction (hypoglycemia) before unconsciousness occurs.
Insta-Glucose (ICN Pharmaceuticals, Inc.)	30.8 grams of liquid glucose. A convenient plastic tube of carbohydrate gel for use by diabetics to treat hypoglycemic symptoms.
Instant Glucose	Available from the Diabetes Association of Cleveland, 2022 Lee Road, Cleveland, OH 44118.
Instant Allergy Desensitization Kits (Lilly)	Contain single-peak pork insulin, single-peak beef insulin, or single-component pork insulin with 0.1% human serum albumin, plus directions for use.
Monojel (Sherwood)	25 G unit dose of 40% dextrose in gel packaged in foil pouches. Used to abort falling blood sugar.
Monocomponent Insulin (various)	Highly purified (99% pure insulin) by diethylaminoethylcellulose chromatography. Commercially available in United States from Lilly, Nordisk and Novo.

[a] Most insulins are available in U–40 (coded red) and U–100 (coded orange). The ultra-pure insulins by Novo and Nordisk and the Iletin II by Lilly are only available in U-100 strengths. Lilly also manufactures a regular (concentrated) Iletin (prescription only) containing 500 units of pork insulin/ml; used in patients with marked insulin resistance.

[b] Insulins with a combination of beef and pork contain 70% beef and 30% pork; B, beef and P, pork.

[c] Biologic response varies greatly in different individuals, so times are approximate.

[d] Purity of insulins is judged on a number of factors, but primarily on the parts per million of proinsulin. Conventional USP insulin can have 20–40,000 ppm. The single-peak insulins that were manufactured in the United States after 1975 contain between 300 and 3,000 ppm. The improved single-peak insulins that are available in the United States after 1980 contain approximately 50 ppm of proinsulin. The purified pork insulins from Novo, Nordisk, and Lilly contain less than 10 ppm of proinsulin.

Insulin Preparations Product Table, continued

e Mix regular with NPH in any proportion; stable for 5 minutes only. With protamine zinc insulin, use at least twice as much regular. Intermix lentes in any proportion. Stable for long periods. Lente plus regular, use within 5 minutes.
f Lente can be mixed with semilente or ultralente in any proportion and is stable for 2–3 months.
g NPH plus regular. Mix in any proportion; stable for 5 minutes only.
hOne part protamine zinc insulin to two parts regular equals NPH. Ultralente 70% plus semilente 30% yields lente. Lentes mix in any proportion, stable for 2–3 months.

Insulin Syringes and Related Products Table

Product (Manufacturer or Supplier)	Sizes Available or Description	Comments
Syringes		
Auto-Syringe AS*6C U-100 Insulin Infusion Pump (Auto-Syringes, Inc.)	9½ ounce, battery-operated infusion pump is small enough to be inconspicuous and uses a 3 cc syringe available from the same company. Requires other equipment also available from the same company.	portable insulin delivery system. Pump may be programmed to operate as an open-loop insulin delivery system for control of diabetes. An adjustable control allows for a constant rate of infused insulin throughout the day. A push button allows a bolus of insulin before meals. This product is recommended for Type I diabetics.
Busher Auto Injector (Becton-Dickinson)	connects to short-type reusable insulin syringe or with an adaptor to long type. Provides quick automatic insertion of the needle at proper depth and angle.	used in past to help patients overcome needle fear. Patients should be trained to overcome emotional factors.
CPI/Lilly Insulin Infusion Pump-Model 9100 (Cardiac Pacemakers, Inc.)	13 oz. battery-operated insulin infusion pump that provides a constant infusion of insulin to the patient. Bolus doses can be given before meals and snacks. Syringes and infusion sets are provided by CPI.	easy to use, does not require mixing of insulin with diluting fluid, has several functions not provided by other pumps. Excellent alarm system, high quality. It provides a summary of insulin units given over a period of time. Manufacturer dependability and support is excellent.
GT Automatic Injector (American Medical Products)	small, well-designed metal device that connects to Plasti-Pak syringes and allows the patient to inject insulin automatically.	speed of needle penetration is 2 to 3 times faster than the manual technique. The needle is hidden and supposedly eliminates psychological fear and apprehension. Well-designed, easy to use.
Injector-Aid (Support Systems)	model BD-1 for Becton-Dickinson disposable syringes, and MJ-1 for Monoject disposable syringes.	injection helper. Useful for handicapped or sightless patients.
Insulin Syringe, Single Use Lo-Dose (Becton-Dickinson)	0.5 cc with 28 G ½″ needle. 30/package and 100/package.	cannot change needle size. Used for patients taking less than 50 units of U-100 insulin. Larger print of calibrations allows more accurate dosing. Can be used up to 3 times.
Med-E-Jet Inoculator (Med-E-Jet)	jet injector powered by carbon dioxide cartridges.	provides a subcutaneous injection of insulin with less trauma. Can be used by sightless patients. Expensive, complicated to use, dosage adjustments in 5-unit increments.
Medi-Jector (Derata Corp.)	high quality needleless jet injector. Can deliver from 1 to 100 units per injection.	powered by a series of springs. Somewhat cumbersome in design. Bottle of insulin attaches to the device and once the dose is selected, it can be easily used by visually impaired diabetics. Dose changes can be made in increments of 1 unit.

Insulin Syringes and Related Products Table, continued

Product (Manufacturer or Supplier)	Sizes Available or Description	Comments
Mill Hill Infuser Insulin Pump (Harvard Apparatus)	10½ ounce battery-operated lightweight insulin infusion pump that uses a 6-ml Monoject disposable syringe. Catheters, needles, battery chargers, and other equipment are also available from the company.	pump designed to administer insulin continuously throughout the day. A bolus of insulin is injected before each meal. Insulin provided by infusion pumps must be diluted, and the patient needs to check his own blood glucose levels periodically. Somewhat larger than competition's product. Recommended for Type I diabetics.
Monoject Insulin Syringe (Sherwood)	1 cc with self-contained 27 G ½″ needle. U-40 and U-100. 30/package or 120/package. 27 G ⅝″ available in U-100. 0.5 cc for patients using 50 units or less of U-100 insulin.	bold numbers, preferred needle gauge, reduced dead space, sterile. 27 G less painful. Sometimes difficult to open, more storage space required. Can be reused up to 3 times.
Plastipak Self Contained Insulin Syringe (Becton-Dickinson)	1 cc with 28 G ½″ in U-40 and U-100. 1 cc with 27 G ⅝″.	no dead space. Excellent for travel. More expensive than reusable but sterile and convenient. Less pain with 27½ G. Can be reused up to 3 times.
Single Use, Long Type (Becton-Dickinson)	2 cc U-100. 30/package, detachable needles.	2 cc useful for patients taking large doses. Detachable needles produce clinically significant dead space if insulin mixing is needed.
Stylex Insulin Syringe (Pharmaseal)	1 cc U-40, and U-100 syringes with 25 G ⅝″ needles.	needles pop off. Significant dead space. Lettering rubs off easily.
Syrijet Mark IV (Mizzy, Inc.)	high-quality jet injector. Up to 34 units/injection.	easy to use but requires education program and physician monitoring. Can be used up to 4 times/day to improve control. Should be used with home blood glucose monitoring. Dosage adjustments in 2-unit increments. Comparatively inexpensive.
Yale Glass Insulin Reusable Short Type Luer Tip Syringe (Becton-Dickinson)	1 cc U-40 red scale 2 cc U-40 red scale.	can use with reusable or disposable needles. Preferred over Luer-Lok. Less expensive. Dual scale yields dose errors. Encourage patients to switch to U-100 disposable.
Yale 0.35 cc Special Insulin Syringe (Becton-Dickinson)	0.35 cc, calibrated up to 35 units.	available for patients using small doses of U-100 insulin.

Aids for Visually Impaired Patients

C-Better Syringe Magnifier (Tri County Rehabilitation Center, Stuart, Fla.)	snap-on magnifier.	magnifies two times. Plastic. Fits different type syringes.
Cemco Syringe Magnifier (Cemco)	unbreakable stainless steel magnifier.	easy to snap on and off. Magnifies bubbles and calibrations on syringe. Not for totally blind.
Char-Mag Syringe Magnifier (Char-Mag Company)	magnifier made of optical quality plastic.	easy to snap on and off. Magnifies bubbles and calibrations on syringe. Not for the totally blind.
Cornwall, Becton-Dickinson Adjustable Positive Stop (American Foundation for the Blind)	metal, complicated device that covers most of syringe. Dose set with plunger springs.	large and bulky. Use only with U-100 glass syringe. Accurate but expensive.
Dos-Aid (American Foundation for the Blind)	plastic tray that adjusts to hold syringe and insulin bottle. Plunger is pulled back to a plunger stop.	uses all types of disposable syringes. Simple to teach; accurate. Can't mix insulins.

Insulin Syringes and Related Products Table, continued

Product (Manufacturer or Supplier)	Sizes Available or Description	Comments
HoldEase (Meditec Inc.)	a plastic guide device that holds both the insulin and syringe. Guide can be compressed, causing the needle to be inserted in vial.	useful in getting needle into vial. Other less expensive products are available.
IDM (Androse Inc.)	plastic scale that attaches to plunger. Can be cut to proper length so when end reaches barrel of syringe correct dose is measured.	inexpensive and simple to use. Can use only with U-100. Not as accurate as Insulgage.
Insulin-Aid (Seabee Enterprises)	device made of plexiglass that magnetically attaches to a metal surface and holds any insulin bottle inverted to make it easier to withdraw insulin into syringe.	useful if one needs an extra hand to withdraw insulin into syringe.
Insulgage (Meditec Inc.)	small plastic gauge that attaches to B-D long or Jelco disposable syringes. Gauge and plunger are pulled back until gauge drops into place between plunger end and barrel.	accurate, simple to teach, can be used with mixed insulins. Available for U-100 disposable syringes and inexpensive.
Insulin Needle Guide (MES 165) (American Foundation for the Blind)	aluminum trough with a V-shaped notch so that the point will align with the center of a bottle of insulin. Can be custom-made to fit any bottle.	will hold any size insulin bottle. Need to send the empty insulin bottle to ensure a custom fit.
Insulin Needle Guide (MES 168) (American Foundation for the Blind)	round aluminum cap to fit the top of an insulin bottle. The inner contour is funnel-shaped and guides the needle into rubber cap.	used for Lilly insulin bottles only. It is small, sturdy, and inexpensive.
Insulin Syringe MES 260 (American Foundation for the Blind)	precision device consisting of a glass barrel inside a 3½″ metal casing. Units drawn up determined by an audible click.	used only with U-40. Syringe expensive but accurate.
Monoject Scale Magnifier (Monoject Inc.)	magnifier made of optical quality plastic.	easy to snap on and off. Magnifies bubbles and calibrations on syringe. Not for totally blind.
Templet Insulin Measuring Device (Greater Detroit Society for the Blind)	insulin measuring device made of stapled and soft adhesive tape that is attached to the plunger.	can be constructed to desired dose and is simple to use, easy to handle, accurate, and inexpensive.
Tru-Set Insulin Syringe Control (American Foundation for the Blind)	metal frame which clips onto the barrel of the syringe. Frame piece can be set with a screw to stop the plunger at the desired level on the syringe.	stable and functional but needs a sighted person to set it. Cannot mix two types of insulin in one syringe.
Vial Center-Aid (George Wright Industries)	device snaps on the insulin bottle, helps to center needle on the top of the vial.	helps avoid bent and blunted needles; made of metal-plated materials that will not scratch; easy to keep clean.

Miscellaneous

Product (Manufacturer or Supplier)	Sizes Available or Description	Comments
Alcohol Swabs and Alcohol Wipes Spongettes (Becton-Dickinson, Sherwood Medical)	70% isopropyl alcohol for single use.	unit dose of alcohol swabs. More expensive but good for travel.
Becton-Dickinson Insulin Travel Kit (Becton-Dickinson)	plastic carrying case for vial of insulin and disposable syringes.	useful for travel.
Diabetic's Wallet (California Wallets)	4″ × 6″ durable, machine-washable cloth wallet that holds eight syringes, two bottles of insulin, alcohol swabs, and ID card.	well-designed device to carry diabetic supplies. Inexpensive.

Insulin Syringes and Related Products Table, continued

Product (Manufacturer or Supplier)	Sizes Available or Description	Comments
Monoject Insulin Users Travel Kit (Monoject Inc.)	durable case that holds two insulin vials, five syringes, and alcohol wipes.	useful for travel.
Needle Sharpener (Aloxite Safety Blade Hone, Carborundum Co. and others)	used to sharpen reusable needles.	patients should be encouraged to use disposable needles.
Northeast Medical Products Diabetics Case (Northeast Medical Products, Inc.)	soft vinyl case with washable liner that allows storage of syringes, two vials of insulin, specimen bottle, and urine testing equipment.	larger than competitors' products.
91% Isopropyl Alcohol (Lilly and various manufacturers)	used for sterilizing needles and syringes and for cleansing skin before injections. Preferred to rubbing alcohol due to less water and not denatured; therefore safer with insulin.	Lilly product is in plastic, nonbreakable bottles.
Ster-Inge (Ster-Inge)	device to sterilize glass syringes and disposable or reusable needles.	simple to operate. Recommended for patients who do not use disposable syringes.
Sugar Babe (Sugar Babe Inc.)	well-constructed doll with specially formulated skin that has a natural feel and assists diabetics in learning to inject insulin. Also contains a carrying case and a guide for insulin-dependent diabetics.	well-designed and useful product to assist in the training of Type I children diabetics.
Syringe and Needle Destroyers (B-D's Destruclip) (Becton-Dickinson)	device to destroy disposable needles after use. Cuts off needle and cuts syringe into parts.	useful in hospitals and nursing homes where large numbers of syringes are used.

Urine and Blood Glucose Test Product Table

Product (Manufacturer)	Product Formulation and Sizes	Active Ingredients	Indication of Product Deterioration	Time Required to Evaluate (seconds)	Drug Interference	Comments[a]
Chemstrip bG (Bio-Dynamics)	strip: 25's	glucose oxidase, peroxidase, *o*-tolidine, tetramethyl-benzidine	darkening of test area	120–180	no false(+), possibly some false(−)	product can easily be used by patients to test glucose in whole blood; requires a drop of blood on both zones of the test strip; requires cotton ball to wipe off blood after 60 seconds; tests are reliable but not as accurate as those read by a machine
Chemstrip G (Bio-Dynamics)	strip: 100's	glucose oxidase, peroxidase, *o*-tolidine	discoloration of test area	60	no false(+), possibly some false(−)	inexpensive; convenient for Type II diabetics; not quantitative

Urine and Blood Glucose Test Product Table, continued

Product (Manufacturer)	Product Formulation and Sizes	Active Ingredients	Indication of Product Deterioration	Time Required to Evaluate (seconds)	Drug Interference	Comments[a]
Clinistix (Ames)	strip: 50's	glucose oxidase, peroxide, *o*-tolidine	tan or dark test area	10	no false(+), some false(−) (levodopa, ascorbic acid, aspirin)	inexpensive, convenient for Type II diabetics; not quantitative
Clinitest (Ames) *5-drop method* *2-drop method*	tablets: 36's, 100's, 250's, 1000's foilwrap: 24's and 500's tablets: 36's	copper reduction	deep blue tablet	15, then shake gently	false(+) in presence of reducing agents, no false(−)	2-drop most reliable at high glucose levels; use for "sliding scale"; use for Type I; inexpensive but inconvenient (requires water, dropper, and test tube); not specific for glucose; only difference in 2-drop and 5-drop method is the amount of urine used
Dextrostix (Ames)	strip: 25's, 100's	glucose oxidase, peroxidase, *o*-tolidine	test area does not resemble "O" on color chart	60 (test for blood glucose)	no false(+), some false(−)	useful in screening; accurate if read by Dextrometer; can use to correlate blood and urine glucose levels; home use improves control; requires a drop of blood
Diastix (Ames)	strip: 50's, 100's	glucose oxidase, peroxidase, potassium iodide, chromogen	variation from light blue or "neg" on color chart	30, dip, remove excess urine, and read	no false(+), some complete false(−) (see Clinistix)	easy to read; relatively expensive; more accurate than TesTape but less than Clinitest; under-reading possible at high glucose levels; for use by both Type I and Type II
Mega-Diastix (with control tablets) (Ames)	strip: 50's, 100's	glucose oxidase, peroxidase, potassium iodide, chromogen	variation from light blue or "neg" on color chart	30, dip, remove excess urine, and read	no false(+), some complete false(−) (see Clinistix)	extra-large strips for visually impaired diabetic; control tablets used to test to see if patient can read accurately
Stat Tek Test Strips (Bio-Dynamics)	strip: 25's	glucose oxidase, peroxidase, *o*-tolidine	test area does not resemble "O" on color chart	120	no false(+), some false(−)	strips can be used only with Stat Tek Colorimeter; useful in monitoring blood glucose levels; requires a drop of blood

Urine and Blood Glucose Test Product Table, continued

Product (Manufacturer)	Product Formulation and Sizes	Active Ingredients	Indication of Product Deterioration	Time Required to Evaluate (seconds)	Drug Interference	Comments[a]
TesTape (Eli Lilly & Co.)	strip: 100 tests/dispenser	glucose oxidase, peroxidase, *o*-tolidine, yellow dye	brown color or doesn't resemble "O" on test with distilled water	60	no false(+), some partial false(−) (see Clinistix)	most inexpensive test; convenient for home and travel; accuracy adequate if all 3+ read as 4+; not as quantitative as Diastix or Clinitest

[a]Protect all products from heat, light, and moisture

Combination Urine Test Product Table

Product (Manufacturer)	Product Formulation and Sizes	Active Ingredients	Indication of Product Deterioration	Time Required to Evaluate (seconds)	Drug Interference	Comments
Chemstrip 8 (Bio-Dynamics)	strip: 50's	glucose oxidase, peroxidase, *o*-tolidine, sodium nitro-ferricyanide	discoloration of test area	0–60 (dip and read)	no false(+) (glucose)	tests for glucose, protein, pH, blood, ketones, bilirubin, urobilinogen, and nitrite; error potential is great; specific individual tests recommended
Chemstrip GK (Bio-Dynamics)	strip: 100's	glucose oxidase, peroxidase, sodium nitro-ferricyanide	discoloration of test area	60	for ketones: false(+) possible but rare, for glucose: no false(+), some possible false(−)	this product is similar to Ketodiastix in that it is useful to monitor glucose and ketones in the urine
Combistix (Ames)	strip: 100's	glucose oxidase	discoloration of test area	30–60 (dip and read)	no false(+) (glucose), some false(−)	test for glucose, protein, and pH
Ketodiastix (Ames)	strip: 50's, 100's	glucose oxidase, nitroprusside	glucose area green; ketone area darkened	15–30 (dip and read)	no false(+) (glucose), some false(−)	useful combination product for glucose and ketones. No need to use this test often, only when passing 4+ glucose often
Labstix (Ames)	strip: 100's	glucose oxidase, nitroprusside	discoloration of test area	30–60 (dip and read)	no false(+) (glucose), some false(−)	test for blood, pH, glucose, acetone and protein; amount of use does not warrant expense for individual patient

Combination Urine Test Product Table, continued

Product (Manufacturer)	Product Formulation and Sizes	Active Ingredients	Indication of Product Deterioration	Time Required to Evaluate (seconds)	Drug Interference	Comments
Multistix (Ames)	strip: 100's	glucose oxidase, peroxidase, o-tolidine, sodium nitro-ferricyanide	discoloration of test area	0–60 (dip and read)	no false(+) (glucose)	same as N-Multistix but does not test for nitrite
N-Multistix (Ames)	strip: 100's	glucose oxidase, peroxidase, o-tolidine, sodium nitro-ferricyanide	discoloration of test area	0–60 (dip and read)	no false(+) (glucose)	tests for glucose, protein, pH, blood, ketones, bilirubin, urobilinogen, and nitrite; error potential is great; specific individual tests recommended
Uristix (Ames)	strip: 100's	glucose oxidase	discoloration of test area	30–60 (dip and read)	no false(+) (glucose), some false(−)	test for glucose and protein; useful to determine if protein in urine (diabetic nephropathy)

Urine Ketone Test Product Table

Product (Manufacturer)	Product Formulation and Sizes	Active Ingredients	Indication of Product Deterioration	Time Required to Evaluate	Drug Interference	Comments
Acetest (Ames)	tablets: 100's, 250's	nitroprusside	darkened brown, tablet	30 seconds (urine), 2 minutes (plasma), 10 minutes (whole blood)	false(+) possible but rare (levodopa)	test for acetone and acetoacetic acid; useful in determining whether or not a diabetic is developing ketoacidosis; patient with 2% or more glucose should test for ketones
Ketostix (Ames)	strip: 50's, 100's	nitroprusside	tan or brown	15 seconds	false(+) possible but rare (levodopa)	test for acetoacetic acid; useful in determining whether or not a diabetic is developing ketoacidosis; patient with 2% or more glucose should test for ketones

Miscellaneous Products Table

Product (Manufacturer)	Description
Autoclix (Sherwood)	a plastic device in which a lancet is inserted through a platform that allows the patient to stick his finger and obtain a drop of blood. Various size platforms are available so that different depths can be obtained. Device is used with Monolets.
Autolet (Ulster Scientific Inc.)	a plastic, push-button device connected to a lancet and platform that is used to prick the finger and makes it easier for diabetics to obtain a drop of blood for testing with Dextrostix, Chemstrip bG, and Stat Tek Strips.
Clinilog (Ames)	a diary for diabetics to record date, urine sugars, urine acetone, and remarks plus a glossary of terms for diabetic patients, plus diet information. Patient should keep track of weight, changes in medication, exercise, diet, infections or emotional stress.
Dextrometer (Ames)	a colorimeter used with Dextrostix that provides accurate blood glucose determinations. Has a digital readout, is lightweight, and has a battery attachment for use when traveling. Can be used by pregnant, unstable, and Type I diabetics to improve control by home blood glucose monitoring.
Glucola (Ames)	100 g of glucose in 7-oz disposable bottle. Requires 0.5 hour to evaluate. Caffeine-free, carbonated cola-flavored preparation. For use as a carbohydrate challenge in glucose tolerance testing.
Glucometer (Ames)	a battery-powered reflectance photometer with digital display and built-in timer. Used with Dextrostix. Less expensive and smaller than a Dextrometer. Easier to calibrate and use.
Monolets (Sherwood)	a plastic-covered lance that is used with Autolet or by itself to assist diabetic patients in getting a drop of blood for blood glucose self-monitoring.
Stat Tek Twin Beam Electronic Photometer (Bio-Dynamics)	a meter used with Stat Tek Strips that provides accurate blood glucose determinations. Larger and more expensive than the Dextrometer. Useful for home blood glucose monitoring in appropriate diabetic patients.
Urine Specimen Jars	pharmacists should keep available for diabetic patients and encourage patients to take urine specimens when seeing their physicians.

14 Infant Formula Products

Michael W. McKenzie, Kenneth J. Bender, and A. Jeanece Seals

Questions to Ask the Parent

What is the child's age and weight?

Is the child under a physician's care?

Are you breast-feeding the child now or has your pediatrician recommended a formula?

Is the child allergic to milk? Are there other dietary restrictions or health problems?

Are you using an iron-fortified formula?

Are you using a multivitamin with minerals formulation for your baby? Was it recommended by your pediatrician?

Is your baby receiving fluoride supplementation?

Does the baby have diarrhea, constipation, or vomiting?

Does the child have a fever, dry skin, or a loss of appetite?

Do you have any questions about mixing the formula?

Milk, alone or in a mixture, is an infant's most important food. Until recently, breast-feeding was the most frequently used method to ensure the nutritional needs of infants. Before the 20th century, few infants not suckled by mothers or wet nurses survived their first year of life.

Substitute feedings for breast milk were made possible by discoveries in biology and medicine in the late 19th century. The starting point of all modern studies on infant metabolism began with the calorimetric feeding method (1). This method made it possible to feed infants according to their caloric (energy) requirements.

The modern era of infant formulas began in 1915 when an artificial milk was developed based on the fat content of human milk (2). Homogenized vegetable and animal fats and oils were added to skim cow's milk to approximate the fatty acid content of human milk. This first formula was named SMA, for synthetic milk adapted. Modifications of this basic formula produced many of the present-day infant formulas.

Before the acceptance of single-formula mixtures, evaporated milk was the most common infant feeding. Evaporated milk was advantageous because it was inexpensive, readily available, and required no refrigeration. By 1960, an estimated 80% of formula-fed infants in the United States were given either evaporated milk or a milk preparation marketed in evaporated form (1).

Advances in the uniformity, convenience, nutritional quality, and safety of infant formulas during the past 20 years established this as the most frequently used method of infant feeding. The popularity of infant formula products is reflected by the fact that commercially prepared milk-based or milk-free formulas account for approximately 68% of the milk and formulas fed to infants (3). Most of these products are purchased as concentrated liquids requiring the addition of water to supply the appropriate calories per fluid ounce. The more expensive, ready-to-use formulas that require no mixing or diluting are also extensively used, while powdered formulas are used less.

The composition of commercial infant formulas is in accordance with guidelines generated from extensive assessment of infant nutritional needs. Formula variation provides the opportunity to select a product that is acceptable to a particular infant and satisfies special nutritional requirements. However, these variations have produced differences in palatability, digestibility, and convenience of administration. The pharmacist, in consultation with the infant's physician, should be able to evaluate indications and advise on the selection of infant formulas.

Physiologic Considerations in Infant Nutrition

The physiologic capabilities of the infant's GI and renal systems are considered in the development of formulas that can adequately substitute for human milk. In early infancy, food must be liquid until coordination between complex tongue movements and mature swallowing reflexes develops. Frequent feedings are necessary since the stomach capacity is small.

Fats, proteins, and carbohydrates can be digested by the newborn. Protein and fat are digested mainly in the infant's small intestine. Infants have lower concentrations of bile acids in the small intestine. Furthermore, the proportion and specific forms of bile acids differ between infants and adults (4). Absorption of fat improves as the infant matures with age. Long-chain saturated fatty acids (butterfat) are not absorbed as well as unsaturated fatty acids (vegetable oils) (5).

Protein digestion does not differ appreciably between infants and adults, even though infants have less active trypsin and chymotrypsin (6, 7). Amino acids from protein digestion are absorbed by active transport mechanisms.

Starch is not absorbed well by infants (8). Lactose is absorbed well due to the presence of greater activity of the enzyme, lactase, in the small intestine of the infant than in the adult (9). Monosaccharides are absorbed well, but the absorptive capacity of infants may not equal that of adults (10–11).

The excess ingestion of electrolytes and minerals, and the metabolic end-products from protein metabolism, constitute the renal solute load. A simple, direct relationship between renal solute loads and dietary concentrations of protein and minerals does not exist. Significant amounts of minerals and protein waste products are excreted through the skin (sweat), lungs (water vapor), and GI tract. In addition, amino acids from protein digestion are used in protein anabolism for tissues. When metabolized, the carbohydrate present in formulas yields essentially no solutes for renal excretion (12).

However, the renal solute load is important because it determines the quantity of water excreted through the kidney. Young infants have less ability than older infants, children, and adults to concentrate or dilute renal solute loads (12, 13, 14). Under normal conditions, infant formulas in proper concentration provide enough water (1.5 ml/kcal/day) for all routes of water loss including urinary excretion. If decreased water intake or excessive water loss occurs, diets with high renal solute loads may stress the limited capacity of the kidney reabsorptive system (12).

Content of Milk and Formulas

The initial comparison to be considered is that between the standard of human milk and cow's milk, which is used as the protein base for most commercial preparations.

Human Milk: Standard of Comparison

Human milk is the standard against which all formulas may be compared. It is more effective than cow's milk in meeting the nutritional requirements of the human infant. The differences in composition reflect the different needs of the human infant and the calf. Although cer-

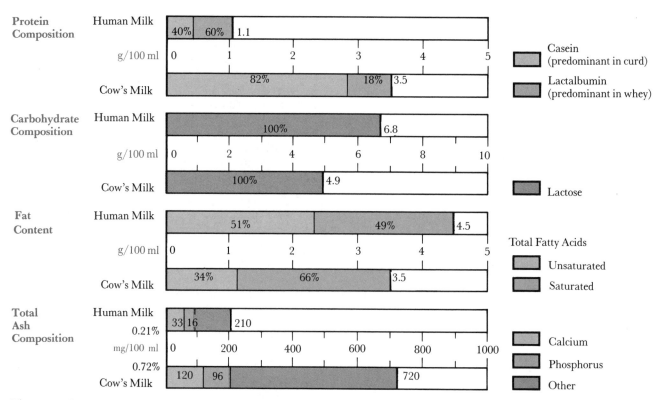

Figure 1. Comparison of human and cow's milk.

tain conditions in the infant may necessitate therapeutic formulas, human milk is the most appropriate diet for most infants.

Cow's milk has about three times the ash and protein normally found in human milk (Figure 1). This difference reflects the calf's larger growth rate and proportionate demand for protein and minerals. The urea formed from protein nitrogen combines with the mineral residue (ash) to create a higher renal solute load for the infant ingesting cow's milk. Although cow's milk usually is diluted with water and carbohydrates, the solute load requiring renal excretion generally remains greater than the load from human milk.

Not only does cow's milk contain a higher percentage of protein than human milk, but the protein differs in composition. The difference in protein composition alters digestibility and may create a milk "sensitivity," making it difficult for the infant to digest a milk-based formula. Compared with human milk, cow's milk has a higher proportion of casein protein (crude protein mixture of alpha-, beta-, gamma-, and kappa-caseins) to lactalbumin protein (primarily alpha-lactoglobulin but includes alpha-lactalbumin). Casein is relatively insoluble and occurs in milk as a "tough" curd; lactalbumin is highly soluble and occurs in milk as whey. The large amount of curd in cow's milk slows the gastric emptying rate and may cause GI distress. Processing cow's milk (acidification, boiling, and treatment with enzymes) reduces the curd tension.

Sensitivity to cow's milk differs from milk allergy in that sensitivity may be relieved by altering the casein to lactalbumin ratio; an allergic reaction requires that all animal milk protein be eliminated. Although heating cow's milk may increase digestibility by reducing curd tension, it will not alter its antigen activity in allergic infants.

The fat in cow's milk differs from that in human milk in two ways. The triglycerides in cow's milk contain primarily short- and long-chain fatty acids (butyric and caproic). Human milk fat includes medium-chain fatty acids (capric and lauric) but not the short-chain group. In addition, human milk contains a majority of monosaturated fatty acids, and cow's milk butterfat consists primarily of saturated fatty acids. Commercial milk-based formulas incorporate the highly digestible, unsaturated, medium-chain triglycerides by replacing butterfat with vegetable oil and special medium-chain triglyceride oils.

The carbohydrate percentage in cow's milk is smaller than that in human milk, and carbohydrate supplementation is often necessary. Honey and other unrefined foods are probably poor choices for carbohydrate supplementation, since they may contain botulism spores that are possible contributors to crib death in susceptible infants (15). Lactose is the carbohydrate source in both cow's milk and human milk. Lactose is absorbed into the brush border of the small intestine and cleaved by the enzyme lactase into galactose and glucose. These sugars are then absorbed actively against concentration gradients.

Cow's milk and human milk differ in absolute and proportionate amounts of calcium and phosphorus. The effect of this difference on calcium absorption is not clear because of the interrelation of additional factors such as vitamin D, fat absorption, and active transport. For the premature infant, an appropriate phosphorus intake is required to minimize renal solute load. An intake too low in phosphorus can lead to rickets in the premature infant.

Evaporated Milk

Evaporated milk is standardized with respect to concentrations of protein, fat, carbohydrate, and major minerals. Cow's milk evaporated to one-half its original volume is preferred over whole cow's milk because it is sterile and convenient and because the curd formed after coagulation by gastric secretions is smaller and softer. Formulas made with evaporated milk, water, and sucrose must take into account that evaporated milk has one-half the fluid content of whole milk and its caloric content is twice as great. For a 3,000-g infant, a formula with 150 ml of evaporated milk, 300 ml of water, and 45 g of sucrose supplies enough fluid (450 ml) and calories (380 kcal) to meet the RDA, although evaporated milk formulas and unmodified cow's milk fail to meet current recommendations for ascorbic acid, vitamin E, and essential fatty acids (16, 17, 18).

Skim Milk or 2% Fresh Pasteurized Milk

Skim milk, from which fat has been removed by centrifugation, generally contains 0.1% fat and does not contain acceptable protein, fat, or carbohydrate ratios. Skim milk is generally not recommended for infants less than 1 year of age. Skim milk has been used in an attempt to prevent obesity and perhaps to aid in preventing atherosclerosis. These proposed benefits have not been proved and remain controversial.

Infants fed skim milk gain somewhat less in weight and slightly, but not significantly, more in length than infants fed whole milk (19). Although this result may seem desirable, considerations of energy balance offer cause for concern.

Infants fed skim milk utilize more of their stores of body fat. Over an extended period, once fat stores have been depleted, the infant's ability to respond adequately to a major illness may be compromised (20). In addition, infants receiving a major percentage of caloric intake from skim milk may receive exceedingly high protein intake and low-fat intake and an inadequate intake of essential fatty acids.

It is important to recognize that, per unit volume, skim milk provides a slightly greater renal solute load than does whole milk. The solute concentration is further increased by water loss during boiling (2).

Two-percent milk is a product from fresh whole and skim milk combined to contain 2% fat. Fat-free milk solids, vitamins, and minerals can be added to this pasteurized and homogenized milk formulation. Two-percent milk has commonly been used in infants after the age of 4 or 5 months. A disadvantage to the use of 2% milk as the only dietary source is the unbalanced percentage of calories supplied from protein, fat, and carbohydrate. Evidence that 2% milk will aid in preventing or correcting obesity is not available.

Goat's Milk

Although not widely used, goat's milk is generally accepted as nutritionally adequate. It contains primarily medium- and short-chain fatty acids and may be digested more readily than cow's milk. Because goat's milk is deficient in folates, daily supplementation of about 50 μg of folate (as folic acid) should be given to prevent megaloblastic anemia in infants fed only with unfortified goat's milk.

Breast-Feeding Considerations

Although not bacteriologically sterile, human milk and breast-feeding provide certain advantages over administering cow's and goat's milk. Because of its lack of opportunity for contamination and its abundance of "host resistant factors" (including bifidus factor, lactoferrin, lymphocytes, lysozyme, macrophages, and secretory IgA), infectious agents such as *Escherichia coli* and poliomyelitis virus that affect or enter the body through the GI tract have less chance of causing an infection (22–26). Protection from *Salmonella* species infection may be afforded by breast-feeding (27). These anti-infective properties of human milk may be lifesaving with poor home hygiene and also provide protective effects in well-sanitized homes (28). *Escherichia coli* and *Klebsiella* species organisms, which may be etiologic in some cases of necrotizing enterocolitis, are very uncommon in the intestine of the infant receiving fresh breast milk from the mother (29, 30). This protective effect has not been demonstrated in infants fed pooled and/or previously frozen breast milk. The protective aspects of breast milk, though effective in preventing several infectious diseases of the GI tract, have not been proved to be effective for neonates at risk for necrotizing enterocolitis. However, the clinical course of infants fed fresh breast milk from the mother is less fulminating if necrotizing enterocolitis does develop (31).

The most common food allergen in infancy is beta-lactoglobulin, a cow's milk protein. Secretory IgA in human milk helps prevent absorption of food allergens. The best prophylaxis against food allergy in infancy is breast-feeding and avoiding semisolid food until 4–6 months of age (32).

The closer contact between mother and infant during breast-feeding with resultant increase in maternal hormone secretion and neonatal somatosensory, olfactory, and auditory stimulation may increase maternal-neonate bonding (33). This intense attachment formed through breast-feeding may be helpful in preventing later psychosocial emotional disturbances, including "disorder of mothering" with subsequent child abuse (33, 34).

Iron from breast milk is absorbed more efficiently by the infant than iron in cow's milk formulas. Even though breast milk contains a small amount of iron, an average of about 50% of the iron in breast milk is absorbed, compared with 12% from unfortified cow's milk formula (35). Bottle-fed infants must receive iron supplementation or iron-fortified formula because nonhuman milks contain little iron. Iron supplementation of breast-fed infants remains controversial. Advocates of iron supplementation cite data indicating that absorption of iron from breast milk averages less than 0.25 mg/day (36). This amount is significantly less than the 0.5 mg of iron/day needed to ensure adequate iron nutritional status (37). Supplementation in infants from the early weeks of life with approximately 7 mg of elemental iron from ferrous sulfate has been recommended (38).

Zinc and perhaps other trace minerals are absorbed more readily from breast milk than other milks (39).

Cretinism may be mitigated by breast-feeding because of significant thyroid hormones in human milk (40). Conversely, breast-feeding may delay the diagnosis of hypothyroidism in an infant.

Low-birth-weight infants also seem to benefit from fresh breast milk. The presence of specific antibodies, the unique characteristics of the protein and fat, and the lower osmolality of human milk have been implicated in the more favorable response of low-birth-weight or prematurely born infants fed breast milk. However, the unique nutritional needs of the premature infant can be therapeutically managed with special low-birth-weight formulas. These formulas contain necessary nutrients, including vitamin D, calcium, and phosphate, that may not be adequately supplied by breast milk alone.

Breast-feeding also prevents the infant from being exposed to emulsifiers, additives such as carrageenan, lecithin, and sodium citrate, thickening agents, antioxidants, and pH adjusters found in commercial formulas. Although these agents generally are not associated with ill effects and are approved by the *Codex Alimentarius* of the Food and Agricultural Organization of the United Nations (41), they are not found in human milk.

Study results demonstrate a greater gain in weight and length of bottle-fed than breast-fed infants (42). Bottle-fed infants generally gain more weight for a specified gain in length than breast-fed infants. Overfeeding may contribute to subsequent obesity because an abnormally large population of adipocytes develops or because a habit of overeating is established. However, a correlation between obesity in infancy and obesity in the adolescent or adult has not been demonstrated conclusively. Some investigators have found no relationship between age of introduction of supplementary foods and development of or persistence of obesity (43).

One minor problem associated with human milk is created by the presence of increased levels of nonesterified fatty acid (44). Abnormal lipolytic activity in the breast milk of some women causes increased levels of nonesterified fatty acid. This results in the inhibition of UDP-glucuronyl transferase and leads to a prolonged unconjugated hyperbilirubinemia in infants. Breast-feeding need not be stopped in most cases of breast milk jaundice (45). The jaundice eventually subsides even if breast-feeding is continued. If the infant appears to be in danger from hyperbilirubinemia itself, a temporary pause in breast-feeding for 1–4 days is usually adequate to reduce the bilirubin to a safe level. Breast feeding can then be resumed.

Many advantages of breast-feeding may not fully apply if it is maintained for only 1–2 months, as is commonly the case, rather than 6 months as recommended (35). Introduction of solid foods before 2 months of age may compromise iron absorption from breast milk (46). Supplemental solid foods should not be administered until after 6 months to ensure adequate iron absorption from breast milk.

Another potential problem in using human milk arises when the mother is taking medication. Drugs excreted in human milk may have undesirable effects on the infant and also may alter breast milk composition (47–49). For example, changes were reported in milk protein, fat, and calcium content in women taking combination-type oral contraceptives (50). Although these contraceptive agents are not specifically contraindicated for nursing mothers, the infant should be observed for adverse effects. Also, lactation is diminished by progesterone-estrogen combinations taken before adequate milk secretion is established (3–4 weeks postpartum) (51).

Many drugs taken by the lactating woman may be found in her milk (48). The degree of drug transfer across the membrane between plasma and milk is influenced by its solubility in lipid and water, by its pKa or degree of ionization, and by selective transport mechanisms. The pH of milk is less than that of plasma; consequently, milk may act as an "ion trap" for basic compounds. Conversely, acidic drugs tend to be inhibited from entering milk.

The following drugs are not recommended for nursing women: anticoagulants, antimetabolites, atropine, most cathartics, dihydrotachysterol, ergot, iodides, metronidazole, radioactive drugs, and tetracycline. In addition, oral contraceptives, lithium carbonate, sulfonamides, reserpine, steroids, propylthiouracil, diazepam, diuretics, nalidixic acid, barbiturates, phenytoin, and cough medicines with codeine should be used only under medical supervision (49).

The Committee on Nutrition of the American Academy of Pediatrics reaffirmed the recommendations for breast-feeding (18). However, the Committee recognized that some disorders make breast-feeding unsuitable:

- Infants with certain genetic disorders, such as galactosemia, are intolerant to human milk.
- Certain drugs that can harm the infant may be concentrated in human milk.
- Some mothers have an inadequate supply of milk.

Caution is needed against issuing dire warnings to mothers who cannot or do not wish to breast-feed. Normal growth and development are possible without it. When breast-feeding is unsuccessful, inappropriate, or ceased early, infant formulas provide the best alternative for meeting nutritional needs during the first year (18).

Standard Formula

The growth rate of infants is faster from birth to 1 year than at any other time. Infants are expected to double their birth weight at 4 months and to triple it at 1 year (52). Because of this rapid growth rate, the nutritional adequacy of an infant's diet is very important.

Three basic nutritional principles should be considered in evaluating an infant formula:

- It should contain adequate, but not excessive, amounts of all essential nutrients.
- It should be readily digestible.
- It should have a reasonable distribution of calories derived from protein, fat, and carbohydrate.

Metabolic studies suggest that 7–16% of the calories should be derived from protein, 30–55% from fat, and 35–65% from carbohydrate (53). Human milk provides 7%, 55%, and 38% of its calories from protein, fat, and carbohydrate, respectively; corresponding figures for whole cow's milk are 20%, 50%, and 30%.

A formulation may be altered by the manufacturer in response to changes in availability of ingredients or modifications in recommended allowances. The carbohydrate source for Lofenalac was changed from a combination of maltose, sucrose, dextrins, and arrowroot starch to corn syrup and tapioca starch when arrowroot starch became unavailable. The fat source of Similac was modified by adding soy oil to the combination of corn and coconut oils in response to the decreased availability and rising cost of corn oil. Accurate listing of current ingredients and quantities may be obtained only by direct communication with the manufacturer.

Physical Characteristics

All infant formulas are emulsions of edible oils in aqueous solutions. Separation of fat rarely occurs in infant formulas. The fat can be redispersed by shaking the container. If separation of fat has occurred because of the lack of stabilizers or with storage beyond shelf life, redispersion by normal shaking may not be possible.

Protein agglomeration may occur if the storage time is excessive. This agglomeration may range from slight, grainy development through increased viscosity and formation of gels, to eventual precipitation of protein (54). Protein agglomeration and fat separation do not affect the safety or nutritional adequacy of the formulas. The objectionable appearance and the greater viscosity of the formula are detriments to their use.

Liquid infant formulas contain thickening and stabilizing agents to provide uniform consistency and to prolong stability. Carrageenan is a stabilizing agent in many infant formulas. Conditions of use are specified in the Code of Federal Regulations (55). Guidelines on maximum levels of use for a number of thickening agents and emulsifiers are provided by the *Codex Alimentarius* Commission. The use of guar gum, locust bean gum, distarch phosphate, acetylated distarch phosphate, phosphated distarch phosphate, hydroxypropyl starch, carrageenan, lecithin, and monoglycerides and diglycerides as stabilizers, thickening agents, and emulsifiers is covered by FDA's food additive regulations and they are generally recognized as safe (56, 57). Infant formulas may contain one or more of these substances; no one formula contains all of them.

Microbiologic Safety

Guidelines of the Infant Formula Council (a voluntary, nonprofit, trade association composed of five companies engaged in the manufacture and marketing of infant formulas) require liquid formulations to be free of all viable pathogens and their spores and other organisms that may cause product degradation (58). Microbiologic contamination may alter the nutritional quality of formulas and result in diarrhea and subsequent fluid and electrolyte imbalances. The quality control measures at every stage of formulation and production provide a sterile product free of microbial effects as long as the container remains intact. Powdered formulas are essentially free of microorganisms, and the required heating during final preparation (as indicated on label directions) destroys most microorganisms introduced during preparation.

Digestibility

Milk produces a precipitate or curd when it comes in contact with hydrochloric acid in the stomach. Curds contain most of the casein and calcium of milk. The whey of milk contains proteins and lactose in the watery portion. Unprocessed milk produces tough curds that are difficult for infants to digest. Human milk contains less casein than cow's milk and produces more digestible curds in the stomach. Homogenization, evaporation, boiling, and drying reduce the curd tension of cow's milk. Infant formulas containing cow's milk are processed to avoid problems with curd production.

Caloric Density, Osmolarity, Osmolality, and Renal Solute Load

Caloric Density

The metabolic calorie [large calorie or kilocalorie (kcal)] is the amount of heat required to raise the temperature of 1,000 g of water from 15°C to 16°C. The recommended daily dietary allowance (RDA), as established by the National Academy of Science/National Research Council, is 117 kcal/kg/day for infants from birth to 6 months and 108 kcal/kg/day from 6 months to 1 year. A term, full-weight infant should have no difficulty in consuming enough of a standard diluted formula (20–30 kcal/oz or 67 kcal/100 ml) to meet these needs. A premature or low-birth-weight infant has a higher caloric need and may require as much as 130 kcal/kg/day (59). An infant recovering from illness or malnutrition also requires more calories (17). Infant formulas with caloric densities significantly lower or higher than 67 kcal/100 ml are regarded as therapeutic formulas for specific management of special clinical conditions and should be used only under medical supervision.

Osmolarity and Osmolality

Osmolarity is the concentration of a solute in a solution per unit of total volume of solution (mOsm/liter of formula). Osmolarity of human milk is approximately 273 mOsm/liter. The Committee on Nutrition recommends that formulas for normal infants may have concentrations of no greater than 400 mOsm/liter without a warning statement on the label. Hyperosmolar formulas have been implicated in causing necrotizing enterocolitis (60, 61).

Osmolality is the solute concentration in a solution per unit of solvent (mOsm/kg of water). The osmolality of a formula is directly related to the concentration of molecular or ionic particles in solution and inversely proportional to the concentration of water (62). The osmolality of human milk is approximately 300 mOsm/kg of water. The osmolarity of 400 mOsm/liter corresponds to an approximate osmolal concentration of 460 mOsm/kg of water (59). Osmolality is related to the carbohydrate and mineral content of the formula.

For dilute solutions, there is little difference in osmolality and osmolarity. However, infant formulas are relatively concentrated solutions; osmolarity may be only 80% of the osmolality [osmolarity (mOm/liter) = osmolality (mOsm/kg of water) × kg of water/liter] (62). It has been suggested that osmolality should be used to report osmotic activities of infant formulas (62). Osmolality is preferred since osmotic activity is a function of a solute-solvent relationship and, secondarily, because values from the laboratory osmometer are osmolal values.

The relationship between osmolality and caloric density is reasonably linear in formulas having a caloric density of 44–90 kcal/100 ml, the range of caloric concentrations usually fed to infants (62). If the osmolality of a 67-kcal/100-ml formula is known, the osmolality of a formula in the 44–90-kcal/100-ml range prepared from a liquid concentrate may be calculated assuming a direct proportion between osmolality and caloric density (an 80-kcal/100-ml formula would have 120% the osmolality of the 67-kcal/100-ml formula) (62).

Renal Solute Load

Renal solute load is related to the protein (urea) and mineral content of the formula. It represents the total amount of water-soluble substances that must be removed from the body by the kidneys. The renal solute loads of human milk and cow's milk are approximately 79 and 228 mOsm/liter, respectively (62). Renal solute loads can be calculated from the sum of milliequivalents of sodium, potassium, and chloride plus 4 mOsm of urea/g of protein in a liter of formula or milk (62).

Osmolality of Infant Formulas

Table 1 cites the results of osmolality determinations on human milk, milk-based formulas, and soy-based formulas (63). The osmolality of a given formula increases with increasing caloric content. There is no meaningful difference in the osmolalities of the commonly used infant ready-to-feed formulas that provide 67 kcal/100 ml (63). The osmolalities of reconstituted concentrated products when diluted to provide 67 kcal/100 ml are not considerably different from the osmolalities of the corresponding ready-to-feed products (63). Directions for diluting concentrated formulas must be followed exactly to prevent hyperosmolal states, such as diarrhea and dehydration, which could harm the infant.

The soybean formulas have lower osmolalities than the milk-based formulas. These formulas contain maltodextrins of higher molecular weight. Soyalac contains a lower carbohydrate concentration than Nursoy, Isomil, or ProSobee (62).

Table 1. Osmolality of milks and selected infant formulas				
	Caloric density		Osmolality[a] (mOsm/kg water)	
Product	kcal/ oz	kcal/ 100 ml	Undi- luted	Diluted 1:1
Breast milk	20	67	286	
Cow's milk	20	67	288	
Ready-to-feed				
Similac	13	43	193	
Similac	20	67	295	
Similac	24	80	362	
Similac	27	90	411	
Enfamil	20	67	288	
SMA	20	67	296	
PM 60/40	24	80	315	
Premature formula	24	80	425	
Isomil	20	67	252	
Nutramigen	20	67	451	
Concentrates				
Similac	20	67	664	287
Enfamil	20	67	665	299
SMA	20	67	671	287
Isomil	20	67	528	252
Nursoy	20	67	572	241
ProSobee	20	67	523	223
Soyalac	20	67	620	273

Excerpted from *Am. J. Dis. Child.*, **131**, 140 (Feb. 1977).

[a] Determined by freezing-point depression method.

Approximate reconstitution of most powdered formulas using the manufacturer-supplied scoops results in formulas with higher osmolalities than the same formulas when reconstituted precisely by weighed measures according to the manufacturer's formulations of the respective products (63). Powdered formulas reconstituted by the scoop method provide more than the desired 67 kcal/100 ml. The final osmolality varies widely when powdered samples from different containers are reconstituted in the same manner. The difference in osmolality between cans of a reconstituted product appears to be due to a large variability in powder composition (63). In addition, powder formulas provide consistently greater osmolality than the same product in the ready-to-feed liquid form.

The standard formulas with 67 kcal/100 ml that are used routinely to feed preterm newborn infants have osmolalities similar to breast milk and pose no apparent increased risk of GI mucosal injury (63). Products for premature infants (Similac 24 LBW, Enfamil, Premature Formula, Similac Special Care) have osmolalities in the normal range.

Nutritional Requirements

The Food and Nutrition Board of the National Research Council established recommended dietary allowances (RDA's) that meet the needs of most healthy infants (64) (Table 2). (See Chapter 12, *Nutritional Supplement, Vitamin, and Mineral Products*.) The Committee on Nutrition of the American Academy of Pediatrics has established standards for formulas prepared for healthy infants from birth (2.5–4.0 kg) to 12 months of age (8–10 kg) (Table 3) (18). The FDA has adopted these recommendations as guidelines for nutrient composition and nutrient levels in infant formulas (65).

Usual dilutions of unmodified cow's milk and evaporated milk do not meet the standards (18). Iron deficiency and hyperphosphatemia are common complications in infants fed only cow's milk. Vitamin C supplementation is necessary in infants receiving only cow's milk. The high salt and saturated fat content of cow's milk may contribute to high blood pressure and coronary artery disease in later life, although this has not yet been proven (66, 67). The high protein and mineral content of cow's milk increases the risk of hypernatremia and dehydration whenever diarrhea or other conditions increase the demand for water.

Nutritional requirements are best expressed as the amounts needed per 100 kcal of total food intake, rather than amounts per kilogram of body weight (Table 3). This system provides a convenient way to reflect the interaction of one nutrient with another, such as vitamin A and unsaturated fatty acids, and it can be applied to formulas of different caloric concentrations (17).

Protein

The RDA for protein is 2.2 g/kg from birth to 6 months and 2.0 g/kg from 6 months to 1 year. Infant formulas must provide a minimum of 1.8 g/100 kcal of protein having a PER (protein efficiency ratio, derived from the weight gain per gram of protein fed) at least 100% that of casein (11). These recommendations apply primarily to formulas; human milk contains 1.5 g/100 kcal and is adequate for the term infant. If a formula has a PER less than 100% of casein, the amount of protein/100 kcal should be increased to compensate for the lower PER. A formula that used a protein with a PER 75% that of casein would have to provide at least 2.4 g of protein/100 kcal (1.8/0.75). No protein with a PER less than 70% that of casein can be used (18).

It is important that the protein source in formulas contain the eight essential amino acids (isoleucine, leucine, lysine, methionine, phenylalanine, threonine, tryptophan, and valine). There is evidence that histidine also is essential for the newborn (68). Both human and cow's milk contain histidine in quantities exceeding estimated infant requirements of 26 mg/100 kcal and may be fed to newborns until the body begins to synthesize histidine (2–3 months after birth). Tyrosine and cystine, as well as histidine, may be essential initially for the premature infant (69, 70).

The protein in a formula may be derived from single or multiple sources and may be supplemented with L-amino acids or acceptable hydrolysates (18). Vegetable protein sources are acceptable. Hydrolysates are enzymatic breakdown products with reduced antigenicity. As measured by weight gain in rats, beef heart is 80% as efficient as casein, soy 70%, and casein hydrolysates 100%

Table 2. Recommended daily allowances of nutrients for normal term infants

Nutrient	RDA (0–6 mo)
Energy (kcal)	570–870
Protein (g)	13.2
Essential fatty acids (% of kcal)	2
Vitamins	
Vitamin A (IU)	1,400 (420 µg)[a]
Vitamin D (IU)	400 (10 µg)[b]
Vitamin K (µg)	12[c]
Vitamin E (IU)	4.5 (3 mg of α-T.E.)[d]
Ascorbic acid (mg)	35
Thiamine (µg)	300
Riboflavin (µg)	400
Pyridoxine (µg)	300
Vitamin B_{12} (µg)	0.5
Niacin (mg) (mg equivalents)[e]	6
Folacin (µg)	30
Pantothenic acid (mg)	2[c]
Biotin (µg)	35[c]
Choline (mg)	
Inositol (mg)	
Minerals	
Calcium (mg)	360
Phosphorus (mg)	240
Magnesium (mg)	50
Iron (mg)	10
Iodine (µg)	40
Zinc (mg)	3
Copper (µg)	500–700[c]
Manganese (µg)	500–700[c]
Sodium (mg)	115–350[c]
Potassium (mg)	350–925[c]
Chloride (mg)	275–700[c]
Fluoride (µg)	100–500[c]
Chromium (µg)	10–40[c]
Selenium (µg)	10–40[c]
Molybdenum (µg)	30–60[c]

National Research Council of the Food and Nutrition Board of the National Academy of Sciences, 1980.

[a] Retinol equivalents. One retinol equivalent equals 3.33 IU of vitamin A activity from retinol.

[b] Cholecalciferol. Ten micrograms of cholecalciferol equal 400 IU of vitamin D.

[c] Estimated safe and adequate daily dietary intakes. Because there is less information on which to base allowances, some figures are provided as ranges of recommended intakes.

[d] T.E., alpha-tocopherol equivalents; 1 mg of *d*-alpha-tocopherol equals 1 α-T.E. The activity of *d*-alpha-tocopherol is 1.49 IU/mg.

[e] One niacin equivalent equals 1 mg of niacin or 60 mg of dietary tryptophan.

(71). Serum albumin levels obtained from infants can be used as a direct measurement of satisfactory protein nutritional status.

Through electrodialysis or ion exchange, casein may be altered to produce a lactalbumin-to-casein ratio resembling that of human milk.

Most commercial formulas use 2.3 g of protein/100 kcal. The minimum quantity and quality of required protein (1.8g/100 kcal) promote growth and development equal to that of human milk (72, 73).

Levels of protein higher than 1.8 g/100 kcal do not confer any advantage when given to normal infants. Low-birth-weight infants may have a higher protein requirement; however, too much protein may overwhelm the ability of the infant kidney to excrete the nitrogenous waste. The Committee on Nutrition states that the maximum protein level should be 4.5 g/100 kcal. Therapeutic formulas such as Meat Base Formula, which have protein levels greater than 4.5 g/100 kcal, should be used only under medical supervision.

Fat and Essential Fatty Acids

Most commercial formulas have replaced butterfat with vegetable oil to obtain an easily digestible fat source. Vegetable oil digestibility is increased with a high proportion of unsaturated fatty acids and decreased with a large amount of long-chain fatty acids. Medium-chain fatty acids (8–10 carbons) that are unsaturated are absorbed most easily. Corn and soy oils are easier to digest than coconut oil, which has a relatively high number of long-chain saturated fatty acids. Commercial formulas have been produced from which about 85% of the fat is absorbed—the absorption rate of fat in human milk (74).

The Committee on Nutrition recommends a minimum of 3.3 g/100 kcal (30% of calories) and a maximum of 6.0 g/100 kcal of fat (18). A normal caloric distribution in an infant's diet derives 30–55% of the calories from dietary fat. Diets that supply more calories from fat may cause ketosis because ketone bodies are formed from excess free fatty acids (53). Fat is an efficient calorie source because of its high caloric density. It contains 9 kcal/g compared with 4 kcal/g for protein and carbohydrate. Fat in a diet increases palatability and enhances the absorption of lipid-soluble vitamins.

Fat also supplies the essential fatty acids not synthesized in the human body. The American Academy of Pediatrics recommends linoleic acid intakes of 300 mg/100 kcal or 2.7% of total calories (18). Linoleic and arachidonic acids enable optimum caloric intake use and proper skin composition; four other fatty acids also are essential (75). Linoleic acid represents the bulk of polyunsaturated fatty acids in infant formulas.

Special formulas free of fat or low in fat are regarded as therapeutic formulas and should be used under medical supervision.

Carbohydrates

Although there is no RDA for carbohydrates, a human infant efficiently uses 35–65% of the total calories from a carbohydrate source (39). Most carbohydrate sources used in infant formulas are monosaccharides or disaccharides, that are digested and absorbed more readily by the infant than polysaccharides (starch). Lactose is the major source of carbohydrate in milk-based formulas. It is hydrolyzed by acids and the enzyme lactase to glucose and galactose. Disaccharide hydrolysis in a newborn may be incomplete, and because lactase activity develops late in fetal life, infants born during the seventh and eighth months of gesta-

Table 3. Infant nutritional recommendations for normal term infants (per 100 kcal)

Nutrient	FDA regulations minimum	Committee on Nutrition Minimum	Committee on Nutrition Maximum
Protein (g)	1.8	1.8	4.5
Fat			
(g)	1.7	3.3	6.0
(% calories)	15.0	30.0	54.0
Essential fatty acids			
(linoleate) (% calories)	2.0	3.0	
(mg)	222.0	300.0	
Vitamins			
Vitamin A (IU)		250.0 (75 μg)[a]	750.0 (225 μg)[a]
Vitamin D (IU)	40.0	40.0	100.0
Vitamin K (g)		4.0	
Vitamin E (IU)	0.3	0.3[b]	
Vitamin C (mg)	7.8	8.0	
B_1 (thiamine) (μg)	25.0	40.0	
B_2 (riboflavin) (μg)	60.0	60.0	
B_6 (pyridoxine) (μg)	35.0	35.0[c]	
B_{12} (μg)	0.15	0.15	
Niacin[d]			
(μg)		250.0	
(μg equivalents)	800.0		
Folic acid (μg)	4.0	4.0	
Pantothenic acid (μg)	300.0	300.0	
Biotin (μg)		1.5	
Choline (mg)		7.0	
Inositol (mg)		4.0	
Minerals			
Calcium (mg)	50.0[e]	50.0[e]	
Phosphorus (mg)	25.0[e]	25.0	
Magnesium (mg)	6.0	6.0	
Iron (mg)	1.0	0.15	
Iodine (μg)	5.0	5.0	
Zinc (mg)		0.5	
Copper (μg)	60.0	60.0	
Manganese (μg)		5.0	
Sodium (mg)		20.0 (6 mEq)[f]	60.0 (17 mEq)[f]
Potassium (mg)		80.0 (14 mEq)[f]	200.0 (34 mEq)[f]
Chloride (mg)		55.0 (11 mEq)[f]	150.0 (29 mEq)[f]

Reprinted from the *Federal Register*, 45, 17206 (1980).

[a]Retinol equivalents.
[b]With 0.7 IU/g of linoleic acid.
[c]With 15 μg/g of protein in formula.
[d]Although expressed as niacin, it is recognized that on the average, 1 mg of niacin is derived from each 60 mg of dietary tryptophan.
[e]Calcium-to-phosphorus ratio must be no less than 1.1 nor more than 2.0.
[f]Milllequivalent for 670 kcal/liter of formula.

tion may be unable to hydrolyze the same amount of lactose that a term infant can generally metabolize. These infants are especially prone to lactose intolerance (manifested by diarrhea, abdominal distention, and cramping) during the first weeks after birth (76). Secondary lactase deficiency is a temporary reduction in intestinal lactase caused by gastroenteritis or malnutrition.

Congenital lactase deficiency is a rare type of milk intolerance that results from an inborn error of metabolism (77). Low levels of lactase in the GI tract of these infants and in low-birth-weight infants can lead to an inability to metabolize the quantity of lactose found in breast milk or infant formulas. This is a temporary adverse reaction that most infants outgrow. The availability of formulas as substitutes for breast milk and those with nutrient sources other than cow's milk affords convenient alternatives where milk intolerances or hypersensitivities are suspected.

Other carbohydrates such as dextrins, maltoses, corn syrup solids, and sucrose are used in infant formulas when milk protein is to be avoided by allergic infants. Formulas that contain sucrose and corn syrup as carbohydrate sources have a sweeter taste than those that contain lactose.

Carbohydrates provide 40–50% of the calories in most infant formulas. If more than 50% of the calories are derived from carbohydrates, an infant's ability to hydrolyze disaccharides may be compromised. The increased passage of disaccharides in the feces creates an osmotic gradient in the colon that results in loose, characteristically acidic, watery stools. The excess lactose in the ileocecal region is fermented by bacteria to produce carbon dioxide and lactic acid. This process irritates the colon and may cause diarrhea, resulting in dehydration and electrolyte imbalance.

Vitamins

Niacin The Committee on Nutrition specifies that infant formulas should contain a minimum of 250 μg of niacin/100 kcal. The FDA has recommended a standard of 800 μg of niacin equivalents/100 kcal. One mg of niacin is derived from each 60 mg of dietary tryptophan, an amino acid precursor of niacin. The protein level in formulas as recommended by the Committee on Nutrition provides the tryptophan that supplies the niacin equivalents.

Pyridoxine The minimum recommendation for pyridoxine (vitamin B_6) is 35 μg/100 kcal. Higher protein intake from certain formulas necessitates an increased amount of pyridoxine. At least 15 μg of pyridoxine for each gram of protein is recommended.

Vitamin A The maximum level of 750 IU/100 kcal of vitamin A (4,800 IU/liter) is recommended. This level is intended mainly for those formulas in which intake is likely to be low:

- Ingestion of only 300–400 ml of formula/day;
- During the first weeks of life;
- For infants who do not absorb fat well.

Vitamin D The Committee on Nutrition recommends a maximum of 100 IU/100 kcal of vitamin D (670 IU/liter of formula). Most formulas contain 62 IU of vitamin D/100 kcal (400 IU/liter). The recommended higher levels of vitamin D would meet the requirements for low-birth-weight infants (2.5–3.5 kg) whose intake is low or whose absorption of fat is poor.

Vitamin K Milk-based formulas contain sufficient quantities of vitamin K to prevent deficiency. Furthermore, the bacterial flora engendered by milk-based formulas in healthy infants contribute to an adequate supply of vitamin K. The minimum level of 4 μg of vitamin K/100 kcal in milk-based formulas is sufficient for normal infants. The Committee on Nutrition recommends that soy isolate and other milk-substitute formulas should contain a minimum of 8 μg of vitamin K/100 kcal.

Vitamin E Vitamin E (tocopherol) is necessary to protect cell membranes from oxidative damage. Premature infants are born with disproportionately small body stores of

vitamin E compared with those of term infants (78). Tocopherol levels are proportional to the oxidants (iron) and oxidizable substrate [polyunsaturated fatty acids (PUFA)] in the diet. Hemolytic anemia was reported in premature infants who received formulas with high levels of polyunsaturated fatty acids supplemented with iron (79–82). Some formulas are supplemented with higher levels of polyunsaturated fatty acids because cow's milk is low in linoleic acid, containing 20–25% as much as human milk (83). The additional oxidant activity of iron (8 mg/kg or more) increases the risk for hemolytic anemia in premature infants with insufficient tocopherol levels.

To avoid hemolytic anemia in premature infants, the ratio of vitamin E intake to polyunsaturated fatty acids (E/PUFA) should not be less than 0.4 (84), where E/PUFA is:

$$\frac{\text{Vitamin E per unit volume (IU of alpha-tocopherol)}}{\text{PUFA per unit volume (grams of linoleic and arachidonic acid)}}$$

Term infants require 0.3 IU of vitamin E/100 kcal and at least 0.7 IU of vitamin E/g of linoleic acid. Most infant formulas are supplemented to provide 0.8 IU/g of polyunsaturated fatty acids, or 13 IU/liter (83).

Biotin, Choline, and Inositol The requirements for these vitamins are not known. The recommendation for biotin is a minimum of 1.5 μg/100 kcal, which approximates that amount commonly used in milk-based formulas. Milk-based formulas provide 7 mg/100 kcal or 45 mg of choline/liter. Inositol is present in most formulas in a concentration of 4 mg/100 kcal or 26 mg/liter.

Electrolytes

The levels of electrolytes and minerals in infant formulas should be near the minimal levels since maximal levels (based on cow's milk) constitute a significant solute load. However, the amount of residue from cow's milk can be excreted in isotonic urine (300 mOsm/liter) by the normal healthy infant (85).

The amount of sodium, potassium, and chloride in infant formulas is based on the minimum levels found in human milk. The levels of sodium, potassium, and chloride in infant formulas should be 6–17, 14–34, and 11–29 mEq/liter, respectively. These minimal levels can be expressed as sodium (20 mg/100 kcal), potassium (80 mg/100 kcal), and chloride (55 mg/100 kcal). These levels are sufficient to meet the growth needs of the infant and leave little residual for excretion in urine.

The ratio of sodium to potassium should not exceed 1.0, and the ratio of sodium plus potassium to chloride should be at least 1.5. The Committee on Nutrition recommends that these ratios should be similar to those in human milk (sodium to potassium, 0.5; sodium plus potassium to chloride, 2.0). These ratios may reduce the possible risk of hypertension in infants at risk from excess sodium (86, 87). No adverse reactions were identified when total sodium intake averaged 3 mEq/kg/day up to 6 months of age (88). Human milk provides about 1 mEq of sodium/kg/day (88). The amount of sodium in the diet of infants less than 6 months of age was reduced from approximately 3 to 2 mEq/kg/day by the reduction or elimination of salt from strained and junior foods (89). This level of sodium intake has not been proven harmful. There is no evidence that intakes up to 9 mEq/kg/day predispose infants to subsequent hypertension (88).

The concentration of chloride should not be lower than 11 mEq/liter. Maintenance of adequate chloride levels in soybean infant formulations is necessary to prevent hypochloremic, hypokalemic alkalosis (89, 90).

Minerals

Calcium and Phosphorus

The ratio of calcium to phosphorus should be no less than 1.1 and no more than 2.0. A ratio of calcium to phosphorus within this range ensures an alkaline ash diet similar to that in human milk. A high phosphate intake has been associated with hypocalcemic tetany (91, 92).

Iron

The Committee on Nutrition recommends that all formulas contain at least the lower level of iron found in human milk (0.15 mg/100 kcal or 1 mg/liter) and that the iron be in a bioavailable form. Infants at risk for iron deficiency should be given formulas supplemented with iron between 1 and 2 mg/100 kcal (approximately 6–12 mg/liter). Most iron-supplemented formulas contain 12 mg/liter.

Iron availability may be less in formulas with higher protein concentration; iron deficiency is more common in infants fed 2.4% protein (3.6 g/100 kcal) than in those fed 1.5% (2.3 g/100 kcal) in a milk formula (93).

Formulas for low-birth-weight infants contain 3 mg of iron/liter. Conservative levels of iron are used because iron supplementation in low-birth-weight infants up to the age of 2 months has been associated with an increased risk of hemolytic anemia. These formulas do not supply enough iron to meet the normal intrauterine accretion rate of iron. The decision to determine if or when iron supplementation is needed for infants fed low-birth-weight formulas should be left to the discretion of the physician.

Zinc, Copper, and Manganese

The minimum requirement for zinc by the infant is approximately 0.5 mg/100 kcal (3.2 mg of zinc/liter). Less zinc may be absorbed in soybean formulas due to the presence of phytate in soy protein (94). The minimum level for copper is 69 μg/100 kcal. The requirement for manganese is unknown. The Committee on Nutrition recommends 5 μg of manganese/100 kcal in the formula.

Vitamin and Mineral Supplements

There is no evidence that supplementation is necessary for the term, formula-fed infant. Likewise, the normal, breast-fed infant of the well-nourished mother has not been shown conclusively to need any specific vitamin and mineral supplement (95). However, iron and vitamin D supplementation has been recommended for term, breast-fed infants.

Vitamin and mineral supplementation may be needed in preterm and low-birth-weight infants and in those whose mothers are inadequately nourished. These infants and those with overt nutritional deficiencies, malabsorptive and other chronic diseases, rare vitamin dependency conditions, inborn errors of vitamin or mineral metabolism, or deficiencies related to the intake of drugs will need vitamin and mineral supplementation directed by a physician (95). Table 4 gives guidelines for supplementation.

Table 4. Guidelines for use of supplements in healthy infants

Infant	Multivitamin/ Multimineral	D	E[a]	Folate	Iron[b]
Term infants					
Breast-fed	0	±	0	0	±
Formula-fed	0	0	0	0	0
Preterm infants					
Breast-fed[c]	+	+	±	±	+
Formula-fed[c]	+	+	±	±	+
Older infants (>6 mo)					
Normal	0	0	0	0	±
High-risk[d]	+	0	0	0	±

Excerpted from *Pediatrics*, 66, 1017 (1980).

Symbols indicate: +, a supplement is usually indicated; ±, it is possibly or sometimes indicated; 0, it is not usually indicated. Vitamin K for newborn infants and fluoride in areas where there is insufficient fluoride in the water are not shown.

[a]Vitamin E should be in a form that is well absorbed by small, premature infants. If this form of vitamin E is present in formulas, it need not be given separately to formula-fed infants. Infants fed breast milk are less susceptible to vitamin E deficiency.

[b]Iron-fortified formula and/or infant cereal is a more convenient and reliable source of iron than a supplement.

[c]Multivitamin supplement (plus added folate) is needed primarily when calorie intake is below approximately 300 kcal/day or when the infant weighs 2.5 kg; vitamin D should be supplied at least until 6 months of age in breast-fed infants. Iron should be started by 2 months of age.

[d]Multivitamin-multimineral preparations including iron are preferred to use of iron alone.

Breast-Fed Infants

The antirachitic properties of the small amount of vitamin D in breast milk seem to be adequate for the normal, term infant of a well-nourished mother. If the mother's nourishment has been inadequate in vitamin D, supplements of 400 IU of vitamin D may be administered (96). Mothers should be encouraged to drink adequate amounts of milk during the breast-feeding period to minimize vitamin and mineral deficiency.

Breast-fed premature infants infrequently may demonstrate rickets (97, 98). This may be due to the low phosphorus content (150 mg/liter) of breast milk, in contrast to approximately 450 mg/liter in formulas (96, 97). This condition is correctable with phosphate supplementation. Vitamin D supplementation is also helpful (99).

Vitamin A deficiency rarely occurs in breast-fed infants; therefore, vitamin A may be omitted from supplements designed to provide vitamin D for infants.

Vitamin E is not needed for the normal, breast-fed term infant.

Vitamin B_{12} deficiency has been reported in breast-fed infants of strict vegetarian mothers (100). This deficiency is relatively rare in the United States. A malnourished nursing mother and her infant should receive multivitamin supplements to prevent megaloblastic anemia.

Breast-fed infants rarely develop iron deficiency anemia before the age of 4–6 months because neonatal stores of iron are adequate. After 6 months, the neonatal stores may be depleted; consequently, in normal, breast-fed term infants, the addition to the diet of iron-fortified cereal is desirable to supply adequate amounts of iron.

The benefit of fluoride supplementation in the breast-fed infant is controversial. The Committee on Nutrition states that fluoride supplements can be initiated shortly after birth in breast-fed infants (101). This approach is based on the possibility that dental caries may be further reduced in breast-fed infants who consume little or no water. This issue is not significant when breast-feeding is only maintained for a few months. However, if an infant is breast fed exclusively for more than 6 months, fluoride administration is warranted. Totally breast-fed infants in a nonfluoridated area should receive fluoride supplementation from birth since this regimen gives additional protection to the calcifying primary teeth with little risk of fluorosis in the permanent dentition (102, 103). In fluoridated areas where infants receive a diet supplemented by additional food and water, fluoride supplementation is not advised to avoid the risk of mild enamel fluorosis (102, 103). Table 5 contains the supplemental fluoride dosage schedule recommended by the Committee on Nutrition.

Formula-Fed Term Infants

Consumption of adequate amounts of commercial milk-based formula by a term infant excludes the need for vitamin and mineral supplementation in the first 6 months of life (18). Proper solid foods after 6 months of age also negate the need for vitamin and mineral supplements. After 4 months, an iron-fortified formula and/or iron-fortified cereal are preferable to iron supplement products (104). Cereal should be of low anigenic potential. Formula intake should be proportionately reduced as cereal is started to minimize overfeeding.

Vitamin and mineral supplements are not needed if an older infant (greater than 6 months) is receiving a diet of milk or formula, mixed feedings, and increased amounts of table food. Cow's milk, if used at this time, should be fortified with vitamin D and cereal should be fortified with iron (98). The diet should include an adequate source of vitamin C. A multivitamin with minerals may be needed in infants at special nutritional risk as a result of intercurrent illness or poverty.

If powdered or concentrated formula is used, fluoride supplements should be administered only if the community water contains less than 0.3 ppm of fluoride. Ready-to-use formulas are manufactured with water low in fluoride; therefore, recommendations for fluoride supplements are similar to those for breast-fed infants (98).

Preterm Infants

Preterm infants need vitamin and mineral supplementation since their nutrient needs are proportionately greater than those of term infants (due to a more rapid growth rate) and because of decreased intestinal absorption (105). Prior to consumption of about 300 kcal/day or reaching a body weight of 2.5 kg, a multivitamin supplement that provides the equivalent of the RDA's for term infants should be administered. The multivitamin should include vitamin E in a form well absorbed by preterm infants, such as *d*-alpha-tocopheryl polyethylene glycol 1,000 succinate (106). Folic acid deficiency has been reported in preterm infants (107). The instability of folic acid excludes its incorporation into liquid multivitamin/mineral preparations. Folate can be added to a multivitamin preparation in a concentration to provide 0.1 mg/day dose (the U.S. RDA). The shelf life should be limited to 1 month, and the label should read "shake well" (98). Iron supplementation should be withheld until after several weeks of life to minimize the

Table 5. Supplemental fluoride dosage schedule (mg/day)

Age	Concentration of fluoride in drinking water (ppm)		
	<0.3	0.3–0.7	>0.7
2 weeks–2 years	0.25	0	0
2–3 years	0.50	0.25	0
3–16 years[b]	1.00	0.50	0

Excerpted from *Am J. Dis. Child.*, *134*, 866 (1980).

[a] 2.2 mg sodium fluoride contains 1 mg of fluoride.

[b] The American Academy of Pediatrics recommends 16, rather than 13, as the termination age. The American Dental Association recommends 13 as the termination age.

possibility of hemolytic anemia in infants with insufficient vitamin E absorption. Iron is required at a dosage of 2 mg/kg/day starting by at least 2 months of age because neonatal iron stores may become depleted earlier than in term infants. Iron-fortified formulas supply sufficient iron to prevent iron deficiency in preterm infants (98).

Vitamin and mineral supplementation (vitamins C, D, and E, folate, and iron) may be needed for preterm and term infants receiving home-prepared evaporated milk or cow's milk formulas. The need for supplements with evaporated milk depends on whether the preparation is fortified.

Types and Uses of Infant Formulas

Formulas for Term Infants

Several studies indicate that growth rates of formula-fed infants are essentially similar to those of breast-fed infants (108–110). Commercial formulas for normal infants are basically milk base, soy base, protein hydrolysate base, or meat base. These formulas must meet the minimum requirements for the various nutrients per 100 kcal as required by the FDA and as recommended by the Committee on Nutrition (Table 3) (18).

Milk-Based Formulas

These formulas are prepared from nonfat cow's milk, vegetable oils, and added carbohydrate (lactose or corn syrup solids). The added carbohydrate is necessary because the ratio of carbohydrates to protein in nonfat milk solids from cow's milk is less than is desirable for infant formulas. Corn syrup solids have been used in some formulations because they are less expensive than lactose and are of equivalent caloric value. Protein provides about 10% of calories, and fat generally provides about 48–50% of calories (111). The most widely used vegetable oils are corn, coconut, and soy. Replacement of the butterfat allows better fat absorption and reduces the sour odor of vomitus from infants. Vitamins and minerals are added in accordance with the guidelines of the Committee on Nutrition. Milk-based formulas are available either without iron or fortified to the extent of 12 mg/liter.

Milk-Based Formulas with Added Whey Proteins

When whey is added in the proper amounts to nonfat cow's milk, the ratio of whey proteins to casein can be made to approximate that of human milk. This ratio of 60% of protein from whey and 40% from casein differs considerably from cow's milk, in which casein accounts for approximately 80% of the protein and whey for about 20% (112). Minerals can be removed from whey by electrodialysis or ion-exchange processes, and then minerals can be added to the formula to approximate the mineral content of human milk. Formulas containing partially demineralized whey proteins are not nutritionally superior to milk-based formulas for the normal infant. The high nutritional quality and relatively low renal solute load of these formulas are assets in the therapeutic management of ill infants (112).

Soy-Based Formulas

These formulas contain protein from water-soluble soy isolates. Originally, soy flour was used as the source of protein, but these formulas produced loose, malodorous stools that stained diapers and not infrequently resulted in excoriation of the diaper area (113). Soy-isolate formulas are white, nearly odorless, and rarely cause loose or malodorous stools (113). Vegetable oils provide the fat content, and corn syrup solids and/or sucrose supply the carbohydrate in these formulas. Vitamin K is added to provide a level of 100 μg/liter. These formulas are used most commonly in the management of infants allergic to milk or who are suspected of milk allergy.

Protein Hydrolysate-Based Formulas

Protein hydrolysate-based formulas contain enzymatically hydrolyzed casein. The nitrogen sources are free amino acids and simple polypeptides. Thus, these formulas can be fed to infants sensitive to intact proteins of milk or other foods. Sucrose and tapioca starch are the carbohydrate source. Other nutrients are added to meet the nutrient requirements established by the Committee on Nutrition.

Meat-Based Formulas

The protein source is prepared from beef heart. Approximately 50% of the fat in the formula is derived from meat, and the remainder comes from sesame oil (114). The carbohydrate is supplied from sucrose and modified tapioca starch. Meat-based formula is relatively high in protein and fat but relatively low in carboyhdrate. Consequently, additional carbohydrate ordinarily is added before feeding.

Therapeutic Formula Use

The therapeutic infant formulas may be deficient in or supplemented with additional quantities of one or more nutrients; therefore, they are not designed to provide adequate amounts of nutrients for normal infants. The use of these formulas is limited to disorders and conditions where the infant is treated on an individual basis by medical specialists. This type of limited use requires that nutrition specialists have flexibility in developing sole source nutrient formulations that meet the specific nutritional needs of the infant (115).

Milk Protein Allergy

Food allergy may occur in infants because the immature digestive and metabolic processes may not be completely effective in converting dietary proteins into nonantigenic amino acids. The incidence of milk intolerance in the first 2 years of life is estimated to be 0.4–7.5% of the infant population (116). The latter figure agrees with skin testing data (117). An overall incidence of 0.5–1% was proposed and seems to be a median figure for infancy (118). The diagnosis of cow's milk allergy is defined as symptomatology involving the respiratory tract, skin, or the GI tract that disappears when cow's milk is removed from the diet and reappears on two separate challenges when cow's milk is given during a symptom-free period (116).

Water-soluble soy isolates (Isomil, ProSobee, and Nursoy) are used in infants with documented or suspected milk allergy. Protein hydrolysate formulas (Nutramigen and Pregestimil) also can be used. The meat-based formula derives its substitute for milk protein from beef heart and may require carbohydrate supplementation.

Fat Restriction

Conditions that may necessitate a low or moderate fat intake include cystic fibrosis, celiac disease, and short bowel syndrome. Cystic fibrosis causes a deficiency of pancreatic enzymes including lipase. Celiac disease is characterized by an intolerance to the gluten protein of wheat and rye and by the transient inability to absorb fat and starch. Formulas with a moderate amount of medium-chain triglyceride oil are helpful in these conditions because their fat is assimilated more easily. The digestibility of medium-chain triglyceride closely approximates that of human milkfat.

Pregestimil and Portagen are examples of formulas used to provide nutrients in infants that need a fat-restricted diet. Pregestimil contains casein hydrolysate, fat as medium-chain triglyceride oil, and carbohydrate, primarily in the form of glucose. Tapioca starch provides 15% of the calories but may not be fully digested by the young infant (114), casuing loose stools. Portagen is useful for patients with chyluria, intestinal lymphangiectasia, and various steatorrheas (114).

Soy-based formulas are not recommended for infants with cystic fibrosis because of the risk of hypoproteinemia since these infants lose substantial amounts of nitrogen through the stools (119).

Carbohydrate Disorders

Disaccharidase deficiency may occur as a congenital defect or secondary to cystic fibrosis or celiac disease. The absence of disaccharidase leads to malabsorption and acidic diarrhea. In these cases the formula CHO-Free, which has no carbohydrates, may be given temporarily. Formulas without the suspect disaccharide then may be tried to reestablish the infant's diet. CHO-Free, when mixed with glucose, can be useful in treating infants with combined deficiency of lactase, maltase, and sucrase (114).

In cases of galactosemia, a relatively rare disorder resulting from a deficiency of either galactose 1-phosphate uridyl transferase or galactokinase, it is necessary to eliminate dietary lactose, so that the body may convert glucose only to the amount of galactose it requires. Galactosemia is characterized in untreated infants by failure to thrive, liver disease, cataracts, and mental retardation. Dietary lactose may be essentially eliminated by using soy-isolates or Nutramigen, which contains only 16 mg of lactose/67 kcal (equivalent to 8 mg of galactose) as a contaminant of its casein protein, or Meat Base Formula, which has only trace amounts of galactose from the heart muscle protein.

Congenital Heart Disease

Infants with congenital heart disease often require a formula with an increased caloric concentration because they may tire in feeding before a volume with sufficient nutrients has been consumed. In addition, an excessive renal load must be avoided.

Lonalac contains a very low amount of sodium (approximately 1 mEq/liter or 1 mEq/667 kcal). Prepared from casein, coconut oil, lactose, minerals, and vitamins, it provides a caloric distribution similar to that of whole milk (114). This formula can be used only for a short time before sodium must be supplemented. The formula presents a relatively high renal solute load (slightly less than that of whole cow's milk), and caution is required in view of the limited liquid volume intake characteristic of the seriously ill heart patient. The relatively low renal solute load and adequate caloric intake of whey-adjusted milk formulas (SMA) permits their use in long-term management of infants with congestive cardiac failure (112).

Phenylketonuria

Phenylketonuria, an inborn error of amino acid metabolism, results from the failure of phenylalanine to be converted to tyrosine in the body. Phenylalanine accumulation alters brain development and leads to mental retardation. Phenylalanine restriction is the only indication for Lofenalac, which may be used to eliminate dietary phenylalanine. It contains an enzyme hydrolysate of casein with various amino acids, including a trace of phenylalanine and supplemented with L-methionine, L-tyrosine, and L-histidine. Lofenalac provides approximately 18 mg of phenylalanine/100 kcal and is inadequate as a sole source of this amino acid (120). Because it is an essential amino acid, phenylalanine then must be supplied in monitored quantities. Formulas are used that have a predominance of whey protein, which has less phenylalanine than casein as a supplementary source of phenylalanine.

Excessive phenylalanine restriction bringing blood levels below 2 mg/100 ml has resulted in retarded bone growth, vacuolization of bone marrow cells, megaloblastic anemia, hypoglycemia, and death (121). Lofenalac, like other therapeutic formulas, should be used only as directed and indicated. Using therapeutic formulas indiscriminately or interchanging them arbitrarily with standard formulas must be avoided.

Low-Birth-Weight

Low-birth-weight infants (less than 2 kg at 3 weeks) or premature infants (born before 37 weeks from the first day of the last menstrual period) need a higher caloric content for growth than full-term infants because of an increased caloric need and decreased ability to consume an adequate volume of formula.

No commercially available formula is completely satisfactory for management of the low-birth-weight infant (<2,500 g) (62). For the very low-birth-weight infant, human milk is deficient in protein, phosphorus, calcium, and vitamin D (122). Modifications of commercially available formulas permit individualization of a dietary regimen for the low-birth-weight infant.

Examples of commercial preparations that provide the required higher caloric concentrations and are used in the hospital setting for these infants are Premature

Formula, Similac Special Care, Similac 24LBW, and specifically concentrated SMA-Improved and Similac PM 60/40 (80 kcal/100 ml).

Enfamil Premature Formula with Whey was developed to provide the types and levels of nutrients suited to the nutritional needs of the rapidly growing low-birth-weight infant. This formula provides a 60% lactalbumin: 40% casein ratio at a level of 3 g/100 kcal, medium-chain triglycerides as 40% of the fat calories, carbohydrates as glucose polymers and lactose, calcium at a level of 117 mg/100 kcal and a calcium-to-phosphorus ratio of 2:1, and an isotonic osmolality (300 mOsm/kg of water) at a dilution of 24 kcal/30 ml or 80 kcal/100 ml.

Formulas that provide sufficient caloric concentration and adequate nutrients for low-birth-weight infants may provide an excessive renal solute load. Individualization of management and careful monitoring of clinical progress and urinary osmolality are necessary.

Problems with Formulas

Infants are particularly susceptible to dehydration because of their high metabolic rate and ratio of surface area to weight and height. Fluid volume depletion by diarrhea may quickly (within 24 hours) produce severe dehydration with fluid electrolyte imbalance, shock, and possibly death. A common etiology of diarrhea in infants is improper dilution of concentrated liquid or powder formula and, therefore, care must be taken to ensure proper formula preparation.

If diarrhea is a problem, the pharmacist should ascertain the severity, frequency of stools, duration, and method of preparing the infant formula. If the diarrhea is serious (many more stools per day than the normal range of one to five) or has continued for 48 hours, or if the infant is clinically sick (fever, lethargy, anorexia, irritability, dry skin, or weight loss), the infant should be referred to a physician for appropriate care.

Medical care should be directed at identifying the cause of the diarrhea as well as correcting the physiologic imbalances. Reducing fat intake, using medium-chain triglyceride sources, or temporarily eliminating lactose may be helpful in determining whether the diarrhea is diet related.

Milk diarrhea of short duration may resolve without medical measures, but the infant should be observed closely. Because improper digestion of the infant's formula may initiate diarrhea and because continuation of a formula while diarrhea persists may yield only marginal nutrient absorption, a temporary (24-hour) discontinuation of usual foods may be helpful. Lytren or Pedialyte may be used cautiously for short-term management of electrolyte loss. However, these solutions should not be used when parenteral rehydration is required, nor should they be used to provide nutritional value. Parents should be reminded that a solution such as Pedialyte is not a new infant formula for the baby after diarrhea has ceased and that resumption of a nutritionally adequate formula should begin under a physician's direction.

Adverse effects of formula or breast milk on the infant's GI tract may range from mechanical obstruction (inspissated milk curds) and effects of osmolality to a hypersensitivity for specific milk proteins. Clinical intolerance to cow's milk is associated most frequently with lactose (as discussed previously) and protein of milk (123). All formulas for normal infants contain protein or hydrolyzed proteins that are immunologically different from proteins of the human body (54). It is estimated that approximately 10% of infants in the United States are fed soy-isolate formulas because of concern over allergy or sensitivity to cow's milk.

Hyperosmolar formulas may adversely affect low-birth-weight infants during their early neonatal period (54). Conflicting data exist on the association of hyperosmolar formula and the incidence of necrotizing enterocolitis in the first week of life (33, 124). Formulas for low-birth-weight infants should not exceed the recommended maximum solute concentration of 400 mOsm/liter (18).

Generally, infant formulas have proved to be nutritionally adequate and safe preparations. Remarkably, relatively few problems with infant formulas have occurred. However, a review of the literature for past problems provides a perspective on safety and reliability of infant formulas. Examples of past nutritional problems with infant formulas include: high phosphate intake from milk-based formulas, associated with hypocalcemic tetany (90, 91); vitamin A deficiency among infants receiving formulas made from defatted soy flour (125); acute epidermal and retinal bleeding episodes in infants fed casein hydrolysate-based or meat-based formulas with low vitamin K levels (126); skin lesions in infants fed milk-based formulas with low linoleic acid levels (127); hemolytic anemia in infants who were receiving iron therapy and fed formulas with high levels of polyunsaturated fats (105); megaloblastic anemia in infants fed formulas with low folic acid levels (128); thiamine deficiency in infants receiving soy formulas with low thiamine levels (129); convulsive seizures in infants receiving formulas with deficient levels of pyridoxine (130); and goiter in infants receiving soy formulas without iodine supplementation (131). All of these past nutritional deficiencies associated with infant formulas have been corrected with appropriate supplementation procedures and technological advances in processing of the formula.

Continued monitoring and careful study are needed to prevent further inadequacies in the nutritional efficacy and safety of infant formulas. Reports are a testimony to this necessity. Rickets has been observed in very low-birth-weight infants who received a soy-isolate formula (132, 133). The poor absorption of calcium, phosphorus, and vitamin D in these infants with immature GI tracts contributed to the development of rickets. Neutropenia and anemia from a nutritional copper deficiency were reported in a premature infant receiving a powder milk formula without supplemental trace metal elements (134). Metabolic alkalosis was noted in infants receiving a soy protein-isolate formula with low levels of chloride (89). The syndrome is characterized by failure to gain weight, loss of appetite, and lethargy as well as the hypokalemic, hyponatremic, hypochloremic metabolic alkalosis. The chloride deficits in these infants were corrected by increasing oral intake of potassium chloride. The above-mentioned nutritional deficits have now been corrected by the manufacturers.

Formula/Bottle Preparation

Infant formula preparation requires careful technique, and the pharmacist should explain the directions adequately to parents to ensure satisfactory nutrition for their infant. There are three forms of infant formulas—ready-to-feed, concentrated liquid, and concentrated powder. The latter two require the addition of water or, to add calories, a water-carbohydrate solution such as water-dextrose. Failure to dilute a concentrated formula properly could result in a hypertonic solution, precipitating diarrhea and dehydration. In an extreme case, overconcentrated formulas produced renal failure, disseminated intravascular coagulation, gangrene of the legs, and coma (135).

Equal amounts of water and concentrated liquid formula provide the necessary 20 kcal/30 ml. The powdered formula requires one packed level measure of powder (1 tbsp) to 60 ml of water. For special dilutions of therapeutic formulas and other modified formulas, the directions on the product should be followed.

Infants are highly susceptible to infections because of insufficient antibody formation and decreasing maternal antibody titer. Until an infant can produce adequate antibodies, it is especially important to sterilize all equipment used in formula preparation. Bottles, nip-

ples, can openers, funnels, caps, and other equipment should be washed with hot soapy water and rinsed thoroughly with hot running water (water should be squeezed through the holes in the nipples) (Table 6).

Formulas may be prepared for individual feedings or for a 24-hour supply, the latter procedure being more advantageous and efficient for milk, water, and carbohydrate mixtures. Formulas may be prepared to prevent bacterial contamination by terminal heating or aseptic technique (136). The American Academy of Pediatrics Committee on the Fetus and Newborn does not recommend the use of washed equipment and hot tap water to prepare formula. The Committee recommends that some method of sterilization (preferably the terminal heating method) with emphasis on the need for 25 minutes of active boiling and the necessity for clean equipment be used before feeding milk mixtures to infants (137).

Although the terminal heating method has been recommended as being the most effective, there are some special formulas, such as CHO-Free liquid and meat-based formulas, that should not be heated terminally because the procedure may cause the ingredients to separate and make feeding difficult. The terminal heating method is more convenient than aseptic technique for preparing a day's supply.

The commercially sterilized liquid formulas and bacteriologically safe powdered formulas may be prepared more conveniently in single bottles. A day's sup-

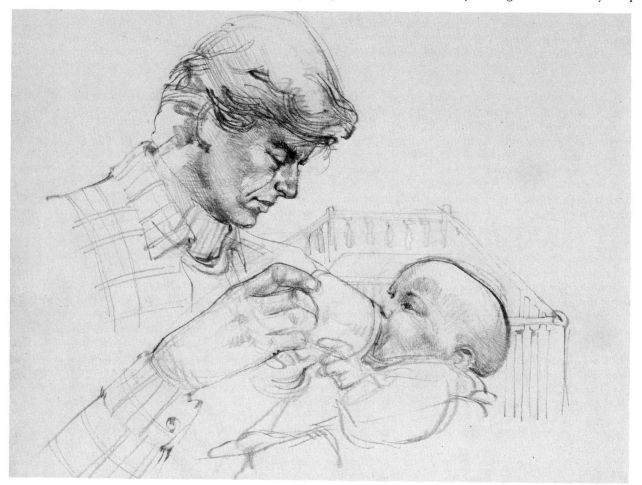

Table 6. Formula preparation

Terminal heating	Aseptic	Single-bottle[a]
1. Rinse the bottle and nipple with cool water immediately after the feeding. Wash the day's supply of bottles, nipples, and caps with hot, soapy water, and rinse well.	1. Rinse the bottle and nipple with cool water immediately after the feeding. Wash the day's supply of bottles, nipples, and caps with hot, soapy water and rinse well.	1. Rinse the bottle and nipple with cool water immediately after the feeding. Wash the day's supply of bottles, nipples, and caps with hot, soapy water and rinse well.
2. Rinse the outside of the formula can and shake the contents well. Open the can with a clean can opener, mix the formula with water, or water-carbohydrate solution if prescribed, and pour the solution into bottles. Attach the nipples and cover them loosely with caps.	2. Boil the bottles, nipples, caps, can opener, and mixing utensils for 5 minutes in a deep cooking utensil with enough water to cover each item. Remove the items with tongs, and place the bottles on a clean towel or rack.	2. For formulas that require water, pour into each bottle the amount of water needed to prepare the feeding. Attach the nipples and cover them loosely with caps. Place the bottles on a rack in a deep cooking utensil containing ~5–8 cm. of water. Bring water to a boil, cover, and allow it to boil gently for 25 minutes. Remove the cooking utensil from the stove, allow it to cool, and tighten the caps and bottles. The bottles may be left inside the cooking utensil until they are needed.
3. Place the bottles on a rack in a deep cooking utensil containing ~5–8 cm of water. Heat water to boiling, and allow it to boil gently for 25 minutes while covered before removing from the stove.	3. While the equipment is being cleaned, boil some water in a covered saucepan or tea kettle for 5 minutes (slightly more water than the prescribed amount should be used to allow for evaporation).	
4. After the sides of the cooking utensil have cooled enough to be touched comfortably, remove the lid and the formula bottles. (Leaving the utensil closed for this period is recommended to prevent formation of milk film on bottles and clogging of nipples.)	4. Remove the boiled water from the stove, allow it to cool, and measure the required amount.	3. For formulas that need no water, boil the bottles, nipples, caps, and can opener for 5 minutes. Put the nipples and caps on the bottles with aseptic care.
5. Warm the bottle of formula to the desired temperature before feeding.	5. Rinse, shake the can well, and add the commercially processed formula or evaporated milk and carbohydrate mixture to the boiled water and stir with a clean spoon. (If bottled milk or other unsterilized milk is used, it should be boiled with the water. Evaporated milk, carbohydrate modifiers, and commercially processed formulas usually are not boiled.)	4. At feeding time, remove the cap and nipple aseptically. Add the appropriate amount of formula and replace the nipple. With the powdered formula, also replace the cap, and shake the bottle vigorously to mix.
	6. Pour the formula into bottles, and attach the nipples and caps with aseptic care. Store them in the refrigerator. Formula should be used within 24 hours.	5. Feed the infant while formula is at room temperature.
	7. Warm the bottle of formula to the desired temperature before feeding.	

Adapted from "Handbook of Infant Formulas," 6th ed., J. B. Roerig, Division of Pfizer, New York, N.Y., 1969, pp. 86, 88, and H. N. Silver, *Pediatrics, 20,* 997 (1957).

[a]For supplementing the diet of breast-fed infant or when traveling.

ply of bottles may be sterilized in advance, adding the formula at feeding time. This practice eliminates the need for refrigeration of bottled formula and prefeeding warming.

The terminal heating method may allow bacterial growth during storage if instructions are not followed or if bottles are not cleaned thoroughly of milk film (138).

Feeding the Infant

The newborn infant may want to be fed at intervals of 2–3 hours. This schedule is permissible, but it does not allow the mother very much rest, and the infant may consume only small amounts (15 ml) of formula at a time. The baby should be encouraged to lengthen the interval to 4 hours as soon as possible. Most infants readily adopt a 4-hour schedule by the time they are 3–4 weeks old, but some prefer a shorter interval for several months (139).

Babies vary considerably in the amount of formula desired. The amount given should be consistent with the RDA for caloric intake (Table 2). Some pediatricians prescribe more formula than babies probably will accept, relying on each baby's own appetite to limit intake. This method works well if the mother does not urge or force the infant to take more than is desired at any one feeding. If an infant finishes a bottle and still seems hungry, another bottle should be offered.

Complaints about an infant's rejection of a formula may be resolved in some cases by examining the specific feeding problem. Spitting up often is caused by improper burping, feeding a large amount too quickly, laying the infant face down too soon after feeding, or having excess mucus in the nasopharynx. During feeding, the infant should be held in a well-supported position at a 45° angle, preferably with the head nestled in the curve of the arm. Infants should not be given a bottle in the crib while lying flat. They should be burped after every 30–45 ml of formula by gently patting or rubbing the back interchangeably. After feeding, the infant should be positioned on the abdomen (on the right side) to prevent regurgitation and aspiration of formula.

Many infants are chronic spitters of formula. If they are growing and gaining weight, there is no reason to be greatly concerned.

Product Selection Guidelines

Pharmacists should be able to discuss with parents the advantages and disadvantages of breast-feeding versus formula-feeding for a term infant. The limitations to breast-feeding should be recognized, such as the presence of certain drugs in breast milk and genetic disorders in infants. Mothers who cannot or do not wish to breast-feed should be reassured that normal growth and development in their infants are possible without breast-feeding.

In recommending the type of infant formula and its method of preparation, the pharmacist should take into consideration the parents' ability to follow directions, their attitudes and preferences, and the sanitary conditions and refrigeration facilities available. Instruction in cleaning techniques may include a step-by-step emphasis on the importance of sanitary conditions. For example, the top of the infant formula container should be cleaned thoroughly before opening, either by rinsing the top with hot tap water or by dipping it in boiling water for about 14 seconds before it is opened. Partially used

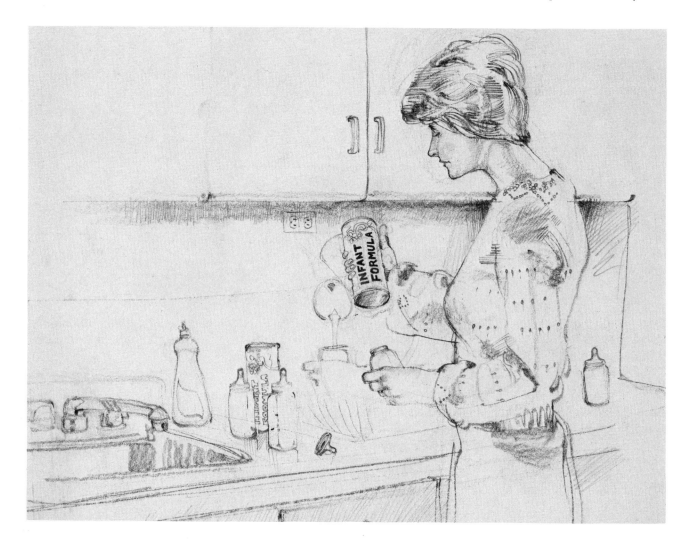

formula cans should be kept covered, placed in the refrigerator, and stored no longer than 48 hours.

For many parents, cost may be a critical factor in the selection of an infant formula. The concentrated formula preparations are less expensive than the ready-to-feed products; powdered preparations range between the two. Convenience is also a consideration. The powder and concentrated liquid formulas require more manipulative functions in preparation and more attention to aseptic technique. A formula that is well tolerated by the infant, convenient to prepare for the parents, and within the family budget should be used.

Summary

Pharmacists can monitor the response of infants to formula by questioning the parents. Detailed information obtained from discussions with parents about the type and severity of symptoms of the infant and complaints by the parents may help the pharmacist make appropriate recommendations: change in feeding procedures, use of a different type of formula, or referral to a physician.

Questions concerning vitamin and mineral supplementation in infants on formulas or breast milk must be answered accurately and completely. Information presented in this chapter and Chapter 12, *Nutritional Supplement, Mineral, and Vitamin Products,* can be useful in making proper recommendations for iron, fluoride, and multivitamin supplementation. Pharmacists can encourage the use of iron-fortified infant formulas to conform with the Committee on Nutrition's recommendations. The use of an iron-fortified formula in young infants does not increase the incidence or severity of GI symptoms compared to infants not receiving iron-fortified formulas (140). The stools of an infant receiving a formula or supplement containing iron may be darker, and the parents should be advised. The use of vitamin supplements should be limited to infants with known problems in fat absorption and those receiving restricted diets because of allergies or metabolic disease (17, 94). Prescribed fluoride supplementation should be based on the knowledge of the amount of fluoride in the water of the community and the type of feedings (breast milk, formula, or table food).

Pharmacists should keep current with the nutritional recommendations proposed by the FDA and the Committee on Nutrition. A thorough understanding of the nutritional requirements of infant formulas can assist pharmacists in allaying the concerns of parents. Compliance with recall announcements for deficient infant formulas is necessary to prevent possible adverse reactions in infants.

References

1. T. E. Cone, Jr., "200 Years of Feeding Infants in America," Ross Laboratories, Columbus, Ohio, 1976, p. 93.
2. H. J. Gerstenberger, H. D. Haskins, H. H. McGregor, and H. O. Ruh, *Am. J. Dis. Child.,* 10, 249 (1915).
3. G. A. Martinez and J. P. Nalezienski, *Pediatrics,* 64, 686 (1979).
4. M. K. Younsozai, in "Infant Nutrition," 2nd ed., S. J. Fomon, Ed., W. B. Saunders, Philadelphia, Pa., 1974, pp. 95–108.
5. E. E. Ziegler, S. J. Fomon, L. J. Filer, and L. N. Thomas, "Proceedings of the International Symposium on Dietary Lipids and Postnatal Development," Milan, Italy, 1972.
6. E. Delachaume-Salem and H. Sarles, *Biol. Gastroenterol,* 2, 135 (1970).
7. B. Borgström, B. Lindquist, and G. Lundh, *Am. J. Dis. Child.,* 99, 338 (1960).
8. T. A. Anderson, S. J. Fomon, and L. J. Filer, *J. Lab. Clin. Med.,* 79, 31 (1972).
9. S. Auricchio, A. Rubino, and G. Mürset, *Pediatrics,* 35, 944 (1965).
10. G. M. Gray and F. J. Ingelfinger, *J. Clin. Invest.,* 45, 388 (1966).
11. W. P. T. James, *Clin. Sci.,* 39, 305 (1970).
12. K. E. Bergmann, E. E. Ziegler, and S. J. Fomon, in "Infant Nutrition," 2nd ed., S. J. Fomon, Ed., W. B. Saunders, Philadelphia, Pa., 1974, pp. 245–265.
13. C. M. Edelman, Jr., H. L. Barnett, and V. Troupkou, *J. Clin. Invest.,* 39, 1062 (1960).
14. L. I. Kleinman, in "Perinatal Physiology," U. Staue, Ed., Plenum Medical, New York, N. Y., 1978, pp. 589–616.
15. S. S. Arnon, T. F. Midura, K. Damus, R. M. Wood, and J. Chin, *Lancet,* 1, 1273 (1978).
16. H. M. Seidel, in "Pediatrics," 2nd ed., M. Ziai, Ed., Little, Brown, Boston, Mass., 1975, p. 209.
17. C. W. Woodruff, *J Am. Med. Assoc.,* 240, 657 (1978).
18. Committee on Nutrition, American Academy of Pediatrics, *Pediatrics,* 57, 278 (1976).
19. S. J. Fomon, in "Infant Nutrition," 2nd ed., W. B. Saunders, Philadelphia, Pa., 1974, p. 80.
20. S. J. Fomon, in "Infant Nutrition," 2nd ed., W. B. Saunders, Philadelphia, Pa., 1974, p. 81.
21. S. J. Fomon, in "Infant Nutrition," 2nd ed., W. B. Saunders, Philadelphia, Pa., 1974, p. 255.
22. A. S. Goldman and C. W. Smith, *J. Pediatr.,* 82, 1082 (1973).
23. L. Gothefors and J. Winberg, *J. Trop. Pediatr. Environ. Child Health,* 21, 260 (1975).
24. *British Medical Journal,* 1, 1167 (1975).
25. M. Béhar, *Bull. Pan Am. Health Organ.,* 9, 1 (1975).
26. O. A. Stoliar, R. P. Pelley, E. Kaniecki-Green, M. H. Klaus, C. C. J. Carpenter, *Lancet,* 1, 1258 (1976).
27. G. L. France, D. J. Marmer, and R. W. Steele, *Am. J. Dis. Child,* 134, 147 (1980).
28. A. S. Cunningham, *J. Pediatr.,* 90, 726 (1977).
29. L. Gothefors, S. Olling, and J. Winberg, *Acta Paediatr. Scand.,* 64, 807 (1975).
30. L. J. Mata and J. J. Urrutia, *Ann. N. Y. Acad. Sci.,* 176, 93 (1971).
31. R. M. Kliegman, *Pediatr. Clin. N. Amer.,* 26, 327 (1979).
32. D. J. Matthew, B. Taylor, A. P. Norman, M. W. Turner, and J. F. Soothill, *Lancet,* 1, 321 (1977).
33. M. H. Klaus, J. H. Kennell, N. Plumb, S. Zuehlke, *Pediatrics,* 46, 187 (1970).
34. M. H. Klaus and J. H. Kennell, "Mother-Infant Bonding: The Impact of Early Separation or Loss on Family Development," C. V. Mosby, St. Louis, Mo., 1976, p. 43.
35. P. R. Dallman, *Am. J. Dis. Child,* 134, 453 (1980).
36. U. M. Saarinen, M. A. Siimes, and P. R. Dallman, *Pediatrics,* 91, 36 (1977).
37. S. J. Fomon, in "Infant Nutrition," 2nd ed., W. B. Saunders, Philadelphia, Pa., 1974, p. 310.
38. S. J. Fomon and R. G. Strauss, *N. Engl. J. Med.,* 299, 355 (1978).
39. K. M. Hambidge, *Pediatr. Clin. N. Amer.,* 24, 95 (1977).
40. H. H. Bode, W. J. Vanjonack, and J. D. Crawford, *Pediatr. Res.,* 11, 423 (1977).
41. D. B. Jelliffe and E. F. P. Jelliffe, *N. Engl. J. Med.,* 297, 912 (1977).
42. S. J. Fomon, in "Infant Nutrition," 2nd ed., W. B. Saunders, Philadelphia, Pa., 1974, p. 79.
43. J. S. Vobecky, P. P. Demers, and D. Shapcott, Western Hemisphere Nutrition Congress VI, Los Angeles, Calif., 1980.
44. R. L. Poland, G. Schultz, and G. Garg, *Pediatr. Res.,* 14, 1328 (1980).
45. R. L. Poland, *J. Pediatr.,* 99, 86 (1981).

46. F. A. Oski and S. A. Landaw, *Am. J. Dis. Child, 134,* 459 (1980).
47. *Medical Letter on Drugs and Therapeutics, 16,* 25 (1974).
48. P. O. Anderson, *Drug Intell. Clin. Pharm., 11,* 208 (1977).
49. C. S. Catz and G. P. Giacoia, in "Dietary Lipids and Postnatal Development," C. Galli, G. Jacini, and A. Pecile, Eds., Raven Press, New York, N. Y., 1972, p. 247.
50. V. M. Barsivala and K. D. Virka, *Contraception, 7,* 307 (1973).
51. C. S. Catz and G. P. Giacoia, *Pediatr. Clin. North Am., 19,* 151 (1972).
52. C. W. Woodruff, *J. Am. Med. Assoc., 240,* 657 (1978).
53. S. J. Fomon, "Infant Nutrition," Medcom, New York, N. Y., 1972, p. 31.
54. S. A. Anderson, H. I. Chinn, and K. D. Fisher, in "A Background Paper on Infant Formulas," Life Sciences Research Office, Bethesda, Md., 1980, pp. 1–33.
55. *Federal Register, 44,* 40343 (1979).
56. *Federal Register, 44,* 40343 (1979).
57. *Federal Register, 44,* 40343 (1979).
58. Infant Formula Council, Manual Registration No. 5674, Atlanta, Ga., 1973.
59. T. A. Anderson, S. J. Fomon, and L. J. Filer, *J. Lab. Clin. Med., 79,* 31 (1972).
60. R. W. Krouskop, E. G. Brown, and A. Y. Sweet, *Pediatr. Res., 8,* 383 (1974).
61. T. V. Santulli, J. N. Schullinger, W. C. Heird, R. G. Gongaware, J. Wigger, B. Barlow, W. A. Blanc, and W. E. Berdon, *Pediatrics, 55,* 376 (1975).
62. R. M. Tomarelli, *J. Pediatr., 88,* 454 (1976).
63. C. L. Paxson, E. W. Adcock, III, and F. H. Morriss, Jr., *Am. J. Dis. Child, 131,* 139 (1977).
64. "Recommended Dietary Allowances," 9th ed., National Research Council, Food and Nutrition Board, Washington, D.C., 1980.
65. *Federal Register, 45,* 17206 (1980).
66. Committee on Nutrition, American Academy of Pediatrics, *Pediatrics, 53,* 115 (1974).
67. Committee on Nutrition, American Academy of Pediatrics, *Pediatrics, 49,* 305 (1972).
68. S. J. Fomon, in "Infant Nutrition," Medcom, New York, N. Y., 1972, p. 121.
69. S. J. Fomon, in "Infant Nutrition," Medcom, New York, N. Y., 1972, p. 121.
70. G. Gaull, J. A. Sturman, and N. C. R. Räihä, *Pediatr. Res., 6,* 538 (1972).
71. S. J. Fomon, "Infant Nutrition," 2nd ed., W. B. Saunders, Philadelphia, Pa., 1974, p. 59.
72. S. J. Fomon, L. N. Thomas, L. J. Filer, Jr., T. A. Anderson, and K. E. Bergmann, *Acta Paediatr. Scand., 62,* 33 (1973).
73. *Lancet, 2,* 1359 (1974).
74. "First After Mother's Milk," Wyeth Laboratories, Philadelphia, Pa., 1971, p. 6.
75. H. Schlenk, *Fed. Proc., 31,* 1430 (1972).
76. S. J. Fomon, in "Infant Nutrition," Medcom, New York, N. Y., 1972, p. 194.
77. A. Holzel, V. Schwarz, and K. W. Sutcliffe, *Lancet, 1,* 1126 (1959).
78. M. Y. Dju, K. E. Mason, and L. J. Filer, Jr., *Etudes Neonatates, 1,* 49 (1952).
79. H. Hassan, S. A. Hashim, T. V. Van Itallie, and W. H. Sebrell, *Am. J. Clin. Nutr., 19,* 147 (1966).
80. F. A. Oski and L. A. Barness, *J. Pediatr., 70,* 211 (1967).
81. J. H. Ritchie, M. B. Fish, V. McMasters, and M. Grossman, *N. Engl. J. Med., 279,* 1185 (1968).
82. S. S. Lo, D. Frank, and W. H. Hitzig, *Arch. Dis. Child., 48,* 360 (1973).
83. D. L. Phelps, *Pediatrics, 63,* 933 (1979).
84. M. W. Dicks-Bushnell and K. C. Davis, *Am. J. Clin. Nutr., 20,* 262 (1967).
85. S. J. Fomon, in "Infant Nutrition," 2nd, W. B. Saunders, Philadelphia, Pa., 1974, p. 253.
86. L. K. Dahl, *Am. J. Clin. Nutr., 21,* 787 (1968).
87. L. J. Filer, Jr., *Nutr. Rev., 29,* 27 (1971).
88. "Sodium Intake by Infants in the United States," Committee on Nutrition, American Academy of Pediatrics, Evanston, Ill., 1979.
89. S. Roy, III, and B. S. Arant, Jr., *N. Engl. J. Med., 301,* 615 (1979).
90. E. H. Garin, D. Geary, and G. A. Richard, *J. Pediatr, 95,* 985 (1979).
91. Committee on Nutrition, American Academy of Pediatrics, *Pediatrics, 62,* 826 (1978).
92. A. Mizrahi, R. D. London, and D. Gribetz, *N. Engl. J. Med., 278,* 1163 (1968).
93. P. R. Dallman, *J. Pediatr, 85,* 742 (1974).
94. A. S. Prasad and D. Oberleas, *Lancet, 1,* 463 (1974).
95. Committee on Nutrition, American Academy of Pediatrics, *Pediatrics, 66,* 1015 (1980).
96. S. Bachrach, J. Fisher, and J. S. Parks, *Pediatrics, 64,* 871 (1979).
97. J. C. Rowe, D. H. Wood, D. W. Rowe, and L. G. Raisz, *N. Engl. J. Med., 300,* 293 (1979).
98. P. O'Connor, *Clin. Pediatr., 16,* 361 (1977).
99. N. Hoff, J. Haddad, S. Teitelbaum, W. McAlister, and L. S. Hillman, *J. Pediatr., 94,* 460 (1979).
100. M. C. Higginbottom, L. Sweetman, and W. L. Nyhan, *N. Engl. J. Med., 299,* 317 (1978).
101. Committee on Nutrition, American Academy of Pediatrics, *Pediatrics, 63,* 150 (1979).
102. W. S. Driscoll and H. S. Horowitz, *Am. Dent. Assoc. J., 96,* 1050 (1978).
103. W. S. Driscoll and H. S. Horowitz, *Am. J. Dis. Child., 133,* 683 (1979).
104. Committee on Nutrition, American Academy of Pediatrics, *Pediatrics, 58,* 765 (1976).
105. Committee on Nutrition, American Academy of Pediatrics, *Pediatrics, 60,* 519 (1977).
106. S. Gross and D. K. Melhorn, *J. Pediatr., 85,* 753 (1974).
107. D. Stevens, D. Burman, M. K. Strelling, and A. Norris, *Pediatrics, 64,* 333 (1979).
108. S. J. Fomon, L. N. Thomas, L. J. Filer, E. E. Ziegler, and N. I. Leonard, *Acta Paediatr. Scand.* (Suppl.), *223,* 1 (1971).
109. R. L. Jackson, R. Westerfield, M. A. Flynn, E. R. Kimball, and R. B. Lewis, *Pediatrics, 33,* 642 (1964).
110. L. J. Filer, Jr., "Abstracts of the Nutrition Foundation, Inc.," Food and Nutrition Liaison Committee, 1980.
111. S. J. Fomon and L. J. Filer, Jr., in "Infant Nutrition," 2nd ed., W. B. Saunders, Philadelphia, Pa., 1974, p. 383.
112. S. J. Fomon and L. J. Filer, Jr., in "Infant Nutrition," 2nd ed., W. B. Saunders, Philadelphia, Pa., 1974, p. 384.
113. S. J. Fomon and L. J. Filer, Jr., in "Infant Nutrition," 2nd ed., W. B. Saunders, Philadelphia, Pa., 1974, p. 387.
114. S. J. Fomon and L. J. Filer, Jr., in "Infant Nutrition," 2nd ed., W. B. Saunders, Philadelphia, Pa., 1974, p. 393.
115. S. A. Anderson, H. I. Chinn, and K. D. Fischer, in "A Background Paper on Infant Formulas," Life Sciences Research Office, Bethesda, Md., 1980, p. 14.
116. J. W. Gerrard, J. W. A. MacKenzie, N. Goluboff, J. Z. Garson, and C. S. Maningas, *Acta Paediatr. Scand.* (Suppl.), *234,* 1 (1973).
117. A. S. Goldman, D. W. Anderson, Jr., W. A. Sellers, S. Saperstein, W. T. Kniker, and S. R. Halpern, *Pediatrics, 32,* 425 (1963).
118. S. Freier and B. Kletter, *Clin. Pediatr., 9,* 449 (1970).
119. P. A. di Sant' Agnese, in "Current Pediatric Therapy," S. S. Gellia and B. M. Kagan, Eds., W. B. Saunders, Philadelphia, Pa., 1973, p. 234.
120. S. J. Fomon, in "Infant Nutrition," 2nd ed., W. B. Saunders, Philadelphia, Pa., 1974, p. 391–392.
121. "Amino Acid Metabolism and Genetic Variation," W. I. Nyhan, Ed., McGraw-Hill, New York, N. Y., 1967, pp. 6–63.
122. G. B. Forbes, *Pediatr. Res., 12,* 434 (1978).
123. C. W. Woodruff, *Nutr. Rev., 34,* 33 (1976).
124. L. S. Book, J. J. Herbst, S. O. Atherton, and A. L. Jung, *J. Pediatr., 87,* 602 (1975).
125. D. Cornfeld and R. E. Cooke, *Pediatrics, 10,* 33 (1952).
126. H. I. Goldman and F. Deposito, *Am. J. Dis. Child, 111,* 430 (1966).
127. W. F. J. Cuthbertson, *Am. J. Clin. Nutr., 29,* 559 (1976).
128. C. D. May, E. N. Nelson, C. U. Lowe, and R. J. Salmon, *Am. J. Dis. Child., 80,* 191 (1950).

129. W. A. Cochrane, C. Collins-Williams, and W. L. Donohue, *Pediatrics*, *28*, 771 (1961).
130. D. B. Coursin, *J. Am. Med. Assoc.*, *154*, 406 (1954).
131. J. D. Hydovitz, *N. Engl. J. Med.*, *262*, 351 (1960).
132. P. B. Kulkarni, R. T. Hall, P. G. Rhodes, M. B. Sheehan, J. C. Callenbach, D. R. Germann, and S. J. Abramson, *J. Pediatr.*, *96*, 249 (1980).
133. R. F. Cifuentes, S. W. Kooh, and I. C. Radde, *J. Pediatr.*, *96*, 252 (1980).
134. Y. Tanaka, S. Hatano, Y. Nishi, and T. Usui, *J. Pediatr.*, *96*, 255 (1980).
135. C. A. L. Abrams, L. L. Phillips, C. Berkowitz, P. R. Blackett, and C. J. Priebe, *J. Am. Med. Assoc.*, *232*, 1136 (1975).
136. H. K. Silver, *Pediatrics*, *20*, 993 (1957).
137. Committee on the Fetus and the Newborn, American Academy of Pediatrics, *Pediatrics*, *28*, 674 (1961).
138. C. C. Fischer and M. A. Whitman, *J. Pediatr.*, *55*, 116 (1959).
139. S. J. Fomon, in "Infant Nutrition," 2nd ed., W. B. Saunders, Philadelphia, Pa., 1974, p. 80.
140. F. A. Oski, *Pediatrics*, *66*, 168 (1980).

Infant Formula Product Table

Product[a] (Manufacturer)	Calories per 30 ml	Calories per 100 ml	Protein (g/100 ml)	Fat (g/100 ml)	Carbo-hydrate (g/100 ml)	Sodium (mEq/ 100 ml)	Potas-sium (mEq/ 100 ml)	Chloride (mg/ 100 ml)	Calcium (mg/ 100 ml)	Phos-phorus (mg/ 100 ml)
Standard Formulas										
Advance (Ross)	16	54	2.0	2.7	5.5	1.3	2.2	1.5	51.0	39.0
Breast Milk	22	75	1.1	4.5	6.8	0.7	1.3	1.1	33.6	16.0
Cow's Milk, whole, fortified	21	69	3.5	3.5	4.9	2.5	3.6	2.7	120.0	96.0
Enfamil (Mead Johnson)	20	68	1.5	3.7	7.0	1.0	1.7	1.4	53.0	44.0
Enfamil with Iron (Mead Johnson)	20	68	1.5	3.7	7.0	1.0	1.7	1.4	53.0	44.0
Evaporated Milk, diluted 1:1, fortified	21	69	3.5	4.0	4.9	2.8	3.9	3.2	134.6	102.5
Goat's Milk, fresh	21	69	3.6	4.0	4.6	1.4	4.6	4.5	128.0	104.9
Similac (Ross)	20	68	1.55	3.6	7.23	1.1	2.0	1.5	51.0	39.0
Similac with Iron (Ross)	20	68	1.55	3.6	7.23	1.1	2.0	1.5	51.0	39.0
SMA Iron-Fortified (Wyeth)	20	68	1.5	3.6	7.2	0.65	1.4	1.0	44.0	33.0
Therapeutic Formulas										
Milk Allergy										
Isomil (Ross)	20	68	2.0	3.6	6.80	1.3	1.8	1.5	70.0	50.0
i-Soyalac (Loma Linda)	20	66	2.1	3.75	6.65	1.5	2.0	1.5	63.4	42.3
Meat Base Formula (1:1 dilution) (Gerber)	20	68	2.7	3.5	6.4	1.2	1.4	1.4	102	68.0
Nursoy (Wyeth)	20	67.6	2.1	3.6	6.9	0.87	1.9	1.0	63.4	44.38
Nutramigen (Mead Johnson)	20	68	2.2	2.6	8.8	1.6	2.0	1.7	63	48
ProSobee (Mead Johnson)	20	68	2	3.6	6.9	1.3	2.1	1.6	63	50
Soyalac (Loma Linda)	20	66	2.1	3.8	6.65	1.5	1.9	1.1	63.4	42.3
Electrolyte Imbalance										
Lytren (Mead Johnson)	9	33	none	none	7.7	3.0	2.5	2.5	8.0	8.9
Pedialyte (Ross)	6	20	none	none	5.0	3.0	2.0	3.0	8.0	none
Medium Chain Triglyceride Requirement										
Portagen (Mead Johnson)	20	68	2.4	3.2	7.8	1.4	2.2	1.6	63	48

Iron (mg/ 100 ml)	Type of Carbohydrate	Source of Protein	Type of Fat	Vit. A (IU/ liter)	Vit. D (IU/ liter)	Thiamine (mg/liter)	Niacin[b] (Equivalent) (mg/liter)	Ascorbic Acid (mg/liter)
1.2	corn syrup, lactose	cow's milk, soy isolate	soy, corn oils	2,400	400	0.75	10.0	50
0.15	lactose	human milk	human milk fat	2,400	5	0.16	3.5	8
0.05	lactose	cow's milk	butterfat	1,850	400	0.29	1.0	10
0.05	lactose	cow's milk	butterfat	1,850	400	0.20	1.0	7
0.1	lactose	goat's milk	goat's milk fat	2,074	24	0.40	1.9	15
0.15	lactose	cow's milk	soy, coconut oils	1,690	420	0.53	8.5	55
1.3	lactose	cow's milk	soy, coconut oils	1,690	420	0.53	8.5	55
0.15	lactose	cow's milk	soy, coconut oils	2,500	400	0.65	7.0	55
1.2	lactose	cow's milk	soy, coconut oils	2,500	400	0.65	7.0	55
1.3	lactose	demineralized whey	safflower oil (blend), soy, coconut oils	2,640	423	0.71	10.1	58
1.2	sucrose, corn syrup	soy protein	soy, coconut oils	2,500	400	0.40	9.0	55
1.3	sucrosa, tapioca dextrins	soy isolate	soy oil	2,113	423	0.53	8.5	63
1.37	sucrose, modified tapioca starch	beef heart	sesame, beef fat	1,808	407	0.60	4.1	61
1.3	sucrose	soy isolate	safflower oil (blend) soy coconut oils	2,640	420	0.71	10.0	58
1.3	sucrose, modified tapioca, starch	hydrolyzed casein	corn oil	1,690	420	0.53	8.5	55
1.3	corn syrup solids	soy isolate	soy oil, coconut oil	2,100	420	0.53	8.5	55
1.3	sucrose, corn syrup	soy extract	soy oil	2,113	423	0.53	8.5	63
none	corn syrup solids, glucose	none	none	none	none	none	none	none
none	dextrose	none	none	none	none	none	none	none
1.3	corn syrup solids, sucrose	casein	corn, MCT[c] oils	5,300	530	1.1	13.7	55

Infant Formula Product Table, continued

Product[a] (Manufacturer)	Calories per 30 ml	Calories per 100 ml	Protein (g/100 ml)	Fat (g/100 ml)	Carbo-hydrate (g/100 ml)	Sodium (mEq/ 100 ml)	Potas-sium (mEq/ 100 ml)	Chloride (mg/ 100 ml)	Calcium (mg/ 100 ml)	Phos-phorus (mg/ 100 ml)
Carbohydrate and/or Fat Restriction										
Pregestimil (Mead Johnson)	20	68	1.9	2.7	9.1	1.4	1.9	1.6	63	42
Skim milk, fortified, market average	11	36	3.6	trace	5.3	2.3	3.6	3.0	122.7	98.0
High Protein and/or Caloric Requirement										
Enfamil Premature Formula (Mead Johnson)	24	81	2.4	4.1	8.9	1.4	2.3	1.9	95	48
Similac PM 60/40 (Ross)	20	68	1.58	3.76	6.88	0.7	1.5	0.7	40.0	20.0
Sodium Restriction										
Lonalac (Mead Johnson)	20	68	3.4	3.5	4.8	0.1	3.3	1.7	116	106
Phenylketonuria										
Lofenalac (Mead Johnson)	20	68	2.3	2.7	8.8	1.4	1.8	1.3	63	48

[a]Values are based on ready-to-use strength and were obtained with cooperation of the Dietary Service, Shands Hospital, Gainesville, Florida, and manufacturers.

Iron (mg/ 100 ml)	Type of Carbohydrate	Source of Protein	Type of Fat	Vit. A (IU/ liter)	Vit. D (IU/ liter)	Thiamine (mg/liter)	Niacin[b] (Equiva- lent) (mg/liter)	Ascor- bic Acid (mg/liter)
1.3	corn syrup solids, modified tapioca starch	hydrolyzed casein	corn, MCT[c] oils	2,100	420	0.53	8.5	55
trace	lactose	cow's milk	none	4,167	400	0.40	trace	19
0.13	lactose, corn syrup solids	cow's milk	corn, MCT[c], coconut oil	2,500	510	0.63	10.1	69
0.26	lactose	demineralized whey, casein	corn, coconut oils	2,500	400	0.65	7.3	55
0.11	lactose	casein	coconut oil	1,000	none	0.42	0.85	none
1.3	corn syrup, modi- fied tapioca starch	hydrolyzed casein	corn oil	1,690	420	0.53	8.5	55

[b] See Table 2 for explanation of niacin equivalent.
[c] MCT, medium-chain triglycerides.

15 Weight Control Products

Glenn D. Appelt

Questions to Ask the Patient

What are your age, height, and weight?

How long have you had a weight problem?

How much overweight do you feel you are?

Is there a family history of obesity? Do either of your parents have a weight problem?

Do you tend to eat excessively when you are anxious, nervous, or tired?

Have you consulted a physician about the problem?

Are you following a diet?

What diet preparations have you used previously? Were they effective?

What attempts have you made in an effort to lose weight? For example, do you belong to a self-help group, such as Weight Watchers?

Do you have a regular exercise program? Does your physician recommend that you exercise?

Are you being treated for any chronic disease, such as hypertension, diabetes, thyroid, or heart disease?

What medicines are you currently taking?

Obesity is the pathologic accumulation of fat, which exceeds that needed for optional body functioning (1). From a practical viewpoint, obesity may be defined as the physical state in which body weight, in relation to height, exceeds the ideal weight by 20%, according to Metropolitan Life Insurance data (Table 1) (2). Although the term "obese" often is associated with "overweight," the terms are not interchangeable. Athletes, for example, may be overweight but not obese. Measurement of skinfold thickness has been suggested to be a practical means of determining the extent of obesity (1). The triceps skinfold, as measured by calipers, has been reported to be the most representative of body fat (3). Daily caloric allowances for persons with moderate physical activity may vary with age and sex (4). Values for average males (weight, 70 kg or 154 lb; height, 1.78 m or 5'10") in a temperate climate range from 3,200 cal at age 25 years to 2,550 cal at age 65 years. Corresponding figures for average females (weight, 58 kg or 128 lb; height, 1.63 m or 5'4") are 2,300 and 1,800 cal. The values for women increase slightly during pregnancy (300 cal) and significantly during lactation (1,000 cal).

It takes 3,500 excess calories to result in 0.454 kg (1 lb) of body fat. Most obesity cases involve overeating, particularly of carbohydrates or fats. The calories ingested beyond those necessary for normal energy requirements usually are deposited and stored as fat. Because the lack of food is rarely a problem in the United States, Americans must decide how much and what type of food to consume. Apparently, many make unwise choices, since obesity is a common American affliction. Obesity is estimated to occur in 24–45% of Americans over 30 years of age (5, 6). In children, the incidence is reported to be from 2–15% (5).

Clinical Considerations

Obesity is a subject of intense study. Many factors enter into metabolic equilibrium. Appetite control is only part of the answer. Psychological components may contribute to or cause overeating, leading to obesity. Often self-therapy groups may help in treating the cause; the use of pharmacologic agents tend to treat only the symptoms. In addition, caloric expenditure by physical activity could promote the maintenance of a nonobese state in the motivated individual.

Etiology of Obesity

The question of why individuals ingest more calories than they expend is complex. The answer may be related to physiologic, genetic, environmental, or psychological factors. Endocrine disorders, such as hypothyroidism or Cushing's syndrome, apparently are rarely involved in obesity. Obesity may result from an anatomical or biochemical lesion in the brain's feeding centers, although this hypothesis has not been proven in humans (7). Another theory suggests that in the obese person there is a deficiency of an enzyme responsible for alpha-glycerophosphate oxidation, resulting in increased availability of this substrate for triglyceride synthesis (8). One hypothesis suggests that prostaglandins are involved in the development of obesity through an effect on lipogenesis (9). Overproduction of prostaglandins in adipose cells may result in an increase in fatty tissue.

Some researchers believe that thin and obese people differ in the degree of thermogenesis after food ingestion (10). Overeating in nonobese subjects causes increased heat production, which tends to dissipate the excess calories. In obese subjects, the dissipation of thermal energy is less pronounced, resulting in fat storage. The thermogenesis theory was expanded to include a specialized form of fat tissue (brown fat), which participates in thermogenesis. The exact role of brown fat is unclear, but it appears to favor increased triglyceride hydrolysis (11).

A biochemical basis for obesity has been suggested that involves adenosine triphosphatase (ATPase) (12). Red blood cells in obese people were noted to have lower levels of ATPase compared with individuals of normal weight. This enzyme facilitates the sodium-potassium pump process in body cells which could result in caloric expenditure (12). In other words, the obese individual with reduced ATPase activity is more likely to add fat since he or she burns fewer calories than the nonobese individual.

The correlation of a primitive "hibernation response" with human obesity has been proposed (13). Adaptive reactions preparing the body for an impending shortage may be predominant in the obese individual. Although humans do not hibernate, an "endomorphic system" representing a relic of the human evolutionary past may be operant and initiate the overeating typical of the obese person. It is suggested that this "hunger reaction" may be initiated by the beta-endorphins.

One belief holds that obese people sleep more than thin people. A connection exists between metabolism and sleep that may be related to obesity (14). Obesity has been correlated with the frequency of an ultra-radian brain rhythm (NREM-REM). This observation lends credence to the proposal that there is a decrease in the amount of sleep in obese people when they lose weight (15). Conversely, it has been observed that there is an increase in the amount of sleep time when anorexic patients gain weight (16).

Another hypothesis relates infantile obesity to excess fat cells during infancy that may predispose the individual to obesity later in life (17). Obese patients have not only larger than normal fat cells but also an increased number of these cells. Apparently, as people lose weight on a low-calorie diet, the size of each fat cell decreases, but the total number of fat cells remains the same; when people return to increased weight levels, the fat cells regain their original size. Obesity in children may result from the addition of new fat cells; "adult onset obesity" may represent an expansion of fat cells already present

Table 1. Desirable weights for men and women, according to height and frame, ages 25 and over

Height (in shoes)*	Weight in pounds (in indoor clothing)		
	Small frame	Medium frame	Large frame
Men			
5' 2"	112–120	118–129	126–141
3"	115–123	121–133	129–144
4"	118–126	124–136	132–148
5"	121–129	127–139	135–152
6"	124–133	130–143	138–156
7"	128–137	134–147	142–161
8"	132–141	138–152	147–166
9"	136–145	142–156	151–170
10"	140–150	146–160	155–174
11"	144–154	150–165	159–179
6' 0"	148–158	154–170	164–184
1"	152–162	158–175	168–189
2"	156–167	162–180	173–194
3"	160–171	167–185	178–199
4"	164–175	172–190	182–204
Women			
4'10"	92– 98	96–107	104–119
11"	94–101	98–110	106–122
5' 0"	96–104	101–113	109–125
1"	99–107	104–116	112–128
2"	102–110	107–119	115–131
3"	105–113	110–122	118–134
4"	108–116	113–126	121–138
5"	111–119	116–130	125–142
6"	114–123	120–135	129–146
7"	118–127	124–139	133–150
8"	122–131	128–143	137–154
9"	126–135	132–147	141–158
10"	130–140	136–151	145–163
11"	134–144	140–155	149–168
6' 0"	138–148	144–159	153–173

Prepared by and reprinted with permission from the Metropolitan Life Insurance Company. Derived primarily from data of the *Build and Blood Pressure Study, 1959,* Society of Actuaries.

*1-inch heels for men and 2-inch heels for women.

(2). Previous experiments suggest that the earlier the onset of obesity, the greater the number of fat cells (18). After the age of 20, obesity is caused almost exclusively by the expansion of existent cells. Accordingly, an overweight child or adolescent may be more susceptible to obesity as an adult.

A child who has one obese parent has a 40% chance of being obese; if both parents are obese, there is an 80% possibility (19). These data suggest a direct genetic component, and although it has not been proven in human obesity, animal studies indicate this relationship (20). In experimental animals, genetic transmission of obesity is associated with modified organ size and composition (21, 22). Human data suggest fundamental relationships between body build and obesity (23, 24). Studies revealed that obese women differed from nonobese women in a morphologic characteristic other than the degree of adiposity. Obese women were more endomorphic than nonobese women: Abdomen mass overshadowed thoracic bulk, all regions were notable for their softness and roundness, and the hands and feet were relatively small.

Obesity may result from environmental influence, such as the widespread advertising of food products. Occupational, economic, and sociocultural factors also may be considered in the broad environmental sense. It now appears that socioeconomic status and related social factors are important in obesity development. Obesity is seven times more common among women of low socioeconomic groups than among those of higher status (25). The mental health indices of the obese subjects in the low socioeconomic group reflected "immaturity," "rigidity," and "suspiciousness" in comparison with those individuals in the same group with normal weight. A defect in impulse control may be suggested by the "immaturity" rating. In addition, obesity was found to be more prevalent in young females of low socioeconomic status than in those of a higher socioeconomic status (26). Another study confirmed the greater incidence of obesity among women of low socioeconomic status and found a similar but less marked trend in men. In addition, suggestive relationships between ethnic and religious factors and obesity were found for both sexes (27).

Obesity has a psychogenic component in 90% of the cases (28). Although the psychologic aspect of caloric excess usually is exemplified by compulsive overeating replacing other gratifications, other factors are also involved. Obesity may be related to physical activity and emotions (29). Decreased physical activity may play a role in the development and maintenance of obesity. This theory involves the aspect of caloric expenditure rather than caloric ingestion and stresses the function of caloric disequilibrium in obesity. Mental depression may not be an incidental occurrence in obese people but rather one of the main reasons for the obesity (29). Another psychological aberration in obese patients is the disturbance in body image, where the body is viewed as "grotesque and loathsome" (30).

Appetite Control

The hypothalamus apparently contains centers that are intimately involved in the food ingestion process. Studies in rats show a "satiety center" and an "appetite center" located in the hypothalamic region (31). Destroying the satiety center leads to marked overeating with subsequent obesity; conversely, obliterating the appetite center results in emaciation. These results indicate that there may be a feedback inhibition of the appetite center by impulses from the satiety center after food is ingested. The glucostatic hypothesis of appetite regulation states that hunger is related to the degree that glucose is used by cells called "glucostats" (32). When glucose utilization by glucostats in the satiety center is low, the inhibitory effect on the appetite center is reduced, favoring eating behavior. Conversely, when glucose utilization is high, the appetite center is inhibited, and the desire for food intake is reduced.

The hypothalamus contains high concentrations of noradrenergic terminals (33). A discrete fiber system that supplies the hypothalamus with most of its norepinephrine-secreting terminals is called the "ventral noradrenergic bundle." Destroying the noradrenergic terminals in the hypothalamus or damaging the ventral noradrenergic bundle results in obesity in animals (34). It has been suggested that this noradrenergic bundle normally mediates satiety and that it may serve as a substrate for amphetamine-induced appetite suppression (35).

The interpretation of visual and chemical food-related stimuli occurs in the cerebral cortex, and acceptance or rejection of the sight, aroma, or taste of foods involves this area of the CNS. An obese person may respond differently from people of normal weight to the appearance, taste, and sight of food (36). Research involving the trigeminal nerve, a pathway relaying sensory input from the oral cavity to the hypothalamus, indicates this system's possible role in food intake. The trigeminal circuit is a system of oral touch, and the excessive nibbling common to obese individuals may be due to their greater sensitivity to this stimulus (37).

Role of Obesity in Other Conditions

Studies have shown a significant association between early mortality and obesity. Cardiovascular diseases account for many early deaths (38). There is evidence that sustained hypertension is more common in overweight people, although the correlation between blood pressure and adiposity is not well established (39). It seems reasonable to suggest that high-risk people, such as those with a positive family history of youthful obesity, reduce their salt intake (40). If a patient cannot control obesity by any reasonable means, the pharmacist may recommend salt intake reduction. Weight reduction due to water loss by reduced sodium intake may be of psychological benefit. However, it should be stressed that this weight loss is not relevant to effects on fat cells. Vascular changes and cerebrovascular diseases have been associated with obesity (41, 42).

The relationship between obesity and diabetes mellitus is well documented (38). An early study revealed that 85% of patients over 40 years old who developed diabetes mellitus were overweight (43). Glucose intolerance commonly occurs with obesity, and relative insulin resistance is noted in obese subjects (39, 44). The hyperinsulinemia that occurs in obesity is related to increased body fat (45). Weight reduction results in improved glucose tolerance in the obese diabetic and reduced hyperinsulinemia in both nondiabetic and diabetic obese persons (46, 47). The severity of diabetes mellitus and the need for insulin or oral hypoglycemic agents often may be decreased by weight reduction. (See Chapter 13, *Diabetes Care Products.*)

In addition to the correlations of obesity with these disease states, obese individuals have larger and more cellular organs (heart and liver) (48). Obesity may also be related to cholesterol gallstone formation, since the level of this compound is characteristically elevated in obesity (49).

Hyperostosis of the spine (formation of bony bridges between the vertebrae) has been associated with hyperglycemia and obesity, although these factors are at least partly independent of each other (50). In addition, excessive obesity may contribute to respiratory stress. Obesity alters pulmonary function resulting in plethora, reduced lung volume, hypercapnia, and pulmonary hypertension (51). The description by Charles Dickens of Joe, the fat boy in *The Pickwick Papers*, reveals a person with marked obesity and somnolence. The description may be the first account of this condition in the literature; the "pickwickian syndrome" describes a person who is obese, exhibits narcoleptic behavior, and has an excessive appetite (52).

Certain skin disorders including candidiasis, tinea infections, furunculosis, pruritus vulvae, and trophic ulcerations occur frequently in obese individuals (53). These conditions have been associated with diabetes mellitus, which may explain the high incidence in obese persons. It should be noted, however, that scabies and psychosomatic skin disorders also occur in significant numbers of the obese. These conditions are not directly related to the diabetic state.

Although obesity generally is caused by overeating, it may not always denote adequate nourishment. Obesity may mask malnutrition. Often the obese individual overconsumes carbohydrates at the expense of omitting other nutrients such as protein, vitamins, and minerals from the diet (54).

Symptoms of Obesity

Common patient complaints regarding obesity are often cosmetic, involving a desire to "look slim." However, remarks such as "I can't tie my shoes without getting out of breath" indicate actual physical discomfort. The obese patient may also complain of persistent backache and varicose veins.

Because obesity may be caused by the inactivity resulting from mental depression, patients who remain obese after prolonged self-medication with nonprescription anorexic products should be referred to a physician (26). A psychogenic component involving inactivity due to depression or a compulsive anxiety reaction related to repeated "snacking" may be involved in such cases. The pharmacist should emphasize that weight loss will not occur unless caloric imbalance is corrected. Chronic use of nonprescription products to correct obesity may indicate a more severe underlying problem.

Treatment

Drug treatment of obesity is of limited value since the only satisfactory means of long-term weight control is calorie reduction and physical activity (55).

Amphetamines have been prescribed for obesity. Amphetamine and related prescription drugs are thought to suppress appetite by an effect on the appetite centers in the hypothalamus (56). Unfortunately, tolerance develops to the amphetamine's appetite suppressant activity, making long-term use undesirable. In addition, subtle or profound depression secondary to withdrawal from the effects of amphetamines can further complicate the effectiveness of other weight control

measures. Because overeating seems to be controlled primarily by psychological behavior factors, overeating will occur as soon as the anorexigenic effects disappear. Amphetamines and other related agents have the potential for abuse and dependence; their value is limited to short-term use (a few weeks) in obesity control as an adjunct to a controlled diet. Amphetamines should be used only when alternative therapy has been ineffective. Amphetamine and related prescription products apparently suppress appetite by stimulating the satiety center in the hypothalamic ventromedial nucleus. This process may occur indirectly on the frontal lobes of the cortex (57).

Human Chorionic Gonadotropin

Human chorionic gonadotropin (HCG) has been used by some clinicians in treating obesity. Several controlled clinical studies have indicated that HCG is no more effective than a placebo injection in weight reduction (58–64). One investigation supports the effectiveness of HCG (65); however, this study had a high dropout rate and uncertain control subjects (66). There appears to be no rationale in claims that HCG contributes to weight reduction regimens by influencing fat distribution, inducing a sense of well-being, or preventing hunger and fatigue in persons on a reducing diet. The Food and Drug Administration has required the following addition to the indications in all HCG labeling (66):

> HCG has not been demonstrated to be effective adjunctive therapy in the treatment of obesity. There is no substantial evidence that it increases weight loss beyond that resulting from caloric restriction, that it causes a more attractive or "normal" distribution of fat or that it decreases the hunger and discomfort associated with calorie-restricted diets.

Phenylpropanolamine

Phenylpropanolamine is a sympathomimetic agent related chemically and pharmacologically to ephedrine and amphetamine. It acts as an indirect sympathomimetic, exerting more prominent peripheral adrenergic effects compared with weak central stimulant actions (67). In the past, controversy has existed as to phenylpropanolamine's effectiveness as an anorexigenic agent (68). Early animal studies indicated its usefulness in diminishing food intake in animals (69, 70). Later clinical studies indicated a possible appetite-suppressant activity. Results from one double-blind study indicated that phenylpropanolamine (25 mg), taken 30 minutes before lunch, reduced intake of a liquid diet (71). In another double-blind study, subjects who received the same dosage reported a significant reduction in their consumption of dinner and snacks (72). A double-blind clinical evaluation of a phenylpropanolamine/caffeine/vitamin combination compared with a placebo and diet showed a significantly greater weight loss over a 4-week period in patients on a 1,200-cal diet who received the same combination product (73).

All authorities, however, do not agree on the effectiveness of phenylpropanolamine as an anorexigenic agent. The *AMA Drug Evaluations* (74) states that weight control products containing phenylpropanolamine are "only minimally effective." A basic pharmacology textbook states that the drug is ineffective as an appetite suppressant (75). In addition, no mention of its use in obesity is made in a standard pharmacy reference (67).

In 1978, the FDA advisory review panel on nonprescription miscellaneous internal drug products found phenylpropanolamine to be generally safe and effective for short-term weight control (76). The use of the drug in long-term weight control was not supported by an independent panel (77).

Although the effects of phenylpropanolamine on the cardiovascular system and CNS are not as potent as those of amphetamine, side effects may occur, particularly if the recommended dosage is exceeded. Nervousness, restlessness, insomnia, headache, nausea, and excessive increase in blood pressure are some of phenylpropanolamine's adverse effects (67). Evidence suggests that the drug may reduce vitamin A levels in experimental animals (82). Early reports indicate adverse reactions, including those affecting the cardiovascular system (78–83).

Hypertensive reactions in previously normotensive individuals have been reported with single oral doses of 85 mg of phenylpropanolamine in the free form (84, 85). In another instance, the same dosage form of phenylpropanolamine, taken with indomethacin, induced a severe hypertensive episode (86, 87). Cerebral hemorrhage has been described in a single case report (88). A double-blind study in young normotensive adults revealed that significant elevations in blood pressure may occur after a single dose of phenylpropanolamine (89). It has been suggested that hypertensive effects are more likely to occur when phenylpropanolamine is in the free form råther than in a sustained-release preparation (90).

Central nervous system stimulation as evidenced by convulsive seizures has been noted (91). Psychotic reactions have been described with phenylpropanolamine 50 mg (in combination with isopropamide and phenyltoloxamine) (92). Mental disturbances have been described in considerable detail and it is evident that the possibility of psychotic episodes exists (93). "Amphetamine-like reactions" to phenylpropanolamine have been reported. Seven cases were reported from emergency room records over a 6-month period. All adverse effects occurred within 1–2 hours after ingestion of a single dose of either phenylpropanolamine alone or phenylpropanolamine in combination with caffeine. These effects included respiratory stimulation, tremor, restlessness, increased motor activity, agitation, and hallucinations (94). Pharmacists can warn patients of the possible CNS effects of phenylpropanolamine. According to some clinicians, phenylpropanolamine "poses a danger to the public" and should be regarded as a drug with potential for abuse (95).

Many phenylpropanolamine products also contain caffeine, which may produce side effects such as nervousness, irritability, and anxiety. Such a combination appears to have an increased propensity to induce CNS stimulation. One study has revealed a relative lack of side effects from orally administered phenylpropanol-amine and phenylpropanolamine with caffeine (96).

Although the FDA advisory review panel on nonprescription cold, cough, allergy, bronchodilator, and antiasthmatic drug products did not review anorectics as such, it concluded that nervousness, insomnia, motor restlessness, and nausea may occur with phenylpropanolamine doses of 50 mg every 3 hours (97). However, these same side effects can occur almost as often with a placebo. The panel also concluded that at oral therapeutic doses the incidence of side effects with phenylpropanolamine is low (98). The use of weight control products in children without the expressed advice or directions of a physician is not rational.

Because phenylpropanolamine is an adrenergic substance, it may elevate blood glucose levels and produce cardiac stimulation. For these reasons, the labels on products containing that agent warn that individuals with diabetes mellitus, heart disease, hypertension, or thyroid disease should seek medical advice before taking this drug.

Phenylpropanolamine has been implicated in "drug-drug" interactions with monoamine oxidase inhibitors (99–101). Severe hypertensive episodes may be more likely when preparations containing phenylpropanolamine in a free form, rather than in a sustained-release form, are ingested by patients already taking monoamine oxidase inhibitors (100, 101).

One report described a subject who had various adverse effects when phenylpropanolamine was ingested concurrently with aspirin and acetaminophen over a 3-week period. These adverse effects included nausea, vomiting, headaches, weakness, malaise, and severe muscle tenderness. Subsequently, brown-colored urine was noted and a percutaneous renal biopsy revealed acute interstitial nephritis (102). A case of fatal ventricular arrhythmia induced by thioridazine was thought to be initiated by phenylpropanolamine administration (103). Severe hypertension has been reported when phenylpropanolamine was taken with methyldopa or oxyprenolol (a beta-blocker similar to propranolol, which is investigational in the United States) (104). There is one report of a positive phentolamine test for pheochromocytoma in hypertension induced by phenylpropanolamine (105). Some nonprescription products contain caffeine and phenylpropanolamine; the possibility of an additive effect with these two cardiac stimulants should be considered (80).

A review of phenylpropanolamine use in short-term weight control reflects the present status of this drug as a nonprescription weight control product (106).

Benzocaine

Benzocaine was first incorporated into a weight-control preparation in 1958 (107). A preparation containing benzocaine and methylcellulose in chewing gum wafers was tried for 10 weeks in 50 patients who were 5.5–46 kg overweight. The patients were instructed to chew one or two wafers, followed by a glass of water, just prior to meals. In addition, they were placed on low-calorie diets and were directed to chew the gum every 4 hours if there was a strong desire to eat. Results showed that 90% of the subjects lost weight. However, the study did not use a placebo control group, and the weight loss could have been caused by benzocaine, methylcellulose, or the diet alone. The benzocaine dose was small, and any marked degree of numbness in the oral cavity was questionable. It is conceivable that subtle effects on taste sensitivity or taste modification may occur, and perceived analgesia or numbness is not necessary for possible appetite suppressant activity. Obese persons may be more sensitive to taste stimuli (37).

Constant snacking is characteristic of the "oral syndrome" in many obese persons. A nontraditional appetite-control plan using benzocaine, glucose, caffeine, and vitamins in a hard candy form was tried (108). The subjects ingested the candies when they wanted a snack and before and after meals. The purpose of this approach was to keep the patients orally active and at the same time elevate their blood glucose levels. The influence of benzocaine was considered to be an essential component of the significant weight reduction in the study group.

Capsules or tablets containing benzocaine are designed to be swallowed, and hence the drug does not come into contact with the oral cavity. Any appetite suppression would depend on an effect on the GI mucosa. However, there are no conclusive clinical data to support such an activity. The FDA advisory review panel on nonprescription miscellaneous internal drug products classified benzocaine as generally effective for short-term weight control (76). Its use in long-term weight control was not deemed appropriate by an independent panel (77).

Although they are rare, cyanotic reactions have been reported following benzocaine administration (109). Methemoglobinemia in infants also has been reported (110–113). These reactions refer primarily to infants and therefore are not specifically relevant to the drug's use in the noninfant obese population. It is important, however, to be aware of potential benzocaine toxicity. A fatal anaphylactic reaction occurred in an adult a few minutes after the ingestion of a throat lozenge containing benzocaine (114). Obese persons taking preparations containing benzocaine over long periods may expose themselves to the consequences of drug-induced hypersensitivity.

Bulk Producers

Typical examples of bulk producers are methylcellulose, carboxymethyl cellulose, psyllium hydrophilic mucilloid, agar, and karaya gum. Bulk-producing laxatives are a common source of these agents. It has been suggested that the bulk-producing activity produces a sense of fullness, reducing the desire to eat. The efficacy of the bulk-forming agents as appetite suppressants in controlling obesity has not been established (115). A radiographic study shows that a methylcellulose mass is almost entirely eliminated from the stomach in 30 minutes. In addition, intestinal peristalsis is actually accelerated by methylcellulose, as evidenced by the fact that most of the methylcellulose mass reaches the ileum in only 30 minutes (116). Therefore, neither bulk production by methylcellulose nor an increase in the rate of gastric transport offers a mechanism to produce satiety.

No experimental evidence exists to support an appetite-suppressant claim. However, bulk-producing substances have been approved for dietary use by the FDA (117).

It is assumed that the benefit of bulk producers in obesity control is related to caloric intake reduction, irrespective of the ingestion of the bulk producer. Bulk producers probably are no more effective than a low-calorie, high-residue diet in a weight reduction program. Moreover, their laxative effect may not always be desirable. Because of the danger of esophageal obstruction with methylcellulose wafers, generous amounts of fluid should accompany ingestion of bulk producers (115). Agents with anticholinergic properties reduce bowel motility. Concurrent use of these agents with bulk producers may be hazardous, because they may produce intestinal obstruction.

Other Products

Vitamins and minerals are present in some nonprescription weight control products. If a dieting patient is not receiving sufficient quantities of vitamins and minerals in the diet regimen chosen, then this addition is warranted. However, in a well-balanced, low-calorie diet, recommended daily allowances for vitamins and minerals are present.

Alginic acid, sodium bicarbonate, and carboxymethyl cellulose are found in some nonprescription products. The carbon dioxide evolved from the sodium bicarbonate combines with the alginic acid and a foamy methylcellulose mass is formed (115). This bulk is purported to relieve the feeling of "emptiness" in the stomach. The alleged properties of grapefruit extract in accelerating fat metabolism have not been substantiated.

Dietary aids such as carbohydrate "candy" type foods and low-calorie nutritionally balanced liquids are not considered drugs but are available as adjuncts in a weight reduction program. In addition, synthetic sweeteners such as saccharin may be valuable in reducing excessive sugar consumption and thus lowering caloric intake.

Caffeine is often included in products marketed as nonprescription weight-control products. Caffeine is a CNS stimulant and may allay fatigue of a dieting individual with a markedly reduced caloric intake (106). It should be recalled that phenylpropanolamine also has the capacity to produce CNS stimulation and combination products of phenylpropanolamine and caffeine are commonly used (118). Caffeine does not possess appetite suppressant properties.

Glucose

Preparations containing glucose and vitamins are claimed to elevate blood glucose levels when taken before meals or at snack time, so that the satiety center exerts an inhibitory influence on the appetite center. This assertion, however, is questionable. A clinical study reported that a glucose load (50 g) taken 20 minutes before lunch suppressed caloric intake relative to control load at lunch ($p < 0.01$) (119). Reactions to a glucose load's oral qualities may constitute the principal factor in the first 20 minutes rather than GI or post-absorptive effects on satiety. However, the efficacy of glucose in long-term weight control programs has not been established.

Low-Calorie Balanced Foods

The "canned diet" products are considered substitutes for the usual diet. One product typical of this group supplies 70 g of protein/day, an amount the manufacturer states "is the recommended daily dietary allowance of protein for normal adults." It also contains 20 g of fat and 110 g of carbohydrate in a daily ration for a total daily calorie intake of 900 calories. Powder, granule, and liquid forms are available, and these products are also formulated as cookies and soups.

These dietary foods are low in sodium. Weight loss in the first 2 weeks is probably caused, in part, by water loss from the tissues. It is questionable whether a weight loss over a short period is significant with regard to the effective long-term treatment of obesity.

The pharmacist should be aware that products that substitute 900 cal/day for the usual diet are usually effective in reducing weight. Moreover, it appears that any diet of 900 cal that supplies adequate protein and lower carbohydrate and fat intake should enable an obese patient to lose weight.

Artificial Sweeteners

Sucrose overuse is common. A sucrose substitute, saccharin, provides no calories and may allow significant calorie reduction in certain patients. Saccharin is about 400 times more potent than sucrose as a sweetener. It produces a bitter taste in some individuals, and it is not heat stable; nevertheless, it is the most popular artificial sweetener, especially since the prohibition of nonregulated use of cyclamates. Saccharin may have considerable importance in reducing caloric intake in some individuals. For instance, if saccharin is used to sweeten a cup of coffee instead of one heaping teaspoonful of sugar, 33 calories are removed from the diet.

In 1972, bladder tumors were discovered in rats fed saccharin in utero and throughout life. The FDA then removed saccharin from the list of food additives generally recognized as safe. Saccharin is presently permitted in products labeled specifically as diet foods or beverages. It may accumulate in fetal tissues and should therefore not be used during pregnancy (120). As of June 1, 1978, pharmacies carrying saccharin-containing products are required to display posters containing the following warning statement (121):

SACCHARIN NOTICE This store sells food including diet beverages that contain saccharin. You will find saccharin listed in the ingredient statements on most foods which contain it. All foods that contain saccharin will soon bear the following warning: Use of this product may be hazardous to your health. This product contains saccharin, which has been determined to cause cancer in laboratory animals. This store is required by law to display this notice prominently.

Human epidemiologic studies have not revealed a clearcut relationship between saccharin consumption and urinary bladder carcinoma (122). One study reported a positive relationship (123) but it has been criticized for deficiencies in design and analysis (124).

Aspartame is a synthetic dipeptide about 180 times as sweet as sugar. The FDA has determined that aspartame has been shown to be safe as a food additive. Products containing aspartame are required to carry the warning: "Phenylketonurics: Contains Phenylalanine." Since phenylalanine is contained in aspartame, individuals with phenylketonuria or patients who should avoid protein foods must be alerted to this fact. In addition, directions not to use aspartame in cooking or baking (the compound loses its sweetness) are required on "table products" of aspartame (125).

Fructose, sorbitol, or xylitol may be employed as alternates to saccharin. These sweeteners contain calories and should not be viewed as being a "sugar-free" diet item. Fructose and xylitol are sweeter than sucrose, and xylitol is less calorigenic and more expensive (126). Apparently, neither sorbitol nor xylitol cause tooth decay and some products containing xylitol have a more pleasant taste (127). However, some evidence implicates xylitol in the development of urinary tract abnormalities, kidney stones, and tumors in laboratory animals (128). Further tests are under way to evaluate this possibility. The ingestion of sufficient amounts of dietetic candies containing sorbitol may result in an osmotic catharsis in small children (129).

There are several naturally occurring compounds that show promise as sucrose substitutes (130). Monellin, thaumatin, and miraculin are proteins from plant sources presently being investigated as possible sucrose substitutes.

Dosage Forms

Nonprescription products for obesity control are available as liquids, powders, granules, tablets, capsules, sustained-release capsules, wafers, cookies, soups, chewing gum, and candy preparations. If candy cubes, wafers, or chewing gum are substituted for high-calorie desserts or "snacks," the candy-like nature of the dosage form may offer patients a psychological aid that is not found when a standard tablet or capsule is used. Ingesting large quantities of diet candy would, of course, contribute significantly to caloric intake.

Adjunctive Therapy

The only real therapy for most cases of obesity is diet alone or in conjunction with other therapeutic measures. The pharmacist should make sure that any diet is being followed under a physician's supervision. Patients having difficulty in losing weight may find reinforcement in self-help groups and behavior modification.

Diet

High-protein, low-carbohydrate diets in the 800–1,000 cal/day range are used frequently in weight reduction programs. Total fasting or semistarvation sometimes is proposed as a means of weight reduction in grossly obese persons (131, 132). Starvation, either total or partial, depletes the body of lean tissue and essential electrolytes in addition to fat (133). The ketosis and ketoacidosis resulting from a fasting state reflect a metabolic alteration. If total fasting is employed as a means of treating obesity, hospitalization is recommended to deal effectively with mood changes or alterations in physiologic functions such as cardiac arrhythmias (134). "Crash" diets involving 500 cal/day for 4–8 weeks have been implicated in the loss of scalp hair (135). This effect apparently reflects the trauma attributed to semistarvation.

Low-carbohydrate diets have been advocated on the basis that an individual may eat as much as he or she desires as long as no carbohydrates are ingested. Fat from food may be deposited as fat in the body, and proteins may be converted to fat. The excess fat metabolized may result in an increased production of ketones to the degree that ketosis, acidosis, and dehydration may occur. Some diets recommend inclusion of large quantities of fat in the diet (1, 136). Although a high-fat diet may suppress fat synthesis it doesn't prevent fat disposition. An additional problem encountered in these diets is the elevation of blood cholesterol.

A carbohydrate-free, high-fat diet does cause an immediate weight reduction due to water loss (dehydration) but it does not affect adiposity. The "drinking man's diet" adds alcohol to this regimen, which tends to add more calories and the increased liability of fat deposition. A high-meat (protein-fat), no-carbohydrate diet presents an extra burden to the kidney due to the resultant increased urea load. In addition, an increase in the uric acid levels in this diet may precipitate gouty arthritis in susceptible persons. A low-protein, low-fat "rice" diet was advocated several years ago. This unbalanced diet could lead to ill health (136).

A diet containing kelp, vinegar, lechithin, and vitamin B_6 has been proposed. Excess kelp, which contains high amounts of iodine, may decrease thyroid function by negative feedback mechanisms. The other ingredients in this diet do not have any established value in weight reduction. The weight loss in this diet is due to the low caloric intake, rather than the use of these specific additives.

The extent of injuries and deaths due to the use of extremely low-calorie protein diets is unclear. However, it is apparent that studies oriented toward geographic incidence, concurrent pathology, age, and other factors need careful scrutiny. The complaints reported to the FDA frequently include nausea, vomiting, diarrhea (liquid preparations), constipation (dry preparations), faintness, muscle cramps, weakness or fatigue, irritability, cold intolerance, decreased libido, amenorrhea, hair loss, dry skin, cardiac arrhythmias, recurrence of gout, dehydration, and hypokalemia (137).

The possibility of "drug-food" interactions with low-calorie protein diets exists. Patients taking prescription medicines such as diuretics, antihypertensives, hypoglycemic agents, insulin, adrenergics, high doses of corticosteriods, thyroid preparations other than those used in replacement therapy, and lithium therapy should not use the liquid protein diet.

The pharmacist should warn the patient not to undertake this type of diet approach without proper medical supervision. The patient's age also should be taken into consideration, since elderly obese persons may be more susceptible to cardiovascular stress and gout, usually prevalent in this age group.

A balanced diet containing not less than 12–14% of protein, no more than 30% fat (unsaturated preferred), and the remainder carbohydrate (low sucrose) is preferable to unbalanced diets of questionable value and potential by dangerous effects (1).

Group Therapy

Group therapy and behavior modification are effective in treating obesity. Groups such as TOPS (Take Off Pounds Sensibly) and Weight Watchers have been successful in the treatment of obesity (138). The group pressure resulting from praise or criticism apparently is an effective deterrent to overeating for many persons. Behavior modification involving eating considered as a "pure" activity (not combined with any other activity), as well as eating more slowly, may be beneficial. In addition, keeping a "diet diary" and using a "unit dose" concept for food may prove helpful in a weight reduction program. Psychotherapeutic approaches also show promise in obesity control (139).

Surgical Intervention

In refractory cases of gross obesity, intestinal bypass operations have been performed (140). This type of procedure is probably the most hazardous measure used to treat extreme obesity and has led to alternative, perhaps safer procedures such as gastric partitioning to control morbid obesity (141).

Product Selection Guidelines

In recommending a nonprescription product for weight control, the pharmacist should stress the importance of a diet plan and/or exercise program. Weight cannot be reduced without a concerted effort to change one's eating and exercise habits and to maintain the new habits. In light of the pharmacist's role in total health care, emphasis should be placed on alternate means of obesity control. The pharmacist should inquire about previous diet control regimens the patient has attempted so that other nonprescription diet management programs may be recommended. The pharmacist may also participate in monitoring the patient's weight-reduction efforts.

As a health care professional, the pharmacist should emphasize the importance of a rational, low-calorie, balanced diet and proper exercise to correct caloric imbalance, as well as the importance of individual effort in maintaining a diet management program. The patient may be referred to a reinforcing group.

The patient should appreciate the caloric value of various food types. A nonprescription obesity control product should be considered only as an adjunct to a planned weight reduction program. Vitamins sometimes are added to such products on the assumption that dieting individuals may not have an adequate vitamin intake. This practice may be justified in individual cases but cannot be applied to all patients. Caffeine is included in some preparations, probably in an effort to allay fatigue, a contributing factor that may lead to an impulsive desire to eat.

Summary

The effectiveness of a weight reduction program depends largely on the patient's education and the acceptance of a regimen necessary to achieve long-term weight control. A patient should recognize the many facets of a successful weight reduction program, including motivation, physical activity, reduced caloric intake, and possibly a pharmacologic "crutch" such as a nonprescription product. The role of the pharmacist as a qualified health professional is to supply pertinent and accurate information regarding these matters.

References

1. R. S. Goodhart and M. E. Shils, "Modern Nutrition in Health and Disease," Lea and Febiger, Philadelphia, Pa., 1980, pp. 721, 736.
2. A. Angel, *Can. Med. Assoc. J., 110,* 540 (1974).
3. C. C. Seltzer, J. Goldman, and J. Mayer, *Pediatrics, 36,* 212 (1965).
4. M. G. Wohl, "Modern Nutrition in Health and Disease," Lea and Febiger, Philadelphia, Pa., 1960, p. 532.
5. U. S. Public Health Service, "Obesity and Health: A Sourcebook of Current Information for Professional Health Personnel," Publ. No. 1485, Washington, D.C., 1966.
6. M. G. Wagner, *J. Am. Diet. Assoc., 57,* 311 (1970).
7. J. Mayer, *Annu. Rev. Med., 14,* 111 (1963).
8. D. J. Galton, *Br. Med. J., 2,* 1498 (1966).
9. P. B. Curtis-Prior, *Lancet, 1,* 897 (1975).
10. D. S. Miller, P. Mumford, and M. J. Stock, *Am. J. Clin. Nutr., 20,* 1223 (1967).
11. R. E. Smith and B. A. Horowitz, *Physiol. Rev., 49,* 330 (1969).
12. M. de Luise, G. Blackburn, and J. Filer, *N. Engl. J. Med., 303,* 1017 (1980).
13. D. Margules, *Psychology Today,* Oct., 136 (1979).
14. K. Adam, *Br. Med. J., 2,* 234 (1977).
15. A. H. Crisp, E. Stonehill, and G. W. Fenton, *Psychother. Psychosom., 22,* 159 (1973).
16. J. H. Lacey, A. H. Crisp, and R. S. Kalucy, *Br. Med. J., 4,* 556 (1975).
17. J. Hirsch and J. I. Knittle, *Fed. Proc., 29,* 1516 (1970).
18. L. B. Salans, S. W. Cushman, and R. E. Weisman, *J. Clin. Invest., 52,* 929 (1973).
19. S. R. Williams, "Nutrition and Diet Therapy," C. V. Mosby, St. Louis, Mo., 1967, p. 477.
20. J. Mayer, *Bull. N. Y. Acad. Med., 36,* 323 (1960).
21. K. J. Carpenter and J. Mayer, *Am. J. Physiol., 193,* 449 (1958).
22. N. B. Marshall, S. B. Andrus, and J. Mayer, *Am. J. Physiol., 189,* 342 (1957).
23. C. C. Seltzer and J. Mayer, *J. Am. Med. Assoc., 189,* 677 (1964).
24. C. C. Seltzer and J. Mayer, *J. Am. Diet. Assoc., 55,* 454 (1969).
25. M. E. Moore, A. Stunkard, and L. Srole, *J. Am. Med. Assoc., 181,* 962 (1962).
26. A. Stunkard, E. d'Aquili, S. Fox, and R. D. L. Filion, *J. Am. Med. Assoc., 221,* 579 (1972).
27. P. B. Goldblatt, M. E. Moore, and A. J. Stunkard, *J. Am. Med. Assoc., 192,* 1039 (1965).
28. "Drugs of Choice 1980–81," W. Modell, Ed., C. V. Mosby, St. Louis, Mo., 1980, p. 296.
29. A. Stunkard, *Psychosom. Med., 20,* 366 (1958).
30. A. Stunkard and M. Mendelson, *J. Am. Diet. Assoc., 38,* 328 (1961).
31. A. W. Hetherington and S. W. Ransom, *Am. J. Physiol., 136,* 609 (1942).
32. J. Mayer, *Ann. N. Y. Acad. Sci., 63,* 15 (1955).
33. V. Vngorstedt, *Acta Physion. Scand. Suppl., 365,* 1 (1971).
34. J. E. Ahlskog and B. G. Hoebel, *Science, 182,* 166 (1973).
35. R. M. Gold, *Science, 182,* 488 (1973).
36. B. G. Hoebel, *Annu. Rev. Physiol., 33,* 533 (1971).
37. H. P. Ziegler, *Psychology Today,* Aug., 62 (1975).
38. H. H. Marks, *Metabolism, 6,* 417 (1957).
39. G. V. Mann, *N. Engl. J. Med., 291,* 226 (1974).
40. J. Stamler, "The Hypertension Handbook," Merck Sharp & Dohme, West Point, Pa., 1974, p. 15.
41. S. L. Wilens, *Arch. Intern. Med., 79,* 120 (1947).
42. S. Heyden, C. G. Hames, A. Bartel, J. C. Cassal, H. A. Tyroler, and J. C. Coroni, *Arch. Intern. Med., 128,* 956 (1971).
43. G. F. Baker, "Clinic and Metropolitan Life Insurance Co.: Diabetes in the 1940's," New York Metropolitan Life Insurance Co. Press, 1940.
44. S. M. Genuth, *Ann. Intern. Med., 79,* 812 (1973).
45. A. Z. El-Khodary, M. F. Ball, I. M. Oweiss, and J. J. Canary, *Metabolism, 21,* 641 (1972).
46. J. H. Karam, G. M. Grodsky, F. C. Pavlatos, and P. H. Forsham, *Lancet, 1,* 286 (1965).
47. R. S. Yalow, S. M. Glick, and J. Roth, *Ann. N. Y. Acad. Sci., 131,* 357 (1965).
48. "The Merck Manual," 13th ed., Merck and Co., Inc., Rahway, N. J., 1977, p. 1180.
49. "Muir's Textbook of Pathology," 9th ed., D. F. Cappell and J. R. Anderson, Eds., Edward Arnold Ltd., London, England, 1971, p. 587.
50. H. Julkunen, O. P. Heinonen, and K. Pyorala, *Ann. Rheum. Dis., 30,* 605 (1971).
51. R. H. L. Wilson and N. L. Wilson, *J. Am. Diet. Assoc., 55,* 465 (1969).
52. C. S. Burwell, E. D. Robin, R. D. Whaley, and A. G. Bickelmann, *Am. J. Med., 21,* 811 (1956).
53. A. M. Mousa, M. M. Solimon, and M. R. I. Hamza, *J. Egypt. Public Health Assoc., 52,* 65 (1977).
54. J. Woodsworth, "Diet Revolution," St. Martin's Press, New York, N.Y., 1977, p. 66.
55. *FDA Drug Bulletin* (December 1972).
56. S. Cole, *Psychol. Bull., 79,* 13 (1973).
57. W. C. Bowman, M. J. Rand, and G. B. West, "Textbook of Pharmacology," Blackwell, Oxford, England, 1968, p. 332.
58. L. S. Craig, R. E. Ray, S. H. Waxler, and H. Madigan, *Am. J. Clin. Nutr., 12,* 230 (1963).
59. S. Carne, *Lancet, 2,* 1282 (1961).
60. E. Sohar, *Am. J. Clin. Nutr., 7,* 514 (1959).
61. B. W. Frank, *Am. J. Clin. Nutr., 14,* 133 (1964).
62. J. M. Harris and E. Warsaw, *J. Am. Ger. Soc., 12,* 987 (1964).
63. B. Hastrup, B. Nielson, A. P. Skouby, *Acta Med. Scand., 168* (fasc. 1) 25 (1960).
64. P. Lebon, *J. Am. Ger. Soc., 14* (2), 116 (1966).
65. W. L. Asher and H. W. Harper, *Am. J. Clin. Nutr., 26,* 211 (1973).
66. *FDA Drug Bulletin, 5* (April–June, 1975).
67. "Remington's Pharmaceutical Sciences," 16th ed., A. Osol, Ed., Mack, Easton, Pa., 1975, p. 830.
68. H. I. Silverman, *Am. J. Pharm., 135,* 45 (1963).
69. M. L. Tainter, *J. Nutr., 27,* 89 (1944).
70. A. Epstein, *Comp. Physiol. Psychol., 52,* 37 (1959).
71. B. G. Hoebel, J. Cooper, M. Kamin, and D. Willard, *Obesity Bariatr. Med., 4,* 192 (1975).
72. B. G. Hoebel, J. Krauss, J. Cooper, and D. Willard, *Obesity Bariatr. Med., 4,* 200 (1975).
73. S. I. Griboff, R. Berman, and H. I. Silverman, *Curr. Ther. Res., 17,* 535 (1975).
74. "AMA Drug Evaluations," 4th ed., American Medical Association, Chicago, Ill., 1980, p. 937.
75. A. Goth, "Medical Pharmacology," 7th ed., Mosby, St. Louis, Mo., 1974, p. 110.
76. *Medical Letter on Drugs and Therapeutics, 21,* 65 (August 10, 1979).
77. P. R. Salmon, *Br. Med. J., 1,* 193 (1965).
78. "Summary Minutes of the FDA OTC Miscellaneous Drug Products Panel," Chevy Chase, Md., August 4–6, 1978.
79. S. R. Shapiro, *N. Engl. J. Med., 280,* 1363 (1969).
80. R. B. Peterson and L. A. Vasquez, *J. Am. Med. Assoc., 223,* 324 (1973).
81. S. Ostern and W. H. Dodson, *J. Am. Med. Assoc., 194,* 472 (1965).
82. P. B. Acosta and P. J. Garry, *Fed. Proc., 37,* 485 (1978).
83. P. H. Livingston, *J. Am. Med. Assoc., 196,* 1159 (1966).

84. D. B. Frewin, P. P. Leonello, and M. E. Frewin, *Med. J. Aust., 2,* 479 (1979).
85. J. D. Horowitz, J. J. McNeil, B. Sweet, F. A. O. Mendelsohn, and W. J. Louis, *Med. J. Aust., 1,* 175 (1979).
86. K. Y. Lee, L. J. Beilin, and R. VanDongen, *Lancet, 1,* 1110 (1979).
87. K. Y. Lee, L. J. Beilin, and R. VanDongen, *Med. J. Aust., 1,* 525 (1979).
88. J. King, *Med. J. Aust., 2,* 258 (1979).
89. J. D. Horowitz, L. G. Howes, N. Christophidis, W. J. Lang, M. R. Fennessy, and M. J. Rand, *Lancet, 1,* 367 (1980).
90. M. F. Cuthbert, *Lancet, 1,* 367 (1980).
91. P. D. Deocampo, *Med. Soc. N.J., 76,* 591 (1979).
92. F. J. Kane and B. Q. Green, *Am. J. Psychiat., 123,* 484 (1966).
93. G. Norvenius, E. Widerlov, and G. Lonnerholm, *Lancet, 2,* 1367 (1979).
94. A. J. Dietz, *J. Am. Med. Assoc. 245,* 601 (1981).
95. A. Blum, Editorial, *J. Am. Med. Assoc., 245,* 1347 (1981).
96. H. I. Silverman, *Curr. Ther. Res., 28,* 185 (1980).
97. "Summary Minutes of the FDA OTC Panel on Cold, Cough, Allergy, Bronchodilator, and Antiasthmatic Drug Products," Washington, D.C., June 19–20, 1973.
98. *Federal Register, 42,* 56756 (1977).
99. C. M. Tonks and A. T. Lloyd, *Br. Med. J., 1,* 589 (1965).
100. A. M. S. Mason and R. M. Buckle, *Br. Med. J., 1,* 875 (1969).
101. M. F. Cuthbert, M. P. Greenberg, and S. W. Morley, *Br. Med. J., 1,* 404 (1969).
102. W. M. Bennett, *Lancet, 2,* 42 (1979).
103. G. Chouinard, A. M. Ghadirian, and B. D. Jones, *Can. Med. Assoc. J., 119,* 729 (1978).
104. E. H. McLaren, *Br. Med. J., 2,* 283 (1976).
105. F. C. Duvernoy, *N. Engl. J. Med., 280,* 877 (1969).
106. G. D. Appelt, *Colo. J. Pharm., 24,* 35 (1981).
107. M. Plotz, *Med. Times, 86,* 860 (1958).
108. C. W. McLure and C. A. Brusch, *J. Am. Med. Women's Assoc., 28,* 239 (1973).
109. B. M. Bernstein, *Rev. Gastroenterol., 17,* 123 (1950).
110. H. deC. Peterson, *N. Engl. J. Med., 263,* 454 (1960).
111. N. Goluboff and D. J. MacFadyen, *J. Pediatr., 47,* 22 (1955).
112. J. A. Wolff, *Pediatrics, 20,* 915 (1957).
113. N. Goluboff, *Pediatrics, 21,* 340 (1958).
114. D. J. Hesch, *J. Am. Med. Assoc., 172,* 62 (1960).
115. "The Pharmacological Basis of Therapeutics," 6th ed., A. G. Gilman, L. S. Goodman, and A. Gilman, Eds., Macmillan, New York, N. Y., 1980, p. 1004, 995.
116. E. J. Drenick, *J. Am. Med. Assoc., 234,* 271 (1975).
117. D. C. Fletcher, *J. Am. Med. Assoc., 230,* 901 (1974).
118. *American Druggist, 52* (Sept. 1980).
119. D. A. Booth, A. I. Campbell, and A. Chase, *Nature, 228,* 1104 (1970).
120. *Medical Letter on Drugs and Therapeutics, 17,* 61 (1975).
121. *Federal Register, 43,* 8793 (1978).
122. R. K. Kalkhoff and M. E. Levin, *Diabetes Care, 1,* 211 (1978).
123. G. R. Howe, J. D. Burch, A. B. Miller, B. Morrison, P. Gordon, L. Weldon, L. W. Chambers, G. Fodor, and G. M. Winsor, *Lancet, 2,* 578 (1977).
124. Editorial, *Lancet, 2,* 592 (1977).
125. *Federal Register, 46* (142), 38284 (1981).
126. J. D. Brunzell, *Diabetes Care, 1,* 223 (1978).
127. W. H. Bowen, *Pharmacy Times, 43,* 25 (January 1977).
128. *Apharmacy Weekly, 16,* 49 (1977).
129. J. R. Gryboski, *N. Engl. J. Med., 275,* 718 (1966).
130. G. D. Appelt, *Colo. J. Pharm., 22,* 50 (1979).
131. W. L. Bloom, *Metabolism , 8,* 214 (1959).
132. S. M. Genuth, J. H. Castro, and V. Vertes, *J. Am. Med. Assoc., 230,* 987 (1974).
133. R. E. Bolinger, B. P. Lukert, R. W. Brown, L. Guevara, and R. Steinberg, *Arch. Intern. Med., 118,* 3 (1966).
134. I. C. Gilliand, *Postgrad. Med. J., 44,* 58 (1968).
135. R. B. Odum and D. K. Goette, *J. Am. Med. Assoc., 235,* 476 (1976).
136. F. Netter, "Fad Diets Can Be Deadly," Exposition Press, Hicksville, N. Y., 1975, pp. 98–103.
137. *FDA Drug Bulletin* (Jan./Feb. 1978).
138. A. Stunkard, H. Levine, and S. Fox, *Arch. Intern. Med., 125,* 1067 (1970).
139. A. Stunkard, *Arch. Gen. Psychiatry, 26,* 391 (1972).
140. H. F. Conn, "Current Therapy," W. B. Saunders, Philadelphia, Pa., 1975, p. 406.
141. W. G. Pace, *Ann. Surg., 190,* 392–400 (1979).

Appetite Suppressant Product Table

Product (Manufacturer)	Phenylpropanolamine Hydrochloride	Bulk Producer	Other Ingredients
Anorexin Capsules (Thompson Medical)	25 mg		caffeine, 100 mg; vitamin A, 1,667 IU; vitamin D, 133 IU; thiamine, 1 mg; riboflavin, 1 mg; pyridoxine HCl, 0.33 mg; cyanocobalamin, 0.33 μg; ascorbic acid, 20 mg; niacinamide, 7 mg; calcium pantothenate, 0.33 mg
Appedrine Tablets (Thompson Medical)	25 mg		caffeine, 100 mg; vitamin A, 1,667 IU; vitamin D, 133 IU; thiamine, 1 mg; riboflavin, 1 mg; pyridoxine HCl, 0.33 mg; cyanocobalamin, 0.33 μg; ascorbic acid, 20 mg; niacinamide, 7 mg; calcium pantothenate, 0.33 mg
Appress (North American)	25 mg		caffeine, 100 mg
Ayd's AM/PM (Jeffrey Martin)	50 mg (AM) 25 mg (PM)		caffeine, 200 mg (AM)
Ayd's Extra Strength (Jeffrey Martin)	75 mg		caffeine, 200 mg
Caffeine Free Extra Strength Dexatrim (Thompson Medical)	75 mg		
Caltrim Diet Plan Capsules (Commerce)		carboxymethyl cellulose sodium, 500 mg	benzocaine, 9 mg; vitamin A, 4,000 IU; vitamin D, 400 IU; thiamine, HCl, 1 mg; riboflavin, 1.2 mg; ascorbic acid, 30 mg; niacinamide, 10 mg; iron, 10 mg; calcium, 87 mg; phosphorus, 45 mg
Caltrim Reducing Plan Tablets (Commerce)	25 mg	carboxymethyl cellulose sodium, 25 mg	caffeine, 100 mg; ascorbic acid, 20 mg; niacinamide, 7 mg; vitamin A, 3.68 mg; tartaric acid, 2 mg; thiamine HCl, 1mg; riboflavin, 1 mg; vitamin D, 0.344 mg; pyridoxine HCl, 0.344 mg; *d*-calcium pantothenate, 0.344 mg; vitamin B_{12}, 0.344 μg
Cenadex (Central)	75 mg		caffeine, 200 mg
Coffee, Tea & A New Me (Thompson Medical)	25 mg		
Control (Thompson Medical)	75 mg		
Dex-A-Diet II (O'Connor)	75 mg		caffeine, 200 mg
Dex-A-Diet Lite (O'Connor)	75 mg		
Dexatrim Capsules (Thompson Medical)	50 mg		caffeine, 200 mg
Diadax Capsules (O'Connor)	50 mg		

Appetite Suppressant Product Table, continued

Product (Manufacturer)	Phenylpropanolamine Hydrochloride	Bulk Producer	Other Ingredients
Diadax Tablets (O'Connor)	25 mg		
Dietac (Menley & James)	37.5 mg		
Dietac Sustained Release (Menley & James)	75 mg		
Diet-Gard (Whitehall)	25 mg		
Diet-Trim Tablets (Pharmex)	NS[a]	carboxymethyl cellulose	benzocaine
Extra Strength Dexatrim (Thompson Medical)	75 mg		caffeine, 200 mg
E-Z Trim Capsules Time Release (Fox)	75 mg		
Gold Medal Diet Caps (Pfeiffer)	50 mg		caffeine, 200 mg
Grapefruit Diet Plan with Diadax Tablets (O'Connor)	10 mg		natural grapefruit extract, 16.6 mg; ascorbic acid, 10 mg; vitamin E, 3.6 mg
Grapefruit Diet Plan with Diadax Vitamin Fortified Continuous Action Capsules (O'Connor)	30 mg		natural grapefruit extract, 50 mg; ascorbic acid, 30 mg; vitamin E, 11 IU
Grapefruit Diet Plan with Diadax Chewable Tablets Extra Strength (O'Connor)	25 mg		natural grapefruit extract, 33 mg; ascorbic acid, 20 mg; vitamin E, 11 mg
Grapefruit Diet Plan with Diadax Extra Strength Vitamin Fortified Continuous Action Capsules (O'Connor)	75 mg		natural grapefruit extract, 100 mg; ascorbic acid, 60 mg; vitamin E, 30 IU
Odrinex Tablets (Fox)	25 mg		caffeine, 100 mg
Prolamine Capsules (Thompson Medical)	35 mg		caffeine, 140 mg
Slim Line Candy (Thompson Medical)			benzocaine, 5 mg; corn glucose syrup; natural and artificial flavoring
Slim Line Gum (Thompson Medical)			benzocaine, 6 mg
Spantrol Capsules (North American)	75 mg	carboxymethyl cellulose sodium, 135 mg	caffeine (anhydrous), 150 mg; benzocaine, 9 mg; ascorbic acid, 30 mg; thiamine HCl, 1 mg; riboflavin, 1.2 mg; niacinamide, 10 mg; pyridoxine HCl, 1 mg; iron, 10 mg
Super Odrinex (Fox)	25 mg		caffeine, 100 mg
Thinz Drops (Alval Amco)	a		fructose, pyridoxine, potassium chloride

Appetite Suppressant Product Table, continued

Product (Manufacturer)	Phenylpropanolamine Hydrochloride	Bulk Producer	Other Ingredients
Thinz Before Meals (Alval Amco)	25 mg		dicalcium phosphate, ascorbic acid, ferrous sulfate, potassium iodide, thiamine HCl
Thinz-Span (Alval Amco)	75 mg		caffeine, riboflavin, ascorbic acid, iron, thiamine HCl, alpha-tocopherol, iodine
Thinz Back-To-Nature (Alval Amco)	75 mg		caffeine, lecithin, kelp cider vinegar, riboflavin, pyridoxine
Thinz Delite (powder meal) (Alval Amco)	a		vitamins A, B, B_2, B_6, B_{12}, C; folic acid; phosphorous; calcium; iodine; copper; pantothenic acid; potassium; zinc; protein; amino acids; lecithin; caffeine; honey; beet powder

a Quantity not specified.

Weight Control Product Table

Product (Manufacturer)	Dosage Form	Calories Supplied	Essential Composition
Bulk Producers			
Diet-Aid (Rexall)	tablet	not stated	alginic acid, 200 mg; carboxymethyl cellulose sodium, 100 mg; sodium bicarbonate, 70 mg
Instant Mix Metamucil plain and orange flavor (Searle)	powder in single-dose packets	4/packet 4½/packet (orange)	psyllium mucilloid, 3.7 g; citric acid; sodium bicarbonate (equiv. to 250 mg sodium); sucrose
Metamucil (Searle)	powder	14/tsp	psyllium mucilloid, 50%; dextrose, 50%
Metamucil Orange Flavor (Searle)	powder	28½/tsp	psyllium mucilloid, 32%; sucrose, 68%
Pretts (Marion)	tablet	4½/tablet	alginic acid, 200 mg; sodium carboxymethyl cellulose, 100 mg; sodium bicarbonate, 70 mg
Reducets (Columbia Medical)	capsule	0	benzocaine, 5 mg; methylcellulose, 100 mg; multivitamins; minerals
Artificial Sweeteners			
Equal (Searle)	packets	4/g	aspartame
Ril-Sweet (Plough)	liquid	0	saccharin sodium, 3.3%
Sucaryl Sodium (Abbott)	tablet liquid	0	saccharin sodium, 16 mg/tablet, 1.21% (liquid)
Sweeta (Squibb)	tablet liquid	0	saccharin sodium, 15 mg/tablet, 7 mg/drop

Weight Control Product Table, continued

Product (Manufacturer)	Dosage Form	Calories Supplied	Essential Composition
Low-Calorie Foods			
Dietene (Doyle)	powder	190/packet	nonfat dry milk, cocoa, carrageenan, artificial flavor, lecithin, polysorbate 80, malt, vitamins, sucrose, calcium caseinate, minerals; sodium, 5.2 mEq/packet
Slender (Carnation)	liquid; powder to be mixed with milk; bar	225/can; 170 mixed with 6 oz. skim milk; 225 mixed with 6 oz. whole milk; 275/2 bar serving	nonfat dry milk, sucrose, vegetable oil, artificial flavors, vitamins, minerals
Low-Calorie Candy			
Ayds (Jeffrey Martin)	candy cube	25/cube	corn syrup, vegetable oils, sweetened condensed skim milk, vitamins, minerals

16 Sleep Aid, Sedative, and Stimulant Products

James P. Caro and Charles A. Walker

Questions to Ask the Patient

Sleep Aid and Sedative Products

How long have you had a sleep problem? Do you have difficulty sleeping every night or only occasionally?

Is the problem related to falling asleep or staying asleep?

Does your sleep problem interfere with your daily routines?

Do you wake up early? If you do, can you fall back to sleep?

Can you relate the sleep problem to a cause such as a change in work shifts, anxiety, or pain?

Are you taking tranquilizers, sleeping tablets, or any other medicine? If so, how often do you take them? What time of day do you take them?

Do you drink coffee, tea, cola, or alcohol? How much do you drink daily? What time of day do you drink them?

Do you have any chronic diseases?

Are you under a physician's care?

Have you used sleep aid products previously? Which ones? Were they effective?

Stimulant Products

How long do you intend to use a stimulant product?

Are you a regular drinker of coffee and other caffeinated beverages?

Have you ever experienced unpleasant reactions to coffee?

Which stimulant products have you used before? How well did they work?

Are you now being treated for a condition that requires the use of other drugs?

Do you have anxiety, nervousness, or any other nervous conditions?

In the United States, almost one-half the population occasionally has problems sleeping. Some people have trouble falling asleep; others awaken in the middle of the night. Sleep disorders can have a psychologic or physiologic origin.

Insomnia may be classified as either difficulty in falling asleep, difficulty in remaining asleep, or too early final wakening (1). Many factors may be involved. The amount of sleep required varies between individuals. Some people sleep very few hours but meet their sleep requirements. They are not candidates for sleep aids.

At the opposite end of the spectrum are individuals who need stimulants to stay awake. Boredom, fatigue, and the tedium of extended periods of monotonous activity such as highway driving may induce sleepiness.

Nonprescription drugs are available to combat both of these disorders. Pharmacists should counsel patients on correct use of sedatives and stimulants and be able to suggest adjunct, nondrug means to solve the problem. Usually a restful sleep pattern may be established without drugs; for example, taking a leisurely walk before bedtime may relax the body enough to facilitate falling asleep. Excessive intake of caffeine either in beverages or as a stimulant is unwise under any circumstances. It may have untoward effects, such as nervousness and irritability, and may contribute to insomnia.

Sleep Aid and Sedative Products

Although many nonprescription preparations have been promoted as providing "safe and restful sleep" or relief from "simple nervous tension," claims for the safety and efficacy of these products are unsubstantiated. Many contain drugs found in prescription medications such as antihistamines, but in much lower doses. It is assumed that these lower doses minimize the adverse effects of these agents. Unfortunately, the sedative effects also are minimal since sedation is usually only a secondary (or side) effect rather than the primary pharmacologic effect of the drug.

The sedative effect of these agents is subject to considerable personal variation; some individuals may even experience a paradoxical state of excitement. The low efficacy of these preparations poses an additional hazard because individuals who do not experience sedation at normal doses may exceed the recommended dose and suffer toxic effects.

The FDA advisory review panel on nonprescription night-time sleep aid and daytime sedative drug products has subjected the active ingredients of these preparations to a thorough review and evaluation (2). As a result, all daytime sedative products were found neither safe nor effective and were withdrawn from the market June 22, 1979, when the final rule was published.

The panel's findings on nonprescription sleep aids are not yet final. Nevertheless, the panel has recommended that most of these agents be eliminated from nonprescription products due to evidence that they are neither safe nor effective. Methapyrilene was previously withdrawn from the marketplace because of reports of carcinogenicity. The tentative conclusions call

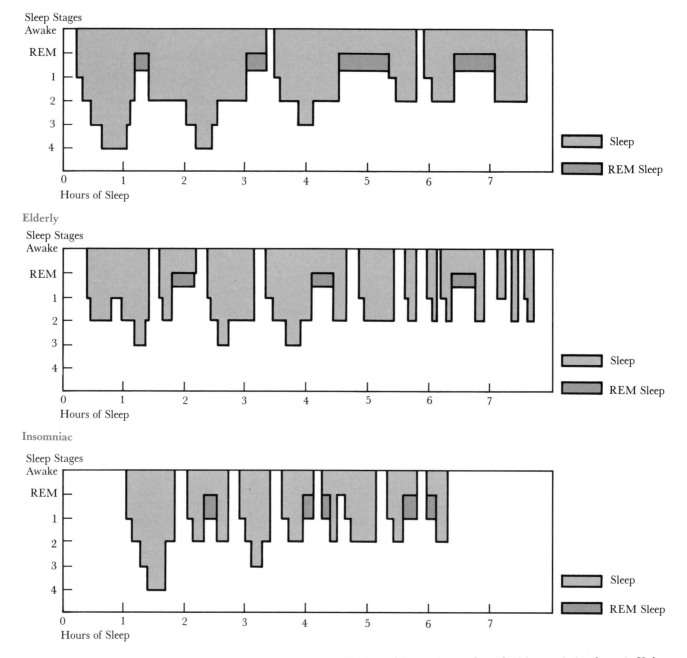

Figure 1. Hours of sleep and sleep stages in young adults, the elderly, and insomniacs. Adapted with permission from A. Kales, *Ann. Intern. Med., 68,* 1078–1104 (1968).

for elimination of all nonprescription sedative agents except doxylamine succinate, phenyltoloxamine citrate, and pyrilamine maleate. These remaining ingredients would be subjected to an additional testing period to determine if Category I status (generally recognized as safe and effective) is indicated. The panel also advocates testing of diphenhydramine as a nonprescription sleep aid. Diphenhydramine is available by prescription only. Nonprescription status is granted only if there is sufficient evidence that the agent can be used safely and at an effective dosage without medical supervision. In the case of nonprescription sleep aids, the FDA panel's recommendations are still tentative and therefore carry no regulatory authority. At this time, the projected publication of the final regulations has not been established.

Physiology of Sleep

The sites and mechanisms of action of sleep-inducing drugs are largely unknown. Neurophysiologic investigations have yielded many theories concerning the influence of brain structures on consciousness and have provided some insight into the complex feedback systems that control consciousness. It is now known that the brain stem coordinates the activity of these systems.

The brain stem contains the reticular activating system (RAS), which monitors and selectively limits all sensory input to the brain. Although the reticular activating system responds to stimuli by arousing the brain, the cerebral cortex discriminates among stimuli even during sleep. For this reason, only selected stimuli will produce arousal from sleep (3).

Sleep is characterized by a decrease of activity in the ascending and descending reticular activating system pathways. This reticular deactivation occurs by passive limitation of sensory input, such as sleeping in a dark, quiet room, and by active influence from the cerebral cortex, medulla, and possibly other structures (4).

Sleep is classified into rapid eye movement (REM), also known as paradoxical sleep, and nonrapid eye movement (non-REM) stages (Figure 1). Non-REM sleep is subdivided into stages I–IV, according to increasing depth of sleep. In young adults, REM sleep constitutes about 25% of a night's sleep. During REM sleep the body is physiologically more active than it is in non-REM stages. In young adults there is an initial awake period (sleep latency) followed by a rapid progression through stages I–IV of non-REM. This sequence is then reversed, followed by the first REM period. This initial sequence of non-REM sleep (REM latency) lasts about 70 minutes. The first REM period is very short and is followed by another cycle. In each successive cycle, less time is spent in stage IV and more time is spent in the other stages, including REM. In the elderly, both sleep latency and REM latency are increased, stage IV may be decreased or absent, and awakenings are more frequent (5).

Etiology of Insomnia

The occasional inability to attain restful sleep is a common problem. It is estimated that about 50% of the population experiences insomnia at some time, and 33% voices it as an ongoing complaint (6). Although insomnia is usually transient and self-limiting, it may be of sufficient duration or severity to interfere with how an individual functions during the waking hours. Severe or chronic insomnia may be a symptom of serious psychologic or physiologic illness.

Situational Stress and Anxiety

These conditions cause difficulty in falling asleep. Usually acute and transient, they include anything that may cause worry or excitement. Situational stress and anxiety are probably the most frequent causes of insomnia in young people.

Difficulty in falling asleep will resolve when the precipitating cause is eliminated. When insomnia is a short-term (less than 1 week) problem that can be attributed to a specific situation, nondrug measures and nonprescription preparations may provide sufficient relief. However, pharmacists should be aware that chronic insomnia is often a symptom of depression. Any patient complaining of insomnia coupled with loss of energy, weight loss or weight gain, severe anxiety, or decreased sex drive should be referred to a physician for a thorough evaluation.

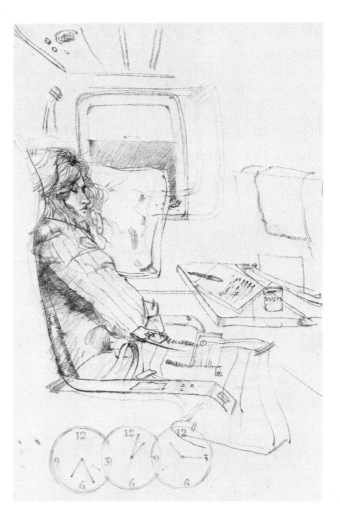

Pain or Physical Discomfort

Pain of any type will disturb sleep. It is important to recognize that the underlying cause of pain needs to be identified and treated. Several disorders including angina, vascular headache, and duodenal ulcer pain may be exacerbated during sleep as a result of increased autonomic activity during REM periods. Patients complaining of insomnia because of pain or discomfort should be questioned closely to determine whether self-treatment or referral to a physician is indicated. (See Chapter 11, *Internal Analgesic Products.*)

Change in Daily Rhythm

A change in work shift and "jet lag" are typical occurrences that may precipitate insomnia.

Age

Elderly individuals are prone to early or frequent awakening because sleep cycles change with age. Moreover, sensitivity to caffeine increases with age so that individuals who previously consumed coffee and colas with impunity may find that these beverages are beginning to disturb sleep (4).

Depression

Some types of depression are associated with awakenings during the night or early morning. If anxiety occurs with depression, the patient may complain of difficulty in falling and remaining asleep. If suspected, referral to a physician is appropriate.

Conditions with Nocturnal Exacerbation

Autonomic nervous system bursts during REM sleep precipitate angina attacks, vascular headaches, and duodenal ulcer distress that disturb sleep. Asthma, epilepsy, and lumbosacral and cervical disc disease also have been implicated in sleep disturbances.

Endocrine Abnormalities

Hypothyroidism and hyperthyroidism as well as other endocrine disorders disturb sleep patterns, but the mechanism is unknown.

Sleep Apnea

This sleep disturbance, which is most common in men over 40, is manifested by loud, irregular snoring. In this syndrome, respiration actually stops for periods of 20–90 seconds many times during the night, resulting in partial awakening and sleep disruption. The patient may be unaware of irregular respiration and may complain only of feeling tired during the day. Researchers believe that sleep apnea is caused by a defect in CNS respiratory control which, in some cases, is complicated by an anatomical upper airway obstruction.

Nocturnal Myoclonus

Nocturnal myoclonus is classified as a form of epilepsy and has been treated with anticonvulsants. This syndrome consists of recurrent, rhythmic movement of one or both legs. Although the patient may not actually awaken, sleep is disrupted and the patient may complain of sleeping poorly or feeling tired during the day.

The patient may be unaware of the nocturnal movement but complaints from a spouse may help identify patients with this syndrome.

Drug Use

Many drugs may cause sleep disturbances. Certain anorexic preparations (prescription and nonprescription) containing CNS stimulants, caffeine, and aminophylline may cause nervousness and prevent sleep in some individuals. Alcohol, amphetamines, barbiturates, diphenhydramine, ethchlorvynol, glutethimide, methyprylon, monoamine oxidase inhibitors, narcotics, scopolamine, and tricyclic antidepressants are drugs that cause sleep disturbances by suppressing REM (7). Amphetamines, barbiturates, benzodiazepines, chloral hydrate, glutethimide, and reserpine decrease stage IV sleep.

Ironically, the widely used benzodiazepine and barbiturate hypnotics disrupt sleep patterns by suppressing REM. In addition, tolerance to the hypnotic effects of these agents develops quickly. As a result of these properties, patients get caught in a vicious cycle of taking more medication to induce sleep which, in turn, causes further disruption of sleep by suppressing REM. When patients try to discontinue the medication after chronic use, the body responds with a compensatory rebound in REM that is accompanied by additional sleep disturbances and nightmares. The patient seeks relief by resuming drug use and the cycle continues until professional intervention is sought.

Patients who describe a history of drug use for insomnia should be referred to a physician for a thorough evaluation of possible causes and treatment.

Pharmacologic Agents

Nonprescription drugs that have been used to treat insomnia include antihistamines, salicylates and salicylamide, and scopolamine (an anticholinergic). None of these drugs has been proven safe and effective and, therefore, they should be used cautiously if used at all. Patients using sedative products containing these agents, particularly pregnant women, should be warned of possible adverse effects. The pharmacist should urge patients to try adjunctive nondrug measures to help them sleep.

Antihistamines

The FDA advisory review panel on nonprescription sleep aid drug products has placed diphenhydramine hydrochloride, doxylamine succinate, phenyltoloxamine citrate, and pyrilamine maleate in Category III, indicating that there are insufficient data to permit final classification.

Antihistamines are classified into five groups according to chemical structure. The ethanolamines, which include diphenhydramine, doxylamine, and phenyltoloxamine, are probably the best suited for use as sleep aids since they have a highly sedative effect. The ethanolamines also have a low incidence of GI side effects.

The ethylenediamines produce less sedation and drowsiness and have a higher incidence of GI effects.

This group includes methapyrilene (withdrawn from market due to potential carcinogenicity) and pyrilamine, which is present in many nonprescription sleep aids as the maleate salt. The alkylamines and piperazine antihistamines produce less sedation and are not suitable for use as sleep aids. Chlorpheniramine and chlorcyclizine are examples of alkylamines and piperazines, respectively.

Antihistamines in the phenothiazine group (promethazine) have been shown to display prominent CNS depressant effects but are not available in nonprescription preparations.

Antihistamines can induce symptoms of both CNS stimulation and depresssion. Drowsiness is the most common side effect of therapeutic doses and excitation may be a symptom of intoxication. However, some people exhibit paradoxical excitation with therapeutic doses. The CNS depressant action of antihistamines also is unpredictable because individuals vary in sensitivity to this effect and tolerance develops with continued use. Patients who use antihistamines should be warned not to drive an automobile or operate hazardous machinery while taking these drugs until their response to the drug is known. Alcohol and other CNS depressants may add to the depressant effect and should be avoided.

The mechanisms by which antihistamines exert their CNS effects are unclear, but similarities between the actions of antihistamines and scopolamine suggest that acetylcholine antagonism in the CNS is common to both (8).

Side effects of antihistamines include dizziness, tinnitus, blurred vision, GI disturbances, and dryness of the mouth and throat. Antihistamines may also cause CNS stimulation, resulting in nervousness and insomnia. However, this effect is uncommon, occurring primarily in children.

Although the antihistamines have a wide margin of safety, potential poisoning with these agents should not be discounted if an acute overdose is taken, especially in combination with alcohol or other CNS depressants. The symptoms observed with intoxication result from the CNS effects and are characteristic of anticholinergic overdose (the pupils become fixed and dilated, fever may be present, sweating may be decreased or absent, and excitement, hallucinations, and convulsions occur). In severe cases, these symptoms are followed by coma and cardiorespiratory collapse. Treatment consists of preventing the drug's absorption, inducing emesis, and providing supportive measures such as assisting ventilation and controlling convulsions. (See Chapter 7, *Emetic and Antiemetic Products.*)

Antihistamines have produced teratogenic effects in animals and therefore should be avoided by pregnant women. High doses may precipitate convulsions and should be used with caution in persons with epilepsy.

The antihistamines commonly used in nonprescription sleep aid products are doxylamine and pyrilamine maleate, alone or in combination. The dose of doxylamine as a sedative is 25–50 mg in a single dose at bedtime. The usual dose of pyrilamine maleate is 25–50 mg in a single dose at bedtime (9).

Salicylates and Salicylamide

Salicylates and salicylamide are included in sleep aid products primarily to relieve minor pain that may hinder sleep. Although salicylamide also has sedative properties, the doses contained in nonprescription preparations (200–400 mg) probably are insufficient to produce sedation (10). In addition, the results of one study indicate that salicylamide's bioavailability is poor because the drug is relatively insoluble and rapidly inactivated in the GI tract and liver (11). Salicylamide is not metabolized to salicylate in the body. The FDA advisory review panel has found no evidence that these ingredients are effective as sleep aids. Additionally, the inclusion of these agents in nonprescription sleep aids is an example of irrational combination therapy. Insomnia is not always a result of pain and should be treated with analgesics only when pain is the causative factor. (See Chapter 11, *Internal Analgesic Products.*)

Salicylates are present in nonprescription sleep aid products as various salts, in doses of 80–200 mg. Salicylamide is included in doses of 200–400 mg.

Scopolamine

Scopolamine previously has been available as an active ingredient in nonprescription sleep aids. The FDA advisory review panel has determined that scopolamine is neither safe nor effective for nonprescription use as a sedative. Although it may be marketed until a final ruling is published, scopolamine has already been removed from most nonprescription products.

Scopolamine, a belladonna alkaloid, is an anticholinergic agent that differs from atropine in that it lacks a CNS stimulant effect. Scopolamine acts as a hypnotic by depressing the cerebral cortex, especially the motor areas (12). Although scopolamine does suppress REM sleep, the dose in nonprescription preparations probably is insufficient to produce "REM rebound." Patients who use these preparations chronically or who exceed the recommended dosage may experience this effect (3).

Scopolamine has been used as a preanesthetic medicine for its sedative action. In obstetrics it was combined with narcotics to produce a state of amnesia and partial analgesia ("twilight sleep"). Although scopolamine is effective in preventing motion sickness, it has been replaced by newer agents such as dimenhydrinate, with fewer side effects.

The most common side effect of scopolamine is dryness of the mouth and throat. Other effects such as blurred vision, photophobia, and urinary retention are uncommon at the dosage provided in nonprescription preparations.

Infants and young children are particularly susceptible to the toxic effects of belladonna alkaloids. The fatal scopolamine dose in children may be as low as 10 mg (13). This dosage would require ingestion of 40 or more dosage units of available nonprescription preparations. Under such circumstances, it is likely that a toxic dose of antihistamine would also be present since scopolamine is only available as a combination product. The symptoms of scopolamine poisoning are delirium, tachycardia, fever, and hot, dry, flushed skin. In severe cases, respiratory depression and coma may result.

Treatment of oral scopolamine poisoning consists of delaying and preventing the drug's absorption by administering milk, inducing emesis, administering activated charcoal, and counteracting its central peripheral effects with physostigmine. In addition, general measures such as reducing fever, controlling convulsions, and maintaining urinary output are used. If scopolamine overdose is suspected, referral to a poison control center, emergency facility, or a physician is indicated.

The amount of scopolamine in nonprescription products may be 0.1–0.5 mg/dose. Scopolamine (as the aminoxide hydrobromide salt) should not be used in children under 12 or in patients with narrow-angle glaucoma, coronary insufficiency, or prostatic hypertrophy. This agent should be used cautiously with other drugs possessing anticholinergic activity (other belladonna alkaloids, phenothiazines, tricyclic antidepressants, and antihistamines) and CNS depressants because concurrent use may enhance the anticholinergic action or the CNS depression.

The FDA advisory review panel has concluded that scopolamine and its salts are ineffective sleep aid ingredients at dosages currently employed. Moreover, the panel has found that therapeutic doses pose a significant hazard of adverse anticholinergic effects. As a result of these findings, scopolamine and its salts have been placed in Category II and will be removed from the market when the recommendations are made final.

L-Tryptophan

This amino acid has been used to treat insomnia, depression, and various dyskinesias. When used in treating insomnia, doses of 1–10 g have been effective in decreasing latency and increasing total sleep time. However, there is also evidence that REM sleep may be suppressed and additional studies are needed to determine the clinical usefulness of this agent. L-Tryptophan is not currently marketed in the United States as a sleep aid, but it is readily available as a nutritional supplement (14).

Adjunctive Measures

Before advising patients on the proper use of nonprescription sleep aid preparations, the pharmacist should recommend the following nondrug measures appropriate to help relieve insomnia:

- Drinking a hot milk beverage at bedtime;
- Participating in stimulating daytime activities;
- Arising at a specific early hour each morning regardless of the previous night's sleep. (After a few nights of poor sleep, improvement may occur and sleep may become more regular.);
- Advising the patient not to worry if unable to sleep since anxiety can contribute to or cause insomnia;
- Abstaining from or decreasing consumption of beverages containing caffeine;
- Avoiding heavy meals several hours before bedtime;
- Avoiding naps during the day;

- Performing light exercise such as taking a leisurely walk before bedtime;
- Avoiding strenuous exercise before bedtime.
- Designating a specific time for sleep;
- Relaxing by engaging in activities such as reading in bed, watching television, or listening to relaxing music;
- Minimizing external stimuli that might disturb sleep (use dark shades over the windows to keep out light and ear plugs to keep out noise).

Stimulant Products

Nonprescription stimulant products, of which caffeine is the only available active ingredient, are used most commonly to induce wakefulness and to relieve the sense of boredom and fatigue associated with performing tedious work for extended periods. For example, it is used to prevent "highway hypnosis" encountered during long periods of continuous driving. Caffeine also is used inappropriately to combat hangover symptoms and to antagonize the depressant properties of alcohol and other sedatives.

Approximately 7 million kilograms of caffeine (1,3,7-trimethylxanthine) are consumed yearly in the United States. The related dimethylxanthines, theophylline and theobromine, are not used therapeutically as stimulants (Figure 2). The caffeine content of nonalcoholic beverages is shown in Table 1.

More than 25 nonprescription analgesic products contain as much as 64 mg of caffeine per dose. Caffeine is considered a relatively safe substance when administered orally in doses of less than 200 mg (15). However, recent evidence suggests that caffeine should not be considered as innocuous a substance as was originally thought (16).

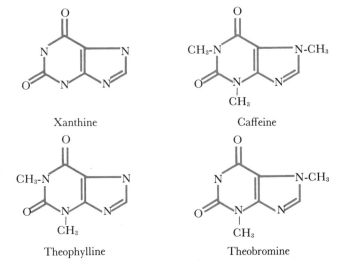

Figure 2. Structure of methylated xanthines.

Table 1. Approximate caffeine content in common substances

Product or substance	Caffeine (mg)
1 cup of brewed coffee	100–150
1 cup of instant coffee	86–99
1 cup of decaffeinated coffee	2–4
12 ounces of cola drink	40–72
1 cup of tea	60–72
1 cup of cocoa	50
1 ounce of milk chocolate	3–6
1 ounce of bittersweet chocolate	25
1 tablet of various cold preparations	30
Nonprescription stimulant tablet	100–200

Adapted from R. G. Martinek and W. Wolman, *J. Am. Med. Assoc., 158,* 1030 (1955), and J. A. Roth, A. C. Ivy, and A. J. Atkinson, *J. Am. Med. Assoc., 126,* 814 (1944), and W. Wolman, *J. Am. Med. Assoc., 159,* 250 (1955).

Caffeine Effects on Nervous System

Indications for stimulant use are drowsiness and fatigue. In a study on driver performance, caffeine improved alertness, but contradictory evidence exists on caffeine's sobering effect. Mental activity was improved by caffeine in tests that involved simple arithmetic, typing, and decoding, especially in long sessions, when fatigue and boredom may have been possible factors (15).

The FDA advisory review panel on nonprescription night-time sleep aid and stimulant drug products considers caffeine to be safe and effective as a stimulant when administered in doses of 100–200 mg no more often than every 3–4 hours (17).

The physiologic consequences of various caffeine doses have been studied in humans. Improvement of skeletal muscle tone is a fundamental property of caffeine useful in combating fatigue (18). This effect is produced mainly by CNS stimulation and in part by the direct action on the voluntary musculature. It is difficult to separate the central from the peripheral influence, but the central effects probably are more important and pronounced. Small doses (50–200 mg) stimulate cerebrocortical areas associated with conscious mental processes; ideas become clearer, thoughts flow more easily and rapidly, and fatigue and drowsiness decrease (19) (Figure 3). Doses larger than 250 mg often cause insomnia, restlessness, irritability, nervousness, tremor, headaches, and, in rare cases, a mild form of delirium manifested as perceived noises and flashes of light. Among investigations of caffeine's objective and subjective effects, one study evaluating the effects of placebo versus caffeine (150–300 mg) on objective performance and mood showed that although caffeine produces a subjective feeling of increased alertness and physical activity, objective performance requiring alertness and psychomotor coordination is not improved (18).

Caffeine is therapeutically effective in treating drug-induced depression of the medullary respiratory center. Injected doses of caffeine larger than 250 mg stimulate vagal respiratory and vasomotor areas of the medulla oblongata (20).

Effects on Cardiovascular System

Xanthines may stimulate the myocardium directly, promoting an increase in cardiac contractile force, rate, and output (21). These cardiac effects may be masked, however, because xanthines, especially caffeine in large doses, also stimulate the medullary vagal nuclei and tend to produce a reflex decrease in heart rate. Large doses (more than 250 mg) may induce cardiac irregularities due to a direct effect on the myocardium (19). Experimentally, caffeine stimulates norepinephrine synthesis and release in the brain and epinephrine release from the adrenal medulla (19).

In humans, caffeine does not cause a consistent decrease in systemic mean blood pressure despite a decrease in peripheral resistance. Generally, with moderate caffeine doses, blood pressure is maintained by increased cardiac output. However, large intravenous doses of caffeine have been shown to cause a transient fall in blood pressure due to medullary vagal nuclei stimulation, which also may result in bradycardia and a slight decrease in cardiac output (19).

Xanthines cause a marked increase in cerebral vascular resistance with an accompanying decrease in cerebral blood flow and in the oxygen tension of the brain. This vasoconstriction action is believed to be responsible for the striking relief of hypertensive headache by caffeine (20).

In an investigation on the effect of 140 mg of caffeine in tea on hemodynamic measures in patients with cardiac disease, there was a significant rise in the cardiac index, stroke index, oxygen consumption, and minute ventilation (22). A small but significant increase in brachial arterial pressure and ventricular filling pressure also occurred. No arrhythmias were seen in any of the patients as a result of drinking tea.

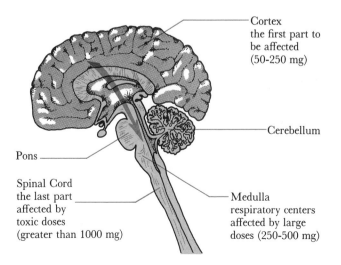

Figure 3. The site of action of caffeine in the central nervous system. (The arrow indicates the progression of the effect.)

There have been conflicting reports of a positive correlation between coronary artery disease and coffee consumption. One study compared the histories of 700 heart attack patients with the histories of 13,000 other patients (23). Patients who drank as much as five cups of coffee/day had a 50% greater risk of heart attack than those who abstained; patients who drank six or more cups/day had a 100% greater risk of heart attack than abstainers. Some investigators believe that caffeine consumption increases the risk of heart attack. These results have been disputed by other studies that failed to show a correlation between coffee consumption, serum lipids, or serum cholesterol, and coronary disease (24, 25).

Other Caffeine Effects

A mild degree of tolerance and physical dependence occurs with habitual caffeine ingestion. Irritability, nervousness, and headache were reported in habitual coffee users (five or more cups/day) following withdrawal from the beverage (26). Although these symptoms do not prove actual caffeine physical dependence, they may indicate psychologic dependence. Another study conducted to determine tolerance to caffeine in healthy subjects provided some information on physiologic changes associated with chronic caffeine administration (27). After caffeine and coffee consumption, the amount of REM sleep was increased for the entire night and was shifted to the early portion of the night. Stages III and IV of non-REM sleep were concentrated later in the night than normal and the amount of each was reduced (28). It was established that 150 mg of caffeine taken at bedtime reduces pulse rate significantly in non-coffee drinkers but not in those who habitually consume caffeinated beverages. The study also indicated that caffeine administration (150 mg) to non-coffee drinkers delays the onset of sleep patterns. On the other hand, chronic coffee drinkers show no symptoms of bradycardia or insomnia (27). Although results indicate possible physical changes in coffee drinkers, it is the general opinion that caffeine tolerance in chronic users occurs because of increased metabolism. Chronic caffeine use may produce a degree of tolerance to caffeine-induced insomnia and a decrease in the mental alertness produced by caffeine (a decrease in caffeine's ability to act as a stimulant) (29).

"Caffeinism" is the syndrome associated with excessive caffeine intake. Ingesting more than 1 g/day of caffeine (about 10 cups of coffee) may produce symptoms similar to those of anxiety neurosis. The CNS symptoms related to excessive stimulation include nervousness, irritability, agitation, headache, tachypnea, tremulousness, and muscle twitches. Sensory disturbances such as hyperesthesia, tinnitus, and visual hallucinations may occur. Insomnia characterized by a delay in sleep onset or by frequent awakenings may be a consequence of caffeinism.

The effects of regular coffee, decaffeinated coffee, and caffeine on gastric acid secretion and lower esophageal sphincter pressure have been investigated in healthy subjects (30). The results of this study suggest that regular and decaffeinated coffee are more potent stimulants of gastric acid secretion than caffeine, that decaffeination diminishes coffee's acid secretory potency only minimally, and that regular and decaffeinated coffee increase lower esophageal sphincter pressure, whereas caffeine alone has only a minimal effect. Clinical recommendations based on the known GI effect of caffeine thus may bear little relation to the actual observed action of regular or decaffeinated coffee (30). Moreover, the effects of caffeine alone may not be similar to the effects of beverages in which caffeine is present. Therefore, decaffeination does not necessarily completely remove undesirable effects of caffeinated beverages.

Caffeine has been shown to cause birth defects in rats. Abnormalities were reported for animals administered caffeine by intubation in doses of 125, 80, and 40 mg/kg. A decrease in fetal weight and crown-rump distance was noted for animals given 40 mg/kg. At 80 mg/kg, 56% of litters contained fetuses with five or more variations; at 125 mg/kg, 100% of the litters contained fetuses with five or more variations (19).

It is not known whether caffeine is teratogenic in humans but caffeine does cross the placenta and pregnant women or those who may become pregnant should be advised to limit their use of caffeine. The FDA has removed caffeine from the list of substances generally recognized as safe. Further studies are required to determine whether caffeine causes birth defects in humans (31).

A positive association has been established between coffee consumption and the incidence of pancreatic cancer (16). Despite this established relationship, more data are needed before a final conclusion can be drawn. It is noteworthy that a similar relationship was not established between cancer of the pancreas and tea consumption. From this report, it is difficult to establish whether or not the causal relation is due to caffeine contents of the coffee or other ingredients in the coffee bean.

Caffeine's value in mixtures for relief of headache and other pain is questionable except in the treatment of vascular headache. One study reported that caffeine in combination with aspirin was no more effective than aspirin alone for headache (33). Caffeine generally is believed to play a minor role in the toxic effects from excessive analgesic use (33, 34).

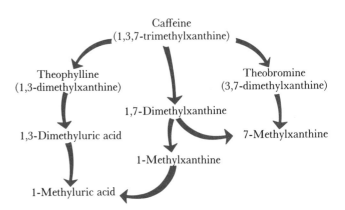

Figure 4. Caffeine metabolism in humans.

Renal irritation and nephrotoxicity may occur following chronic abuse of caffeine-containing analgesic drug mixtures. One study reported a significant number of renal tubular cells and red blood cells in the urine of 10 healthy volunteers following the ingestion of 1.2 g/day of caffeine for 5 days (35, 36).

Caffeine taken with analgesics may, by its stimulant properties, act as a mood enhancer when pain is accompanied by minor depression; however, the rationale for fixed combinations of caffeine and analgesics is questionable.

Caffeine has a hyperglycemic effect and may elevate blood glucose levels. The hyperglycemic effect of caffeine is mediated through its effect on cyclic AMP and large doses will induce the release of adrenal catecholamines (37, 38). This in turn stimulates glycolysis and glucose formation in the liver, thereby raising blood glucose levels.

Caffeine or its metabolites interfere in vanillylmandelic acid 4-hydroxy-3-methoxymandelic acid (VMA) determination. The test is used to detect elevated adrenal or sympathetic catecholamine levels as seen in pheochromocytoma or neuroblastoma. An increase in urinary catecholamine levels may be detected following caffeine ingestion (39).

Figure 4 shows the human metabolism of caffeine, after which approximately two-thirds of the drug is excreted in the urine as monomethylxanthine or dimethyluric acid. Although coffee and preparations containing caffeine often are prohibited in individuals suffering from gout, this prohibition may not be justified (19). Uric acid is not formed following caffeine ingestion, and the methylxanthines and methyluric acids that do appear as metabolites do not provoke attacks of gout. Therefore, it is doubtful that therapeutic doses of caffeine aggravate the disease. However, caffeine ingestion may produce high readings of serum uric acid when the Bittner assay is used (40).

In a study of caffeine use in hyperkinetic children, it was concluded that caffeine may have a place in the therapeutic management of children with minimal brain dysfunction syndrome and consequent hyperkinetic impulse syndrome (35).

Medical Aspects of Caffeine Consumption

The use of coffee, tea, or drugs containing caffeine is important for individuals with different types of diseases. In hypertension, caffeine beverages are often denied. If the patient is not over excited by coffee or tea, the denial of these drinks may not be warranted. However, in cases of hypertension, overconsumption of caffeine beverages or caffeine drugs is not advisable since caffeine can increase cardiac output through its direct effect on the heart muscle and the possible potentiation of hypertension. The overusage of caffeine drugs in susceptible individuals may give rise to palpitation and tachycardia. Repeated stimulation of the CNS produces vexation, fretfulness, and malaise. These reactions may be accompanied by insomnia, all of which aggravate the circulatory symptoms and premature systole may ensue.

Moderate doses of caffeine in humans result in prolonged augmentation of gastric secretion (41). In view of the responsiveness of the human gastric mucosa to caffeine, cognizance must be taken of the ubiquitous use of caffeine beverages drugs in the pathogenesis of peptic ulcers and the management of ulcer patients. In nervous insomnia, caffeine beverages are wisely contraindicated.

Caffeine Toxicity

Fatal caffeine poisoning is extremely rare. Death has been reported in only a few cases following intravenous injection or oral administration. In adults the lethal intravenous dose of caffeine was reported to be 3.2 g; the reported oral lethal dose range is 18–50 g (39). The administration route influences the severity of toxic manifestations. Peak blood levels occur within 2 hours after oral administration (42). The average half-life is 3–3.5 hours in smokers and 6 hours in nonsmokers (39). Smoking induces the hepatic enzymes required to metabolize the chemicals absorbed from tobacco smoke, resulting in the faster metabolism of some drugs including caffeine. The clearance of caffeine is 55% higher in smokers than nonsmokers, which may contribute to the higher coffee consumption of smokers and to their ability to better tolerate coffee close to retiring (30). Children are very susceptible to caffeine toxicity; caffeine-containing drugs should be kept out of their reach.

In adults, doses of more than 10 g ingested orally are needed to induce convulsions (19). In cases of oral overdosage, the stomach should be emptied by inducing emesis or by using gastric lavage. Depressants, such as barbiturates, have been used to control caffeine-induced convulsions.

The following treatment of caffeine overdosage is suggested:

- Emesis with syrup of ipecac;
- Ingestion of aluminum hydroxide gel as an antacid and protective agent against GI irritation;
- Oxygen inhalation;
- Short-acting barbiturates injected cautiously to control neuromuscular irritability and convulsions;
- Intravenous fluids to combat dehydration;
- Antibiotics for complicating infections;
- Evacuation.

Potential Interactions

Caffeine may interact with other drugs. It was observed in experimental animals that isoniazid and meprobamate enhance the caffeine effect (43, 44). Meprobamate may increase caffeine concentration in the brain by 55% and may decrease it in the liver and kidney (45). It is important for the pharmacist to be cognizant of possible caffeine interactions in patients taking these specific medications.

Summary

Patient Assessment

The pharmacist should determine through direct observation and a series of questions whether or not a stimulant is appropriate. The pharmacist should determine if the patient is a heavy coffee or tea consumer; if GI problems or hyperactivity occur following coffee or caffeine intake, if any other unpleasant reactions occur, or, if the patient is a heavy coffee drinker, whether the patient becomes hyperactive when deprived of caffeine; and whether the patient normally suffers from anxiety, nervousness, or specific cardiovascular problems. If the patient is pregnant, the pharmacist should assess the stage of pregnancy and degree and frequency in terms of the planned use of the stimulants or caffeine. The pharmacist should assess whether the patient is using sedatives or hypnotics and socially antagonizing their effects with stimulants. If so, the specific drugs being used should be determined as well as to what extent problems are experienced or inherent with these practices.

Patient Education

The pharmacist should educate the patient regarding the use of stimulant products. It should be emphasized to stimulant users that following the ingestion of caffeine, a period of behavioral and mental depression ensues. This may be relevant in automobile accidents that sometimes occur after caffeine ingestion. When driving long distances, frequent stops are effective in combating fatigue. If the weather is conducive, driving with windows down to allow fresh air can help one stay awake. The patient should always be cognizant of the side effects due to caffeine ingestion. He or she should remember that some tolerance as well as psychologic dependence may develop to the use of caffeine.

Nonprescription stimulant usage should be held to a minimum. It is a mistake to fight fatigue by indulgence in stimulants. Patients should recognize that fatigue is a symptom that might be related to a disease. Sufficient time for recovery from fatigue must be allowed, especially after infectious diseases. For simple fatigue, rest is the sovereign remedy. But in cases of chronic fatigue, professional help may be needed and great effort may have to be exerted to determine its cause.

Sleep Aid and Sedative Product Use

Insomnia usually is a transient, self-limiting condition caused by stress or change of location or schedule. Patients who request nonprescription sleep aid or sedative products should be informed that these products are only for occasional use at recommended dosages and their effectiveness in long-term use has not been established. Scopolamine preparations should not be recommended because they are ineffective at recommended doses and higher doses may precipitate toxicity. The antihistamines are the most satisfactory ingredients of nonprescription sleep aid and sedative products. The FDA advisory review panel on sleep aid drug products has recommended additional testing of these agents at doses greater than those presently used and is recommending the introduction of diphenhydramine as a nonprescription sleep aid.

The temporary use of an antihistamine product along with nondrug measures is probably the most rational advice a pharmacist can give a patient suffering from insomnia. Patients using any nonprescription sleep aid product should be cautioned that their ability to drive an automobile or operate hazardous machinery may be impaired and that concurrent use of these products with alcohol or other CNS depressants will intensify the CNS depression.

Stimulant Product Use

The pharmacist should advise caffeine product users of the possible side effects and dangers of overconsumption of these compounds. Because of caffeine's possible interactions with other drugs, caffeine intake should be reduced during the treatment of specific diseases, especially cardiovascular, psychological, or renal problems. The use of analgesic combinations that contain caffeine is not advisable for patients with rheumatoid arthritis or other conditions that require large doses (10–30 tablets/day) of medicine because in these amounts there is danger of caffeine toxicity. Caffeine consumption should be avoided prior to blood or urine analysis.

The pharmacist should caution against caffeine overuse. Habitual use may lead to sleep deprivation. The CNS stimulants may facilitate the ability to ignore the sensation of tiredness, but they do not replenish depleted energy. Continuous use of coffee or caffeine tablets does not allay emotional fatigue. Neither coffee nor caffeine tablets taken after alcohol consumption induce sobriety, but the degree of CNS depression is lessened, and somnolence is diminished or eliminated. In other words, a person may still be inebriated without feeling sleepy.

References

1. C. C. Brown, E. L. Hartmann, G. L. Usdin, E. D. Weitzman, D. J. Greenblatt, and L. E. Hollister, *Patient Care, 10,* 98 (1976).
2. *Federal Register, 43* (1978).
3. "The Anatomy of Sleep," Roche Laboratories, Nutley, N.J., 1966, pp. 39–59.
4. "The Nature of Sleep," G. E. W. Wolstenholme and M. O'Conner, Eds., Little, Brown, Boston, Mass., 1961, pp. 86–102.
5. K. L. Melmon and H. F. Morrelli, "Clinical Pharmacology—Basic Principles in Therapeutics," 2nd ed., Macmillan, New York, N.Y., 1978, pp. 886–887.
6. J. Moriarity, *Dis. Nerv. Syst., 36,* 279 (1975).
7. G. Fass, *Am. J. Nurs., 71,* 2316 (1971).
8. R. H. Dreisbach, "Handbook of Poisoning," 8th ed., Lange Medical, Los Altos, Calif., 1974, pp. 606–608.
9. *Federal Register, 43,* 25584–87 (1978).
10. "The Pharmacological Basis of Therapeutics," 6th ed., A. G. Gilman, L. S. Goodman, and A. Gilman, Eds., Macmillan, New York, N.Y., 1980, p. 369.
11. L. Fleckenstein, G. R. Mundy, R. A. Horovitz, and J. M. Mazzulo, *Clin. Pharmacol. Ther., 19,* 451 (1976).
12. "Martindale: The Extra Pharmacopoeia," 26th ed., N. W. Blacow, Ed., Pharmaceutical Press, London, England, 1972, p. 295.
13. R. H. Dreisbach, "Handbook of Poisoning," 8th ed., Lange Medical, Los Altos, Calif., 1974, p. 305.
14. "Martindale: The Extra Pharmacopoeia," 26th ed., N. W. Blacow, Ed., Pharmaceutical Press, London, England, 1972, p. 82.
15. "Drill's Pharmacology in Medicine," 4th ed., J. R. Dipalma, Ed., McGraw-Hill, New York, N.Y., 1971, p. 537.
16. B. MacMahon and S. Yen, *N. Engl. J. Med., 304,* 630 (1981).
17. *Federal Register, 43,* 25597 (1978).
18. A. Goldstein, S. Kaizer, and R. Warren, *J. Pharmacol. Exp. Ther., 150,* 146 (1965).
19. "The Pharmacological Basis of Therapeutics," 6th ed., A. G. Gilman, L. S. Goodman, and A. Gilman, Eds., Macmillan,

New York, N.Y., 1980, p. 592.

20. "The Pharmacological Principles of Medical Practice," 7th ed., J. C. Krantz and C. J. Carr, Eds., Williams and Wilkins, Baltimore, Md., 1969, pp. 256–260.
21. L. Rosenberg, D. Stone, S. Shapiro, D. W. Kaufman, P. D. Stalley, and O. S. Mietinen, *Am. J. Epidemiol., 111,* 675 (1980).
22. L. Gould, M. K. Gofwami, C. V. Reddy, and R. F. Gomprecht, *J. Clin. Pharmacol., 13,* 469 (1973).
23. Boston Collaborative Drug Surveillance Program, *Lancet, 2,* 1278 (1972).
24. S. Heyden, *Z. Ernaehrung, 9,* 388 (1969).
25. J. A. Little, H. M. Shanoff, A. Csima, and R. Yano, *Lancet, 1,* 732 (1966).
26. J. F. Greden, P. Fontain, M. Lubersky, and K. Chamberlaine, *Am. J. Psychiat., 135,* 96 (1978).
27. T. Colton, R. E. Gosselin, and R. P. Smith, *Clin. Pharmacol. Ther., 9,* 31 (1968).
28. I. Karacan, J. I. Thornby, and A. M. Anch et al., *Clin. Pharmacol. Ther., 20* (6), 682–689 (1976).
29. K. H. Pieper, *Arzneim. Forsch., 13,* 585 (1963).
30. S. Cohen and G. H. Booth, *N. Engl. J. Med., 293,* 897 (1975).
31. *Federal Register, 45,* 205 (1980).
32. C. G. Moertel, D. L. Ahmann, W. F. Tyler, and N. Schwartau, *J. Am. Med. Assoc., 229,* 55 (1974).
33. L. J. Cass and W. S. Fredrik, *Curr. Ther. Res. Clin. Exp., 4,* 583 (1962).
34. M. Grotten, S. Dikstein, and F. G. Sulman, *Arch. Int. Pharmacodyn. Ther., 155,* 365 (1965).
35. R. C. Schnackenber, *Am. J. Psychiat., 130,* 796 (1973).
36. *FDA Drug Bulletin, 10* (3), 19–20 (1980).
37. E. W. Sutherland, G. A. Robinson, and R. W. Butcher, *Circulation, 37,* 279 (1968).
38. D. Robertson, C. Jurgen, M. Frolich, R. K. Carr, J. T. Watson, J. W. Hollifield, G. D. Shand, and J. A. Oates, *N. Engl. J. Med., 298,* 181 (1978).
39. C. Landis, in "Problems of Addiction and Habituation," Vol. 13, P. H. Hoch and J. Zubin, Eds., Grune and Stratton, New York, N.Y., pp. 37–48.
40. F. H. Myers, E. Jawetz, and A. Goldfein, "Review of Medical Pharmacology," 4th ed., Lange Medical, Los Altos, Calif., 1974, p. 678.
41. H. T. Debas, M. M. Cohen, I. B. Holubitsky, and R. C. Harrison, *Scand. J. Gastroenterol., 6,* 453 (1971).
42. J. Axelrod and J. Reichenthal, *J. Pharmacol. Exp. Ther., 107,* 519 (1953).
43. M. Inselvini and H. Casier, *Arch. Int. Pharmacodyn. Ther., 122,* 163 (1959).
44. E. M. Boyd, *Toxicol. Appl. Pharmacol., 1,* 258 (1959).
45. V. J. M. Dimaio and J. C. Garriott, *J. Forensic Sci., 3,* 275 (1975).

Sleep Aid and Sedative Product Table

Product (Manufacturer)	Antihistamine	Other Ingredients
Alva Taranquil-Span (Alval Amco)	chlorpheniramine	potassium bromide, potassium salicylate, L-tryptophan, niacin, niacinamide, thiamine
Alva Tranquil (Alval Amco)	chlorpheniramine	potassium bromide, potassium salicylate, L-tryptophan, niacin, niacinamide, thiamine
Compoz Tablets (Jeffrey Martin)	pyrilamine maleate, 25 mg	
Nervine Capsule-Shaped Tablets (Miles)	pyrilamine maleate, 25 mg	
Nytol Capsules and Tablets (Block)	pyrilamine maleate, 25 mg/tablet 50 mg/capsule	
Quiet Tabs (Commerce)	pyrilamine maleate, 25 mg	
Quiet World Tablets (Whitehall)	pyrilamine maleate, 25 mg	aspirin, 227.5 mg; acetaminophen, 162.5 mg
Relax-U-Caps (Columbia Medical)	pyrilamine maleate, 25 mg	
Sedacaps (Vitarine)	pyrilamine maleate, 25 mg	
Sleep-Eze Tablets (Whitehall)	pyrilamine maleate, 25 mg	
Sominex (J. B. Williams)	pyrilamine maleate, 25 mg	
Somnicaps (Amer. Pharm.)	pyrilamine maleate, 25 mg	
Tranquil Capsules (North American)	pyrilamine maleate, 25 mg	
Unisom (Leeming)	doxylamine succinate, 25 mg	

Stimulant Product Table

Product (Manufacturer)	Caffeine	Other Ingredients
Amostat Tablets (North American)	100 mg	
Caffedrine Capsules (Thompson Medical)	200 mg (timed release)	
Nodoz Tablets (Bristol-Myers)	100 mg	
Pep-Back (Alval Amco)	not stated	salicylamide
Quick-Pep Tablets (Thompson Medical)	150 mg	
Summit (Pfeiffer)	100 mg	acetaminophen, 325 mg
Tirend Tablets (Norcliff Thayer)	100 mg	
Valerianets Dispert (Alvin Last)		extract valerian, 50 mg
Vivarin Tablets (J. B. Williams)	200 mg	dextrose, 150 mg
Wakoz (Jeffrey Martin)	200 mg	

17 Menstrual Products

Barbara H. Korberly, Catherine A. Sohn, and Renee P. Tannenbaum

Questions to Ask the Patient

When was your last period? Was it late or early?

Do you use any contraceptive measures?

When does your pain occur in relation to the onset of your menstrual period?

How do your present symptoms vary from those of your normal cycle (flow, duration, and intensity)?

Are you under the care of a physician?

Do you have any vaginal discharge accompanied by pain, itching, pus, blood, or foul odor?

What have you already done to treat this problem?

Do you have any known drug allergies (aspirin)?

Are you taking any medicine for another condition?

Do you use tampons or sanitary napkins?

Menstruation (menses) is a regular physiologic condition in women during their childbearing years. In addition to the blood loss, many women experience unpleasant symptoms during various phases of the menstrual cycle, such as headaches, fluid retention, breast tenderness, irritability, anxiety, backache, abdominal pain and cramping, and depression.

The presence and intensity of these symptoms vary widely from one woman to another. The pharmacist should be able to interview and assess a woman's symptoms to determine their severity and whether physician referral is warranted. In addition, the pharmacist should be able to evaluate the many nonprescription preparations so that effective therapy and adjunctive measures can be recommended to help alleviate the patient's premenstrual or menstrual discomfort.

Recent recognition of the illness toxic shock syndrome has focused attention on the use of tampons, the risk associated with their use, and recommendations for their correct use.

Menstrual Cycle

The reproductive years of the female are characterized by monthly rhythmic changes in rates of secretion of female hormones necessary for reproduction. This rhythmic pattern is called the female sexual cycle or menstrual cycle. Two functions of the menstrual cycle are to release a mature ovum (egg) from an ovary and to prepare the uterine endometrium for implantation of the embryo should the ovum be fertilized during its course through the fallopian tube. In the absence of fertilization, the degenerated ovum is discarded along with the endometrial lining of the menstrual flow (menstruum) that passes through the cervix, down the vaginal canal, and out of the body (Figure 1A)(1).

Menstruation is this periodic, physiologic discharge of blood, mucus, and cellular debris from the uterine mucosa, which occurs at more or less regular intervals from puberty to menopause, except during pregnancy and lactation. The normal menstrual cycle is coordinated with the ovarian cycle and depends on the integrated functions of the endocrine and nervous system. Menarche, the occurrence of the first menstrual period, is a function of the maturation process of the young female. It is preceded by the development of required organ systems, a growth spurt, and early signs and appearance of secondary sex characteristics. It usually occurs at the end of the pubertal process.

The average age at which menstruation begins is between 12 and 13 years, but its onset may be as early as the 10th and as late as the 16th year. The onset of menstruation depends on such variables as race, genetic factors, environmental temperature conditions, and nutritional status. Menopause is the cessation of menstrual function and occurs on the average at 47 years of age, with a range of between 45 and 55 years of age. There are wide variations in the age at which menopause begins.

The duration of the normal female menstrual cycle averages 28 days. The first day of menstrual flow is considered to be day 1 of each new cycle. Each cycle may be as short as 20 days or as long as 45 days in normal, healthy women. There is, however, great variation among women and within the cycle of any individual woman. Variations in the menstrual cycle occur in relation to the woman's age, physical and emotional well-being, and environmental factors.

The duration of menstrual flow is also variable. The usual duration is between 3 and 7 days, but it can vary from as short as 2 days to as long as 8 days. For any

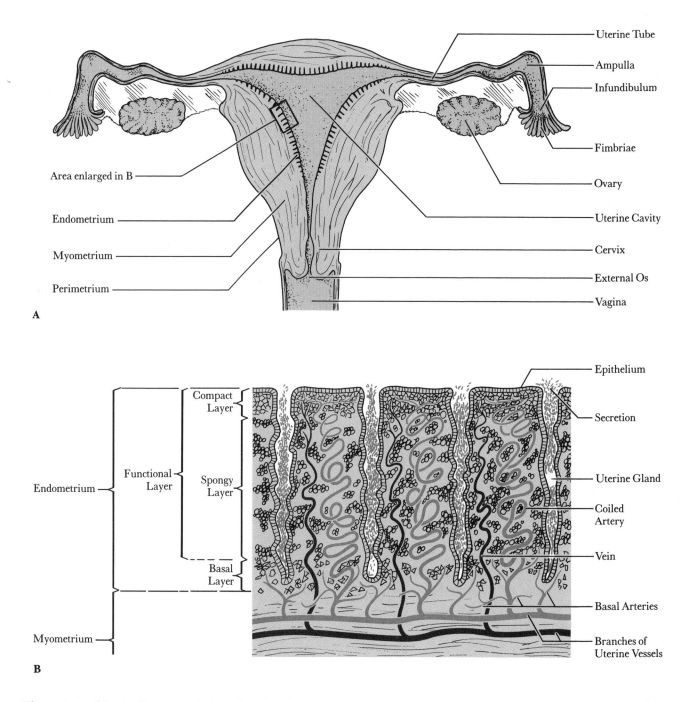

A

B

Figure 1A and B. A, diagrammatic frontal section of the uterus and uterine tubes. The ovaries and vagina are also indicated. **B**, enlargement of the area outlined in A. Modified from K. L. Moore, *The Developing Human:* "Clinically Oriented Embryology," 2nd ed., 1977, courtesy of W. B. Saunders Co.

individual woman, the menstrual flow is fairly constant. The amount of blood and tissue debris lost in menstruation averages about 70 ml, but many women lose considerably more (2). Women under 35 tend to lose more blood than those over 35 years of age. Although it is difficult to quantitate the amount of blood lost, studies indicate that a slight lowering of hemoglobin may occur even in healthy women with adequate diets. The total body fluid loss during menstruation may range from 60 to 200 ml. In the presence of malnutrition, poor dietary habits, and anemias of different etiologies, the significance of this menstrual blood loss on the development of iron deficiency anemia can be great (3).

The menstrual discharge has a characteristic dark reddish color due to the blood and mucosal breakdown products. The offensive odor of the menstruum is attributable to decomposed blood elements and the vulvar sebaceous gland secretions. In addition to the blood elements, the flow contains cervical mucus, vaginal mucosa, numerous bacteria, and degenerated endometrial particles. The odor and secretions of menstruation must be differentiated from the foul-sweet odor of *Trichomonas* species infections and the heavy, creamy secretions of vaginal yeast infections. (See Chapter 19, *Personal Care Products*.) These conditions usually warrant physician referral for prescription treatment.

Physiology

Hormone release is regulated by complex neuroendocrine feedback systems that are not yet fully understood.

The hypothalamus releases luteinizing hormone-releasing hormone (LH-RH). Under the influence of LH-RH, the anterior pituitary gland releases luteinizing hormone (LH) and follicle stimulating hormone (FSH). Luteinizing hormone and FSH are also called gonadotropic hormones. Under the influence of LH and FSH, the ovaries secrete estrogens and progesterone.

As previously stated, the primary results of the female sexual cycle are maturation of an ovum and development of the uterine endometrium to provide a life support system for a fertilized ovum (embryo). Maturation of the ovum is a function of the ovarian cycle and preparation of the uterus is the function of the endometrial cycle.

The ovarian cycle is regulated by cyclical increases and decreases in the levels of the gonadotropic hormones LH and FSH (Figure 2). At the beginning of each month of the female sexual cycle, at about the onset of menstruation, the concentration of FSH starts to increase. This hormonal increase causes follicles to develop within the ovary (follicular phase) (Figure 3), stimulating the maturation of an ovum as well as the release of estrogen from the ovary. The higher levels of estrogen trigger the release of LH from the anterior pituitary. Luteinizing hormone causes final maturation of the follicle and release of the mature ovum (ovulation) on day 14. The high levels of LH also cause the empty follicle to develop into the corpus luteum (luteal phase), which over the next 11–12 days secretes increasing levels of progesterone and estrogen (Figure 3). As the corpus luteum regresses on about the 26th day of the fe-

male cycle, the anterior pituitary gland begins to secrete FSH again (Figure 2), initiating new growth of a follicle and maturation of an ovum.

The endometrium, under the influence of the two ovarian hormones, estrogen and progesterone, exhibits characteristic cyclic changes that can be divided into a proliferative phase (estrogenic or follicular phase), the secretory phase (progestational or luteal phase), and the menstrual phase.

The proliferative phase of the endometrial cycle takes place from about day 5 to day 14 of the typical 28-day cycle (Figure 3). During menstruation (days 1–5) much of the endometrium is sloughed, leaving a thin endometrial lining. Under the influence of estrogens secreted by the ovaries, the stromal cells, epithelial gland cells, and blood vessels of the endometrium proliferate

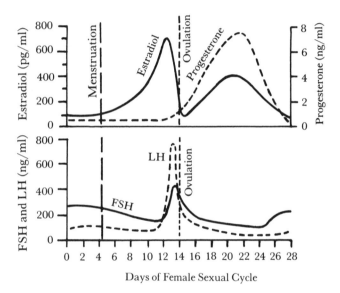

Figure 2. Plasma concentrations of the gonadotropins and ovarian hormones during the normal female sexual cycle. Reprinted with permission from A. C. Guyton, "Textbook of Medical Physiology," 6th ed. W. B. Saunders, Philadelphia, 1981, p. 1006.

rapidly (Figure 1B). By the time ovulation takes place on day 14, the endometrium is 2–3 mm thick (1).

During the secretory phase (days 15–27), progesterone from the newly formed corpus luteum of the ovary causes marked swelling and secretory development of the endometrium. The glandular cells begin to secrete small amounts of epithelial fluid, lipid and glycogen stores increase significantly in the stromal cells, and the blood supply increases in proportion to the secretory activity. The thickness of the endometrium approximately doubles during the secretory phase so that toward the end of the monthly cycle the endometrium has a thickness of 4–6 mm (1).

On approximately day 27, estrogen and progesterone levels decrease sharply due to regression of the corpus luteum. Tissue fluid and secretions decrease, as does the thickness of the endometrium. During the 24 hours preceding menstruation (day 28), the blood vessels leading to the mucosal layers of the endometrium become vasospastic, causing the endometrial tissues to become ischemic. It is thought that prostaglandins, primarily the PGF alpha group, cause the intense arterial spasm and smooth muscle contraction that occur just before menstruation (1). Necrosis and small vessel hemorrhage begins to develop, causing the outer layers of the endometrium to separate from the uterus. The sloughed tissue and blood in the uterine cavity initiates further uterine contractions that expel the uterine contents, starting the menstrual flow (day 1 of the new cycle) (1).

Menstrual Abnormalities

Dysmenorrhea

Dysmenorrhea is a term used to describe painful menstruation, one of the most common gynecologic disorders in nulliparous women. About 50% of women are affected by mild cramp-like symptoms that occur at the onset of menses and disappear within 1–2 days without restricting normal activities. About 10% of women experience severe cramping pain strongest over the lower abdomen, which is often accompanied by systemic symptoms including nausea, vomiting, diarrhea, head-

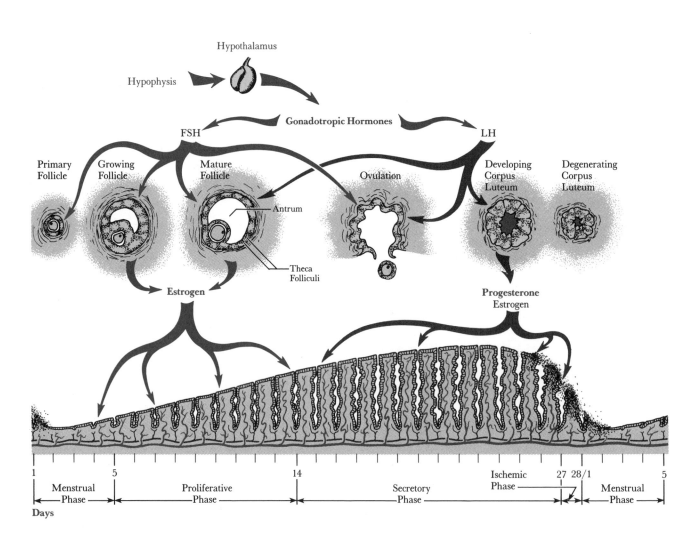

Figure 3. Schematic drawing illustrating the interrelations of the hypothalamus, hypophysis (pituitary gland), ovaries, and endometrium. One complete menstrual cycle and the beginning of another are shown. Changes in the ovaries, called the ovarian cycle, are promoted by the gonadotropic hormones (FSH and LH). Hormones from the ovaries (estrogens and progesterone) then promote changes in the structure and function of the endometrium. Thus, the cyclical activity of the ovary is intimately linked with changes in the uterus. K. L. Moore, *The Developing Human*; "Clinically Oriented Embryology," 2nd ed., 1977, courtesy of W. B. Saunders Co.

ache, and dizziness. This group is usually incapacitated by the pain that occurs most often during the first few days of menses.

When dysmenorrhea occurs in the absence of any pelvic disease it is referred to as primary dysmenorrhea. When dysmenorrhea occurs because of an underlying condition, such as endometriosis, fibroids, or pelvic inflammatory disease, it is termed secondary dysmenorrhea.

In the past, many theories have attempted to explain or associate primary dysmenorrhea with psychological factors. Although psychogenic factors may affect the assessment of pain, there has been no evidence that these factors are important in the etiology of dysmenorrhea. Evidence suggests that endogenous prostaglandins may play a role in primary dysmenorrhea (4). The intrauterine production of prostaglandins at menstruation may be regulated by ovarian steroid hormones, such as estradiol, which is at high levels after ovulation and before the development of menstruation. Evidence of increased concentrations of prostaglandins and prostaglandin metabolites have been found in the menstrual fluid, endometrium, and peripheral circulation of women with primary dysmenorrhea. Since endogenous prostaglandins may play a role in primary dysmenorrhea, any drug that inhibits their synthesis may be effective in reducing pain and other systemic symptoms.

Intrauterine devices (IUD's) used for contraception may cause severe uterine bleeding and/or pain. This is generally due to the degree of endometrial compression and myometrial distention caused by the IUD. It has been postulated that endometrial trauma induced by the presence of the IUD may enhance the biosynthesis of prostaglandins, which would be the etiology for secondary dysmenorrhea. These problems are often a common cause for removal of the device.

Amenorrhea

Amenorrhea is the lack of menstruation. Amenorrhea is classified as primary if the female has never menstruated and secondary if there is a cessation of menses for longer than 3 months. Primary amenorrhea usually refers to the failure of menses to occur before the 18th birthday and is usually associated with chromosomal, pituitary, or ovarian dysfunction (3).

The most common causes of secondary amenorrhea are pregnancy, lactation, and menopause. Menstruation does not occur in pregnancy due to the secretion of progesterone and estrogen from the corpus luteum and later due to the formation of the placenta, which secretes tremendous amounts of progesterone to maintain the endometrium during pregnancy. Menstruation stops at menopause due to failure of the ovary to respond to gonadotropins.

Breast feeding will inhibit ovulation and menstruation in about 50% of nursing mothers. It is hypothesized that the same nervous signals from the breasts to the hypothalamus that cause prolactin secretion during suckling simultaneously inhibits LH-RH by the hypothalamus, thus inhibiting release of the gonadotropic hormones, LH and FSH (1). Although continual (round-the-clock) breast feeding provides some protection against pregnancy, it cannot be relied upon as a contraceptive measure (5).

When evaluating amenorrhea in a patient who is not pregnant, lactating, or postmenopausal, ovarian function should be determined. A common cause of amenorrhea in a woman of childbearing age is the cessation of oral contraceptive therapy. Such cases usually require physician supervision but rarely reflect any serious problem. Less common causes of amenorrhea include genetic defects (Turner's syndrome), primary disorders of the uterus, hypothalamic disorders, adrenal disorders, and primary ovarian or pituitary failure. These patients should be evaluated based on the age of onset and duration of symptoms.

Intermenstrual Pain and Bleeding

Intermenstrual pain (termed "mittelschmerz") usually occurs at mid-cycle and may last from a few hours to a few days. The pain may be accompanied by various amounts of bleeding.

There appears to be a relationship between intermenstrual pain, bleeding, and ovulation. The etiology of the pain is unknown but may be inflammation of the ovulatory site itself or peritoneal irritation from follicular fluid released at ovulation (3). The bleeding may occur due to a temporary decrease in estrogen levels and, if slight, no treatment is necessary. If bleeding is severe, diagnostic measures should be employed to rule out other etiologies such as intrauterine lesions.

Premenstrual Syndrome

Many woman suffer from a recurrent complex of symptoms known as premenstrual syndrome. Although symptoms usually begin 2–3 days before the onset of menses, they may also occur toward the end of menses. The onset of symptoms varies among women but is usually constant in the cycle of any one woman.

The premenstrual syndrome encompasses a variety of symptoms with severity ranging from mild to incapacitating. Questionnaire data indicate that 70–90% of women admit to recurrent premenstrual symptoms, with 20–40% reporting some degree of temporary mental or physical incapacitation (5). Symptoms of premenstrual tension include the following:

- **Psychological**—irritability, lethargy, depression, anxiety, sleep disorders, crying spells, hostility;
- **Neurologic**—headache (migraines usually occur the week preceding menstruation), dizziness, fainting, seizures (occur rarely in epileptic patients);
- **Breasts**—tenderness, swelling;
- **Gastrointestinal**—constipation, abdominal bloating, abdominal cramping, craving for sweets;
- **Extremities**—edema;
- **Urinary**—less frequent urination;
- **Skin**—acne.

The most common psychological symptom of premenstrual syndrome is tension, hence the term "premenstrual tension." Its onset often is heralded by sudden mood swings and is characterized by depression, irritability, and lethargy. An increased thirst or appetite accompanied by a craving for sweets and salty foods is common.

One of the most common physical symptoms experienced by women is premenstrual edema or bloating, especially apparent as enlarged, tender breasts, abdominal swelling, swollen feet or ankles, and a puffy face. If severe, weight gain of up to 9 lb may result. However, the majority of women gain no more than 5 lb. Once menstruation has begun, there is noticeable polyuria and rapid disappearance of edema.

The pathogenesis of the premenstrual syndrome remains speculative; however, evidence suggests that it is associated with the cyclic nature of the hypothalamic-pituitary-ovarian axis (6). It has been suggested that the premenstrual syndrome results from the precipitous drop in progesterone levels that occurs at the time of menstruation or from elevated estrogen levels. Others suggest that high levels of prolactin, deficiencies in vitamin B_6 or vitamin A, or hypoglycemia may produce the symptoms. Many have suggested an underlying psychogenic disorder. Another hypothesis suggests that since water retention is so common, premenstrual edema may be a manifestation of an underlying neuroendocrine disorder involving estrogen, aldosterone, vasopressin, prolactin, and/or dopamine (6). However, it appears that symptoms result from changing levels of prostaglandins and neurotransmitters that ultimately affect mood. Increased prostaglandin levels may be responsible for many symptoms seen in the premenstrual syndrome such as joint pains, breast tenderness, headaches, and nausea (7). One hypothesis concerning the premenstrual syndrome suggests that the intermediate lobe of the pituitary gland may be involved through effects of melanocyte-stimulating hormone and endorphins (6). No one hypothesis has yet explained the full spectrum of symptoms composing the premenstrual syndrome.

Patient Assessment

Most women who purchase nonprescription menstrual cycle products are otherwise healthy females, who are experiencing midcycle or premenstrual fluid retention, headache, or abdominal cramping characteristic of the premenstrual syndrome. Before recommending any product for a patient, the pharmacist should establish whether the symptoms are related to normal functional menstrual discomforts, similar to symptoms of previous cycles, or if they are unusually severe for her typical menstrual pattern.

Any irregularities concerning the frequency, volume, or character of the menstrual discharge or any comments of unusually pronounced pain and/or fluid retention indicate the need for immediate referral to a gynecologist.

If evaluation indicates that the discomfort is related to the woman's normal menstrual cycle, the pharmacist should inquire about products previously taken for relief of symptoms so as to avoid recommending any product that has failed to give her relief. It is most important to determine whether the patient was taking a full therapeutic dose of an agent because so many nonprescription products promoted for menstrual and premenstrual symptoms contain doses of ingredients that would be subtherapeutic if given alone. The presence or absence

of salicylate allergy (aspirin allergy) should always be verified. Recommendations for any nonprescription product should be accompanied by appropriate patient counseling regarding proper use and dosing and any other adjunctive measures.

Dysmenorrhea

Before recommending any product for a patient, it is important for the pharmacist to establish the onset of pain in relation to menses. Primary dysmenorrhea produces pain that occurs before or during the first 2 days of menses. Pain that occurs during the first few days of menses and increases in severity throughout menses may suggest underlying pathology; these patients with secondary dysmenorrhea should be referred to a physician for evaluation.

Therapy for primary dysmenorrhea should begin with therapeutic doses of nonprescription analgesics such as aspirin or acetaminophen. Ideally, the drug should be started 1 day before the onset of the menses. There are no clinical data that document the superiority of advertised menstrual products over plain aspirin or acetaminophen. Should patients not obtain relief of symptoms from these analgesics, physician referral for a therapeutic trial of nonsteroidal anti-inflammatory agents can be recommended based on clinical studies demonstrating efficacy in their ability to inhibit prostaglandins.

Amenorrhea

Any patient developing primary or secondary amenorrhea must be evaluated by a physician. The most common causes of secondary amenorrhea are pregnancy, lactation, menopause, and withdrawal of oral contraceptives. Other etiologies that must be considered are disorders of the hypothalamus, pituitary gland, adrenal gland, ovaries, and uterus.

Intermenstrual Pain and Bleeding

Many women experience pain and bleeding for brief periods between menses. This discomfort is generally associated with ovulation. Therapeutic doses of analgesics such as aspirin or acetaminophen may be recommended for relief of pain of less than 2 days' duration. If pain is severe, or bleeding continues for more than 2 days, the patient should be referred to a physician (8).

Premenstrual Syndrome

The premenstrual syndrome is a recognized clinical entity affecting a large portion of the female population (6). Because no single etiology has been established, many treatment alternatives have been proposed based on anecdotal reports. Oral contraceptives have been shown to relieve dysmenorrhea but not to alleviate other associated symptoms of abdominal bloating and fluid retention. Reports using various vitamin therapies remain unsubstantiated by double-blind trials and are regarded as placebo therapy.

Treatment

Pharmacologic Agents

There are several types of nonprescription pharmacologic agents available for the treatment of dysmenorrhea and premenstrual syndrome.

Analgesics

In the treatment of primary dysmenorrhea, the first objective of therapy is to rule out secondary dysmenorrhea. Selection of a drug for primary dysmenorrhea should begin with the nonprescription analgesics. Most nonprescription products contain either aspirin or acetaminophen as the analgesic. Aspirin is an inhibitor of prostaglandin synthesis. The exact effect of acetaminophen on prostaglandin synthesis is unclear. Aspirin and acetaminophen have equivalent analgesic efficacy for headache and other minor pains (9). Equivalence and efficacy in menstrual pain has not yet been determined. However, both agents are routinely used for menstrual pain and are rated as safe when taken in the recommended nonprescription doses of 325–650 mg every 4 hours, not to exceed 4,000 mg in 24 hours for not more than 10 days (9).

Before recommending aspirin, the pharmacist should question the patient regarding aspirin allergy; disease states that may preclude the use of salicylates such as bleeding disorders, ulcers, and asthma; and any current medicines that may interact with these compounds such as anticoagulants, probenecid, phenytoin, and oral hypoglycemic agents. The pharmacist should caution patients to use acetaminophen within the recommended dosages because of its potential for hepatotoxicity in massive overdose. (See Chapter 11, *Internal Analgesic Products*.)

The nonprescription products available for the relief of menstrual pain have never been shown to be more effective than aspirin or acetaminophen alone. Whenever possible, the pharmacist should suggest either aspirin or acetaminophen in the recommended doses as the first approach to the therapy of primary dysmenorrhea.

Clinical trials have shown that nonsteroidal prostaglandin inhibitors (flufenamic acid, ibuprofen, indomethacin, mefenamic acid, naproxen, and tolmetin sodium) provide significant relief of primary dysmenorrhea. These agents have been shown to be more effective than aspirin or acetaminophen with minimal adverse effects. However, the safety of long-term, intermittent use of these agents has not been established. Referral to a physician for a trial with these agents is warranted when nonprescription analgesics are not effective.

Since primary dysmenorrhea occurs in ovulatory cycles, oral contraceptives that suppress ovulation and lower the prostaglandin concentration have been used. Both the nonsteroidal anti-inflammatory agents and oral contraceptives require the recommendation and supervision of a physician.

Antihistamines

Many menstrual products contain various amounts of antihistamines such as pyrilamine maleate. Pyrilamine is an antihistamine included in many premenstrual products for the relief of symptoms associated with the premenstrual syndrome. It has been rated as safe and effective, although patients should be warned of possible drowsiness from the antihistamine.

Sympathomimetic Amines

Phenylpropanolamine hydrochloride, ephedrine sulfate, and cinnamedrine hydrochloride are sympathomimetic amines found in products used in the treatment of premenstrual syndrome. Sympathomimetic amines do have a relaxant effect upon the uterus, but clinical studies have not been completed to indicate whether phenylpropanolamine or ephedrine are effective for this purpose (10). The manufacturer using cinnamedrine in its product cites unpublished studies to support its claims for use, but the real value of cinnamedrine has not been established, and it has been placed in category III (11).

Adverse effects associated with the use of sympathomimetic amines include nervousness, restlessness, and headache, all symptoms associated with "premenstrual tension." Before recommending products containing sympathomimetic amines, the pharmacist must ascertain that the patient is not being treated with prescription products containing reserpine, guanethidine, methyldopa, propranolol, or monoamine oxidase inhibitors, or nonprescription products containing sympathomimetic amines or ammonium chloride (12). Urinary acidification by ammonium chloride enhances urinary excretion of sympathomimetic amines with reduced therapeutic activity (12). In addition, these products should be used with caution in patients with diabetes mellitus, heart disease, hypertension, or thyroid disease. (See Chapter 10, *Asthma Products*, and Chapter 15, *Weight Control Products*.)

Diuretics

Many menstrual products contain doses of diuretic agents that would be subtherapeutic if taken individually; they have been approved as safe and effective when used in combination. The most frequently used agents include ammonium chloride, caffeine, and pamabrom.

Ammonium Chloride Ammonium chloride is an acid-forming salt with limited value (1–2 days' duration) in promoting diuresis. There are no large-scale studies of the use of this diuretic alone in premenstrual syndrome. However, one double-blind crossover clinical trial compared the effectiveness of ammonium chloride (325 mg) and caffeine (100 mg) with placebo for the relief of symptoms associated with premenstrual weight gain in 22 women. The ammonium chloride and caffeine combination induced a statistically significant greater reduction in weight compared with placebo [mean weight change of ≤ 1.5 lb. (0.7 kg)]. Subjective evaluation indicated a more favorable attitude in subjects given ammonium chloride and caffeine compared with those given placebo (13).

The FDA has concluded that ammonium chloride in combination with caffeine is rational since the diuretic mechanisms of action are different and adjunctive.

Large doses of ammonium chloride (4–12 g/day) are associated with GI symptoms including nausea and vomiting, even when administered after meals. Central nervous system toxicity, including headache, hyperventilation, drowsiness, and mental confusion, may occur. The drug is contraindicated in patients with impaired renal and liver function because metabolic acidosis may result.

Caffeine   Caffeine is incorporated in various nonprescription products to alleviate the mental and physical fatigue that commonly accompanies water retention during the premenstrual period.

Doses of caffeine between 100 and 200 mg taken not more than every 3–4 hours have been classified by the FDA advisory review panel on nonprescription stimulant drug products as safe and effective for use as a stimulant (14). It is approved as safe and effective in menstrual products as a diuretic for the relief of symptoms associated with the menses.

As a member of the xanthine family, caffeine promotes diuresis by inhibition of renal tubular reabsorption of sodium and chloride. However, documented effectiveness of caffeine as a diuretic is lacking. Doses above 100 mg may provoke gastric irritation by augmenting gastric secretions. Coffee, cola, or tea drinkers should consider this when taking caffeine-containing products.

Pamabrom   Pamabrom is marketed in combination with analgesics and antihistamines for the relief of the premenstrual syndrome. As a derivative of theophylline, pamabrom has weak diuretic properties, and is approved as safe and effective as a diuretic in menstrual products. Manufacturers' recommendations suggest that combination products be taken for 4–7 days before the onset of menstruation. Daily doses of pamabrom should not exceed 200 mg.

Miscellaneous Ingredients

Various agents such as uva ursi, zea mays, buchu, and triticum (common couch grass) are included for a "diuretic" action in some of the combination menstrual products. There are no clinical data to support their efficacy as diuretics for the treatment of dysmenorrhea. These agents should not be recommended.

Other ingredients are found in various menstrual products, but their value is questionable. Homatropine methylbromide and atropine sulfate are present in subtherapeutic dosages. Even at these doses, however, patients with glaucoma should not use products containing these anticholinergic agents.

Alternative Therapy

A rational, professional approach to treating premenstrual syndrome consists of dietary modification to prevent edema formation through salt restriction and avoidance of salt-rich foods before menstruation. Since premenstrual edema is generally asymptomatic and self-limiting, more potent prescription diuretics are seldom necessary. In addition, the potential side effects, such as electrolyte imbalance, may outweigh the psychological benefit of diureses for the majority of patients.

However, for a patient significantly troubled with premenstrual edema, the pharmacist may refer the patient to her physician for prescription of a limited quantity of a mild diuretic.

Related Menstrual Products

Feminine Cleansing Products

The pharmacist should be familiar with the available feminine hygiene products and should know what, if anything, to recommend under a given set of circumstances. (See Chapter 19, *Personal Care Products.*)

Feminine Napkins and Tampons

Feminine napkins are pads that are used to absorb menstrual or other vaginal discharges. They are made of absorbent cotton, synthetic, or cellulose material (derived from wood pulp) and covered with a lightweight paper gauze to decrease irritation. A layer of cellulose or thin plastic is incorporated into the side of the pad worn away from the perineum to minimize leakage and soiling of undergarments.

Feminine napkins are available in a wide variety of sizes and absorbencies. Some require a belt to hold them in place on the perineum so they can effectively absorb the menstruum, but most newer styles are held in place with adhesive strips on the underside of the pad, which affixes to the woman's undergarment.

Since most women experience their heaviest menstrual flow on day 2 of the menstrual cycle, "super" napkins or "maxi" pads may be used at this time. The napkins should be changed frequently to minimize the development of unpleasant odors arising from the breakdown of blood products and vaginal secretions. During days of heaviest flow, napkins may need to be changed every 2–4 hours, while changing every 4–6 hours may be adequate for days of lesser menstrual flow. Frequent changing of sanitary pads also helps to minimize the degree of irritation or chafing of the upper inner thigh associated with napkin use. Dusting this area with a talcum powder may also alleviate chafing. The goal is to allow maximum absorption of discharged fluid and to minimize odor and risk of irritation and infection.

"Mini" or "light" pads and "junior" or "teen" napkins are designed to accommodate the smaller anatomy and lighter flow of the adolescent female. The narrower width of the pads may reduce chafing and irritation. Many women prefer the new, less cumbersome light pads for the first and last days of their cycles. These light pads or the new, thin shields also may be used to protect undergarments from being stained by vaginal cream, suppository leakage, or normal vaginal secretions.

Tampons are intravaginal inserts, made of cellulose or synthetic materials, designed to absorb menstrual or other vaginal discharge. They have the advantage over feminine napkins of being worn internally, which lessens chafing, odor, bulkiness, and irritation. Until reports associated tampon use with toxic shock syndrome, marketing data estimated that 70–80% of menstruating women in the United States used tampons (15). Some women use both a tampon and napkin on days of heavy menstrual flow or on days when they know their schedule will not permit frequent changing. However, this prolonged wearing should be discouraged, in light of evidence associating this practice with a higher risk of microvaginal ulceration and infection (16).

Tampons labeled "deodorant" have been renamed by the FDA as "scented" since none of the available products contains an effective antimicrobial agent (17). Some fragrance materials may cause local irritation and allergic reactions, such as allergic contact dermatitis, because mucosal surfaces readily absorb these materials.

Before 1977, all tampons were made of rayon or rayon and cotton materials. Since then, 44% of tampon products (65% of the estimated market) have contained newer, more absorbent synthetic materials. Both absorbency types have been documented to cause vaginal mucosal drying, epithelial changes, and microulcerations; however, the incidence is much higher in women using the superabsorbent tampons. Most microulcerations are asymptomatic and resolve spontaneously, but some were still present in preovulatory phase in up to 31% of women examined. Tampon use over a period of several months to years has also been associated with cervicovaginal ulcerations. The immediate and long-term clinical significance of these findings has yet to be demonstrated.

The FDA's advisory review panel in the division of obstetrics and gynecology evaluated femine napkins and tampons and classified unscented menstrual pads into performance Class I. This classification indicates that the device meets only the general controls applicable to all devices. The FDA advisory review panel has classified "scented" menstrual pads and both unscented and scented menstrual tampons into performance Class II, which requires the future development of standards to ensure the safety and efficacy of the products (17).

Toxic Shock Syndrome

Toxic shock syndrome (TSS) is an illness that can develop in young, otherwise healthy, women in association with tampon use during menstruation (15, 18, 19). The disease complex is characterized by the sudden onset of

- High fever (102° or greater);
- Diffuse erythematous, macular, sunburn-like rash that subsequently desquamates, most notably on the palms and soles;
- Low systolic blood pressure of < 90 mm Hg in an adult (shock or hypotension).

In addition, the patient with TSS may present with at least four of the following symptoms:

- Nausea, vomiting, or diarrhea;
- Severe myalgias;
- Sore throat;
- Renal failure (decrease in urinary output);
- Low platelet counts, bruising, and/or bleeding;

- Hepatic failure (rise in level enzymes and bilirubin);
- Irritability, disorientation, and/or coma;
- Hypotension, shock, arrhythmias, and/or adult respiratory distress syndrome.

Steps should be taken to rule out meningococcemia, Rocky Mountain spotted fever, or bacterial sepsis. Ninety-five percent of TSS cases occur in women during or within 48 hours of ending their menstrual period (especially days 2–4). Blood and throat cultures are negative for bacteria; however, vaginal cultures are frequently positive.

From January 1 through October 16, 1980, 408 cases of TSS were reported to the Center for Disease Control (CDC), with a mortality of 10%. The estimates of a woman's risk for development of TSS range from 3 to 6.2 cases/100,000 women of menstruating age (12–49 years)/year. Risk was determined to be highest in women using tampons continually throughout menstruation (15). The etiologic agent is suspected to be a select type of *Staphylococcus aureus*, colonizing the skin or vagina, which produces an enterotoxin that subsequently is absorbed and is responsible for the systemic complex of symptoms. A large number of cases of TSS occurred in women using the new, superabsorbent synthetic cellulose tampons, marketed under the brand name Rely (Procter and Gamble); however, TSS has been documented with all brands in a study reported to the CDC including (in decreasing order of frequency) Rely (used by 71% of patients), Playtex (19%), Tampax (5%), Kotex (2%), and o.b. (2%) (20). The Rely brand tampons were removed from the market by the manufacturer under a consent agreement with the FDA, although it had not been documented that the increased rate of occurrence was directly related to the Rely product. It has been proposed that the different frequency of occurrence could be due to greater use of Rely product in the population at risk. However, the risk factors for TSS remain controversial because subsequent studies by the CDC failed to demonstrate a significant difference in occurrence in patients who developed TSS versus control subjects who did not, based on brand of tampon, degree of absorbency, inclusion of a deodorant (fragrance) ingredient, or frequency of tampon changing (18).

The unacceptably high mortality, in otherwise young, healthy women, initially reported to be between 3% and 10%, has most frequently been associated with severe hypotensive shock. Successful treatment may necessitate administration of large volumes of intravenous fluids to maintain circulation and cardiac output. Occasionally, dialysis has been reported to be necessary for management of transient uremia and renal failure. The use of beta-lactamase-resistant antibiotics such as nafcillin or a cephalosporin has not affected the outcome of severity of individual cases of TSS, but has reduced the rate of recurrence (19).

Current recommendations to patients regarding TSS include

- Women who use tampons and who have not had TSS are at a very low risk of TSS and need not change their pattern of tampon use; however, they may decrease an already small risk by avoiding the use of tampons entirely.

- Tampons should be changed 4–6 times/day.
- Intermittent use of tampons and sanitary napkins (using tampons for only a portion of the menstrual cycle or use of sanitary napkins at night if tampons are worn during the day).
- Any patient developing sudden onset of high fever, sunburn-like rash, hypotension, vomiting, and diarrhea should immediately remove tampon and seek emergency medical treatment (fluids may be required for shock and possible beta-lactamase-resistant antibiotics for vaginal *Staphylococcus aureus*).
- Women who have had TSS are at a much higher risk (up to 45% in one study) of developing recurrences, and should not use tampons for several menstrual cycles after their illness unless eradication of *Staphylococcus aureus* from vaginal flow has been documented.

The pharmacist is in a unique setting to evaluate the data on TSS and educate patients on current recommendations. The FDA advisory review committee is evaluating proposals for product labeling and consumer information inserts on tampon use and TSS. The proposed warning statement required on packages of menstrual tampons, as of October 21, 1980, reads (20):

WARNING Tampons have been associated with toxic shock syndrome, a rare disease that can be fatal. You can almost entirely avoid the risk of getting this disease by not using tampons. You can reduce the risk by using tampons on and off during your period. If you have a fever of 102° or more and vomit or get diarrhea during your period, remove the tampon at once and see a doctor right away.

Summary

Premenstrual and menstrual pain is a frequent problem in the majority of women. In most cases, nonprescription analgesics such as aspirin and acetaminophen are efficacious. In some women, nonsteroidal anti-inflammatory agents for pain and prescription diuretics for premenstrual edema may be required. The pharmacist should remember that menstruation is a normal physiologic process. Although it has been characterized as an "emotional monthly upheaval," it is not for the majority of women who function normally and require little to no pharmacologic intervention during this time.

Specific problems identified in this chapter, such as dysmenorrhea, amenorrhea, and significant premenstrual edema, require careful evaluation and physician referral in most instances.

References

1. A. C. Guyton, "Textbook of Medical Physiology," 6th ed., W. B. Saunders, Philadelphia, Pa., 1981, pp. 1005–1016.
2. R. C. Benson, "Handbook of Obstetrics and Gynecology," Lange Medical, Los Altos, Calif., 1980, pp. 28–37.
3. "Harrison's Principles of Internal Medicine," 9th ed., G. W. Thorn, R. D. Adams, E. Braunwald, K. G. Isselbacher, and R. G. Petersdorf, Eds., McGraw-Hill, New York, N.Y., 1980, pp. 224–229.
4. O. Ylikorkala and M. Y. Dawood, *Am. J. Obstet. Gynecol., 130,* 833 (1978).
5. "Current Obstetric and Gynecologic Diagnosis and Treatment," Ralph C. Benson, 3rd ed., Lange Medical, Los Altos, Calif., 1980, pp. 112–119.
6. R. L. Reid and S. S. Yen, *Am. J. Obstet. Gynecol., 135,* 85 (1981).
7. P. W. Budoff, "No More Menstrual Cramps and Other Good News," Putman and Sons, New York, N.Y., 1980, pp. 53–75.
8. E. R. Novak, G. S. Jones, and H. W. Jones, "Novak's Textbook of Gynecology," 9th ed., Williams and Wilkins, Baltimore, Md., 1976, pp. 58–96.
9. *Federal Register, 43,* 35346 (1977).
10. "Martindale, The Extra Pharmacopoeia," 27th ed, The Pharmaceutical Press, London, England, 1978, p. 11.
11. R. W. Soller, Glenbrook Laboratories, New York, N.Y. Personal communication, September 8, 1981.
12. P. D. Hansten, "Drug Interactions," 4th ed., Lea and Febiger, Philadelphia, Pa., 1979, pp. 22, 266.
13. J. J. Hoffman, *Curr. Ther. Res., 26,* 575 (1979).
14. *Federal Register, 43,* 25561 (1978).
15. J. P. Davis, P. J. Chesney, P. J. Wand, and M. LaVenture, *N. Engl. J. Med., 303,* 1429 (1980).
16. E. G. Friedrich and K. A. Siegesmund, *Obstet. Gynecol., 55,* 149 (1980).
17. *Federal Register, 45,* 12713 (1980).
18. K. N. Shands, G. P. Schmid, B. B. Dan, D. Blum, J. Guidotti, N. T. Hargrett, R. L. Anderson, D. L. Hill, C. V. Broome, J. D. Bond, and D. W. Fraser, *N. Engl. J. Med., 303,* 1436 (1980).
19. *Morbidity and Mortality Weekly Report, 30,* 25 (1981).
20. *Federal Register, 45,* 69840 (1980).

Menstrual Product Table

Product[a] (Manufacturer)	Analgesic	Diuretic	Antihistamine	Caffeine	Other Ingredients
A-Nuric (Alvin Last)		buchu powdered extract, 65 mg couch grass powdered extract hydrangea powdered extract			
Aqua-Ban (Thompson Medical)		ammonium chloride, 325 mg		100 mg	
Cardui (Chattem)	acetaminophen, 325 mg	pamabrom, 25 mg	pyrilamine maleate, 12.5 mg		
Diurex (Alval Amco)	potassium salicylate	uva ursi buchu		not stated	salicylamide juniper berries methylene blue magnesium trisilicate
Diurex-2 (Alval Amco)	potassium salicyclate	uva ursi buchu		not stated	salicylamide iron juniper berries methylene blue magnesium trisilicate
Diurex Long Acting (Alval Amco)	potassium salicylate	uva ursi buchu		not stated	riboflavin
Femcaps (Buffington)	acetaminophen				ephedrine sulfate, 8 mg atropine sulfate, 0.03 mg
Flowaway Water 100's (DeWitt)		uva ursi extract, 98 mg buchu leaves extract, 24 mg		20 mg	potassium nitrate, 171 mg
Fluidex (O'Connor)		buchu powdered extract, 65 mg couch grass powdered extract, 65 mg corn silk powdered extract, 32.5 mg hydrangea powdered extract, 32.5 mg			
Fluidex-Plus with Diadax (O'Connor)		buchu powdered extract, 65 mg couch grass powdered extract, 65 mg corn silk powdered extract, 32.5 mg hydrangea powdered extract, 32.5 mg			phenylpropanolamine hydrochloride, 25 mg
Humphrey's No. 11 (Humphrey's Pharmacal)					cimicifuga, 3X pulsatilla, 3X sepia, 3X
Lydia E. Pinkham Tablets (Cooper Vision Pharmaceuticals, Inc.)					extract of Jamaica dogwood pleurisy root licorice dried ferrous sulfate, 75 mg

Menstrual Product Table, continued

Product[a] (Manufacturer)	Analgesic	Diuretic	Antihistamine	Caffeine	Other Ingredients
Lydia E. Pinkham Vegetable Compound Liquid (Cooper Vision Pharmaceuticals, Inc.)					extract of Jamaica dogwood pleurisy root licorice alcohol, 13.5%
Midol (Glenbrook)	aspirin, 454 mg			32.4 mg	cinnamedrine, 14.9 mg
Odrinil (Fox)		buchu powdered extract, 32.4 mg uva ursi powdered extract, 32.4 mg corn silk powdered extract, 32.4 mg juniper powdered extract, 16.2 mg		50 mg	
Pamprin (Chattem)	acetaminophen, 325 mg	pamabrom, 25 mg	pyrilamine maleate, 12.5 mg		
Sunril (Schering)	acetaminophen, 300 mg	pamabrom, 50 mg	pyrilamine maleate, 25 mg		
Trendar (Whitehall)	acetaminophen, 325 mg	pamabrom, 25 mg			
Tri-Aqua (Pfeiffer)				100 mg	

[a] Tablet unless specified otherwise.

18 Contraceptive Methods and Products

Luis Hernandez

Questions to Ask the Patient

Have you spoken with your physician or a family-planning service regarding the best type of contraceptive method for you? If so, what was recommended?

Are you presently using a contraceptive method or product? If so, what do you use and why do you wish to use another method?

Have you had any problems such as irritation, allergies, or inconvenience that you feel may be related to the contraceptive method/product you have been using?

Promoting family planning and reducing the incidence of sexually transmitted disease are among the objectives established by the U.S. Department of Health and Human Services for improving the health of people living in the United States during the 1980's (1).

Improvement in the public health is expected to be accomplished primarily through education and information measures, utilizing practicing professionals and health educators. Pharmacists can play an important role by providing information and counseling on nonprescription contraceptive methods. The pharmacist may be the only professional contact for people who use nonprescription contraceptives (2).

The role of the pharmacist in providing this information takes on greater significance in light of the controversy surrounding the most effective prescription agents, the oral contraceptives and the intrauterine device (IUD). In recent years, questions concerning the safety of these agents have led to a decline in their use and a return to the safer, barrier methods of contraception.

Family planning is a health measure intended to improve maternal and infant health and the emotional and social well-being of both individuals and the family unit. Although the current trend is for smaller, planned families [by 1976, 68% of married couples in the United States were using contraception (1)], contraceptive information and methods still are not fully available to the groups at highest risk of morbidity, mortality, and socioeconomic adverse effects related to pregnancy. These high-risk groups include teenagers, unmarried women, and women over the age of 34.

Illegitimate births and unwanted pregnancies are frequent occurrences (3, 4); unmarried women contribute 14.2% of all births, and 14 million unplanned pregnancies occur each year (5). More than 750,000 unmarried teenagers become pregnant each year (6).

Teenage pregnancies present a special problem due in part to the epidemic proportions in which they are occurring. In the past decade, the rate of illegitimate births among women 15–17 years old increased 49% (7).

Pharmacists are the most accessible health professionals, not only because of the informal nature of the pharmacy consultation, but because of the relative anonymity that such an informal encounter provides. Many teenagers are embarrassed and often are anxious that their parents will be contacted. The pharmacist can provide this group with professional advice and may be the only professional contact a teenager feels is available to him or her. It is especially important when advising all patients that the pharmacist provide an atmosphere of understanding and privacy and accurate, unbiased information on contraception.

The pharmacist can provide another service to teenaged patients and, indeed, to all patients. The only product that effectively prevents the spread of venereal diseases is the condom and the pharmacist can provide counsel on its proper use. The incidence of venereal disease, like teenage pregnancy, has reached epidemic proportions in the United States. Patient education and condoms can play a major role in preventing the spread of sexually transmitted diseases.

Sexually transmitted diseases include gonorrhea, syphilis, *Chlamydia,* genital herpes, condyloma acuminata, trichomoniasis, hepatitis A and B infections, and several others (8, 9). Specific health risks associated with sexually transmitted disease are pelvic inflammatory disease, infant pneumonia, infant death, birth defects, mental retardation, and sterility.

The pharmacist who provides information on contraception and the prevention of veneral disease is providing a very important service to the community and one that directly affects the lives and well-being of his or her patients.

Conception

Conception (impregnation) is the union of an ovum (egg) from the female and a spermatozoon (sperm) from the male. Contraception is the voluntary prevention of pregnancy. Anything that blocks any part of the fertilization process in the male or female or prevents or even delays the union of a sperm with the egg can prevent conception and is called a contraceptive agent, device, or method.

After ovulation, the egg remains fertilizable for about 6–24 hours, possibly as long as 48 hours. (See Chapter 17, *Menstrual Products*.) After ejaculation, sperm retain their ability to fertilize an egg for about 24–48 hours, although normal sperm life may be 72 hours in the presence of cervical mucus and as long as 4 days or more under optimal conditions. In general, to result in conception, sexual intercourse must take place within the 4-day period including 2 days before the egg's release, the day of ovulation, and 1 day afterward.

A major consideration in preventing conception is the survival time of sperm during which they can fertilize the egg. Although sperm may remain active (maximum duration of motility is 48–60 hours), they may no longer be able to fertilize an egg (10–13). Sperm remain viable in the vagina for 2.5 hours, in the cervix for perhaps 48 hours, in the uterus for 48 hours, and in the fallopian tube, where they can fertilize an egg, for a maximum of 48 hours (10). The time periods are not additive.

Contraception

Contraception is accomplished by preventing the semen containing sperm from entering the vagina or the cervical canal, by immobilizing sperm that have entered the vaginal canal, by preventing follicular development and altering ovum transport, by preventing attachment of a mature egg to the endometrium, or by limiting intercourse to times when a mature egg is not available for fertilization. The ideal method should be effective, safe, simple, easy to use, inexpensive, reversible, and aesthetically acceptable.

Selection of a contraceptive method is extremely personal and should be individualized. The key to success of any method is motivation; if a couple strongly wishes to prevent conception, nearly any properly used contraceptive method will be reasonably successful (14). It is the responsibility of the pharmacist to provide complete information on the various contraception methods to allow the patient to determine which method or combination of methods is best suited to the patient's specific needs.

Contrary to popular belief, many persons in the United States do not understand the basic principles of reproduction and conception (15, 16). Family-planning services generally are lacking or unused at colleges and universities; although some elementary and secondary schools attempt to provide sex education and birth control programs, they are frequently inadequate, underfunded, or instituted after patterns of sexual activity have been established (17–22). Fortunately, these inadequacies are overcome as more people become positively concerned and involved.

Methods of Contraception

Nonprescription Contraceptive Products

Contraceptive agents are available without prescription for both men and women. The pharmacist should be familiar with the various types of condoms, jellies, creams, foams, vaginal tablets, and vaginal suppositories. Physician consultation should be recommended to the patient whenever the interview uncovers evidence of an underlying medical problem or the existence of a disease state.

Condoms

Condoms (which may be called bags, balloons, French letters, prophylactics, protectives, rubbers, safes, sheaths, or skins) are among the most effective, and most practical of all nonprescription contraceptives. However, it is estimated that less than 10% of high-risk sexually active men and women use condoms (1). They are simple to use, harmless, inexpensive, easy to purchase, and do not require a physical examination or physician's advice. They are the only contraceptive used by males and are relatively effective. The condom provides a mechanical barrier that collects the seminal fluid and prevents sperm from entering the uterus and fertilizing the ovum. Properly used, condoms are considered the only method, other than abstinence, to avoid acquiring or transmitting venereal diseases.

Offering dual protection against pregnancy and venereal disease (it is the only contraceptive method that offers protection against venereal disease), the condom today is a carefully produced, rigorously tested, and highly effective contraceptive product readily available (23–25). In the United States, more than 300 million condoms are purchased each year, with sales increasing 15% annually. Eighty-four percent of the purchases are made in pharmacies with about one-third being made by women (26).

Condoms are made of rubber (or latex) or collagenous tissue (frequently obtained from lamb cecum). These materials are elastic, strong, and thin. The skin condom, the first type developed, generally is considered a luxury. It is more costly than rubber or latex condoms and is preferred by some users since the natural material transmits heat and sensation more readily. Rubber condoms are used more frequently; however, some people are allergic to them.

The psychologic and physiologic needs of the potential condom user are met by a wide choice of styles (opaque, transparent, colored, plain-ended, reservoir-ended, rippled or pagoda shaped, strictured or contoured, flocked with a rough rubber surface, dry, or lubricated with a water-soluble substance or silicone). Condom thickness appears better correlated with durability (and therefore effectiveness) than with other features. Condoms usually are thicker toward the closed end.

Although condoms provide a high degree of protection against conception, tearing or rupturing during intercourse as a result of improper use is a major cause of failure (27).

Two techniques help to ensure the integrity of the condom; if it is plain-ended, it should be unrolled on the erect penis with about ½–¾ inch of space left at the end to accommodate the ejaculate; if the natural moisture in the women's genital tract is scant, the outside of the condom should be lubricated with a contraceptive cream or jelly to prevent tearing on insertion (28). A water-soluble jelly is preferable owing to ease of cleansing. Petroleum jelly, liquid petrolatum, and other oils should not be used as lubricants because they may cause the rubber to deteriorate and increase the probability of rupture.

An often overlooked reason for inadvertent impregnation is improper use of the condom, probably due to lack of knowledge. First, prior to ejaculation, sperm in the urethral secretions may cause conception. Second, due to loss of erection following ejaculation, semen may leak out the open end of the condom, or the condom may slip off while the penis is still in the vagina or while being withdrawn. For best contraceptive effectiveness, the condom must be put on before the penis comes in contact with the vagina and must be worn throughout coitus. Following ejaculation, the penis should be withdrawn immediately. Accidents may be avoided if the ring (or open end) at the top of the condom is held securely to prevent spillage during withdrawal. As an added protection, the condom may be coated with a vaginal contraceptive (foam, cream, or jelly) or used with a vaginal spermicide before intercourse. This method provides lubrication and a secondary defense against spilled semen. If the condom does tear during use, a vaginal spermicide should be inserted by the woman as soon as possible.

The reservoir-ended condom is less likely to burst because there is more space to hold the ejaculated semen. The lubricated condom has the advantage of easier insertion. The lubricated, reservoir-ended condom is the recommended type; however, the user may prefer another type.

Vaginal Contraceptives

Except for condoms, all other nonprescription contraceptive agents are designed for use by the woman. The products in general use all contain a chemical spermicide and are formulated as creams, jellies, aerosol foams, suppositories, and foaming tablets.

Following a 7-year review of the safety and effectiveness of nonprescription vaginal contraceptive drug products, the FDA advisory panel on nonprescription contraceptives and other vaginal drug products published its final recommendations (29). The panel considered the effectiveness and safety of all marketed products for which spermicidal or contraceptive claims

had been made (Table 1). Based on its evaluation of the available data, only three chemical agents, all of which are nonionic surfactants, have been determined to be safe and effective for nonprescription use as vaginal spermicides. These chemicals are menfegol, nonoxynol-9, and octoxynol (octoxynol-9). Chemicals that have been categorized as generally not safe and effective are phenylmercuric acetate and phenylmercuric nitrate. Because of the unavailability of sufficient data, dodecaethylene glycol monolaurate (PEG 600 monolaurate), Laureth-10S, and the combination of methoxypolyoxyethyleneglycol laurate-550 and nonoxynol-9 were not classified, and an additional 2 years is being allowed for submission of supportive data.

The four criteria for determining safety and effectiveness of spermicides were rapid and complete killing of all sperm on contact or rendering the sperm incapable of fertilization, no evidence of systemic toxicity or irritation to the vaginal and penile mucosa, no effect on the development of the embryo or fetus, and no adverse long-term toxicity (30).

The nonionic surfactants appear to exert their spermicidal effect through direct action on the lipid layer protecting the surface of spermatozoa that results in a loss of motility and fructolytic power and altered permeability. Survival of sperm depends on the metabolism of fructose (31).

Vaginal contraceptive products intended for use with a diaphragm are formulated to provide less spreading and contain a lower concentration of spermicide chemical. The products intended to be used alone, in addition to a higher spermicide content, are formulated to spread over the cervical os and form a protective barrier.

The method of use of the creams, jellies, and foams is fairly simple. The preparation must be inserted into the upper portion of the vagina. The applicator furnished with the product is used to deposit the required amount of vaginal spermicide near the cervix. It should be inserted approximately 3–4 inches into the vagina before the applicator is emptied. Coital movements aid in distributing the agent throughout the vagina and over the cervix.

Table 1. FDA categorization of active ingredients of vaginal contraceptives

Ingredient	Category
Dodecaethyleneglycol monolaurate	III
Laureth-10S	III
Menfegol	I
Methoxypolyoxyethyleneglycol laurate-550 and nonoxynol-9	III
Nonoxynol-9	I
Octoxynol-9	I
Phenylmercuric acetate and phenylmercuric nitrate	II

Federal Register, 45, 82017 (1980)

Creams, jellies, and foams should be inserted not more than 1 hour, preferably 10–30 minutes, before intercourse and should be reapplied if intercourse is repeated. Douching should not be carried out for 6–8 hours after intercourse since it will dilute and/or remove the spermicidal agent, without necessarily removing the remaining viable sperm.

The incidence of side effects with the creams, jellies, and foams is very low and limited to local irritation of the vagina and penis in sensitive individuals. When this occurs the use of the product should be discontinued immediately and another type or method of contraception used.

Creams and Jellies   Choice depends on individual preference. The cream provides greater lubrication during intercourse; the jelly affords easier removal and dissipation because of its water-soluble characteristics. Jellies tend to spread unevenly in the vagina and over the cervix and therefore may be relatively less effective than creams. For this reason their use should be recommended only in combination with a diaphragm.

When used properly, the diaphragm-spermicide combination is among the more effective methods of contraception. In a study of 2,168 women conscientiously using the diaphragm and jelly, accidental pregnancies in the first 12 months of use ranged from 1.9/100 woman-years for women under 18 years to 3.0/100 woman-years for women in the 30–34 age group (32). Even though less effective, jellies and creams used alone are simpler to use and do not require a medical examination or a prescription.

Aerosol Foams   Foams are one of the most effective vaginal contraceptive methods with a reported pregnancy rate of only 3.98/100 woman-years (33). An aerosol dispenser is used to load an applicator with the foam, which is basically a spermicidal cream. Good adherence to the vaginal walls and tenacious covering of the cervical os contribute to the effectiveness of foams. Applicators, which may be prefilled by the user for up to 7 days prior to use, are available.

Although foams do not contribute any appreciable lubrication, they offer the advantage of being almost totally undetectable during use.

Vaginal Suppositories   Two types of suppositories are available that contain nonoxynol-9 as the active spermicidal agent.

One type (S'Positive) utilizes a vegetable oil base that melts at body temperature to form a protective barrier over the entrance to the cervix. The manufacturer recommends that the suppository be inserted at least 20 minutes before intercourse to allow for complete melting and distribution.

The second type of suppository (Encare, Intercept, and Semicid) utilizes a base that foams on contact with vaginal moisture to form a protective barrier. The manufacturers recommend insertion 10 minutes before intercourse.

The pharmacist should be familiar with differences in recommendations for use and claims for the length of time the product will be effective. In general, the suppositories are claimed to be effective only 1 hour after insertion. If intercourse does not take place within that time, a second suppository should be inserted, as it should be if intercourse is to be repeated. Douching should be avoided for at least 6 hours after intercourse to avoid interference with spermicidal action. If local irritation of the vagina and/or penis occurs, the use of the product should be discontinued.

Adequate controlled studies comparing the relative effectiveness of vaginal inserts with foams, creams, or jellies have not been published.

Douching   Flooding and flushing out the vagina mechanically (with water or with a spermicidal agent) immediately after coitus to remove the semen has been practiced for years to avoid pregnancy. Unfortunately, this after-the-fact method is totally unreliable for conception control. Douching is not a contraceptive method and must be discouraged.

The practice is based on the concept that a quick and thorough douching washes the semen from the vagina before the sperm can enter the uterus, thus preventing conception. However, if no other means of contraception is used, douching cannot be effective because direct cervical insemination occurs before douching. Sperm may reach the cervix within 90 seconds of ejaculation. Immediate postcoital tests revealed active spermatozoa in the endocervix within 1.5–3 minutes after coitus, and spermatoza have been recovered from the fallopian tubes 30 minutes after insemination (34). It is highly improbable that douching can be initiated quickly or thoroughly enough to remove all traces of semen, and therefore all sperm, from the vagina.

The method is mentioned only because douching apparently is practiced widely and several commercial douche products are available. There is no convincing evidence to show that douching with or without added chemicals is an effective contraceptive.

Toxicity Potential

The active ingredients in many spermicidal preparations are potentially toxic if they are ingested in pure form, but the toxic agents are present only in small percentages (35). Signs and symptoms of toxicity vary depending on the ingredient ingested. The possibility remains remote that a child or adult would ingest enough toxic agent to cause overt signs and symptoms of acute toxicity; nevertheless, contraceptive preparations should be kept out of the reach of children.

Nonpharmaceutical Methods

Rhythm

The rhythm methods (fertility awareness methods) involve abstinence from sexual relations during the fertile period of the female cycle. Rhythm is one of the least effective methods, although some couples find it satisfactory. Its effectiveness is enhanced if the woman has a regular menstrual cycle. Anyone choosing this approach should be instructed on its use by a trained counselor or physician.

The major, relatively simple techniques for establishing the time of ovulation are the calendar method (Ogino-Knaus), the thermal or temperature method (basal body temperature, or BBT), and the cervical mucus method (ovulation method or Billing's method) (36). The calendar method predicts ovulation on the basis of probabilities calculated from a woman's menstrual history. The thermal method and Billing's method detect ovulation on the basis of a specific physiologic change that occurs during the menstrual cycle.

If ovulation could be determined accurately, rhythm undoubtedly would become a more acceptable method of contraception. Theoretically, if intercourse were avoided for 2 days before ovulation, the day of ovulation, and 1 day after ovulation, conception would not occur. These 4 days constitute the fertile (unsafe) phase of the menstrual cycle. The intermenstrual days occurring before and after the 4 fertile days are the infertile (safe) phase. The alternation of the fertile phase with the preceding and succeeding infertile phases is called the rhythm (37). Unfortunately, the widely differing lengths of most women's menstrual cycles make it nearly impossible to determine precisely when ovulation takes place (Table 2) (38, 39).

When ovulation begins, a woman's basal body temperature drops slightly, followed by a rise of about 0.5°F (0.28°C) over 24–72 hours. After 3 days of elevated temperature, the safe period begins. The temperature fluctuation and a meticulous graphical record of at least 1 year's menstrual cycles form the basis for predicting ovulation and using the rhythm method. For added safety, intercourse should be avoided several days before and after the unsafe period.

The basal thermometer, specifically designed to check basal body temperature, records 96–100°F (35.6–37.8°C) with 0.1°F intervals, allowing detection of small changes in body temperature. Better accuracy is achieved from a rectal recording of 5 minutes taken immediately upon awakening and before arising (40). The thermometer should be shaken down the night before and placed at the bedside (to prevent physical exertion on awakening, which causes rise in temperature). Charts for recording the basal body temperature during the menstrual cycle are available.

The cervical mucus method depends on observation of the changes in the character and appearance of the cervix and cervical secretions that occur just before ovulation in some women. Just before ovulation, the cervical os (opening to the cervix) expands. During ovulation, the cervical secretions change in character from the viscous, slightly yellowish mucus normally present during the pre- and postovulatory phase to a clear, slippery discharge resembling raw egg white. This change is due to the increasing levels of estrogen present during the ovulatory phase. (See Chapter 17, *Menstrual Products*.)

Additional symptoms such as abdominal swelling, rectal pain or discomfort, or lower abdominal pain also may accompany ovulation.

Before adopting the cervical mucus method for contraception, a woman should observe her secretions and record her observations on a calendar for at least 3–4 months. She should avoid intercourse for the 4 days be-

Table 2. How to calculate the interval of fertility			
If your shortest cycle has been (no. of days)	Your first fertile (unsafe) day is	If your longest cycle has been (no. of days)	Your last fertile (unsafe) day is
21*	3rd day	21	10th day
22	4th	22	11th
23	5th	23	12th
24	6th	24	13th
25	7th	25	14th
26	8th	26	15th
27	9th	27	16th
28	10th	28	17th
29	11th	29	18th
30	12th	30	19th
31	13th	31	20th
32	14th	32	21st
33	15th	33	22nd
34	16th	34	23rd
35	17th	35	24th

Reprinted with permission from R. A. Hatcher, G. K. Stewart, F. Stewart, F. Guest, P. Stratton, and A. H. Wright, "Contraceptive Technology 1980/1981," 10th ed., Irvington, New York, N.Y., 1980, pp. 100–115.

*Day 1, first day of menstrual bleeding.

fore the mucosal changes are expected to occur and the 3 days after their appearance. Other mucus-like substances such as semen, lubricants, spermicides, and discharges due to infections should be considered. Women who practice douching cannot use the mucus method for contraceptive purposes since the secretions are washed away and cannot be observed. This method is more effective if combined with the basal body temperature method (39).

For Roman Catholic patients, pharmacists should be aware that the methods of contraception approved by the Catholic Church are abstinence and rhythm (36). The patient should be fully informed of the risks and difficulties inherent in practicing rhythm.

Coitus Interruptus (Withdrawal)

Coitus interruptus involves the removal of the erect penis from the vagina and the area of eternal genitalia before ejaculation. The problem with this method is that sperm in the urethral secretions released before ejaculation may fertilize the egg. Moreover, there has been little success, if any, in the long-term at maintaining this form of physical control during sexual excitement.

Contraceptive Effectiveness

The reliability of a contraceptive method is in direct proportion to the motivation and intent of the user. Any contraceptive method works better than none at all, but even the most effective method must be used consistently. Effectiveness depends on acceptability and suitability to a couple's needs at a particular time (Table 3).

Table 3. Pregnancy rates of various contraceptive methods

Method	Number of pregnancies/100 women during first year of use	
	Theoretical	Actual
Hysterectomy	0.0001	0.0001
Tubal ligation	0.04	0.04
Vasectomy	0.15	0.15
Oral contraceptive (combined)	0.34	4–10
Low-dose oral progestin	1–1.5	5–10
Intrauterine device	1–3	5
Condom	3	10
Diaphragm with spermicide	3	17
Coitus interruptus	9	20–25
Rhythm (calendar)	13	21
Rhythm (cervical mucus)	2	25
Rhythm (thermal)	7	20

Reprinted with permission from R. A. Hatcher, G. K. Stewart, F. Stewart, F. Guest, P. Stratton and A. H. Wright, "Contraceptive Technology 1980/1981," 10th ed., Irvington, New York, N.Y., 1978, p. 4.

Theoretical contraceptive effectiveness relies on the assumption that the method is used according to instructions. Actual effectiveness is reduced by inconsistent or incorrect use (41). Besides biologic efficiency, effectiveness in use depends on factors such as personal preference, the mores of the social group, availability, cost (initial and long range), storage, use (ease, frequency, and propensity), timing in relation to intercourse, interference with intercourse, requirements for medical consultation, and side effects. The overall effectiveness of a contraceptive method is determined essentially by its ability to reduce the probability of conception, by consistency of use, and continuation of use (42).

Among women who use no method of contraception, 80% may expect to become pregnant within 1 year.

Pregnancy Testing

The first laboratory test for the detection of pregnancy, a bioassay developed by Ascheim and Zondek in 1928, was based on the observation that urine from a pregnant woman contained high levels of human chorionic gonadotropin (HCG). When the urine was injected into mice or rats, it caused corpus luteum formation with accompanying swelling and hemorrhaging. The test required 5 days for results. A year later, Friedman developed a similar test that used a rabbit as the test animal and required only 48 hours. Other bioassays for pregnancy include production of ovarian hyperemia in the rat, extrusion of eggs in the frog, and extrusion of sperm in the toad following injection of HCG-containing urine from pregnant women.

Currently, immunoassay is the most widely used method for pregnancy testing. Two techniques are utilized. One involves inhibition of hemagglutination in a test tube, and the other involves inhibition of latex particle agglutination on a slide. The slide test requires only 2 minutes to perform, but should be done at least 18–20 days after the last menstrual period for accurate test results. The hemagglutination inhibition test performed in a test tube requires about 2 hours to perform and is the method used for the home early pregnancy tests now being marketed in the United States. The kits all work on the same principle of measuring the amount of HCG in a woman's urine. The manufacturers' instructions indicate that the test may be performed after the ninth day after the day on which the period was expected to begin. However, the FDA has stated that product accuracy claims are based on tests performed 15 or more days after a missed period (43).

The home pregnancy test kits include a test tube containing dried sheep red blood cells on which HCG has been adsorbed and sufficient HCG antiserum to prevent agglutination of these cells when suspended in the water provided in the kit. If the urine contains HCG, it reacts with the available HCG antiserum and permits visible agglutination of the sheep red cells. In performing the test, exactly 3 drops of first-morning urine are added carefully to the tube containing the

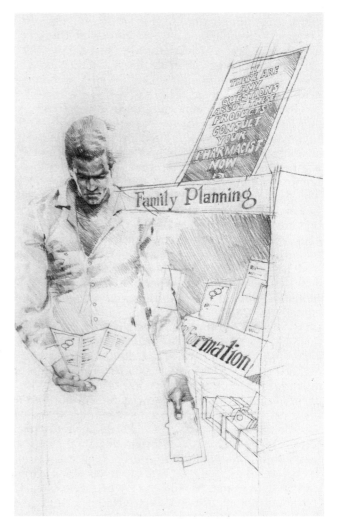

HCG-red blood cells and HCG antiserum. The pre-measured water then is added, and the tube is stoppered and shaken for at least 10 seconds. The tube then is placed in the holder provided and left undisturbed for 2 hours. It is important to avoid any vibration during this time as well as direct sunlight. After 2 hours a positive test produces a dark brownish, doughnut-shaped ring (agglutination), and a negative test reveals an evenly dispersed brownish deposit (no agglutination).

The accuracy of this test when performed at home was observed to be about 97% for positive readings and 80% for first negative readings (44). The test is intended to be sensitive to HCG urine levels at 23 days or more after ovulation in pregnant women (9 days after the missed menstrual period). If a negative result is obtained with the first test and menses does not occur in 7 days, the manufacturers recommend that the test be repeated. The accuracy of the negative test results increases to 91% on these second tests. If the second test is negative, a physician should be consulted.

The FDA advises that, in addition to jarring the test solution while the test is in progress and exposure to sunlight, other factors can adversely affect accuracy. Contaminated urine samplers or containers and reading the results too early or too late will produce inaccurate results. Recent pregnancies may produce false-positive results. Urine must be free of excess sugars, blood, or other contaminants (43). The color and thickness of the ring may vary depending on the kit used and the amount of HCG in the urine.

False-positive results may be observed in menopausal patients, since the test does not distinguish pituitary from chorionic gonadotropin, in patients taking phenothiazines or methadone, and in the presence of proteinuria. False-negative results may occur in ectopic pregnancies and threatened abortions (45, 46).

Contraceptive Counseling

Interest in barrier methods of contraception is increasing because of the continuing health risk controversy surrounding oral contraceptives and the IUD. Nonprescription contraceptive agents offer a high degree of safety to the user along with high theoretical effectiveness rates. The low-use effectiveness rates that have been observed seem to be a direct result of inconsistent or incorrect use (40). The pharmacist is the most likely source of information and instruction on the use of nonprescription contraceptive agents.

Although there have been legal and psychological barriers to displaying and discussing contraceptive agents with patients, they have largely been set aside by a June 1977 U. S. Supreme Court ruling. This ruling allows the sale of nonprescription contraceptives to minors and permits both advertising and display of prescription and nonprescription contraceptive agents by persons and companies licensed to sell these products.

As a first step in establishing an organized and ongoing consultation service, a specific area in the pharmacy should be designated for the stocking and display of nonprescription contraceptive agents. A full line of agents should be made available and complimentary family planning information included in this product section.

Equally important is the availability of a patient consultation area that affords privacy and comfort. Patient information on contraceptive products and methods should be used to reinforce and supplement verbal counseling conducted in this area. Various sources of information on family planning are included in the appendix to this chapter.

The pharmacist should keep in mind the right of the patient to request or refuse counseling. The service should be promoted with discretion and professionalism. An informational pamphlet describing the service could be developed and distributed to patients at the same time that a history is taken for the patient profile. The pharmacist should always remember that contraception is a very personal issue and the patient's right to privacy must be protected.

Certain other tools are needed by the pharmacist to provide effective counseling. Knowledge about the physiology of conception, various methods of contraception that are available, and the mechanisms of action, effectiveness, reasons for failure, relative costs, risks, and side effects of the various methods and agents is essential.

For this purpose, a basic library of references on relevant subjects is valuable as is a directory of family-planning counseling services and clinics available in the geographic area. Included in the directory should be names of physicians known to be knowledgeable and interested in contraceptive counseling.

Acceptability to the user of a contraceptive method is the key to dedicated use resulting in a high rate of effectiveness. The patient must decide which method of conception control best suits his or her needs.

Summary

It is apparent that there is an unfulfilled need for contraceptive method counseling for a large number of people. The practicing pharmacist can and should be integrally involved with other health professionals in supplying information on all methods of conception control. Although the function of the pharmacist in this activity may center on agents that do not require the services of a physician, knowledge of all methods is essential.

The pharmacist can provide a further service to the patient through physician referrals and consultation regarding observed side effects and untoward reactions resulting from contraceptive use.

References

1. "Promoting Health/Preventing Disease, Objectives for the Nation," U.S. Department of Health and Human Services, Public Health Service (Fall 1980).
2. T. Gorman, *Drug Topics, 123,* 65 (April 6, 1979).
3. M. Zelnik and J. J. Kanter, *Fam. Plann. Perspect., 6,* 74 (1974).
4. J. Sklar and B. Berkov, *Fam. Plann. Perspect., 6,* 80 (1974).
5. "Statistical Abstract of the United States," 98th ed., U.S. Government Printing Office, Washington, D.C., 1977.
6. "Teen Pregnancy: The Problem That Won't Go Away," Alan Guttmacher Institute, 1981.

7. S. Kweskin, *Patient Care, 12,* 108 (Sept. 30, 1978).
8. *American Pharmacy, NS20,* 29 (1980).
9. K. F. Breen, *Drug Topics, 124,* 50 (November 21, 1980).
10. W. J. Dignam, in "Birth Control: A Continuing Controversy," Charles C Thomas, Springfield, Ill., 1967, pp. 142–151.
11. G. Pincus, "The Control of Fertility," Academic, New York, N.Y., 1965, p. 96.
12. B. J. Duffy and M. J. Wallace, "Biological and Medical Aspects of Contraception," University of Notre Dame Press, Notre Dame, Ind., 1969, pp. 83–85.
13. H. Balin and S. Glasser, "Reproductive Biology," Excerpta Medica, Amsterdam, 1972, p. 350.
14. R. W. Kistner, *J. Am. Med. Assoc., 215,* 1162 (1971).
15. T. Crist, *Obstet. Gynecol. News,5,* 16 (Dec. 15, 1970).
16. E. M. Nash and L. M. Louden, *J. Am. Med. Assoc., 210,* 2365 (1969).
17. G. Hollis and K. Lashman, *Fam. Plann. Perspect., 6,* 173 (1974).
18. N. N. Wagner, P. R. Millard, and R. J. Pion, *J. Am. Pharm. Assoc., NS10,* 258 (1970).
19. B. N. Fujita, N. N. Wagner, and R. J. Pion, *Am. J. Obstet. Gynecol., 109,* 787 (1971).
20. N. N. Wagner, N. Perthou, B. Fujita, and R. J. Pion, *Postgrad. Med., 46,* 68 (1969).
21. S. O. Gustavus and C. A. Huether, *Fam. Plann. Perspect., 7,* 203 (1975).
22. M. L. Finkel and D. J. Finkel, *Fam. Plann. Perspect., 7,* 256 (1975).
23. I. A. Dalsimier, P. T. Piotrow, and J. J. Dumm, *Popul. Rep. H,* H/1 (1973).
24. J. J. Dumm, P. T. Piotrow, and I. A. Dalsimer, *Popul. Rep. H,* H/21 (1974).
25. "The Condom: Increasing Utilization in the United States," M. H. Redford, G. W. Duncan, and D. J. Prager, Eds., San Francisco Press, San Francisco, Calif., 1974.
26. *Drug Topics, 124,* 50 (June 2, 1980).
27. C. Tietze, "Family-Planning Programs: An International Survey," Basic Books, New York, N.Y., 1969, pp. 183–191.
28. A. F. Guttmacher, W. Best, and F. S. Jaffe, "Planning Your Family," Macmillan, New York, N.Y., 1964, pp. 41–42.
29. *Federal Register, 45,* 82014–49 (Dec. 12, 1980).
30. R. McConnell, *Acta Endocrinologica (Supplement),* 85, pp. 373–386 (1974).
31. T. Mann, "The Biochemistry of Semen," Methuen, London, pp. 46, 57, 151 (1954).
32. M. E. Lane, R. Arceo, and A. J. Sobrero, *Fam. Plann. Perspect., 8,* 81 (1976).
33. G. S. Bernstein, *Contraception, 3,* 37 (1971).
34. C. C. Marcus and S. L. Marcus, in "Progress in Infertility," Little, Brown, Boston, Mass., 1968, pp. 21–62.
35. R. E. Gosselin, H. C. Hodge, R. P. Smith, and M. N. Gleason, "Clinical Toxicology of Commercial Products: Acute Poisoning," 4th ed., Williams and Wilkins, Baltimore, Md., 1976, Sect. II, pp. 1–273; Sec. V, pp. 1–799.
36. C. Ross and P. T. Piotrow, *Popul. Rep., I,* I/1 (1974).
37. J. Rock, in "Manual of Family Planning and Contraceptive Practice," 2nd ed., M. S. Calderone, Ed., Williams and Wilkins, Baltimore, Md., 1970.
38. L. Mastroianni, Jr., *Fam. Plann. Perspect., 6,* 209 (1974).
39. R. A. Hatcher, G. K. Stewart, F. Stewart, F. Guest, P. Stratton, and A. H. Wright, "Contraceptive Technology 1980/1981," 10th ed., Irvington Publishers, New York, N.Y., 1980, pp. 100–115.
40. B. J. Pisani, in "Manual of Family Planning and Contraceptive Practice," 2nd ed., M. S. Calderone, Ed., Williams and Wilkins, Baltimore, Md., 1970.
41. C. Tietze, in "Manual of Family Planning and Contraceptive Practice," 2nd ed., M. S. Calderone, Ed., Williams and Wilkins, Baltimore, Md., 1970, pp. 268–269.
42. C. Tietze and S. Lewit, *Fertil. Steril., 22,* 508 (1971).
43. *FDA Consumer,* June 1979.
44. N. B. Ryder, *Fam. Plann. Perspect., 5,* 133 (1973).
45. Warner Chilcott, Studies 2CO814 and 2CO815, Morris Plains, N.J.
46. *Medical Letter on Drugs and Therapeutics, 20,* 39 (1979).

Appendix:
Family-Planning Information

- Planned Parenthood Federation of America, Inc.
  810 Seventh Avenue
  New York, N.Y. 10019

  Offers family planning services, infertility therapy, pregnancy counseling, abortion and sterilization services or referral for such services, education for marriage and sex education, prenatal care, and a variety of special programs. Patient-level pamphlets cover all methods or individual ones (some in Spanish). Teaching aids, posters, and subscription periodicals are offered.

- The Population Council
  Publications and Information Office
  1 Dag Hammarskjold Plaza
  New York, N.Y. 10017

  Publishes the monthly "Studies in Family Planning" and "Population and Development Review," as well as books and monographs. The Council endeavors to advance knowledge in the broad field of population control by fostering research, training, and technical consultation and assistance in the social and biomedical sciences.

- Zero Population Growth
  1346 Connecticut Avenue, N.W.
  Washington, D.C. 20036

  Activities aimed at population education and political action to remove laws that inhibit or restrict individual freedom of choice of medically approved contraception techniques. Advocates an end to population growth in the United States through its population policy.

- The Alan Guttmacher Institute
  515 Madison Avenue
  New York, N.Y. 10022

  Publishes "Family Planning Perspectives" (bimonthly), "International Family Planning Perspectives and Digest" (quarterly), "Family Planning/Population Reporter," and "Planned Parenthood Washington Memo." The Institute has prepared a detailed two-volume manual, *Developing Statewide Family Planning Programs: A Planning Handbook* (available for $50), to assist administrators and program officials in developing a statewide approach to family planning programs that will meet federal and state requirements. The Institute also has published *Contraceptive Services for Adolescents: Each State and County, 1975,* a nationwide study (available for $5.00).

- Population Information Program
  The Johns Hopkins University
  624 N. Broadway
  Baltimore, Md. 21205

  Publishes "Population Reports," an excellent series that provides an accurate and authoritative overview of important developments in the population field.

- The Population Program
  The Rockefeller Foundation
  1133 Avenue of the Americas
  New York, N.Y. 10036

  Strives toward the goal of population stabilization through support of research, training, and experimental programs in a broad range of fields related to population.

- Special Programs of Research, Development and
    Research Training in Human Reproduction
  World Health Organization
  Avenue Appia
  1211 Geneva 27, Switzerland

  The objectives are geared to meet the expressed needs of member states for technology for family planning and infertility that is safer, more effective, and better adapted to the needs of their populations, and to focus on the development of new methods and service approaches that emphasize ease of provision through primary health care, simplicity of use, and low cost.

Spermicide Product Table

Product (Manufacturer)	Dosage Form	Spermicide	Other Ingredients
Anvita (A. O. Schmidt)	suppositories	phenylmercuric borate, 1:2,000	boric acid, aluminum potassium sulfate, thymol, chlorothymol, aromatics, cocoa butter
Because (Schering)	foam	nonoxynol 9, 8%	benzethonium chloride, 0.2%
Conceptrol (Ortho)	cream gel	nonoxynol 9, 5% nonoxynol 9, 4%	
Dalkon (Robins)	foam	nonoxynol 9, 8%	benzethonium chloride, 0.2%
Delfen (Ortho)	foam	nonoxynol 9, 12.5%	
Emko (Schering)	foam	nonoxynol 9, 8%	benzethonium chloride, 0.2%; stearic acid; triethanolamine; glyceryl mono-stearate; poloxamer 188; polyethylene glycol 600; substituted adamantane; dichlorodifluoromethane; dichloro-tetrafluoroethane
Encare (Eaton-Merz)	suppository	nonoxynol 9, 2.27%	
Intercept (Ortho)	suppository	nonoxynol 9, 100 mg	
Koromex (Holland-Rantos)	foam	nonoxynol 9, 12.5%	propylene glycol, isopropyl alcohol, laureth-4, cetyl alcohol, polyethylene glycol stearate, fragrance, dichlorodi-fluoromethane, dichlorotetrafluoro-ethane
Koromex II-A Jelly (Holland-Rantos)	gel	nonoxynol 9, 2%	propylene glycol, cellulose gum, boric acid, sorbitol, starch, simethicone, fragrance
Ramses 10 Hour (Schmid)	jelly	nonoxynol 9, 5%	
Semicid (Whitehall)	suppository	nonoxynol 9, 100 mg	
S'Positive (Jordan-Simner)	suppository	nonoxynol 9, 5.67%	vegetable oil base benzethonium chloride

Vaginal Spermicides Used With a Diaphragm

Product (Manufacturer)	Dosage Form	Spermicide	Other Ingredients
Koromex II (Holland-Rantos)	jelly cream	octoxynol, 1% octoxynol, 3%	
Ortho-Creme (Ortho)	cream	nonoxynol 9, 2%	
Ortho-Gynol (Ortho)	jelly	octoxynol, 1%	
Ortho-Gynol II (Ortho)	jelly	nonoxynol 9, 2%	

Condom Product Table

Brand Name (Supplier)	Type
Conceptrol Shields, Lubricated (Ortho Pharmaceutical)	rubber-shaped and/or ribbed, packaged with lubricant
Conceptrol Shields, Non-lubricated (Ortho Pharmaceutical)	rubber-shaped and/or ribbed, packaged dry
Conture (Akwell)	rubber-shaped and/or ribbed, packaged with lubricant
Excita Sensitol (Schmid)	rubber-shaped and/or ribbed, packaged with lubricant
Fetherlite (Schmid)	rubber-plain end, packaged dry rubber-plain end, packaged with lubricant
Fiesta Sensi-Color (Schmid)	rubber-reservoir end, packaged with lubricant
Fourex (Schmid)	lamb cecum-regular end, packaged with lubricant
Guardian (Youngs)	rubber-reservoir end, packaged with lubricant
Naturalamb (Youngs)	lamb cecum-regular end, packaged with lubricant
Nuda (Akwell)	rubber-reservoir end, packaged with lubricant
Nuform Sensi-Shape, Lubricated (Schmid)	rubber-shaped and/or ribbed, packaged with lubricant
Nuform Sensi-Shape, Non-lubricated (Schmid)	rubber-shaped and/or ribbed, packaged dry
Prime (Akwell)	rubber-reservoir end, packaged with lubricant
Prime, Non-Lubricated (Akwell)	rubber-reservoir end, packaged dry
Ramses (Schmid)	rubber-plain end, packaged dry
Ramses Sensitol (Schmid)	rubber-plain end, packaged with lubricant
Sheik Plain End (Schmid)	rubber-plain end, packaged dry
Sheik Reservoir End, Lubricated (Schmid)	rubber-reservoir end, packaged with lubricant
Sheik Reservoir End, Non-lubricated (Schmid)	rubber-reservoir end, packaged dry
Stimula (Akwell)	rubber-shaped and/or ribbed, packaged with lubricant
Tahiti (Akwell)	rubber-reservoir end, packaged with lubricant
Trojan-Enz, Lubricated (Youngs)	rubber-reservoir end, packaged with lubricant

Condom Product Table, continued

Brand Name (Supplier)	Type
Trojan-Enz, Non-lubricated (Youngs)	rubber-reservoir end, packaged dry
Trojans (Youngs)	rubber-plain end, packaged dry
Trojans Plus (Youngs)	rubber-shaped and/or ribbed, packaged with lubricant
Trojans Ribbed	rubber-shaped and/or ribbed, packaged with lubricant

19 Personal Care Products

Donald R. Miller and Stephen G. Hoag

Questions to Ask the Patient

Feminine Cleansing Products

Have you noticed an abnormal vaginal discharge? Are you experiencing pain or itching?

Are there any sores in the vaginal area?

Have you ever had this condition before?

How long has the condition been present?

Have you ever seen a physician or treated this condition yourself before?

Do you douche? How frequently?

Are you taking any prescription drugs? Are you using any nonprescription feminine cleansing or deodorant products?

Do you have an IUD?

Are you pregnant?

Do you have any medical problems such as diabetes?

Antiperspirant and Deodorant Products

Do you wish to purchase an antiperspirant or a deodorant or a combination of both types?

Do you perspire heavily even in cool temperatures? Do you perspire heavily when you are nervous and excited?

Do you feel that you need an extrastrength product? Why?

Do the palms of your hands and the soles of your feet perspire heavily?

Has the amount of perspiration changed lately?

Skin Bleaching Agents

Have you been using a skin bleaching product? If so, for how long?

For what type of freckle or "skin spot" do you use it?

How long has it been present?

Has it changed color or increased in size?

Do you have any medical problems?

Is there any possibility that you are pregnant?

Are you taking any medicines, including birth control pills?

Depilatories

Why do you want to use a depilatory?

Are you presently taking any medicines?

Is your skin very sensitive?

Have you used depilatories before?

Nonmedicated Shampoos

What special problems do you have with your hair (oily, dry, tangles easily)?

In what age group is the primary user? (Young children need a decreased irritant; teens need shampoos for oily hair.)

American society today is probably unsurpassed in history in its concern for cleanliness, personal hygiene, and elimination of body odors. The many products promoted are intended to keep us clean and odor-free from head to toe. Included among these are feminine cleansing and deodorant products, skin bleaching products, antiperspirants and deodorants, depilatories, and nonmedicated shampoos. Many of these products are intended to affect processes that are physiologically normal. Therefore, the pharmacist must consider use of such products from the cosmetic as well as medical point of view.

Feminine Cleansing and Deodorant Products

Feminine toiletry and cosmetic products are used for general cleansing of the vaginal or perineal areas, for deodorizing, for relief of itching, burning, erythema, and edema, for removing secretions or discharge, and for psychological reasons, such as producing a soothing and refreshing feeling. Some of these feminine products, such as douches, may be prescribed by physicians for altering vaginal pH to affect microscopic flora.

Many gynecologists believe that the healthy vagina cleanses itself and that the perineal area may be cleaned adequately with soap and water. Others seem to feel that douching, done properly, promotes healthy vaginal tissues. The value of feminine deodorant sprays is also controversial. Their efficacy as deodorants is often questioned, and possible adverse effects, such as irritation of vaginal mucous membranes, have come to light since the sprays first appeared.

The word "hygiene" is not used here in connection with these products because most of the products do not possess medicinal properties, especially the deodorant sprays. Their action and benefit are cosmetic. Furthermore, the few douche preparations that do have therapeutic properties should not be recommended for self-medication in the presence of disease; their use may delay the user from seeking medical attention. Nonprescription vaginal cleansing and deodorant products should always be used as cosmetics and toiletries unless a physician or pharmacist is supervising their use for therapeutic purposes.

Physiology of the Vaginal Tract

The important physiologic considerations concerning feminine cleansing and deodorant product use include vaginal epithelial thickness and glycogen content, normal bacterial flora, vaginal pH, production of secretions and discharge, and production of objectionable odor. Vaginal surfaces are lined with squamous epithelium, and estrogens are mainly responsible for controlling the thickness of this lining. Epithelial cell height increases at menarche and decreases at menopause. Before menarche and after menopause the vaginal epithelium is apparently less resistant to infection. Glycogen content of vaginal epithelium is increased during the childbearing years.

Vaginal health depends on pH, normal bacterial flora, epithelial cellular height, and epithelial glycogen content. The normal vaginal bacterial flora include Döderlein's bacillus (a strain of *Lactobacillus*), diphtheroids, *Staphylococci*, *Bacteroides*, and anaerobic *Streptococci* species (1). Döderlein's bacillus metabolizes epithelial glycogen to lactic acid. Vaginal pH is normally alkaline before menarche and after menopause but is normally acid during the childbearing years as a result of this metabolic production of lactic acid by bacteria. The vaginal pH ranges from 3.0 to 6.1; the average range is usually 3.5–4.2 (2–4). The acidic vaginal pH and the presence of normal flora usually preclude pathogen growth, but a pH shift toward alkalinity may render the area more susceptible to infection. Preg-nancy and the pseudopregnancy produced by oral contraceptives cause increases in vaginal pH and glycogen content (5).

Vaginal mucous secretion is composed in part of the endocervical mucus as well as bacteria and desquamated vaginal epithelium. This discharge is a natural cleansing mechanism, but in the absence of personal cleanliness the discharge or secretion may accumulate on external genital surfaces and produce an odor. The vulvoperineal area contains sebaceous, apocrine, and eccrine glands, each producing minimal secretions, as well as Bartholin's glands, which secrete a very small amount of mucus during sexual stimulation. In addition, there is a clear, alkaline transudate in the vagina during sexual excitement. Vaginal discharge may increase noticeably during periods of emotional stress and ovulation.

The mucous, sebaceous, and apocrine perineal secretions and the vaginal discharge are subject to bacterial decomposition if left on the skin for long periods. This bacterial decomposition of normal secretions is the main cause of objectionable odor. Other causes of odor include semen, old blood, infection, copper IUD's, and forgotten foreign bodies, such as tampons or portions of tampons (6).

Vaginitis

Etiology and Classification

Besides cosmetic and deodorant considerations, the most common reasons for using douches and other feminine cleansing products are probably vulvar pruritus (and/or a burning sensation) and excessive vaginal discharge (leukorrhea). One of the most frequent causes of these symptoms is vaginitis, an inflammation of vulvar and vaginal epithelium usually caused by disturbances of the normal flora or by pathogenic microorganisms. A classification of vaginitis is given in Table 1, but most cases may be placed in one of four categories: *Trichomonas vaginalis* vaginitis, *Candida albicans* (monilial) vaginitis, nonspecific vaginitis, or atrophic vaginitis. Because there are no nerve endings in the vagina to perceive pain and pruritus, the patient has no symptoms until the external genitalia become involved in the infection.

Trichomonal and monilial vaginitis are the most common types in women of childbearing age. Prolonged tetracycline use, steroid therapy (including oral contraceptives), cancer, pregnancy, and diabetes are among the factors possibly predisposing to the overgrowth of monilial organisms *(C. albicans)* (7). Nonspecific vaginitis is frequently due to an infection by *Gardnerella vaginale* (formerly *Hemophilus vaginalis* and *Corynebacterium vaginale*) (8, 9). Atrophic vaginitis occurs after menopause when vaginal epithelium thins. *Proteus* may be implicated in a significant number of chronic cases of atrophic vaginitis. Although childhood vulvovaginitis is relatively uncommon, it usually has the same cause and manifestations as atrophic vaginitis. Monilial and trichomonal infections may occur simultaneously, and both organisms may be present in the normal, healthy vagina (10, 11). Trichomonal and *Gardnerella* vaginitis are transmitted primarily by sexual contact.

Table 1. Classification of vaginitis

Type	Organism	Age group affected
Infectious		
Atrophic (senile)	Coliforms *Staphylococci* *Streptococci*	Postmenopausal (prepubertal, rarely)
Gonorrhea	*Neisseria gonorrhoeae*	Adult
Herpes II	Herpes II	All
Monilial	*Candida albicans*	Adult (especially if pregnant or diabetic)
Mycoplasma	*Mycoplasma*	All
Nonspecific	*Gardnerella vaginale*[a] Coliforms *Staphylococci* *Streptococci*	All
Preadolescent (childhood vulvovaginitis)	Helminths Coliforms *Staphylococci* *Streptococci*	Prepubertal
Trichomonal	*Trichomonas vaginalis*	Adult (prepubertal, rarely)
Tuberculous	*Mycobacterium tuberculosis*	All
Noninfectious		
Allergic and chemical		All (when foreign chemicals are instilled vaginally)
Postirradiation		All (when irradiation is used for treatment of cervical carcinoma)
Traumatic		All

[a] *Gardnerella vaginale* (formerly *Hemophilus vaginalis* and *Corynebacterium vaginale*) is frequently considered by itself because it is the most frequent pathogen in nonspecific bacterial vaginitis.

Symptoms

The symptoms of vaginitis, leukorrhea and pruritus, may cause a woman to seek medical attention or to self-medicate. Offensive odor may be caused by discharge associated with trichomonal or *Gardnerella* organisms. The description of a purulent vaginal discharge should alert the pharmacist to the possibility of vaginitis and the need for a specific diagnosis and prescribed therapy. In postmenopausal women, a thin watery discharge accompanied by pruritus indicates possible atrophic vaginitis or malignancy. The pharmacist should determine whether vaginitis symptoms are present, how long they have persisted, and whether predisposing factors exist. The patient also should be asked whether any previous attempts at self-treatment have been made, because

symptoms may be due to an adverse reaction to a non-prescription product.

Depending on the specific diagnosis of vaginitis, the physician may prescribe antitrichomonal, antimonilial (antifungal), or antibacterial therapy. In atrophic vaginitis, however, systemic or local estrogenic hormone therapy may be prescribed because estrogen stimulates vaginal epithelium, increasing its thickness and resistance to infection. Nonprescription feminine cleansing and deodorant products should be used in cases of vaginitis only on a pharmacist's or physician's advice.

Pruritus with or without a malodorous discharge may occur in conditions other than vaginitis such as cystitis, urethritis, chemical irritation, venereal disease, and carcinoma of the cervix, endometrium, or vagina. Regardless of the cause, these symptoms are an indication for diagnostic evaluation by a physician, especially if they are persistent, severe, or recurrent. Patients should be told not to bathe or douche immediately before visiting a physician for an examination for vaginitis (12).

Vaginal Douches

Douches may exert cleansing effects by lowering surface tension and promoting mucolytic and proteolytic action; standards for evaluating these effects have not been established (11). Douche products are available as liquids, liquid concentrates to be diluted in water, powders to be dissolved in water, and powders to be instilled as powders. (The term "douche" is not limited to a stream of water.) Within the past few years, premixed douche liquids in disposable applicators have become available and are widely advertised. Disposable applicators are convenient to use and do not require the care and cleaning procedures that nondisposable douche equipment requires.

Ingredients

Recommended concentrations for many ingredients in feminine cleansing and deodorant products are listed in Table 2, but many manufacturers do not list concentrations.

Antimicrobial Agents Most antimicrobial agents in douche products are present in concentrations that provide preservative properties to the product but no therapeutic activity. They include benzethonium and benzalkonium chlorides, chlorothymol, hexachlorophene, and parabens. Other compounds, such as boric acid, cetylpyridinium chloride, eucalyptol, menthol, oxyquinoline, phenol, sodium perborate, and thymol may be included for purported antiseptic or germicidal activity. However, the value of these ingredients as antimicrobials is questionable, depending in some cases on the concentration used. Because many manufacturers do not list concentrations of ingredients when the products are considered cosmetics, it is impossible to assess their efficacy.

Boric acid (5%) under physician supervision is an effective antimicrobial for treating monilial vaginitis, and povidone-iodine is an effective antimicrobial agent for adjunctive therapy in monilial and trichomonal vag-

Table 2. Recommended concentrations for components of feminine cleansing and deodorant products

Agent	Recommended concentration	Activity	Agent	Recommended concentration	Activity
Alum	0.5–5.0%[a]	Astringent	Methyl salicylate	10–25%[a]	Counterirritant Deodorant
Aluminum (micronized powder)		Astringent	Oxyquinoline	1:1,000 vaginally or externally	Antiseptic
Benzalkonium chloride	1:5,000–1:2,000 vaginally 0.02–0.2% externally	Antimicrobial	Papain		Proteolytic
			Parabens (total)	0.05–0.3%[a]	Antimicrobial
			Phenol	0.5–1.0%[a]	Antiseptic Counterirritant
Benzethonium chloride	1:750[a]	Antimicrobial	Phenylmercuric acetate	0.02% on mucous membranes 0.2% externally 0.002–0.125% as a preservative	Antimicrobial
Benzocaine	1.0–20%[a]	Local anesthetic			
Boric acid[b]	1.0–4.0%[a]	Buffer			
Cetylpyridinium chloride	1:10,000–1:2,000 on mucous membranes	Antiseptic surfactant	Povidone-iodine[d]	10% (0.5–3.0% of available iodine)[a]	Antimicrobial
Chloramine-T	1:1,000–1:100 externally	Antimicrobial	Resorcinol	2.0–20%[a]	Antimicrobial
Citric acid		Buffer	Salicylic acid	2.0–20%[a]	
Eucalyptol		Antiseptic Counterirritant Deodorant	Sodium bicarbonate		Antiseptic Buffer
			Sodium perborate		Antiseptic Buffer
Hexachlorophene	0.2%[c]	Antimicrobial			
Lactic acid		Buffer	Thymol	1.0%	Antiseptic Counterirritant
Menthol	0.1–2.0%[a]	Antiseptic Counterirritant			
			Zinc oxide	15–25%[a]	
Methylbenze-thonium chloride	1:10,000–1:100[a]		Zinc sulfate	0.25–4.0%[a]	Astringent

Adapted from Remington's Pharmaceutical Sciences, 14th ed., A. Osol and J. E. Hoover, Eds., Mack, Easton, Pa., 1970.

[a]Recommendation does not specify difference in concentration between external skin and mucous membranes and should be viewed cautiously because mucous membranes may be more sensitive.

[b]From T. E. Swate and J. C. Weed, *Obstet. Gynecol., 43*, 893 (1974).

[c]Present legal FDA maximum allowable concentration in nonprescription products (From FDA Minutes of the OTC Panel on Contraceptives and Other Vaginal Drug Products.)

[d]From J. J. Ratzan, *Calif. Med., 110*, 24 (1969).

initis (13, 14), although questions of safety have arisen (15). The possibility of local irritation or sensitization exists with many antimicrobial agents found in douches, and if these effects are encountered, the patient should be instructed to discontinue use of the product and to consult a physician.

Counterirritants Counterirritant compounds such as eucalyptol, menthol, phenol, methyl salicylate, and thymol are included in douche products for their anesthetic or antipruritic effects; however, the efficacy of these agents has not been substantiated. Eucalyptol and methyl salicylate may mask odors by their fragrances. Aromatic agents (chlorothymol, eucalyptol, menthol, thymol, or methyl salicylate) may be added for the general effect of producing a soothing and refreshing feeling. (See Chapter 27, *External Analgesic Products.*)

Astringents Astringent substances such as ammonium and potassium alums and zinc sulfate are included in some douches to reduce local edema, inflammation, and exudation. Micronized aluminum powder also has been used as an astringent douche (3). The astringent concentration is important because many astringents are irritants in moderate or high concentrations (16).

Proteolytics At least one proteolytic agent, papain, is used in a douche product to remove excess vaginal discharge. Papain may elicit allergic reactions.

Surfactants Docusate sodium, nonoxynol 4, and sodium lauryl sulfate are used to facilitate the douche's spread over vaginal mucosa and penetration of mucosal folds (rugae) (2). Cetylpyridinium chloride, benzalkonium chloride, and benzethonium chloride also have surface-active properties.

Substances Affecting pH   Many vaginal douche products are buffered or contain substances that purposely render them either acidic or alkaline. For example, sodium perborate and sodium bicarbonate provide alkalinity, and lactic acid and citric acid provide acidity. The significance of pH and buffering is discussed in the section on advisability of douching.

Miscellaneous Ingredients   Other ingredients occasionally found in douches are emollients, emulsifiers, keratolytics, and substances intended to raise the preparations' osmolarity. Liquid vehicles are alcohol, propylene glycol, water, or combinations of these substances. Talc is used as a vehicle for douche powders intended to be instilled as powders (insufflations). Lactose may be added as a bacterial nutrient, but the reason for its inclusion is unclear. Many gynecologists feel that a simple douche consisting of small amounts of white vinegar and tap water (2 tbsp of vinegar/quart water) is as good as commercially available products. Premixed vinegar douches have been made available commercially.

Types of Syringes
Several types of syringes are used for douching. The combination water bottle-syringe (fountain syringe) and the folding feminine syringe are held above hip level while the douche liquid is instilled into the vagina by gravity. These syringes are supplied with the necessary tubing and tips for use with douches or with enemas. Patients should be advised of the difference between douche and enema tips and that they are not interchangeable. Interchanging douche and enema tips may lead to infection. The main advantage to the combination (fountain) and folding feminine syringes is that fluids are instilled with gentle gravity force only, thereby minimizing the chance of excessive fluid force.

Bulb-type feminine syringes also may be used with douche liquids by gentle squeezing of the bulb. The main advantage of bulb-type feminine syringes is ease of handling, since it is not necessary to use tubing or to hold the syringe at an elevated level. Care must be exercised, however, to avoid excessive squeezing and excessive fluid force on instillation of the douche. Excessive force may introduce fluid into the cervix, which may cause an inflammatory response, depending on the degree of uterine involvement.

Techniques of Douching
To avoid the possible dangers of improper douching, several investigators recommend procedures to ensure safe instillation (7, 17–19):

- Douches should never be instilled with excess pressure. The force of gravity is sufficient if a bag, tube, and nozzle are used. The douche bag should not be more than 60 cm (about 24 inches) above the hips. If a syringe is used, minimum pressure should be applied.
- Most douches should be instilled while the patient is lying down, the knees drawn up and the hips raised.
- Water used to dilute powder or douche solutions should be lukewarm, not hot.
- Douching equipment should be cleaned thoroughly before and after use. Sterilization by boiling is also recommended. (The use of disposable douche products eliminates this inconvenience.)
- Douches should not be used during pregnancy.
- Douches should not be used when using the cervical mucus method of contraception, so that test results are not altered. (See Chapter 18, *Contraceptive Methods and Products*.)

Recommendations concerning the frequency of douching vary widely. One study found that 175 women douching daily had higher vaginal epithelial glycogen concentrations than 199 women douching less often than daily, implying that the group douching more frequently experienced a beneficial effect. Water and a medicinal powder douche were used, but the ingredients and nature of the medicinal powder were not stated (20).

Some studies recommend avoiding routine douching altogether (15, 18, 21). A common recommendation, however, is that a woman who prefers routine douching should not do so more than twice per week unless otherwise advised by the physician or pharmacist. The potential for harm from frequent douching depends in part on the formulation and the technique of instillation, both of which may be incorrect. Properly prepared and properly instilled, a douche used twice per week should cause no harm, but it has not been proven that twice-weekly or even less frequent douching is necessary at all.

An alternative self-bathing method for vaginal and perineal areas has been studied for benefits and possible adverse effects in more than 500 women, including 180 with symptoms or diagnosis of vaginitis. The technique involves gentle washing, with the fingers, of the vulvar, perineal, and anal regions and the vagina, using only lukewarm water and a mild soap. The technique was effective as a cleansing practice and was 94% effective in clearing the symptoms of vaginitis, whose recurrence rate was slightly more than 5% (22).

Patient Consultation
Evaluating whether or not a woman should use a douche for routine vaginal cleansing is quite difficult; both sides of the conflict are well represented in the literature. The FDA position regarding safety and efficacy of vaginal douching is that there are no standards for evaluating or substantiating claims (23).

Adverse effects of douches on vaginal pH, flora, and cytology have been cited as potential hazards of routine douching. However, the effects of acid, alkaline, and vinegar douches on vaginal pH and vaginal mucosal cytology are not significant (4, 24). An alkaline douche is said to be more effective than an acid douche for removing vaginal discharge and relieving pruritus, and it is effective as adjunctive therapy in vaginitis (24–26).

Other reports also support douching as a safe, effective cleansing mechanism that does not alter vaginal pH significantly if the douche preparation is unbuffered (2,

3, 27); acidic rather than alkaline douches are advised, however, because shifts toward alkalinity may inhibit normal flora and promote pathogen growth (2, 3). Of course, care should be taken that the douche is not excessively acidic, causing irritation or injury.

In one study, douching caused no significant alterations in normal vaginal flora. Moreover, significant increases in vaginal epithelial glycogen content were observed in women who douched and it was concluded that douching was not only harmless but even beneficial to vaginal and cervical epithelium (20). Others also have attested to the safety of routine douching carried out according to physician instructions (28, 29). No evidence was found that douche ingredients may be absorbed systemically in significant quantities. Boric acid and phenylmercuric acetate may be absorbed but not in toxic amounts (13, 15).

On the other hand, there is good evidence that povidone-iodine is absorbed from the vagina in significant amounts (30). This poses a particular hazard to pregnant women, in whom amniotic fluid may contain total iodine levels 10–150 times control values (31). It seems unlikely that a single application of povidone-iodine during pregnancy would affect the fetus; however, repeated application may result in iodine-induced goiter and hypothyroidism in the fetus, with sequelae such as airway obstruction, mental and physical retardation, and neurologic disturbances (30). The vagina is a highly absorptive organ, and during pregnancy it becomes hyperemic, having the potential for exaggerated absorption of toxic substances. Therefore it seems wise to avoid douching with anything that contains potentially toxic chemicals during pregnancy. Pregnant women may also be at risk for fetal complications or other hazards of douching.

A significant number of case reports described adverse effects, suggesting that douching may be unwise without specific indication. Five cases were studied in which salpingitis, endometritis, or pelvic inflammatory disease was associated with douching. Instillation pressure of the douche fluid was implicated in each case (19).

Ninety percent of 101 patients with pelvic inflammatory disease were reported as being "vigorous" douchers (32). Other conditions linked to douching are infection, hemorrhage, trauma, embolism, and chemical peritonitis (17, 18, 22, 33).

Perhaps the most frequent adverse affects of douches are direct, primary mucosal/dermal irritation or allergic contact sensitivity from specific ingredients. No well-controlled clinical studies of these effects on vaginal mucosa after douching could be found, but many ingredients of douche preparations have been implicated in these dermal effects. Dermal irritants or sensitizers may affect the vaginal epithelium similarly. Compounds incorporated into douche products that cause direct chemical effects, especially allergic contact sensitivity, include benzalkonium and benzethonium chlorides, benzocaine, chlorhexidine hydrochloride, chloroxylenol, parabens, phenol, propylene glycol monostearate, and triethanolamine (34–39).

Potential hazards must be weighed against the questionable value of routine douching in the absence of symptoms. According to one investigator, despite reported adverse effects, "a douche properly prepared and administered is harmless" (19). The key words in this statement are "properly prepared and administered." This is where the pharmacist can help by proper counseling.

Douche products should not be considered contraceptive agents. Douches of normal volume, properly instilled, are ineffective in removing seminal fluid for contraceptive purposes (21). Precoital douches also are ineffective as contraceptives (19). Postcoital douching is preferred by some women, but the benefits are probably psychological or placebo because the superiority of douching over cleansing with soap and water has not been demonstrated conclusively. Douching should be done no sooner than 6–8 hours after the use of a vaginal spermicide because spermicidal agents may be removed in the douching process.

Feminine Deodorant Sprays

Feminine deodorant sprays are aerosol products in mist or powder form intended for use on the external genital area to reduce or mask objectionable odor. A typical formula includes an antimicrobial agent, an emollient carrier, a perfume, and a propellant. Talc is added to spray powders. The FDA considers these products cosmetics and prohibits references to "hygiene" by manufacturers (40). The sprays do not possess therapeutic or medicinal properties. They may be used as deodorants or simply for their placebo effect.

Ingredients

Some concentrations of feminine deodorant spray ingredients may be safe for external skin but not necessarily for vaginal mucosa.

Perfumes   Fragrances or perfumes, the main ingredients of feminine deodorant sprays, are responsible for deodorant activity. They should be selected with care because some may be irritating to perineal and vaginal mucosa (41). Fragrances are characterized as mild or strong, short- or long-lasting, sweet, medicinal, and floral, among other categories (42). Some products contain encapsulated perfumes that are released slowly on contact with moisture.

Antimicrobials   Antimicrobial compounds in sprays include benzalkonium and benzethonium chlorides, chloroxylenol, and hexachlorophene. These and similar compounds are preservatives rather than therapeutic agents. Although a deodorant action may be achieved by inhibiting or eradicating vulvoperineal bacteria, the sprays do not deodorize by this mechanism. Properly used, they do not alter normal vulvovaginal flora (43). Holding the spray too close to the body may result in an excessively high surface concentration of the antimicrobial agent or may cause the agent to enter into the vagina, where the concentration also may be excessive.

Emollients   A number of emollient substances are included in these formulations as vehicles and for their soothing effect on the skin. The most commonly used are fatty alcohols, esters such as isopropyl myristate, and polyoxyethylene derivatives of fatty esters. Unfortunately, some of these substances also may be sensitizers (35, 37, 41).

Propellants If the spray is held too close to the body and the propellant reaches the skin, the chilling effects or even tissue freezing when the spray evaporates may cause irritation and edema (44, 41, 45). With proper application, propellants are not likely to be irritants. The fluorinated hydrocarbon propellants previously used have largely been replaced by aliphatic hydrocarbons such as propane and isobutane. These have low toxicity potential and a vapor pressure similar to fluorocarbons (46).

Proper Application of Sprays

Most manufacturers recommend that sprays be held at least 20 cm (about 8 inches) from the body when applying. By following this direction, premarketing evaluations of sprays consistently demonstrate safety. The most frequent adverse effect resulting from applying a spray held too closely is irritation as a result of evaporation and "chilling" from propellants inappropriately reaching the skin, excessive concentrations of ingredients on cutaneous surfaces, or accidental penetration of ingredients into the vagina from the force of the spray (ingredients are intended only for external use).

The relationship between frequency of use and the incidence of adverse effects has not been described well in the literature. It is reasonable to assume, however, that frequent application, perhaps several times/day, may elicit more frequent local reactions than less frequent use. If women are fully informed of the possibility and nature of side effects, they can, with the help of the pharmacist, determine a desirable frequency of application for themselves.

Patient Consultation

As with douche products, the advisability and benefits of using feminine deodorant sprays are controversial. Their efficacy even as deodorants has been questioned, and adverse effects have been reported (47). When the sprays are used as directed, however, manufacturers report that extensive testing fails to demonstrate adverse effects.

A feminine deodorant spray was evaluated in 1,400 women after more than 200,000 test applications by direct application and patch testing (48). However, the results of the study are difficult to evaluate because many details were not provided. The study findings supported the position that the sprays were nonirritating and nonsensitizing. It was also reported that, in one group of 300 women, 8% of the control group experienced erythema from soap and water, but only 3% of those using the spray experienced this effect. The study results provided no other explanations for consumer complaints of vulvar irritation after the use of these sprays. It was suggested that close-fitting and/or nonabsorbent undergarments caused vulvar irritation even if no spray was applied; that the symptoms might appear if sprays are used immediately after intercourse; or that the sprays were held too close to the body when applied.

Despite reports that these aerosol products are not hazardous when evaluated in controlled studies and when properly used, there is evidence that hazards do exist. Physicians in private practice reported vulvar irritation in some of their female patients, and feminine deodorant sprays were strongly suspected as being the cause (49, 50). The FDA receives many reports of adverse local reactions, all locally severe and all attributed to the use of these products (51). In most of these cases, systemic steroid treatment was required even when the sprays were discontinued. The specific ingredients responsible for adverse effects, however, were not identified. Four positive patch-test reactions to specific ingredients were reported after 30 women and 2 men were tested with the individual ingredients in 12 different sprays (41). The ingredients eliciting positive responses were benzethonium chloride, chlorhexidine, isopropyl myristate, and perfume. Ingredients in douches that cause either direct primary irritation or allergic contact sensitization also are found frequently in feminine deodorant sprays. Women who use sprays immediately before sexual intercourse also may exhibit local reactions (41).

Most evidence criticizing feminine deodorant spray use is from case reports or complaints received by manufacturers, physicians, and the FDA; most evidence in defense of these products is cited by the authors as the findings of controlled studies. However, in controlled studies, subjects are given instructions on proper application. The use of sprays throughout the population is uncontrolled, and it is especially difficult to assess the incidence of improper application. It seems that feminine deodorant sprays are harmless to most users, but reports of adverse effects are too frequent to be ignored, and the significant potential hazards must be considered. Furthermore, the superiority of these sprays over soap and water has been questioned (52, 53). In the absence of conclusive demonstrations of prominent adverse effects, feminine deodorant sprays continue to be marketed.

Miscellaneous Products

Although their uses and ingredients are similar to the douche or spray formulations, some nonprescription vaginal products are available as suppositories, premoistened towelettes, and local anesthetic creams.

The antimicrobial agents used in vaginal antiseptic suppositories are chloramine-T and phenylmercuric acetate, each contained in a greaseless, water-dispersible suppository base. Both compounds are effective antimicrobial agents in vitro, but subjective appraisal of their clinical efficacy is impossible because the agents' concentration in the vagina following dispersion is unknown (54). Both chloramine-T and phenylmercuric acetate may produce local irritation in sufficient concentration or in sensitive individuals. Because these suppositories are used for purposes similar to those for douches, the same considerations concerning benefits and risks apply.

Premoistened towelettes are used for their deodorant, cleansing, and/or cosmetic properties. Except for the propellants in sprays, ingredients of these towelettes are similar to those of aerosols. Women who are sensitive to aerosol propellants might be informed of the towelette formulations. Direct irritation or sensitization from other towelette ingredients may occur.

One vaginal product contains benzocaine as the local anesthetic and resorcinol for antimicrobial effects. Concentrations of benzocaine and resorcinol in this cream are not provided, so efficacy cannot be readily determined. Both ingredients may cause local irritation or sensitization (16, 34, 35). The intended purpose and use of this product present another significant hazard: the masking of vaginitis symptoms. In the presence of symptoms possibly indicating vaginitis, the pharmacist should not recommend a vaginal cream or similar local anesthetic vaginal product without concurrent recommendation by the woman's physician.

A new nonprescription hydrocortisone cream is now being advertised. There is a possibility of increased mucosal absorption of the hydrocortisone. Patients should be instructed to use hydrocortisone products with caution since could mask vaginitis symptoms.

Product Selection Guidelines

The pharmacist should determine persistence, recurrence, and severity of any symptoms or ascertain signs of infection or disease before attempting to recommend a product. If infection or disease is suspected, the patient should be referred to a physician. Patient history or medication profiles may reveal predisposing factors to vaginitis such as pregnancy, diabetes, and chronic use of steroids (including oral contraceptives) or antibiotics (especially tetracyclines). If local infection or other systemic diseases are suspected, specific diagnosis and medical treatment are always indicated.

When satisfied that a nonprescription product may be used safely, the pharmacist should make the following recommendations:

- Douches used routinely in the absence of symptoms should probably be acidic or as nearly physiological as possible.
- If a douche is used to remove excessive discharge, an alkaline douche may be more effective.
- Douches and sprays should be avoided before coitus.
- Douches are not contraceptive and should be used after coitus only for cleansing. If spermicidal jelly, cream, or foam is used, douching should be delayed a minimum of 6–8 hours following intercourse.
- Proper application techniques should be followed.
- If irritation occurs, the product should be discontinued.
- Regardless of the reasons for seeking a vaginal product, thorough cleansing with soap and water may be equally or more effective.

Antiperspirants and Underarm Deodorants

Commercial products to alleviate body odor have been sold since the late 1800's. Today, Americans spend more than three-quarters of a billion dollars annually on products to decrease or prevent underarm odor and wetness (55). Nearly every adult in North America uses one of the variety of antiperspirants, deodorants, or deodorant soaps available. However, many consumers are unaware of the difference between antiperspirants and deodorants, and they may buy one product expecting the other's effect. Therefore, pharmacist input into the selection of a product is desirable.

Anatomy and Physiology of Sweat Glands

Commercial products may be aimed at affecting the products of two types of sweat glands—eccrine and apocrine. Eccrine, or true sweat glands, are simple coiled tubular glands lying deep in the dermis, unrelated to hair follicles. They are distributed over most of the skin surface, but particularly on the palms, soles, face, and axillae. Eccrine glands consist of a secretory coil in the lower dermis and subcutaneous tissue and a duct that travels in a helical manner to the skin surface (Figure 1). The duct contains an intraepidermal unit that modifies composition of the sweat. Constituents of eccrine secretion are water, sodium, potassium, chloride, urea, lactate, and very small amounts of glucose. The secretion is hypotonic and has a pH of 4–6.8.

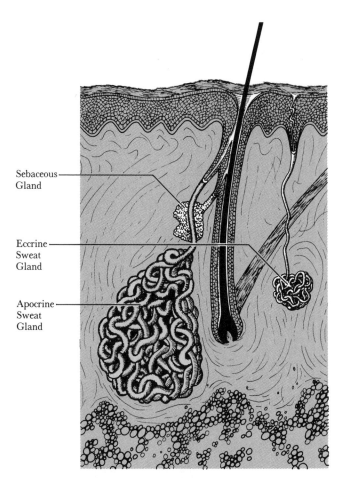

Figure 1. Glandular appendages of the epidermis.

Adequate eccrine gland function is vital to maintenance of normal body temperature. Heat can be dispelled by evaporation of moisture on the skin surface. However, the cooling function of sweat is provided by glands all over the body and therefore inhibition of sweating in just one area, such as the axillae, is not harmful (56). Although perspiration contains "waste products" such as urea and lactate, perspiring is not important in purification of the blood. People who live in cool environments do not suffer from lack of perspiration (56).

The eccrine glands are unusual in being cholinergic in function but supplied with sympathetic nerves. Intact innervation is necessary for function. Activity of the glands' nervous stimulation is controlled by three stimuli: Thermal stimulation produces sweating mainly on the face and upper trunk; emotional stimulation causes perspiration mainly on the palms, soles, and axillae; and sensory stimulation can produce local perspiration (hot, spicy food causes sweating around the face). Thermal stimulation has a latent period before sweating starts, but emotional and sensory stimulation cause an immediate response. In the normal adult, the quantity of eccrine perspiration varies from negligible under basal conditions to 12 liters in 24 hours at maximal stimulation (56). The average production is about 1 liter/day, but this varies with race, age, sex, conditioning, and acclimatization to heat. Eccrine sweat is normally odorless, although food and drug substances may be excreted with it.

Apocrine glands produce a scanty, milky substance that is odorless upon secretion but becomes odoriferous upon bacterial decomposition. Apocrine glands are confined mainly to the axilla, the areola, groin, and perineum. They are poorly developed in children and begin to enlarge at puberty. Each consists of a coiled secretory tubule and a duct that normally opens into the neck of the hair follicle above the sebaceous gland (Figure 1). The secretion serves no known useful purpose but it may have evolved as a mechanism for sexual attraction (56). Apocrine secretion is intermittent and produced at a very slow rate. There are differences in apocrine activity between races. Secretion rate is indifferent to thermal stimulation but responds to emotional stress and mechanical stimulation.

Disorders of Sweat Glands

Some underarm moisture (hidrosis) or odor (bromhidrosis) is normal but is ingrained into our culture as being offensive. Excess wetness may be embarrassing as well as damaging to clothes. Odor and wetness are related but distinct problems. Wetness is caused by eccrine glands, while odor is primarily caused by bacterial decomposition of apocrine secretion. It is hard to determine what causes more concern since the problems are usually considered by laity to be inseparable (55).

Wetness is due to water being secreted faster than it evaporates. The axillae normally retain moisture because evaporation is retarded there. Transient hyperhidrosis is a physiologic response to heat or emotion. Pathologic hyperhidrosis may be caused by certain medical disorders like thyrotoxicosis, anxiety and fever,

abnormalities in the autonomic system, or disorders of the sweat glands themselves (57). Hyperhidrosis due to disorders of the sweat glands usually presents as a symmetrical problem involving the axillae, soles, or palms (people with moist handshakes). Hyperhidrosis more often affects young women (54).

In contrast to hyperhidrosis, anhidrosis may occur due to hypothermia, local lesions in the autonomic nervous system, or malfunction of the sweat gland itself. Compensatory hyperhidrosis occurs in the remaining normal sweat glands when those elsewhere are not functioning (58).

Prickly heat (miliaria rubra) involves closure of the pore of the eccrine sweat gland and blockage of sweat delivery. Closure of the pore causes sweat to enter the surrounding epidermis with consequent irritation.

The immediate cause of body odor is the growth of bacteria in the secretion of apocrine sweat glands. The odor of freshly collected perspiration may be mild but not generally objectionable. It varies with the individual, activity, emotional state, and diet (59). Both eccrine and apocrine secretions are sterile and initially odorless. When left to stand, perspiration undergoes considerable change, mainly due to bacterial degradation of apocrine secretions (60). It is not clear what component actually causes the odor, but degradation of apocrine secretions produces short-chain fatty acids like caproic and butyric acids, mercaptans, indoles, ammonia, amines, and hydrogen sulfide. The presence of hair increases axillary odor since it acts as a collecting site for secretions, debris, and bacteria. Wetness from eccrine secretion promotes bacterial growth and dispersion of apocrine secretion.

It is also not known which organisms produce the odor or in what numbers they must be present. Differences of 100-fold have been observed in the healthy axillae of the same persons at different times without noticeable odor (56). Such observations may not have differentiated between resident bacteria, whose normal habitation is the skin, and transient bacteria which are deposited incidentally from the atmosphere and clothing. Conditions that favor retention of apocrine secretion on the skin or which favor bacterial multiplication should be conducive to the development of odor, but the latter assumption in particular remains unproved. In most cases body odor is not due to biologic dysfunction but is a matter of personal hygiene. Presence of sebum, perspiration, and debris greatly increase axillary odor. Regular removal of debris by bathing will reduce odor but washing alone does not remove all products of degraded perspiration and cannot remove many of the resident bacteria on the skin. Thus, for some individuals additional measures must be employed.

In assessing the appropriate method of dealing with perspiration problems, the pharmacist must first determine whether the person is more concerned about a wetness problem or an odor problem. Second, the pharmacist should determine if the problem is psychological or pathologic. In pathologic hyperhidrosis, patients will complain of constant heavy perspiration inappropriate to the climate and situation and more frequently complain of palmar or plantar sweating than axillary (57).

Nonprescription antiperspirants are not adequate to relieve pathologic hyperhidrosis. Patients with such a problem should be referred to a physician for diagnosis and treatment.

Wetness problems that do not respond to nonprescription products may be treated in several ways. Stronger concentrations of aluminum chloride in absolute ethanol (Drysol and Xerac-AC) are available on prescription. These preparations are applied to the hyperhydrotic areas at bedtime; the area may be covered with a plastic wrap, then the residue is washed off in the morning (61). Systemic anticholinergics may be prescribed to reduce perspiration flow. Rarely, in refractory cases of hyperhidrosis, radiotherapy or various operative procedures, including sympathectomy, excision, or curettage of eccrine glands, and cryotherapy, may be attempted (57).

Treatment of Perspiration Problems

Disorders of perspiration can be approached in multiple ways. A substance can be applied to reduce the amount of eccrine perspiration secreted (no product can reduce apocrine secretion). Such substances are labeled antiperspirants, and are classified as drugs by the FDA because they are intended to influence a physiologic body process. In addition, a substance may prevent, mask, or change perspiration odor without attempting to block its flow. These preparations are termed deodorants and are regarded as cosmetics. Deodorants may contain perfumes to mask odor, germicides to inhibit bacterial growth, or powders to absorb moisture. Many commercial products are combinations of antiperspirants and deodorants. However, any product labeled as a "deodorant" cannot make any antiperspirant claims.

The fact that numerous products are marketed for these purposes speaks for their popularity. Plain antiperspirants tend to be the least acceptable since their action is relatively hard to notice, while the failure of a deodorant product to do its job is much more obvious.

Another approach to preventing odor is good hygiene. In addition to a regular bathing, shaving the affected area is valuable. This removes hair that serves to retain moisture, which acts as a substrate for bacteria.

Pharmacologic Agents

The FDA advisory review panel on nonprescription antiperspirant drug products issued a tentative monograph in October 1978. It found that aluminum chlorohydrates, aluminum chloride, buffered aluminum sulfate, and aluminum zirconium chlorohydrates (other than in aerosol form) were safe and effective as topical antiperspirants, in the appropriate concentration. However, due to concerns for their safety, the panel has recommended that all aerosol antiperspirants be studied further (61).

Currently used ingredients have evolved from the empirical use of astringent metal salts, many of which were tried and discarded due to undesirable properties like staining or irritation. Although their action in reducing flow of eccrine perspiration can be measured objectively, their mechanism of action has been a subject of

intense debate that is still unresolved. The oldest theory attributes their action to simple astringency, causing shrinkage of the pore. It was speculated that antiperspirants acted on sweat glands to produce inflammation and swelling around the duct, thereby contracting its orifice. However, a number of chemicals that are strong astringents have minimal antiperspirant activity. Another theory was that antiperspirants increased the permeability of the sweat duct, causing reabsorption of sweat (the "leaky hose" theory) (62).

One study has indicated that a physically demonstrable obstruction of the duct accounts for anhidrosis (63). After stripping the stratum corneum from the skin, antiperspirant activity still remains; thus obstruction is more than superficial. A plug may be caused by keratin precipitated by the antiperspirant. However, the keratin plug is probably a late, nonspecific reaction to injury, while the initial plug is caused by an amorphous, aluminum-containing cast that extends down the length of the duct. There is no inflammation (63). The individual sweat duct remains physically occluded until it is replaced by normal cell renewal in 2–3 weeks. Thus, antiperspirants have a prolonged action (56). The degree to which antiperspirants decrease wetness is relatively feeble and could not be enough to cause an appreciable decrease in odor (56). Antiperspirants are also strong antibacterials and, therefore, may be effective deodorants (61, 64).

For maximum decrease in wetness, prescription products must be used. Ideally, the product should be applied at night when sweat glands are inactive, and after application, the affected area should be occluded for 2–8 hours. A high degree of acidity may be desirable to help deposit the aluminum salts deep in the epidermis. Dry skin also enhances penetration (57, 65).

Because acidity is irritating to the skin and damaging to clothing, nonprescription antiperspirant formulations may be buffered by the addition of urea or glycine in 5–10% concentrations. Buffers do not appreciably increase the pH of a preparation or act as alkalis to precipitate aluminum hydroxide, which would reduce antiperspirant activity. However, at ironing temperatures, urea decomposes to ammonia and neutralizes acidity to protect clothing (59).

The adverse effects of nonprescription antiperspirants are mostly skin irritation (tingling, stinging, or burning) and are due to chemical reaction with the skin; sensitization is very rare (56). Normally irritation can be reduced by decreasing the frequency or amount used. Antiperspirants should not be applied to freshly shaved skin. If erythema or papules develop, discontinuation of the product should be advised for a few days. During this period, a deodorant can be applied instead. The patient can usually return to the same antiperspirant later, using it in lesser amounts. In case the user is sensitive to a specific ingredient, content of all products are fully labeled so that a different formulation can be used.

There is no evidence that antiperspirants cause permanent harm to sweat glands. Normal sweating resumes a week after discontinuing use. There also is no evidence of systemic toxicity caused by topical application of antiperspirants (56).

Aluminum Chloride

Aluminum chloride, $AlCl_3$, hydrolyzes in water to aluminum hydroxide and hydrochloric acid, forming strongly acidic solutions. This characteristic tends to cause damage to fabrics in contact with treated skin and makes it very irritating to the skin at higher concentrations. Therefore the FDA advisory review panel on nonprescription antiperspirant drug products has recommended that only concentrations of 15% or less should be considered both effective and safe. Solutions of aluminum chloride show significantly greater efficacy compared to less irritating antiperspirant compounds (56).

Aluminum Chlorohydrates

Aluminum chlorohydrates are available commercially in several different forms that differ in the ratio of aluminum to chlorine. The empirical formulas of the most widely used ingredients are $Al_2(OH)_4Cl_2$ and $Al_2(OH)_5$-Cl, which are known as 2/3 basic and 5/6 basic aluminum chloride, respectively. Aluminum chlorohydrates are available also as polyethylene glycol or propylene glycol complexes. These complexes are formulated to provide greater alcohol solubility and do not affect the safety or efficacy of the salts from which they are prepared (56). The advantage of chlorohydrate salts over aluminum chloride is their lower acidity. The greater the aluminum-to-chlorine ratio in the salt, the less acidic is the solution.

The panel found that aluminum chlorohydrates are safe and effective when applied topically to the underarms in concentrations of 25% (anhydrous) or less. These concentrations have produced very little skin irritation, either in patch testing or in market experience.

Aluminum Zirconium Chlorohydrates

Salts of zirconium enjoyed a brief period of popularity until they were discovered to cause skin and lung granulomas. However, they apparently are safer when combined with aluminum salts. Aerosol products containing zirconium have already been banned (66). Skin changes have been found in rabbits injected with zirconium aluminum glycine complex, but the panel did not consider this serious enough to disallow nonprescription use in nonaerosol form (56).

Aluminum zirconium salts vary in their ratio of aluminum to zirconium to chlorine. These complexes are also acidic, with solutions having a pH around 4. They are recommended for nonprescription use in concentrations of not more than 20% anhydrous weight, applied topically to the axillae.

Buffered Aluminum Sulfate

Aluminum sulfate itself produces a high degree of irritation. However, it is available as an 8% solution buffered with 8% sodium aluminum lactate. This preparation is effective and virtually nonirritating (56).

Glutaraldehyde

Glutaraldehyde 2% in buffered solution is available without prescription. It is used to treat hyperhidrosis of the palms and soles, but not the axillae (67). It is thought to act by occluding the sweat ducts.

Antibacterials

Deodorants may use perfumes and colognes to cover up body odor or they may try to prevent it by inhibiting bacterial action. It is not known what bacteria need to be inhibited or to what numbers they must be reduced in order to prevent odor, but this has not prevented a variety of compounds from being tried.

The antibiotic neomycin has excellent broad spectrum topical activity. However, it may sensitize the skin to further applications. Boric acid has also been used but it can be absorbed through the skin and cause toxicity. Quaternary ammonium compounds such as benzalkonium chloride have a broad spectrum of activity. However, they are swiftly inactivated by the skin and are incompatible with soaps or anionic surfactants.

The phenolic compounds are longer lasting and compatible with soaps. Hexachlorophene was the most widely used before being banned from nonprescription use. Triclosan and trichlorocarbanilide are frequently found in deodorants and deodorant soaps such as Dial and Coast. The astringent aluminum salts also have antiseptic properties. Compounds of metals other than aluminum are used as deodorants. Zinc phenolsulfonate is useful in liquid products; zinc oxide, peroxide, or stearate are used in powders (59).

Dosage Forms

The ideal antiperspirant or deodorant should apply conveniently, dry quickly, not stain clothing, be nonirritating, and last all day after a single application. The variety of products available indicates that they are far from ideal.

Creams were the first available form of antiperspirant but were largely abandoned for more elegant and convenient forms. Aerosols became immensely popular in the 1960's, capturing up to 85% of the market. However, their use plummeted after publicity about adverse effects on the lung and on the environment. Furthermore, their effectiveness is low.

All dosage forms are not equally effective. Table 3 gives the range of perspiration reduction in laboratory hot rooms based on data submitted to the FDA. Several points are illustrated by these data:

- No nonprescription product inhibits wetness completely; during normal use only 20–40% reduction can be expected (56).
- Minor variations in formulation may have a critical effect on a product's activity (68); thus two similar products may be quite different in effectiveness.
- There is extreme individual variability in response to antiperspirants; some subjects actually perspire more after some applications (66).

The FDA advisory review panel felt that a 20% reduction in wetness was the minimum required to be noticeable by the user. Therefore, FDA has suggested that an average reduction of 20% be ensured for each final formulation.

Powders are not listed in Table 3, as these are generally deodorants that absorb moisture. To be active, antiperspirant ingredients must be in solution (59). Sodium bicarbonate is a time-honored deodorant; besides

Table 3. Efficacy of antiperspirant application forms

Application form	Average sweat reduction
Aerosols	20–33%
Creams	35–47%
Roll-ons	14–70%
Lotions	38–62%
Liquids	15–54%
Sticks	35–40%

Reprinted from the *Federal Register, 43,* 46694 (1978).

absorbing moisture, its alkalinity may be inhibitory to bacteria.

Labeling Claims

The panel felt there were insufficient data on non-prescription antiperspirants for certain label claims to be allowed. Unless appropriate data are submitted for each product, the FDA would prohibit claims of "long lasting" or "all day" effectiveness, and claims of being effective for "emotional" or "troublesome" perspiration. Claims about "extra strength" would be disallowed entirely since concentration does not necessarily correlate with effectiveness. However, a product could be labeled "extra effective" if it caused an average 30% reduction in wetness.

Patient Consultation

The pharmacist should be sure that the consumer understands the difference between deodorants and antiperspirants. Deodorants are not a substitute for cleanliness; their use should follow bathing. Antiperspirants reduce but do not stop wetness, especially during thermal or emotional stress. Antiperspirants are not effective immediately after application. Repeated applications over time are needed to achieve the maximal effect (56).

When applying antiperspirants, the user should let his or her underarm dry. This reduces discomfort by reducing the hydrolysis of aluminum salts to hydrochloric acid by moisture. In addition, the antiperspirant effect is completely abolished if the subject is perspiring during application (63). Application should be avoided on open, broken, abraded, or freshly shaved skin.

Finally, the patient should be advised of the marked variation in response to antiperspirants from person to person and product to product. If one product does not perform satisfactorily it is quite reasonable to try others.

Skin Bleaching Products

Hyperpigmentation of the skin may result from a variety of causes. It is usually asymptomatic and of no medical consequence, although it occasionally may signify systemic illness. Hyperpigmentation, particularly on the face, however, can be a source of cosmetic disability

and mental distress. Thus, agents that can bleach away excess pigment when applied topically have a large market around the world. Most of the skin bleaching products are available without a prescription.

Physiology of Skin Pigmentation

Normal skin color is contributed by melanocytes in the basal layer of the epidermis which produce pigment granules called melanosomes (Figure 2). These pigment granules contain a complex protein called melanin, a brown-black pigment. Melanocytes can be viewed as tiny one-celled glands with long projections to pass pigment particles into the keratinocytes which synthesize skin keratin. As keratinocytes migrate upward they carry the pigment with them and deposit it on the surface of the skin as they die. (See Chapter 28, *Topical Anti-infective Products.*) Melanocytes are also present in the hair bulb cells and pass pigment granules onto the hair (69).

Melanin is the most efficient sunscreen known. It acts to prevent damaging ultraviolet rays from the sun from entering deeper parts of the skin. When ultraviolet

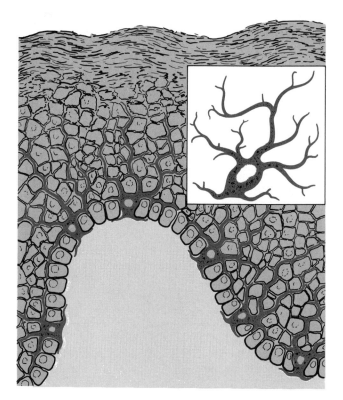

Figure 2. Melanocytes in the epidermis. The melanin-forming cells are situated among the basal cells. They have long branching cell processes of tubes through which the pigment granules are carried to be injected into the remaining nonmelanin-forming cells of the epidermis. The melanin often forms a supranuclear cap of pigment granules in the basal cells. The inset shows a single melanocyte with its elaborate branches. Adapted with permission from D. M. Pillsbury, "A Manual for Dermatology," W. B. Saunders, Philadelphia, Pa., 1971, pp. 22, 30.

light strikes the skin, not all of it is absorbed. Some reaches the deeper layers and may cause sunburn. Solar radiation also stimulates melanocytes to provide more melanin. This results in the gradual skin darkening or a "tan." The various human races have roughly the same number of melanocytes but dark-skinned peoples have more active ones.

Hyperpigmentation Syndromes

Certain systemic diseases and skin diseases cause pigment cells to become overactive resulting in darkening of the skin or to become underactive with resultant lightening of the skin.

Endocrine imbalances, such as Addison's disease, Cushing's disease, hyperthyroidism, pregnancy or estrogen therapy (including oral contraceptives), and skin cancer (melanoma) will affect skin pigmentation. Metabolic alterations affecting the liver and certain nutritional deficiencies can be associated with diffuse melanosis (70). Physical trauma or inflammatory dermatoses may cause a postinflammatory pigmentation. Also, certain drugs like chlorpromazine and hydroxychloroquine have an affinity for melanin and may cause hyperpigmentation. Thus, the pharmacist must inquire about concurrent drug therapy and systemic illnesses before recommending a nonprescription product. Diffuse pigmentation disorders and those caused by systemic factors should never be self-medicated without prior evaluation by a physician.

There are several causes of hyperpigmentation that are amenable to self-medication (69–71). These include freckles, melasma, and lentigines. Freckles are simply spots of uneven pigmentation that are exacerbated by the sun. Melasma (also called chloasma) is a condition in which blotchy patches occur on the face, usually due to hormonal imbalance; it is often caused by pregnancy ("the mask of pregnancy") or oral contraceptives, and sun exposure is necessary for its development. Lentigines are hyperpigmented spots that may appear at any age anywhere on the skin or mucous membranes and are due to an increased deposition of melanin and an increased number of melanocytes. They are darker than freckles and not induced by ultraviolet radiation. Solar or "senile" lentigines, commonly but incorrectly known as "liver spots," appear on the exposed surfaces of fair-skinned people and are induced by ultraviolet radiation.

Treatment

The intensity of localized hyperpigmentation on freckles, melasma, lentigines, or postinflammatory pigmentation may be decreased by topical nonprescription skin bleaching agents. Specific systemic therapy is required for diffuse systemic pigmentation disorders.

Nonprescription products are directed at suppression of melanin formation within the skin. The importance of avoiding excessive contact with sun, and the use of sunscreen agents or protective clothing needs to be emphasized to patients.

Physician-directed management of hyperpigmentation may include more effective prescription agents such as ointments formulated with 0.1% tretinoin, 5% hydroquinone, and 0.1% dexamethasone (74). Monobenzone should not be used because it produces irreversible depigmentation of normal as well as darkened skin. Light cryosurgical freezing with liquid nitrogen may also be used.

Pharmacologic Agents

Historically, a number of topical agents have been used in skin bleaching preparations. These have included hydroquinone, the monobenzyl and monomethyl ethers of hydroquinone, ammoniated mercury, ascorbic acid, and peroxides (72) Only preparations containing hydroquinone were submitted to the FDA advisory review panel on nonprescription skin bleaching agents for their review (70)

Hydroquinone

The panel has recommended that hydroquinone (p-dihydroxybenzene) in concentrations of 1.5–2% be available for nonprescription use. Hydroquinone and its derivatives are extensively used by industry as antioxidants.

Hydroquinone produces reversible depigmentation of the skin and hair of mice, guinea pigs, or humans by a complex mechanism of action. Hydroquinone and its derivatives are oxidized by tyrosinase to form highly toxic, free radicals that cause selective damage to the lipoprotein membranes of the melanocyte, thereby reducing conversion of tyrosine to dopa and subsequently to melanin (73). However, experiments on guinea pigs also indicate that it has toxic effects at the subcellular level in both follicular and nonfollicular melanocytes. It disrupts membranous cytoplasmic organelles, affecting formation, melanization, and degradation of melanosomes.

Several studies demonstrated that topical preparations of 2–5% hydroquinone are effective in producing cutaneous depigmentation (70). The 2% concentration is safer and has produced results equal to higher concentrations (74).

The effectiveness of hydroquinone varies among patients. The results are best on lighter skin and on lighter lesions. In blacks the response to hydroquinone depends on the amount of pigment present (75). The earlier it is used to treat minor skin blemishes, the more likely results will be satisfactory. When depigmentation does occur, melanin production is reduced by about one-half (70). Hyperpigmented areas fade more rapidly and completely than surrounding normal skin (71). Treatment may not lead to complete disappearance of hypermelanosis, but results are often satisfactory enough to reduce self-consciousness about hyperpigmentation.

When beginning treatment, melanin excretion may transiently increase. A decrease in skin color usually becomes noticeable in about 4 weeks; however, the time of onset varies from 3 weeks to 3 months. Eighty percent of patients with melasma improve within 8 weeks (71). Depigmentation lasts for 2–6 months but is reversible. Darker lesions repigment faster than lighter lesions. As the ability of the sun to darken lesions is much greater than that of hydroquinone to lighten them, strict avoidance of sunlight is imperative. Although sunscreens may help, even visible light will cause some darkening, and sun protection should preferably be opaque (71). Some hydroquinone products are available in an opaque base (Eldopaque) or together with a sunscreen (Ambi).

Side effects of topical hydroquinone are mild when used in low concentrations. Tingling or burning on application and subsequent erythema and inflammation were observed in 8% of patients using a 2% concentration and 32% of patients using a 5% concentration of hydroquinone (74). Higher concentrations frequently irritate the skin and if used for prolonged periods cause disfiguring effects including epidermal thickening and colloid milium (yellowish papules associated with colloid degeneration) (70).

In some cases lesions become slightly darker before fading. A transient inflammatory reaction may develop after the first few weeks of treatment. Occurrence of inflammation makes subsequent lightening more likely, although inflammation can occur without depigmentation developing. Appearance of mild inflammation need not be considered an indication to stop therapy except in the patient whose reaction increases in intensity (sensitization should be considered). Topical hydrocortisone may be used temporarily to alleviate the reaction. Contact with the eyes should be avoided.

If hydroquinone is accidentally ingested, it seldom produces serious systemic toxicity (70). However, oral ingestion of 5–12 g doses has produced tremor, convulsions, and hemolytic anemia (76).

Hydroquinone is easily oxidized in the presence of light and air. Any discoloration or darkening of the cream is an indication of deterioration in the strength of available hydroquinone (70). Thus, the preferable method of packaging it is in small squeeze tubes.

The dosage of hydroquinone is a thin application of 1.5–2% concentration rubbed into affected areas twice daily. Due to lack of safety data, it is not recommended for children under 12, except with the supervision of a physician. If no improvement is seen within 2 months, the use of hydroquinone should be discontinued and the advice of a physician sought. Once the desired benefit is achieved, hydroquinone can be applied as often as needed to maintain depigmentation.

Ammoniated Mercury

Ammoniated mercury, also known as ammoniated mercuric chloride, was in common use as a skin bleaching agent before monobenzone became available. No products with this ingredient were submitted for review by the panel, probably due to recognized concern for its safety. Chronic application can cause systemic mercury intoxication, and sensitization is common. There also is a lack of efficacy data. Therefore, the panel on skin bleaching products has recommended that ammoniated mercury not be made available on a nonprescription basis.

Monobenzone

The monobenzyl ether of hydroquinone is restricted to prescription only use. Its actions and onset time are similar to hydroquinone except that depigmentation may be permanent. Monobenzone should never be used

to treat hyperpigmentation because it permanently depigments both the hyperpigmented and the normal skin (71). Its use is restricted to depigmenting residual areas of normal skin in patients with extensive vitiligo (condition resulting in patches of depigmentation possibly with hyperpigmented borders).

Secondary Ingredients

Since hydroquinone is oxidized by contact with air, additional antioxidants such as sodium bisulfite may be added to the formulation. Hydroquinone is incompatible with alkali or ferric salts due to the ease of oxidation (76). Iodochlorhydroxyquin or oxyquinolone sulfate may be added as antimicrobial preservatives (70).

The inclusion of a sunscreen agent, such as an aminobenzoic acid ester, is rational and appropriate, provided that combination products are advertised as skin bleaching agents with added sunscreen and not primarily as sunscreens.

Patient Consultation

Before selecting a nonprescription product, be sure that a physician has confirmed the need for using it. Skin bleaching products are intended to lighten only limited areas of hyperpigmented skin. If the product is effective it should be noticeable within 2 months. It will not permanently injure the skin. Hydroquinone may be test-applied to a small area of unbroken skin and assessed for 24 hours to observe for irritation or allergic reactions. It should never be applied near the eyes or to cut, abraded, or sunburned skin.

Depilatories

Although the biologic significance of hair is minute, its cosmetic importance is considerable. Any discrepancy between cosmetic standards and normal biological range may prove to be embarrassing. Excessive growth of facial or body hair has been a common complaint among women for centuries (77). Some remedies used in the past for hair removal include arsenic trisulfide ointment, hot leeches, ants' eggs, and the blood of yellow frogs (77, 78).

Physiology of Normal and Abnormal Hair Growth

Racial and cultural factors affect both the type of normal hair growth and people's attitude about it. In American culture any hair except on the scalp is considered a masculine trait. However, the growth of upper lip and preauricular hair soon after puberty is a normal racial characteristic among females of some ethnic groups. It is attributed to sensitivity of the skin to androgens (78). Excess hair growth of essentially normal distribution is termed hypertrichosis, while a change in hair growth distribution inconsistent with sex and racial background is called hirsutism (78). Either may be due to a change in one of two distinct features of hair growth: its cycle or pattern.

The hair growth cycle comprises successive stages of growth (anogen) and rest (telogen). During the rest period, the fully developed hair is retained in the follicle for a while and then shed. If the rest phase is long and hair is shed well before the next growth phase for that follicle, the skin appears relatively hairless. If the rest phase is short, the succeeding hair appears in the follicle shortly after or even before the earlier hair is gone, and the skin appears hairy. Androgens influence the growth cycle by increasing the length of the growth phase at the expense of the rest phase.

The hair growth pattern refers to the type of hair made by the follicle, either "vellus" or "terminal." Follicles over most of the body produce only fine, fuzz-like vellus hair; however, follicles can be transformed to produce longer, coarser, pigmented terminal hair. In both sexes, androgens cause terminal hair to replace vellus in the pubic area and axillae. Additional androgen stimulation causes transformation of follicles on the face, chest, and abdomen.

Hirsutism can usually be traced to an endocrine origin (78). It may be due to the virilizing effects of excess androgen or progestin production, or to excessive adrenal corticosteroids. Hypertrichosis may be caused by drugs such as acetazolamide, chlorpromazine, diazoxide, minoxidil, penicillamine, or phenytoin (79–80). The central issue is determining whether self-medication is advisable in separating the infrequent instances of endocrine or drug-induced disease from the vast majority of cases in which excess hair is purely a cosmetic problem. Whenever other signs of virilization are present, the patient should be referred to a physician for assessment. The menstrual history can be valuable. If menstruation is completely normal, the patient is unlikely to have serious endocrinopathy.

Methods of Hair Removal

Medical demands for hair removal are rare. Occasionally ingrown beard hairs need to be removed and surgeons still remove hair from operative sites (81). However, when patients desire the removal of hair for cosmetic reasons, no amount of dissuasion can usually change their minds.

There is no way to increase or decrease the number of hair follicles in the skin; these are fixed at birth. However, hair can be removed either at the surface (depilation) or at the roots (epilation). Since epilation removes the hair at a deeper point it has to be repeated less often. All practical methods except electrolysis are temporary (Table 4).

Women often shave hair from their legs and trunk, but find shaving the face repugnant. There is no evidence that shaving makes hair grow faster or coarser (77, 78). Local epilation by plucking is usually not harmful and probably the best method of removing a few strong hairs. Provided that removal of the hair is complete and includes the hair bulb, hair is not noticeable again for 3–6 weeks. However, damage to the follicles may sometimes cause infection.

Wax epilation is essentially a form of mass plucking. A wax of low melting point (or adhesive semisolid applied on a backing material) rapidly solidifies and enmeshes hair. It is then pulled quickly off the skin, against the direction of hair growth, along with embedded hairs. If not done skillfully this technique can be painful to use, and allergic reactions to the adhesives

Table 4. Methods of hair removal	
Method	**Implement or process**
Depilation (action on the hair shaft)	
Shaving	Razor or electric shaver
Abrasion	Pumice or fiber
Dissolving	Chemicals, enzymes
Bleaching	Peroxides, organic acids
Epilation (action on the hair root)	
Extraction	Tweezers, wax, adhesives
Toxins	Metabolic—endocrine or nutritional disorders
	Disease—infection, immune deficiency
	Poison—metals, drugs
Destruction	Electrolysis—galvanic
	Cautery—short-wave
	Chemical—phenol, acid
	Ionization—X-rays or gamma rays

Reprinted with permission from H. B. Spoor, *Cutis, 21,* 283 (1978).

can occur. The patient should be cautioned to make sure that the wax is not too hot prior to use. Moreover, hair should be allowed to grow for several weeks prior to waxing to prevent irritation.

Permanent removal of hair by electrolysis (galvanic or short-wave diathermy) can be very tedious and expensive, even on facial hair, because only a few nonadjacent hairs should be done at one time. Galvanic electrolysis is less traumatic but slower than wax epilation (81). Even with good technique, 15–25% of hairs regrow and the operation has to be done again. Although somewhat painful (the needle must be inserted into the bulb of the hair shaft), some dermatology experts feel that competent operators can produce excellent results (82). However, self-operated electrolysis is not advisable because significant scarring occurs if the follicle is not destroyed correctly.

Depilatory creams and lotions are thus a logical and convenient alternative for hair removal. Most chemical depilatories are based on substituted mercaptans used in the presence of alkaline-reacting materials (calcium thioglycolate with calcium hydroxide). This combination has generally supplemented the sulfides of barium, strontium, and calcium, which are faster acting but are poisonous and have strong odors.

Chemical depilatories act by reducing disulfide bonds between cystine molecules in hair keratin. Increasing osmotic pressure within the hair fiber results in swelling and deterioration to a soft plastic mass which is easily wiped off the skin in 5–15 minutes. To some extent skin is subject to the same degradation as hair but thioglycolate preparations seldom cause skin reactions. When they do, the reaction is usually irritant rather than allergic. Hair that is regrowing is less bristly than after shaving so there is less itching during regrowth. Coarse, highly pigmented hair is tougher to remove than vellus hair. Chemical depilatories also have bactericidal properties (83).

Pharmacologic Agents

Thioglycolates

These make up the large majority of commercial preparations. A 2–4% concentration is sufficient; higher concentrations do not work appreciably faster (84). Increasing the concentration of alkali increases the depilation rate but also increases skin irritation. Thioglycolates are safe topically and have little systemic toxicity if absorbed (84); they have only a mild odor. These preparations are oxidized by air and therefore should not be kept too long and they should be kept in a tightly covered container.

Alkaline Sulfides

Barium, calcium, or strontium sulfides act two to three times faster than thioglycolate (84) but are more irritating. They have a strong odor due to hydrolysis to hydrogen sulfide and are poisonous if ingested.

Application

The depilatory may be tested by applying it to a small patch of normal skin for 15 minutes and then washing off. Wait 24 hours to see if hypersensitivity develops. If no reaction occurs, apply a thick layer with the enclosed plastic glove or applicator against the direction of hair growth. Leave on for 5–15 minutes and then remove with a spatula or tissue (avoid contact with water to minimize odor). Wash the skin with soap and water. If necessary, 1% hydrocortisone cream can be applied to counteract irritation. The treatment is repeated as needed, normally every 2–4 weeks.

Nonmedicated Shampoos

In contrast to body hair, scalp hair has long been a source of beauty and social distinction. Interestingly, it has only been in this century that much attention has been paid to cleaning it (85).

Originally, shampoos were made of soaps; today synthetic detergents are used almost exclusively in commercial products. The success of modern shampoos is based on their being not only cleansers, but also cosmetics that impart luster, beauty, and manageability to hair. A good shampoo makes hair feel clean, provides it with a gloss or sheen, and does not leave it "frizzy" or unmanageable (does not adversely affect its physical properties). Shampoos are often formulated to emphasize special properties, such as minimizing eye sting, conditioning, adding body, or having an appealing fragrance.

Hair

Hair has three layers: the medulla, which receives nourishment from the root; the cortex, which contains pigment; and the cuticle, which is a thin translucent layer that lets color shine through to the outside. Normal hair varies in thickness (texture) from coarse to fine.

Hair soil includes natural skin secretions, skin debris, dirt from the environment, and residue of hair grooming products. The scalp normally secretes enough oil to keep hair glossy and scalp comfortable. However, a build-up of oil between shampoos makes it limp and stringy. On the other hand, too little oil makes hair dull, lifeless, "flyaway," and easily breakable.

Specialty Shampoos

Today's shampoos may stress any number of special components or properties. However, their main benefit is still cleansing. Manufacturers must be careful about therapeutic claims because such products would be considered drugs by the FDA.

A conditioner is a product applied to hair to restore oils, sheen, elasticity, and manageability. It is useful on dry, damaged, or over-processed hair. Many shampoos include conditioners in the formulation.

A cream rinse is a product used after a shampoo to smooth the cuticle, eliminate tangles, and make hair manageable.

Protein shampoos are excellent for fine, limp, or damaged hair. Hair strands can be increased in bulk with a protein shampoo, by conditioning, or by coloring. They are not necessary for normal hair; they don't help dry hair and can make oily hair limp sooner after shampooing. The protein does not become a permanent part of hair; it is only adsorbed temporarily and washed off again at the next shampoo.

Herbal shampoos contain saponins from natural products, such as quillaja bark or soaproot, that foam well and have good cleaning properties.

Ingredients

Soaps are salts of fatty acids. Unfortunately, they tend to form insoluble mineral salts due to the presence of the carboxyl group at the end of the long-chain hydrocarbon. This leaves a dulling scum on hair. Over the years, however, it has been possible to formulate soap-based shampoos with a mixture of natural oils and alkanolamines to obtain a desirable product. Also sequestering agents can be added to bind calcium and magnesium ions. Oils with primarily short-chain fatty acids (coconut oil) tend to yield better foaming shampoos and work well even at low temperatures. However, they do not perform well in hard water.

Synthetic detergents have the carboxyl group of the fatty acid replaced with another hydrophilic group, thus avoiding their negative properties. Detergents tend to be classified by their hydrophilic groups. By far the most widely used detergent in shampoos is the anionic agent, sodium lauryl sulfate (a sulfated derivative of lauryl alcohol). It and other alkyl sulfates are completely effective in hard water, provide excellent foam, and leave hair feeling smooth and soft. They also are perfumed easily, easily rinsed out, and do not become rancid (85). Originally, sodium salts were used but now ammonium or tri- and diethanolamine salts are often used because they are less drying to hair.

Nonionic detergents also are popular. They have low foaming properties and are especially mild to the eyes. Many shampoos contain combinations of soaps and detergents to balance their desirable characteristics.

Additives

As perusal of any label will verify, many secondary ingredients are routinely added to shampoos.

Conditioning agents are added to coat hair with a very small amount of lubricating material because most surfactants clean hair so well that it becomes unmanageable. These are emollients such as lanolin and its derivatives, glycerol, propylene glycol, and lauryl or octyl sarcosines. Cationic materials are added to reduce the electrostatic charge on hair (but are irritating to the eyes). They are adsorbed onto hair and retained after rinsing.

Foam builders and stabilizers (lauryl monoethanolamide) make the product more pleasing to use. Thickeners, which may be simple salts (NaCl) or methylcellulose derivatives, also make the product more aesthetically acceptable. Sequestering agents prevent formation of calcium, magnesium, and iron soaps. These include ethylenediaminetetraacetic acid (EDTA), citric acid, and pyrophosphates. Short-chain alcohols act as clarifying agents and increase rinsability. In creams and lotions, stearate and palmitate salts are added as opacifying agents. Finally, the formulation may include preservatives, antioxidants, buffering agents, perfumes, and dyes.

Formulations

Shampoos are available in clear liquids, lotions, pastes, and gels, allowing for great latitude in physical and performance capabilities. Dry shampoos are valuable to ill or incapacitated persons who cannot wet their hair. Dry shampoos are mixtures of absorbent powders and mild alkalis that pick up soil from hair and scalp. After leaving them in hair for a period, they are brushed or combed out.

Product Selection Guidelines

Most modern shampoos work very well, with little to choose between them in consumer acceptability (86). Those who shampoo more regularly should choose a gentle shampoo. Teenagers tend to have oily hair, and they should avoid conditioning shampoos, although a cream rinse will aid combing and manageability. Shampoos for dry or oily hair vary in the amount of detergent in the formulation.

One sudsing and rinse is enough for frequent shampoos. Hair should be rinsed very well to remove all traces of shampoo. For best results, it should be gently dried with a towel or blow dryer set at low temperatures.

Summary

The psychological benefits of using personal care products are unquestionable. However, such products may be misused in terms of frequency of use, selection of a product, or technique of application. Many products can cause direct contact irritation or allergic sensitivity, but perhaps the greatest hazards are with the user and inadequate counseling, rather than with the product. The incidence of adverse effects is small, but, in almost all cases, the benefits are only cosmetic.

The available literature is not convincing that vaginal cleansing and deodorant products are advisable for routine use. Antiperspirants and underarm deodorants, skin bleaching agents, depilatories, and nonmedicated shampoos are appropriate for routine use provided that the user understands what reasonably can be expected from the product. The advice of a pharmacist in product selection and education can be of great value.

References

1. C. Y. Kawada, *Am. J. Hosp. Pharm.*, *37*, 1061 (1980).
2. K. J. Karnaky, *Am. J. Surg.*, *101*, 456 (1961).
3. K. J. Karnaky, *Am. J. Obstet. Gynecol.*, *115*, 283 (1973).
4. R. Glynn, *Obstet. Gynecol.*, *20*, 369 (1962).
5. H. J. Palacios, *Ann. Allergy*, *37*, 110–113 (1976).
6. *Drug and Therapeutics Bulletin*, *18*(14), 55–56 (1980).
7. F. Sadik, *J. Am. Pharm. Assoc.*, NS12, 565 (1972).
8. F. J. Fleury and R. W. Roller, in "Current Therapy," H. F. Conn, Ed., W. B. Saunders, Philadelphia, Pa., 1981, pp. 914–918.
9. M. E. Levison, *Drug Ther.*, *9*(1), 171–180 (1979).
10. T. D. De and N. V. Tu, *Am. J. Obstet. Gynecol.*, *87*, 92 (1965).
11. L. A. Gray and M. L. Barnes, *Am. J. Obstet. Gynecol.*, *92*, 125 (1963).
12. R. Landesman, *Drug Ther.*, *9*(1), 185–186 (1979).
13. T. E. Swate and J. C. Weed, *Obstet. Gynecol.*, *43*, 893 (1974).
14. J. J. Ratzan, *Calif. Med.*, *110*, 24 (1969).
15. "Summary Minutes of the FDA OTC Panel on Contraceptives and Other Vaginal Drug Products," Rockville, Md., Feb. 7–8, 1975.
16. "Remington's Pharmaceutical Sciences," 16th ed., A. Osol, Ed., Mack, Easton, Pa., 1980, p. 720.
17. J. Barnes, *Practitioner*, *184*, 668 (1960).
18. J. F. Byers, *Am. Fam. Physician*, *10*, 135 (1974).
19. D. V. Hirst, *Am. J. Obstet. Gynecol.*, *64*, 179 (1952).
20. J. H. Long, M. L. Carey, A. E. Hellegers, and M. P. Pentecost, *West. J. Surg. Obstet. Gynecol.*, *71*, 122 (1963).
21. H. A. Kaminetzky, *J. Am. Med. Assoc.*, *191*, 154 (1965).
22. L. McGowan, *Am. J. Obstet. Gynecol.*, *93*, 506 (1965).
23. "Summary Minutes of the FDA OTC Panel on Contraceptives and Other Vaginal Drug Products," Rockville, Md., Sept. 20–21, 1974.
24. R. Glynn, *Obstet. Gynecol.*, *22*, 640 (1963).
25. M. H. Gotlib and D. N. Adler, *Med. Times*, *96*, 902 (1968).
26. R. S. Cohen, L. S. Polsky, C. A. Straniero, and C. Brown, *Curr. Ther. Res.*, *15*, 839 (1973).
27. W. A. Abruzzi, *J. Am. Med. Women's Assoc.*, *21*, 406 (1966).
28. R. J. Stock, M. E. Stock, and J. M. Hutto, *Obstet. Gynecol.*, *42*, 141 (1973).
29. C. A. D. Ringrose, *N. Engl. J. Med.*, *295*, 1319 (1976).
30. H. Vorherr, U. F. Vorherr, P. Mehta, J. Ulrich, and R. Messer, *J. Am. Med. Assoc.*, *244*, 2628 (1980).
31. N. Etling, F. Gehin-Fouque, and J. P. Vielh, *Obstet. Gynecol.*, *53*, 376 (1979).
32. H. H. Neumann and A. DeCherney, *N. Engl. J. Med.*, *295*, 789 (1976).
33. G. F. Egenolf and R. McNaughton, *Obstet. Gynecol.*, *7*, 23 (1956).
34. F. H. Downer and C. J. Stevenson, *Adverse Drug React. Bull.*, *42*, 136 (1973).
35. C. D. Calnan, *Proc. Roy. Soc. Med.*, *55*, 39 (1962).
36. *Medical Letter on Drugs and Therapeutics*, *10*, 27 (1968).
37. A. A. Fisher, F. Pascher, and N. B. Kanof, *Arch. Dermatol.*, *104*, 286 (1971).
38. A. A. Fisher and M. A. Stillman, *Arch. Dermatol.*, *106*, 169 (1972).
39. E. Schmunes and E. J. Levy, *Arch. Dermatol.*, *106*, 169 (1972).
40. *Federal Register*, *40*, 8926 (1975).
41. A. A. Fisher, *Arch. Dermatol.*, *108*, 801 (1973).
42. G. Carsch, *Soap Chem. Spec.*, *47*, 38 (1971).
43. J. Meyer-Robin and V. Kassebart, *Kosmetologie*, *4*, 159 (1971).
44. F. Sadik, *Pharmindex*, *22*, 11 (1980).
45. J. A. Cella, *Am. Cosmet. Perfum.*, *86*(10), 84 (1971).
46. P. A. Saunders, in "Modern Pharmaceuticals," G. S. Baker and C. T. Rhodes, Eds., Marcel Dekker, New York, N.Y., 1979, pp. 591–647.

47. G. McBride, *J. Am. Med. Assoc.*, *219*, 449 (1972).
48. G. S. Kass, J. A. Cella, and N. H. Sloan, "Feminine Hygiene Deodorant Sprays," Paper presented at XIV International Congress of Dermatology, Venice, Italy, May 22, 1972.
49. A. Kantner, *Am. Cosmet. Perfum.*, *87*, 31 (1972).
50. B. A. Davis, *Obstet. Gynecol.*, *36*, 812 (1970).
51. J. M. Gowdy, *N. Engl. J. Med.*, *287*, 203 (1972).
52. *Medical Letter on Drugs and Therapeutics*, *12*, 88 (1970).
53. M. Morrison, *FDA Consumer*, *7*, 16 (1973).
54. A. E. Elkhouly and R. T. Yousef, *J. Pharm. Sci.*, *63*, 681 (1974).
55. I. L. Chavkin, *Cutis*, *23*, 24 (1979).
56. *Federal Register*, *43*, 46694 (1978).
57. W. J. Cunliffe and S. G. Tan, *Practitioner*, *216*, 149 (1976).
58. W. B. Shelley and R. Florence, *N. Engl. J. Med.*, *263*, 1056 (1960).
59. S. Plechner in "Cosmetics: Science and Technology," 2nd ed., Vol. 2, M. S. Balsam and E. Sagarian, Eds., Wiley-Interscience, New York, N.Y., 1972, pp. 373–416.
60. W. B. Shelley, H. J. Hurley, and A. C. Nichol, *Arch. Dermatol. Syphilol.*, *68*, 430 (1953).
61. *Medical Letter on Drugs and Therapeutics*, *19*, 20 (1977).
62. C. M. Papa and A. M. Kligman, *J. Invest. Dermatol.*, *49*, 139 (1967).
63. E. Holzle and A. M. Kligman, *J. Soc. Cosmet. Chem.*, *30*, 279 (1979).
64. W. B. Shelley and H. J. Hurley, *J. Am. Med. Assoc.*, *244*, 1956 (1980).
65. E. Holzle and A. M. Kligman, *J. Soc. Cosmet. Chem.*, *30*, 357 (1979).
66. *Federal Register*, *42*, 41374 (1977).
67. "AMA Drug Evaluations," 4th ed., American Medical Association, Chicago, Ill., 1980, pp. 1016, 1017.
68. P. A. Majors and J. E. Wild, *J. Soc. Cosmet. Chem.*, *25*, 139 (1974).
69. J. A. Parrish, "Dermatology and Skin Care," McGraw-Hill, New York, N.Y., 1975, pp. 29–31.
70. *Federal Register*, *43*, 51546 (1978).
71. K. A. Arndt, "Manual of Dermatologic Therapeutics," 2nd ed., Little, Brown, Boston, Mass., 1978, pp. 118–126.
72. S. S. Bleehan, *J. Soc. Cosmet. Chem.*, *28*, 407 (1977).
73. K. Jimbow, H. Obata, M. A. Pathak, and T. B. Fitzpatrick, *J. Invest. Dermatol.*, *62*, 436 (1974).
74. K. A. Arndt and T. B. Fitzpatrick, *J. Am. Med. Assoc.*, *194*, 965 (1965).
75. M. C. Spencer, *J. Am. Med. Assoc.*, *194*, 962 1965).
76. "American Hospital Formulary Service," American Society of Hospital Pharmacists, Washington, D.C., 1978, 84:50:04.
77. *Lancet 1*, 488 (1967).
78. J. H. Casey, *Aust. N.Z. J. Med.*, *10*, 240 (1980).
79. R. N. Earheart, J. Ball, D. D. Nuss, and J. L. Seling, *South. Med. J.*, *70*, 442 (1977).
80. A. McQueen, in "Iatrogenic Diseases," 2nd ed., P. F. D'Arhy and J. P. Griffin, Eds., Oxford University Press, New York, N.Y., 1979, pp. 77–91.
81. H. B. Spoor, *Cutis*, *21*, 283 (1978).
82. *Medical Letter on Drugs and Therapeutics*, *23*, 44 (1981).
83. S. J. Powis, T. A. Waterworth, and D. G. Arkell, *Br. Med. J.*, *2*, 1166 (1976).
84. R. H. Barry, in "Cosmetics: Science and Technology," 2nd ed., Vol. 2, M. S. Balsam and E. Sagarian, Eds., Wiley-Interscience, New York, N.Y., 1972, pp. 39–72.
85. D. H. Powers, in "Cosmetics: Science and Technology," 2nd ed., Vol. 2, M. S. Balsam and E. Sagarian, Eds., Wiley-Interscience, New York, N.Y., 1972, pp. 73–116.
86. *Consumer Reports*, *33*, 529 (1968).

Personal Care Product Table

Product (Manufacturer)	Antimicrobial	Local Anesthetic/ Antipruritic/ Counterirritant	Other Ingredients
Betadine Douche (Purdue Frederick)	povidone-iodine		
Bo-Car-Al (Beecham Products)		phenol menthol methyl salicylate eucalyptol thymol	potassium aluminum sulfate sodium chloride polyethylene glycol
Cortef Feminine Itch Cream (Upjohn)			hydrocortisone, 0.5%
Demure (Vicks)	benzethonium chloride		lactic acid
Femidine Douche (A.V.P.)	povidone-iodine		
Gynecort Creme (Combe)			hydrocortisone, 0.5%
Jeneen (Norwich)			lactic acid sodium lactate octoxynol 9 propylene glycol
Lysette (Lehn & Fink)			triethanolamine dodecylbenzene sulfonate alcohol, 31%
Massengill Disposable Douche (Beecham Products)	cetylpyridinium chloride		alcohol lactic acid octoxynol fragrance
Massengill Douche Powder (Beecham Products)		methyl salicylate phenol thymol	ammonium aluminum sulfate berberine sodium chloride
Massengill Liquid (Beecham Products)			alcohol lactic acid sodium bicarbonate octoxynol aromatics
Massengill Medicated Disposable Douche (Beecham Products)	povidone-iodine		
Massengill Vinegar & Water Disposable Douche (Beecham Products)			citric acid sodium benzoate vinegar
Norforms (Norwich-Eaton)	methylbenzethonium chloride		Peg-20, Peg-6 Peg-20 palmitate methylparaben lactic acid
Nylmerate II (Holland-Rantos)			alcohol, 50% acetic acid boric acid, 0.7% polysorbate, 20% nonoxynol 9 sodium acetate

Personal Care Products Table, continued

Product (Manufacturer)	Antimicrobial	Local Anesthetic/ Antipruritic/ Counterirritant	Other Ingredients
PMC Douche Powder and Disposable Douche (Thomas & Thompson)	boric acid, 82%	thymol, 0.3% phenol, 0.2% menthol	ammonium aluminum sulfate, 16% eucalyptus oil peppermint oil
Povi-Douche (North American Pharmacal)	povidone-iodine, 7.5%		
Summer's Eve Disposable Douche (Personal Laboratories)			sodium citrate citric acid quaternium-15 fragrance
Summer's Eve Medicated Disposable Douche (Personal Laboratories)	potassium sorbate, 1%		
Summer's Eve Vinegar & Water Disposable Douche (Personal Laboratories)	sorbic acid		vinegar
Stomaseptine (Berlex)		menthol eucalyptol thymol } 2%	sodium perborate, 18% sodium chloride, 28% sodium borate, 25% sodium bicarbonate, 25%
Trichotine Liquid and Powder (Reed and Carnrick)			sodium perborate (powder) sodium borate (liquid) aromatics sodium lauryl sulfate alcohol, 8% (liquid)
Trichotine-D (Reed and Carnrick)			sodium lauryl sulfate trisodium EDTA
V.A. (Norcliff Thayer)	boric acid, 78% 8-hydroxyquinoline citrate, 2%		zinc sulfate, 7.5% alum, 12%
Zonite (Norcliff Thayer)	benzalkonium chloride, 0.2%	menthol thymol } 0.08%	propylene glycol, 5% buffer

20

Otic Products

Keith O. Miller

Questions to Ask the Patient

Earache

Do you have an earache?

Is the pain sharp and localized or dull and generalized?

How long have you had the earache?

Is it a constant pain or is it made worse by chewing or pulling on the ear?

Do you have a cold or the flu?

Do you have a fever?

Have you been swimming in the past few days?

Have you attempted to clear your ears recently to remove ear wax? If so, what method did you use?

Have you had similar symptoms in the past?

What have you already done to treat your earache?

Do you wear dentures or have any dental problems?

Hearing Loss

How long have you noticed that your hearing is not as good as it used to be?

Do you have a cold or the flu?

Have you been swimming in the past few days?

Have you been traveling in an airplane recently or been in any places where the air pressure has changed suddenly (fast elevators)?

Are you taking any prescription medicines, even for other medical problems?

Tinnitus

Are the sounds continuous or intermittent?

Are you taking aspirin or any medicines that your physician has prescribed or that you have purchased without a prescription?

Discharge

Could you describe the appearance and amount of the discharge?

Was your ear itchy before the discharge appeared?

Did you have any pain after the discharge appeared?

Did you have pain before the discharge started?

Have you taken aspirin or tried to rinse out the ear?

Do you have diabetes or any other medical problems?

Do you have a problem with dandruff?

Ear disorders are very common and in most cases cause discomfort. Patients usually complain of "earache," "impacted ear," "running ear," "cold in the ear," or a combination of these symptoms. Before recommending any nonprescription product to patients with ear disorders, the pharmacist should have a clear picture of the symptoms of ear disorders and their corresponding pathophysiology. This information will help the pharmacist understand the recommended treatment plans and permit an accurate evaluation of the patient's problem.

Ear disorders may be caused by a disease of the auricle, external auditory meatus (external ear canal), or middle ear or by a disease in another area of the head or neck. A traumatic or pathologic condition of the tongue, mandibles, oropharynx, tonsils, or paranasal sinuses may cause referred pain to the ear and may appear to the patient as an "earache." These conditions often are caused by some underlying disease process that requires accurate diagnosis and treatment by a physician. Therefore, self-medication may be unwise.

Home remedies and nonprescription drugs usually are restricted to self-limiting disorders related only to the external ear. Self-medication should be reserved for minor conditions. In addition, it may be used effectively for prophylaxis to aid the normal body defenses and to improve the integrity of the skin lining the auricle and external auditory canal.

Ear Anatomy and Physiology

The external ear is composed of the auricle (pinna) and the external auditory meatus (Figures 1). The auricle is the external appendage consisting of cartilage (elastic type) covered by a thin layer of normal skin that is highly vascularized except for the lobule, which is mainly fatty tissue. The auricle is a flattened, irregular oval structure that is considered an extension of the cartilaginous ear canal. A thin tissue layer called the perichondrium covers both the cartilaginous auricle and the outer cartilaginous half of the external auditory canal (1). The periosteum, a specialized connective tissue, covers the inner bony half of the external auditory canal.

The external auditory meatus is tubular, forming a channel for sound waves to pass to the tympanic membrane (ear drum) and protecting the membrane from injury. In adults, the external auditory canal is about 24 mm long and has a volume of about 0.85 ml (17 drops) (2). Both the auricle and the external auditory canal show much individual variation in size and shape. The auditory meatus is the only epidermal-lined cul-de-sac in the body.

The channel narrows about 7 mm from the tympanic membrane; this area is called the isthmus (3). Proximal to the isthmus, the canal floor dips downward to the junction of the annular ring of the tympanic membrane to the canal wall, forming a depression termed the "tympanic recess." Excess water and fluids in the tympanic recess may cause a feeling of fullness in the ear. Their removal is accomplished by having the patient tilt the head on the side with the affected ear down. This position permits the excess fluid to drain out of the ear by gravity. To permit direct visual examination of the tympanic membrane, it may be necessary to straighten the canal by applying upward and backward traction on the auricle.

The auricular skin is continuous and lines the entire auditory meatus and the outer covering of the tympanic membrane (4). The skin covering the cartilaginous portion is thicker than the skin covering the bony portion. The skin of the cartilaginous part of the canal contains hair follicles, large sebaceous glands, which open either to the skin surface or into the hair follicle lumen, and ceruminous glands (2). There are 1,000–2,000 ceruminous glands in the average ear, although older people may have fewer (2). The hairs appear to fulfill a protective function, evidenced by their ability to trap foreign bodies in their waxy network. No hair follicles or glands (sebaceous and ceruminous) are found in the inner half of the external auditory canal.

Cerumen (earwax) is derived from the watery secretions of the apocrine glands and the oily secretions of the sebaceous glands (2). Collectively these glands are referred to as ceruminous glands. These glands are abundant in the skin of the cartilaginous portion of the canal but are absent from the skin of the bony portion of the canal. This colorless, watery-like fluid secretion is com-

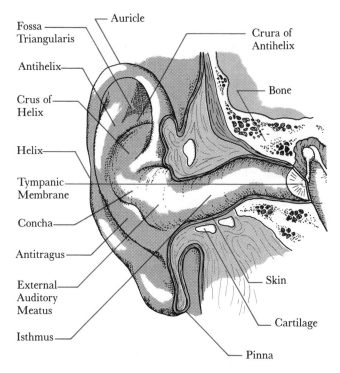

Figure 1. Anatomy of the auricle and external ear.

posed of polypeptides, lipids, fatty acids, amino acids, and electrolytes (2, 5). Cerumen turns brown when it mixes with desquamated epithelial cells and dust particles. The cerumen lubricates the skin and traps foreign material entering the external auditory canal, providing a protective barrier (3, 4, 6). Under normal conditions, the cerumen forms small, round droplets and dries into a semisolid. It then is expelled unnoticed by epithelial migration. This migration is the movement of epithelial cells across the surface of the tympanic membrane and the epithelial lining of the external auditory meatus to the outside during the process of mastication. The skin of the normal external auditory meatus is acidic with a pH between 5.0 and 7.2 (2). This "acid mantle" provides a protection against opportunistic bacteria and fungi (4).

The tympanic membrane is pearl-gray, egg shaped, semitransparent, and about 0.1 mm thick and 8–9 mm wide (the narrow portion is at the bottom) (2). Its outer epithelial layer is continuous with the epidermis of the external auditory canal; the middle layer is tough, fibrous tissue; and the innermost layer is a mucous membrane continuous with the tympanic cavity lining (7). In adults, the membrane forms approximately a 45° angle with the external meatus floor, and is almost horizontal in infants (2). It provides protection to the middle ear from external foreign material and also aids in transmitting airborne sound waves into the middle ear. Anatomically, the tympanic membrane is considered with the external auditory canal because it is attached to the canal's medial terminal end (Figure 1). Functionally, it is considered with the middle ear (tympanic cavity) (3).

Etiology of Ear Conditions

Predisposing factors often lead to the breakdown of natural barriers of the normal ear canal; hairs in the outer half of the meatus, the size of the ear canal and its isthmus, and cerumen collectively prevent the introduction of foreign material that may cause injury or infection. The integrity of the skin layers and the acid pH of the canal provide protection against infection. Infection usually is preceded by an alteration of the protective acid pH of the canal.

An inherited narrowed ear canal, a malformation of the mandible, and/or excess hair growth in the canal may impair the normal cleansing process and decrease the efficiency of the epithelial migration. Hyperactive ceruminous glands may cause excessive wax production to accumulate and become impacted. Black people have shorter and straighter ear canals, and external otitis occurs less frequently in blacks than in nonblacks (8).

Certain conditions and activities contribute to the breakdown of natural barriers of the normal ear canal. Warm humid climates, inside environments with intense heat and humidity, accompanied by sweating, and exposure to water (swimming and diving) during the summer months have been implicated. The increased exposure to moisture may result in tissue maceration that breaks down the protective barrier of the skin, alters the pH of the skin, and predisposes the ear canal to infection (4). There is a positive correlation between the amount of water exposure in the ear canal and the incidence of external otitis (8).

The etiology of ear disorders may be due to a variety of trauma-induced causes. Improperly cleaned or poorly fitted ear plugs may cause trauma and/or maceration of the skin in the ear canal. They also may be sensitizing. Poorly fitted aids may be another source of trauma-induced injury.

Patients commonly use an instrument, a cotton applicator, or other device to clean their ears; such use is likely to push the ear wax deeper in the ear canal and cause it to become tightly impacted, increasing the difficulty of subsequent removal. Its subsequent removal or

modification of protection by the cerumen may increase the predisposition for bacterial or fungal infection in the ear canal. This cleaning process often causes trauma to the skin covering the ear canal and predisposes the ear to infection. Mechanical cleaning of the ear decreases the ear's normal natural cleaning process. The normal healthy ear cleans itself, thus negating any need for cleaning with mechanical devices or instruments.

After the protective layer of the skin of the ear canal has been compromised, a preinflammatory stage occurs; the patient most likely will involuntarily scratch the ear or rub the auricle in response to an itch (9). These involuntary maneuvers further abrade the skin, causing deep fissures in the epidermis of the cartilaginous portion of the ear canal. A full inflammatory reaction follows this fissure formation, causing edema, pain, swelling, and redness of the affected areas. This area becomes a good culture medium for bacteria or fungi, making subsequent infection likely.

Neurodermatitis sometimes occurs in middle-aged patients and is a cause of involuntary rubbing, scratching, or cleaning the ear canal in response to vague itch or a feeling of fullness (4, 10). Overproduction of cerumen may produce similar symptoms. In some people under conditions of high emotional tension and excessive heat, the ceruminous glands respond excessively and can alter the normal chemical composition and acid nature of the ear canal skin.

Common Problems of the Ear

Many disorders of the ear are minor and easily resolved. However, the pharmacist should keep in mind that the pain associated with even minor disorders can be significant. Some untreated ear problems can result in hearing loss. The pharmacist can assist the patient by helping evaluate the disorder, by discussing the proper course of action (self-treatment or referral to a physician) and by recommending an efficacious nonprescription product, if appropriate (Table 1).

Table 1. Symptoms of otic disorders

	Boil	Otomycosis	Bacterial external otitis	Nonsuppurative otitis media	Impacted cerumen	Suppurative otitis media
Pain[a]	Often	Possibly	Often	Rarely	Rarely	Usually
Hearing deficit	Rarely	Possibly	Possibly	Possibly	Often	Possibly
Purulent discharge	Rarely	Rarely	Often	Rarely	Rarely	Occasionally and indicative of perforation
Bilateral symptoms	Rarely	Rarely	Possibly	Often	Rarely	Occasionally
Appropriateness of self-medication	Auricle only	Never	Never	Never	Never	Never

[a]Pain is increased with chewing, traction on the auricle, and medial pressure on the tragus except in otitis media, where it is knife-like and steady.

Table 2. Interpretation of physical findings of the external ear

Physical findings	Probable appearance	Physiologic basis	Example
Enlarged lymph node	Swollen, tender to touch, pre- and postauricular	Inflammation of lymph node; spread of infection outside the ear	Mastoiditis, otitis media
Tophus	Hard, pale node on helix, chalk-like dust upon rupture	Urate crystals	Gout
Sebaceous cyst	Swollen, erythematous postauricle lesion in the skin of the ear	Inflammation of sweat gland	Skin infection
Cerumen	Red-orange paste-like discharge	Normal secretion of wax	Normal finding
Blood	Red-blue discharge	Ruptured blood vessel	External otitis
Serous fluid	Clear discharge	Blocked eustachian tube	Chronic (purulent) otitis media
Pus	Yellowish discharge	Acute inflammation	Acute suppurative otitis media

Adapted with permission from *Drug Intell. Clin. Pharm., 11*, 657 (1977).

Disorders of the Auricle

The disorders associated with the auricle, the part of the ear not within the head, are generally minor and involve lacerations, boils, and dermatitis. These conditions are generally self-limiting. Table 2 gives examples of some common physical findings related to disorders of the external ear.

Trauma

Lacerations, including scrapes and cuts, involving only the auricle skin usually heal spontaneously. A wound that does not heal normally should be checked by a physician. Deep wounds that may involve injury to the cartilage also require examination by a physician. Injury to the auricle that does not perforate the subperichondrium may cause subcutaneous bleeding and produce a hematoma. A hematoma requires aspiration or incision by a physician, since the red-blue swelling may obliterate normal auricular contours and frequently results in inflammation and in perichondritis or "cauliflower ear." The swelling can also cause local pruritus and pain upon touch.

Boils

Boils (furuncles) are usually localized infections of the hair follicles. The etiology is uncertain. Fatigue and emotional stress appear to predispose to furuncles. Anemia and diabetes mellitus as well as malnutrition have been found to be predisposing factors in some populations. In a high percentage of cases in young adults, no specific causative or predisposing factor has been established. Poor body hygiene is generally contributory to boils (11).

Boils often involve the anterior external auditory meatus. They usually begin as a red papule and may progress into a round or conical superficial pustule with a core of pus and erythema around the base. The lesion gradually enlarges, becomes firm, then softens and opens spontaneously (after a few days to as long as 2 weeks), discharging the purulent contents. Because the skin is very taut, minimal swelling may cause severe pain.

Boils are usually self-limiting; however, they may be severe, autoinoculable, and multiple. Deeper lesions may lead to perichondritis (inflammation of the connective tissue). The pus-producing organism found in boils is usually *Staphylococcus aureus* (9).

Small boils may be treated by good hygiene combined with topical compresses. Hot compresses of saline solution may be applied to the auricle and the side of the face. Cases in which boils do not respond rapidly to topical dressings should be referred to a physician. In addition, patients with recurring boils should be referred to a physician for evaluation and possible systemic antibiotic therapy.

Perichondritis

Perichondritis is an inflammation involving the perichondrium (the fibrous connective tissue surrounding the auricular cartilage) usually following a poorly treated or untreated burn, injury, hematoma, or local infection.

The onset of perichondritis is characterized by a sensation of heat and stiffness of the auricle with pronounced pain. As the condition progresses, an exudate forms and the auricle becomes dark red, diffuse, and swollen. The entire auricle becomes shiny and red with uniform thickening caused by edema and inflammation. The lesions usually are confined to the cartilaginous tissue of the auricle and external canal. Constitutional disturbances may include generalized fever and malaise.

Perichondritis frequently results in severe auricular deformity, and atresia (a pathologic closure) of the external auditory canal may occur. A patient suspected of having perichondritis symptoms should be seen by a physician.

Dermatitis of the Ear

An inflammatory condition of the skin may result from an abrasion of the auricle and, if untreated, may develop into an infection of these skin layers. Inflammatory conditions such as seborrhea, psoriasis, and contact dermatitis (poison ivy and poison oak) also may affect the skin of the auricle and the external ear canal. Contact dermatitis also may be caused by an allergic response to jewelry, cosmetics, detergents, or topical drug applications. The lesions may spread to the auditory canal, neck, and facial areas (9).

The symptoms of dermatitis of the ear usually include itching and local redness followed by vesication, weeping, and erythema. The lesions form scales and yellow crusts on the skin (7, 10). They may spread to adjacent unaffected areas, and excessive scratching may cause them to become infected. Topical drugs should be used cautiously with dermatitis because of their potential allergenicity, which could exacerbate the condition. Seborrheic dermatitis of the ear is usually associated with dandruff. Treatment with dandruff-control shampoos is recommended (9). Cases that are difficult to control and generalized around the ear should be referred to a physician.

Itching or Pruritus of the Ear

An itchy ear canal is a common symptom and may mask the preinflammatory stages of acute external otitis. Itching can also occur without visible lesions of the ear. Patients with chronic external otitis experience itching due to dry ears often because of the absence of cerumen. Itching is a very common complaint with chronic external otitis (10). Itching may be due to eczema of the skin around the ears, infections, allergic seborrheic dermatitis, psoriasis, contact dermatitis, or neurodermatitis (4).

Itching commonly begins an annoying itch-scratch cycle that results in trauma, infection, epidermal barrier destruction, and inflammation of the affected areas. Ear scratching has been known to be a nervous habit that may be addictive (9). Careful observation to determine the cause of itching often is helpful prior to any attempt to afford symptomatic relief and to correct the problem.

Aural Drainage

Any patient with a discharge or drainage from the ear should be referred to a physician for proper diagnosis and treatment. The drainage or discharge may be blood, watery fluid (serum), or purulent or mucoid material. Head trauma may cause leakage of cerebrospinal fluid. The origin of the fluid may be due to an infection of the external ear canal. A ruptured tympanic membrane usually produces a bloody serum-like fluid. Any trauma to the ear canal may cause bleeding and, if infected, the ear may exude a pus-like fluid from which the causative organisms may be cultured and appropriate antibiotics chosen.

The FDA advisory review panel on nonprescription topical analgesic, antirheumatic, otic, burn, and sunburn treatment drug products concluded that for drainage due to any cause, self-medication is inappropriate and not safe.

Disorders of the External Auditory Canal

Boils

Boils of the external auditory canal are pathologically similar to those found on the auricle and external auditory meatus. Symptoms include pain of the infected site, which is usually exacerbated by mastication. The auditory meatal opening may be partly occluded by swelling; however, hearing is impaired only if the opening is completely occluded. Edema and pain over the mastoid bone directly behind the auricle may occur. Traction of the auricle or the tragus is very painful. Patients with boils in the external auditory canal should be referred to a physician because unresolved conditions may lead to a generalized infection of the entire external auditory canal.

Otomycosis

Otomycosis, external fungal infection of the ear, is more common in warmer, tropical climates than in mild, temperate zones. *Aspergillus* species and *Candida* species are the most common causative agents (4, 9). Antibiotic treatment of a bacterial ear infection, with resultant suppression of normal bacterial flora, may predispose an individual to a mycotic external ear infection (9).

A superficial mycotic infection of the external auditory meatus is characterized by pruritus with a feeling of fullness and pressure in the ear. Pain may be present, increasing with mastication and traction on the pinna and the tragus. The fungus forms a mass of epithelial debris, exudate, and cerumen and, in the acute state, may clog the external auditory meatus. Hearing may be impaired.

Depending on the nature of the fungus, the color of the mass may vary. The skin lining the external auditory canal and the tympanic membrane becomes beefy-red and scaly and may be eroded or ulcerated (2). A scant, colorless mucoid discharge is common. Otomycosis is particularly serious in diabetic patients because of the microangiopathy and associated cutaneous manifestations common to diabetes mellitus (4). Mycotic ear infections must be treated by a physician.

Keratosis Obturans

This condition is rare, and its etiology is unclear (4). Wax accumulates in the deeper parts of the external auditory canal and, with adjacent epithelial cells that contain cholesterol, forms a mass and exerts pressure on the surrounding tissue. The mass is a shiny, white plug-like occlusion of the external auditory canal. It may cause a ring of pressure and erosion of the epithelial tissues surrounding it, forming a potential entrance for organisms to initiate a bacterial infection (1). The infection may form abscesses in the subcutaneous tissue and mastoid bone tissue.

Pain in the ear and decreased hearing are common symptoms. A discharge and tinnitus (ringing in the ear) also may occur. Mechanical removal of the obstruction is necessary but often difficult. Removal should be reserved for a physician; patients should not attempt to remove the obstruction themselves.

Foreign Objects in the Ear

Young children often use the ear canal for inserting small items such as beans, peas, marbles, pebbles, or beads. If the objects become lodged in the ear canal, they may cause significant hearing loss. Vegetable seeds, such as dried beans or dried peas, lodged in the external auditory meatus swell when moistened during bathing or swimming and become wedged in the bony portion of the canal, causing severe pain. Furthermore, if an obstruction of the external auditory meatus is not removed promptly, acute bacterial external otitis may result. Insects may enter the meatus and cause distress by beating their wings and crawling.

Foreign objects lodged in the ear canal may not cause symptoms and may be found only during a routine physical examination. Usually, a hearing deficiency or pain is observed with pressure in the ear during mastication. An exudate may form because of secondary bacterial infection. Mechanical removal should be reserved for a physician because unskilled attempts at removal often result in damage to the skin surrounding the external auditory meatus.

Impacted Cerumen

The accumulation of cerumen in the external auditory meatus may be caused by any of three factors: overactive ceruminous glands, an abnormally shaped external auditory meatus, or abnormal cerumen secreted by the ceruminous glands. Overactive ceruminous glands cause cerumen to accumulate in the external auditory canal. A tortuous or small canal or abnormal narrowing of the canal may not permit normal migration of the cerumen to the outside, allowing cerumen to accumulate. Abnormal cerumen may be drier or softer than normal cerumen and may interfere with the normal epithelial migration. It is often packed deeper into the external auditory meatus by repeated attempts to remove it, which is the most common cause of impacted cerumen. In general, there usually is no cerumen in the inner half of the external auditory canal unless it has been pushed there. In elderly persons, cerumen is frequently admixed with long hairs in the external auditory canal, preventing normal expulsion and forming a matted obstruction in the ear.

External Otitis

External otitis (inflammation of the skin lining the external auditory canal often due to infection) is one of the most common diseases of the ear. It is very painful and annoying. The external auditory canal is considered a blind canal lined with skin. It is a dark, warm cul-de-sac that is well suited for collecting moisture. Prolonged exposure to moisture tends to disrupt the continuity of the epithelial cells, causing skin maceration and fissures, which provide a fertile area for bacterial growth. Additionally, this prolonged exposure to moisture tends to raise the normal skin pH, improving the growth me-

dium for bacteria. Factors contributing to susceptibility to external otitis include race, heredity, age, sex, climate, diet, and occupational background (9). The most common causative organisms of external otitis include *Pseudomonas* species, also *Staphylococcus* species, *Bacillus* species, and *Proteus* species. Fungi may be identified (9).

There is very little subcutaneous tissue between the skin tightly bound to the perichondrium on the cartilaginous portion and the periosteum on the bony portion of the external auditory canal. Consequently, there is disparity between the size of the visible swelling and the amount of pain associated with the condition. The lack of space available for expansion increases skin tension. Inflammation causing edema provokes severe pain in the inflamed skin that is out of proportion to visible swelling. As the inflammation increases, pain may be increased significantly during mastication. Symptoms often develop following attempts to clean the ear of foreign debris (with cotton swabs, hairpins, matchsticks, pencils, fingers, or other objects) or to scratch the ear to relieve itching. The instruments may traumatize and damage the horny skin layer, forming an opening that allows invasion of organisms.

A normal, healthy external auditory canal is impervious to pathologic organisms. Generally, individuals must be susceptible to bacterial infections, and the skin integrity must be interrupted before an organism can produce an infected lesion.

Another type of trauma-induced external otitis is called "swimmer's ear," or desquamative external otitis (9). Excessive moisture in the external auditory meatus may cause water to accumulate in the tympanic recess, resulting in tissue maceration because of water absorption into the stratum corneum. This excessive moisture accumulation may be important in predisposing the ear canal to infection. After bathing or swimming, patients frequently attempt to clear the ear canal of water with objects that cause abrasions or lacerations of the skin lining. Also, cerumen accumulated in the external auditory meatus absorbs water and expands. The trapped water provides a medium for infection (3). Within a few hours to 1 day following exposure to excess water, symptoms of itching, pain, and possible draining from the ear with partial occlusion occur. In many cases, this condition is related to climatic conditions where the relative humidity and temperature are high or where dust and sand storms occur (3).

A bacterial infection of the external auditory canal leads to inflammation and epidermal destruction of the tympanic membrane (4). The infection may progress through the fibrous layer of the tympanic membrane and cause perforation and spreading of the infection into the middle ear, resulting in intense pain and discomfort. External otitis due to infection, like otomycosis, is particularly difficult to control in diabetics (4, 12).

Symptoms of acute external otitis are related to the severity of the pathologic conditions. There usually is mild or moderate pain that becomes pronounced by pulling upward on the auricle or by pressing on the tragus. There may be a discharge. Hearing loss may occur if the ear canal is obstructed by swelling and edema or by debris.

Chronic external otitis usually is caused by the persistence of predisposing factors. The most common symptom is itching, which prompts patients to attempt to scratch the ear canal to reduce or relieve the itch. This scratching can cause the skin to become obliterated or broken (10).

In allergic external otitis and dermatitis of the external auditory canal caused by seborrhea, a common symptom is itching, burning, or stinging of the lesions. Often the complaints seem excessive compared with the visible signs.

Chronic cases and those cases with symptoms of severe pain, lymphadenopathy, discharge, possible hearing loss, and fever should be referred to a physician (3). Tender nodes may be felt anterior to the tragus, behind the ear, or in the upper neck just below the pinna. Minor cases and chronic and allergic external otitis, especially swimmer's ear otitis, often may be treated adequately with nonprescription products. All progressive symptoms of disease processes pertaining to the external ear canal or auricle should be treated only under physician supervision.

Disorders of the Middle Ear

Disorders involving the middle ear should not be treated with nonprescription otic products. However, a brief overview of the common conditions involving the middle ear will aid the pharmacist in evaluating symptoms. Although some symptoms of middle ear disorders are the same as those of external ear disorders, others are not (Table 3). All bacterial infections of the middle ear should be promptly evaluated and treated by a physician. The usual treatment is systemic antibiotics.

Otitis Media

Otitis media is an inflammatory condition of the middle ear that occurs most often during childhood. Conditions that interfere with the eustachian tube function, such as upper respiratory tract infection, allergy, adenoid lymphadenopathy, and cleft palate, predispose individuals to otitis media (4). Blockage of the eustachian tube allows the oxygen in the middle ear cleft to be absorbed. This leaves a relative negative pressure or vacuum that results in a transudation (movement) of fluid into the middle ear cleft. Nose blowing and sneezing against occluded nostrils may worsen the condition and therefore should be avoided (13, 14). If the serous fluid in the middle ear cavity remains sterile, the condition is referred to as serous otitis media and is most often of viral origin; if it becomes infected, it is called purulent otitis media and is most often of bacterial origin.

Children often experience repeated episodes of eustachian tube obstruction caused by masses of adenoids that become endematous and block the eustachian tube openings, resulting in otitis media. Adenoidectomy usually prevents future incidence. In adults, recurrent otitis media may be caused by a nasopharyngeal tumor.

The most common symptoms in the acute phase of purulent otitis media are pain, hearing loss, and constitutional disturbances such as fever, often as high as 104° F (40° C), and malaise (15). As noted by one investigator, "the strategic location of the middle cleft and

Table 3. Some abnormal physical findings of the middle ear

Physical findings	Probable appearance	Interpretation
Perforation	Dark, thin, oval discoloration	Rupture of the eardrum
Acute purulent otitis media	Yellowish pus behind eardrum; bulging, hyperemic membrane; light reflex absent	Acute infection of the middle ear
Chronic serous otitis media	Amber-like fluid behind eardrum; observable fluid level with air bubbles; retraction of handle of malleus	Blockage of eustachian tube

Reprinted with permission from *Drug Intell. Clin. Pharm. 11*, 661 (1977).

mastoid cells separated from the sigmoid sinus and meninges by a mere thin shell makes every infection of the middle ear capable of intracranial infection" (4). Severity of symptoms increases as the condition worsens. Pain arises from the pressure of the fluids in the middle ear. This causes an outward tension on the tympanic membrane, which is innervated with sensory nerves. The rapid production of fluid and tension in a short period is responsible for the acute pain described as sharp, knife-like, and steady. The pain usually does not increase with mastication or when traction is applied to the auricle or tragus. Excessive nose blowing especially against occluded nostrils may force additional purulent mucus into the eustachian tube, perpetuating the condition.

If patients are not treated promptly, the pressure inside the middle ear may increase, leading to distention and bulging of the tympanic membrane. As bulging increases, so does necrosis, leading to perforation and escape of the purulent material from the middle ear. The mucopurulent discharge may cause a secondary bacterial external otitis infection. The appearance of a discharge is usually accompanied by a lessening of pain due to the decreased tension on the tympanic membrane. The initial discharge may be bloodstained, followed by a foul-smelling, purulent, serous fluid (7). The tympanic membrane usually loses its pearl-gray luster and appears yellow to orange-pink to rusty purple, another important diagnostic factor. Ear drops do not assist in the resolution of acute otitis media while the tympanic membrane is intact. The use of nonprescription otic drugs for the treatment of any form of otitis media is not recommended.

Serous otitis media symptoms include a sensation of fullness in the ear accompanied by hearing loss (16). The condition worsens as the fluid accumulates and fills the middle ear cleft. The sensation of fullness is associated with voice resonance, a congested feeling in the ears, a hollow sound, or a popping or cracking noise in the ears especially during swallowing or yawning. These symptoms usually are not present in external otitis.

Chronic Otitis Media

In chronic serous otitis media, the fluid in the middle ear may be thin and serous or thick and viscous ("glue ear") (4). Chronic serous otitis media occurs most often in small children. It may be caused by inadequate treatment of previous acute otitis media episodes or by recurrent upper respiratory tract bacterial or viral infections associated with eustachian tube dysfunction.

The most common symptom is impaired hearing, but the onset is often insidious, and the child may have no acute symptoms (17). Frequently, parents accuse the child of being inattentive and disobedient. Pain is usually absent. The diagnosis is performed by visual inspection of the tympanic membrane. The tympanic membrane appears yellow to orange and lusterless, and its flexibility is lost. It is not perforated but often appears to be retracted. Often long-standing fluid becomes more and more viscous, thus the term "glue ear."

Treatment often involves evacuation of the fluid by aspiration through an incision in the tympanic membrane (myringotomy) and implantation of a temporary, pressure-equalizing tube (16). This procedure usually is performed bilaterally and is especially useful in patients who do not have hypertrophied adenoids and when an adenoidectomy is not beneficial. After the middle ear cleft has been evacuated and the pressure-equalizing tubes permit the atmospheric pressure to equalize with that in the middle ear, hearing returns to normal. It is not uncommon for children during the first 10 years of life to wear the tubes for 6–12 months. Usually during this time, the tubes are extruded spontaneously, and repeated implantation of the pressure-equalizing tubes is usually unnecessary.

The tubes are especially helpful during acute or persistently frequent episodes of acute eustachian tube obstruction (a frequent episode of acute serous otitis media or barotrauma). The ventilation tubes permit normal atmospheric environmental changes in the middle ear cavity and allow for changes in air pressures to occur that are not dependent on the eustachian tube. The mucosal and epithelial linings are then permitted to return to normal function.

Chronic purulent otitis media is usually secondary to a persistent tympanic membrane perforation. With exacerbation, the patient may exhibit the symptoms of acute purulent otitis media as well as mucopurulent discharge.

Tympanic Membrane Perforation

The most common causes of traumatic perforation of the tympanic membrane are water sports, such as diving or water-skiing (7). Any corrosive agent introduced into the ear canal may produce tympanic membrane perforation. Other causes of perforation include blows to the head with a cupped hand, foreign objects entering the ear canal with excessive force, and forceful irrigation of the ear canal. At the moment of injury, the pain

is severe, but it decreases rapidly. Hearing acuity usually diminishes. An untreated injury may lead to otitis media. Other complications may include tinnitus, nausea, and vertigo, and may progress to mastoiditis. Any patient suspected of having an acute perforated tympanic membrane should be examined thoroughly by a physician.

Barotrauma (Acute Aero-otitis Media)

Barotrauma occurs during quick descent from high altitude (10, 16). The middle ear fails to ventilate, resulting in a negative pressure in the middle ear. This negative pressure causes a suction and forces the tympanic membrane to retract, causing pain. In addition, edema is formed, with transudation and hemorrhage into the middle ear space. Barotrauma may also occur in individuals who fly and have an upper respiratory tract infection or any condition associated with impaired eustachian tube ventilation.

Upon examination, the tympanic membrane appears inflamed and retracted and is similar to that seen with acute otitis media, causing differential diagnosis to be unclear.

Pretreatment with antihistamines and/or decongestants may help to avoid serious symptoms during air travel for patients susceptible to barotrauma. Treatment of acute episodes consists of oral decongestants, antihistamines, and autoinflation of the eustachian tube (Valsalva's maneuver) (4, 16).

Hearing Disorders

Obstructive Hearing Loss

Accumulated cerumen is a common cause of hearing loss, especially in persons with overactive cerumen glands. The accumulated cerumen causes an obstruction and produces a feeling of fullness or diminished hearing. A hearing impairment may occur when the cerumen occludes the canal, impairing the transmission of sound waves to the tympanic membrane. Impacted cerumen can be removed only by direct manipulation; the procedure should not be attempted by the patient or untrained personnel. Following swimming or bathing, water can be entrapped in the ear canal. The trapped water is absorbed by a cerumen mass that occludes the canal, causing a hearing deficit. A temporary hearing impairment may result from any external otitis due to excessive edema, which with accumulated cerumen and debris, may occlude the canal.

Serous otitis media, external otitis, acute otitis media, and chronic otitis media seldom produce tinnitus as the sole or predominant complaint. Most patients have sensory insult from loud noise exposure, ototoxicity, head concussions, Meniere's disease, or acoustic neuroma (16).

Tinnitus

Tinnitus may be associated with hearing loss, exposure to high noise levels or acoustic trauma, or may be a symptom of a systemic disease or a drug toxicity (18). Disequilibrium (vertigo) may be of otic origin. It may be due to drug toxicity, intracranial or neurologic diseases, infection, hyperventilation, or severe ceruminal impaction (18). Tinnitus sometimes can be very annoying to the patient. It can be constant or intermittent. Tinnitus has been described as sounding like steam escaping from a small pipe, ringing, roaring, pulsating, crickets, and humming (19). The intensity of the apparent disturbance varies from patient to patient, and patients' reactions may vary from minor distraction to severe mental depression. Tinnitus can arise from a variety of causes often involving the inner ear. It may be the result of blockade of the ear canal, or the eustachian tube and middle ear cavity, which is easily corrected following proper diagnosis.

Patients with tinnitus caused by such drugs as salicylates (arthritis patients), quinidine (heart patients), and quinine (malaria patients or patients with leg cramps) usually will notice a decrease of the intensity of the tinnitus symptoms following the discontinuation of the medication. Any patient who experiences any symptom of tinnitus should receive a medical examination and evaluation. Nonprescription ear drops are not effective and are not recommended for the treatment of tinnitus.

Assessment

To choose realistically between self-treatment and physician referral, the pharmacist must be able to assess the nature and severity of the patient's otic condition by evaluating the signs and symptoms (Table 1). The most common complaints may include one or more of the following symptoms: localized pain, itchiness in the ear canal, a feeling of fullness, hearing loss, lymphadenopathy, fever, and malaise.

Ear Pain

Pain in the ear commonly expressed by the patient as an earache may be caused by a variety of disorders; careful inspection with proper instrumentation by trained personnel often is necessary to determine the etiology of the pain. External otitis, foreign material (cerumen) packed against the tympanic membrane, and acute otitis media and its possible complications (mastoiditis or abscess) are all common causes of ear pain. Referred pain to the ear from the sinuses, nasopharynx, the tongue, the hypopharynx, the larynx, the temporomandibular joint or the muscles of mastication on the lower molars, loose-fitting dentures, and eruption of molar teeth may appear to the patient as ear pain. Improper treatment may delay successful therapy. Proper diagnosis and determining the etiology of the pain preclude self-medication.

Applied pressure on the pinna or the tragus increases pain in external otitis, which is important for differential diagnosis (20). Patients with otitis media rarely report increased pain with pressure on the pinna or tragus. Sometimes mastication may cause increased pain in patients with either external otitis or otitis media and is another important consideration in diagnosis.

Boils

The signs and symptoms of a boil in the ear canal include a localized, burning pain that increases when the patient chews, when traction is applied to the auricle, and when the tragus is pressed medially. A red, inflamed, raised lesion can be seen along the ear canal. The skin around the affected area is intact and not broken, providing the patient has not attempted to scratch it. The patient's subjective hearing is usually intact. If lymphadenopathy, fever, malaise, or severe pain is present, the patient should be seen by a physician.

Foreign Objects

The signs and symptoms of a foreign object in the ear usually include a feeling of fullness with hearing loss from the affected ear. Pain may be present and increased by chewing, traction on the auricle, and pressure applied medially on the tragus. Lymphadenopathy, fever, or malaise does not occur acutely but may develop later with a foul-smelling discharge from the affected ear. Collectively, these characteristics indicate a secondary infection. All patients with foreign objects in the ear with or without secondary infection should be seen and treated by a physician.

External Otitis

The only conclusive means by which bacterial or fungal external otitis may be ruled out is by microbiologic culture. However, culture is not always practical, nor is it always needed. Pain and swelling localized in the ear canal usually are the motivating symptoms that cause the patient to seek professional help. A bacterial infection may be characterized by increased pain with chewing, traction applied on the auricle, and pressure applied medially on the tragus. Lymphadenopathy and a feeling of fullness may be additional characteristics with possible febrile condition and associated malaise. Otoscopic examination is painful and reveals a swollen inflamed ear canal and an inflamed tympanic membrane. A purulent, foul-smelling discharge may block visual inspection of the tympanic membrane. Any foul-smelling mucopurulent discharge indicates a bacterial infection. Patients with external otitis should be referred to a physician for thorough cleansing and inspection of the ear canal.

Hearing Loss

Hearing loss is subjective unless diagnosed and evaluated by an audiologist. Acute hearing loss without pain may be due to impacted cerumen, which may be observed during direct visualization of the ear canal. Impacted cerumen in the ear canal obstructs the tympanic membrane and prevents its visualization.

Patients with impacted cerumen without secondary complications may be treated safely with nonprescription cerumen-softening agents. Patients with hearing loss without pain, and whose tympanic membrane is visible and not obstructed, should be evaluated and treated by a physician. A perforated tympanic membrane results in decreased hearing. Usually, the patient has experienced a sharp pain of short duration at the time of injury. Treatment for a perforated tympanic membrane includes repair and medical therapy to prevent infection in the middle ear.

Otomycosis

Patients with otomycosis usually complain of itching and a feeling of fullness in the affected ear. A colorless discharge may or may not be present. Pain usually is not present but may occur in severe cases. The pain increases with chewing, traction on the auricle, and pressure applied medially on the tragus. Constitutional disturbances usually occur only in severe cases, which often are due to secondary bacterial infections with obstruction of the ear canal causing a hearing loss.

Otitis Media

The only conclusive means of diagnosing otitis media is a complete physical examination, using a pneumatic otoscope, and a complete patient history. In most cases, otitis media is caused by eustachian tube dysfunction. It is found most commonly in children. Patients may be asymptomatic or may complain of occasional fullness and "cracking" or a "hollow sound" in the ears. The effect is usually bilateral. Otoscopic findings are specific and may demonstrate typical changes in tympanic membrane mobility consistent with the symptoms and degree of severity of the disorder.

A complication of prolonged serous otitis media is caused by bacteria and viruses extending along the eustachian tube causing suppurative otitis media. Pneumatic otoscopic findings are specific and demonstrate a bulging, poorly resilient tympanic membrane. Deformation of the tympanic membrane is caused by the pus and exudate that accumulate behind the tympanic membrane. The patient usually experiences pain that is dull and throbbing at first and then rapidly progresses to a sharp, knife-like agonizing pain. These symptoms usually follow an upper respiratory tract infection. Constitutional symptoms include chills, fever, and malaise. A purulent discharge occurs only after tympanic membrane perforation, at which time the patient experiences sudden and welcome relief of pain. A bloody, purulent, smelly drainage flows from the ear. The fever rapidly returns to normal.

Treatment is aimed at reventilating the middle ear space, reducing nasopharyngeal and eustachian tube edema, and managing the infection. Patients with any of these symptoms should be evaluated and treated by a physician because middle ear disorders are often associated with an underlying cause and require thorough diagnostic evaluation and treatment.

Treatment

Normally, the skin lining the external auditory meatus provides adequate protection against bacterial or fungal infection; cerumen provides a lubricant to the skin to maintain its integrity. The hair helps shield the meatus from dust and debris. Cerumen provides a continuing, self-cleaning process that removes particulate matter and debris from the external auditory meatus. An infection of the auricle or external auditory meatus is a skin infection and should be treated as such.

Progressive symptoms of otic disease should be evaluated and treated only under physician supervision. Cerumen-softening and cerumenolytic agents only soften and loosen cerumen to enable its easy removal by a physician. These agents do not remove cerumen. Effective mechanical removal by irrigation or instrumentation should be reserved for the physician. Surgical intervention may be necessary for deep cuts, bruises, or abrasions of the ear. Severe infections often require both systemic and local antibiotics.

Self-treatment of boils may be instituted by applying heat followed by an antibiotic ointment to the affected area. A soft cotton applicator is useful to apply the ointment over and around the boil. The antibiotic ointment may be used even if the boil ruptures. The lesion usually is self-limiting and clears after several days of frequent applications. Resistant lesions require incision and drainage by a physician.

Treatment of external otitis usually includes antibiotic and hydrocortisone drops applied in the ear canal. When cellulitus and lymphadenopathy are present, oral antibiotics are effective. Trauma to the ear should be avoided. The ear canals should be kept clean and dry at all times. Following swimming or bathing, the ear canals may be filled for 1–2 minutes with alcohol, glycerine, propylene glycol, or water acidified to a pH of 4–5 to help restore the normal acidic pH to the ear canal (4). An acidified aluminum acetate (Burow's) solution may be used for its astringent effect to obtain rapid resolution of edema and crusting. External otitis should be treated promptly for a satisfactory outcome. If not treated properly, external otitis is likely to spread to the mastoid bone or to the middle ear cavity, causing severe patient disability. Permanent hearing loss may occur.

Minor symptoms of otomycosis (rare) may be treated prophylactically with alcohol, propylene glycol, glycerin, or water that has been acidified. Aluminum acetate solution also may be used for its astringent effect. These ingredients have been demonstrated to be safe and effective for maintaining a clean, dry ear canal and promoting aural hygiene (4). The choice of the product depends on availability. Patients with severe otomycosis and impacted mycotic debris should have their ear canals cleaned and treated by a physician.

Primary Nonprescription Pharmacologic Agents

Nonprescription products used for palliative treatment of auricular ear disorders should include selective products useful for the treatment of skin disorders.

Salicylic acid when applied to the skin is a mild irritant and continuous application may cause dermatitis (21). The use of salicylic acid in topical preparations applied to the ear canal is considered undesirable unless supervised by a physician.

Antibiotic ointments, such as neomycin and bacitracin ointments, alone or in combination with polymyxin-B sulfate, are adequate for treating minor lesions of the auricle. Antibiotics cannot penetrate into abscesses because of the intrinsic tendency of abscesses to wall themselves off.

Acetic Acid Solutions

Weak acetic acid solutions are used to treat mild forms of external otitis. A concentration of 2–2.5% may be made easily in the pharmacy from glacial acetic acid or from white distilled household vinegar, which is usually 5% acetic acid. A 50:50 mixture of distilled household vinegar with either water, propylene glycol, glycerin, or rubbing alcohol (70% isopropyl alcohol or 70% ethanol) may be used (22). (Patients should be cautioned that denaturants in 70% rubbing alcohol formulations may cause sensitization.) The mixture is conveniently made and inexpensive. Acetic acid increases the acidity of the normal skin of the external auditory canal, creating an undesirable environment for the growth of bacteria, especially *Pseudomonas* species (6, 22). Alcohol is a local anti-infective and provides a local drying effect for prophylaxis against swimmer's ear (7, 20, 23).

Aluminum Acetate (Burow's Solution)

External otitis or local itching of the external ear caused by external ear dermatitis may be treated with an astringent such as 1:20 or 1:40 aluminum acetate solution (3, 22, 24, 25). One tablet or packet dissolved in 500 ml of water yields a concentration of 1:40. Aluminum acetate solution is used widely for conditions involving the external ear. Its major value is its acidity, which restores the normal antibacterial pH of the ear canal. Applied locally as protein precipitants, astringents dry the affected area by reducing the secretory function of the skin glands (25). Contraction and wrinkling of the affected tissue may be seen; astringents also toughen the skin to prevent reinfection.

A wet compress of aluminum acetate solution may be used with a gauze dressing on the auricle (3). Drops may be instilled into the external auditory meatus. The usual dose is 4–6 drops every 4–6 hours until itching or burning subsides. The drops also may be used prophylactically against swimmer's ear to help clean and dry the ear canal after swimming or bathing. Aluminum acetate solution is suitable for children and adults. Used properly, it is nonsensitizing and well tolerated (21). Adverse reactions are rare.

Antipyrine

The FDA advisory review panel on nonprescription topical analgesic, antirheumatic, otic, burn, and sunburn treatment drug products concluded that antipyrine is neither safe nor effective for nonprescription use as a topical otic analgesic and anesthetic and should be used only under the advice and supervision of a physician (26). The clinical effectiveness and safety of antipyrine in treating otic disorders has not been substantiated.

Benzocaine

The usefulness of benzocaine or other local anesthetics for local analgesia in the ear canal is not clear. The FDA advisory review panel concluded that benzocaine is neither safe nor effective for nonprescription use as a topical analgesic and suggested that benzocaine is ineffective topically as an analgesic and/or anesthetic on the tissue of the tympanic membrane and ear canal (25). Hypersensitivity to benzocaine is considered a general contraindication to its topical use in the ear or elsewhere applied to the skin.

Benzocaine is a topical, local anesthetic commonly used for pain, discomfort, or pruritus associated with skin ulcers, wounds, mucous membranes, hemorrhoids, and skin irritations, including sunburn and insect bites. Benzocaine is poorly soluble in water, very slowly absorbed through the skin, and relatively nontoxic. The localized anesthesia produced is not complete but is long acting because of benzocaine's poor solubility and its slow absorption.

Benzocaine has been used as a local anesthetic to treat pain associated with external otitis and other disorders of the auricle and/or ear canal. Its application to weeping wounds of fulminating infections usually is not effective because an adequate concentration cannot be achieved due to drainage of body fluids away from the wound. Symptomatic pain relief in such cases may be undesirable, because it may disguise the symptoms of an exacerbating infection.

The topical application of any local anesthetic may produce the same untoward effects as those following parenteral administration. Reactions or complications are usually avoided by applying the minimal effective dose. Special caution should be exercised in patients with known drug sensitivity and in those with severe trauma and/or sepsis of the applied areas.

Boric Acid

Boric acid is an ingredient in several ear preparations. It is a weak, local anti-infective, and is nonirritating to intact skin in a dilute solution of 1–5%. Supersaturated alcoholic boric acid solutions have improved the antibacterial action over alcohol itself (either 99% isopropyl or 70% ethyl alcohol). Acetic acid and boric acid increase the acidity of dosage forms, increasing the normal acidity of the skin (6, 22). Because of its toxicity, boric acid should be used with caution, particularly with children and on open wounds, where the potential for systemic absorption is high (25).

Camphor

Camphor is used in eardrops and earwax softeners as a weak antiseptic and a mild anesthetic intended to suppress itching. However, its effectiveness in the concentrations used has not been substantiated.

Carbamide Peroxide

The antibacterial properties of carbamide peroxide (urea hydrogen peroxide) are due to its release of nascent oxygen, and its main value is to clean wounds. The effervescence caused by the oxygen release mechanically removes debris from inaccessible regions. In otic preparations, the effervescence disorganizes wax accumulations. Carbamide (urea) helps debride the tissue. These actions soften the residue in the ear, and removal of the liquefied cerumen may be assisted by warm water irrigation.

The FDA advisory review panel concluded that 6.5% carbamide peroxide solution in anhydrous glycerin instilled into the affected ear is safe and effective for nonprescription use as an earwax-softening agent (27). The panel recommends the solution be instilled into the affected ear and allowed to remain at least 15 mintues with the head tilted (the affected ear up) before the wax is removed by gently washing with lukewarm water and using a soft rubber syringe. The process may be repeated a second time, if necessary. It is not recommended for children under 12 years of age.

Chloroform

Chloroform is an irritant and preservative used in some eardrops. It is volatile and evaporates on exposure to the air. Its effectiveness for treating ear disorders has not been substantiated.

Glycerin

Glycerin may be used as a solvent, a vehicle, or an emollient, and also as a humectant because of its hydroscopicity. Glycerin is widely used as a solvent and a vehicle in many otic preparations (prescription and nonprescription). It is safe and nonsensitizing when applied to open wounds or abraded skin.

The FDA advisory review panel on topical analgesic, antirheumatic, otic, burn, and sunburn treatment drug products recommends that glycerin be used as a cerumen-softening agent in an aqueous solution containing 95% glycerin or greater (27). Dehydrated glycerin contains no less than 98.5% glycerin. Glyercin USP contains no less than 95% glycerin (it may contain a maximum of 5% water) (29).

Ichthammol

Ichthammol is a weak antiseptic and irritant with demulcent and emollient properties. Its primary contribution is as an emollient, not as an antiseptic. Ichthammol ointment (10%) is used for treating local inflammation associated with minor boils or an abscessed wound. Ichthammol is used with glycerin in external otitis and cellulitis. Evidence to support effectiveness and efficacy is not available (11).

Menthol

Menthol, which is included in some earwax softeners, is an antipruritic and counterirritant and provides localized coolness when applied to the tissues. Menthol's clinical effectiveness in treating ear disorders has not been substantiated.

Olive Oil (Sweet Oil)

Olive oil, a fixed oil containing mixed glycerides of oleic acid (about 83%), is used as an emollient and topical lubricant (29). Often it is instilled into the ear canal to alleviate itchiness and burning and may be used for softening earwax (12).

Phenol in Glycerin

Phenol in glycerin (5–10%) was formerly prescribed to treat pain caused by ear disorders (30). Its use is not recommended because of its inherent dangers of necrosis and perforation of the tympanic membrane (31, 11). Phenol is a potent, but toxic bactericide. It is absorbed by the skin and has caused severe toxic effects and death when used in excess (11).

Propylene Glycol

Propylene glycol is a solvent that has preservative properties and is a useful humectant. Used in both prescription and nonprescription otic preparations, propylene glycol is a clear, colorless, nonirritating, viscous liquid. Its viscosity provides increased contact time to the tissues of the external auditory meatus. Adding acetic acid to propylene glycol increases the solution's acidity, enhancing its anti-infective properties (32).

Thymol

Thymol, a phenol obtained from thyme oil, has a more agreeable odor than phenol. It has antibacterial and antifungal properties in a concentration of 1% (25). In the presence of large amounts of proteins, its antibacterial activity is greatly reduced. It has been used traditionally in topical preparations partly because of its deodorant properties. Its clinical effectiveness for ear disorders has not been substantiated.

Other Cerumen-Softening Products

Other products used to soften earwax include light mineral oil, a mixture of warm water and 3% hydrogen peroxide in a ratio of 1:1, and a 3% hypertonic sodium chloride solution (22). The use of undiluted 3% hydrogen peroxide and the indiscriminate use of aqueous hydrogen peroxide (1:1 ratio) instilled in the ear canal are unwise, since they may cause maceration of the skin and predispose it to infection (9). Cerumen-softening agents only soften the hardened, impacted cerumen. They do not and should never be expected to both soften and remove cerumen. The impacted cerumen can be removed only by irrigation or mechanical means and only by a physician.

Removal of the cerumen, desquamated debris, and dried secretions often is best accomplished by suction or use of a small cotton-tipped applicator. (This method should be performed only by trained personnel.) Gentle irrigation with an ear syringe or a forced water spray should be performed only if the tympanic membrane is known to be intact. Direct visualization of the ear canal is important for the patient's safety. In patients who have difficulty with hard, impacted cerumen, the occasional instillation of olive oil, mineral oil, glycerin, diluted hydrogen peroxide solution, or propylene glycol in the ear may soften the cerumen and promote normal removal.

The patient may irrigate the ear canal with warm water, normal saline, a mixture of 20–30% alcohol and water, or aluminum acetate solution to help prevent cerumen buildup (22). If the tympanic membrane is perforated or if it is not known whether or not the tympanic membrane is intact, these cerumen-softening drug products should be used only under a physician's direct supervision.

More than 90% of all cases of external otitis may be treated properly with aluminum acetate solution or acetic acid (2%) in either 70% alcohol or propylene glycol, 4–6 drops every 4–6 hours. This treatment is preferred except in diabetic patients and in unusually severe cases of external otitis. In severe cases, these solutions may be used to irrigate the debris from the ear canal to improve the effectiveness of topical antibacterial otic drops (4). Patients with a known tympanic membrane perforation should not use otic preparations without their physicians' consent.

All nonprescription otic preparations may be contraindicated because of local irritation and hypersensitivity caused by the ingredients. Patients should be advised that if a rash, local redness, or other noticeable adverse symptom occurs, the medication should be discontinued.

Product Selection Guidelines

Patient Considerations

The pharmacist's evaluation of the patient's present health status must be based on information in the medical and drug history, including current symptoms. This information should include the presence of chronic diseases that may impair healing, such as diabetes mellitus (patients taking insulin or oral hypoglycemics), or conditions, such as dandruff, that may influence the patient's response to self-medication.

Other considerations include deformities or ear scars. An earache due to otitis media, secondary to an upper respiratory tract infection, should be ruled out

before the pharmacist considers initiating treatment of an external ear disorder. A history of pressure in or referred pain to the ear may be caused by a tumor in the area around the ear. Recent injury or trauma in the head or neck regions also may cause referred pain to the ear. Adults with recurrent otitis media may respond very poorly to treatment.

Management of ear disorders often may be difficult because of underlying diseases or predisposing factors. The skin of patients with diabetes mellitus is more prone to infection (bacterial and fungal), especially when the diabetes is uncontrolled. Infections in diabetics tend to clear up more slowly and to recur more frequently. The increased predisposition to infection is related to circulatory skin impairment, increased glucose concentrations, and abnormalities in immunologic responses. Ear disorders, especially external otitis, are difficult to treat in diabetic patients. Rigid control of diabetes cannot be overemphasized for favorable outcome of treatment.

The pharmacist should ask specific questions regarding the patient's medical history, such as whether the patient has experienced similar symptoms previously and, if so, when and how they were treated. The pharmacist should ask the patient to describe the symp-

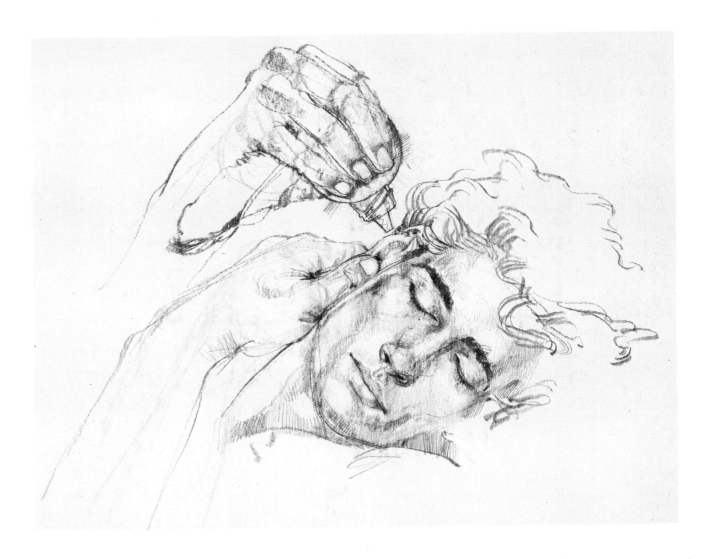

toms. The patient's history should reveal underlying disease states and predisposing factors, including allergies, that may influence the response to self-medication.

The pharmacist first should consider whether the patient can be treated appropriately with nonprescription drugs. Health professionals (pharmacists and nurses) properly trained to visualize the tympanic membrane and ear canal with a suitable otoscope and those properly instructed in aural hygiene may, in most cases, perform irrigation safely with an ear syringe or a forced water spray. Pharmacists may assess the severity of the otic disorder and either provide appropriate nonprescription medication with instructions or refer the patient to a physician. Appropriately selected nonprescription drug products can be relied upon to provide a suitable therapeutic response. Proper selection and instruction by the pharmacist require a clear knowledge of the symptoms of the patient and the pathophysiology of the illness. Referral to medical treatment by a physician requires an ability to recognize the severity of the illness or the potential or actual complications associated with the condition. The patient should always be referred to a physician if any of the following symptoms exist: severe pain, lymphadenopathy, discharge from the ear, possible hearing deficit, or a fever.

Patient Consultation

Many physicians feel that cleansing procedures and self-medication for treating ear disorders should not be delegated to the patient or to anyone who is not properly trained. Patients must be evaluated for their ability to understand the hazards of inappropriate self-medication. The pharmacist with proper instruction in aural visualization and irrigation procedures can usually make these judgments.

The use of nonprescription drugs for the ear should be supervised like other drug products dispensed by the pharmacist (34). The proper use of medicine droppers for administering eardrops into the ear and ear syringes for irrigating the ear should be understood fully by the patient. Eardrops should be warmed to body temperature by holding the medication container in the palm of the hand or in a vessel of warm water for a few minutes before administration.

A cotton plug may be inserted gently to help maintain the medication in the ear canal. Cotton wicks, however, usually require insertion with instrumentation and should be used only by trained personnel. Pulling the auricle back may allow the medicine to reach a greater depth in the ear canal. In addition, patients should be advised that if the symptoms persist or increase in severity within a few days following the initiation of self-medication, a physician should be consulted. Symptoms usually begin to subside within 1–2 days if self-medication is appropriate. If symptoms persist or if an adverse reaction to the medicine occurs, the patient should be referred to a physician.

Summary

Otic disorders affect both young and old people, and their visible signs are not always proportional to the amount of pain suffered. Nonprescription products are available for treatment of disorders in both the auricle and the external auditory canal. Disorders involving the middle ear should not be treated with nonprescription products.

By assessing the complaint and reviewing the patient's history, the pharmacist should be able to judge whether symptoms may be self-treated or referral to a physician is indicated. Health professionals trained in otic procedures may examine the tympanic membrane with an otoscope and irrigate the ear canal gently with a syringe or a forced water spray. This procedure should be performed only if the tympanic membrane is known to be intact and there are no underlying disorders.

Objects such as hairpins, pencils, matchsticks, cotton swabs, or other sharp instruments should never touch the external auditory canal, and objects smaller than a finger draped with a clean washcloth should never enter the external auditory canal. Good personal hygiene, especially of facial and neck areas, should be maintained. Dandruff and dirty hair may be controlled with appropriate shampoos and washing. A skin infection must not be neglected because an infection may be transferred very easily to uninfected areas.

Most nonprescription otic products have been shown to be safe and effective, and the choice of a specific product generally depends on availability and patient preference. The pharmacist should advise the patient to consult a physician if symptoms do not subside within 1–2 days after treatment is initiated or if adverse reactions occur.

References

1. I. Hall and B. Colman, "Diseases of the Nose, Throat and Ear," 10th ed., Williams and Wilkins, Baltimore, Md., 1973, pp. 278, 315, 324.
2. I. Friedman, "Pathology of the Ear," Blackwell Scientific Publications, London, England, 1974, pp. 10, 14, 15, 27.
3. D. Deweese and W. Saunders, "Textbook of Otolaryngology," 4th ed., C. V. Mosby, St. Louis, Mo., 1973, pp. 235, 245, 272–274, 327, 328, 336, 337, 346.
4. M. M. Paparella and D. A. Shumrick, "Otolaryngology," Vol. 2, W. B. Saunders, Philadelphia, Pa., 1980, pp. 31, 1345–1349, 1393, 1412, 1413, 1419, 1445.
5. S. Riegelman and D. L. Sorby, in "Dispensing of Medication," 7th ed., E. W. Martin, Ed., Mack, Easton, Pa., 1971, p. 908.
6. G. L. Adams, R. L. Boies, Jr., and M. M. Paparella, "Fundamentals of Otolaryngology," 5th ed., W. B. Saunders, Philadelphia, Pa., 1978, pp. 181, 184.
7. "Disease of the Nose, Throat and Ear," 12th ed., J. J. Ballenger et al., Eds., Lea and Febiger, Philadelphia, Pa., 1977, pp. 609, 784, 786, 787, 789, 820.
8. *Federal Register, 42,* 1977, p. 63559.
9. S. R. Mawson and H. Ludman, "Diseases of the Ear," 4th ed., Yearbook Medical, Chicago, Ill., 1979, pp. 252, 257, 261, 267.
10. B. H. Senturia, M. D. Marcus, and F. E. Lucente, "Diseases of the External Ear, An Otologic-Dermatology Manual," 2nd ed., Grune and Stratton, New York, N.Y., 1980, pp. 79, 80.
11. A. Rook, D. S. Wilkinson, and F. J. G. Ebling, "Textbook of Dermatology," Blackwell Scientific Publications, Oxford, 1979, pp. 443, 553.
12. A. Cohn, *Arch. Otolaryngol., 99,* 138 (1974).
13. J. Bossi and J. Jackman, *Drug Intell. Clin. Pharm., 11,* 665 (1977).
14. G. D. L. Smyth, "Chronic Otitis Media in Otolaryngology," Vol. 1, G. M. English, Ed., Harper and Row, Hagerstown,

Md., 1976, p. 2.

15. D. Elliott, E. Mortimer, and L. Rutledge, *Patient Care, 5*, 20 (1971).

16. K. J. Lee, "Differential Diagnosis, Otolaryngology," Arco, New York, N.Y., 1978, pp. 91, 94, 115.

17. G. R. Fraser, "The Causes of Profound Deafness in Childhood," Johns Hopkins University Press, Baltimore, Md., 1976, p. 268.

18. R. P. Wood and F. L. Northern, "Manual of Otolaryngology," Williams and Wilkins, Baltimore, Md., 1979, pp. 39, 42.

19. L. J. Bradford and W. G. Hardy, "Hearing and Hearing Impairment," Grune and Stratton, New York, N.Y., 1979, pp. 106–107.

20. D. Wright and F. Alexander, *Arch. Otolaryngol., 99*, 16–18 (1974).

21. A. Wade and J. E. Reynolds, "Martindale, The Extra Pharmacopoeia," 27th ed., Pharmaceutical Press, 1979, pp. 212, 272.

22. "AMA Drug Evaluations," 4th ed., American Medical Association, Chicago, Ill., 1980, pp. 432, 433.

23. D. Wright and M. Dinen, *Arch. Otolaryngol., 95*, 245 (1972).

24. "Drugs of Choice," W. Modell, Ed., C. V. Mosby, St. Louis, Mo., 1974, p. 603.

25. "Remington's Pharmaceutical Sciences," 14th ed., Mack, Easton, Pa., 1970, pp. 768, 775, 1191.

26. *Federal Register, 42*, 63564 (1977).

27. *Federal Register, 42*, 63562–63 (1977).

28. "The United States Pharmacopoeia," 20th ed., Mack, Easton, Pa., 1980, p. 353.

29. "The United States Dispensatory," 27th ed., A. Osol and R. Pratt, Eds., J. B. Lippincott, Philadelphia, Pa., 1973, pp. 199, 804.

30. M. S. Ersner, in "Diseases of the Nose, Throat and Ear," 1st ed., C. Jackson and C. L. Jackson, Eds., W. B. Saunders, Philadelphia, Pa., 1945, p. 266.

31. L. R. Boies, "Fundamentals of Otolaryngology," W. B. Saunders, Philadelphia, Pa., 1950, pp. 66, 67.

32. *Medical Notes of External Otitis*, Burroughs Wellcome Co., 1972.

33. R. D. Stride, *J. Laryngol. Otol., 73*, 48 (1959).

34. "Self-Medication," J. A. D. Anderson, Ed., University Park Press, Baltimore, Md., 1979, pp. 49, 68.

Otic Product Table

Product (Manufacturer)	Ingredients
Aqua-Otic-B (Ortega)	aluminum acetate; boric acid, 1%; acetic acid, 1%; propylene glycol; benzyl alcohol, 0.5%
Auro-Dri (Commerce)	glycerin, 5% in isopropyl alcohol, 97.25%
Auro Ear Drops (Commerce)	carbamide peroxide, 7.15%; propylene glycol, 92.45%
Debrox Drops (Marion Laboratories)	carbamide peroxide, 6.5%; anhydrous glycerol
Dents Ear Wax Drops (C. S. Dent)	glycerin, 96%
Dri Ear Drops (Pfeiffer)	boric acid, 2.75%; in isopropyl alcohol
Ear Drops by Murine (Abbott)	carbamide peroxide, 6.5%; anhydrous glycerin
Ear-Dry (Scherer)	boric acid, 2.75%; isopropyl alcohol
E.R.O. (Scherer)	glycerin, 95%; propylene glycol, 5%
Kerid Ear Drops (Blair)	glycerin, 30%; urea, 0.1%; propylene glycol
Oil for Ear Use (DeWitt)	cajuput oil, 1.6%; white thyme oil, 1.6%; camphor, 0.5%; menthol, 0.3%
Pfeiffer Ear Drops (Pfeiffer)	glycerin, 99.75% (v/v); camphor; cajeput oil; eucalyptus oil; thyme oil
Swim-Ear (Fougera)	boric acid, 2.75%; isopropyl alcohol

21 Ophthalmic Products

Dick R. Gourley and Michael C. Makoid

Questions to Ask the Patient

Is your vision blurred? Is your eye painful as opposed to itching or stinging?

How long have these symptoms been present? What were you doing when you noticed them? Have you had a similar problem before?

Have you used a nonprescription eye product recently? Which one(s) did you use? For what symptoms?

Have your eyes been exposed recently to irritants such as smog, chemicals, or sun glare? Have you used any pesticides or fertilizers recently?

Do you have any other eye problems (double vision, discharge, or twitch)?

Do you have chronic diseases such as diabetes, glaucoma, or hypertension?

Are you taking any prescribed medicines?

Do you wear contact lenses? Hard or soft lenses? What contact lens products do you use?

Do you have any allergies?

Have you recently had a head cold or sinus problem?

Do you use eye cosmetics? Do you use hair spray or spray deodorants?

As the most available member of the health care team, the pharmacist often must deal with a patient having ocular discomfort. In deciding between physician referral and self-medication, the pharmacist should have a thorough understanding of common eye problems. Minor symptoms may signal the beginning of a more serious problem that requires evaluation and treatment by a physician.

Nonprescription ophthalmic products are basically safe and effective only to relieve minor symptoms such as stinging, itching, tearing, "tired eyes," or "eye strain." These problems are usually self-limiting. Self-medication should be discouraged in patients experiencing pain and/or blurred vision. These patients should be referred to a physician. A dilemma with the use of nonprescription ophthalmic products is that the diagnosis of conditions for which these products can be used is generally a self-diagnosis, based on a hit-or-miss approach. If the patient makes the wrong self-diagnosis and administers inappropriate therapy, an exacerbation of symptoms and possibly a worsening of the problem itself may occur. Moreover, nonprescription products may cause allergic reactions due to the active ingredients or to preservatives in the final product. The disorders and symptoms for which self-medication is indi-

cated and may be effective or for which physician referral is indicated, as recommended by the FDA advisory review panel on nonprescription ophthalmic drug products, are listed below.

Ocular disorders amenable to treatment with nonprescription products (1)

- Tear insufficiency—keratoconjunctivitis sicca and dry eye in the elderly (professional medical diagnosis is indicated even if treatment is with nonprescription drugs);
- Corneal edema (professional medical diagnosis is indicated, even if treatment is with nonprescription agents);
- Inflammation and irritation of the eye—presence of loose foreign material in the eye, irritation from airborne pollutants and chlorinated water, and allergic conjunctivitis.

Ocular disorders for which self-medication may be effective (1)

- Hordeolum (stye);
- Blepharitis;
- Conjunctivitis.

Ocular disorders for which physician referral is indicated (1)

- Embedded foreign body;
- Uveitis;
- Glaucoma;
- Flash burns;
- Tear duct infections;
- Corneal ulcers.

Eye Anatomy and Physiology

The eye is divided into three general areas: the eyelids, the external eye, and the internal eye (Figure 1).

Eyelids

The eyelids are movable folds of tissue that protect the eye and distribute tears over the surface of the globe. The eyelids are covered anteriorly (externally) with skin, and lined posteriorly (internally) with conjunctiva, a thin transparent mucous membrane terminating at the corneal-scleral junction. Four types of glands are present in the lids: the meibomian glands, the glands of Zeis and Moll, and the accessory lacrimal glands of Kraus and Wolfring. The meibomian glands are long sebaceous glands that secrete an oily substance that helps maintain the integrity of the tear film by preventing rapid evaporation. The glands of Zeis are smaller modified sebaceous glands associated with eyelash folli-

cles; Moll's glands are modified sweat glands. The accessory lacrimal glands of Kraus and Wolfring supply most of the needed moisture to the conjunctival sac and cornea.

External Eye

The external eye, the area immediately in front of the cornea, consists of the lacrimal apparatus and the cul-de-sac that contains the lacrimal fluid. In the normal human eye, tears are constantly produced and removed, maintaining a resident volume of 7 μl (2). The lacrimal fluid keeps the cornea and conjunctiva moist, protects the eye, clears away foreign materials from the eye (maintains a smooth optical surface), and inhibits the growth of microorganisms. Once formed, tears are conveyed across the corneal surface by the movement of the eyelids, finally collecting in the lower cul-de-sac for eventual drainage through the nasolacrimal duct into the nose.

Lid movement influences the drainage rate and thus physical movement of topically instilled drugs (2). The drainage apparatus begins at the punctum and ends in the nose. The passageway is a highly vascularized mucous membrane and consequently offers an extremely facile route for systemic absorption of topically instilled drugs, giving rise to the potential for systemic side effects (3–5).

Tear turnover in the precorneal area is rapid [16%/min in humans (2)], and any additional instilled fluid also drains away rapidly, with a rate constant proportional to the volume instilled (4). This process usually accounts for the loss of more than 90% of an instilled dose (6, 7); as a result, maintaining a high drug concentration for a prolonged period in the precorneal area is difficult.

Internal Eye

The eyeball (or globe) may be considered as a three-layered sac divided into three compartments and filled with three fluids. The three layers of the eye are an outer fibrous layer, consisting of the sclera (white of the eye) and the cornea; the middle vascular layer (uveal tract), consisting of the iris, ciliary body, and choroid; and the inner photoreceptor layer, consisting of the pigmented epithelium and retina. The three compartments are the anterior chamber, the space between the iris and the cornea; the posterior chamber, the space between the iris and the lens; and the vitreous cavity, the space posterior to the lens. The three intraocular fluids are the aqueous humor, found in both the anterior and posterior chambers; the vitreous humor, found in the vitreous cavity; and the blood, found in the uveal tract, which includes the iris, ciliary body, and choroid.

The sclera makes up about 85% of the globe surface. Anteriorly, it joins with the cornea. The cornea is a smooth, nearly circular, layered structure averaging 1.0 mm thick in adults. The cornea consists of five distinct layers including the epithelium, Bowman's membrane, the stroma, Descemet's membrane, and the endothelium. The corneal epithelium is lipophilic and will allow the passage of fat-soluble substances. Disruption of the corneal epithelium may alter the transport of topi-

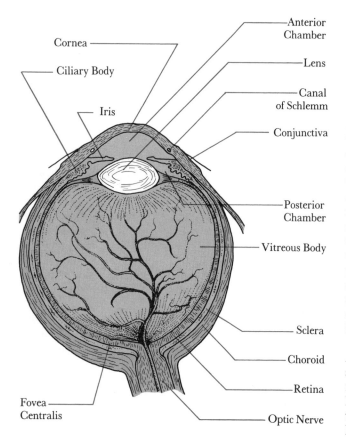

Figure 1. Horizontal cross section showing the anatomy of the eyeball.

Labels: Cornea — Ciliary Body — Iris — Anterior Chamber — Lens — Canal of Schlemm — Conjunctiva — Posterior Chamber — Vitreous Body — Sclera — Choroid — Retina — Optic Nerve — Fovea Centralis

cally applied drugs. The corneal stroma is hydrophilic and allows passage of water-soluble substances. The penetration of topically applied drugs through the cornea depends upon phase solubility. The endothelium, and to a lesser degree the epithelium, provide a barrier to excessive corneal hydration. Damage to either tissue may lead to corneal edema and decreased transparency.

The iris, a thin, circular disk in front of the lens, regulates the amount of light reaching the retina, using two muscles, the sphincter pupillae and the dilator pupillae. Surrounding the globe just posterior to the limbus, where the cornea and sclera join, is the ciliary muscle. The ciliary body is composed of the ciliary muscles and the ciliary epithelium. The ciliary epithelium is important in the production of aqueous humor. The ciliary muscle changes the shape of the lens, enabling the eye to focus on near objects (accommodation). The choroid, which is mainly composed of blood vessels, supplies blood to the retinal pigment epithelium and the external layers of the retina (rods, cones, and inner nuclear layer). The internal layers of the retina are supplied by the central retinal artery.

The anterior chamber, the space between the iris and the cornea, is encircled by the trabecular meshwork, the outflow channel for aqueous humor via the canal of Schlemn. The canal of Schlemn is a circular modified venous structure in the anterior chamber angle. The meshwork consists of multiple perforated sheets (8–10). The aqueous humor is actively secreted by the ciliary epithelium of the ciliary body and flows from the posterior chamber through the pupillary opening into the anterior chamber.

The aqueous humor fills the anterior and posterior chambers. Its main functions are maintenance of the intraocular pressure and nourishment of the avascular lens and cornea. The aqueous humor turnover rate is 1–1.4%/min, or about 2.75 μl/min, of which about 80% exists via the canal of Schlemn (11–13). The bulk flow of aqueous humor is a primary means of drug removal in the internal eye (14).

The lens is a biconvex structure located in the posterior chamber behind the iris. Its function is to focus light rays upon the retina. Behind the lens is the vitreous cavity. Light passing through the cornea and lens converges in this space. The vitreous humor is a transparent jelly-like substance that fills the vitreous cavity, offers support to the structures within the eye, and helps maintain the transparency of the eye because it is impervious to cells and debris.

The retina is a sensory structure that contains cells that respond to visual stimuli by a photochemical reaction. The 10 recognizable layers of the retina are the retinal pigment epithelium, the rods, the cones, the external limiting membrane, the inner and outer nuclear layers, the inner and outer plexiform layers, the ganglion cell layer, and the nerve fiber layer.

Etiology of Ocular Disorders

Ocular inflammation and/or discomfort may be due to several conditions, including anatomical anomalies (such as incomplete closure of the eyelids), abnormal physiologic conditions (such as dry eye syndrome, also referred to as keratoconjunctivitis sicca or KCS), allergic response, infection, and irritants (including excessive ultraviolet radiation, drying winds, volatile chemical components of smog, and chemicals in fertilizers, pesticides, cleaning agents, and cosmetics). Table 1 provides a guide to the differential diagnosis of common causes of the inflamed eye.

Conditions due to physical causes (such as burns, lacerations, and concussions) or conditions associated with specific disease states should be referred immediately to a physician.

Conditions of the Eyelids

The skin layer covering the eye is very thin and, consequently, very delicate. Patients with injured or inflamed eyelids should be referred to a physician. For immediate treatment of so-called "black eye," cold compresses in the initial 24 hours after injury followed by warm applications are helpful. These patients should be referred to their physician to rule out any other ocular injury.

Irritation

Irritation may range from slight inflammation to severe chemical burns. Chemical burns of the eyelids or external ocular tissues must be treated immediately by copious irrigation with sterile water or saline. If these are not available, tap water should be used. The offending agent must be diluted and removed quickly before extensive tissue damage occurs. Flushing should be continuous until the patient sees the ophthalmologist or is in the emergency room. Patients should be referred to an ophthalmologist or the emergency room as soon as possible after injury for follow-up evaluation and treatment.

Inflammation of only the lid margins (blepharitis) may result from associated seborrheic dermatitis of the scalp; *Staphylococcus aureus*; contact dermatitis due to chemical fumes, such as smog; drugs used to treat ocular inflammation; or irritation from eye strain caused by improper refraction or rubbing of the eyes. Assessment should be based on careful study of the patient's history. Symptoms are hyperemia of the lid margins and associated skin scaling. The main complaint is redness of the lids, burning and itching of the eyes, and photophobia, concomitant with conjunctivitis. Vision usually remains normal. Symptomatic treatment with nonprescription decongestants is not satisfactory. Symptoms will recur unless the underlying problem is effectively treated.

Infections

Hordeolum (stye) is an acute suppurative inflammation of the eyelash follicle or sebaceous or sweat gland. As with pustules anywhere in the body, the most common cause is *Staphylococcus aureus*. The principal symptoms are pain, acute tenderness in the area around the hordeolum, and localized redness and swelling. Touching or squeezing the stye may cause the infection to spread and should be avoided. Hordeola usually are self-limiting and respond well to warm moist compresses of tap water or a 3% boric acid solution applied 3 or 4 times/day for 10–15 minutes (which help bring

Table 1. Differential diagnosis of common causes of inflamed eye

	Acute conjunctivitis	Acute iritis[a]	Acute glaucoma[b]	Corneal trauma or infection
Incidence	Extremely common	Common	Uncommon	Common
Discharge	Moderate to copious	None	None	Watery or purulent
Vision	No effect on vision	Slightly blurred	Markedly blurred	Usually blurred
Pain	None	Moderate	Severe	Moderate to severe
Conjunctival injection	Diffuse; more toward fornices	Mainly circumcorneal	Diffuse	Diffuse
Cornea	Clear	Usually clear	Steamy	Change in clarity related to cause
Pupil size	Normal	Small	Moderately dilated and fixed	Normal
Pupillary light response	Normal	Poor	None	Normal
Intraocular pressure	Normal	Normal	Elevated	Normal
Smear	Causative organisms	No organisms	No organisms	Organisms found only in corneal ulcers due to infection

From D. Vaughan and T. Asbury, *General Ophthalmology*, 9th ed., Lange Medical, Los Altos, Calif., 1980.

[a]Acute anterior uveitis.
[b]Angle-closure glaucoma.

styes to a "head," leading to drainage). Antibiotic ointment may be applied under a physician's care or supervision.

Cosmetic agents frequently become contaminated with microorganisms, the occurrence of contamination being associated with length and frequency of use, personal habits, product formulations, and presence or absence of preservatives (15). The incidence of cross-inoculation is high, particularly among adolescents or anyone who shares cosmetics (15–17). Because cosmetics are a source of ocular infection, patients should be advised to avoid wearing eye makeup for at least 1 week before ocular surgery. Mascara should not be used to hide blepharitis because it may aggravate and prolong the condition. Women with symptoms of blepharitis or conjunctivitis should be interviewed carefully by the pharmacist to ascertain whether eye cosmetics are used routinely.

Foreign Bodies

Foreign bodies are the most frequent cause of eye injury. Lint, dust, and similar objects can be removed from the eye by flushing with normal saline or water. However, metallic or nonmetallic foreign bodies that are blown into the eye may cause serious problems if not removed. If the foreign body is small and not readily seen with the naked eye, fluorescein may be used to outline the particle. If the foreign body is lodged in the conjunctival area, it should be removed by the physician in the office or emergency room. If the foreign body is deeply placed, it may require removal in the operating room. The pharmacist should refer the patient to the emergency room or to a physician when in doubt about a foreign body, or if instrumentation is necessary for removal of the foreign body.

External Ocular Disorders

Disorders affecting the external eye are chemical burn, conjunctivitis, and conditions of the lacrimal system. Conjunctivitis may be due to causes ranging from a foreign body to an allergic reaction; careful and accurate patient assessment is essential. Many cases require physician referral. Table 2 gives a differential diagnosis of conjunctivitis.

Conjunctivitis

Conjunctivitis (inflammation of the conjunctiva) is a common external eye problem. Its symptoms are a diffusely reddened eye with a purulent or serous discharge accompanied by itching, smarting, stinging, or a scratching, "foreign body" sensation. If the patient has not experienced pain or blurred vision, conjunctivitis is a likely diagnosis.

Conjunctivitis may be caused by foreign bodies, contusions or lacerations, or parasitic infestations. Most foreign bodies may be removed easily with irrigation or a cotton-tipped applicator provided no damage has occurred to deeper structures. If removal is difficult, the patient should be referred to a physician; the eye may have been irritated by rubbing, causing corneal epithelial abrasions subject to infection. Patients with contusions or lacerations of the conjunctiva should be referred to an ophthalmologist for assessment of possible trauma to the globe or conjunctiva.

Clinical findings and cytology	Viral	Bacterial	Chlamydial	Atopic (allergic)
Itching	Minimal	Minimal	Minimal	Severe
Hyperemia	Generalized	Generalized	Generalized	Generalized
Tearing	Profuse	Moderate	Moderate	Moderate
Exudation	Minimal	Profuse	Profuse	Minimal
Preauricular adenopathy	Common	Uncommon	Common only in inclusion conjunctivitis	None
In stained scrapings and exudates	Monocytes	Bacteria, PMNs	PMNs, plasma cells, inclusion bodies	Eosinophils
Associated sore throat and fever	Occasionally	Occasionally	Never	Never

Table 2. Differentiation of the common types of conjunctivitis

From D. Vaughan and T. Asbury, *General Ophthalmology*, 9th ed., Lange Medical, Los Altos, California, 1980.

PMNs, polymorphonucleocytes.

Conjunctival irritation due to foreign bodies, chemical irritants, or allergies generally is treated by removing the cause and administering nonprescription decongestants. A clue to chemical conjunctivitis, caused by airborne irritants such as smoke, smog, or garden sprays, is that both eyes are involved. Allergic conjunctivitis usually occurs on warm, windy days in the spring and during hay fever season. Typical symptoms, such as swelling, congestion, stinging, watering, and itching, affect both eyes.

Bacterial conjunctivitis usually is self-limiting and does not impair vision. If the patient awakens with the eyelids stuck together by dried exudate or if there is discharge or signs of swelling of the preauricular lymph node, the etiology is probably bacterial. In such cases, nonprescription ophthalmic products have only limited efficacy (18). Referral to a physician is needed, since recovery may be hastened with an appropriate prescription drug, such as a sulfonamide or another antibiotic-containing ophthalmic product. Without treatment, most bacterial conjunctivitis lasts 10–14 days, although *Staphylococcus* and *Moraxella* species infections may become chronic. The more common forms of bacterial conjunctivitis (staphylococcal or diplococcal) are characterized by a purulent discharge. Corneal infections may exhibit symptoms similar to those of bacterial conjunctivitis. These infections are more serious and may obliterate vision rapidly. An accurate diagnosis is important. Pinkeye, a moderately contagious bacterial infection of the conjunctiva caused by *Hemophilus* species in warm climates and *Pneumococci* species in temperate climates, is characterized by an acute onset of conjunctival hyperemia, and a moderate amount of mucopurulent discharge. If there is pain or photophobia, the cornea may be affected (19).

Viral conjunctivitis may resemble chemically induced conjunctivitis; symptoms may include red, perhaps swollen, watery, itching eyes and swollen preauricular lymph nodes. Unlike chemical irritations, however, viral conjunctivitis often is accompanied by systemic symptoms. Systemic symptoms may be present in some types of viral conjunctivitis. In Newcastle disease conjunctivitis, a rare disorder that occurs in poultry workers, veterinarians, or laboratory helpers working with live virus, the patient may develop an influenza-like syndrome with symptoms including mild fever, headache, and arthralgia (18, 19). By careful patient questioning, the pharmacist may discover that the patient also has influenza. The reddened eyes in such cases suggest viral conjunctivitis, which is not amenable to specific drug therapy.

Lacrimal Disorders

The therapy of dacryoadenitis (inflammation of the lacrimal gland) is determined by etiology. Assessment should be made by a physician.

Decreased tear production may be associated with aging, physical trauma, and infection (trachoma). Symptoms are burning and constant foreign body sensation and reddened and dry eyes. Treatment is tear replacement with artificial tears.

Continued self-medication of a dry eye syndrome without professional diagnosis may cause an exacerbation of the underlying condition due to the delay in medical treatment. The FDA advisory review panel on nonprescription ophthalmic drug products concluded that "directions suggesting long-term use [of artificial tear products] should be limited to professional labeling and should not be a part of the OTC labeling. While these products are intended to serve as tear substitutes and are used on an ongoing basis, safeguards against the [long-term] unsupervised use of tear substitute preparations for long periods must be established through proper labeling, warning that professional consultation should be sought if symptoms persist for more than 72 hours" (20).

Some allergic reactions may cause excessive tearing and watery eyes. Cold water compresses and cool, clean air are beneficial for symptomatic relief, as are nonprescription vasoconstrictors. If, as in hay fever, the causative agent cannot be removed, oral antihistamines may be useful.

Internal Eye Conditions

Internal eye disorders may have far greater consequences than conditions of the external eye. Early diagnosis may help prevent partial or total loss of vision. The pharmacist should emphasize the importance of physician referral.

Glaucoma

Glaucoma is characterized by increased intraocular pressure, causing degeneration of the optic disk and defects in the visual field (18, 21). It may be classified as either primary (including open-angle, narrow-angle, or hypersecretion glaucoma), congenital, or secondary. The most common form is primary open-angle glaucoma. Initial treatment of open-angle and secondary glaucoma may be medical; narrow-angle and congenital glaucoma treatment is generally surgical. Most chronic open-angle glaucoma sooner or later requires surgical intervention (22).

Primary open-angle glaucoma occurs as a result of decreased outflow (drainage) of aqueous humor from the anterior chamber of the eye. In patients with this disorder, the chamber angles appear normal. The decreased outflow is most likely caused by degenerative changes in the trabecular meshwork and canal of Schlemn. Open-angle glaucoma causes no early symptoms, and some loss of vision usually occurs late in the progress of the disease. Both eyes are nearly always involved, although one eye may be more severely affected (21).

Secondary glaucoma also occurs due to increased outflow. Foreign bodies or tumors obstructing the trabecular meshwork, ocular inflammation, ocular trauma, hemorrhage, and topical corticosteroid therapy are causes of secondary glaucoma.

Narrow-angle glaucoma (angle-closure or acute glaucoma) is characterized by a sudden onset of blurred vision followed by excruciating pain that may be accompanied by nausea and vomiting. It occurs with sudden increase in intraocular tension due to a block of the anterior chamber angle by the root of the iris, which cuts off all aqueous outflow. The chamber angle is anatomically closed. Any abnormal dilation of the pupil (for example, from mydriatics) or swelling of the iris or lens may produce this obstruction. There is no pain with open-angle glaucoma. Narrow-angle glaucoma can be very dangerous and requires immediate referral to a physician or medical center.

Cataracts

Approximately 15% of the individuals in the United States who are considered legally blind have cataracts as an underlying cause. A cataract is an opacity of the crystalline lens. At present, drug therapy is not a treatment for cataracts but only an aid for certain symptoms. The treatment of cataracts involves surgical removal of the opacity. However, the pharmacist may be questioned by patients concerned with cataracts. Many patients are under the misconception that there are medications available without a prescription for treatment of cataracts. No medications, glasses, diet, or exercise will reduce the effect of a cataract once it is formed. The only way to improve the vision in an eye with a cataract is to remove the lens surgically (23).

Uveitis

Uveitis is a general term for inflammatory disorders of the uveal tract. Causes include infection, trauma, anatomical abnormalities such as cataracts and systemic inflammatory disease. One or all three portions of the uveal tract may be involved simultaneously. *Anterior uveitis* is the term used for an inflammation of the iris (*iritis*) and/or of the ciliary body (*iridocyclitis*), and *posterior uveitis* is the term used for an inflammation of the choroid (*choroiditis*) and/or of the retina (*chorioretinitis*) (18).

Treatment

Most nonprescription ophthalmic products are promoted for relief of noninfectious conjunctivitis. If an irritant has not been sprayed or instilled directly into the eye and if the cornea is not abraded, nonprescription decongestants are useful in relieving the discomfort. It may be advisable to discontinue topical application of cosmetics while using a nonprescription decongestant. Nonprescription decongestants should not be used with other topical ophthalmic drugs since the pharmacokinetic characteristics of the drugs may be changed.

The following list gives specific recommendations for treatment of conditions that may be amenable to self-medication (1).

- **Tear insufficiency**—Keratoconjunctivitis sicca and dry eye in the elderly may be treated with natural tears products. The products with the more viscous vehicles, such as methylcellulose or polyvinyl alcohol, provide a longer contact time. Tear replacement is the first treatment; however, if this is not successful, other therapeutic measures such as ocular inserts, soft contact lens therapy, or other methods are used. Product selection of a natural tears product will depend upon patient acceptance as well as product quality (24). In addition, the patient should be advised to consult a physician.
- **Corneal edema**—If corneal edema is due to eye strain and not due to other causes, such as elevated intraocular pressure, endothelial damage, or epithelial damage, self-medication may be helpful. Hypertonic solutions such as sodium chloride 5% (drops or ointment) may provide a sufficient dehydrating effect. The ocular decongestants may also be beneficial. If the condition persists for more than 24 hours, the patient should be referred to a physician.
- **Inflammation and irritation of the eye**—Presence of loose foreign material in the eye such as dust or lint may be removed by flushing the eye with water or using a collyrium (eyewash). The use of a medicated product is usually not necessary. Irritation from airborne pollutants and/or chlorinated water are amenable to treatment with nonprescription products. Ocular decongestants used after swimming will give relief, and in some cases use of natural tear products may be helpful. Allergic conjunctivitis may be treated

with ocular decongestants to give symptomatic relief. If the symptoms do not resolve within 3 days, the patient should be referred to his or her physician.

Conditions for which self-medication may be effective include hordeolum, blepharitis, and conjunctivitis (1).

Eye patches are used in occlusion therapy of amblyopia, thereby forcing the patient to depend on the amblyopic eye for vision. The use of eye patches in the treatment of certain ocular conditions in young children includes eye patches applied for 1 or 2 days after treatment of corneal abrasion, removal of a foreign body, or an ultraviolet sunlamp burn. Eye patches should not be used unless recommended by a physician. In some cases (young children), eye patches may induce strabismus or amblyopia (24).

Ophthalmologists occasionally use steroids to treat allergic conjunctivitis. Pharmacists should watch for evidence of chronic steroid use (repeated requests for prescription renewal) because long-term use may cause glaucoma and/or cataracts and exacerbate herpetic corneal ulcers.

Patients experiencing pain or blurred vision should be referred to a physician. The pharmacist may suggest oral analgesics as an interim measure to relieve the pain until a physican can be contacted.

Pharmaceutical Agents

In general, nonprescription ophthalmic products must be initially sterile and must have bacteriostatic additives to maintain sterility. They should be buffered, optically clear, and free from particles, filaments, and fibers. In addition, they must not contain any extraneous excipients such as coloring agents or fragrance, and they should approximate the tonicity and pH of tears as nearly as possible.

All ophthalmic products should have an expiration date and should be used or discarded within 3 months from the date of opening. Another hazard associated with all ophthalmic solutions is the introduction of drug crystals into the eye as a result of drug crystallization on the lip of the bottle or the dropper tip. However, microbial contamination is a more serious problem. Consequently, the patient should be warned not to touch the tip of the dispenser and to keep it tightly closed when not in use. All ophthalmic solutions that are cloudy, discolored, or have been open for more than 3 months or that contain foreign particles should be discarded.

Nontherapeutic substances in nonprescription ophthalmic preparations include antioxidants, stabilizers, buffers, wetting or clarifying agents, bacteriostatic preservatives, tonicity adjusters, vehicles for ointments, and viscosity-increasing agents. Because the eye is a sensitive organ, the FDA advisory review panel on nonprescription ophthalmic drug products reviewed inactive as well as active compounds. It noted that some agents considered traditionally inactive as formulation aids could be active in certain situations, such as agents used as emollients and demulcents. The panel ruled that labeling claims of this activity in the product necessitated classification of that agent as an active ingredient; if no

claim was made for that activity, the agent was considered to be inactive (25).

Antioxidants and Stabilizers

Edetic acid (sodium salt), sodium bisulfite (0.1%), sodium metabisulfite (0.1%), sodium thiosulfate (0.2%), and thiourea (0.1%) were classified as acceptable for use in ophthalmic solutions by the FDA advisory review panel on nonprescription ophthalmic drug products. Edetic acid acts as a chelator of metal ions that catalyze redox reactions; other agents are oxidized preferentially instead of the active component.

Buffers

Agents used as buffer components in nonprescription ophthalmic solutions include acetic acid, boric acid, hydrochloric acid, phosphoric acid, potassium bicarbonate, potassium borate and tetraborate, potassium carbonate, potassium citrate, the potassium phosphates (mono-, di-, and tribasic), sodium acetate, sodium bicarbonate, sodium biphosphate, sodium borate, sodium carbonate, sodium citrate, sodium hydroxide, and sodium phosphate. All are accepted by the FDA, although choice of a specific buffer depends on the drug used in the product being formulated.

Tears have a pH of 7.4; consequently, tear substitutes and all ophthalmic products should approximate this level. The acceptable pH range for ophthalmic products is 6.0–8.0 (26); products outside this range may be irritating. In an animal study, products outside the range of 4.0–10.0 with a strong buffer capacity caused corneal damage (27). The eye is able to tolerate products outside the acceptable range if the buffering capacity is low since the tears can overcome the buffer and return the eye to the physiologic level. This enables drug products to be formulated with a low pH for stability purposes and still allow the product to be relatively nonirritating. The buffer system contributes to the tonicity of the ophthalmic product. The tonicity of the entire formulation should approximate 0.9% sodium chloride solution to be isotonic with lacrimal fluid.

Wetting or Clarifying Agents

Polysorbate 80 (1.0%), polysorbate 20 (1.0%), poloxamer 282 (Pluronic L-92) (0.25%), and tyloxapol (Triton WR-1339) (0.25%) reduce surface tension, and thereby allow the solution to better wet the eye. However, they may decrease phenylmercuric nitrate antibacterial activity. Tyloxapol is used for in-situ cleaning of artificial eyes.

Preservatives

Preservatives prevent growth or destroy microorganisms accidentally introduced into the container after opening. The pharmacist should discuss proper instillation technique with the patient to lessen the opportunity for contamination.

Several preservatives have been classified by the FDA as Category I (Table 3). Benzalkonium chloride and benzethonium chloride are accepted as preservatives, although claims of effectiveness as cleaning agents or antibacterials have not been satisfactorily substanti-

Table 3. Classification of ophthalmic product preservatives

Compound	Concentrations (%)[a]	Category
Benzalkonium chloride	0.0013	I
Benzethonium chloride	0.01	I
Cetylpyridinium chloride	0.02	III
Chlorhexidine hydrochloride		III
Chlorobutanol	0.05	I
Edetic acid	0.1	II
Edetic acid–benzalkonium chloride	0.1–0.01	I
Parabens	0.01	II
Phenylethyl alcohol	0.5	III
Phenylmercuric acetate	0.004	I
Phenylmercuric nitrate	0.004	I
Sodium benzoate		III
Sodium propionate	0.75	III
Sorbic acid		II
Thimerosal	0.01	I

Reprinted from the *Federal Register, 45*, 30034 (1980).

[a]Allowed in ophthalmic products intended for instillation in the eye.

ated. When concentrations of benzalkonium chloride higher than 0.013% (0.017, 0.033, and 0.10%) were applied experimentally to rabbit eyes, corneal damage was reported. Benzalkonium chloride (0.02%) is available for instillation into the cul-de-sac to clean artificial eyes in situ. This product is not for use in the intact eye.

Benzalkonium chloride may be present in nonprescription products as a 0.013% concentration alone or in combination with edetic acid or an edetate salt. This concentration may be used safely within the eye.

Benzethonium chloride may be present in products intended for instillation into the human eye in concentrations up to 0.01%. Products that are not intended for instillation directly in the eye may contain benzethonium chloride in a maximum concentration of 0.02%.

Chlorobutanol is another commonly used preservative. This agent hydrolyzes above pH 5–6 and also permeates plastic; it is effectively removed from solution if stored in a plastic container.

Edetic acid is not effective alone as a preservative but enhances the action of benzalkonium chloride against *Pseudomonas* species. It is a weak primary sensitizer, and products containing this agent have been implicated in allergic reactions.

The mercurial preservatives (phenylmercuric acetate, phenylmercuric nitrate, and thimerosal) are moderately effective bacteriostats. However, they have a slow kill rate and may induce allergic reactions. Thimerosal may be a contact allergen due to the thio or mercuric radical. Thimerosal is used as an antiseptic in ophthalmic ointments used for conjunctivitis and corneal ulcers, and to prevent infection following removal of foreign

bodies. However, the panel has not assessed the effectiveness of the compound as an antiseptic in the concentrations employed.

Several other agents are being investigated by the panel, but there is insufficient evidence concerning their safety and efficacy. Cetylpyridinium chloride is classified in Category III becasue of its extensive binding capabilities.

Data are lacking on chlorhexidine hydrochloride and gluconate because they are not used routinely in the United States in ophthalmic products that are instilled into the eye. However, they are used in contact lens products that are not instilled. Parabens (methyl and propyl *p*-hydroxybenzoic acid) (aromatic preservatives) are efficient only at the limit of solubility, and at that concentration they are irritating. In addition, they are known sensitizers and a source of carbon for *Pseudomonas aeruginosa*.

Phenylethyl alcohol is slow acting and potentially irritating, but it may be useful in combination with other preservatives. However, it has not been widely used in the last several years; consequently, no studies have been provided to prove safety and effectiveness.

Sodium propionate is a fungistat and is of questionable use in ophthalmics. Sodium benzoate and sorbic acid, either alone or in combination with other agents, have not been shown to be safe and effective preservatives for ophthalmic use even though they have been used by the food, drug, and cosmetic industries for years.

Tonicity Adjusters

Products of 0.9 ± 0.2% sodium chloride equivalence may be considered isotonic and comparable to natural tears in tonicity. The eye tolerates 0.6–1.8% sodium chloride equivalence without damage (26–28). In addition to the danger of ocular damage, solutions at nonphysiologic tonicity may elicit excessive blinking or tearing. This severely hampers the product's bioavailability, due to early washout by eye fluids (14). Agents used to adjust tonicity in ophthalmic preparations are dextran 40, dextran 70, dextrose, glycerin (1%), potassium chloride, propylene glycol (1%), and sodium chloride, in addition to those agents used as buffers.

Vehicles in Ophthalmic Ointments

Many types of vehicles (petrolatum, vegetable oils, mineral oils, lanolin, and lanolin substitutes such as polyethylene glycols) are used in ophthalmic ointments. Some of these substances are used as adjuncts to modify the product's consistency. These agents are considered to be safe and effective for lubricating the eye, providing an emollient effect, or as drug delivery systems. Consideration must be given to the preservatives necessary to maintain sterility because the significant increase in retention time could result in corneal damage by these agents.

Viscosity-Increasing Agents

The viscosity-increasing agents are used primarily for their physical characteristics rather than for a specific chemical action. Many of the polymers may influence interfacial tension, lowering surface tensions of saline from 72.2 dynes/cm to about 50 dynes/cm (42–66 dynes/cm) when present in a 1% concentration. They aid in wetting the eye by decreasing the contact angle of the solutions and therefore increasing the liquid's tendency to spread (30). They are virtually nontoxic in the concentrations used in ophthalmic products. Many of the polymers are film formers and may build up on contact lenses. The following agents are acceptable for use to increase viscosity in ophthalmic products:

- **Cellulose derivatives**—carboxymethyl cellulose sodium, hydroxyethylcellulose (HEC), hydroxypropyl methylcellulose (HMPC), methylcellulose (MC);
- **Dextran 70;**
- **Gelatin (1%);**
- **Liquid polyols**—glycerin, polyethylene glycol 300, polysorbate 80, propylene glycol, polyvinyl alcohol (PVA) 2%, povidone.

There is insufficient evidence on acetylated polyvinyl alcohol, and it has been placed in Category III.

Viscosity inducers may be used for their wetting, adhesive, and/or lubricating properties, specifically in dry eye treatment (artificial tears). Increased viscosity moderately increases the bioavailability of therapeutic agents by increasing retention time (7, 31).

There are no apparent differences among artificial tear products. In general, products containing viscosity agents are retained about twice as long as saline solution (several minutes). The retention time depends on the viscosity and the drainage rate, not on the concentration of the polymer (31). Methylcellulose solutions, as formulated, are more viscous than polyvinyl alcohol solutions and tend to form crusts on the eyelids, which may be annoying to some patients. However, the methylcellulose solutions are retained longer than the polyvinyl alcohol solutions, due to their higher viscosity for a given concentration. Products containing polyethylene glycol polymers are claimed to possess a mucomimetic property similar to gelatin and bovine mucin. In the presence of these substances, wetting of the corneal surface is facilitated.

Patients should not use alkaline borate products concomitantly with products containing polyvinyl alcohol because gummy deposits may result.

Medicinal Agents

Therapeutic agents contained in nonprescription ophthalmic products include antipruritics, anti-infectives, astringents, and decongestants/vasoconstrictors. Few of these drugs have been proven safe and effective. Many are contraindicated in specific conditions.

Antipruritics

Antipyrine (0.1–0.4%), camphor, and menthol (peppermint oil) are present in some nonprescription ophthalmic medications because of their mild local analgesic and cooling effect. Such products are considered generally unsafe because the local analgesia produced may mask the presence of foreign bodies, leading to severe corneal abrasions.

Anti-infectives

There is no acceptable nonprescription ophthalmic anti-infective available for treatment of minor external eye infections. Boric acid is weakly effective at best and at worst may be dangerous because systemic absorption may result in boron toxicity, especially in small children. Silver protein products are effective but lack patient acceptability because of their staining properties. Yellow mercuric oxide has been marketed in the past; however, there is insufficient evidence of its efficacy. Further study has been recommended for all of these products before they can be considered both safe and effective.

The FDA advisory review panel has reviewed sulfacetamide 10% (available only on prescription) for deregulation to nonprescription standing to treat surface infections of eyelids and conjunctiva. Evaluation of the data suggest that it would not be safe for nonprescription use due to its irritating and allergic potential. In addition, indiscriminate use could lead to overgrowth of resistant strains of organisms (32).

Astringents

Astringents are applied locally to precipitate proteins and reduce local edema and inflammation. In high concentrations, many astringents are irritating or caustic; therefore, they must be formulated in concentrations low enough to be nonirritating. Barberine, hydrastine, peppermint oil, rose geranium oil, and infusion of rose petals were promoted as astringents in ophthalmic products. These products were judged unacceptable by the FDA advisory review panel because there was no substantive evidence of safety and/or effectiveness (33).

The only astringent recommended by the FDA advisory review panel for use in nonprescription ophthalmic products is zinc sulfate (0.25%). The dosage for adults and children is 1–2 drops of a 0.25% solution instilled in the affected eye up to 4 times/day. Zinc salts have no decongestant action; however, they may be used in combination with a vasoconstrictor. They are mild vasodilators in the concentrations used. Zinc sulfate is indicated for temporary relief from minor eye irritations.

Decongestants/Vasoconstrictors

Vasoconstrictors are effective in the symptomatic treatment of allergic conjunctivitis. Reddened eyes usually are rapidly whitened by vasoconstrictors that limit the local vascular response by constricting the blood vessels. The vasoconstrictors, which are all sympathomimetic amines, not only affect the vascular receptors but also stimulate other receptors such as the nerves that control pupillary size.

These agents generally are contraindicated in known narrow-angle glaucoma patients. They are designed specifically for short-term, primarily cosmetic use and should not be used on a regular basis. They are potentially hazardous in that they may mask symptoms of a serious problem, delaying necessary medical treatment.

If an ophthalmic decongestant is used when there is disease of the globe interior, no relief can be expected, and complications from the lack of primary treatment may occur. Furthermore, bacterial or other infections also may be masked by the use of symptomatic treatment. If an ocular condition persists for more than 48 hours, the patient should be referred to a physician. Drugs used as decongestants/vasoconstrictors are ephedrine hydrochloride, naphazoline hydrochloride, phenylephrine, and tetrahydrozoline (34).

Ephedrine is similar to epinephrine in that it is short acting and produces rebound congestion. However, it is more stable than epinephrine.

The imidazoline derivatives, naphazoline and tetrahydrozoline, are more stable and have a longer duration of action than epinephrine (2–3 hours). They are buffered to pH 6.2. Naphazoline is used in prescription ophthalmic solutions at a concentration of 0.1%; however, this high concentration is not considered safe for nonprescription use. Naphazoline hydrochloride is available as a 0.012% solution in nonprescription products. Tetrahydrozoline is used at a concentration of 0.05%.

Untoward effects occurring after use of imidazoline class drugs have been reported, particularly CNS stimulation after accidental ingestion by children. Although rebound congestion was reported after prolonged intranasal use of naphazoline, it has not been reported after ophthalmic use.

Phenylephrine is the vasoconstrictor used most commonly in nonprescription ophthalmic products. Its effectiveness is variable due to its relative instability. Solutions usually are effective initially, but with continued use, oxidation may reduce the product's activity significantly although no evidence of discoloration is present. Furthermore, phenylephrine products in polyethylene containers may be less stable than those packaged in glass. Oxygen diffuses through the polyethylene and hastens oxidation of the amine unless an oxygen-resistant coating is put over the plastic bottle. Patients allergic to epinephrine may show cross-sensitivity to phenylephrine.

Rebound congestion may occur following the prolonged use of vasoconstrictors in the eye. The tissues become more congested and edematous as the vasoconstriction of the drug subsides. The phenomenon causes a vicious cycle because it leads to more frequent use of the drug that causes it.

Hypertonic Agents

Symptomatic relief of corneal swelling may be produced by hypertonic solutions. The only acceptable hypertonic agent is sodium chloride in a concentration of 2–5%. Sodium chloride is available for nonprescription use as a sterile solution or ointment. The dosage for adults and children is 1–2 drops of a 2–5% concentration instilled in the affected eye(s) every 3–4 hours or as directed by a physician. Pharmacists should warn the patient of transient stinging and burning. Although available for nonprescription use, it should be used under the advice of a physician.

Pharmacokinetic Considerations

Properties of the drug, its formulation, and the eye itself influence the pharmacokinetics of topical ophthalmic products. Pharmacists should take these factors into consideration when recommending a nonprescription preparation.

The physical drug properties that probably have the most effect on transport of the drug into and through the eye are lipid solubility and water solubility (35). Protein-binding of drugs in the tear fluids may further reduce the amount of free drug available for absorption and thus adversely affect its bioavailability. Metabolism in the precorneal area and absorption by tissues other than the cornea also are potential drug loss mechanisms (35–38). Because the conjunctiva and nasolacrimal duct are highly vascularized, drugs may be absorbed into the bloodstream and lost from the target site (39). Moreover, since drugs in the eye are eliminated primarily by bulk flow, elimination may be either enhanced or retarded by a drug's pharmacologic effect. In a glaucomatous eye, the reduction of intraocular pressure brought about by increased outflow could lessen the duration of action of the drug (14).

The concentration, volume instilled, and contact time also are important variables that may affect a drug's ocular availability and effectiveness. High concentrations may cause irritation, which in turn causes tearing and thus flushing of the precorneal area, removing the drug from the absorption site (14). Since the nasolacrimal drainage rate also is a function of instilled volume, it is desirable to administer the smallest volume of product possible. In addition, patients instilling more than one medication into the eye should wait at least 3–5 minutes between drops. This procedure ensures that the first drop is not flushed away by the second drop or, conversely, the second drop is not diluted by the first. Both conditions would reduce bioavailability (4, 40).

The eye is a unique system relative to biopharmaceutics and pharmacokinetics. Several factors not dependent on the drug molecule itself greatly influence the activity of the applied drug. The absorption and elimination rate constants used to explain the kinetics of drug transport are a complication of the various processes going on in the whole system, dominated by an apparent parallel elimination in the precorneal area, distribution in the aqueous humor, and bulk flow from the aqueous humor (14).

Product Selection Guidelines

The following general guidelines should help the pharmacist in selecting a suitable nonprescription ophthalmic product:

- Nonprescription ophthalmic products should only be used in situations where vision is not threatened and should not be used for longer than 48 hours without medical referral, unless a stye is involved; treatment with a nonprescription product would normally take 3–4 days before the stye would subside.
- Nonprescription ocular medications should not be recommended to patients who have demonstrated an allergy to any of the active ingredients, preservatives, or other agents in the product.

- Patients with narrow-angle glaucoma should not use sympathomimetic amines, and patients with open-angle glaucoma should use these drugs only on the advice of a physician.
- Patients already using a prescription ophthalmic product should use nonprescription ophthalmic products only after consulting with a pharmacist or a physician.

The pharmacist should instruct the patient on the proper use of ophthalmic products (41). Before administration, the hands should be washed and the product inspected for expiration date, contamination, discoloration, and/or other problems.

Ophthalmic drops should be administered to the patient with the head tilted back and up. The skin below the eye just above the cheekbone should be pulled down, and the fluid dropped into the lower conjunctival sac away from the tear ducts. To avoid contamination, the dropper tip should not touch the eye or lid. Suspension fluids should be shaken well before instillation.

For ophthalmic ointments the patient should assume the same position. A thin line of ointment should be applied along the conjunctival surface of the lower lid. The patient should be instructed to close the eyes for a short period to allow the medication to be dispensed throughout the eye. Gently massaging the eye to distribute the ointment over the cornea is helpful. The tip of the ointment tube should not touch the eye, and the cap should be replaced immediately.

Eyecups should be discouraged as a method for administering ophthalmic solutions. They may harbor bacteria that cause infections.

Summary

The eye is one of the most sensitive areas of the human body and may be subject to many types of disorders. Pharmacists often are the first health care professionals to be informed of a patient's ocular condition. The decision to recommend self-medication with a nonprescription product or physician referral rests with the pharmacist. Ocular problems lasting more than 48 hours should be referred. Usually nonprescription ophthalmic preparations relieve symptoms only; they do not treat the disorder. Self-medication by the patient is generally trial and error with the possibility of a wrong guess leading to exacerbation of symptoms. The pharmacist should exercise professional judgment when suggesting ophthalmic products for ocular disorders such as tear insufficiency, corneal edema, and minor inflammation and irritation of the eye including some minor external infections such as hordeolum, blepharitis, and conjunctivitis. Patients with ocular disorders such as an embedded foreign body, uveitis, glaucoma, flash burns, tear duct infections, and corneal ulcers should be referred to a physician. Symptoms of these conditions would include pain, blurred vision, and/or mucopurulent discharge.

References

1. "Ophthalmic Drug Products for Over-the-Counter Human Use," *Federal Register*, Part II, Department of Health, Education, and Welfare, *45*, May 6, 1980, pp. 3006-12.
2. S. Mishima, A. Gasset, S. D. Klyce, and J. L. Baum, *Invest. Ophthalmol., 5*, 264 (1966).
3. J. J. Greco and D. C. Kelman, *Ann. Ophthalmol., 5*, 57 (1973).
4. S. S. Chrai, M. C. Makoid, S. P. Eriksen, and J. R. Robinson, *J. Pharm. Sci., 63*, 333 (1974).
5. E. Epstein, *Ann. J. Ophthalmol., 59*, 109 (1965).
6. L. Harris and M. Galin, *Arch. Ophthalmol., 84*, 105 (1970).
7. S. S. Chrai, T. F. Patton, A. Mehta, and J. R. Robinson, *J. Pharm. Sci., 62*, 1112 (1973).
8. A. Bill and B. Svedbergh, *Acta Ophthalmol., 50*, 295 (1972).
9. D. G. Cole and R. C. Tripathi, *Exp. Eye Res., 12*, 25 (1971).
10. A. Bill, *Invest. Ophthalmol., 14*, 1 (1975).
11. P. Ellis and D. Smith, "Handbook of Ocular Therapeutics and Pharmacology," 4th ed., C. V. Mosby, St. Louis, Mo., 1975, pp. 83-85.
12. J. G. Daubs, *Am. J. Ophthalmol., 49*, 1005 (1972).
13. E. Weigelin, F. Sayegh, W. von Kilitzing, and A. Fawrmounti, *Eye Ear Nose Throat Mon., 54*, 13 (1975).
14. M. C. Makoid and J. R. Robinson, *J. Pharm. Sci., 68*, 435 (1979).
15. L. A. Wilson, A. J. Julian, and D. G. Ahern, *Am. J. Ophthalmol., 79*, 596 (1975).
16. S. Aronson and E. Yamamoto, *Invest. Ophthalmol., 5*, 75 (1966).
17. B. D. Zuckerman, *Am. J. Ophthalmol., 62*, 672 (1966).
18. D. Vaughan, R. Cook, and T. Asbury, "General Ophthalmology," 7th ed., Lange Medical, Los Altos, Calif., 1974, pp. 49-53, 69-95, 192-204.
19. *Medical Letter on Drugs and Therapeutics, 18*, 70-72 (1976).
20. *Federal Register, 45*, 30044 (1980).
21. T. H. Roy, "Practical Management of Eye Problems: Glaucoma, Strabismus, Visual Fields," Lea and Febiger, Philadelphia, Pa., 1975, pp. 9-17.
22. A. M. Potts, *Am. J. Ophthalmol., 86*, 743 (1978).
23. D. R. Gourley and R. E. Records, *U.S. Pharmacist, 5*, 7 (1980).
24. "Manual of Ocular Diagnosis and Therapy," D. Pavan-Langston, Ed., Little, Brown, Boston, Mass., 1980, pp. 99-100.
25. *Federal Register, 45*, 30023 (1980).
26. "Remington's Pharmaceutical Sciences," 16th ed., Mack Publishing, Easton, Pa., 1980, p. 1506.
27. J. M. Conrad and J. R. Robinson, *J. Pharm. Sci., 66*, 219 (1977).
28. J. E. Hoover, "Dispensing of Medications," 8th ed., Mack Publishing, Easton, Pa., 1976, p. 236.
29. G. S. Banker and C. T. Rhodes, "Modern Pharmaceutics," Marcel Decker, New York, N.Y., 1979, p. 505.
30. M. A. Lemp and F. J. Holly, *Ann. Ophthalmol., 4*, 15 (1972).
31. T. F. Patton and J. R. Robinson, *J. Pharm. Sci., 64*, 1312 (1975).
32. *Federal Register, 45*, 30028 (1980).
33. *Federal Register, 45*, 30037 (1980).
34. *Federal Register, 45*, 30033-35 (1980).
35. K. D. Swan and N. G. Shite, *Ann. J. Ophthalmol., 25*, 1043 (1942).
36. S. Y. Butelho, *Sci. Am., 211*, 78 (1964).
37. N. Ehlera, *Acta Ophthalmol. Suppl., 81* (1965).
38. O. F. Erickson, *Am. J. Ophthalmol., 43*, 295 (1957).
39. T. F. Patton and J. R. Robinson, *J. Pharm. Sci., 65*, 1295 (1976).
40. C. Asseff, R. Weisman, B. Becker, and R. Podos, *Am. J. Ophthalmol., 75*, 212 (1973).
41. H. Wedemeyer and D. R. Gourley, in "Handbook for Institutional Pharmacy Practice," M. C. Smith and T. R. Brown., Eds., Williams and Wilkins, Baltimore, Md., 1978, pp. 273-282.

Ophthalmic Decongestant Product Table

Product (Manufacturer)	Viscosity Agent	Vasoconstrictor	Preservative	Buffer	pH	Other Ingredients
Adsorbonac (Burton Parsons)	povidone, 1.67%		edetate sodium, 0.1% thimerosal, 0.004%		NS[a]	sodium chloride, 2%, 5%
Clear Eyes (Abbott)		naphazoline hydrochloride, 0.012%	benzalkonium chloride, 0.01% edetate disodium, 0.1%	boric acid sodium borate	6.0	
Collyrium Drops (Wyeth)		ephedrine, 0.1%	thimerosal, 0.002%	boric acid, 0.4% sodium borate, 3%	6.8	antipyrine, 0.4% sodium salicylate, 0.056%
Degest 2 (Barnes-Hind)	hydroxy-ethyl-cellulose	naphazoline hydrochloride, 0.012%	benzalkonium chloride, 0.0067% edetate disodium, 0.02%	sodium citrate	NS[a]	
Eye Cool (Milroy)		phenylephrine hydrochloride, 0.08%	edetate disodium, 0.05% thimerosal, 0.002%	sodium borate boric acid	7.0–8.0	eucalyptus oil menthol sodium chloride sodium bisulfite
20/20 Eye Drops (S.S.S.)		naphazoline hydrochloride, 0.012%	thimerosal, 0.005%	boric acid, 1.25% sodium carbonate, 0.004%	6.0–6.5	potassium chloride, 7.4% zinc sulfate, 0.06%
Isopto-Frin (Alcon)	hydroxy-propyl methyl-cellulose, 0.5%	phenylephrine hydrochloride, 0.12%	benzethonium chloride	sodium citrate sodium phosphate sodium biphosphate	7.3	
Murine (Abbott)			benzalkonium chloride, 0.01% edetate sodium, 0.05%	mono- and dibasic sodium phosphate	6.0	glycerin sodium chloride potassium chloride
Murine Plus (Abbott)		tetrahydrozoline hydrochloride, 0.05%	benzalkonium chloride, 0.01% edetate sodium, 0.1%	boric acid sodium borate	6.0	
Naphcon (Alcon)		naphazoline hydrochloride, 0.012%	benzalkonium chloride, 0.01%		6.3	
Optigene III (Pfeiffer)		tetrahydrozoline hydrochloride, 0.05%	benzalkonium chloride, 0.01% edetate disodium, 0.1%	boric acid sodium borate	5.8–6.5	sodium chloride
Phenylzin (Cooper Vision)	hydroxy-propyl methyl-cellulose, 0.1%	phenylephrine hydrochloride, 0.12%	benzalkonium chloride, 0.01% edetate disodium, 0.01%	boric acid sodium carbonate	6.6	sodium bisulfite potassium chloride zinc sulfate, 0.25%
Prefrin Liquifilm (Allergan)	polyvinyl alcohol, 1.4%	phenylephrine hydrochloride, 0.12%	benzalkonium chloride, 0.004%	sodium phosphate sodium biphosphate	NS[a]	antipyrine, 0.1%
Prefrin Z (Allergan)	polyvinyl alcohol, 1.4%	phenylephrine hydrochloride, 0.12%	thimerosal, 0.005%	sodium hydroxide sodium citrate	NS[a]	zinc sulfate, 0.25% sodium chloride sodium bisulfite

Ophthalmic Decongestant Product Table, continued

Product (Manufacturer)	Viscosity Agent	Vasoconstrictor	Preservative	Buffer	pH	Other Ingredients
Soothe (Burton Parsons)		phenylephrine hydrochloride, 0.15%	edetate sodium, 0.1% thimerosal, 0.004%		NS[a]	isotonic buffered vehicle
Tear-efrin (Cooper Vision)	hydroxy-propyl methyl-cellulose, 0.5%	phenylephrine hydrochloride, 0.12%	benzalkonium chloride, 0.01% edetate disodium, 0.01%		4.1	sodium bisulfite sodium chloride
Vaso Clear (Cooper Vision)		naphazoline hydrochloride, 0.02%	benzalkonium chloride, 0.01% edetate sodium, 0.03%		6.2	lipiden poly-meric system
Visine (Leeming)		tetrahydrozoline hydrochloride, 0.05%	benzalkonium chloride, 0.01% edetate disodium, 0.1%	boric acid sodium borate	NS[a]	sodium chloride
Visine A.C. (Leeming)		tetrahydrozoline hydrochloride, 0.05%	benzalkonium chloride, 0.01% edetate disodium, 0.1%	boric acid sodium borate	NS[a]	zinc sulfate, 0.25%
Zincfrin (Alcon)		phenylephrine hydrochloride, 0.12%	benzalkonium chloride, 0.01%	barbital barbital sodium	7.5	zinc sulfate, 0.25%

[a] pH not stated

Artificial Tear Product Table

Product (Manufacturer)	Viscosity Agent	Preservative	pH	Other Ingredients
Adsorbotear (Burton Parsons)	hydroxyethylcellulose, 0.44%	edetate disodium, 0.1% thimerosal, 0.004%	NS[a]	povidone
Hypotears (Cooper Vision)		benzalkonium chloride, 0.01% edetate disodium, 0.03%	6.6	
Isopto Alkaline (Alcon)	hydroxypropyl methylcellulose, 1%	benzalkonium chloride, 0.01%	NS[a]	
Isopto Plain (Alcon)	hydroxypropyl methylcellulose, 0.5%	benzalkonium chloride, 0.01%	NS[a]	
Lacril (Allergan)	hydroxypropyl methylcellulose, 0.5% gelatin A, 0.01%	chlorobutanol, 0.5%	NS[a]	
Liquifilm Forte (Allergan)	polyvinyl alcohol, 3.0%	edetate disodium thimerosal, 0.002%	NS[a]	
Liquifilm Tears (Allergan)	polyvinyl alcohol, 1.4%	chlorobutanol, 0.5%	NS[a]	sodium chloride
Lyteers (Barnes-Hind)	hydroxyethylcellulose, 0.2%	edetate sodium, 0.05% benzalkonium chloride, 0.01%	NS[a]	potassium chloride, sodium chloride

Artificial Tear Product Table, continued

Product (Manufacturer)	Viscosity Agent	Preservative	pH	Other Ingredients
Milroy Artificial Tears (Milroy)	methylcellulose	benzalkonium chloride, 0.002%	8.0–8.6	boric acid sodium borate
Murocel Ophthalmic Solution (Muro)	methylcellulose, 1%	methylparaben propylparaben	NS[a]	sodium chloride
Muro Tears (Muro)	hydroxypropyl methylcellulose dextran	benzalkonium chloride	NS[a]	boric acid potassium chloride sodium borate sodium chloride
Neo Tears (Barnes-Hind)	hydroxyethylcellulose polyvinyl alcohol	edetate disodium, 0.02% thimerosal, 0.004%	NS[a]	polyethylene glycol 300 sodium biphosphate sodium phosphate
Tearisol (Cooper Vision)	hydroxypropyl methylcellulose, 0.50%	benzalkonium chloride, 0.01% edetate disodium, 0.01%	7.5	boric acid potassium chloride sodium carbonate
Tears Naturale (Alcon)	water-soluble polymeric system	benzalkonium chloride, 0.01% edetate disodium, 0.05%	7.0	
Tears Plus (Allergan)	polyvinyl alcohol, 1.4% povidone	chlorobutanol, 0.5%	NS[a]	
Ultra Tears (Alcon)	hydroxypropyl methylcellulose, 1%	benzalkonium chloride, 0.01%	7.5	

[a]pH not stated

Eyewash Product Table

Product (Manufacturer)	Buffer	pH	Preservative	Other Ingredients
Blinx (Barnes-Hind)	boric acid sodium borate	NS[a]	phenylmercuric acetate, 0.004%	
Collyrium (Wyeth)	boric acid, 0.4% sodium borate, 3%	6.8	thimerosal, 0.002%	antipyrine, 0.4% sodium salicylate, 0.056%
Dacriose (Cooper Vision)	sodium phosphate	NS[a]	benzalkonium chloride, 0.01% edetate disodium, 0.3%	potassium chloride sodium chloride
Enuclene (Alcon)		6.5	benzalkonium chloride, 0.2%	tyloxapol, 0.25%
Eye-Stream (Alcon)	sodium acetate sodium citrate	7.0	benzalkonium chloride, 0.013%	calcium chloride magnesium chloride potassium chloride sodium chloride
Lauro Eye Wash (Otis Clapp)	boric acid sodium borate	7.0		sodium chloride
M/Rinse (Milroy)	boric acid sodium borate	NS[a]	edetate disodium, 0.1% thimerosal, 0.004%	potassium chloride sodium chloride
Murine (Abbott)	sodium biphosphate sodium phosphate	7.4	benzalkonium chloride, 0.01% edetate disodium, 0.05%	potassium chloride sodium chloride
Op-thal-zin (Alcon)		7.5	benzalkonium chloride, 0.01%	zinc sulfate, 0.25%
Trisol Eye Wash (Buffington)	boric acid sodium borate	7.0		sodium chloride

[a]pH not stated

22 Contact Lens Products

James W. Seig

Questions to Ask the Patient

What types of problems are you having with your lenses? Are they related to eye irritation or changes in vision?

What type of lenses do you wear? Hard or soft?

How long have you been wearing lenses? When did the problems arise?

What medicines are you currently taking?

Have you become pregnant or begun using oral contraceptives since you were fitted for lenses?

How many hours per day do you wear your lenses before problems arise?

Do you remove your lenses during the course of the day?

How long ago did you see your optometrist or ophthalmologist?

Hard Lens Wearers

Do you soak your lenses when not in use?

How often do you replace solutions in your lens storage container?

How often do you clean your lenses?

What products do you use? Do you use a combination-type solution?

How often do you clean your storage container? Does it need to be replaced?

Soft Lens Wearers

Do you clean your lenses prior to disinfection?

What method of disinfection do you use?

How often do you disinfect your lenses?

Do you use commercial saline solution or do you mix your own? How often do you replace it?

Do you use any cosmetic or medicines (nonprescription or prescription) that are applied to the eye area?

The first corneal plastic contact lens was introduced in the United States in 1948, but it was not until the advent of the contour fitting principle in 1955 that lens use among the general population began to gain wide acceptance. "Contour-fitting" means the use of lenses with multiple inside radii rather than a single posterior curve, and it soon became standard practice to tailor lenses for the individual cornea. So successful were these early lenses that they rapidly boomed in popularity to the extent that today more than 10% of patients requiring corrective lenses choose contact lenses. Furthermore, of this group, nearly 90% use contact lenses to correct vision of the otherwise healthy eye. This use means that much of the motivation to wear contact lenses must be considered to be cosmetic. It has been well established that corneal contact lenses, even when expertly fitted, produce some degree of alteration of the ocular tissues and changes in the corneal metabolism. This alteration makes it imperative that both the user and the health professional be aware of the proper methods for care, maintenance, and safe use of these products.

More than 60 nonprescription contact lens-related products are available. Several reviews of contact lens usage and contact lens solutions have been published (1–3). Selection of products is dependent upon their compatibility with each other as well as with the specific lens device. These considerations place a direct responsibility upon the pharmacist to understand this area of professional practice and act as an effective, up-to-date information consultant to the contact lens wearer.

Indications for Contact Lens Usage

One important consideration in contact lens usage is that the decision to wear lenses is sometimes based upon therapeutic necessity (4–6). Keratoconus is a gradual thinning of the central cornea, and satisfactory vision is usually unattainable with ordinary eyeglasses. This condition responds only to contact lenses or corneal transplantation (7, 8).

Aphakia is a condition that results when the crystalline lens of the eye is removed (9). A typical example is that of an otherwise visually sound eye that has been rendered sightless due to an opacified lens arising from progressive cataracts. Aphakic individuals characteristically show improved quality of vision with cataract contact lenses compared with cataract spectacles. Extended-wear contact lenses are particularly important for such patients because of the difficulty in insertion and removal due to poor visual acuity when the lenses are not in place.

Visual aberrations arising from corneal scarring are also often better corrected by contact lenses (10). The close proximity of the lens actually transforms the corneal topography rather than simply correcting refractive error by changing the direction of incident light, as in the case of spectacles.

Other indications for the use of contact lenses include myopia ("nearsightedness") and hypermetropia ("farsightedness"). Herein lies the opportunity for the individual patient to, in most cases, choose between contact lenses or eyeglasses.

Perhaps the main reason for choosing contact lenses among many wearers is the perceived improvement in personal appearance. Other strongly influencing factors favoring contact lens wear include: no obstruction of vision due to supportive eyeglass frames (11–13), greater clarity in the peripheral visual field, no fogging of lenses due to sudden temperature changes, and more freedom of motion during vigorous activity. Although it has been demonstrated that there is no substantial difference in visual acuity between contact lenses and eyeglasses, a number of factors give rise to a subjective perception of improvement by the contact lens wearer (14). Increased sensitivity to light and improved quality of the retinal image often occur with contact lens wear (15, 16). With eyeglasses, the myope sees a smaller than normal image whereas the hypermetropic individual sees a larger than normal image. Both individuals see objects in nearly their true sizes with contact lenses and for high myopes the image size increase with contact lenses is significant and decidedly beneficial.

Contraindications to Contact Lens Usage

The successful wearing of contact lenses depends upon adequate tear production. Because the cornea is avascular, tears provide oxygen and remove waste products in addition to providing lubrication and serving as a barrier to microorganisms.

Absolute Contraindications

Certainly, contact lenses are not for everyone. Many individuals who require vision correction cannot and/or should not wear contact lenses. Contraindications are often based upon lifestyle as well as medical history.

Occupational conditions that may prohibit the wearing of contact lenses include exposure to dust and particulate matter, wind, glare, molten metals, irritant chemicals, and chemical fumes (3). Chemical fumes, in particular, can be hazardous due to concentration of irritants under the lens or inside the lens in the case of soft lenses. The lens device prolongs contact of such substances with the cornea and can lead to corneal toxicity.

Corneal contact lenses should not be used for cosmetic reasons if a patient has active pathologic intraocular or corneal conditions, although they may be used in cases of open-angle glaucoma (7).

Medical reasons that contraindicate contact lens wear include chronic conjunctivitis, blepharitis, recurrent viral or bacterial infections, poor blink rate or incomplete blink, and insufficient or abnormal tear production (17). An obstructed nasolacrimal duct, anatomical or physiologic abnormalities, and various clinical conditions, such as herpes simplex, are all contraindications to contact lens use (17). Diabetics are often advised against wearing contact lenses because of retarded healing processes and the tendency toward prolonged corneal abrasion with such use. Chronic common colds as well as allergic conditions such as hay fever and asthma may make lens wear extremely uncomfortable or impossible.

Dry spots on the cornea, often found in postmenopausal women, prevent the successful use of lenses (18). These spots, possibly caused by the absence of the precorneal film, are often identified with lacrimal insufficiency due to subclinical hypothyroidism.

Relative Contraindications and Cautions

Contact lenses should be used with caution in patients with epilepsy, diabetes mellitus, high blood pressure, heart disease, or severe arthritis. The corneal topography may be altered by pregnancy or by oral contraceptives (17, 18). The fluid-retaining properties of estrogen may lead to edema of the cornea and eyelids as well as decreased tear production. They should be used with caution by elderly persons, because of possible lacrimal insufficiency, and by individuals with arthritis, which may restrict the movement and dexterity needed to insert lenses.

Diseases secondary to contact lens wear have been described (19). Lens wearers moving from a low to a high altitude may encounter hypoxia, or metabolic deficiency, resulting in irritation and corneal abrasions (20).

Many systemic medications, such as diuretics, oral contraceptives, and tricyclic antidepressants, affect the eyes and therefore may reduce lens tolerance (17, 18, 21). Microedema caused by hormonal therapy as well as premenstrual edema may also cause problems in the use of contact lenses (22). Orally administered antihistamines and decongestants may decrease tear production and cause a mild keratitis, interfering with lens wear (23, 24).

During the adaptive period to contact lenses the eyelids may become hyperemic; this condition may lead to blepharitis, especially in the upper lid (25). Short pseudoblinks, often found with new wear of hard lenses, may cause irritation of the conjunctiva of the upper eyelid. A poor blinker or nonblinker may be helped by a fenestrated (windowed) lens (UF-9) or an otherwise adapted one (26). Chin elevation and squinting may result from irritating lenses (25).

Cosmetics and Contact Lenses

Cosmetics must be chosen with care (27). Women should be advised to insert lenses before applying make-up, and care should be taken so as not to touch the lens with eyeliner or mascara. Nearly all eye cosmetics have an oily base and cause greasy smudges that can be difficult to remove. It is best to use those with an aqueous base since oil-based products may cause blurred vision and irritation if they are deposited on the lens. Powders may also be irritating if small particles become lodged under the lens. Mascara should be applied only to the very tips of the lashes. Hair sprays, in particular, must be used with caution. Irritation may occur if some of the spray particles are trapped in the tear layer beneath the lens, and some sprays may actually damage the lens. Nail polish, hand creams, and perfumes should be applied only after the lens has been inserted. Men frequently contaminate their lenses with hair preparations; special care must be taken to clean hands thoroughly before handling contact lenses. Thorough washing of the hands prior to inserting lenses is advised, but consideration of the type of soap is often neglected. Soaps containing cold cream or deodorants should be avoided since they can leave a film on the fingers after

rinsing. This residue is readily transferred to a soft lens and causes blurred vision. Hard lenses are not as prone to such problems due to the protective action of the wetting solution.

Lens Choice: Hard or Soft?

Contact lenses are often broadly classified into two distinct groups based upon the chemical make-up and physical properties of the lens. Lenses that are relatively inflexible, do not appreciably absorb water, and that retain their shape when removed from the eye are commonly termed "hard" lenses. Lenses that are moderately to highly flexible, absorb and retain a high percentage of water, and conform to the shape of a supporting surface are commonly called "soft" lenses.

The choice between hard and soft lenses is influenced by a number of factors that vary from individual to individual. Patients may base their selection on advice from friends or relatives who have had experiences with one type of lens or another, or promotional claims through media advertising or recommendations of a vision care specialist with respect to the specific optical requirements of the eye itself. In many instances, the final choice may very well be strongly influenced by the very connotations of the words "hard" and "soft" with respect to a perception of comfort on the part of the would-be wearer.

Table 1. FDA-approved soft contact lenses

Proprietary lens name	Generic names	Manufacturers	Water in saline (%)
Accugel	droxifilcon A	Strieter Laboratories	46.6
Amsof	deltafilcon A	Lombard Lenses	43.0
AoSoft	tetrafilcon A	American Optical Corp.	42.5
Aquaflex	tetrafilcon A	UCO Optics Inc.	42.5
AquaSoft	deltafilcon A	Aquarius Inc.	43.0
CustomFlex	deltafilcon A	Custom Labs Inc.	43.0
DuraSoft	phemfilcon A	Wesley-Jessen Inc.	30.0
Flexlens	hefilcon A	Flexlens Inc.	45.5
Gelflex	dimefilcon A	Dow Corning Ophthalmics	35.5
Hydrocurve	hefilcon A	Continuous Curve Contact Lenses Inc.	45.5
Hydrocurve II	bufilcon A	Continuous Curve Contact Lenses Inc.	45.0
Hydro-Marc	etafilcon A	Frontier Contact Lenses Inc.	43.0
Hydron	polymacon	American Hydron	38.6
Naturvue	hefilcon A	Bausch & Lomb Inc.	45.5
Permalens	perfilcon A	CooperVision Optics Inc.	71.0
Sauflon	lidofilcon B	Heyer-Schults Medical Optics Center	79.0
Sof-Form	deltafilcon A	Salvatori Ophthalmics	43.0
Soflens	polymacon	Bausch & Lomb Inc.	38.6
Softcon	vifilcon A	American Optical Corp.	55.0
Softics	deltafilcon A	Advance Contact Inc.	43.0
Softsite	hefilcon A	Paris Contact Lenses Inc.	45.5
Tresoft	ocufilcon A	Alcon Optics	46.0
Tri Pol 43	deltafilcon A	Capitol Contact Lenses Inc.	43.0

Reprinted with permission from J. Z. Krezanoski, *Am. Pharm.*, *NS21*, 15 (1981).

Table 2. Extended-wear soft lenses

Company	Trade name	Material	Hydration (%)
Continuous Curve	Hydrocurve	Copolymer of hydroxyethyl-2-methacrylate *n*-(1, 1-dimethyl-oxybutyl) and methacrylic acid	55
Cooper Labs	Permalens	Terpolymer of 2-hydroxyethyl methacrylate *n*-vinyl-2-pyrrolidone and methacrylic acid	71
Hyer-Schulte Medical Optics Center	Sauflon P.W.	Copolymer of PMMA, *n*-vinyl-2-pyrrolidone	79

Reprinted with permission from "Physicians' Desk Reference For Ophthalmology," Medical Economics Co., Oradell, N.J., 1980/81, p. 28.

Hard lenses are polymerized products of esters of acrylic acid or methacrylic acid (28). The most common plastic found in hard lenses is polymethylmethacrylate (PMMA), also known as Lucite or Plexiglas.

Contact lenses made of PMMA are hydrophobic (29). However, PMMA possesses many characteristics that make it ideal for an on-the-eye corrective lens:

- Lenses are very light, due to a specific gravity of 1.18–1.20.
- The refractive index, 1.49–1.50, is similar to glass spectacle lenses.
- They allow a light transmission of 90–92%.
- Lenses are not affected by weak alkalis or weak acids.
- The plastic does not cause sensitivity reactions when placed onto the cornea.

The "hardness" of these hard lenses is less than that of glass, however, and reasonable care must be exercised so as not to scratch or chip them.

The main chemical difference between the hydrophobic hard lens and the hydrophilic soft lens is that the soft lens contains hydroxyl or hydroxyl and lactam groups that cause it to absorb and hold water. Table 1 lists some representative soft lenses that were approved by the FDA for distribution in the United States on May 1, 1980. Nearly all are composed of 2-hydroxyethylmethacrylate (HEMA) with small amounts of cross-linking agents that form a hydrophilic gel (hydrogel) network (30). The degree of cross-linking determines lens hydrophilicity. Greater cross-linking means less hydrophilic groups available for interaction with water which, in turn, produces a less flexible, less hydrated lens than those originally available (31).

Water content varies among soft lenses with values ranging from 30% to 79%. Extended-wear soft lenses generally require at least 55% water for long-term comfort and some typical lenses are listed in Table 2. One such extended-wear lens, Hydrocurve II, was approved for general use in January 1981. All extended-wear lenses had previously been approved by the FDA only for use by patients who had undergone cataract surgery.

The water content of nonspecialty soft lenses has gradually decreased since they were introduced. The water content of a HEMA-type lens can vary between 5% and 90%, but the theoretical "ideal" value would be 75–78%, which matches the hydration level of the corneal stroma.

Reasons for the reductions from this ideal water content can be summarized as follows: Highly hydrated lenses are more comfortable, but they are also more fragile and susceptible to cuts and tears from fingernails during insertion and removal. Lowering the water content produces a more damage-resistant lens.

In addition, decreasing the water content produces a less flexible lens, which increases the amount of astigmatism that can be corrected with a soft lens. When a soft lens is placed on the cornea, its shape is transformed by the corneal topography. Unlike a hard lens that can be formed to a permanent curvature, the soft lens is severely limited in its ability to correct irregular corneal curvature (corneal astigmatism). Soft lenses have a 97% light transmission with a diameter of 0.75 mm. A soft lens with a water content of 60% can be fitted to eyes with an upper limit of astigmatism of about 1.00 diopters. A diopter is a unit of refracting power used as a quantitative measure of the abnormal refraction of light at a surface such as the cornea. Reducing the water content to around 40% extends the limit to about 1.7 diopters (7).

Furthermore, reducing the percentage of water in a soft HEMA lens also reduces the thickness of the hydrated lens. This reduction gives a lens with more lid comfort.

Soft lenses in the nonhydrated (dry) state are rigid and extremely brittle. They should never be handled in the dry state by the wearer. When hydrated, they expand as water is absorbed into the gel matrix (32). They are most comfortable when they are at least the diameter of the cornea, have thin edges, and undergo little movement on the eye. A lens with a water content of around 80% will have a thickness of 0.5–0.6 mm. If this percentage is dropped to around 50–60%, the average thickness will be 0.3–0.4 mm. When the percentage is reduced to 35–40%, the average thickness decreases to 0.2–0.3 mm. Many patients find that they cannot tolerate lenses with a thickness above 0.4 mm because of lid discomfort. For patients who cannot tolerate regular soft lenses at all, several ultrathin soft lenses are available with a thickness as low as 0.07 mm. However, these lenses are extremely fragile and must always be handled with great care.

A semihard contact lens has been approved for use in a wide variety of visual problems such as astigmatism and hypermetropia. Patients suffering decreased visual acuity from corneal edema have been helped after only a few hours of wearing the lens. The lens, previously described as "flexible but dry," is made of cellulose acetate butyrate (CAB). These lenses are not as dry as hard lenses because the surface tension of CAB is 38% lower than PMMA. Cellulose acetate butyrate has optical qualities and durability similar to PMMA, the material used for hard lenses. In addition, thermal conductivity is 28% greater than PMMA, and this permits more rapid heat dissipation (33). The CAB lens is more flexible than PMMA but less flexible than the HEMA (soft) lenses. The semihard lens is being investigated for use in extended wear, since it appears that the extended wear of CAB lenses provides excellent visual results with only minimal effects on corneal thickness (34,35).

A relatively new soft lens under FDA review is made of a cross-linked dimethyl polysiloxane, hydrocarbon-substituted rubber (silicone). This extremely hydrophobic lens absorbs only 0.5% water by weight—less than the conventional hard lenses—and is not permeable to most liquids. Silicone is chemically and physiologically inert, flexible, and rubbery, but it has a certain innate rigidity. It is pliable in the dry state, and fingernails can penetrate it. The lens is less flexible than the hydrogel lens, has a refractive index of 1.439, and permits light transmission of 86% in the dry state and 91% when wet (36–39). Silicone lenses are being investigated for their use in extended wear.

Silicone has excellent optical properties. The silicone does not conform to the cornea but maintains its shape and provides more stability than the thinner soft lenses. At least one new drug application for this lens has been submitted to the FDA.

Advantages of Soft Lenses

Soft lenses provide certain advantages that make them more attractive to the first-time lens wearer. They are considerably more comfortable than hard lenses, and this effect is most apparent during the initial break-in period (40, 41). Photophobia is not likely to occur with soft lenses and glare is reduced significantly. As with hard lenses, however, flare around the periphery may be noticed at night, particularly in individuals who have large pupils (42). This flare is caused by refracted light entering the eye through the edge margin of the contact lens.

Soft lens wearers can change more easily from lenses to eyeglasses after a specific period of wear. A common problem among hard lens wearers is "spectacle blur," or "contact blindness." Nonpathologic spectacle blur is simply a refractive change due to the corneal curvature modifying effect of a hard lens. It may last for a short time or up to hours or days. The net result is unclear vision after a patient has removed contact lenses and put on eyeglasses. For this reason, a hard lens wearer who wishes to obtain a prescription for eye-

glasses is usually advised to refrain from wearing lenses for at least 2 weeks prior to scheduled eye examinations. The average soft lens patient does not usually experience spectacle blur.

Soft lenses are also lost less frequently because they do not dislodge or fall out as often as hard lenses (43). They are better suited for occasional wear and sports, but, like hard lenses, they must be removed prior to swimming as they will float off the cornea. Soft lenses do not allow dust particles, eyelashes, or other foreign material to get caught under the lens as easily as hard lenses.

Disadvantages of Soft Lenses

Although many patients prefer the comfort of soft lenses, it has been shown that not all soft lens wearers can achieve good visual acuity (44,45). The hydration of the lens may change either in or out of the eye (particularly with extremes of temperatures and low relative humidity) and this change can decrease the quality of the visual image (44). Since a soft lens conforms in large part to the corneal shape, it is difficult to predict the degree of vision improvement prior to actually placing the lens on the eye. Also, since soft lenses cannot be precisely tailored to the specific requirements of an individual cornea, the fitting process is less exact than with hard lenses. As a result, the overall quality of vision with soft contact lenses usually does not equal that of a properly fitted pair of hard lenses. Fortunately, these differences are small and should be no cause for concern to the average wearer. The major consequence of these differences is only seen when a lens wearer switches from hard to soft contact lenses. In some cases, the decrease in vision quality is unacceptable to the established hard lens wearer. Many specialists in vision care advise against this transition for this reason, particularly with patients who do quite well with their hard lenses.

Unlike hard lenses, soft lenses can absorb chemical compounds of topical ophthalmic solutions (46–50). Ocular irritation may result, and the lens may be damaged. Drugs such as epinephrine can enter the hydrogel and discolor it due to colored oxidative breakdown products. Other drugs may bind to the matrix and cause oxidative breakdown of the plastic (51). All manufacturers of soft lenses emphasize that no solutions, with the exception of a few specially formulated rewetting solutions, should be placed into the eye with the soft lens in place. If a drug solution is placed into the eye prior to lens insertion, the wearer must wait until the drug solution has cleared from the precorneal (conjunctival) pocket. For most drug solutions, 20–30 minutes is adequate. There may be instances in which the ophthalmologist prefers that lenses are worn while a prescription medication is instilled in the eye so that the lens may serve as a reservoir for the drug. If no instructions accompany the prescription, the pharmacist should contact the physician. Pharmacists must emphasize that this is especially true for any nonprescription ophthalmic product not especially designed for use with contact lenses. In the case of topical ophthalmic ointments, the lenses should not be worn at all.

Soft lenses also cannot be marked to identify left from right positioning the eyes. The usual method for hard lenses is to incorporate a small colored dot marker on one hard lens to identify it as a left or right lens. This marker, located at the outer periphery of the lens, is not perceived by the wearer when the lens is on the cornea. A soft lens wearer who is uncertain of the positional identity of the lenses may have to see a vision specialist for proper determination.

Soft lenses are generally more costly than hard lenses (52). While the initial cost of acquiring soft lenses has been decreasing with the increased number of new users, the overall cost is greater due to more frequent replacement requirements. In addition to replacement necessitated by changes in the refractory requirements of the eye, soft lenses are less durable.

The care given to contact lenses varies considerably in the hands of the wearer. Inadequate care or neglect of hard lenses may lead to corneal problems and/or wearer discomfort, but the lens will still maintain its optical qualities. However, soft lenses rapidly degenerate to useless pieces of plastic if they are neglected. When used with a conscientious care and cleaning program, soft lenses can be expected to have an average life of 18–24 months compared with a 9–12-year life expectancy for a similarly used hard contact lens (53).

Although a particular prescriber may recommend a specific type or brand of soft lens routinely, this use does not necessarily suggest a testament to the optical quality of that product. Rather, most prescribers limit themselves to a particular lens only because their experience in fitting that lens improves the quality of the fit in their patients. As has been stated before, the fitting of soft lenses is a less precise procedure than for hard lenses. Good visual acuity is more dependent upon the fit of the lens than upon small differences in optical quality among brands. Most prescribers will stay with a particular lens for this reason. Likewise, many prescribers will recommend a specific regimen for lens care since this limits the variables involved in assessing the performance of soft lenses among patients.

Contact Lenses and Blinking

The normal blink rate in humans is considered to be about 20 times/minute. This value will vary among individuals and often even within the same individual depending upon activity. It is characteristic for the blink rate to decrease dramatically during reading or deep thought.

The presence of a contact lens in the eye also tends to inhibit blinking. This tendency is usually manifested by a false, or incomplete, blink. The pressure of the lens on the lid causes incomplete lid closure and normal tear distribution under the lens is adversely affected. This effect can lead to corneal edema and complaints of burning, irritation, and dryness by the lens wearer, especially after an extended session of reading or stressed mental activity.

Blinking also plays a role in cleaning the contact lens as well as the cornea, so that incomplete blinkers often cite chronic blurry vision due to smudged lenses as well. Some patients can be counseled to blink properly

and subsequently adapt to lenses quite well. Others may require more extensive measures such as drilling holes in the lens (fenestrating) to improve tear distribution (54). This technique has achieved only limited success, however, since the holes quickly become plugged with mucin or other protein and lipid substances normally present in the tears.

Corneal Effects of Hard and Soft Lenses
Corneal Hypoxia and Edema

The process of oxidative metabolism in the human cornea consumes from 5 to 6 μl of oxygen/sq cm/hour (55). Nearly all of this oxygen is transferred to the avascular cornea from the tears. This process means that an adequate supply of oxygen can be provided only if the cornea is continuously bathed with fresh tears (55–58). A contact lens interferes with normal oxygen uptake because the presence of the lens reduces the effective tear volume available to the cornea. Additionally, because both hard and soft lenses are nearly impermeable to oxygen (the exceptions are the several extended wear types), it becomes crucial that lenses be fitted so as to maximize tear movement between the lens and the cornea (32). Even when properly fitted, both hard and soft lenses produce a progressive hypoxia of the cornea during the time in which the lenses are in place (54–59).

One major effect of this hypoxia is edema of the corneal tissues (25, 54, 60–62). Although tear flow is inhibited more by the presence of a soft lens, it also has been demonstrated that corneal thickness is increased to a greater extent by hard lenses (61–63). After approximately 16 hours of continuous wear, hard or soft lenses cause the glycogen content of the cornea to fall to a level that results in significant edema. If the lenses are then removed for 6 hours, the glycogen levels return to approximately 93% of the normal value and about 98% in 8 hours. The best procedure to follow is to prevent edema from reaching this extent. A good approach is to remove lenses for a 1-hour "rest period" after 7–9 hours of continuous wear. The lenses may then be reinserted for up to 8 hours if necessary. Wearing regular hard or soft lenses uninterrupted for 14–18 hours once or twice a week will usually cause no problems, but continuing such a practice on a daily basis should be avoided. Most patients eventually develop painful abrasions due to improper fit during the edematous state.

Oral contraceptives have been implicated in persistent corneal edema (17, 64). Patients taking oral contraceptives for at least 6 months prior to fitting of contact lenses generally do much better than those who begin use of oral contraceptives after regular contact lens use. Likewise, a lens wearer who stops using oral contraceptives may develop problems with lens fit due to changes in the cornea (decreased microedema).

Corneal Abrasions

Corneal abrasions are surface defects in the acutely sensitive epithelial layer of the cornea. The causes range from poorly fitted lenses or simple overwear to scratches caused by entrapment of foreign bodies such as dust, make-up, or eyelashes under the lens. The cornea is sensitive to pain upon abrasion, so that blepharospasm (reflex lid closure), lacrimation, and raising of the hands to the affected eye are immediate. Rubbing of the eye, although almost reflexive, must be avoided since it can cause more extensive damage while the lens remains in the eye.

Fortunately, the pain associated with corneal abrasion is usually of greater magnitude than the damage that is present. The epithelium regenerates very quickly so that most minor epithelial defects (2 mm in diameter or less) heal within 12–24 hours. A pressure dressing is usually all that is required to prevent infection. The lens is usually left out for about a week and then the wearer may proceed using a modified break-in schedule suggested by the vision specialist. More extensive abrasions may require pressure dressing and application of 5% homatropine hydrobromide to neutralize ciliary spasm. Systemic analgesics may be useful in such cases.

Signs and Symptoms of Lens Problems

A "symptom" may be defined as a subjective patient complaint; a "sign" is an objective measurement or observation by a trained practitioner. Patients may encounter various problems initially in adapting to lenses, particularly hard lenses, and even long-time wearers occasionally experience difficulties of one type or another. The following listing provides a perspective for counseling a lens wearer who seeks advice. Many of these problems arise from different causative factors, and the identification and resolution of a specific problem may require a trained vision specialist. Most of this information is particularly applicable to hard lens wear.

- **Deep aching of eye**—This pain persists even after the lens is removed and may be caused by poorly fitted lenses (too tight). The lenses must be loosened or their diameter increased.
- **Bubbles under lens**—Bubbles are caused by trapped air due to a lens that is too tight (stagnation of circulation). They may cause "dimples" in the epithelium but they usually disappear 3–4 hours after the lens is removed.
- **Blurred vision**—Several factors may produce this effect:
  Improper refractive power;
  Tear film buildup—surface scratches, cosmetics, and surface scratches on the outer face of the lens anchor a stagnant tear film rich in lipid or proteinaceous material. (Repeated removal and cleaning of the lens may provide only temporary relief, often for only a few minutes after reinsertion);
  Cosmetic film buildup—Eye make-up and cosmetics can be transferred to the lens from the fingers;
  Switched lenses;
  Corneal edema—Edema may be a problem especially when blurring occurs after a few hours of wear. The patient may think that the lenses are dirty and may remove and clean them. Vision improves temporarily because edema has decreased while the lenses are out of the eye. Edema also causes haloes (rainbows) around lights, redness, burning, and itching;
  Oral contraceptive use.

- **Excessive tearing**—Several factors contribute to excessive tearing:
  Tearing is a normal symptom when lens wear is first initiated;
  Poorly fitted lens (too tight causes poor circulation, too loose causes excessive contact with lids);
  Chipped, rough edges.
- **Fogging** ("misty vision," "smoky vision") can be caused by two factors:
  Corneal edema, from lenses that are too tight, resulting in poor circulation;
  Overwearing of contact lenses.
- **Itching**—This problem may be caused by allergic conjunctivitis and may be treated with short-term topical steroids.
- **Lens falls out of eye**—Poorly fitted lenses are probably the cause.
- **Inability to wear lenses in morning:**
  Cornea and lids are slightly swollen in the morning; (closed lids create favorable conditions for bacteria to multiply in the conjunctival sac).
  Mild conjunctivitis.
- **Photophobia:**
  Normal symptom initially—use sunglasses;
  Poorly fitted lenses—lens is too tight or too loose or lens fits too close to apex of cornea (most sensitive part);
  Scratched lens;
  Oral contraceptive use.
- **Pain after removal of lens**—This effect is usually due to corneal abrasion. The presence of the lens anesthetizes the cornea; sensation returns after 4–6 hours and pain develops. For this reason, the cause may not be linked directly to the lenses by the wearer.
- **Sudden pain in the eye**—A foreign body or chipped lens may be the problem.
- **Squinting**—This effect is caused by excessive lens movement. The wearer squints to center optical portion of lens over the pupil.

Hard Lens Care Products

For the cornea to sustain a normal metabolic balance and maintain proper refractory characteristics for optical clarity, it must have relatively constant exposure to the atmosphere during waking periods (56, 57). This exposure permits atmospheric oxygen to dissolve in the precorneal fluid and transfer to the cornea. This precorneal fluid also must constantly bathe the corneal surface; this process is aided by blinking. The presence of a hard contact lens impairs these normal processes. For this reason, the insertion of a contact lens must be considered to be an abnormal alteration of the corneal environment. To minimize the stresses of this environment, hard contact lens wear must be supported with concurrent use of special accessory solutions. When properly formulated, such solutions aid the wearer by providing comfort and safety.

Cleaning Products

Normal tears are composed of secretions from many specialized glands lining the lacrimal apparatus, conjunctiva, and lids. Many components are somewhat hydrophobic and tend to adhere to the surface of a hard lens during normal daily wear. This residue, primarily proteinaceous debris and oils, acts as a growth medium for bacteria. If this material is not removed routinely by daily cleaning, it may harden to form tenacious deposits that create an irregular surface on the lens. This residue will eventually cause irritation to the lids and corneal epithelium and may progress to corneal abrasions and infection. Decreased visual acuity and wear time are likely consequences due to a cloudy lens and/or corneal edema.

Typical cleaning solutions contain nonionic surfactants that emulsify oils and aid in solubilizing other debris. Proteins and lipids are soluble in highly alkaline media, but a high pH can cause lens decomposition. Weakly alkaline solutions may be helpful in dislodging deposits from the lens in conjunction with the surface tension lowering properties of the surfactants.

Lenses should be rinsed thoroughly after cleaning as residual cleaning agents may lead to ocular irritation. For this reason, ordinary shampoos and dishwashing detergents should not be used for cleaning. Detergents may accumulate on the lens and their strong surfactant action may cause physical changes in the polished surface of the lens. Lenses should never be wiped dry with tissue as this will also cause surface scratches.

Hard lenses should be cleaned immediately after removal. Routine daily removal of accumulated deposits will do much to ensure a clear, comfortable lens. Many complaints of lens discomfort or unclear vision can be traced to inadequate or improper cleaning procedures.

There are four basic techniques for cleaning hard lenses, some of which do not rely entirely upon specially formulated solutions.

Friction Rubbing

A contact lens cleaning solution or gel is applied to the inside and outside surfaces of the lens. The lens is then rubbed between the thumb and forefinger, or alternatively, between the forefinger and palm of the opposite hand. This method is least desirable since it may result in scratched and warped lenses if rubbing is too vigorous.

Spray Cleaning

The lenses are placed into a perforated holder and held under a stream of running water from an ordinary faucet. The pressure of the water flow dislodges debris that has been loosened by overnight soaking in the storage case.

Hydraulic Cleaning

The lenses are placed into separate baskets in a plastic container that permits an upward and downward pumping action by a hand-operated plunger. The unit may be filled with a special cleaning solution to assist in removal of deposits.

Ultrasonic Cleaning

The lenses are placed into a water bath through which ultrasound waves are passed. These specialized cleaning units effectively dislodge tenacious deposits, but their cost limits their use to in-office cleaning by the practitioner.

Wetting Solutions

The functions of an ideal wetting solution are

- To convert the hydrophobic lense surface to a hydrophilic surface by means of a uniform film that does not wash away easily (65, 66, 67);
- To increase comfort by providing a cushioning and lubricating effect between the corneal surface and the inner surface of the lens, and between the lens and the inner surface of the eyelid (66, 68);
- To establish a viscous coating on the lens to protect it from oily deposits on the fingers during insertion;
- To stabilize the lens on the fingertip to facilitate insertion, particularly for individuals with poor manual dexterity or unsteady hands.

The term "contact lens" is a misnomer because when properly positioned the lens does not actually contact the corneal surface. Rather, a hard lens should float freely and relatively friction free on a layer of tears and rotate due to blinking. For this to occur, the tear fluids must "wet" the hydrophobic lens surface.

If the lens is cleaned thoroughly prior to insertion, the lacrimal fluid could wet the lens adequately due to natural wetting elements. However, the wetting action of these proteins and well-hydrated polysaccharides does not occur immediately, and 5–15 minutes of discomfort and a pronounced foreign body sensation is usually experienced by the patient following insertion (29).

Wetting is the uniform spreading of a liquid over a solid surface. The surface tension of the liquid, in part with the relationship of the cohesion force (the attraction of liquid molecules for each other) and adhesion (the attraction of the liquid molecules and the molecules of the solid), determines whether the liquid remains as discrete drops or spreads on the surface. Surface-active agents displace liquid molecules from the droplet surface and thereby reduce surface tension. When the surface tension of the liquid is equal to or less than the "critical surface tension" of the solid, the liquid wets the surface. Additionally, for two liquids to mix well, their surface tensions should be similar.

The corneal surface tension is 31 dynes/cm². Normal tear surface tension is 46.3 dynes/cm² and the value of a hard (PMMA) lens is 39 dynes/cm². It does not appear that even normal tears will wet the cornea; however, additional secretions make this possible. The secretions of the accessory glands of the conjunctiva act to transform the cornea surface tension to about 46 dynes/cm². This change permits optimal wetting of the cornea by the tears and demonstrates the important role of normal eye secretions in maintaining a healthy precorneal environment.

The desirable surface tension for a contact lens wetting solution is 39–46 dynes/cm². If the solution is so formulated, it simultaneously mixes well with tears, wets the corneal surface, and adequately spreads across the surfaces of a hard contact lens.

The basic wetting solution is comprised of components selected from four main functional categories:

- Cushioning agents, such as viscosity-inducing additive(s); usually cellulose gum derivatives such as methylcellulose or hydroxypropyl methylcellulose;
- Wetting agents, such as polyvinyl alcohol;
- Preservatives, such as benzalkonium chloride or thimerosal;
- Buffering agents, for pH and tonicity.

The cushioning effect of a wetting solution is due to the presence of hydrophilic polymers that position between the lens and the corneal surface. Cellulose gum derivatives are often employed because they are effective lubricants as well. However, although compounds such as methylcellulose possess a degree of surfactant activity, it is not of sufficient magnitude to promote uniform wetting of a PMMA lens. For this reason, polyvinyl alcohol frequently is used in combination with these agents to decrease surface tension and increase viscosity.

The concentration of the cushioning polymer in wetting solutions affects both the comfort of the lens in the eye and the quality of vision immediately following insertion. In some individuals, a concentration that is too low causes discomfort after only a short period of lens wear. In others, a high polymer concentration raises complaints of blurry vision due to poor mixing of the viscous solution with the tears. In addition, overspill of solution onto the lids and eyelashes causes crusting as the solution dries and this residue can become a source of foreign material falling into the eye. In one study of subjective patient comfort, the optimal viscosity range was 15–20 centipoise (69).

Soaking Solutions

A soaking solution is used to store a hard contact lens whenever it is removed from the eye. The solution serves to maintain the lens in a constant state of hydration for maximum comfort and visual acuity. It also aids in the removal of organic deposits that accumulate on the lens during wear (70). Another function is to maintain lens sterility to prevent transfer of microorganisms to the eye by a contaminated lens.

A PMMA lens absorbs between 1% and 3% moisture by weight. Upon exposure to air, the lens dehydrates and then subsequently rehydrates when placed into contact with a soaking solution or the lacrimal fluid (71). Placing a dehydrated lens into the eye, with or without a wetting solution, causes discomfort as the lens absorbs tears from the precorneal area (72). In addition, a dehydrated lens is flatter than a hydrated lens and this factor causes problems with both comfort and visual acuity until the lens' moisture content stabilizes (73, 74).

Absorption of tears into a PMMA lens during normal wear results in an accumulation of deposits. If the lens is allowed to dry out during overnight storage, these deposits become hard and difficult to remove by normal cleaning procedures. Thorough cleaning of the lens after removal and subsequent storage in a well-formulated soaking solution virtually eliminates the likelihood of deposit buildup.

At one time there was a vigorous controversy over "wet" and "dry" storage of hard contact lenses. Dry storage refers to removal of the lens and storing it in a dry, sealed case or in a special ventilated case. Soaking solution is not added and lenses are inserted the next day with or without a wetting solution. Wet storage consists of cleaning the lens after removal and placing it into a leak-proof case filled with soaking solution. In the morning, the lenses are thoroughly rinsed and inserted with the aid of a wetting solution. Proponents of dry storage based their arguments on the assumption that a dry lens cannot support bacterial growth. Studies were reported that linked storage solutions with bacterial contamination of lenses and dry storage was recommended as the only safe method (75–78). However, numerous subsequent studies showed that pathogens can be cultured from 3% to 5% of lenses from patients who use either method, and as high as 50% from lenses subjected to dry storage (66, 79, 80). Due to hydration by the lacrimal fluid while in the eye, a "dry" lens is not really dry at all and retains enough moisture to support bacterial growth (81). The use of a soaking solution containing suitable preservatives prevents this growth. While it is true that ocular infections have been caused by patient failure to replace old solution in their storage cases, the safest and most comfortable method of lens storage is wet storage with a daily change of soaking solution (29).

Storage solutions use essentially the same preservatives as wetting solutions to maintain sterility. The main difference is that the concentration can be somewhat higher since the soaking solution is rinsed from the lens prior to insertion. However, preservative levels are selected carefully since higher levels do not necessarily give increased effectiveness and may lead to impaired wetting and/or corneal irritation due to the adsorption of preservatives onto the lens (82, 83)

Multifunctional Products

There has been a trend toward the use of combination solutions for the cleaning, soaking, and wetting of hard contact lenses. Initially, all manufacturers recommended three different solutions, specifically formulated, for these functions. Then, solutions claimed to be effective for both wetting and soaking, or for soaking and cleaning, were introduced. Some manufacturers offer a single solution claimed to be effective for all three basic procedures.

The major problem with an all-purpose solution is that to some extent the ingredients required in the formulation perform different and somewhat incompatible functions. For example, high concentrations of benzalkonium chloride are necessary for killing bacteria in soaking solutions, but these same concentrations cause ocular irritation and wetting problems due to the interaction of the preservative with the PMMA lens surface.

If lenses are stored overnight in a solution containing a high concentration of polymers for cushioning and wetting, the lenses may become "gummy" and cause discomfort. Likewise, if the lenses are stored overnight in a cleaning solution containing an anionic detergent, the detergent may eventually build up on the lens and cause irritation. While there is a need for a single agent that will perform all three basic functions adequately, no such agent exists. The all-purpose solutions at present should be considered to be a compromise. They may be considered to be marginally effective, but they cannot be considered to perform as well as the separate solutions. Some patients will do quite well with an all-purpose solution, but others will undoubtedly do better with a multiple solution approach to lens care. This can only be determined by trial for each individual.

Rewetting Products

These solutions are intended to clean and rewet the contact lens while the lens is in place on the eye (84). They depend upon the use of surfactants to loosen deposits and removal is assisted by the natural cleaning action of blinking. Examples of agents that may be used to promote this action are polyoxyl 40 stearate and polyethylene glycol 300. Although these products function well to recondition the in-situ lens, the benefit to the cornea is lacking compared with actual removal, cleaning, and rewetting of the lens. Removal of the lens for even a brief time during the normal wear period allows the cornea to recover some of its depleted glycogen levels. The use of an in-the-eye rewetting solution, although expedient, does not provide this needed respite.

Miscellaneous Lens Care Products

Preinsertion Solutions

Preinsertion solutions are used to prepare the cornea for lens insertion. These products are generally high viscosity polymer solutions that further cushion placement of the lens on the cornea. They may be especially useful during the initial break-in period for individuals with particularly high corneal sensitivity. The high viscosity of these solutions may cause blurred vision for a little while after insertion and some patients may find this annoying.

Conditioners

Conditioners are recommended when tears do not supply a sufficient wetting action or cushioning effect. They also are used to clear the eye of potential debris-forming substances prior to lens insertion, and they can be applied to the eye as frequently as 3 or 4 times/day while the lens is being worn (84).

Contact Lens Remover

The DMV Contact Lens Remover is sometimes recommended to elderly patients. The pharmacist must be aware that good patient instructions are needed. The contact lens remover uses a suction cup, and if the patient places the cup on the cornea instead of the lens, corneal damage may result. Patients should be instructed to clean these removers before and after each use, since they may harbor bacteria. They can be cleaned by using a lens cleaning solution and rinsing them off before use.

Contact Lens Cases

Several devices are available for mailing, soaking, cleaning, and storing hard contact lenses. Standards for these have been recommended, and their relative effectiveness varies from product to product (85).

Other Products

Other ophthalmic products are available to the hard lens wearer for occasional use. Some, such as artificial tears and ocular decongestants, are not recommended for use with the lenses in place. Artificial tears can be used to soothe the eye by virtue of their emollient and lubricating effect. Ocular decongestants relieve mild conjunctivitis associated with prolonged lens wear. Routine use of these products should be avoided. If symptoms requiring their use persist, a visit to a vision specialist is advised to determine the cause. (See Chapter 21, *Ophthalmic Products.*)

Formulation Considerations

In 1968, the FDA classified all contact lens devices as drugs. However, hard contact lenses and their accessory solutions were automatically accepted without provision since their safety and efficacy had been established prior to that time. Even though contact lens solutions are not considered drug products, formulation considerations still apply. The formulation of a contact lens product must be guided by the knowledge that a contact lens solution may be used daily for months or even years. The potential for cumulative effects on the ocular tissues or on the lens device is significant. Since these products are often used by inexperienced people with minimal counseling, all ingredients must be effective and provide a high margin of safety.

The basic considerations for a well-formulated contact lens solution include isotonicity with tears, pH, viscosity, stability, sterility, and provision for maintenance of sterility (bactericidal action).

The pH range for comfort is not well defined because tear pH varies among individuals. The average range of normal tear pH is 7.2–7.4. For instance, if the normal tear pH of one individual is 6.8 and a strongly buffered solution of 7.4 is instilled, some discomfort will likely result. On the other hand, if a weakly buffered solution of 7.4 is instilled, there may be little or no discomfort. It is best to have a weakly buffered solution that can readily adjust to any tear condition. However, as in the case of therapeutic ophthalmic solutions, the stability of the solution components takes precedence over comfort. For this reason, many contact lens solutions are formulated with pH values above or below the value of 7.2–7.4, some as much as 3 full pH units (86). However, these systems are weakly buffered and are well tolerated by the eye.

Routine daily use of any contact lens solution means that the likelihood of bacterial contamination is high. Depending on the individual's specific lens care procedures, a single container may well last for a month or more. For this reason, the solution must contain a suitable bactericidal agent that is both effective over the long-term and nonirritating with daily use in the eye. There are few preservatives that fulfill these criteria (87, 88). The most commonly used agents are benzalkonium chloride, chlorobutanol, thimerosal, and phenylmercuric nitrate; however, these agents are not free from irritation potential, depending upon concentration and patient sensitivity. Solutions from different manufacturers should not be mixed since a precipitant may result. For instance, a product containing alkaline borate buffers forms a gummy, gel-like precipitate on lenses if mixed with a wetting solution containing polyvinyl alcohol.

Soft Lens Care Products

The hydrophilic soft lenses dictate that extreme caution be exercised with regard to the types of chemicals to which they are exposed. These chemicals, many of which penetrate and bind with the lens material, come from cosmetics, environmental pollutants, and nonprescription and prescription ophthalmic products (46, 47). Conventional hard lens solutions are contraindicated for use with soft lenses because absorption of the ingredients causes lens damage and/or ocular irritation (49, 57, 89, 90). Since soft lenses contain a high percentage of water, they are more prone to bacterial contamination (91). Lens sterility must be maintained to prevent ocular infection and also to prevent damage of the lens material by bacteria and fungi (92). Actually, the term "sterility" is a misnomer since maintaining true sterility of a soft lens, especially while being worn in the eye, is not possible. A more appropriate term is "disinfection" since this reflects more accurately the routine procedures used to eliminate bacterial contamination before it increases to harmful levels in the lens.

Like hard lenses, soft lenses require a basic regimen of care to keep them comfortable and optically sound. This regimen centers mainly around cleaning and disinfection and several approaches have been developed. Caution should be advised in selecting products for these procedures since some products are only intended for use with a particular type of soft lens. The pharmacist should be mindful of this and should be able to counsel the soft lens wearer who expresses a desire to alter a regimen of care.

Cleaning Products

The most troublesome aspect of soft lens wear is the accumulation of deposits on the lens. The nature of these deposits is varied, but generally they consist of proteins and lipids originating in the wearer's lacrimal secretions. The rate at which these deposits accumulate is dependent upon the lens and the tears. Deposits are a greater problem with the more highly hydrated lenses. However, patient complaints of dirty lenses are still highly individual. Some wearers experience little difficulty and may wear soft lenses for long periods without significant buildup. Others may show deposits in as little as 2–3 days. Whatever the cause or the accumulation rate, the end result is an uncomfortable lens of poor optical quality (93–95). Specific cleaning procedures have been developed to help the wearer maintain clear lenses for a prolonged period (96–100).

Surface Acting Cleaners

The most common method of cleaning soft lenses involves the use of surface-active materials and friction rubbing. Several drops of a cleaning solution are placed onto the lens surface and the lens is gently rubbed between the thumb and forefinger. An alternate method is to place the lens in the palm of the hand and rub gently with a fingertip. With either method, care must be used so as not to cut the soft lens with a fingernail. Soft lens cleaning solutions generally contain a nonionic detergent, a wetting agent, a chelating agent, buffers, and preservatives. Friction cleaning usually takes about 20–30 seconds and the cleaner must then be thoroughly rinsed from the lens. Rinsing is an essential part of soft lens care, and it should be carried out using a sterile isotonic buffered solution.

Enzymatic Cleaners

The surface-active cleaners generally are quite effective in removing lipid deposits. They are less successful in removing protein debris. Enzyme tablets are an additional cleaning aid that can solve this problem. The lenses are soaked in an enzyme solution (papain) for about 4 hours; this solution effectively loosens protein deposits. The lenses should then be cleansed to remove all traces of enzyme from the lens surface to prevent eye irritation. It is usually sufficient to use enzyme cleaning as a once-a-week supplement to daily cleaning with surface-active chemicals.

Disinfection of Soft Lenses

The FDA requires "sterilization" of soft contact lenses and two methods are currently approved for use: thermal and chemical. Studies have shown that bacteria such as *Pseudomonas aeruginosa* do not enter the matrix of the hydrogel (101, 102), but surface contamination of the lens could lead to ocular infection (103, 104). Both disinfection methods are reliable and lenses must be cleaned and thoroughly rinsed prior to insertion with either technique.

Thermal Disinfection

The basic method of thermal disinfection involves placing the cleaned lenses into separate compartments of a storage case filled with a saline solution. The case is then placed into a heating unit and the temperature is increased to a specific level for a prescribed time (105). Originally, the lenses were disinfected by raising the temperature up to the boiling point for about 20 minutes. Units that use lower temperatures (about 80°C) for a longer time are available. This process is as effective as boiling and has the advantage that it prolongs lens life. Daily boiling of a soft lens weakens the lens and accelerates loss of optical quality. Some practitioners now advise soft lens wearers who use thermal disinfection to disinfect them 2 or 3 times/week and to store the lenses in the refrigerator in the interim.

It is important that protein debris be removed completely from the lenses prior to heating, since denaturing by heat transforms proteins to hard, tenacious deposits (48). After heating and cooling, the lenses are removed from the unit and rinsed with a saline solution prior to insertion. Lens cases for use with the thermal units should be inspected routinely for cracks or leaks and replaced at the first sign of a problem.

Chemical Disinfection

Chemical disinfection may also be termed "cold" sterilization since heat is not used to kill microorganisms. The lenses are stored for at least 4 hours in a solution containing bactericidal agents such as thimerosal and chlorhexidine (90). Chemical disinfection is more costly than thermal methods, but one advantage is the likelihood of longer lens life. A disadvantage is a higher incidence of ocular irritation.

Patients may freely switch from thermal disinfection to chemical methods, but the switch from chemical to thermal may present problems. Lenses that have been subjected to a chemical disinfecting solution must be completely free from all traces of the chemicals or else the lens becomes opaque upon heating. Prolonged soaking in several changes of saline is recommended to purge the lens before using a heating unit.

Insertion

When soft lenses are ready for insertion, a careful process should be followed:

- Wash the hands with noncosmetic soap, and rinse thoroughly. Dry the hands with a lint-free towel.
- Remove the lens for the right eye from its storage container.
- Squeeze the lens gently between thumb and forefinger. If the edges move toward each other, the lens is in correct position.
- Examine the lens for cleanness. If necessary, clean it again.
- Insert the lens on the right eye.
- Repeat the process for the left eye.

Saline Solution

The saline solution for disinfection and rinsing can be purchased premixed, or it can be prepared using salt tablets. A controversy ensued between 1978 and late 1980 over the safety of unpreserved salt tablets for the preparation of soft lens solutions. The FDA maintained that control of water quality and salt concentration was not possible when left to the patient. The FDA acknowledged that daily use of a disinfection unit would prevent overgrowth of bacteria on lenses rinsed with nonsterile saline, but it was argued that many patients do not use the units every day. Salt tablets disappeared from the market for a time, but then reappeared when the FDA advisory review panel ruled that no proof existed that the tablets were an imminent health hazard. It is advised that these tablets should only be used with distilled water labeled "USP" and that the container be refrigerated. A fresh batch of solution should be prepared daily and it should never be reused. Daily use of a thermal or chemical disinfecting procedure is highly recommended when salt tablets are used.

Premixed saline is available from several sources and it is usually preserved with thimerosal. Unpreserved sterile saline solutions are available for individuals sensitive to preservatives. They are packaged in disposable vials land are more costly than their preserved counterparts.

Other Soft Lens Products

Accessory solutions for use with soft lenses have been formulated to permit cleaning, lubricating, and rewetting of the lens in the eye. These solutions typically contain a low concentration of a nonionic surfactant to promote cleaning and a polymer to lubricate the lens surface, along with buffering agents. They are particularly useful to patients with highly hydrated lenses, such as the extended-wear type. Exposure of lenses to wind and high temperature causes a degree of dehydration even with the lens in place in the eye (44). The resulting discomfort can be relieved readily by 1 or 2 drops of these solutions. These solutions can add still another measure of comfort to soft lens wear.

Preservatives Used in Contact Lens Solutions

Benzalkonium Chloride

Benzalkonium chloride is a surface-active agent and germicide effective against a variety of gram-positive and gram-negative bacteria (106–108). In sufficient concentration, it is also effective against perhaps the most worrisome ocular pathogen, *P. aeruginosa*. Several properties of benzalkonium chloride require that care be exercised with respect to its concentration in a hard lens solution.

High concentrations of benzalkonium chloride interfere with the proper wetting of PMMA lenses. The surfactant adsorbs to the lens in such a way as to create another hydrophobic surface. This is a special case where a surface-active agent can actually inhibit rather than promote the wetting process.

High concentrations cause ocular damage, either directly by instillation into the eye or indirectly by adsorption onto the lens (109). The maximum tolerable concentration is probably around 0.03% (1:3,000), with solutions of 0.02% having been shown to be tolerated up to several times a day (110). However, most solutions for direct instillation into the eye contain concentrations well below this.

Weak concentrations are not effective in providing rapid, dependable bactericidal activity. Studies showed that higher concentrations are necessary for activity against *P. aeruginosa* (111). Concentrations of about 1:5,000 can preserve a lens solution effectively, although the presence of foreign material (soaps, metallic ions, and phospholipids) inactivate the preservative (70, 112, 113).

Some patients using a solution preserved with benzalkonium chloride develop ocular irritation due to a buildup of the surfactant on their lenses. Switching to a solution with a lower benzalkonium chloride concentration may alleviate this, but a change to a solution with a completely different preservative/cleaning agent may be required.

Chlorobutanol

Chlorobutanol is a slow-acting germicide that has several disadvantages. The compound is volatile and the concentration falls below the effective level after repeated exposure of the container contents to air. It is also unstable to heat and alkaline media, so that it cannot be used in solutions with a pH higher than 6. However, it does possess some degree of synergism when used with benzalkonium chloride and the two are sometimes used together for this reason (114, 115). When used alone, it probably has no advantage over benzalkonium chloride.

Thimerosal

Thimerosal, or sodium ethylmercurithiosalicylate, was introduced as an alternative to benzalkonium chloride. It is effective against *P. aeruginosa*, but it is slow to act since it depends upon sustained release of mercurial ion which penetrates the bacterial cell (116, 117, 118). Since it is a basic salt, it may cause a precipitate if used with benzalkonium chloride or if its solutions are mixed with solutions containing benzalkonium chloride. Being a mercurial, it may also cause sensitization in some individuals after repeated application. In practice, this problem has not been significant. Like benzalkonium chloride, it acts by interfering with cell metabolism, glycolysis, and respiration.

Phenylmercuric Nitrate

Phenylmercuric nitrate also is a mercurial preservative and similar in action to thimerosal. It is usually used in dilute concentration and it is not precipitated in an acidic pH. When used alone, however, it is not very effective against *P. aeruginosa* (119, 120). At one time, a serious problem existed due to contamination of diagnostic fluorescein solutions preserved with this agent, especially with multidose containers used in clinical office practice. The disposable paper fluorescein strip was introduced for this reason. Organic mercurials can be effective preservatives, but their usefulness in ophthalmic solutions is severely limited by their slow action (118).

Sodium Edetate

Sodium edetate (tetrasodium ethylenediaminetetraacetate) is often used in lens solutions because it disrupts the integrity of bacterial cell walls. As such, it enhances the action of other preservatives (121). Sodium edetate may decrease the action of mercurials (122). It also complexes with other substances, such as metallic ions, that might reduce benzalkonium chloride activity.

Product Selection Guidelines

Hard Lens Products

The variety of accessory solutions available to hard lens wearers poses a puzzling selection problem for many patients. The availability of single- and multiple-task products within the same product line further frustrates and confuses the wearer. This situation means that selection of contact lens products is a prime area where the pharmacist can perform a much needed role as a consultant. Unfortunately, information available to the pharmacist is not sufficient to provide a complete foundation for patient consultation in all aspects of lens wear. Product labeling is often incomplete or limited to

general information. Preservative concentration is usually listed adequately in terms of the specific agent(s) and concentration(s), but concentrations of cushioning and lubricating polymers are usually absent. This makes it extremely difficult for the pharmacist to recommend a specific product for a patient who may require a solution of lower or higher viscosity. Furthermore, other ingredients are often listed simply as "cleaning agents" or "buffers," making alternate selections a random process for patients with sensitivities to these components. The situation is further complicated by the fact that some products are incompatible when used together. More information is therefore needed to enable the pharmacist to counsel the hard lens wearer effectively. Complete product labeling would allow every pharmacist to use his or her knowledge about pharmaceutical systems and components and thereby make selections based upon specific information and patient needs.

The pharmacist must assist the lens wearer in selection of a lens care regimen that the patient will use regularly. A patient who does not carefully follow a regimen using separate solutions may do much better when directed to a combination product. Others may benefit from supplemental products such as rewetting products or conditioners to increase comfort and wear time. However, the pharmacist should be always mindful that frequent use of ocular decongestants or supportive solutions may indicate a more fundamental lens problem, such as improper fit or surface imperfections, that requires referral of the patient to a vision specialist.

A very important question to ask a hard lens wearer who is experiencing ocular irritation is how long the lenses are worn each day. The pharmacist should keep in mind that the presence of a hard lens on the cornea reduces corneal sensitivity to the extent that the wearer may not be aware of overwear abrasion or edema until several hours after the lenses are removed. Often, many cases of burning, itching eyes can be solved by suggesting short periods of lens removal ("rest periods") for patients who must routinely wear their lenses for long hours during the day and evening.

Soft Lens Products

Although most soft lens care regimens are initially recommended by the prescriber, the pharmacist can assist patients who experience difficulty or express dissatisfaction. Often, lifestyle can create problems with soft lens care. A salesperson who spends much time traveling may find thermal disinfection an inconvenience. Switching to a chemical procedure may increase both satisfaction and compliance. Similarly, some premixed saline solutions are bulky and troublesome. Salt tablets may be more acceptable to some patients since the saline solution can be prepared in smaller quantities. The saline can be purchased in 8-oz containers that fit into a shaving kit or make-up bag.

Selection of proper solutions for use with a specific lens material is also a concern for the pharmacist. It should not be assumed that patient selection of a particular product has been guided by this requirement. In addition, counseling in the use of other ocular solutions, suspensions, or ointments is essential for the soft lens wearer.

Many problems associated with soft lens wear arise from the way in which patients handle their lenses. Unsatisfactory results with soft lens products may stem from improper procedures rather than an inadequate product. Specific questions about the care and maintenance regimen used by a wearer can often bring these problems to light. Compatibility of lifestyle and lens care regimen is particularly essential for comfortable and trouble-free soft lens wear.

Patient Counseling

The general instructions for successful contact lens wear are as follows:

- The hands should be washed and rinsed thoroughly before the contact lenses are handled.
- When handling the lenses over a sink, the drain should be covered or closed to prevent loss of the lens.
- Contact lenses are fitted to each eye exactly. To avoid mixing the lenses, it is helpful to always work with the same lens first (always insert or remove the right lens first and then the left). Hard lenses may be marked to help avoid confusion.
- The contact lens wearer should avoid using oily cosmetics or shampoos while the lenses are being worn. Bath oils or soaps with a bath oil or cream base may leave an oily film on the hands that will be transferred to the lenses. These should be avoided also.
- Aerosol cosmetics, such as hair sprays or spray deodorants, damage the lens and should be applied before lens insertion.
- The lenses should be removed before working with strong household chemicals such as paint remover or cleaning fluid. This is especially important if these chemicals are in an aerosol form.
- If the eyes are irritated or red, the patient should not insert the lenses. If the eyes become irritated while wearing the lenses, the lenses should be removed until the irritation subsides.
- Chronic eye irritation may be indicative of a more serious problem. Patients suffering from chronic irritation should be referred to their physician.
- Contact lenses must not be worn while sleeping. Damage to the eye may result. Extended-wear lenses are an exception.
- Lenses should not be worn while sitting under a hair dryer if excessive dryness of the eyes results.
- Contact lenses should not be worn outside on windy days unless eye protection is worn. Windblown soot and other particles may become trapped under the lens and scratch the cornea.
- Contact lenses should not be worn while the patient is participating in contact sports unless additional eye protection is worn.
- Contact lenses should always be stored in a proper lens case when not in use. This prevents lens loss or damage.
- Contact lens care instructions should be followed exactly.
- Soaking solutions should be replaced daily or as di-

rected on the product label. Lenses should not be stored in tap water.
- Contact lenses should be cleaned only with agents specifically made for that purpose. Household cleaners will damage contact lenses.
- Hard contact lenses should only be cared for with products made specifically for hard contact lenses; soft contact lenses should only be cared for with products made specifically for soft contact lenses.
- Contact lens care products from different manufacturers may not be chemically compatible and should not be mixed.
- Contact lens care products should be discarded if the labeled expiration date has passed.
- Contact lenses should not be worn when swimming unless special lenses for this purpose are being used.
- Dropper tips or the tips of lens care product containers should not be touched to prevent contamination.
- Contact lenses and contact lens care products should be kept out of the reach of children.
- Never use saliva to wet contact lenses. This is a dangerous practice and may result in serious, vision-damaging infections.

The following special instructions should be given for successful hard contact lens wear:

- The eyes should not be rubbed while the lenses are in place. Rubbing could result in corneal cuts or abrasion.
- The contact lenses should not be rinsed with very hot or very cold water since temperature extremes may warp the lenses.
- If a lens remover is used, the patient should be instructed in how to use the remover properly since improper use can damage the eye.

The following special instructions shall be given for successful soft contact lens wear:

- Saline solutions should be prepared exactly according to manufacturers directions. Only salt tablets specifically designed for contact lens use should be used. Tablets should be dissolved in the exact amount of fluid recommended by the manufacturer. Saline solutions should be prepared fresh every day; the unused portion should be discarded each day.
- Only distilled or purified water should be used in the soft lens care regimen. Water should be refrigerated to inhibit the growth of microorganisms. It is best to buy only small quantities of water and replace it often.
- Boiling and soaking solutions should be changed daily.
- Soft contact lenses must be thoroughly clean before heat disinfection.
- Hydrogen peroxide or iodophor disinfectants must be completely neutralized before proceeding.
- Enzyme cleaner tablets should be discarded if any discoloration has appeared.
- There are many different types of soft lenses and each requires a specific care regimen. Only care products recommended for the patient's type of soft lens should be used. A physician should be consulted before changing or substituting products.

- Care must be taken when handling soft lenses. They are very fragile and can easily be cut with a fingernail.
- Soft contact lenses should be removed before the installation of any ophthalmic preparation that is not specifically intended for concurrent use with soft contact lenses. The patient should wait at least 20–30 minutes before reinserting the lenses unless directed othewise by his or her physician. Lenses should not be worn at all when a topical ophthalmic ointment is being used.
- Soft contact lenses should not be worn in the presence of irritating fumes or chemicals.

Summary

The continued growth of contact lens use for both cosmetic and therapeutic reasons further increases the need for the practicing pharmacist to keep up-to-date with all aspects of lens products, lens materials, and care and maintenance programs. The pharmacist also should consider contact lens wear as an essential component of the patient profile. Specific information regarding the type of lens, medical reasons for use (if any), and patient sensitivities to formulation ingredients should be included on the profile. Concurrent use of any systemic or topical medication should always be considered when counseling a lens wearer about health care, and particular attention should be given to the possible effects of prescription medications on lens comfort.

The wide variety of products for lens care usually precludes the possibility that the pharmacist can stock every available item, but careful selection of stock can provide a complete care program for most wearers. When a product line is chosen, it is important to stock all products in that line to prevent forcing the patient to choose products from different manufacturers. When approached in a conscientious and knowledgeable manner, the area of contact lens care can provide an important and needed service to the patient and a satisfying benefit to the pharmacist.

References

1. R. A. Koetting, *J. Am. Pharm. Assoc.*, NS15, 575 (1975).
2. D. R. Gourley, *U.S. Pharm.* 2 (2), 40 (1977).
3. O. H. Dabezies, J. M. Dixon, G. P. Halberg, *Patient Care, 12,* 98 (1978).
4. J. N. Buxton and C. R. Locke, *Am. J. Ophthalmol., 72,* 532 (1971).
5. *British Medical Journal, 2,* 655 (1977).
6. A. R. Gasset and L. Lobo, *Ann. Opthalmol., 8,* 843 (1977).
7. L. J. Girard, in "Corneal Contact Lenses," L. J. Girard, Ed., C. V. Mosby, St. Louis, Mo., 1972, pp. 107–120.
8. J. Hartstein, in "Questions and Answers on Contact Lens Practice," C. V. Mosby, St. Louis, Mo., 1973, pp. 68–76.
9. J. Hartstein, in "Questions and Answers on Contact Lens Practice," C. V. Mosby, St. Louis, Mo., 1973, pp. 60–67.
10. C. Thranberend, *Klin. Monatsbl. Augenheilkd., 164,* 509 (1974).
11. F. Dickenson, *Contacto, 11,* 12 (1967).
12. C. H. May, *Contacto, 4,* 41 (1960).
13. T. F. Gumpelmayer, *Am. J. Optom., 47,* 879 (1970).
14. J. A. Baldone, *Trans. Am. Acad. Ophthalmol. Otol., 78,* OP-406 (1974).
15. M. Millodot, *Arch. Ophthalmol., 82,* 461 (1969).
16. "Contact Lens Practice," R. B. Mandell, Ed., Charles C Thomas, Springfield, Ill., 1974, pp. 83–116.
17. L. J. Girard, in "Corneal and Scleral Contact Lenses," L. J. Girard, Ed., C. V. Mosby, St. Louis, Mo., 1967, pp. 40–48.
18. L. J. Girard, in "Corneal and Scleral Contact Lenses," L. J. Girard, Ed., C. V. Mosby, St. Louis, Mo., 1967, pp. 1–17.
19. M. Rubin, *Lancet, 1,* 138 (1976).
20. J. C. Casebeer, *Am. J. Ophthalmol., 76,* 165 (1973).
21. H. M. Rosenwasser, *Opt. J. Rev. Optom., 100,* 41 (1963).
22. K. Dalton, in "Contact Lenses, A Textbook for Practitioner and Student," 2nd ed., Vol. 1, J. Stone and A. J. Phillips, Eds., Butterworth's, Boston, Mass., 1980, pp. 179–180.
23. O. W. Cole, *Contacto, 15,* 5, (1971).
24. "Contact Lens Practice," R. B. Mandella, Ed., Charles C Thomas, Springfield, Ill., 1974, pp. 108–109.
25. "Symposium on Contact Lenses," C. V. Mosby, St. Louis, Mo., 1973, pp. 1–12.
26. "Symposium on Contact Lenses," C. V. Mosby, St. Louis, Mo., 1973, pp. 42–52.
27. G. Mulrooney, *Can. J. Optom., 33,* 74 (1971).
28. "Modern Plastics Encyclopedia," Vol. 1, Breskin, New York, N.Y., 1947, p. 129.
29. O. H. Dabezies, in "Corneal and Scleral Contact Lenses," L. J. Girard, Ed., C. V. Mosby, St. Louis, Mo., 1967, pp. 347–361.
30. "Soft Contact Lens," A. R. Gasset and H. E. Kaufman, Eds., C. V. Mosby, St. Louis, Mo., 1972, pp. 233–239.
31. "Soft Contact Lens," A. R. Gasset and H. E. Kaufman, Eds., C. V. Mosby, St. Louis, Mo., 1972, pp. 175–183.
32. F. B. Hoefle, *Trans. Am. Acad. Ophthalmol. Otol., 78,* OP-386 (1974).
33. G. E. Garcia, *Ophthalmology, 86,* 332 (Feb. 1979).
34. G. E. Garcia, *J. Con. Intra. Lens Med., 2,* 29–34 (1976).
35. B. A. Kaplan and C. J. Trimber, *Ophthalmology, 87,* 292 (April 1980).
36. "Symposium on the Flexible Lens," J. L. Bitonte and R. H. Keates, Eds., C. V. Mosby, St. Louis, Mo., 1972, pp. 73–79.
37. "Symposium on the Flexible Lens," J. L. Bitonte and R. H. Keates, Eds., C. V. Mosby, St. Louis, Mo., 1972, pp. 519–522.
38. A. B. Rizzuit, *Ann. Ophthalmol., 6,* 596 (1974).
39. "Soft Contact Lens," A. R. Gasset and H. E. Kaufman, Eds., C. V. Mosby, St. Louis, Mo., 1972, pp. 126–138.
40. "Contact Lens Practice," R. B. Mandell, Ed., Charles C Thomas, Springfield, Ill., 1974, pp. 437–454.
41. "Symposium on the Flexible Lens," J. L. Bitonte and R. H. Keates, Eds., C. V. Mosby, St. Louis, Mo., 1972, pp. 35–51.
42. "Soft Contact Lens," A. R. Gasset and H. E. Kaufman, Eds., C. V. Mosby, St. Louis, Mo., 1972, pp. 83–86.
43. *Optometric Weekly, 63,* 25 (1972).
44. "Contact Lens Practice," R. B. Mandell, Ed., Charles C Thomas, Springfield, Ill., 1974, pp. 83–116.
45. R. L. Sutherland and W. N. Van Leeuwen, *Can. Med. Assoc. J., 107,* 49 (1972).
46. "Symposium on Contact Lenses," C. V. Mosby, St. Louis, Mo., 1973, pp. 174–180.
47. "Soft Contact Lenses," A. R. Gasset and H. E. Kaufman, Eds., C. V. Mosby, St. Louis, Mo., 1972, pp. 199–209.
48. J. Z. Krezanoski, *J. Am. Optom. Assoc., 43,* 305 (1972).
49. W. R. Bailey, *Contact Lens Society Am., 6,* 33 (1972).
50. M. J. Sibley and G. Yung, *Am. J. Optom., 50,* 710 (1973).
51. J. Sugar, *Arch. Ophthalmol., 91,* 11 (1974).
52. "Symposium on the Flexible Lens," J. L. Bitonte and R. H. Keates, Eds., C. V. Mosby, St. Louis, Mo., 1972, pp. 30–32.
53. *British Medical Journal, 3,* 254 (1972).
54. L. J. Girard, in "Corneal Contact Lenses," L. J. Girard, Ed., 2nd ed., C. V. Mosby, St. Louis, Mo., 1970, pp. 18–24.
55. F. H. Adler, in "Physiology of the Eye," 4th ed., C. V. Mosby, St. Louis, Mo., 1965, pp. 48–49.
56. I. Fatt, *Contact Lens, 14,* 3 (1972).
57. R. M. Hill and I. Fatt, *Am. J. Optom., 35,* 873 (1964).
58. J. F. Hill, *Optom. Weekly, 64,* 943 (1973).
59. R. M. Hill and I. Fatt, *Am. J. Optom., 41,* 678 (1964).
60. "Symposium on Contact Lenses," C. V. Mosby, St. Louis, Mo., 1973, pp. 65–81.
61. S. G. El Hage, C. C. Hughes, K. R. Schauer, and R. L. Harrell, *Am. J. Optom. Physiol. Optics, 51,* 24 (1974).
62. D. R. Korb, *J. Am. Optom. Assoc., 44,* 246 (1973).

63. L. Krejei and H. Krejcova, *Br. J. Ophthalmol., 57,* 675 (1973).
64. L. J. Girard, in "Corneal and Scleral Contact Lenses," L. J. Girard, Ed., C. V. Mosby, St. Louis, Mo., 1967, pp. 40–48.
65. I. J. Szekely, *S. Pharm. J., 52,* 17 (1960).
66. H. L. Gould, *Eye Ear Nose Throat Mon., 41,* 359 (1962).
67. *Contacto, 3,* 262 (1959).
68. H. W. Hind and I. J. Szekely, *Contacto, 3,* 66 (1959).
69. B. F. Rankin, *Optom. Weekly* (May 25, 1961).
70. "Soft Contact Lens," A. R. Gasset and H. E. Kaufman, Eds., C. V. Mosby, St. Louis, Mo., 1972, pp. 61–71.
71. J. C. Neil and J. J. Hanna, *Contacto, 7,* 10 (1963).
72. C. E. Watkins, *Optom. World* (Oct. 1964).
73. R. A. Koetting, *Optom. Weekly* (Oct. 1963).
74. R. A. Koetting, *Optom. Weekly, 57,* 52 (1966).
75. M. F. Obear and F. C. Winter, *Am. J. Ophthalmol., 57,* 441 (1964).
76. C. H. Winkler and J. M. Dixon, *Arch. Ophthalmol., 72,* 817 (1964).
77. J. M. Dixon, E. Lawaczeck, and C. H. Winkler, *Am. J. Ophthalmol., 54,* 461 (1962).
78. F. M. Kadetansky, T. Suie, A. D. Gracy, J. L. Bitonte, *Am. J. Ophthalmol., 57,* 255 (1964).
79. O. H. Dabezies, *Am. J. Ophthalmol., 59,* 684 (1965).
80. J. W. Bettman, Jr., *Am. J. Ophthalmol., 56,* 77 (1963).
81. F. Kapetansky, *Contacto, 9,* 6 (1965).
82. O. H. Dabezies, *Eye Ear Nose Throat Mon., 45,* 78 (Oct. 1966).
83. O. H. Dabezies and T. Naugle, *Eye Ear Nose Throat Mon., 50,* 378 (Oct. 1971).
84. M. J. Sibley and D. E. Lauck, *Contact Lens J., 8,* 10 (1974).
85. "Prescription Requirements for First Quality Contact Lenses," American National Standards Institute, New York, N.Y., 1972.
86. H. L. Gould and R. Inglima, *Eye Ear Nose Throat Mon., 43,* 39, (1964).
87. D. A. Norton, D. J. G. Davies, N. E. Richardson, B. J. Meakin, and A. Keall, *J. Pharm. Pharmacol., 26,* 841 (1974).
88. S. R. Kohn, L. Girshenfeld, and M. Barr, *J. Pharm. Sci., 52,* 967 (1963).
89. R. E. Phares, *J. Am. Optom. Assoc., 43,* 308 (1972).
90. J. Z. Krezanoski, *Ophthal. Optician, 12,* 1035 (1972).
91. "Symposium on the Flexible Lens," J. L. Bitonte and R. H. Keates, Eds., C. V. Mosby, St. Louis, Mo., 1972, pp. 205–212.
92. G. L. Cureton and N. C. Hall, *Am. J. Optom. Physiol. Optics., 51,* 406 (1974).
93. M. F. Refojo and F. J. Holly, *Contact Intracular Lens Med. J., 3,* 23 (1977).
94. J. S. Cumming and H. Karageozian, *Contacto, 19,* 8 (July 1975).
95. G. E. Lowther, *Am. J. Optom. Physiol. Optics, 54,* 76 (1977).
96. J. Z. Krezanoski, *Contact Lens Soc. Am. J., 7,* 9 (1974).
97. J. A. Baldone, *Contact Lens Med. Bull., 4,* 9 (1971).
98. J. Z. Krezanoski, *Ont. Optician, 5,* 9 (1974).
99. W. Sagan and K. N. Schwaderer, *J. Am. Optom. Assoc., 45,* 266 (1974).
100. M. S. Favero, L. A. Carson, W. W. Bond, and N. J. Peterson, *Science, 173,* 836 (1971).
101. B. R. Matas, W. H. Spencer, and T. L. Hayes, *Arch. Ophthalmol., 88,* 287 (1972).
102. "Symposium on the Flexible Lens," J. L. Bitonte and R. H. Keates, Eds., C. V. Mosby, St. Louis, Mo., 1972, pp. 222–234.
103. A. M. Charles, *J. Am. Optom. Assoc., 43,* 661 (1972).
104. A. J. Milauskas, *Am. Acad. Ophthal. Otolaryngol. Trans., 76,* 511 (1972).
105. J. C. Busschaert, J. M. Szabocsik, and R. C. Goud, *J. Am. Optom. Assoc., 45,* 700 (1974).
106. Z. Baker, R. W. Harrison, and B. R. Miller, *J. Exp. Med., 73,* 249 (1941).
107. C. G. Dunn, *Am. J. Surg., 41,* 268 (1938).
108. C. G. Dunn, *Proc. Soc. Exp. Biol. Med., 37,* 661 (1938).
109. K. C. Swan, *Am. J. Ophthalmol., 27,* 1118 (1944).
110. *Contacto, 15,* 20 (1971).
111. C. A. Lawrence, *J. Am. Pharm. Assoc. Sci. Ed., 44,* 457 (1955).
112. C. A. Lawrence, *J. Am. Pharm. Assoc. Sci. Ed., 37,* 57 (1948).
113. G. E. Meyers and C. Lefebvre, *Canad. Pharm. J., 94,* 55 (1961).
114. N. C. Hall and J. Z. Krezanoski, *N. Engl. J. Optom., 14,* 229 (1963).
115. J. H. Wakely, N. C. Hall, and J. F. Krezanoski, *Bull. Parent. Drug Assoc., 21,* 124 (1967).
116. D. P. Bixler, *Am. J. Ophthalmol., 62,* 324 (1966).
117. S. Riegelman, *Am. J. Ophthalmol., 64,* 485 (1967).
118. S. Riegelman, D. G. Vaughan, Jr., and M. Okumoto, *J. Am. Pharm. Assoc. Sci. Ed., 45,* 93 (1956).
119. H. W. Hind and F. M. Goyan, *J. Am. Pharm. Assoc. Sci. Ed., 36,* 33 (1947).
120. P. P. Hopf, *Manuf. Chemist, 24,* 444 (1953).
121. D. R. McGregor and P. R. Elliker, *Can. J. Microbiol., 4,* 499 (1958).
122. J. C. McDonald and S. Brubaker, *Am. J. Ophthalmol., 72,* 139 (1971).

Hard Lens Product Table

Product (Manufacturer)	Suggested Use	Viscosity Agent	Preservative	Other Ingredients
Adapettes (Alcon Optics)	rewetting	adsorbobase povidone	thimerosal, 0.004% edetate disodium, 0.1%	
Adapt (Alcon Optics)	preinsertion	adsorbobase hydroxyethylcellulose	thimerosal, 0.004% edetate disodium, 0.1%	
All-In-One (Rexall)	cleaning wetting soaking		edetate disodium, 0.1% thimerosal, 0.004%	
Blink-N-Clean (Allergan)	cleaning wetting	polyoxyl 40 stearate polyethylene glycol 300	chlorobutanol, 0.5%	
Cleaning and Soaking Solution (Barnes-Hind)	cleaning soaking		edetate disodium, 0.2% benzalkonium chloride, 0.01%	buffering and cleaning agents
Clean-N-Soak (Allergan)	cleaning soaking		phenylmercuric nitrate, 0.004%	cleaning agent[a]
Clens (Alcon Optics)	cleaning		benzalkonium chloride, 0.02% edetate disodium, 0.1%	cleaning agents
Clerz (Cooper Vision Pharmaceuticals)	cleaning rewetting lubricating	hydroxyethylcellulose	thimerosal, 0.001% edetate disodium, 0.1%	poloxamer 407, salts, buffers
Contactisol (Cooper Vision Pharmaceuticals)	cleaning wetting	hydroxypropyl methylcellulose, 0.7%	benzalkonium chloride, 0.01% edetate disodium, 0.01%	nonoxynol 15 salts buffers
Contique Cleaning Solution (Alcon)	cleaning		benzalkonium chloride, 0.02%	
Contique Clean-Tabs[a] (Alcon)	cleaning			cleaning agents
Contique Soaking Solution (Alcon)	soaking		benzalkonium chloride, 0.01% edetate disodium, 0.01%	
Contique Soak-Tabs[a] (Alcon)	soaking		thimerosal, 0.08% benzethonium chloride, 4%	
Contique Wetting Solution (Alcon)	wetting	hydroxypropyl methylcellulose	benzalkonium chloride, 0.004% edetate disodium, 0.025%	
d-Film Gel (Cooper Vision Pharmaceuticals)	cleaning		benzalkonium chloride, 0.025% edetate trisodium, 0.25%	poloxamer 407
duo Flow (Cooper Vision Pharmaceuticals)	cleaning soaking		edetate trisodium, 0.25% benzalkonium chloride, 0.013%	poloxamer 188
Gel Clean (Barnes-Hind)	cleaning		thimerosal, 0.004%	nonionic surfactant
hy-Flow (Cooper Vision Pharmaceuticals)	wetting	polyvinyl alcohol, 1.0% hydroxyethylcellulose, 0.6%	edetate disodium, 0.025% benzalkonium chloride, 0.01%	sodium chloride potassium chloride
LC-65 (Allergan)	cleaning		edetate disodium thimerosal, 0.001%	cleaning agents
Lens Lubricant (Bausch & Lomb)	lubricating rewetting	adsorbobase povidone	thimerosal, 0.004% edetate disodium, 0.1%	

Hard Lens Product Table, continued

Product (Manufacturer)	Suggested Use	Viscosity Agent	Preservative	Other Ingredients
Lensine 5 (Cooper Vision Pharmaceuticals)	cleaning wetting soaking	hydroxyethylcellulose polyvinyl alcohol	edetate disodium, 0.05% benzalkonium chloride, 0.01%	poloxamer 407
Lensine Extra Strength Cleaner (Cooper Vision Pharmaceuticals)	cleaning	povidone	edetate disodium, 0.1% benzalkonium chloride, 0.01%	cleaning agents
Lens-Mate (Alcon)	cleaning wetting soaking	polyvinyl alcohol hydroxypropyl methylcellulose	benzalkonium chloride, 0.1% edetate disodium, 0.01%	
Liquifilm Tears (Allergan)	wetting	polyvinyl alcohol, 1.4%	chlorobutanol, 0.5%	sodium chloride
Liquifilm Wetting Solution (Allergan)	wetting	hydroxypropyl methylcellulose polyvinyl alcohol	benzalkonium chloride, 0.004% edetate disodium	sodium chloride potassium chloride
One Solution (Barnes-Hind)	cleaning wetting soaking	not specified	edetate disodium, 0.1% benzalkonium chloride, 0.01%	cleaning agents
Ova-Nite (Milroy)	cleaning soaking		benzalkonium chloride, 0.02% edetate disodium, 0.25%	nonionic surfactant
Pre-Sert (Allergan)	wetting	polyvinyl alcohol, 3%	benzalkonium chloride, 0.004%	
Soaclens (Burton Parsons)	soaking wetting		thimerosal, <0.004% edetate disodium, 0.1%	
Soakare (Allergan)	soaking		edetate disodium, 0.25% benzalkonium chloride, 0.01%	
Soquette (Barnes-Hind)	soaking	polyvinyl alcohol	edetate disodium, 0.2% benzalkonium chloride, 0.01%	
Titan (Barnes-Hind)	cleaning		benzalkonium chloride edetate disodium	nonionic cleaner buffers
Total All-in-one Contact Lens Solution (Allergan)	cleaning wetting soaking	polyvinyl alcohol hydroxypropyl methylcellulose	benzalkonium chloride edetate disodium	sodium chloride potassium chloride dextrose
Visalens Soaking/Cleaning (Leeming)	cleaning soaking		benzalkonium chloride, 0.02% edetate disodium, 0.10%	sodium borate/boric acid buffer
Visalens Wetting Solution (Leeming)	wetting	polyvinyl alcohol hydroxypropyl methylcellulose	benzalkonium chloride, 0.01% edetate disodium, 0.10%	sodium chloride potassium chloride
Wet-Cote (Milroy)	wetting	polyvinyl alcohol hydroxyethylcellulose	edetate disodium, 0.25% benzalkonium chloride, 0.01%	sodium chloride potassium chloride
Wet-N-Soak (Allergan)	wetting soaking	polyvinyl alcohol	edetate disodium, 0.004% benzalkonium chloride, 0.004%	
Wetting and Soaking Solution (Barnes-Hind)	wetting soaking	polyvinyl alcohol povidone hydroxyethylcellulose	benzalkonium chloride, <0.005% edetate disodium, 0.1%	
Wetting Solution (Barnes-Hind)	wetting	polyvinyl alcohol, 2%	edetate disodium, 0.02% benzalkonium chloride, 0.004%	sodium chloride
Wetting Solution (Rexall)	wetting		edetate disodium, 0.01% benzalkonium chloride, 0.004%	

ᵃTablet must be dissolved in water.

Plate 1

Color Plates

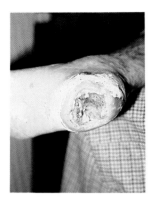

1-1 **Gangrene** of the foot is a serious and common complication of diabetes due to trauma that has gone unrecognized due to neuropathy (loss of sensation) or to vascular lesions. Eventually, trauma may lead to gangrene when the dead (necrotic) skin is removed and ulceration results (as shown). (See Chapter 13, *Diabetes Care Products.*)

1-2 **Chronic gingivitis,** an early stage of periodontitis, is an asymptomatic inflammation of the gingiva (gums) at the necks of the teeth. The gingiva is erythematous and may have areas where it is swollen and glossy in appearance. There may be mild hemorrhage when the person brushes the teeth. Gingivitis is most often due to poor oral hygiene. (See Chapter 23, *Oral Health Products.*)

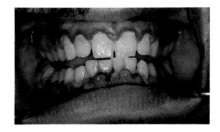

1-3 **Chronic periodontitis (pyorrhea)** is an inflammation of the tissues surrounding the teeth, including the gingiva, periodontal ligaments, alveolar bone, and the cementum (bony material covering the root of a tooth). It is due to plaque accumulation resulting from poor oral hygiene. The gingiva may be erythematous and swollen and may recede from the necks of the teeth. It is not painful and usually is accompanied by halitosis, loosening of the teeth, and mild hemorrhage when the teeth are brushed. (See Chapter 23, *Oral Health Products.*)

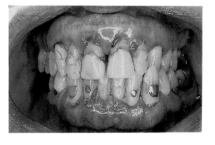

1-4 **Aphthous ulcers (canker sores)** are recurrent, painful, single or multiple ulcerations of bacterial origin. The central ulceration is sharply demarcated, often has a yellow to white surface of necrotic debris, and is surrounded by an erythematous margin. (See Chapter 23, *Oral Health Products.*)

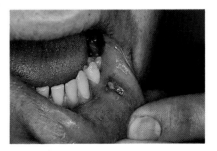

1-5 **Candidiasis (candidosis; moniliasis; thrush)** is an infection due to overgrowth of *Candida albicans.* This condition tends to occur in people with debilitating or chronic systemic disease or those on long-term antibiotic therapy. It commonly appears as a whitish-gray to yellowish, soft, slightly elevated pseudomembrane-like plaque on the oral mucosa (often described as having a "curdled-milk" appearance). A dull burning pain often is present. If the membrane is stripped away, a raw bleeding surface remains. (See Chapter 23, *Oral Health Products.*)

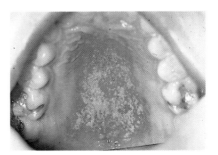

Plate 2

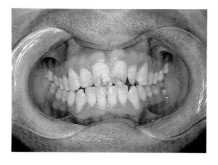

2-6 **Dental fluorosis (mottled enamel)** is due to the long-term ingestion of drinking water containing fluoride at greater than 1 ppm concentration during the time of tooth formation. The appearance of the teeth varies, depending upon the level of fluoride in the water, ranging from white flecks or spots, to brownish stains, small pits, or deep irregular pits that are dark brown in color. (See Chapter 23, *Oral Health Products*.)

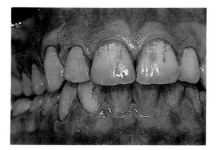

2-7 **Disclosing agents**, which stain mucinous film and plaque on teeth, are helpful to the patient in evaluation of the effectiveness of their brushing and flossing efforts. These agents, such as erythrosin (FD&C Red No. 3), will reveal the presence and extent of deposits on the teeth, which would otherwise appear clean. (See Chapter 23, *Oral Health Products*.)

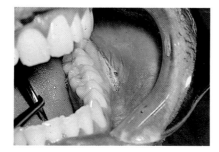

2-8 **Aspirin burn** results from the topical use of aspirin to relieve toothache. An aspirin tablet is placed against the tooth where it is held in place by pressure from the buccal (cheek) mucosa. The mucosa becomes necrotic and is characterized by a white slough that rubs away revealing a painful ulceration. (See Chapter 23, *Oral Health Products*.)

2-9 **Insect bites** are often characterized as itchy red papules in small clusters. A small overlying superficial vesicle may be present. (See Chapter 24, *Insect Sting and Bite Products*.)

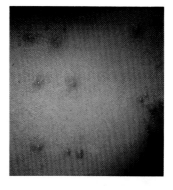

2-10 **Ticks** can attach to human skin and burrow into superficial layers. The back of the organism is usually visible on the surface with careful examination. They are vectors of several systemic diseases. (See Chapter 24, *Insect Sting and Bite Products*.)

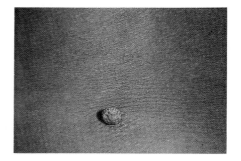

Plate 3

3-11 **Scabies** is caused by a small mite that burrows under the superficial layers of the skin. Small linear blisters, which cause intense itching, can be seen between the finger webs, inner wrists, axilla, around the areola (nipple) of the breast, and on the genitalia. (See Chapter 24, *Insect Sting and Bite Products.*)

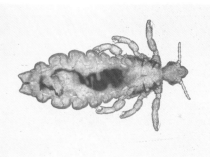

3-12A

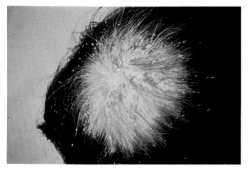

3-12B

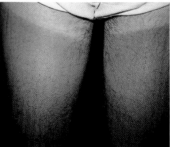

3-12 A and B **Pediculosis capitis** is a louse infestation of the scalp. Examination of the scalp hair in this infestation shows tiny nit eggs attached to the hair shaft (**A**). The organism shown is only occasionally seen (**B**). (See Chapter 24, *Insect Sting and Bite Products.*)

3-13 **Sunburn** presents as erythema (redness), reaching a peak 4–6 hours after excessive sun exposure. Severe burns can result in large blister formation. Photoprotection can be achieved for susceptible patients by proper sunscreen application. (See Chapter 25, *Burn and Sunburn Products.*)

3-14 **Cosmetic-induced photosensitivity** can be caused by ingredients in certain topical colognes and perfumes. They produce erythema (redness) locally, which leaves characteristic postinflammatory pigmentation. (See Chapter 25, *Burn and Sunburn Products.*)

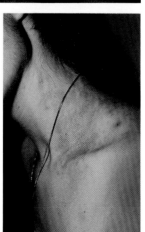

3-15 **Drug-induced photosensitivity** is a reaction that occurs on sun-exposed surfaces of the head, neck, and dorsum (back) of the hands. The erythema (redness) spares photoprotected areas (under the nose and chin, behind the ears, and between the fingers). (See Chapter 25, *Burn and Sunburn Products.*)

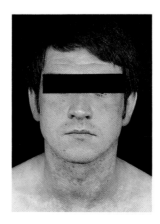

Plate 4

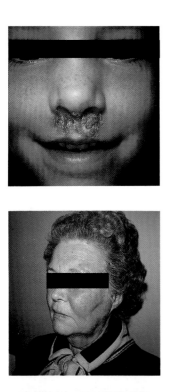

4-16 **Impetigo** is a bacterial infection identified by honeycomb crusts on erythematous bases. A bullous (blistering) form can also be seen. (See Chapter 28, *Topical Anti-infective Products.*)

4-17 **Erysipelas** is a streptococcal infection often involving the face or extremities. The infected area is red and raised with local warmth and edema. The margins are rapidly changing, often in serpiginous (irregular) patterns. (See Chapter 28, *Topical Anti-infective Products.*)

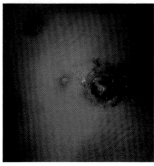

4-18 **Infections of the hair follicles** can be superficial (folliculitis). Deeper involvement is called a furuncle (small boil). A carbuncle forms when adjacent hair follicles are involved. They are usually caused by staphylococcal or streptococcal organisms. (See Chapter 28, *Topical Anti-infective Products.*)

4-19 **Paronychia** is caused by overexposure of the nails to water, causing cuticle loss and inflammation around the nail folds. About 50% of cases have candidal infection. (See Chapter 28, *Topical Anti-infective Products.*)

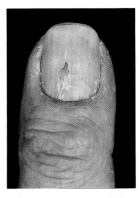

4-20 **Tinea capitis** is a fungal infection of the scalp. There is erythema (redness) and scale on the scalp with local breaking or loss of hair. (See Chapter 28, *Topical Anti-infective Products.*)

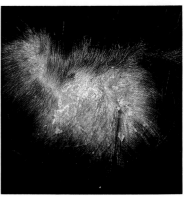

Plate 5

5–21B

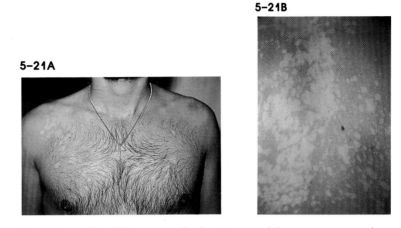

5–21A

5–21A and B **Tinea versicolor** is caused by a yeast organism that overgrows locally, resulting in hyperpigmentation or hypopigmentation (**A**). These mildly scaling eruptions characteristically occur on the chest, upper back, and arms (**B**). (See Chapter 28, *Topical Anti-infective Products.*)

5–22 **Herpes simplex** lesions of the mouth and the eye usually start as a small cluster of vesicles (tiny blisters) that subsequently heal over with a serosanguinous (blood-tinged) crust. Local stinging, burning, and pain often herald the onset of lesions. Eye involvement should always be referred to an ophthalmologist. (See Chapter 28, *Topical Anti-infective Products.*)

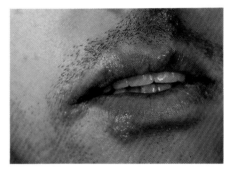

5–23B

5–23A

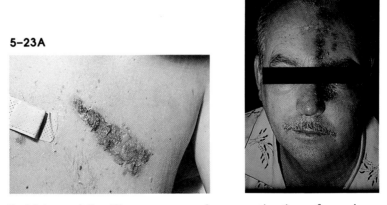

5–23A and B **Herpes zoster** is a reactivation of previous chickenpox virus that has remained latent in the nerve roots. Pain precedes small clusters of vesicles (blisters) on an erythematous base along the distribution of the infected nerve (**A**). It characteristically stops in the midline (**B**). (See Chapter 28, *Topical Anti-infective Products.*)

Plate 6

6-24 Comedonic acne (noninflammatory) occurs when follicles become plugged with sebum, forming a comedone on the surface. The black color is due to oxidation of lipid and melanin, and not dirt, as is commonly believed. (See Chapter 29, *Acne Products.*)

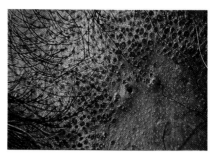

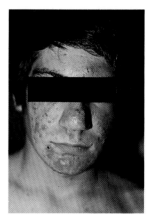

6-25 Pustular acne (inflammatory) presents as inflamed papules, which are formed when a superficial hair follicle is plugged and ruptures at a deeper level. Superficial inflammation results in pustules. Deep lesions cause large cysts to form, resulting in scars. (See Chapter 29, *Acne Products.*)

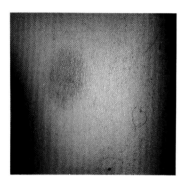

6-26 Fixed drug reaction is an adverse reaction that can appear as erythematous (red) oval patches, which recur in the same site on re-exposure to the causative drug. They resolve with characteristic tan-brown pigmentation. (See Chapter 30, *Dermatitis, Dry Skin, Dandruff, Seborrhea, and Psoriasis Products.*)

6-27A

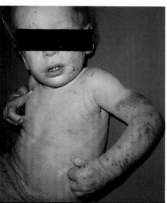

6-27A, B, and C Atopic dermatitis (eczema) is an itchy condition that occurs on the outer aspect (extensor) surface of the elbows and knees (**A**) during the first year of life and then involves predominantly the flexors (**B**). The hands, feet, and face are often involved as well as with erythema, scale, increased skin surface markings, small blisters, and crusting (**C**). Secondary infection is common. (See Chapter 30, *Dermatitis, Dry Skin, Dandruff, Seborrhea, and Psoriasis Products.*)

6-27B

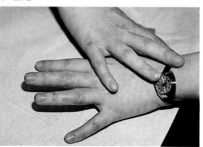

6-27C

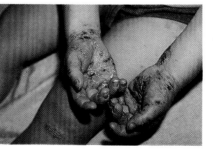

Plate 7

7-28 **Seborrhea (seborrheic dermatitis)** is a red scaling condition of the scalp, midface, and upper midchest of adults. Characteristic greasy yellow scale is seen in the eyebrows and around the folds of the nose. (See Chapter 30, *Dermatitis, Dry Skin, Dandruff, Seborrhea, and Psoriasis Products.*)

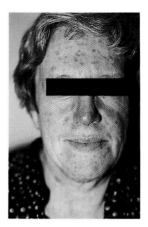

7-29A

7-29A, B, and C **Psoriasis** is a scaling condition in which erythematous plaques (red raised areas) are covered by a thick adherent scale. The borders of the lesions are well defined and vary from guttate (very small plaques) to large plaque types. **A,** guttate (small drop size); **B,** medium-sized plaques; **C,** large plaques. (See Chapter 30, *Dermatitis, Dry Skin, Dandruff, Seborrhea, and Psoriasis Products.*)

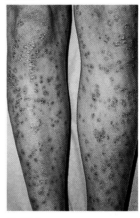

7-29B

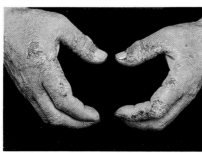

7-29C

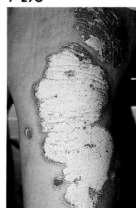

7-30A

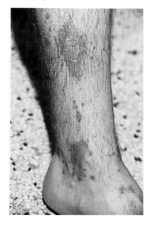

7-30B

7-30 A and B **Poison ivy** causes a linear erythema that can develop large blisters (**A,B**). Similar reactions can also be caused by poison oak and poison sumac. (See Chapter 31, *Poison Ivy and Poison Oak Products.*)

Plate 8

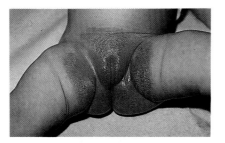

8-31 **Diaper dermatitis** presents as erythema of the groin (crease area around the genitals) and is common in infants. This case was due to a contact allergen. Contact irritants such as urine and feces along with bacterial and yeast infection may also cause problems in this area. (See Chapter 32, *Diaper Rash and Prickly Heat Products.*)

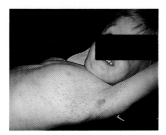

8-32 **Miliaria rubra (heat rash)** is an obstruction of sweat glands. Superficial involvement only results in a tiny vesicle (blister) on the skin surface (miliaria crystallina). When deeper inflammation is also present, the surrounding erythema (redness) is characteristic of miliaria rubra. (See Chapter 32, *Diaper Rash and Prickly Heat Products.*)

8-33 **Calluses** are thickened scales often found over pressure areas. This callus appears on the plantar surface of the foot. (See Chapter 33, *Foot Care Products.*)

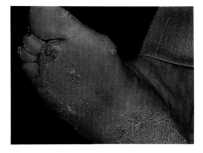

8-34 **Common warts** are lesions caused by a virus. There is a localized rough accumulation of keratin (hyperkeratosis) containing many tiny furrows. If the surface is pared, small bleeding points can be seen. (See Chapter 33, *Foot Care Products.*)

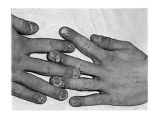

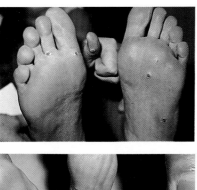

8-35 **Plantar warts,** caused by a viral infection, can often be found on the plantar surface of the foot and present with hard localized accumulations of keratin. The punctate bleeding points seen when the lesions are pared are not found in calluses. (See Chapter 33, *Foot Care Products.*)

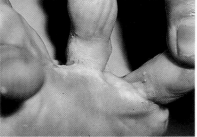

8-36 **Tinea pedis** infection of the toes characteristically starts between the fourth and fifth web space and spreads proximally. Scaling can progress to maceration with resultant small fissures. (See Chapter 33, *Foot Care Products.*)

Soft Lens Product Table

Product (Manufacturer)	Suggested Use	Viscosity Agent	Preservative	Other Ingredients
Adapettes (Alcon Optics)	lubricating rewetting	adsorbobase povidone	thimerosal, 0.004% edetate disodium, 0.1%	
Adsorbonac (Burton Parsons)	thermal disinfection			sodium chloride, 2% and 5%
BoilnSoak (Alcon Optics)	rinsing storing thermal disinfection		thimerosal, 0.001% edetate disodium, 0.1%	boric acid sodium borate sodium chloride, 0.7%
Cleaning & Disinfecting Solution (Allergan)	chemical disinfection		thimerosal, 0.002% tris (2-hydroxyethyl) tallow ammonium chloride, 0.013%	polysorbate 80 sodium bicarbonate propylene glycol sodium phosphate
Clerz (Cooper Vision)	lubricating rewetting	hydroxyethylcellulose	sorbic acid, 0.1% thimerosal, 0.001% edetate disodium	sodium chloride potassium chloride sodium borate
Daily Cleaner (Bausch & Lomb)	cleaning	hydroxyethylcellulose polyvinyl alcohol	thimerosal, 0.004% edetate disodium, 0.2%	tyloxapol sodium phosphate sodium chloride
Disinfecting Solution (Bausch & Lomb)	rinsing storage chemical disinfection		thimerosal, 0.001% chlorhexidine, 0.005% edetate disodium, 0.1%	sodium chloride sodium borate boric acid
Flex-Care (Alcon Optics)	rinsing chemical disinfection		thimerosal, 0.001% edetate disodium, 0.1% chlorhexidine, 0.005%	sodium chloride sodium borate boric acid
Flexsol (Alcon Optics)	chemical disinfection	povidine	thimerosal, 0.001% chlorhexidine, 0.005% edetate disodium, 0.1%	sodium chloride sodium borate boric acid polyoxyethylene polyoxypropylene
Hydrocare (Allergan)	thermal disinfection rinsing storing		edetate disodium, 0.01% thimerosal, 0.001%	soidum chloride boric acid sodium borate
LC-65 (Allergan)	cleaner		edetate disodium thimerosal, 0.001%	
Lens Lubricant (Bausch & Lomb)	lubricating rewetting	adsorbobase povidone	thimerosal, 0.004% edetate disodium, 0.1%	sodium chloride polyoxyethylene
Lensrins (Allergan)	thermal disinfection rinsing		thimerosal, 0.001% edetate disodium, 0.1%	sodium chloride, 0.85%
Normol (Alcon Optics)	rinsing chemical disinfection		thimerosal, 0.001% edetate disodium, 0.1% chlorhexidine, 0.005%	sodium chloride sodium borate boric acid
Permasol (Cooper Vision)	thermal disinfection rinsing		sorbic acid, 0.1% thimerosal, 0.001% edetate disodium	boric acid sodium borate sodium chloride potassium chloride poloxamer 407

Soft Lens Product Table, continued

Product	Use			
Pliagel (Cooper Vision)	cleaning		sorbic acid, 0.25% edetate trisodium	poloxamer 407 sodium chloride potassium chloride
Preflex (Alcon Optics)	cleaning	hexylethylcellulose polyvinyl alcohol	edetate disodium, 0.02% thimerosal, 0.004%	sodium phosphate sodium chloride tyloxapol
Preserved Saline Solution (Bausch & Lomb)	thermal disinfection rinsing storing		thimerosal, 0.001% edetate disodium, 0.1%	boric acid sodium borate sodium chloride
Saline Solution (Allergan)	thermal disinfection rinsing		thimerosal, 0.001% edetate disodium	boric acid sodium borate sequestering agent
Salt Tablets (Blairex)	thermal disinfection rinsing			sodium chloride
Soflens Tablets (Allergan)	weekly protein cleaner			stabilized papain
Soft Care (Barnes-Hind)	rinsing storage chemical disinfection	povidone	thimerosal, 0.001% edetate disodium, 0.1% chlorhexidine gluconate, 0.005%	sodium chloride borate buffer octylphenoxyethanols
Soft Mate Cleaning Solution (Barnes-Hind)	cleaning	hydroxyethylcellulose	thimerosal, 0.004% edetate disodium	sodium chloride tyloxapol
Soft Mate Disinfecting Solution (Barnes-Hind)	chemical disinfection storage	povidone	thimerosal, 0.001% edetate disodium, 0.1% chlorhexidine gluconate, 0.005%	sodium chloride octylphenoxyethanols
Soft Mate Rinsing Solution (Barnes-Hind)	rinsing with chemical disinfection		thimerosal, 0.001% edetate disodium, 0.1% chlorhexidine gluconate, 0.005%	sodium chloride borate buffer
Soft Mate Thermal (Barnes-Hind)	rinsing storage thermal disinfection		thimerosal, 0.001% edetate disodium, 0.1%	sodium chloride boric acid sodium borate
Unisol (Cooper Vision)	rinsing thermal disinfection			sodium chloride sodium borate boric acid
Unpreserved Saline Solution (Alcon Optics)	rinsing storage thermal disinfection			sodium borate boric acid sodium chloride

23 Oral Health Products

John A. Walker and Dennis K. Helling

Questions to Ask the Patient

How long have you had this dental problem? Have you seen a dentist about the problem? When?

Is the problem painful or severe? Is the pain continuous, dull, and/or deep? Is it triggered by hot and cold substances or chewing?

Are there any prior events such as trauma associated with the pain?

Are there any other symptoms associated with the pain? Do you have a cold or sinus or ear infection?

Are your teeth loose? Do your gums bleed when you brush your teeth?

Does the condition produce continuous bad breath?

How do you clean your teeth or dentures? How often? Do you use dental floss?

How often do you see your dentist? Do you use supplemental fluoride in one form or another? Is your water fluoridated?

Do you wear dentures? Are your dentures loose? Do they cause sore spots?

Is the sore visible, and is there a pus discharge? Do you have a fever? Is the sore white in color?

Do you suffer from any chronic medical illnesses such as diabetes mellitus, rheumatic heart condition, asthma, epilepsy, or high blood pressure? Do you have a pacemaker?

What medication(s) are you taking?

Do you have any allergies to foods or medicines? What are they?

In 1976, the Department of Health, Education, and Welfare's Committee on Nutrition indicated that dental caries is the most prevalent disease of all age groups beyond infancy (1). Periodontal disease causes the greatest loss of teeth in the United States and accounts for approximately 70% of tooth loss; caries, direct trauma, and orthodontic extraction account for only 30% of tooth loss. It has been estimated by the U.S. Health Interview Survey that more than 22.6 million people in the United States are edentulous (without natural dentition). In addition, approximately 1 billion dollars are spent annually on oral hygiene products in the United States (2). It becomes clear from these statistics that dental disease is one of the most frequently encountered health care problems in the United States, and a great deal of health care dollars are spent on prevention as well as treatment of dental disease.

The American Dental Association considers the professional pharmacist an integral team member in the prevention and treatment of dental disease (3). The pharmacist sees more patients with dental problems than the average dentist (4). It should be a common goal of dentistry and pharmacy to reduce tooth loss and dental disease and to eliminate these conditions by patient education and improved therapies.

This chapter provides pharmacists with basic information concerning common dental problems, patient counseling, when to make necessary referrals to dentists, and when to recommend appropriate nonprescription dental hygiene and treatment products. Specific dental problems to be discussed include: caries, periodontal disease, oral and perioral ulcers, damaged or misfitting prosthesis and teeth, and other common oral disorders.

Dental Anatomy and Physiology

The teeth and supporting structures are necessary for the normal functions of mastication and articulation and for esthetic appearance. Normally, people are provided with two sets of teeth—the primary or deciduous dentition, followed by the permanent dentition. The primary dentition first appears at approximately 6 months of age with the eruption of the mandibular (lower jaw) central incisor and is usually complete with the eruption of the upper second molars by approximately 24 months (Figure 1). There are 20 deciduous teeth, 10 in each arch. Generally, the permanent dentition initially appears with the eruption of the mandibular first molar behind the deciduous second molar at approximately 6 years and continues in a regular pattern replacing shedding deciduous teeth. The last permanent teeth to erupt into the oral cavity are the permanent third molars (wisdom teeth) between 17 and 21 years of age.

Anatomically, the teeth are grossly viewed as having two parts, the crown and the roots (Figure 2). The roots are normally below the gingival (gum) line and are essential for support and attachment of the tooth with the surrounding tissues. The crown is above the gingival line and is the part of the tooth responsible for mastication. The teeth are comprised of four basic components that make up the crown and root. These are the enamel, the dentin, the cementum, and the pulp.

Enamel is comprised of very hard, crystalline calcium salts (hydroxyapatite) and covers the crown of the tooth to the cementoenamel junction. Enamel protects the underlying tooth structure and serves as the surface material of the crown that withstands the wear of mastication. Dentin lies beneath the enamel and comprises the largest part of the tooth structure. Dentin is softer than enamel. Its tubules enable transport of nutrients from the dental pulp. The dentin protects the dental pulp from mechanical, thermal, and chemical irritation.

The pulp occupies the pulpal cavity and is continuous with the tissues surrounding the tooth by means of

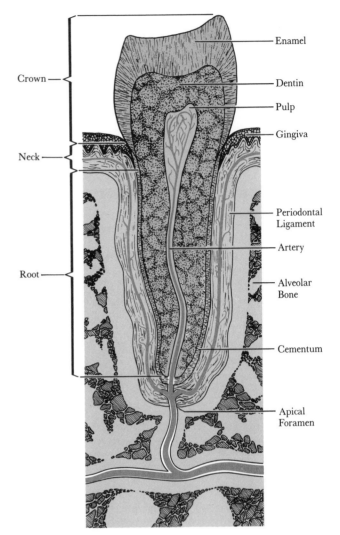

Figure 2. Anatomy of the tooth.

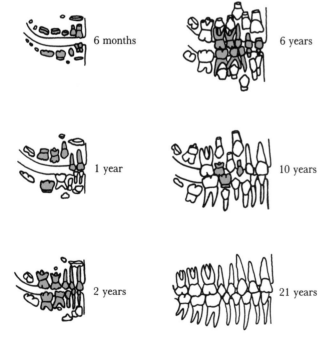

Figure 1. Stages of formation and eruption of deciduous and permanent dentition.

an opening at the apex of the root called the apical foramen. The pulp consists of mostly vascular and neural tissues. The only type of nerve endings in the pulp are free nerve endings; any type of stimulus to the pulp is interpreted as pain.

The bone-like cementum is softer than dentin and covers the root of the tooth, extending from the cementoenamel junction. The major function of cementum is to provide attachment of the tooth with the periodontal ligament via periodontal fibers. The cementum is considered to be one of the four major components of the periodontium or supporting tooth structures.

The periodontium includes the cementum, periodontal ligament, the encompassing alveolar bone, and the gingiva. The periodontal ligament is connective tissue and provides attachment of the tooth to surrounding alveolar bone and gingival tissue. The four functions of the periodontal ligament are supportive, formative, sensory, and nutritive.

The alveolar bone forms the sockets of the teeth. Alveolar bone is thin, spongy bone and attaches to the principal fibers of the periodontal ligament.

Gingiva (gum tissue) is the soft tissue surrounding the teeth and is firmly attached to the underlying alveolar bone. It is normally pink and is keratinized. The gingiva is attached to the cementum by the gingival group of periodontal ligament fibers.

Dentistry is concerned not only with the dentition and its immediately surrounding and supporting tissues, but also with the other oral and extraoral tissues involved in pathologic processes of the head and neck. A thorough dental exam often includes examination of all intraoral tissue including the pharynx, tongue, hard and soft palates, floor of the mouth, vestibule (between the alveolar ridge and cheek), buccal (cheek) tissue, and salivary glands.

The mucosa covering the pharyngeal region, soft palate, floor of the mouth, vestibule, and cheeks is normally more pinkish-red than the gingiva. The outer surface of the mucosa is stratified squamous epithelium but does not have a keratinized stratum corneum outer layer as does the gingiva, which accounts for the difference in color.

The tongue is important in the function of mastication, swallowing, taste, and articulation of speech. The dorsal or upper surface of the tongue is usually irregular and rough in appearance. Taste buds are usually small, oval-shaped organs of flat epithelial cells surrounding a small opening (taste pore). Taste buds are in fungiform papilla, on the surface of and surrounding circumvallate papilla at various locations of the tongue. The epithelium covering the tongue is keratinized, especially at the crest of the filiform papilla.

The major salivary glands are the parotid, submaxillary, and sublingual salivary glands. They are responsible for secretion of saliva, which is an alkaline, slightly viscous, clear secretion containing enzymes (lysozymes and ptyalin), serum albumin, epithelial mucin (a mucopolysaccharide), immune globulin, leukocytes, and minerals. Normal salivary gland function is essential for good oral health.

The dental practitioner is also trained to examine perioral and extraoral tissues, such as the lips, the angles of the mouth, the symmetry of the head and neck, and palpation of the lymph nodes of the region (Figure 3).

Etiology and Pathophysiology of Common Oral Problems

Dental Caries

Dental caries formation requires growth and implantation of cariogenic microorganisms (*Streptococcus mutans, Streptococcus sanguis, Lactobacillus casei,* and *Actinomyces viscosus*) on exposed surfaces. If oral hygiene is neglected, dental plaques containing these organisms remain on the tooth surfaces, allowing the carious process to continue.

Diet and other personal habits constitute other factors in caries development. Foods with a high concentration of refined sugar (sucrose) are strongly cariogenic. Sucrose is converted by bacterial plaque into volatile acids (lactic, pyruvic, acetic, propionic, and butyric acids), which attack, dissolve, and solubilize the calcium salts found in tooth structure (5). Unfortunately, sugar-containing foods are highly popular with the young age group in which the greatest susceptibility to caries occurs. Saccharin-containing food substitutes probably help in this regard, but because of safety questions concerning saccharin, their future use is questionable. Other sugar substitutes may help to curb sugar-hungry appetites (6).

Excessive sugar intake is not the only source of dental caries. Other types of fermentable carbohydrates, such as fructose (found in fruit) and lactose (found in milk), also are cariogenic but to a far lesser extent than sucrose (7). Also, except during pregnancy and childhood, ingesting dairy products or other calcium-rich foods has little or no effect on prevention of caries in fully developed teeth.

The pathophysiology of dental caries is basically one of demineralization caused by organic acids, such as lactic acid, produced (usually anaerobically) by microorganisms resident in dental plaque. This demineralization is actually chronic in nature with a carious lesion starting slowly on the enamel surface and initially exhibiting no clinical symptoms. Once the demineralization progresses through the enamel to the softer dentin, the destruction is much more rapid and becomes clinically evident as a carious lesion. At this point, the patient can become aware of the process by visualization or by symptoms of sensitivity (toothache) to stimuli, such as heat, cold, or percussion. If untreated, the carious lesion can result in damage to the dental pulp itself (with continuous pain as a common symptom) and eventually necrosis of the vital pulp tissue. Since an opening exists between the pulp and surrounding supporting tissues via the apical foramen, the infectious process can progress apically and result in bone loss, abscesses, cellulitis, or osteomyelitis.

Plaque

The accumulation of dental plaque is very much associated with dental caries and periodontal disease. Plaque is thought to start with the formation of acquired pellicle on a clean tooth surface. Pellicle appears to be a thin, acellular, glycoprotein-mucoprotein coating that adheres to the enamel within minutes after cleaning a tooth. Its source is thought to be saliva. The pellicle seems to serve as an attachment for cariogenic bacteria that produce, along with acids, long-chain polymers such as dextrans and levans that adhere to the pellicle and tooth surface. This sticky adherent mass is called dental plaque.

Food residue after meals may be incorporated into plaque by bacterial degradation. Left unchecked, the plaque thickens and bacteria proliferate (4). Dental plaque, if not removed within 24 hours, calcifies (calculus, or tartar) by calcium salt precipitation from the saliva; calculus is removable only by professional dental cleaning (8). Plaque is commonly recognized as the source of microbes that cause caries and periodontitis;

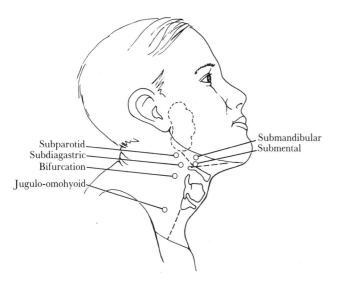

Figure 3. Major lymph node areas of the neck.

thus plaque buildup is related to incidence of oral disease.

The best way to promote dental health is to remove plaque buildup by mechanical means, mainly by brushing and flossing regularly. Chewing gum or eating fibrous foods, such as celery or carrots, does not prevent plaque accumulation or aid in its removal (9).

Fractured Dentition, Restorations, and Dentures

Broken natural dentition is correctable only by a dental practitioner. Besides being esthetically unappealing (especially if it involves an anterior tooth), broken teeth can result in pulp exposure, irritation to adjacent soft tissues, pain, malocclusion, rapid carious breakdown, compromised mastication, or infection. If a tooth's crown is chipped to a minor degree, restorative materials and techniques can often repair the defect adequately. However, a large fracture may require endodontic treatment (root canal therapy), difficult restorative procedures, or extraction of the tooth.

Fractured or Misfitting Restorations and Dentures

Loose, displaced, or broken dental restorations (fillings) and nonremovable prostheses (crowns and bridges) can be evaluated and treated adequately only by a dentist. Loss of normal function, tooth breakdown, and malocclusion are just some consequences of fillings or crowns and bridges in need of repair.

Loose, misfitting, or broken removable dental prosthesis (partial or full dentures) likewise cause serious consequences. Ill-fitting or broken dentures can contribute to the following list of sequelae: accelerated bone loss, ulceration, irritation, tumorous growths, and compromised oral function. To refit, reline, or repair dentures to ensure proper functioning requires professional dental treatment.

Periodontal Disease

Gingivitis and periodontitis have been classified many different ways (10). Only the more common forms of chronic gingivitis and periodontitis are discussed.

Chronic Gingivitis

Chronic gingivitis (inflammation of the gingiva) left untreated is a common precursor to the more advanced inflammatory condition of chronic destructive periodontal disease or periodontitis. Periodontitis is the inflammation and destruction of the periodontium. The etiology of chronic gingivitis is thought to be associated with the presence of microorganisms in the plaque in the gingival sulcus (space between the gingiva and tooth). These organisms are capable of producing harmful products such as acids, toxins, and enzymes that damage cellular and intercellular tissue. Dilatation of gingival capillaries, proliferation of capillaries, and increased blood flow with resultant erythema (redness) of the gingiva are found in early stages of chronic gingivitis. (See *Plate 1-2*.) In time, the capillaries become engorged, venous return is slowed, and localized anoxemia causes a bluish hue to areas of the reddened gingiva. The gingiva may also increase in size, appear swollen, and change shape as a result of the inflammation. The presence of red cells in extravascular tissue and the breakdown of hemoglobin also deepen the color of the gingival tissue. The gingiva may bleed readily when probed or during toothbrushing. The progression of these events is usually slow and often painless to the patient.

Chronic gingivitis may be localized to one or several teeth or generalized, meaning the gingiva around all of the teeth is involved. The inflammation may involve just the marginal gingiva (the border of the gingiva surrounding the neck of the tooth) or may be more diffuse and involve all of the gingival tissue surrounding the tooth. Changes in gingival color, size, shape, and ease of gingival bleeding are common indications of chronic gingivitis that the patient as well as the pharmacist can recognize.

Gingival Disease in Pregnancy

Gingival disease in pregnancy or "pregnancy gingivitis" is caused by local factors as in nongravid patients. No significant gingival changes are seen in pregnancy when oral hygiene is good and local irritants are absent. Pregnancy is thought to modify gingivitis but is not causal. Gingivitis usually becomes more severe in the second or third month of pregnancy and is most severe by the eighth month. Inflammatory edema and discoloration of gingiva increase during pregnancy, and there is an increased tendency for the gingiva to bleed. The condition is usually painless. The severity of the gingivitis will decrease post partum, returning to prepregnancy levels after approximately 1 year.

Acute Necrotizing Ulcerative Gingivitis

Acute necrotizing ulcerative gingivitis (ANUG), also referred to as "Vincent's stomatitis" and "trench mouth," is characterized by necrosis and ulceration of the gingival surface with underlying inflammation. The disease most commonly starts in the gingiva between teeth and displays "punched out" papilla (the raised interproximal gingiva). Spirochete and fusiform bacteria proliferate and invade the gingiva (11). The interdental and marginal gingiva exhibit a necrotic and grayish slough, while the adjacent gingiva usually exhibits marked erythema. The disease may involve a single tooth or group of teeth, or the entire oral cavity. Accompanying symptoms often include severe pain, bleeding gingival tissue, halitosis, foul taste, and increased salivation. Lymphadenopathy, fever, and malaise accompany the disease less frequently.

Acute necrotizing ulcerative gingivitis is seen most frequently in the United States in teenagers and young adults (12). Several predisposing factors have been associated with the disease: anxiety and emotional stress, smoking, malnutrition, and poor oral hygiene (12). The association between the disease and these predisposing factors is not clear. Contrary to some articles in the literature, acute necrotizing ulcerative gingivitis has not been demonstrated to be communicable (12, 13). The precise cause of acute necrotizing ulcerative gingivitis is not known; however, it seems to be associated with spirochete and fusiform organisms (12, 13). Although acute necrotizing ulcerative gingivitis has been reported to go into remission spontaneously without treatment, it can result in progressive tissue destruction, septicemia, and serious systemic sequelae (13).

Periodontitis

Chronic destructive periodontal disease can be classified as periodontitis, trauma from occlusion, and periodontal atrophy (10). Periodontitis is subdivided into simple, compound, and juvenile. Juvenile periodontitis can either be generalized or localized (periodontosis).

Periodontitis is the most common type of periodontal disease and usually results from chronic gingivitis. Simple periodontitis is associated with inflammation alone and commonly features erythematous and chronically inflamed gingiva, periodontal pocket formation (a pathologic deepening of the sulcus), and alveolar bone loss around the tooth. Teeth may become mobile and migrate (move from their normal position). As in gingivitis, simple periodontitis may involve a single tooth, groups of teeth, or all teeth. (See *Plate 1-3.*) Advanced stages of simple periodontitis occur most frequently between 50 and 70 years of age, although the disease may occur at any age (10). Simple periodontitis is often painless but may exhibit sensitivity or pain to thermal changes, food, tactile stimulation, or impaction of debris into the periodontal pockets. Throbbing and acute, severe pain in conjunction with periodontitis results from periodontal abscesses or pulpitis secondary to carious destruction of exposed root surfaces (10).

Compound periodontitis is clinically similar to simple periodontitis. However, compound periodontitis usually progresses more rapidly, exhibits angular rather than horizontal bone loss, exhibits widening of the periodontal ligament space more commonly, and exhibits tooth mobility earlier than simple periodontitis. Compound periodontitis is thought to result not only from inflammatory responses associated with dental plaque, as in simple periodontitis, but also from traumatic occlusion (harmful forces exerted on teeth from teeth in the opposing dental arch).

The juvenile forms of periodontitis are much less common and are poorly understood. Generalized juvenile periodontitis has been associated with childhood systemic conditions, such as Papillon-Lefevre syndrome, Down's syndrome, agranulocytosis, leukemia, and diabetes. Clinically, it exhibits gingival inflammation and purulent exudate, which results in bone loss around the entire dentition, tooth mobility, and migration.

Localized juvenile periodontitis is also referred to as periodontosis. The underlying etiology is unknown. There are, however, microbiologic and immunologic differences and striking clinical differences between periodontosis and adult periodontitis (14, 15). Clinically, periodontosis usually affects patients between puberty and 25 years of age (10). Incisors in both dental arches are affected first and most severely, but destruction can become generalized. Often there is minimal gingival inflammation, but there is rapid and severe vertical bone loss, deep pocket formation, and mobility and migration of incisors and first molars. Later symptoms secondary to exposed root surfaces include periodontal abscesses and regional lymphadenopathy (swelling of lymph nodes in the area). Teeth are often exfoliated (fall out) as a result of the destruction of supportive tissues.

Common Oral Sores

Canker Sores

"Canker sores," also referred to as recurrent aphthous ulcers (RAU) or recurrent aphthous stomatitis (RAS), affect approximately 20–50% of Americans (16). The cause of aphthous ulcers is unknown; however, evidence suggests that the ulcers may result from a hypersensitivity to antigenic components of pleomorphic *Streptococcus sanguis* (17–21). Evidence also suggests that cell-mediated immunity may play a role in causing aphthous ulcers. Lymphocytes from patients with aphthous lesions are cytotoxic to mucosal epithelial cells in vitro (21–23). There appears to be a familial factor in aphthous ulcers. Offspring with one or both parents with a history of aphthous ulcers are more likely to suffer from aphthous ulcers themselves (21). Emotional and physiologic factors also have been associated with exacerbations and remissions of oral aphthous ulcers (24), but these relationships are poorly understood and not universal.

Symptomatically, aphthous lesions can appear on any nonkeratinized mucosal surface in the mouth, such as the lips, buccal mucosa, tongue, floor of the mouth, or soft palate (25). Patients may experience a burning or itching sensation preceding the actual appearance of an aphthous lesion. Patients may experience a single lesion or as many as 30 or more. Most aphthous lesions persist for 10–14 days and heal without scarring (20).

Canker sores usually range from 3 to 5 mm in diameter; however, several lesions may coalesce to form larger, irregularly shaped lesions. Individual aphthous lesions are usually round or oval in shape and are either flat or crater-like in appearance. (See *Plate 1-4.*) The color is usually gray to grayish-yellow with an erythematous halo of inflamed tissue surrounding the ulcer. The lesions can be very painful and can inhibit normal eating, drinking, talking, and swallowing functions. Though many patients have recurrent episodes of oral lesions with periods of remission (no lesions), some patients may chronically experience one or more lesions in the mouth for very long periods. There usually is no fever or lymphadenopathy with aphthous lesions although these symptoms arise if the ulcerations become secondarily infected.

Cold Sores

"Cold sores" or "fever blisters" are caused by the herpes simplex type 1 virus and are referred to as herpes simplex labialis because they most commonly occur on the lip or areas bordering the lip. They are recurrent, often arising in the same location repeatedly. The lesions are painful and cosmetically objectionable. Patients who suffer from herpes labialis are thought to have been primarily infected with herpesvirus (21, 25). Patients may or may not relate a history of primary herpetic stomatitis. Most primary oral infections of herpes seem to be subclinical and, therefore, most patients are unaware of the previous primary exposure (25). The primary infection, historically, has been reported most frequently in childhood; however, it is now estimated that 15% of adults experience the primary infection (21). After the primary infection, the virus apparently remains in host cells. These "resident" viruses are thought to be responsible for recurrent herpes labialis.

Symptomatically, cold sores often are preceded by a prodrome, when the patient notices burning, itching, or numbness in the area of the forthcoming lesion. The lesion first becomes visible as small red papules of fluid-containing vesicles 1–3 mm in diameter. Often many lesions coalesce to form a much larger area of involvement. An erythematous border around the vesicles may or may not be present. A mature lesion often has a crust over the top of many coalesced, burst vesicles. The base of the lesion is erythematous. The presence of pustules or pus under the crust of a cold sore may indicate a possible secondary bacterial infection. Cold sores are self-limiting and heal without scarring, usually within 10–14 days. The recurrence rate and extent of lesions vary greatly from patient to patient. Some patients may experience several large lesions every few weeks; other patients may only have a single small lesion perhaps once a year. Patients often will associate predisposing factors such as sun or wind exposure, fever, systemic disease (colds and flu), or trauma with the onset of cold sores.

Herpesvirus type 1 is contagious and thought to be transmissible by direct contact since the virus does not live outside the host environment (26). Saliva, stratum corneum cells, and mucosal secretions may serve to transmit the virus from patient to patient (21, 26). Herpes simplex type 2 virus, which is the cause of genital lesions and a very common venereal disease, has been demonstrated in herpes lesions of the lip (27).

Common Oral Infections

Dentopyogenic Infections

Dentopyogenic infections are pus-producing infections that are associated with a tooth or its supporting structures (gingiva, periodontal ligament, cementum, and alveolar bone) (24). The symptoms of these infections vary greatly, from mildly symptomatic to fever, malaise, swelling, erythema, warmth at the infection site, and septic shock. The symptoms and severity of these infections are determined by several factors. The anatomic features of the infection site, local and systemic host resistance, virulence of the causative organism(s), and time between onset of infection and treatment all play a part in the clinical presentation. Dentopyogenic infections range in severity from small, well-localized abscesses with no systemic signs of infection to a diffuse, rapidly spreading cellulitis or osteomyelitis with a high morbidity and mortality. Patients with severe symptoms associated with dentopyogenic infections usually seek dental attention as soon as possible; however, patients with minimal symptoms may unwisely delay dental treatment and try self-treatment.

There are four common dental abscesses: periapical abscess, periodontal abscess, pericoronal abscess, and subperiosteal abscess. A periapical abscess, located around the apex of a tooth root, originates from a necrotic, infected dental pulp and gains access to the periapical area by the apical foramen. The two most common causes of dental pulp infection and necrosis and a subsequent periapical abscess are dental caries that expose the pulp to oral bacteria and trauma that causes a decrease or stoppage of blood flow to and/or from the pulp.

A periodontal abscess is usually a result of periodontitis. Periodontitis leads to destruction of supporting tooth structures and the subsequent formation of deep periodontal pockets. The bacteria associated with periodontitis move toward the apex of the tooth within the deepening pocket. The accumulated bacteria within this pocket form an abscess in surrounding tissue if host resistance decreases or if the bacteria are forced into the surrounding tissue from occlusion of the pocket or trauma.

Pericoronal abscesses are most frequently associated with mandibular third molars (lower wisdom teeth). Mandibular third molars in the process of erupting or those that do not fully erupt often have gingiva covering a portion of the crown. This gingival tissue can be traumatized by the opposing upper third molar when the patient bites down. Food, bacteria, and debris also collect beneath this flap of gingiva, and an abscess in the tissue surrounding the lower molar results.

A subperiosteal abscess is a bone abscess located beneath the thin connective tissue covering (periosteum) of the bone surrounding or underlying a tooth socket. These infections are most common after extraction of a tooth.

Dentopyogenic abscesses are usually mixed bacterial infections containing more than one species of microorganisms (24, 28–30). Hundreds of different organisms have been isolated from oral abscesses. The most frequently occurring organisms isolated have been facultative gram-positive cocci (*viridans* group *Streptococcus* species and others) and anaerobic gram-negative rods (including *Bacteroides* species) (24, 28–29).

These oral abscesses, even if well-localized and seemingly not serious, may progress to more severe acute or chronic infections. They usually require dental surgical intervention with or without antibiotic therapy.

Candidiasis

Candida is a true fungus and is found as normal flora in the GI tract and oral cavity in a high percentage of patients (32, 33). *Candida albicans* is by far the most common opportunistic pathogen associated with oral infections. There are three morphologic forms: the yeast cell, hypha, and mycelium. The mycelial form is the pathologic form found in oral candidiasis infections.

Symptomatically, oral candidiasis appears commonly in one of four forms: acute pseudomembranous candidiasis, acute atrophic candidiasis, chronic hyperplastic candidiasis, or chronic atrophic candidiasis (22). The acute pseudomembranous form is often referred to as "thrush" and is characterized by white, "milk curd"-appearing plaques that are attached to the oral mucosa. These plaques usually can be detached easily, displaying erythematous, bleeding, sore areas beneath them. (See *Plate 1-5.*) "Thrush" is most common in infants, pregnant women, and debilitated patients.

Acute atrophic candidiasis, sometimes referred to as "antibiotic tongue" or "antibiotic sore mouth," is characterized by erythematous, painful, sometimes bleeding areas of the mouth. The entire upper surface of the tongue or the entire oral cavity may be involved. This form is thought to be similar to the thrush form but without the white plaques.

Chronic hyperplastic candidiasis most commonly appears as firm, well-attached, persistent, white plaques on the cheeks, tongue, palate, or lips. Unlike the thrush form, these plaques cannot be detached, are resistant to treatment, and are usually painless. This form of oral candidiasis is sometimes referred to as "Candida leukoplakia" or "speckled leukoplakia" (35).

Chronic atrophic candidiasis, sometimes referred to as "denture stomatitis" or "denture sore mouth," is commonly found in patients with full or partial dentures (36). Symptomatically, this form is characterized by generalized inflammation of the denture-bearing area. The tissue may be erythematous and edematous with soreness or a burning sensation, or the tissue may be granular in appearance (34). Inflammation secondary to the trauma of ill-fitting dentures is usually localized to the specific area of trauma; inflammation secondary to *Candida* is generalized to the entire denture-bearing tissue area. It appears that the *Candida* organisms adhere to the denture material or reside in pores of the denture material (37–41). Failure to remove the denture at bedtime and to clean the denture regularly worsens this condition. Angular cheilitis (inflammation of the corners of the mouth) is commonly associated with chronic atrophic candidiasis and other forms of oral candidiasis (34, 36). Cultures of these angular cheilitis lesions frequently are positive for *Candida albicans* and *Staphylococcus aureus* (36, 42, 43).

Candidiasis is often called "the disease of the diseased" because it appears in debilitated patients and patients taking a variety of drugs. Associated predisposing factors include:

- **Physiologic factors**—early infancy, pregnancy, and old age;
- **Endocrine disorders**—diabetes mellitus, hypothyroidism, hypoparathyroidism, and hypoadrenalism;
- **Malnutrition and malabsorption syndromes**—iron-deficiency anemia, pernicious anemia, postgastrectomy, and alcoholism;
- **Malignant diseases**—leukemias and agranulocytopenia and granulocytopenia;
- **Drugs causing depression of defense mechanism**—immunosuppressives, corticosteroids, and cytotoxics and radiation therapy;
- **Drugs commonly causing xerostomia**—anticholinergics, antidepressants, antipsychotics, antihypertensives, and antihistamines;
- **Other changes in host environment**—trauma, chemical damage, postoperative states, radiation therapy, and antibiotics and anti-infectives.

Halitosis

Halitosis, also called fetor oris, is an offensive odor emanating from the oral cavity. Unlike caries, periodontal disease, ANUG, and the other oral pathology in this section, halitosis is a symptom of a disease process or problem. Foul breath can be a useful diagnostic aid, as in the case of ANUG. The sources of halitosis are many, and it should be determined if the source is oral or nonoral. Common oral causes of halitosis include odoriferous food particles, debris, or plaque-coated tongue. These can be the result of poor oral or denture hygiene, ANUG, caries, postsurgical states, extraction wounds, purulent infections, chronic periodontitis, and smoking. Common nonoral sources of halitosis include pulmonary disease such as purulent lung infections, tuberculosis, bronchiectasis, sinusitis, tonsillitis, and rhinitis. Other common nonoral causes of halitosis include the elimination of chemical substances from the blood through the lungs upon exhalation. Examples include alcoholic breath, acetone breath in severely hyperglycemic diabetics, and foul breath from dimethyl sulfoxide use.

Oral Cancer

Oral cancer is of major concern even though it occurs less frequently than periodontitis, caries, aphthous ulcers, and other oral problems. Among the many types of oral and perioral neoplasms are squamous cell carcinomas, basal cell carcinomas, melanomas, sarcomas, spindle cell carcinomas, and carcinoma in situ. Clinically, these carcinomas can appear as red or white lesions, ulcerations, or tumors. As with other carcinomas, the cause of oral and perioral carcinomas is unknown. However, the use of alcohol and tobacco (cigarettes, cigars, pipes, chewing tobacco, and snuff) have been shown to increase the risk of oral cancer.

Patient Assessment

Pharmacists should be able to recognize common oral problems and give appropriate guidance to patients. An effort to determine the severity or potential severity of oral complaints must be made when helping and advising patients. To assess an oral problem and aid in proper treatment, the pharmacist can use visual observation and the patient's verbal history to evaluate signs and symptoms. The pharmacist needs to gather as much useful information as possible from the patient concerning the oral problem and evaluate this information with his or her knowledge of oral conditions before counseling the patient.

Pain is one symptom that can accompany all common oral problems. Questioning the patient about pain and associating it with other symptoms helps the pharmacist better understand the problem. Tooth pain triggered or worsened by heat, cold, or percussion is often indicative of a pulpal response to deep carious lesions or a cracked or broken tooth. Continuous tooth pain may indicate pulpal infection and necrosis, an abscess, or serious periodontal disease. Continuous "soreness" or pain, associated with soft tissues of the mouth and which is more severe upon eating or drinking, is a common complaint with canker sores and acute atrophic candidiasis. Pain along the gingival ridge under a denture indicates the common problems of ill-fitting dentures or denture stomatitis candidiasis. These different features of pain indicate different underlying problems.

Visual signs are helpful in evaluating a patient's oral complaint. The color, shape, and location of various anomalies help in assessing the oral problem. Some examples of color changes include the white plaques of thrush, the erythema associated with the margins of canker and cold sores, and the gingival erythema associated with periodontitis. The irregular shape of coalesced cold sore vesicles, the swelling and asymmetrical shape of a patient's face due to an oral abscess, and the large defect left by a dislodged dental restoration are examples of changes in shape that can aid in evaluating an oral problem. Recurrent oral sores on nonkeratinized oral mucosa (such as canker sores), recurrent vesicular sores on the skin bordering the lip (cold sores), and inflammation under seldom-cleaned dentures (denture stomatitis) are examples of locational clues that can help define oral problems.

Patients' oral hygiene habits and frequency of dental care should be evaluated. If patients admit to poor oral hygiene and infrequent dental care, this can greatly increase the likelihood of dental caries, periodontal disease, misfitting dentures, broken dentures, infection, and other oral problems. Bleeding gingiva, the presence of plaque and calculus on teeth, and loose teeth are sometimes noticed by patients during brushing and flossing and should be investigated. Halitosis commonly results from poor oral hygiene, acute necrotizing ulcerative gingivitis, and dentopyogenic infections, and it merits inquiry.

Other signs and symptoms such as fever, purulent matter (pus), malaise, xerostomia (dry mouth), and changes in taste help identify an oral problem and determine its severity.

An important area of inquiry and evaluation by the pharmacist is the patient's medical and drug history. If available, the patient's medication profile should be reviewed. The pharmacist should seek information concerning past or current medical conditions or disease states, such as rheumatic heart disease, diabetes mellitus, prosthetic joints, and hematologic disorders. The pharmacist should also inquire about any medicines the patient has recently taken or is presently taking. The medical and drug history may suggest to the pharmacist potentially serious dental, as well as medical, complications, such as endocarditis secondary to an oral abscess in a patient with rheumatic heart disease. These historical data also alert the pharmacist to predisposing factors of suspected oral conditions. Examples include a patient with signs and symptoms of oral candidiasis taking an antihistamine that drys the mouth, an orally inhaled steroid that decreases the immune response in the mouth, or a broad spectrum antibiotic that results in superinfection.

Product Selection Guidelines

Oral Hygiene Products

Plaque Removal Products

Toothbrushes are the most effective nonprescription product available to remove dental plaque and maintain good oral hygiene. There are no specific recommendations as to which is the best type of toothbrush to use. Dentists recommend toothbrushes based on the patient's manual dexterity, oral anatomy, and periodontal health. In general, soft, rounded, nylon bristle brushes are preferred by many dentists and dental hygienists. Natural hog bristle brushes are recommended to some patients; however, these brushes are more abrasive and are more likely to abrade tooth surfaces and damage gingival tissue if the patient is overzealous in brushing.

The proper frequency of brushing and method of brushing have not been established and may vary from patient to patient. Thoroughness of brushing without trauma is more important than the method of brushing (43, 44). The proper method and frequency of brushing are best taught to each individual patient by the dentist or dental hygienist after evaluating the patient. In general, patients should brush thoroughly at least once a day, and preferably twice daily, taking time to clean commonly neglected areas such as interdental surfaces, areas behind the back molars, and all sulcular areas (45). Gentle brushing of the upper surface of the tongue is often recommended since it too accumulates plaque. Toothbrushing alone has not been shown to remove plaque adequately from proximal surfaces of teeth (43). Toothbrushing will not remove dental calculus (43). Calculus removal must be done by dentists or dental hygienists.

Specialty brushes and aids are available to remove plaque from difficult-to-clean areas and dentures. Such specialty aids include narrowly shaped interdental brushes, soft wooden tips, rubber tips, denture brushes, and clasp brushes. These products are recommended to patients with specific problems of plaque removal. Electric toothbrushes have not been proven superior to properly manipulated manual toothbrushes (43). However, electric toothbrushes may benefit patients lacking manual dexterity, patients who require someone else to clean their teeth, some patients with orthodontic appliances, and patients motivated by the "novelty" of a powered toothbrush (46). Electric toothbrushes are available from numerous manufacturers and utilize many brush-head motions to clean. Best results can be obtained, in general, if a patient uses a brush carrying the American Dental Association seal of acceptance and follows the specific directions of a dentist or dental hygienist.

Pediatric Toothbrushes

As with adult toothbrushes, no specific size or shape of toothbrush is uniformly recommended for children. In general, the size of the child's toothbrush is smaller than an adult toothbrush and needs to be individualized according to the size of the child's mouth. Children can usually remove plaque more easily with a brush having shorter and narrower bristles than available in most adult toothbrushes.

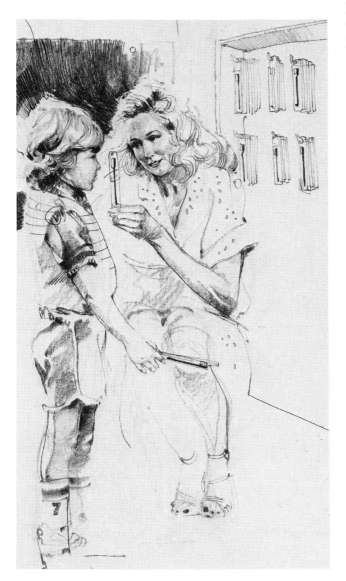

Oral Irrigating Devices

Oral irrigators cannot be viewed as substitutes for the toothbrush, floss, or other plaque-removing devices. At best, they can be considered adjuncts in maintaining oral hygiene (47). Studies have shown that oral irrigators are able to remove only a minimal amount of plaque from tooth surfaces (47, 48). The American Dental Association views these devices as potentially useful for "removing loose debris from those areas that cannot be cleaned with the toothbrush such as around orthodontic bands, fixed bridges, and periodontal pockets" (47). Some periodontal groups, however, have stated that "there is no scientific justification for recommending them as an aid in oral hygiene"; in view of the risks of bacteremia and traumatic lesions, the drawbacks may outweigh the device's value (48). Oral irrigation devices have been reported to cause bacteremia and may be considered contraindicated in patients predisposed to bacterial endocarditis. Patients with significant periodontal disease should use these devices only under the supervision of a dentist (47).

Two types of oral irrigation devices are available—pulsating (intermittent low and high water pressure) and steady stream (constant water pressure). Neither type has shown superior ability to remove debris or plaque. In general, steady-stream types are less expensive than pulsating models. The American Dental Association has evaluated and given its seal of acceptance to several brands of irrigating devices including Dento Spray, Hydro Dent, and Pulsar.

Oral irrigators should be operated with warm or tepid water within recommended water pressure levels. Operating these devices parallel to the long axis of the teeth may cause soft tissue trauma or impact food within a periodontal pocket.

Dentifrices

Dentifrices are products that are used with a toothbrush for cleaning accessible tooth surfaces. Dentifrices are available in three forms—powders, pastes, or gels. The gels and pastes commonly contain a surfactant, humectant, suspending agents, flavoring agents, abrasive, and sometimes fluoride. The powders commonly contain an abrasive and flavoring and sometimes a surfactant. Dentifrices enhance the removal of stain and dental plaque by the toothbrush (49).

Abrasives are generally thought to be the component in dentifrices responsible for physically removing plaque and debris. The ideal abrasive would maximally aid in cleaning and minimally abrade and damage tooth surfaces. Unfortunately, because of the variance in patient brushing techniques and oral conditions, the ideal dentifrice abrasive does not exist. Abrasives in dentifrices have not been shown to damage dental enamel appreciably (50). However, exposed root surfaces (cementum) and dentin can be damaged by toothbrushes and abrasives and may lead to tooth hypersensitivity (50).

Dentifrice abrasives are pharmacologically inactive and insoluble compounds. Common abrasives include silicates, dicalcium phosphate, sodium metaphosphate, calcium pyrophosphate, calcium orthophosphate, calcium carbonate, magnesium carbonate, and aluminum oxides (50). Dentifrices vary greatly in abrasiveness (50). In general, patients might best be advised to use a low-abrasive dentifrice unless advised otherwise by their dentist. Certainly, patients with periodontal disease and exposed root surfaces should use a low-abrasive dentifrice.

Surfactants are incorporated into most dentifrices to aid in removing debris by their detergent action and because the "foaming" they cause is desirable to most patients. The most common surfactants are sodium lauryl sulfate and sodium *N*-lauroyl sarcosinate (50–52). There is no evidence that surfactants in dentifrices possess anticaries activity or reduce periodontal disease, and they are presently considered inactive ingredients by the FDA (53).

Humectants and suspending agents are used in paste and gel dentifrices. The humectants prevent drying out of the preparation and usually include sorbitol, glycerin, and propylene glycol (50, 52). The suspending agents suspend and stabilize the various ingredients and often thicken the preparation. Common suspending agents include methylcellulose, carboxymethyl cellulose, Veegum, bentonite, tragacanth, karaya gum, and sodium alginate (50, 52).

Flavoring and sweetening agents are incorporated in these preparations to make them more appealing. Most dentifrices contain saccharin, sodium saccharin, or sorbitol as sweeteners; however, small amounts of sucrose or corn syrup are found in some preparations. Flavoring agents include a host of essential oils and other flavorings.

Fluoride in the form of stannous fluoride and sodium monofluorophosphate in some dentifrice formulations has been accepted by the American Dental Association as demonstrating a significant decrease in caries incidence compared with similar nonfluoride dentifrices (54). The dentifrices that have shown this anticaries effect carry the American Dental Association Council on Dental Therapeutics' seal on the packaging. There is evidence that sodium fluoride is an effective anticaries topical agent (55). Dentifrices containing sodium fluoride have been accepted by the American Dental Association as effective anticaries agents (56, 57).

Fluorides are anticariogenic because they replace the hydroxyl ion in hydroxyapatite with fluoride ion to form fluorapatite. Fluorapatite in the outer surface of dental enamel is harder and more resistant to acids than hydroxyapatite and, therefore, the enamel is less susceptible to carious breakdown (58). In addition to the formation of fluorapatite, topical fluoride preparations also have been shown to have an antibacterial and antienzyme effect on plaque bacteria resulting in decreased acid production (58–60). Fluoride-containing dentifrices are thought to be of greatest benefit when used by children in areas with a nonfluoridated water supply; however, they can even help reduce caries incidence in patients residing in communities with a fluoridated water supply (54). Fluoride-containing dentifrices do not cause dental fluorosis. (See *Plate 2-6.*)

Three different dentifrices are marketed for the treatment of hypersensitive teeth. These preparations utilize formaldehyde, strontium chloride, or sodium citrate as antihypersensitive ingredients. None of these dentifrices has been shown to be clinically effective for tooth hypersensitivity, and they are not accepted by the American Dental Association Council on Dental Therapeutics (50).

Dental Floss

Many interproximal spaces between teeth are too narrow for even small interdental brushes or other cleaning aids to gain access and remove plaque effectively. Therefore, dental floss or tape is used to physically remove plaque from these areas. Dental floss and tape are available from various manufacturers in waxed and unwaxed forms. The preference of waxed or unwaxed floss remains argumentative (47). Supervised brushing and flossing have been shown to decrease plaque and gingival inflammation in patients (47). Flossing, however, has not been conclusively shown to achieve a reduction in dental caries (47). Teeth should be flossed interproximally with an up-and-down motion five or six times down to the gingiva but not into the space between the gingiva and the tooth. Waxed floss may pass interproximally between tight-fitting teeth easier than unwaxed floss and without shredding. If contacts at the crowns of teeth are too tight to force floss interdentally, then floss threaders can often be used to pass floss between teeth and beneath fixed budges. Floss threaders are usually thin plastic loops or soft plastic, needle-like appliances and should be used cautiously so as not to traumatize the gingiva physically. One manufacturer offers special precut floss with a stiff "floss threader" at the end of the floss (Superfloss).

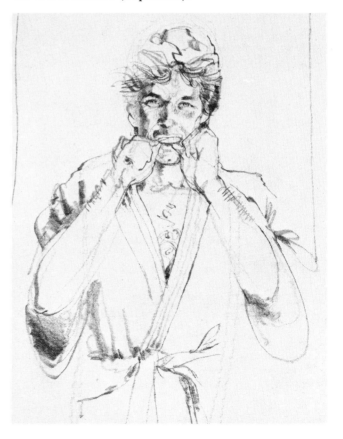

Miscellaneous Hygiene Products

Disclosing Agents

Disclosing agents are used as aids in visualizing dental plaque. They are used both at home by the patient and in the dental office. By staining the dental plaque and making it more easily visible, patients can better evaluate their oral hygiene efforts and detect areas of needed improvement. (See *Plate 2-7.*) In this way, it is hoped that the patient will become better motivated to improve oral hygiene.

Disclosing agents are available for home use as either a solution or chewable tablet. They are intended for occasional use as an indicator and not for continuous long-term use. Disclosing products should be expectorated completely (not swallowed), the mouth should be rinsed with water, and the water expectorated. Solutions are often preferred because they can be applied with a cotton-tipped applicator to a handicapped patient's dentition easily by another person and they can be diluted with water. In addition, solutions are often more acceptable than the tablets in small children. The FDA has found FD&C Red No. 3 and FD&C Green No. 3 safe when used at approved dosages and expectorated. Most nonprescription disclosing products contain FD&C Red No. 3 as a single agent since it has the advantage of staining red (matching oral soft tissues) and not markedly staining hard tissues. However, FD&C Red No. 3 does have the disadvantage of not differentiating plaque well at the gingival margin (47). A mixture of FD&C Red No. 3 and FD&C Green No. 3 has shown the ability to color differentiate between thick and thin plaque (61). This mixture has the advantage of demonstrating areas of rapidly accumulating plaque or areas which the patient neglects during oral hygiene. Fluorescein dye also has been recommended as a dental plaque disclosing agent (48, 61). It is readily taken up by plaque, basically colorless in normal light, and fluoresces with a strong yellow color under 4,800 Å (ultraviolet light). Fluorescein has the disadvantages of being costly (especially when an ultraviolet light source is required) and has the potential for possible tissue damage secondary to ultraviolet light overexposure.

Mouthwashes

Mouthwashes are solutions that often contain breath-sweetening, astringent, demulcent, detergent, or germicidal agents used for freshening and cleaning the oral cavity by gargling (62). They may be cosmetic or may contain a therapeutically effective agent.

Cosmetic Mouthwashes

Most commercially available mouthwashes, even those that claim to "kill germs," are cosmetic in that they may freshen breath and help clean some debris. There is no conclusive evidence that these mouthwashes are effective as oral antiseptic agents or effective in treating oral infections (50). Commonly used germicidal agents in mouthwashes include phenol, phenolic compounds, ammonia compounds, alcohols, volatile oils, and iodide compounds.

An important consideration with the use of mouthwashes is the potential for these agents to disguise and delay treatment of pathologic conditions such as acute necrotizing ulcerative gingivitis, purulent oral infections, periodontitis, and respiratory infections (50). The American Dental Association Council on Dental Therapeutics suggests that "if marked breath odor persists after proper toothbrushing, the cause should be investigated" and not masked with mouthwash (50). These common "medicated" mouthwashes should be considered nontherapeutic and are not included in the Council on Dental Therapeutics' acceptance program (50).

Fluoridated Mouthwashes

Several mouthwashes that contain fluoride are commercially available for nonprescription use. These preparations include 0.05% sodium fluoride in a mouthrinse solution and stannous fluoride in effervescent tablets to make a 0.1% solution for immediate rinsing. These mouthwashes are therapeutic in that the fluoride is a proven pharmacologically active anticaries agent. Several of the 0.05% sodium fluoride mouthrinses have been accepted as effective anticaries agents by the Council on Dental Therapeutics and carry the acceptance seal on their packaging.

Studies in which subjects used 0.05% sodium fluoride rinse once daily have demonstrated a significant reduction in caries incidence (16–49%), especially when used in children living in an area with a nonfluoridated water supply (55, 63, 64). Likewise, a daily 0.1% stannous fluoride aqueous rinse significantly decreases caries incidence in school children living in a community with a fluoridated water supply (65). These mouthrinses are intended to be used once daily, after brushing and flossing the teeth. They should be expectorated and the patient instructed not to rinse, eat, or drink for one-half hour after their use.

Miscellaneous Mouthwashes

Dental practitioners may suggest to patients the use of oxygenating mouthrinses or salt water (saline) as an adjunctive treatment of specific conditions or as a postoperative aid to cleaning and relief of discomfort. Oxygenating mouthrinses, such as 3% hydrogen peroxide diluted in half with warm water and sodium perborate solution, have been used in treatment of acute necrotizing ulcerative gingivitis and as a cleaning agent (66). The efficacy of these mouthrinses in killing oral anaerobic bacteria in vivo in the treatment of infections and periodontitis and as oral cleaning agents has not been established (66). With prolonged use, these rinses may cause soft tissue irritation, decalcify tooth surfaces, and result in development of black hairy tongue (66). The oxygenating rinses should not be used for extended periods (66). Warm salt water solutions can be used safely as a mouthwash for cleaning and may afford some relief of discomfort to some areas in the mouth.

Denture Products

Denture Cleaners

Denture cleaners are used to remove stain, dental plaque, and debris from denture surfaces. Denture cleaners are either chemical or abrasive in their cleaning action. The abrasive cleaners are available in the forms of pastes or powders, with the latter generally being more abrasive. There are several types of chemical cleaners, including dilute acids, alkaline hypochlorites, alkaline peroxides, detergents, and chelating agents. The American Dental Association has found no form of denture cleaning device or product superior to proper cleaning with a denture brush (67). If denture soaking cleansers are used, they should not preclude the use of a denture brush. In general, a denture brush and not a toothbrush should be used to clean a denture, as should a low-abrasive denture cleanser and not a toothpaste. A brush or cleanser that is too abrasive or brushing that is too vigorous damages the denture tooth or base material (68). Patients should not use scouring powders to clean dentures.

There are disadvantages to some soaking agents. Alkaline hypochlorite solutions bleach (lighten) the denture material and corrode stainless steel or colbalt-chromium components of the denture (68, 69). Likewise, dilute acid solutions corrode cobalt-chromium denture materials (68, 69). Alkaline peroxide solutions do not remove certain stains as well as dilute acids or hypochlorites do (68). Patients should not use strong hypochlorite solutions, such as bleach or strong acids, to clean dentures because of the likelihood of damage to the denture material. Patients should not soak or clean dentures in hot water or hot soaking solutions. This may cause distortion or warping of the denture. Stains that are resistant to proper denture brushing and soaking in available solutions should be evaluated by a dentist. All denture products should be rinsed off the denture completely before insertion. Contact of these products with oral or other mucous membranes results in tissue irritation or, more seriously, in severe chemical burns from the alkaline or acid products (70). All denture cleaning products should be kept out of the reach of children.

Denture Adhesives, Reliners, and Cushions

Denture Adhesives   Denture adhesives may be the most overused dental products purchased by patients. Chronic bone resorption of the mandibular and maxillary ridges that support a denture is a consequence of even the best-fitting denture. Periodic dental examinations are necessary to evaluate bone resorption and ensure proper denture fit. Although denture adhesives may increase denture retention in some patients, the need for adhesives increases as the quality of the denture adaptation to underlying soft tissues deteriorates (71, 72). These patients should probably see a dentist. Furthermore, pathologic changes in soft tissue under the denture, such as ulcers and fibrous lesions, and accelerated bone resorption have been reported with the inappropriate use of denture adhesives and ill-fitting dentures (71, 72).

Denture adhesive products are available in powder and paste forms. The adhesive components commonly found in these products include methylcellulose, carboxymethyl cellulose, karaya gum, gelatin, and ethylene oxide polymers. The American Dental Association Council on Dental Materials and Devices has accepted some denture adhesive products with the understanding that the labeling indicate their use only temporarily or with the recommendation of a dentist. All accepted denture adhesives contain the following warning label:

> [Product name] is acceptable as a temporary measure to provide increased retention of dentures. However, an ill-fitting denture may impair your health—consult your dentist for periodic examination.

Denture Reliners and Cushions   Extended use of reliners or cushions for dentures results in damage to both the patient and denture. Denture reliners and cushions have been associated with bone resorption, tumors, traumatic ulcers, and gingival inflammation of the denture-bearing tissues (73, 74). In addition, these products change the positioning of the denture, which can result in denture distortion, malocclusion, temporomandibular joint problems, decreased mastication function, and altered aesthetics (75). Some dentists requested that the sale of these products be halted (73, 76). The American Dental Association does not accept any of these products and discourages their use. The FDA Bureau of Medical Devices requires the following warning label on these products.

> **WARNING** For temporary use only. Long-term use of this product may lead to faster bone loss, continuing irritation, sores, and tumors. For use only until a dentist can be seen.

In general, any patient who is considering purchasing a denture reliner or cushion because of actual or perceived denture problems should see his or her dentist as soon as possible.

Denture Repair Kits   Broken dentures, like natural dentition, can only be evaluated and repaired by a dentist. Initial fitting and periodic refitting of dentures requires extensive dental knowledge and skill. Once a denture is cracked, broken, or distorted, it is, for all practical purposes, impossible for a patient to repair it properly at home. Denture repair kits usually contain methacrylate or other types of glue or acrylic materials. The American Dental Association, as in the case of reliners and cushions, strongly discourages their use (77). The FDA requires the following label on these products:

> **WARNING** For emergency repairs only. Long-term use of home-repaired dentures may cause faster bone loss, continuing irritation, sores, and tumors. See your dentist without delay.

The pharmacist should strongly discourage the use of denture repair kits.

Products for Cold Sores and Canker Sores

Many nonprescription products are available for treatment of cold sores and canker sores. Some of these products provide symptomatic relief, some are irrational and may involve more risk than benefit, and none has been shown conclusively to decrease the recurrence rate of lesions or be curative. Many products are intended for extraoral use only and are not for intraoral use.

Canker Sore Treatment

The main goals in treating canker sores are to control discomfort and to promote healing, so that the patient can eat, drink, and function normally. Topical oral protectants such as Orabase or denture adhesives can be effective in covering lesions and affording symptomatic relief (21, 78). These can be applied as needed.

Topical application of local anesthetic pastes or gels also affords temporary pain relief. Benzocaine and butacaine are the most common local anesthetics in nonprescription products. Benzocaine is a known sensitizer (allergen) and should not be used by patients with a history of problems with other benzocaine-containing products (51, 79). The American Dental Association has accepted topical local anesthetic products containing benzocaine and butacaine as safe and effective, and the acceptance seal can be found on the packaging. Products containing eugenol, phenol, camphor, and menthol as anesthetic, counterirritant, or antiseptic treatments for canker sores should be discouraged. These may cause tissue irritation and damage or systemic toxicity, especially if overused (80). None of these products has been accepted as safe and effective by the American Dental Association for treating canker sores. The value of nascent oxygen-releasing compounds (carbamide peroxide, hydrogen peroxide, and perborates) as effective antiseptics and cleansers of aphthous lesions (small ulcers) has not been established, and tissue irritation and black hairy tongue have been reported (66). Oral aspirin or acetaminophen as systemic analgesics afford additional relief of discomfort. Aspirin should not be retained in the mouth before swallowing or placed in the area of the oral lesions due to the high risk of severe chemical burns with necrosis (81). (See *Plate 2-8.*)

Cold Sore Treatment

The primary goal in treating cold sores, as with canker sores, is to control discomfort and promote healing of these self-limiting lesions. The cold sore should be kept moist to prevent drying and fissuring. This "cracking" of the lesions may render it more susceptible to secondary bacterial infection, may delay healing, and usually increases discomfort. Therefore, products that are highly astringent are best avoided. Bland emollient creams, petrolatum, or protectants such as Orabase can aid in moistening and protecting cold sores (8, 21). If there is evidence of secondary infection of a cold sore, topical application of bacitracin and/or neomycin ointments is recommended along with systemic antibiotics when indicated (8). Allergic reactions to topical neomycin have been reported. Topical local anesthetics in nondrying bases aid in decreasing pain (21). Oral aspirin or acetaminophen also are effective in controlling discomfort. Patients who associate occurrence of cold sores with sun exposure may benefit from the application of a sunscreen containing 5% para-aminobenzoic acid in the form of a lipstick.

Numerous other products available to patients have been proposed in the treatment of cold sores. Evidence demonstrating efficacy, however, is lacking. *Lactobacillus acidophilus* preparations have not shown any conclusive efficacy in the treatment of cold sores or any other oral lesions (21). Nonoxynol 9, a surfactant-spermicidal agent available in nonprescription contraceptive products, has shown "uniformly enthusiastic" results in one clinical trial (82). However, no well-controlled studies have been conducted to demonstrate its efficacy. The essential amino acid L-lysine in oral doses from 300 to 1,200 mg has been touted as "accelerating recovery" and "suppressing recurrence" of cold sores (83). However, subsequent work has shown that L-lysine had no effect on the recurrence rate of cold sores (84). Topical application of caustic or escharotic agents such as phenol or silver nitrate are considered contraindicated by the American Dental Association (80). Topical counterirritants, such as camphor, are of unproven efficacy and are not accepted by the American Dental Association. Topical application of 0.5% hydrocortisone creams or ointments or other corticosteroids are contraindicated according to the American Dental Association (8). Although some investigators consider topical steroids of benefit for herpes infections, others question their efficacy due to the possibility of spreading lesions (21, 26).

Products for "Toothache"

Nonprescription medicines for toothache commonly contain eugenol or benzocaine. Eugenol and clove oil are accepted by the American Dental Association for professional use by the dentist. However, these agents are not accepted as safe and effective nonprescription drugs for toothache. They are generally ineffective in the hands of the patient for toothache and can cause soft tissue damage. Benzocaine also is not accepted as a safe and effective self-treatment for toothache. Toothache is usually an indication of pathology involving tooth substance, dental pulp, or the supporting periodontium. Even if aspirin or acetaminophen are effective in relieving toothache, the patient should seek professional dental help as soon as possible.

Products for Teething

Teething is the eruption of the deciduous teeth through the gingival tissues. Usually this process is uneventful. However, when teething causes sleep disturbances or irritability, symptomatic treatment should be considered. Topical local anesthetics, such as benzocaine and frozen teething rings, may provide symptomatic relief, although the efficacy of these products is unproven. The American Dental Association has not accepted any product for teething. When teething is accompanied by fever or malaise, a dentist or physician should be contacted to rule out an infectious process.

Patient Consultation

After assessing a patient's oral complaint or problem, the pharmacist can advise the patient on the appropriate treatment with a nonprescription product or refer the patient to a dentist. The pharmacist should be able to inform a patient when an oral complaint is usually self-limiting and not severe, or when a problem is likely to be progressive and have serious consequences. An unconcerned patient asking advise about nonprescription medications to treat an oral abscess with accompanying fever, malaise, swelling, lymphadenopathy, and purulent exudate should be referred to a dentist immediately. On the other hand, a concerned patient seeking advice about nonprescription products for a small recurrent cold sore can be reassured that it is usually a self-limiting problem that will remit with proper self-treatment.

The pharmacist is often the first, last, or only health care professional to advise a patient. The patient must know what nonprescription medications not to use and why, despite the advertising claims. Examples include advising against a "whitening" toothpaste to clean a denture because of excess abrasiveness, and advising against applying camphor or phenolic compounds to canker sores because of possible irritation, tissue damage, or systemic toxicity. When counseling a patient on rational self-medication, the pharmacist should do more than just recommend a product. The patient should be informed on how to use the product properly, how long to use the product, what to expect from the product, cautions with the use of the product, and what to do if the product is ineffective. For example, when recommending a sodium fluoride mouthrinse, the patient should know that the fluoride rinse should be used after cleaning the teeth, should be expectorated, and that nothing should be taken by mouth for one-half hour after use; that the mouthrinse can benefit the patient for as long as the patient has natural dentition; that the fluoride is preventive in action and will not cure already carious teeth; and that the product should be kept out of the reach of children because of possible ethanol or fluoride toxicity (55, 85).

What to expect from a nonprescription medicine is more than merely explaining if a product is preventive, curative, or symptom relieving in its action. The patient should realize that nonprescription drugs should improve the condition being treated. If the drug results in no change, worsens the condition, or causes another problem, the product should be discontinued and professional help sought. For instance, a properly used benzocaine product applied to canker sores should afford a reasonable amount of symptomatic relief. However, if the canker sores get progressively more inflamed and painful after application of the product, the patient should be informed to stop using the product because of possible benzocaine allergy. Even nonprescription dental products routinely used by millions of patients and rarely associated with adverse effects should not go unsuspected by the pharmacist when assessing a problem and counseling the patient. Dentifrices, one of the most widely used nonprescription drug products, have been documented as causing desquamation, irritation, and allergic reactions (51, 52). Patients experiencing one of these infrequent effects secondary to a dentifrice should be advised to discontinue use of commercial dentifrices, substitute baking soda or salt water, see if the problem resolves, or see their dentist.

Summary

Since dental disease is the most frequently encountered health care problem in the United States, and because pharmacists see more dental patients than dentists, to-day's pharmacist needs a sound knowledge of dental products and dental therapeutics. The pharmacist-dentist team can improve oral health. With useful references such as *Accepted Dental Therapeutics*, awareness of ongoing FDA and American Dental Association evaluation of dental products, and open lines of communication with dental practitioners, pharmacists can better serve their role as dental health consultants and members of the dental health care team.

References

1. "Nutritional Disorders of Children: Prevention, Screening, and Follow-up," DHEW Publication #HSA 76-5612, 1976, p. 82.
2. International Conference on Research in the Biology of Periodontal Disease, College of Dentistry, University of Illinois, 1977, pp. 443–444.
3. L. A. Saporito, *Pharm. Times* (letter), *39*, 31 (1973).
4. American Dental Association/American Pharmaceutical Association Liaison Committee, "The Dentist and the Pharmacist," American Dental Association, Chicago, Ill., 1970, p. 1.
5. D. A. M. Geddes, *Arch. Oral Biol., 17*, 537 (1972).
6. "Accepted Dental Therapeutics," 37th ed., American Dental Association, Chicago, Ill., 1979, p. 242.
7. R. G. Campbell and D. D. Zinner, *J. Nutr., 100*, 11 (1970).
8. "Oral Microbiology," W. Nolte, Ed., C. V. Mosby, St. Louis, Mo., 1968, pp. 9–21.
9. "Accepted Dental Therapeutics," 37th ed., American Dental Association, Chicago, Ill., 1979, pp. 285–286.
10. F. A. Carranza, Jr., "Glickman's Clinical Periodontology," 5th ed., W. B. Saunders, Philadelphia, Pa., 1979, pp. 194–207.
11. "International Conference on Research in the Biology of Periodontal Disease," College of Dentistry, University of Illinois, 1977, p. 227.
12. "International Conference on Research in the Biology of Periodontal Disease," College of Dentistry, University of Illinois, 1977, pp. 247–249, 402.
13. F. A. Carranza, Jr., "Glickman's Clinical Periodontology," 5th ed., W. B. Saunders, Philadelphia, Pa., 1979, pp. 135–147.
14. M. G. Newman and S. S. Socransky, *J. Periodont. Res., 12*, 120 (1977).
15. J. D. Manson and T. Lehner, *J. Periodontol., 45*, 636 (1974).
16. "Canker Sores and Other Oral Ulcerations," PHS No. 1329, U.S. Government Printing Office, Washington, D.C., 1965, pp. 1–14.
17. E. A. Graykowski, M. F. Barile, and H. R. Stanley, *J. Am. Dent. Assoc., 69*, 118 (1964).
18. M. F. Barile, T. C. Francis, and E. A. Graykowski, in "Microbial Protoplasts, Spheroplasts, and L-Forms," L. B. Guze, Ed., Williams and Wilkins, Baltimore, Md., 1967, pp. 444–456.
19. R. N. Shore and W. B. Shelby, *Arch. Dermatol., 109*, 400 (1974).
20. T. C. Francis, *Oral Surg., 30*, 476 (1970).
21. N. G. Popovich and J. G. Popovich, *U.S. Pharm. 3*, 36 (1978).
22. R. S. Rogers, III, W. M. Sams, Jr., and R. G. Shorter, *Arch. Dermatol., 109*, 361 (1974).
23. A. E. Dolby, *Immunology, 17*, 709 (1969).
24. C. B. Sabiston and W. R. Grigsby, *CRC Crit. Rev. Clin. Lab. Sci., 8*, 213 (1977).
25. N. K. Wood and P. W. Goaz, "Differential Diagnosis of Oral Lesions," 2nd ed., C. V. Mosby, St. Louis, Mo., 1980, pp. 101–104.
26. E. B. Smith, *J. Am. Med. Assoc., 235*, 1731 (1976).
27. R. S. Griffith, A. L. Norins, and C. Kagan, *Dermatologica, 156*, 257 (1978).
28. C. B. Sabiston, Jr., and W. A. Gold, *Oral Surg., 38*, 187 (1974).
29. C. B. Sabiston, Jr., W. R. Grigsby, and N. Segerstrom, *Oral Surg., 41*, 430 (1976).
30. G. Feldmann and O. Larje, *Acta Odontolog. Scand., 24*, 129 (1966).
31. M. H. Goldberg, *J. Am. Dent. Assoc., 80*, 1048 (1970).
32. T. B. Aufdemonte and M. A. McPherson, *Oral Surg., 46*, 776 (1978).
33. T. M. Arendorf and D. M. Walker, *Arch. Oral Biol., 25*, 1 (1980).

34. L. Cohen, *J. Oral Med., 27,* 7, (1972).
35. A. Jepsen and J. E. Winther, *Acta Odontolog. Scand., 23,* 239 (1965).
36. W. P. Holbrook and G. D. Rodgers, *Oral Surg., 49,* 122 (1980).
37. R. P. Masella, C. T. Dolan, and W. R. Laney, *J. Prosthet. Dent., 33,* 250 (1975).
38. W. H. Douglas and D. M. Walker, *Br. Dent. J., 135,* 55 (1973).
39. L. P. Samaranayake and T. W. MacFarlane, *Arch. Oral Biol., 25,* 603 (1980).
40. L. P. Samaranayake, J. McCourtie, and T. W. MacFarlane, *Arch. Oral Biol., 25,* 611 (1980).
41. D. L. Hall, R. Ettinger, J. A. Walker, and C. B. Sabiston, Prevention of Denture Colonization by *Candida albicans,* paper presented at Iowa Section of the American Division of the International Association of Dental Research Meeting, February 28, 1978, Iowa City, Iowa.
42. T. W. MacFarlane, M. M. Ferguson, and D. MacKenzie, *Br. Dent. J., 144,* 199 (1978).
43. "Accepted Dental Therapeutics," 37th ed., American Dental Association, Chicago, Ill., 1979, p. 308.
44. F. A. Carranza, Jr., "Glickman's Clinical Periodontology," 5th ed., W. B. Saunders, Philadelphia, Pa., 1979, p. 729.
45. F. A. Carranza, Jr., "Glickman's Clinical Periodontology," 5th ed., W. B. Saunders, Philadelphia, Pa., 1979, p. 748.
46. F. A. Carranza, Jr., "Glickman's Clinical Periodontology," 5th ed., W. B. Saunders, Philadelphia, Pa., 1979, p. 728.
47. "Accepted Dental Therapeutics," 37th ed., American Dental Association, Chicago, Ill., 1979, p. 309.
48. International Conference on Research in the Biology of Periodontal Disease, College of Dentistry, University of Illinois, 1977, pp. 325–326, 371.
49. "Accepted Dental Therapeutics," 37th ed., American Dental Association, Chicago, Ill., 1979, p. 339.
50. "Accepted Dental Therapeutics," 37th ed., American Dental Association, Chicago, Ill., 1979, pp. 340–343.
51. W. C. Rubright, J. A. Walker, U. L. Kaulsson et al., *J. Am. Dent. Assoc., 97,* 215 (1978).
52. A. A. Fisher, *Cutis, 6,* 554 (1970).
53. *Federal Register, 45,* 20670 (1980).
54. "Accepted Dental Therapeutics," 37th ed., American Dental Association, Chicago, Ill., 1979, pp. 329–332.
55. "Accepted Dental Therapeutics," 37th ed., American Dental Association, Chicago, Ill., 1979, pp. 323–324.
56. W. A. Zacherl, *J. Dent. Res., 60,* 577 (1981).
57. B. B. Beiswanger, C. W. Gish, and M. E. Mallatt, *J. Dent. Res., 60,* 577 (1981).
58. "Nutritional Disorders of Children: Prevention, Screening, and Follow-up," DHEW Publication #HSA 76-5612, 1976, p. 87.
59. W. W. Briner and M. D. Francis, *Arch. Oral Biol., 7,* 541 (1962).
60. W. J. Loesche, R. J. Murray, and J. R. Mellberg, *Caries Res., 7,* 283 (1973).
61. "Accepted Dental Therapeutics," 37th ed., American Dental Association, Chicago, Ill., 1979, p. 310.
62. *Federal Register, 45,* 20671 (1980).
63. A. J. Rugg-Gunn, P. J. Holloway, and T. G. H. Davies, *Br. Dent. J., 135,* 353 (1973).
64. P. Torell and Y. Ericsson, *Acta Odontolog. Scand., 23,* 287 (1965).
65. "Accepted Dental Therapeutics," 37th ed., American Dental Association, Chicago, Ill., 1979, p. 328.
66. "Accepted Dental Therapeutics," 37th ed., American Dental Association, Chicago, Ill., 1979, pp. 344–345.
67. "Guide to Dental Materials and Devices," 7th ed., American Dental Association, Chicago, Ill., 1974/1975, p. 152.
68. D. J. Neill, *Br. Dent. J., 124,* 107 (1968).
69. M. MacCallum, G. D. Stafford, W. T. MacCulloch, and E. C. Combe, *Dent. Practitioner, 19,* 83 (1968).
70. A. Abramson, *Med. World News,* June 28 (1974).
71. K. K. Kapur, *J. Prosthet. Dent., 18,* 550 (1967).
72. D. J. Neill and B. J. Roberts, *J. Dent., 1,* 219 (1973).
73. J. B. Woelfel and R. L. Curry, *J. Am. Dent. Assoc., 71,* 603 (1965).
74. C. R. Means, *J. Prosthet. Dent., 14,* 1086 (1964).
75. J. B. Woelfel and J. A. Kreider, *J. Prosthet. Dent., 20,* 319 (1968).
76. B. W. Thurgood and L. F. DeCounter, *J. Prosthet. Dent., 36,* 17 (1976).
77. American Dental Association/American Pharmaceutical Association Liaison Committee, "The Dentist and the Pharmacist," American Dental Association, Chicago, Ill., 1970, p. 9.
78. "Accepted Dental Therapeutics," 37th ed., American Dental Association, Chicago, Ill., 1979, p. 297.
79. "Accepted Dental Therapeutics," 37th ed., American Dental Association, Chicago, Ill., 1979, p. 120.
80. "Accepted Dental Therapeutics," 37th ed., American Dental Association, Chicago, Ill., 1979, p. 230.
81. "Accepted Dental Therapeutics," 37th ed., American Dental Association, Chicago, Ill., 1979, p. 152.
82. H. J. Donsky, *N. Engl. J. Med., 300,* 371 (1979).
83. R. S. Griffith, A. L. Norins, and C. Kagan, *Dermatologica, 156,* 257 (1978).
84. N. Milmer, J. Scheibel, and O. Jessen, *Acta Dermatovener. [Stockh.], 60,* 85 (1978).
85. E. R. Weller-Fahy, L. R. Berger, and W. G. Troutman, *Pediatrics, 66,* 302 (1980).

Toothpaste Product Table

Product (Manufacturer)	Abrasive Ingredients	Therapeutic Ingredients	Foaming Agents	Inert and Miscellaneous Ingredients
Aim (Lever Bros)	hydrated silica	sodium monofluorophosphate	sodium lauryl sulfate	alcohol, sorbitol, polyethylene glycol 32, saccharin sodium, sodium benzoate, cellulose gum, flavor
Amosan (Coopercare)				sodium peroxyborate monohydrate, sodium bitartrate
Aqua-Fresh (Beecham Products)	silica, calcium carbonate, calcium glycerophosphate	sodium monofluorophosphate	sodium lauryl sulfate	sorbitol, polyethylene glycol 8, cellulose gum
Caroid Tooth Powder (Winthrop)	magnesium carbonate, sodium bicarbonate, calcium carbonate			papain
Chloresium (Rystan)	calcium carbonate, dicalcium phosphate	chlorophyllin	sodium lauryl sulfoacetate	glycerin, sorbitol, carrageenan, mineral oil, methylparaben, flavor
Close-Up (Lever Bros)	hydrated silica; sodium phosphate; disodium phosphate		sodium lauryl sulfate	sorbitol, polyethylene glycol 32, alcohol, saccharin sodium, cellulose gum, sodium benzoate, flavor
Colgate with MFP (Colgate-Palmolive)	dicalcium phosphate dihydrate	sodium monofluoro-phosphate, 0.76%	sodium lauryl sulfate	glycerin, cellulose gum, sodium benzoate, tetrasodium pyrophosphate, saccharin sodium, flavor
Crest (Procter & Gamble)	calcium pyrophosphate, stannous pyrophosphate	sodium fluoride, 0.243%		cellulose gum, glycerin, sorbitol, flavor
Denquel (Vicks)	calcium carbonate, silica, magnesium aluminum silicate	potassium nitrate	sodium lauryl sulfate	glycerin, sorbitol, cellulose gum, sodium saccharin, flavor
Extar (Extar)	magnesium oxide, calcium carbonate, sodium polymetaphosphate, silica gel		sodium lauryl sulfate	tragacanth, saccharin sodium, spralene mint, mint oil, flavor, menthol
Extar Dentifrice Powder (Extar)	sodium polymetaphosphate, sodium phosphate			sequestrene, saccharin sodium
Gleem (Procter & Gamble)	calcium pyrophosphate	sodium fluoride, 0.22%	blend of anionic surfactants	glycerin, sorbitol, cellulose gum, flavor
Kolynos (Whitehall)	dicalcium phosphate		sodium lauryl sulfate	methyl salicylate
Listerine (Warner-Lambert)	dicalcium phosphate			
Macleans Fluoride Toothpaste (Beecham Products)	calcium carbonate, 38%; magnesium aluminum silicate	sodium monofluoro-phosphate, 0.76%	sodium lauryl sulfate, 1.15%	glycerin, 26%
Pearl Drops Tooth Polish (Carter)	dicalcium phosphate, aluminum hydroxide			sorbitol, cellulose gum
Pepsodent (Lever Bros)	alumina, hydrated silica, dicalcium phosphate		sodium lauryl sulfate	sorbitol, glycerin, polyethylene glycol 32, cellulose gum, titanium dioxide, saccharin sodium, sodium benzoate, flavor

Toothpaste Product Table, continued

Product (Manufacturer)	Abrasive Ingredients	Therapeutic Ingredients	Foaming Agents	Inert and Miscellaneous Ingredients
Pepsodent Ammoniated Tooth Powder (Lever Bros)	sodium metaphosphate, tricalcium phosphate		sodium lauryl sulfate	diammonium phosphate, urea, polyethylene glycol 32, carrageenan, saccharin, flavor
Pepsodent Tooth Powder (Lever Bros)	sodium metaphosphate; dicalcium phosphate; magnesium trisilicate		sodium lauryl sulfate	polyethylene glycol 32, carrageenan, saccharin, flavor
Pycopay Tooth Powder (Block)	sodium chloride, sodium bicarbonate, calcium carbonate, magnesium carbonate, tricalcium phosphate			flavor
Revelation Tooth Powder (Alvin Last)	calcium carbonate		soap	menthol, methyl salicylate
Sensodyne (Block)				strontium chloride
Thermodent (Leeming)	diatomaceous earth, silica	strontium chloride hexahydrate	sodium methyl cocoyltaurate	sorbitol, glycerin, titanium dioxide, hydroxyethyl cellulose, flavor, preservative
Topol Smoker's Toothpolish (Jeffrey Martin)	dicalcium phosphate, magnesium aluminum silicate		sodium lauryl sulfate	sorbitol, propylene glycol, sodium saccharin, methylparaben, propylparaben, cellulose gum, flavor
Topol Smoker's Toothpolish with Fluoride (Jeffrey Martin)	insoluble sodium metaphosphate; dicalcium phosphate, magnesium aluminum silicate	sodium fluoride	sodium lauryl sulfate	sorbitol, glycerin, sodium carrageenan, flavor, silica, cellulose gum, sodium saccharin, methylparaben, propylparaben, titanium dioxide
Ultra Brite (Colgate-Palmolive)	hydrated silica alumina	sodium monofluoro-phosphate, 0.76%	sodium lauryl sulfate	glycerin, cellulose gum, sodium benzoate, titanium dioxide, saccharin sodium, flavor

Denture Cleanser Product Table

Product (Manfacturer)	Ingredients
Complete (Vicks)	calcium carbonate, glycerin, sorbitol, cellulose gum, sodium lauryl sulfate, silica, magnesium aluminum silicate, flavor
Denalan (Whitehall)	sodium peroxide, 9.5%; sodium chloride, 90%
Efferdent Tablets (Warner-Lambert)	potassium monopersulfate, sodium borate perhydrate, sodium carbonate, sodium lauryl sulfoacetate, sodium bicarbonate, citric acid, magnesium stearate, flavor
Effervescent Denture Tablets (Rexall)	sodium bicarbonate, citric acid, sodium perborate, sodium acid pyrophosphate, sodium benzoate, trisodium phosphate, sodium lauryl sulfate, poloxamer 188, sorbitol, silica, peppermint oil, povidone

Denture Cleanser Product Table, continued

Product (Manfacturer)	Ingredients
Extar Denture Cleanser (Extar)	sodium polymetaphosphate, saccharin sodium, methylparaben, propylparaben, peppermint, sodium phosphate, sequestrene, lactose
K.I.K. (K.I.K. Co.)	sodium perborate, 25%; trisodium phosphate, 75%
Kleenite (Vicks)	sodium chloride, trisodium phosphate, sodium perborate, sodium dichloroisocyanurate dihydrate, sodium lauryl sulfate, edetate disodium, flavor
Mersene Denture Cleaner (Colgate-Palmolive)	troclosene potassium, sodium perborate, trisodium phosphate
Polident Denture Cleanser Powder (Block)	sodium perborate, potassium monopersulfate, sodium carbonate, sodium tripolyphosphate, surfactant, sodium bicarbonate, flavor
Polident Tablets (Block)	potassium monopersulfate, sodium perborate, sodium carbonate, surfactant, sodium bicarbonate, citric acid, flavor

Toothache/Cold Sore/Canker Sore Product Table

Product (Manfacturer)	Anesthetic	Other Ingredients
Anbesol (Whitehall)	benzocaine, 6.3%	phenol, 0.5%; povidone iodine (0.04% available iodine); alcohol, 70%
Anbesol Gel (Whitehall)	benzocaine, 6.3%	phenol, 0.5%; alcohol, 70%
Baby Orajel (Commerce)	benzocaine 7.5%	viscous water-soluble base
Benzodent (Vicks)	benzocaine, 20% eugenol, 0.4%	hydroxyquinoline sulfate, 0.1%; denture adhesive-like base
Betadine Mouthwash/ Gargle (Purdue Frederick)		povidone-iodine, 0.5%; alcohol, 8.8%
Blistr Klear (Miller-Morton)	camphor	alcohol, 37%, lanolin
Blistex Ointment (Blistex)		camphor, 1%; phenol, 0.4%; spirits of ammonia; peppermint oil; lanolin and petrolatum base
Butyn Dental Ointment (Abbott)	butacaine, 4%	not stated
Campho-Phenique (Winthrop)	phenol, 4.7%	camphor, 10.8%
Cankaid (Becton Dickinson)		carbamide peroxide, 10%; anhydrous glycerol; flavor
Cold Sore Lotion (DeWitt)		gum benzoin, 1.2%; alcohol, 90%; menthol, 0.3%; camphor, 3.7%; phenol, 0.3%
Cold Sore Lotion (Pfeiffer)		gum benzoin, 7.0%; alcohol, 85%
Dalidyne (Dalin)	benzocaine	methylbenzethonium chloride; tannic acid; camphor; chlorothymol; menthol; benzyl alcohol; alcohol, 61%; aromatic base
Dental Poultice (Dent)	benzocaine, 16.6%	oleoresin capsicum, 0.25%; oxyquinoline, 1.82%; thymol, 0.91%

Toothache/Cold Sore/Canker Sore Product Table, continued

Product (Manfacturer)	Anesthetic	Other Ingredients
Dents Toothache Drops (Dent)	eugenol, 7.5%	denatured alcohol, 60%; chlorobutanol, 0.09%
Dents Toothache Gum (Dent)	benzocaine, 5.06%; eugenol, 5.06%	
Double-Action Kit (Dent)	eugenol, 7.5%	denatured alcohol, 60%; chlorobutanol, 0.09%; acetaminophen tablets, 325 mg
Dr. Hands Teething Gel and Lotion (Roberts)	clove oil, menthol	tincture of pellitory; hamamelis water; alcohol, 10%
Gum-Zor (DeWitt)	benzocaine, 5.6%	propylene glycol, 44%; glycerin, 29%; benzyl alcohol, 2.5%; tincture of myrrh; alcohol, 22%
Jiffy (Block)	benzocaine, eugenol	alcohol, 56.5%
Kank-a Viscous liquid (Blistex)	benzocaine, 1%	cetylpyridinium chloride, 0.5%; compound benzoin tincture
Lotion-Jel (Dent)	benzocaine, 5%	
Numzident (Purepac)	benzocaine, clove oil	peppermint oil
Numzit (Purepac)	benzocaine, menthol	glycerin; alcohol, 10%; gel vehicle
Orabase Plain (Hoyt)		pectin, gelatin, carboxymethyl cellulose sodium, polyethylene glycol, mineral oil
Orabase with Benzocaine (Hoyt)	benzocaine	pectin, gelatin, carboxymethyl cellulose sodium, polyethylene glycol, mineral oil
Orajel (Commerce)	benzocaine, 10.0%	polyethylene glycol-like base, 62.7%
Ora-Jel CSM (Commerce)	benzocaine, 10%	tannic acid, 6%; benzalkonium chloride, 0.125%
Ora-Jel-D (Commerce)	benzocaine, 7.5%; clove oil, 0.2%	benzyl alcohol, 1.0%; adhesive base
Ora-Jel Extra-Strength (Commerce)	benzocaine, 20%	
Proxigel (Reed & Carnrick)		carbamate peroxide, 11%; water-free gel base
Rexall Cold Sore Lotion (Rexall)	phenol, menthol	benzoin; camphor; alcohol, 90%
Rexall Cold Sore Ointment (Rexall)	phenol, menthol	benzoin; camphor; alcohol, 30%; viscous base
Rid-A-Pain Dental Drops (Pfeiffer)	benzocaine, 2.5%	cetalkonium chloride, 0.02%; alcohol, 20%
Rid-A-Pain Gel (Pfeiffer)	benzocaine, 10%	alcohol, 7.5%
Tanac (Commerce)		benzalkonium chloride, 0.4%; tannic acid, 2.858%

Toothache/Cold Sore/Canker Sore Product Table, continued

Product (Manfacturer)	Anesthetic	Other Ingredients
Tanac Liquid (Commerce)	benzocaine, 10%	tannic acid, 6%; benzalkonium chloride, 0.125%
Tanac Roll-On (Commerce)	benzocaine, 5%	tannic acid, 6%; benzalkonium chloride, 0.125%
Tanac Solid (Commerce)	benzocaine, 7.5%	tannic acid, 6%; benzalkonium chloride, 0.125%; allantoin
Teething Lotion (DeWitt)	benzocaine, 5.6%	propylene glycol, 44%; glycerin, 29%; benzyl alcohol, 2.5%; tincture of myrrh, 4.5%; alcohol
Toothache Drops (DeWitt)	benzocaine, 5.01%; clove oil, 9.98%	beechwood creosote, 4.83%; flexible collodion (base); alcohol, 20%

Denture Adhesive Product Table

Product (Manufacturer)	Ingredients
Brace (Norcliff Thayer)	cellulose gum, 25%; methyl vinyl ether–maleic anhydride and/or acid copolymer, 15%; povidone, 10%; petrolatum, 34.9%; mineral oil, 14.9%; flavor, 0.2%
Confident (Block)	carboxymethyl cellulose gum, 32%; ethylene oxide polymer, 13%; petrolatum, 42%; liquid petrolatum, 12%; propylparaben, 0.05%
Corega Powder (Block)	karaya gum, 94.6%; water-soluble ethylene oxide polymer, 5%; flavor, 0.4%
Effergrip Denture Adhesive Cream (Warner-Lambert)	carboxymethyl cellulose sodium, 39%; cationic polyarylamide polymer, 10%
Fasteeth (Vicks)	karaya gum, sodium borate
Fixodent (Vicks)	calcium sodium poly(vinyl methyl–ether maleate), petrolatum base, carboxymethyl cellulose sodium
Orafix (Norcliff Thayer)	karaya gum, 51%; petrolatum, 30%; mineral oil, 13%; peppermint oil, 0.08%
Orafix Medicated (Norcliff Thayer)	benzocaine, 2%; allantoin, 0.2%; karaya gum, 51%; petrolatum, 28%; mineral oil, 13%; peppermint oil, 0.08%
Orafix Special (Norcliff Thayer)	cellulose gum, 25%; methyl vinyl ether–maleic anhydride and/or acid copolymer, 15%; povidone, 10%; petrolatum, 34.9%; mineral oil, 14.9%; flavor, 0.2%
Orahesive Powder (Hoyt)	gelatin, 33.3%; pectin, 33.3%; carboxymethyl cellulose sodium, 33.3%
Polident Dentu-Grip (Block)	carboxymethyl cellulose gum, 49%; ethylene oxide polymer, 21%; flavor, 0.4%
Poli-Grip (Block)	karaya gum, 51%; petrolatum, 36.7%; liquid petrolatum, 9.4%; magnesium oxide, 2.7%; propylparaben; flavor
Staze (Commerce)	karaya gum, 46.23%; petrolatum, 48.4%

Denture Adhesive Product Table, continued

Product (Manufacturer)	Ingredients
Sea-Bond (Combe Inc.)	ethylene oxide polymer, sodium alginate
Wernet's Cream (Block)	carboxymethyl cellulose gum, 32%; petrolatum, 42%; liquid petrolatum, 12%; ethylene oxide polymer, 13%; propylparaben, 0.05%; flavor, 0.5%
Wernet's Powder (Block)	karaya gum, 94.6%; water-soluble ethylene oxide polymer, 5%; flavor, 0.4%

Mouthwash Product Table

Product (Manfacturer)	Antiseptic	Anesthetic	Astringent	Other Ingredients
Astring-O-Sol (Winthrop)	alcohol, 65%		zinc chloride	myrrh, methyl salicylate
Cépacol (Merrel Dow)	alcohol, 14%; cetylpyridinium chloride, 1:2,000			phosphate buffers, aromatics
Cépastat (Merrell-Dow)	phenol, 1.4%	eugenol		menthol, glycerin
Cherry Chloraseptic Mouthwash and Gargle (Norwich-Eaton)	phenol, sodium phenolate (total phenol 1.4%)			cherry flavor
Chloraseptic Mouthwash (Norwich-Eaton)	phenol, sodium phenolate (total phenol 1.4%)			menthol
Fluorigard (Colgate-Palmolive)				sodium fluoride, 0.05%
Forma-Zincol Concentrate (Ingram)	formaldehyde		zinc chloride	anise oil, menthol
Gly-Oxide (Marion Laboratories)	carbamide peroxide, 10%			anhydrous glycerin, flavor
Greenmint Mouthwash (Block)	alcohol			chlorophyll, sorbitol, surfactant, flavor
Isodine Mouthwash Gargle Concentrate (Blair)	alcohol, 35%; povidone-iodine, 7.5%			
Kasdenol Powder (Kasdenol)	available chlorine 5–6% (as oxychlorosene)			not stated
Lavoris (Vicks)	alcohol	clove oil	zinc chloride	glycerin, polysorbate 80, citric acid, flavors, poloxamer 407
Listerine (Warner-Lambert)	alcohol, 26.9%			menthol, methyl salicylate, eucalyptol, thymol, poloxamer 407, caramel, benzoic acid
Listermint (Warner-Lambert)	alcohol, 12.8%		zinc chloride	glycerin, poloxamer 407, saccharin sodium, sodium citrate, citric acid, flavor, sodium lauryl sulfate

Mouthwash Product Table, continued

Product (Manfacturer)	Antiseptic	Anesthetic	Astringent	Other Ingredients
Mouthwash and Gargle (McKesson)	cetylpyridinium chloride, alcohol, 14%			saccharin; D & C Green #5
Odara (Lorvic)	phenol, 2%; alcohol, 48%		zinc chloride, 1.1%	glycerin, potassium iodide, methyl salicylate, eucalyptus oil, myrrh tincture
Oral Pentacresol (Upjohn)	secondary amyltricresols, 1 mg/ml; alcohol, 30%			sodium chloride, 8.61 mg/ml; calcium chloride, 0.33 mg/ml; potassium chloride, 0.299 mg/ml
Proxigel (Reed & Carnick)	carbamate peroxide, 11%			water-free gel base
Scope (Procter & Gamble)	cetylpyridinium chloride, domiphen bromide, 0.005%; alcohol, 18.5%			glycerin, saccharin, polysorbate 80, flavor
S.T. 37 (Calgon)	hexylresorcinol, 0.1%			glycerin

24 Insect Sting and Bite Products

Farid Sadik and Jeffrey C. Delafuente

Questions to Ask the Patient

Have you developed hives, excessive swelling, dizziness, vomiting, or difficulty in breathing since being bitten or stung?

Do you have a personal or family history of allergic reactions such as hay fever?

Have you previously had severe reactions to insect stings or bites?

How extensive are the stings or bites on your body?

If the patient is a child, what is his/her age and approximate weight?

Have you ever had adverse reactions to topically applied products?

Medical literature is replete with articles on allergic reactions to insect stings and bites. Many people die and many more are treated for severe systemic reactions as a result of insect stings. Accurate statistics on the number of Americans who die yearly due to insect bites and stings are lacking. An estimated 30–50 Americans die annually from systemic reactions to insect stings, and approximately 1–2 million patients are at risk because of severe stinging insect allergy (1). Data gathered from death certificates may be low because death caused by insect stings may be attributed to other causes, such as heart attacks, strokes, or unknown causes. For example, a 42-year-old man became unconscious 3 minutes after he was stung on the forehead, neck, and underarms by yellow jackets. Five minutes later he was dead. In spite of this, the county coroner reported the death as "natural—cause unknown" (2).

An insect sting or bite is an injury to the skin caused by penetration of the stinging or biting organ of an insect. The reactions that follow are produced mainly by substances contained in the venom of stinging insects or in the saliva of biting insects. Although the pain associated with the skin penetration by stinging or biting is brief, the aftereffects vary considerably.

Types of Injuries

Stinging Insects

Stinging insects belonging to the order Hymenoptera (membranous wings) are most frequently responsible for insect sting hypersensitivity. Among the three families commonly involved are the Apidae, including the honeybee (genus *Apis*); the Vespidae, including wasps (genus *Polistes*); yellow jackets and hornets (genus *Vespula*); the imported fire ants (genus *Solenopsis*); and harvester ants (genus *Pogonomyrmex*). Although they are small, these insects have a venom that is as potent as that of snakes. Death caused by an insect sting results from an anaphylactic reaction and usually comes within minutes; death from snake bite usually is not associated with hypersensitivity and occurs within 3 hours to several days.

The stinging insects inject the venom into their victims through a piercing organ (stinger), a specialized ovipositor delicately attached to the rear of the female's abdomen. (Males do not have an ovipositor and consequently are stingless.) The stinger consists of two lancets, made of highly chitinous material, separated by the poison canal. The venom flows through the canal from the venom sac attached to the stinger's dorsal section. The tip of the stinger, which is directed posteriorly, has sharp barbs, and the base enlarges into a bulb-like structure. Most species of bees and wasps have two types of venom glands under the last abdominal segment. The larger gland secretes an acidic toxin directly into the venom sac; the smaller one, at the base of the sac, secretes a less potent alkaline toxin.

Honeybees

When the honeybee stings, it attaches firmly to the skin with tiny, sharp claws at the tip of each foot, then arches its abdomen, and immediately jabs the barbed stinger into the skin. Because of the barbs, the stinger remains firmly embedded and, when the honeybee pulls away or is brushed off, the entire stinging apparatus (stinger, appendages, venom sac, and glands) is detached from the bee's abdomen. The disemboweled bee later dies. The abandoned stinger, driven deeper into the skin by rhythmic contractions of the venom sac's smooth muscle wall, continues to inject venom.

Wasps, Hornets, Yellow Jackets, and Bumblebees

The stinging mechanism of these insects resemble that of the honeybee, with the main difference being that their stingers are not barbed. The stingers can be withdrawn easily after injecting the venom, enabling these insects to survive and sting repeatedly.

Ants

Ants use their mandibles to cling to the skin of their prey, then bend their abdomen, sting the flesh, and empty the contents of their poison vesicle into the wound (3). Because they use their mandibles, it is often believed that the bite causes the reaction.

Biting Insects

Insects such as mosquitoes, fleas, lice, bedbugs, ticks, and chiggers ("red bugs") bite their prey. They insert their biting organs into the skin to feed by sucking blood from their hosts. (See *Plate 2-9.*)

Mosquitoes

Mosquitoes usually attack exposed parts of the body (face, neck, forearms, and legs). They can, however, bite through thin clothing. When a mosquito alights on the skin, it cuts through the skin with its mandibles and maxillae. A fine, hollow, needle-like, flexible structure (proboscis) is introduced into the cut and probes the tissue for a blood vessel. Blood is sucked directly from a capillary lumen or from previously lacerated capillaries with extravasated blood (4). During feeding the mosquito injects into the wound a salivary secretion containing antigenic components, which cause the itching.

Fleas

Fleas are tiny (1.5–4 mm long), bloodsucking, wingless parasites with strongly developed posterior legs used for leaping. They are found throughout the world (including Arctic regions) but breed best in warm areas with relatively high humidity. Fleas bite covered parts of the body: Bites usually are multiple and grouped and cause intense itching. Each lesion is characterized by an erythematous region around the puncture. Fleas not only are annoying but are responsible for transmitting diseases such as bubonic plague and endemic typhus. They may survive and multiply without food for several weeks. Places that have been vacant for weeks may be heavily infested, partly due to the hatching of eggs.

Bedbugs

Bedbugs have a short head and a broad, flat body (4–5 mm long and 3 mm wide). Their mouth parts consist of two pairs of stylets used to pierce the skin. The outer pair has barbs that saw the skin, and the inner pair is used to suck blood and to allow salivary secretions to flow into the wound. These insects normally hide during the day, become active at night, and bite their victims as they sleep. They usually hide and deposit their eggs in crevices of walls, floors, picture frames, bedding, and other furniture. Persons may be bitten in subdued light by day while sitting in theaters and other public places. A bedbug can engorge itself with blood within 3–5 minutes, thereafter seeking its hiding place. Depending on the severity of the reaction and subsequent bullous papules, itching and an occasional small dermal hemorrhage are present at the puncture site.

Ticks

Ticks are parasites that feed on the blood of humans and domestic animals. During feeding, the tick's mouth parts are introduced into the skin, enabling it to hold firmly. If the tick is removed, the mouth parts are torn from the tick and remain embedded, causing intense itching and nodules. (See *Plate 2-10.*) If the tick is left attached to skin, it becomes fully engorged with blood and remains as long as 10 days before it drops off.

Chiggers

Chiggers are prevalent in southern parts of the United States mainly during summer and fall. Only the larvae, which are nearly microscopic, attack the host by attaching to the skin and sucking blood. Once in contact with the skin, the larvae insert their mouth parts into the skin and secrete a digestive fluid that causes cellular disintegration of the affected area and intense itching. Chiggers do not burrow in the skin; however, as a result of the injected fluid, the skin hardens and a tube is formed in which the chigger lies and continues to feed until engorged, after which it drops off and changes to the adult.

Scabies

The mite causing scabies neither bites nor stings. Scabies, commonly called "the itch," is a contagious parasitic skin infestation caused by the mite *Sarcoptes scabiei,* which burrows beneath the stratum corneum. Characterized by secondary inflammation and intense itching, this infestation is associated with poor hygiene, crowded conditions, and venereal disease. The immunology of scabies is interesting since it takes at least 1 month for the symptoms (primarily itching) to be noted in previously uninfested persons (5). The female mite, which is responsible for causing scabies, is transmitted readily by close personal contact with an infected person. Once on the skin, the impregnated female burrows into the stratum corneum with her jaws and the first two pairs of legs, forming tunnels in which she lays eggs and excretes fecal matter. In a few days, the hatched larvae form their own burrows and develop into adults. They copulate, and the impregnated females burrow into the stratum corneum to start a new life cycle. The most common infestation sites are the interdigital spaces of the fingers, the flexor surface of the wrists, the external male genitalia, the buttocks, and the anterior axillary folds. (See *Plate 2-11.*) The head and neck are not affected, except in infants.

Lice

Lice are wingless parasites with well-developed legs. Each leg has a claw that helps the louse cling firmly to the skin while sucking blood. Three types of lice attack humans: head lice (*Pediculus humanus capitis*), body lice (*Pediculus humanus corporis*), and pubic lice (*Phthirus pubis*). Although head lice usually infest the head, they can be found on other hairy parts of the body as well. The female deposits 50–150 eggs (nits), which become glued to the hair and hatch in 5–10 days. Body lice live, hide, and lay their eggs in clothing, particularly in seams and folds of underclothing, and generally infest crowded environments. Pubic lice, commonly called crab lice because of their crab-like appearance, may be encountered in patients with high standards of hygiene. They infest the pubic area, armpits, and occasionally eyelashes, mustaches, beards, and eyebrows.

Lice cause an immediate wheal around the bite in sensitive individuals. A local, delayed papular reaction appears within 24 hours. Itching and scratching result in excoriation or secondary pyogenic infections.

Head lice infestation has reached near epidemic proportions in classrooms (6). It can be diagnosed by observation with the naked eye. Although both the louse and the nit or egg are visible, diagnosis is made most often by visualization of nits. Some adult lice may occasionally be seen moving through the hair. (See *Plate 3-12A and B*.)

The nits are immobile, gray oval bodies attached to the hair shaft. The eggs are laid on the shaft close to the scalp. As the hair grows, the nit or egg is moved away from the scalp. Since hair grows at a relatively constant rate, approximately ½ inch per month, the duration of infestation may be estimated by measuring the distance of the nit from the scalp surface.

Head lice infestation often causes itching. Scratching the irritation may result in excoriation of the scalp tissue. In some instances, pyoderma results, characterized by erythema, crusting, and oozing on the scalp and hair margins.

Head lice infestation is especially prevalent among school children who are often in close contact with each other and may share clothing or toilet articles. Lice also can be spread by contact with seats on buses and in theaters. Good personal hygiene and careful grooming unfortunately cannot prevent infestation, only stopping the organism can. Awareness of health officials, school authorities, and parents can be effective in this regard.

Allergic Reactions to Stinging Insects

Over the last decade significant progress has been made in understanding the pathogenesis of allergic reactions from the Hymenoptera order of insects. Venoms from these insects have been purified and analyzed. Their mechanisms for causing severe reactions have been investigated, and they are now being used for diagnosis and treatment of stinging insect allergies. Reactions from stinging insects can be more severe than those from biting insects. Therefore, stinging insect allergies are discussed here in more detail.

A gamut of reactions from insect stings occur. Reactions range from small local reactions, limited to the sting site, to systemic reactions leading to death. Reactions may be divided into three categories: anaphylactic, local, and unusual.

Anaphylactic Reactions

These reactions are immunologically mediated, usually occurring within 15 minutes after a sting. The majority of anaphylactic reactions from insect stings are cutaneous in nature. Symptoms include erythema, pruritus, urticaria (hives), or angioedema. The most serious sequelae from stings are systemic anaphylactic reactions. In severe reactions hypotension, laryngeal edema, bronchospasm, and respiratory distress may occur, leading to a shock-like state. If not treated promptly, death may ensue. Less common anaphylactic reactions may cause nausea, vomiting, or diarrhea. Mechanisms of anaphylaxis are discussed below.

Local Reactions

These reactions occur at the sting site. The manifestations are erythema and varying amounts of pain with symptoms lasting from several hours to several days. Swelling may extend from the sting site covering an extensive area. Immune mechanisms have been implicated as the cause of the reaction in some patients. However, not all patients studied have evidence of immunologically mediated reactions (7).

Unusual Reactions

There have been occasional reports of unusual reactions following insect stings. These have included neurologic reactions, renal involvement, serum sickness reactions, encephalopathy, and delayed hypersensitivity skin reactions. The mechanisms for these reactions have not been clearly elucidated, but immunologic causes have been implicated in some cases (8, 9).

Reactions to Biting Insects

Reactions to biting insects are usually local. The pathogenesis of these reactions has not been well characterized (8). Some species of mosquitoes have agglutinin and anticoagulant agents in their salivary secretions; others have neither (10).

Many attempts have been made to identify the antigenic factors in mosquito bites by studying whole mosquito extracts. Extracts from *Aedes aegypti* were shown by paper chromatography to contain at least four fractions that can produce skin reactions (11). Eluates of each constituent caused positive reactions in sensitized individuals (12). Eighteen amino acids have been identified in the extracts of all species of mosquitoes (13).

Reactions to mosquito bites vary in intensity. Wheal formation, erythema, papular reaction, and itching are characteristic. Scratching causes papule and nodule formations that may persist and lead to secondary infections such as impetigo, furunculosis, or infectious eczematoid dermatitis. The bite site may influence reaction intensity; bites on the ankles and legs are more severe than elsewhere on the body because of the relative circulatory stasis in the legs. Consequently, the tendency toward vesiculation, hemorrhage, eczematization, and ulceration is greater in these areas (14). Systemic reactions such as fever and malaise also are common.

Intense itching due to scabies, especially at night, occurs at the infestation site. The burrow (< 1 cm long) is visible to the naked eye and appears as a narrow, slightly raised dark line. Unrestrained scratching may cause secondary bacterial infections, such as impetigo, furuncles, or cellulitis, and excoriation. Scabies diagnosis may be made by identifying the mite under a microscope and by the burrows in the skin.

Pathogenesis of Anaphylaxis

Anaphylactic reactions are mediated by IgE antibodies that bind to the specific antigens (allergens) causing the reaction. The antigens involved in insect stings are proteins and glycoproteins contained in insect venom. After an initial exposure to certain antigens, the body responds by making IgE antibodies against the antigens. These IgE antibodies bind to tissue mast cells and blood basophils. Mast cells are primarily located in lung tissue, bronchial smooth muscle, and vascular endothelium. Once these IgE antibodies are bound to the cells, the person is considered "sensitized."

When a sensitized person is exposed to antigens to which he or she is sensitive, under the appropriate circumstances, IgE on mast cells or basophils will bind the antigen. When this occurs, IgE receptors on the cells are bridged together and the cells release active substances from their granules (15). Active substances released by degranulation include histamine, serotonin, slow-reacting substance of anaphylaxis (SRS-A), eosinophil-chemotactic factor of anaphylaxis (ECF-A), and bradykinin.

Histamine is a bioactive amine that increases capillary permeability, contracts bronchial and vascular smooth muscle, and increases nasal and bronchial mucous gland secretion. Serotonin increases vascular permeability in mice, but its role in human anaphylaxis is unknown. The peptide SRS-A contracts smooth muscle. Unlike histamine, which is preformed in the cell granules, SRS-A is formed after the IgE-antigen interaction occurs, and is then released from the granules. Antihistamines are ineffective at reversing the effects of SRS-A, but epinephrine will terminate muscle contractions induced by SRS-A. ECF-A is also released by mast cells and causes eosinophils to accumulate in the area of the allergic reaction. Eosinophils can release an enzyme, arylsulfatase-B, which inactivates SRS-A. Bradykinin contracts vascular and bronchial smooth muscle, increases vascular permeability, increases mucous secretion, and stimulates pain fibers.

The severity and type of anaphylactic reaction depends upon the location and number of cells degranulating their mediators. Degranulation in specific target organs produce local anaphylaxis. If the reaction is limited to the gastrointestinal tract, diarrhea may occur; release of mast cell mediators in the nasal mucosa may produce rhinorrhea; if the mediators are limited to skin, hives may be the only prominent sign.

Systemic degranulation of mast cells and basophils lead to severe systemic symptoms and is responsible for shock and death occurring after an insect sting. Large amounts of mediators released can cause a marked increase in capillary permeability, leading to leakage of intravascular fluids and hypotension. This shock-like state can be further compounded by mediator-induced laryngeal edema and bronchoconstriction resulting in respiratory distress or failure.

Several theoretical factors may explain why a local reaction occurs in one instance, and a systemic reaction in another (16). The dose of venom injected at each sting may vary, thereby varying the amount of antigen entering the body. The location of the sting may also influence the type of reaction. Head and neck stings may be responsible for more laryngeal edema, while stings on extremities may produce only local reactions. A sting that limits the venom to the intradermal space may present as a local reaction; a sting on a capillary or venule would allow for systemic injection of the venom, and a systemic reaction.

Components of Hymenoptera Venom

Hymenoptera venom contains a number of allergenic proteins, as well as several pharmacologically active molecules. There are variations in the contents of venoms among different families within the Hymenoptera order. Therefore, venoms will be discussed in general terms.

The major antigenic proteins are the enzymes hyaluronidase and phospholipase A (17,18). Hyaluronidase breaks down hyaluronic acid, which is a binding agent in connective tissue. By altering tissue structure, hyaluronidase acts as a spreading factor allowing for better penetration of venom substances. Phospholipase A attacks phospholipids in cell membranes. In addition, phospholipase A contracts smooth muscle, causes hypotension, increases vascular permeability, and is destructive to mast cells.

Studies have shown that 50–100% of individuals with a history of local or systemic reactions to insect stings will have demonstrable IgE antibody to venom constituents (7, 16). The variability in detecting IgE among studies may be due to differences in laboratory techniques and lack of positive identification of the insect eliciting the reaction. Studies further show that the presence of venom-specific IgE in the sera of patients with local reactions correlates with the duration of the reaction (7). Whether venom-specific IgE is directly responsible for local reactions has not been ascertained.

Other venom components include histamine, melitin, apamin, and mast cell degranulating peptide (MCD-peptide) (19, 20). Of these substances, only melitin is antigenic, and not all individuals make antibodies against it (16). While these mediators do not directly contribute to insect sting anaphylaxis, they do affect the rate at which venom antigens become available to the systemic circulation following a sting. These molecules have direct and indirect effects on mast cell mediator release, vascular permeability, and smooth muscle contraction. Table 1 summarizes the pharmacologic actions of the venom constituents.

Prophylactic Treatment

Individuals with stinging insect hypersensitivity should take precautions to avoid exposure to these insects. Foods and odors tend to attract insects; therefore, outdoor activities such as picnicking should be done cautiously. Keeping garbage contained and food covered will help keep insects away. Shoes should always be worn in grass and fields. In addition, perfumes and brightly colored clothes attract stinging insects and should not be worn while outdoors. A common-sense approach will lower the risk of stings and subsequent adverse reactions.

Venom Immunotherapy

Hymenoptera venom is used prophylactically to treat patients who have had reactions to stings. Venom immunotherapy, also known as desensitization, is done by subcutaneous injection of small amounts of venom at regularly scheduled intervals. The dose of the venom is gradually increased over many weeks until a predetermined maintenance dose is reached. The optimal doses, frequency of injections, and duration of maintenance therapy are still being investigated (21, 22, 23).

Immunotherapy causes a decrease in venom-specific serum IgE levels, with a rise in venom-specific serum IgG "blocking antibody" levels. It is believed that production of blocking antibody offers protection against anaphylactic reactions (17, 23), although unequivical proof is lacking (22, 24). Blocking antibody competes with IgE antibody for binding of venom antigens, preventing the antigens from reacting with mast cell–bound IgE. Other factors may also be responsible for successful immunotherapy.

Lyophilized venom extracts are now available for diagnosis and treatment of stinging insect allergy. Greater than 95% of patients treated with these venoms in recommended doses and regimens are protected against serious reactions when restung (22, 24, 25). The remaining 5% are partially protected (24, 25). Before the use of venom extracts, whole-body extracts of insects were used for immunotherapy. Whole-body extracts have been shown to be no better than placebo treatment, and should not be used (8, 23).

For diagnosis by skin testing, a kit of individual venoms of stinging insects is available. The same individual venoms or mixed venoms from yellow jackets, white-faced hornets, and yellow hornets are used for immunotherapy. Mixed venoms are used because some individuals develop cross-sensitivity among vespids. These injections can be dangerous if improperly administered. Thus, the following warning is stated in the package insert (1):

> **WARNING** Hymenoptera venom preparations should be used only by physicians experienced in administering allergens to the maximum tolerated dose and/or after allergy consultation.

Because of the possibility of severe systemic reactions, the patient should be fully informed by the physician of the risks involved and should be under constant supervision. The venom preparations should be used only in settings where emergency resuscitative equipment and trained personnel are immediately available to treat such reactions. Treatment with Hymenoptera venom preparations should be restricted to patients who have previously experienced a potentially life-threatening systemic reaction, due to an immediate hypersensitivity reaction following the sting of the honeybee, yellow jacket, hornet, or wasp. In addition, Hymenoptera venom preparations should only be given after venom hypersensitivity has been confirmed by venom skin testing. Patients receiving whole body Hymenoptera insect immunotherapy should be completely re-evaluated (history and venom skin testing) before treatment with these venom preparations is instituted. All patients receiving venom immunotherapy should have instruction on the procedure of emergency self-injection of subcutaneous epinephrine. These patients should be advised to carry an emergency epinephrine kit during the Hymenoptera season, even while receiving venom immunotherapy. Before administering these venom preparations, physicians should be thoroughly familiar with the information concerning adverse reactions, treatment of overdosage, and precautions for use during pregnancy.

Table 1. Properties of Hymenoptera venom components

	Histamine	Melitin	Apamin	MCD-peptide	Hyaluronidase	Phospholipase A
Pain production	+	+	?	?	O	?
↑ Capillary permeability	+	+	+	+	I	+
Smooth muscle contraction	+	+	O	O	O	+
Histamine release	O	+	O	+	O	+
Cellular damage	O	+	?	+	O	+
Antigenic	O	+	?	?	+	+

+, occurs; O, does not occur; ?, not demonstrated; I, indirectly.

Active Treatment

Because of the wide range of reactions to insect stings and bites, treatment usually depends on the symptoms. Nonprescription drugs are of no value in systemic reactions; such cases need the prompt medical attention. For local reactions, a nonprescription product that minimizes scratching by relieving discomfort, itching, and pain may be recommended. Prophylactic products, such as insect repellants, also are available.

Physician-directed medical treatment (acute or prophylactic) is important in many cases. Because hypersensitive reactions to insect stings and bites occur rapidly and may be severe, the sooner medical attention is given, the better the chances for recovery.

Systemic reactions caused by insect stings and bites are considered emergencies for which aqueous epinephrine, 1:1000, 0.3–0.5 ml, subcutaneously or intramuscularly, should be administered immediately. Aqueous epinephrine, 1:1000, 0.1–0.3 ml, may also be injected directly into the sting site in order to delay absorption of the venom. Sublingual isoproterenol should not be administered simultaneously because it may induce serious arrhythmia. Parenteral antihistamines may be used for persistent urticaria, angioedema, or laryngeal edema in patients who do not respond to epinephrine. Pressor agents may be used if shock persists. Parenteral corticosteroids administered through the systemic route may be used for patients with protracted anaphylaxis and delayed reactions (26). Respiratory support should be available if needed; in severe cases, a tracheotomy may be necessary (27).

For hypersensitive individuals, the pharmacist should recommend the following:

- If symptomatic, the victim must seek medical attention immediately after an insect sting or bite.
- Basic first-aid measures, such as applying ice to the sting and removing the stinger, are generally helpful.
- The directions and the benefits to be gained from using an insect sting emergency kit should be explained carefully. The pharmacist should emphasize that epinephrine is the drug of choice for anaphylactic reactions.
- Receiving injections of venom extract for protection against systemic reactions (desensitization) is useful.

First Aid

Basic first-aid measures are helpful until medical help is available. Prompt application of ice packs to the sting site helps to slow absorption and reduce itching, swelling, and pain (28). Removal of the honeybee's stinger and venom sac, which usually are left in the skin, is another measure that should be offered or explained, particularly to allergic individuals. The stinger should be removed before all venom is injected; it takes approximately 2–3 minutes to empty all of the contents from the honeybee's venom sac. The sac should not be squeezed; rubbing, scratching, or grasping it releases more venom (27). Scraping the stinger with tweezer or a fingernail minimizes the venom flow. After the stinger is removed, an antiseptic should be applied.

Emergency Kits (Prescription Only)

Insect sting emergency kits for hypersensitive individuals may be obtained by prescription. In addition to tweezers for removing the honeybee stinger, the typical kit may include epinephrine hydrochloride and antihistamines.

Epinephrine Hydrochloride

Because of its potent and rapid action, epinephrine hydrochloride 1:1000 injection is preferred to counteract the bronchoconstriction associated with anaphylaxis. It should be administered subcutaneously immediately after stinging. Some insect sting emergency kits have a preloaded (0.3 ml) sterile syringe. Generally, a 0.25-ml dose is injected subcutaneously and, after waiting 15 minutes, another dose may be necessary. For individuals with cardiovascular disease, diabetes, hypertension, or hyperthyroidism, the injection should be administered with caution.

The FDA encourages physicians to prescribe kits containing epinephrine injections for patients who are allergic to insect stings and for individuals responsible for those who may be exposed to insect stings such as scout leaders, camp counselors, and paramedical personnel. These individuals should be trained to administer epinephrine injections. In some states, specially trained nonphysicians may legally administer epinephrine to individuals suspected of having an anaphylactic reaction to insect stings (localized or generalized urticaria, difficult breathing, wheezing, abdominal pain, weakness, confusion, lowered blood pressure, cyanosis, collapse, and unconsciousness). The FDA opposes the over-the-counter sale of epinephrine kits because of possible misuse or deliberate abuse of the material in the kit (29).

Antihistamines

Although they are slow in onset of action and may be ineffective in severe reactions, antihistamines often are used in conjunction with epinephrine hydrochloride. They are administered orally or parenterally.

Ingredients in Nonprescription Products

Most nonprescription products that are used for symptomatic relief of insect stings and bites contain one or more pharmacologic agents, which fall into one of three main categories: external analgesics, skin protectants, and antibacterials.

External Analgesics/Antipruritics

This category is subdivided further into three groups: agents with analgesic activity derived from stimulation of cutaneous sensory receptors (counterirritants), from depression of cutaneous sensory receptors (anesthetics and antihistamines), and from reduction of inflammation (hydrocortisone). These agents are considered safe and effective when used as recommended for adults and children more than 2 years of age. There is no recommended dosage for any of these agents when used for children less than 2 years old except under the advice or supervision of a physician.

Counterirritants

Counterirritants reduce pain and itching by stimulating cutaneous sensory receptors to provide a feeling of warmth, coolness, or milder pain, which obscures the more severe pain of the injury. The activity of these agents is dependent on the concentration. In low concentrations, they may depress the cutaneous receptors and result in an anesthetic effect. (See Chapter 27, *External Analgesic Products*.)

Ammonia Solution This solution has a pungent characteristic odor. Ammonia is lost rapidly upon exposure to air. A 1–2.5% solution of ammonia is applied to the affected area no more than 3–4 times/day.

Camphor At concentrations of 0.1–3%, camphor depresses cutaneous receptors, thereby relieving itching and irritation. At concentrations of 3–11%, camphor acts as a counterirritant because it stimulates cutaneous receptors at higher concentrations. Camphor is safe and effective for use as an external analgesic at these concentrations when applied to the affected area no more than 3–4 times/day.

Camphor-containing products can be very dangerous if ingested. Patients should be warned to keep these (and all drugs) out of the reach of children and to contact a physician or Poison Control Center immediately if ingestion is suspected.

Cresol Camphor complex (camphorated metacresol) is used to reduce pain. The FDA advisory review panel on nonprescription external analgesic drug products concluded that there are insufficient data available to permit final classification of the safety and effectiveness of this drug for use as a nonprescription external analgesic.

Menthol In concentrations of > 1.25%, menthol acts as a counterirritant and excites cutaneous sensory receptors. However, in concentrations of < 1%, it depresses cutaneous receptors and exerts an analgesic effect. Menthol is considered to be a safe and effective antipruritic when applied to the affected area in concentrations of 0.1–1%.

Methyl Salicylate Methyl salicylate stimulates cutaneous receptors when used in concentrations ranging from 10% to 60%.

Peppermint and Clove Oils When applied externally, these oils act as mild counterirritants causing a sensation of warmth.

Ichthammol Ichthammol has bacteriostatic and irritant properties. However, it is difficult to assess its effectiveness in concentrations used in nonprescription products for insect stings.

Local Anesthetics

The FDA advisory review panel on nonprescription external analgesic drug products concluded that the local anesthetics used in insect sting and bite products, benzocaine and dibucaine, are safe and effective when used according to label directions. Dermatitis resulting from topically applied local anesthetics, including benzocaine, has been reported (30). Although adverse reactions from topical applications are often blamed on allergy to local anesthetics, allergy is actually an infrequent cause of reaction (31). The dermatitis that may occur requires frequent contact and patients should be warned against continued applications for prolonged periods. (See Chapter 25, **Burn and Sunburn Products**.)

Phenol Phenol exerts topical anesthetic action by depressing cutaneous sensory receptors. It is caustic when applied in undiluted form to the skin. Phenol aqueous solutions of > 2% are irritating and may cause sloughing and necrosis. Phenol is considered safe and effective as nonprescription external analgesic when applied to the affected area no more than 3–4 times/day in concentrations of 0.5–2% for adults and children 2 years of age and older. Nonprescription products that contain phenol should include the following specific warning: "Do not apply this product to extensive areas of the body or under compresses or bandages" (32).

Benzocaine Benzocaine was found to be safe and effective for use by adults and children over 2 years of age when applied to the affected area no more than 3 or 4 times/day. The concentrations of benzocaine available in nonprescription products range from 5% to 20%.

Cyclomethycaine Sulfate The FDA advisory review panel on nonprescription external analgesic drug products concluded that cyclomethycaine sulfate is safe and effective but that there are insufficient data available to permit final classification of its effectiveness for use as a nonprescription external analgesic.

Dibucaine Dibucaine is another local anesthetic found in insect sting and bite products. Although in the same class as benzocaine, dibucaine products carry specific additional labeling:

> **WARNING** Do not use in large quantities, particularly over raw surfaces or blistered areas.

This is because of the danger of systemic toxicity. Convulsions, myocardial depression, and death have been reported from systemic absorption (33). The recommended dosage for adults and children over 2 years of age is a 0.25–1.0% solution applied to the affected area no more than 3 or 4 times/day.

Antihistamines

Topical antihistamines are considered to be safe and effective external analgesics. These ingredients relieve pain and itching by depressing cutaneous sensory receptors. Although some absorption occurs through the skin, they are not absorbed in sufficient quantities to cause systemic side effects even when applied to damaged skin. However, antihistamines are capable of acting as haptens, producing hypersensitivity reactions.

Continued use of these agents over 3–4 weeks increases the possibility of sensitization. In addition, there is question as to its antipruritic action over a period of time. With this in mind, the FDA advisory review panel on nonprescription external analgesic drug products recommended that these agents be used for no longer than 7 days except under the advice of a physician. These agents are not recommended for children of less than 2 years of age.

Diphenhydramine   Recommended dosage is the application of a product containing this ingredient in a concentration of 1–2% 3 or 4 times/day.

Tripelennamine   Tripelennamine may be applied 3 or 4 times/day in concentrations of 0.5–2.0%.

Both local anesthetics and antihistamines carry the following labeling as recommended by the FDA advisory review panel: "For the temporary relief of pain and itching due to minor burns, sunburn, minor cuts, abrasions, insect bites, and minor skin irritations."

Hydrocortisone

Hydrocortisone is an anti-inflammatory agent that is capable of preventing or suppressing the development or the regression of edema, capillary dilation, swelling, and tenderness accompanying inflammation. It relieves pain and itching by reducing inflammation. Preparations containing hydrocortisone in concentrations from 0.25–0.5% are considered to relatively safe and effective for use as a nonprescription antipruritic. These preparations should be applied 3 or 4 times/day for adults and children 2 years of age and older. Patients should be warned against using topically applied hydrocortisone in the presence of scabies, tinea, bacterial infections, and moniliasis. Not only may the underlying condition be worsened, but hydrocortisone may mask these disorders, making accurate diagnosis difficult (36).

Products containing hydrocortisone or its acetate salts carry specific labeling as follows: "For the temporary relief of minor skin irritations, itching, and rashes due to eczema, dermatitis, insect bites, poison ivy, poison oak, poison sumac, soaps, detergent, cosmetics, and jewelry, and for itchy genital and anal areas." (See Chapter 31, *Poison Ivy and Poison Oak Products*.)

Aspirin

The topical use of aspirin for insect stings has been reported to be effective in reducing the wheal reaction and the subsequent itching and irritation (34). The FDA advisory review panel on nonprescription external analgesic drug products concluded that aspirin is safe but there are insufficient data available to permit final classification of its effectiveness for use as a nonprescription external analgesic (35). It possesses no direct topical anesthetic activity. Therefore, it exerts no anesthetic, analgesic, or antipruritic effect on the skin.

Skin Protectants: Zinc Oxide and Calamine

These ingredients are used in lotions, ointments, creams, and sprays for their cooling, slightly astringent, antiseptic, antibacterial, and protective actions. Calamine is a mixture of zinc oxide and ferrous oxide. The ferrous oxide acts only as a coloring agent and is not an active ingredient. Zinc oxide and calamine tend to absorb fluids from weeping rashes. The FDA review panel on nonprescription skin protectant drug products concluded that zinc oxide and calamine are safe and effective in the nonprescription concentration range of 1–25% and for use as a nonprescription skin protectant (37). Topical dosage for adults, children, and infants is its application to the affected areas as needed.

Titanium Dioxide

Titanium dioxide has an action similar to that of zinc oxide. Its safety and effectiveness have not been established.

Hamamelis Water

Hamamelis water (witch hazel) possesses astringent properties and may act as a hemostatic for small superficial wounds.

Glycerin

The FDA advisory review panel on nonprescription skin protectant drug products concluded that glycerin is safe and effective for nonprescription use as a skin protectant due to its absorbent, demulcent, and emollient properties. In addition, glycerin is widely used for its solvent properties.

Antibacterials

The most commonly used antibacterial agents in nonprescription products for insect stings and bites are benzalkonium chloride, benzethonium chloride, and methylbenzethonium chloride. These medications are included to prevent and treat secondary infection that may result from scratching. The aforementioned quaternary ammonium compounds are classified as safe and effective for first-aid use. (See Chapter 28, *Topical Anti-infective Products*.)

Chloroxylenol

This drug is a bacteriostatic agent that primarily acts against gram-positive bacteria. Evaluation and safety of chloroxylenol in topical preparations could not be made by the FDA advisory review panel on nonprescription antimicrobial drug products because of insufficient data.

8-Hydroxyquinoline Sulfate

This chemical is included in topical preparations for its antibacterial effect.

Chlorothymol

Chlorothymol acts as an antibacterial and antifungal agent. However, it is irritating to mucous membranes.

Cresol

Cresol has a similar action to phenol. It is frequently used as a preservative.

Salicylic Acid

At concentrations ranging from 2% to 20%, salicylic acid acts as a keratolytic. In addition, it exerts a slight antiseptic action.

Scabies and Lice Treatment

Scabies and lice are controlled by using gamma-benzene hexachloride; benzyl benzoate is effective only against scabies and other mites. Both products are available by prescription only. The patient should bathe, vigorously scrubbing the infested area. Then a 25% emulsion of benzyl benzoate or 0.5–1% cream of gamma-benzene hexachloride is applied to the entire body except the face. It should remain on the skin for 24 hours, after which the patient may bathe. A second application is recommended 1 week after the first one to destroy the hatched eggs. Additional applications should be avoided because contact dermatitis may occur. If itching is not relieved immediately after treatment, a soothing lotion such as calamine lotion with menthol and camphor may be used.

Most nonprescription products are based on pyrethrums, which are natural pesticides derived from chrysanthemum plants. They are safe and effective as pesticides. According to product claims, pyrethrum-based products are pediculocidal for head, body, and pubic lice (and the nits) on contact. Pyrethrums are active by way of toxicity to the insects' nervous systems. Most pyrethrum-containing products also contain piperonyl butoxide, which blocks detoxification of the pyrethrums by the insect.

Pyrethrum-based products containing piperonyl butoxide have a low order of toxicity when ingested by mammals. Some pyrethrum-based products are formulated in deodorized kerosene, which has more potential for toxicity when ingested than the active ingredients. These products are irritating to the eyes and product information includes a warning against permitting contact with mucous membranes.

Patients who seek advice concerning treatment of *P. pubis* infestation of the eyelashes may be advised to apply petrolatum ophthalmic ointment thickly to the eyelashes twice daily for 8–10 days, with the remaining nits being mechanically removed (38).

Nonprescription products are more efficacious and safer than many home remedies such as kerosene. Nonprescription products are recommended for active treatment of patients with documented infestations rather than prophylaxis against lice. Duration of effectiveness of nonprescription treatment will be related to environmental conditions connected with the possibility for reinfestation.

To prevent subsequent reinfection of lice, washing or drycleaning of all clothing is necessary. Animals do not become infested by human head lice; therefore, household pets can be spared treatment (6).

Insect Repellents

Insect repellents do not kill insects but keep them away from treated areas. When applied to the skin, repellents discourage the approach of insects and, thus, protect the skin against insect bites. Most repellents are volatile, and when they are applied to skin or clothing, their vapor tends to prevent insects from alighting.

Oils of citronella, turpentine, pennyroyal, cedarwood, eucalyptus, and wintergreen were previously used in insect repellent formulations. However, after World War II, investigations showed that these agents were relatively ineffective. Although more than 15,000 compounds have been tested, only a few are effective and safe enough to use on the skin. An insect repellent should be relatively safe. It should have an inoffensive odor, protect for several hours, be effective against as wide a variety of insects as possible, to withstand all weather conditions, and have an aesthetic feel and appearance.

The best all-purpose repellent is *N, N*-diethyl-*m*-toluamide. Ethohexadiol dimethyl phthalate, dimethyl carbate, and butopyronoxyl are effective repellents, but they are not as effective against as many kinds of insects as *N, N*-diethyl-*m*-toluamide. However, a mixture of two or more of these repellents is more effective against a greater variety of insects than any one repellent. Repellents may be toxic if they are taken internally. People who are sensitive to these chemicals may develop skin reactions such as itching, burning, and swelling. Repellents cause smarting when they are applied to broken skin or mucous membranes. They should be applied carefully around the eyes because they may cause a burning sensation.

Product Selection Guidelines

Medication often is requested after symptoms appear, thus, it is important to determine the nature of symptoms following the sting or bite, how soon the symptoms appeared, the severity of the symptoms, and what other drugs are being used concurrently.

Nonprescription products are of minimal value to hypersensitive individuals. The pharmacist should record all information on hypersensitive individuals and should recommend that the person wear a tag or carry a card showing the nature of the allergy. If the symptoms, such as localized irritation, itching, or swelling, are minor, an appropriate nonprescription product may be recommended. Topical lotions, creams, ointments, and sprays are the main nonprescription products used for symptomatic relief of local reactions to insect stings and bites. The main considerations in product selection are reducing the possibility of additional stings or bites, providing proper protection to the affected skin, preventing secondary infection in the affected area, and relieving itching and irritation.

In spite of being capable of producing topical or systemic adverse reactions, external analgesics and antipruritics are considered to be relatively safe and effective. These nonprescription products are for adults and children 2 years of age and older and should be applied no more than 3 or 4 times/day. For children under 2 years of age, there is no recommended dosage except under the advice and supervision of a physician.

The label on external analgesic nonprescription products should indicate the ingredients and their concentrations, the manner of usage and frequency of applications, and the indications for use. The FDA advisory review panel on nonprescription external analgesic drug products recommended that the labeling should include the following warnings:

- For external use only.
- Avoid contact with eyes.
- If condition worsens, or if symptoms persist for more than 7 days, discontinue use of this product and consult a physician.

- Do not use for children under 2 years of age except under advice and supervision of a physician.

Summary

Stings of honeybees, bumblebees, yellow jackets, hornets, wasps, and ants may cause pain, discomfort, illness, and severe local and systemic reactions. In normal individuals, stinging and biting insects cause local irritation, inflammation, swelling, and itching that provoke rubbing and scratching. In hypersensitive individuals, anaphylactoid reactions may pose serious emergency problems. Papules or nodules from bites or stings may form and persist for months. Potential secondary infections may lead to impetigo, furunculosis, or eczematoid dermatitis. Topical nonprescription products that contain hydrocortisone, calamine, benzocaine, antihistamines, benzalkonium chloride, benzethonium chloride, camphor, and menthol may relieve or prevent these symptoms.

People sensitized to insect venom may react violently when they are stung. They need immediate, active treatment such as the administration of epinephrine hydrochloride. Partial desensitization may be accomplished by insect venom immunotherapy. The pharmacist can play a significant role by advising hypersensitive individuals on emergency procedures for insect stings and bites.

References

1. *FDA Drug Bulletin, 9* (3), 15 (1979).
2. H. G. Rapaport, *Drug Therapy, 23,* May (1975).
3. N. A. Weber, *Am. J. Trop. Med., 17,* 765 (1937).
4. R. M. Gordan and W. Crewe, *Ann. Trop. Med. Parasitol., 42,* 334 (1948).
5. Y. Felman and J. A. Nikites, *Cutis, 25,* 32 (1980).
6. L. C. Parish and J. A. Witkowski, *Drug Therapy, 10,* 145 (1980).
7. A. W. Green, R. E. Reisman, and C. E. Arbesman, *J. Allergy Clin. Immunol., 66,* 186 (1980).
8. R. E. Reisman, in "Allergy and Clinical Immunology," R. F. Lockey, Ed., Medical Examination, Garden City, N. J., 1979.
9. W. C. Light, R. E. Reisman, M. Shimizu, and C. E. Arbesman, *J. Allergy Clin. Immunol., 59,* 391 (1977).
10. W. R. Horsfall, "Medical Entomology," Ronald Press, New York, N.Y., 1962, p. 182.
11. J. A. McKiel and J. C. Clunie, *Can. J. Zool., 38,* 479 (1960).
12. A. Hudson, J. A. McKiel, A. S. West, and R. K. Bourns, *Mosq. News, 18,* 249 (1958).
13. D. W. Micks and J. P. Ellis, *Proc. Soc. Exp. Biol. Med., 78,* 69 (1951).
14. H. V. Allington and R. R. Allington, *J. Am. Med. Assoc., 155,* 240 (1954).
15. T. Ishizaka, *J. Allergy Clin. Immunol., 67,* 90, (1981).
16. D. R. Hoffman, *Ann. Allergy, 41,* 278 (1978).
17. A. K. Sobotka, R. M. Franklin, N. F. Adkinson, M. Valentine, H. Baer, and L. M. Lichtenstein, *J. Allergy Clin. Immunol., 57,* 29 (1976).
18. B. R. Paull, J. W. Yuninger, and G. J. Gleich, *J. Allergy Clin. Immunol., 59,* 334 (1977).
19. D. R. Hoffman, W. H. Shipman, and D. Babin, *J. Allergy Clin. Immunol., 59,* 147 (1977).
20. E. Habermann, *Science, 177,* 314 (1972).
21. D. B. K. Golden, A. K. Sobotka, M. D. Valentine, and L. M. Lichtenstein, *J. Allergy Clin. Immunol., 67,* 370 (1981).
22. D. B. K. Golden, A. K. Sobotka, M. D. Valentine, and L. M. Lichtenstein, *J. Allergy Clin. Immunol., 67,* 482 (1981).
23. R. E. Reisman, *J. Allergy Clin. Immunol., 64,* 3 (1979).
24. D. B. K. Golden, M. D. Valentine, A. K. Sobotka, and L. M. Lichtenstein, *Ann. Intern. Med., 92,* 620, (1980).
25. L. M. Lichtenstein, M. D. Valentine, and A. K. Sobotka, *J. Allergy Clin. Immunol., 64,* 5 (1979).
26. J. Parrino and R. Lockey, in "Current Therapy," W. B. Saunders, Philadelphia, Pa., 1980, p. 602.
27. M. D. Ellis, "Dangerous Plants, Snakes, Arthropods and Marine Life of Texas," U. S. Department of Health, Education, and Welfare, 1975, p. 175.
28. R. E. Arnold, "What to Do About Bites and Stings of Venomous Animals," Collier Books, New York, N.Y., 1973, p. 9.
29. *FDA Drug Bulletin, 10*(2), 12 (1980).
30. *Federal Register, 44,* 69833 (1979).
31. H. Wilson, *Practitioner, 197,* 673 (1966).
32. J. Adriani, *J. Am. Med. Assoc., 196,* 119 (1966).
33. *Federal Register, 44,* 69807 (1979).
34. R. J. von Witt, *Lancet, 2,* 1379 (1980).
35. *Federal Register, 44,* 69845 (1979).
36. A. Kligman and K. Kaidberg, *Cutis, 22,* 232 (1978).
37. *Federal Register, 43,* 34641 (1978).
38. M. Nienhuis and B. Rowles, *U.S. Pharm., 9,* 41 (1980).

Insect Sting and Bite Product Table

Product (Manufacturer)	Application Form	Other Ingredients
A-200 Pyrinate (Norcliff Thayer)	liquid gel	pyrethrins, 0.165% (liq.), piperonyl butoxide; 0.333% (gel); 2% (liq.), 4% (gel); deodorized kerosene, 0.5%
Americaine (American Critical Care)	aerosol	benzocaine, 20%; water dispersible base
Americaine First Aid Spray (American Critical Care)	spray	benzocaine, 10%; benzethonium chloride, 0.1%; alcohol, 25%
Bactine (Miles)	spray	benzalkonium chloride; lidocaine, 2.5%
Barc (Commerce)	liquid cream	isobornyl thiocyanoacetate, 4.1%; related compounds, 0.9%
Bevill's Lotion (Bevill)	lotion	alcohol, 68%; ether, 8%; methyl salicylate, 1%; salicylic acid
Chiggerex (Scherer)	ointment	benzocaine, 2.0%; camphor, 0.008%; olive oil, 0.008%; menthol, 0.005%; peppermint oil, 0.005%; methylparaben, 0.002%; clove oil, 0.002%
Chiggertox Liquid (Scherer)	liquid	isopropyl alcohol, 53%; benzyl benzoate, 21.4%; soft soap, 21.4%; benzocaine, 2.1%
Cuprex (Beecham Products)	liquid	tetrahydronaphthalene, 30.97%; copper oleate, 0.03%
Derma Medicone (Medicone)	ointment	zinc oxide, 137.3 mg/g; benzocaine, 20.0 mg/g; 8-hydroxyquinoline sulfate, 10.5 mg/g; ichthammol, 10.0 mg/g; menthol, 4.8 mg/g; petrolatum; lanolin; perfume
Dermoplast (Ayerst)	spray	polyethylene glycol 400 monolaurate; benzocaine, 20%; methylparaben, 2%; menthol, 0.5%; polysorbate 80
Di-Delamine Double Antihistamine (Commerce)	gel	tripelennamine hydrochloride, 0.5%; diphenhydramine hydrochloride, 1.0%
Di-Delamine Double Antihistamine (Commerce)	spray	tripelennamine hydrochloride, 0.5%; diphenhydramine hydrochloride, 1.0%; benzalkonium chloride, 0.125%
Mediconet (Medicone)	saturated medical pads	hamamelis water, 50%; glycerin, 10%; ethoxylated lanolin, 0.5%; methylparaben, 0.15%; benzalkonium chloride, 0.02%; perfume
Nupercainal Cream (Ciba)	cream	dibucaine, 0.5%; acetone sodium bisulfite, 0.37%; water-washable base
Nupercainal Ointment (Ciba)	ointment	dibucaine, 1%; acetone sodium bisulfite, 0.5%
Obtundia Surgical Dressing (Otis Clapp)	liquid	cresol–camphor complex
Pyribenzamine (Ciba)	cream ointment	tripelennamine, 2%; water-washable base (cream); petrolatum base (ointment)
Rexall First Aid Spray (Rexall)	spray	benzocaine; methylbenzethonium chloride; tyloxapol; chlorothymol; isopropyl alcohol, 4%; camphor
RID (Pfipharmecs)	liquid	pyrethrins, 0.3%; piperonyl butoxide, 3%; petroleum distillate, 1.2%
Surfadil (Lilly)	cream lotion	diphenhydramine hydrochloride, 19%; cyclomethycaine, 0.5%; titanium dioxide, 5% (lotion)
Triple X (Younds Drug)	liquid	pyrethrins, 0.3%; piperonyl butoxide, 3%; petroleum distillate, 1.2%
Tucks and Tucks Take-Alongs (Parke-Davis)	medical pads	hamamelis water, 50%; glycerin, 10%; methylparaben, 0.1%; benzalkonium chloride, 0.003%

25 Burn and Sunburn Products

Chester A. Bond

Questions to Ask the Patient

What caused the burn—chemicals, sun exposure, or heat?

How severe is the burn? Is the skin broken and/or blistered?

How long ago did the burn occur?

Where is the burn? Does it affect the eyes, genitalia, face, hands, or feet?

Is the burn oozing?

Is the burn painful?

How large is the burned area?

How old is the patient?

Does the patient have any other medical problems?

Are there any other injuries?

What treatments have been used?

Each year in the United States there are an estimated 5.6 million fire-related incidents (1), resulting in approximately 2 million burn accidents (2). Of these burn accidents, 100,000 require hospitalization with over 2 million days spent in hospitals (3). Annually, 6,000 deaths are secondary to burn-related accidents (2). Burn injuries can be broken down by age: under 17 years of age (33%), between 17 and 44 years (45%), 45 years and older (23%). Adjusting the number of burns for the population shows that serious burns are most common in those individuals under 17 years old. Although these figures appear high, the mortality/ 100,000 people has decreased slowly since 1920, with a rapid reduction since 1950 (1). This decrease in mortality emphasizes the effectiveness of fire control measures, flame retardant clothing, and improved safety standards for housing. The decrease in mortality can be attributed directly to improved systemic and topical therapies, better understanding of the pathophysiology of the burn wound, and the establishment of easily accessible specialized burn centers.

Confronted with a patient having a small minor burn or sunburn, the pharmacist should render basic first aid, if necessary, and assess whether to recommend physician referral or self-medication to the patient.

Etiology of Burns

Most burn injuries occur in the home or from industrial accidents. Of 400 cases admitted in 1 year to the burn unit at the Birmingham Accident Hospital, 75% of the burns occurred in the home, and 25% were due to industrial accidents (4). In another review, of 789 patients admitted to the burn unit of the University Hospital, Uppsala, Sweden, the most common cause of injury was scalding (34%), fire (32%), hot objects (17%), electricity (7%), and chemical agents (4%) (5). In children under 3 years of age, the most common cause of a severe burn is scalding. In children 3–14 years old, flame burns due to ignited clothing predominate; in persons 15–60 years old, industrial accidents account for the largest percent of burns; in those over 60 years, accidents associated with momentary blackouts, smoking in bed, or house fires are the most common causes of burns. With conventional military warfare, 10–30% of all combat casualties are secondary to thermal injuries (6).

Of the 2 million burn-related accidents occurring annually in the United States, less than 5% of these are severe enough to require hospitalization. Over 80% of minor burns occur in the home with scalds, contact, and fabric burns accounting for 89% of household burns (6). Sixty-three percent of household burns are on the hands and arms, and 34% are on the face and legs. Most of these burns do not require medical assistance and may be managed by the patient with appropriate care and nonprescription products. Of the minor burns that occur outside the home, sunburn is the most common. Sunburn has been underrated in most burn surveys since the public often does not consider sunburn in the same context as thermal burns.

Skin Anatomy and Physiology

The skin is the largest organ in the human body and constitutes approximately 17% of the average person's body weight. Figure 1 depicts a cross-section of the normal anatomy of the skin and the depth of burns in thermal damage. The major function of the skin is to protect the underlying organ systems from trauma, temperature variations, harmful penetrations, moisture, humidity, radiation, and invasion by microorganisms. In addition, the skin produces secretions from its exocrine glands, is involved in carbohydrate, protein, fat, and vitamin D metabolism, operates its own delayed hypersensitivity reactions, and provides the body with the sense of touch. (See Chapter 27, *Topical Anti-infective Products.*)

Pathophysiology of Burns

Burn damage to skin causes cellular death, capillary injury to varying degrees, and coagulation of protein. Capillary injury is manifested by capillary permeability, resulting in the wet or weepy appearance of second- and third-degree burns. Immediately after a moderate to severe burn, there is cessation of blood flow to the affected area, which is caused primarily by thrombosis and which persists for 3–4 weeks in full-thickness burns. In partial-thickness burns after initial occlusion, arterial and venous circulation is restored within 48–72 hours. Should drying of the wound or infection occur, circulation is not re-established, and a partial-thickness burn can be converted to a full-thickness burn (7, 8). Therefore, drying of the burn wound should be prevented if at all possible. When the blood supply is interrupted, delivery of systemically administered antibiotics to the infection site is prevented and both humoral and cellular defense mechanisms are effectively impeded, thus increasing the risk of infection.

With large deep burns, large amounts of body fluids and electrolytes leave the vascular compartment to extravascular spaces. This fluid redistribution is compounded by the loss of large amounts of body fluids and electrolytes through the burn wound itself. As a result, the cardiac output falls and the patient may go into shock. To prevent this, massive amounts of colloids and intravenous fluids are required during the first 2–4 days of hospitalization. Should the patient experience respiratory burn from inhaled hot gases, endotracheal intubation and mechanical ventilatory assistance may be required. Complete re-epithelialization following burns depends on burn depth, the immediate care given to the wound, and whether an infection ensues (9, 10).

Categorization of Burn Injuries

Determining the area and degree of the burn is not simple even for burn specialists. The American Burn Association has identified three treatment categories for burn patients (30):

- **Major burn injuries**—second-degree burns with a body surface area greater than 25% in adults (20% in children); all third-degree burns with a body surface of 10% or greater; all burns involving hands, face, eyes, ears, feet, and perineum; all inhalation injuries; electrical burns; complicated burn injuries involving fractures or other major trauma; and all poor-risk patients (elderly patients and those with an intercurrent disease);
- **Moderate, uncomplicated burn injuries**—second-degree burns with a body surface area of 15–25% in adults (10–20% in children); third-degree burns with a body surface area of less than 10%, and burns not involving eyes, ears, face, hands, feet, or perineum;
- **Minor burn injuries**—second-degree burns with a body surface area of less than 15% in adults (10% in children); third-degree burns with a body surface area of less than 2%; and burns not involving eyes, ears, face, hands, feet, or perineum; excludes electrical injuries, inhalation injuries, and all poor-risk patients.

Determination of Burned Area

The percentage of the body area that has been burned can be estimated by the "Rule of Nines" (Figure 2)

Level

Depth of Burn

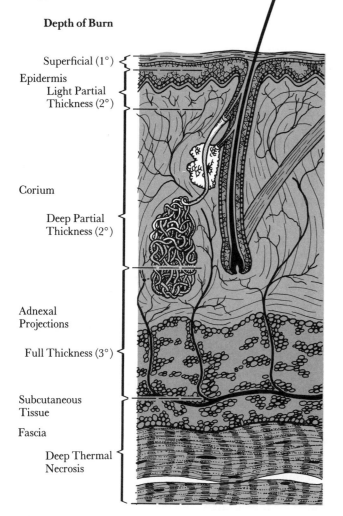

Superficial (1°)

Epidermis

Light Partial Thickness (2°)

Corium

Deep Partial Thickness (2°)

Adnexal Projections

Full Thickness (3°)

Subcutaneous Tissue

Fascia

Deep Thermal Necrosis

Figure 1. Cross-section of skin showing depth of burns.

where the body is divided into 11 areas with each area representing about 9% of the total. For children under 10 years of age, the Rule of Nines must be adjusted since their bodies have different proportions. Generally, the child's head is 19% of the body surface area at birth and decreases by 1% each year, the difference being added in equal amounts of each of the lower limbs.

As a rule of thumb, the area of one side of the hand is 1% of the body surface area of an adult. This quick method estimates the surface area covered by a burn. If the burn is second degree or greater and covers more than 1% of the body surface area, a physician should be consulted.

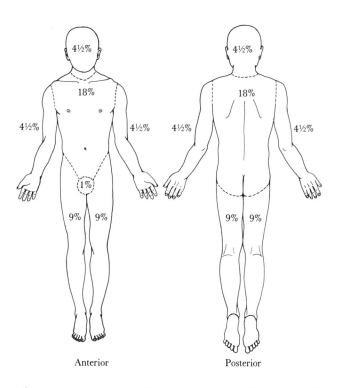

Anterior   Posterior

Figure 2. Rule of nines, first devised by E. J. Pulaski, M.D., and C. W. Dennison, M.D., is a rapid method of estimating the percentage of the body surface burned. It has been widely accepted. For example, an adult with a burn area of one arm (9%), the front of the trunk (18%), and half of one leg (9%) would total 36% burn. Adapted with permission from "The Guide to Fluid Therapy," Baxter Laboratories, Division of Travenol Laboratories, Inc, Deerfield, Ill., p. 111, 1969.

Determination of Clinical Severity

Determining the severity of the burn is a matter of clinical judgment depending on the burn thickness (Table 1).

- **First-degree burns**—These burns affect the epidermis and are characterized by erythema and pain, but no blistering. First-degree burns generally heal within 1 week with no scarring.

- **Second-degree burns**—These are burns that affect the epidermis and some dermis tissue. They are characterized by erythema, blistering, and more severe pain. If the second-degree burn is superficial, healing will occur within 3 weeks with no scarring. If the second-degree burn is deep, a firm, thick scar with loss of hair, sweat glands, and skin pigmentation will occur. Healing may take 1 month or more.

- **Third-degree burns**—These injuries affect the full-skin thickness, do not blister, have a leathery, white mottled appearance, and are less painful than first- and second-degree burns. Pain often is absent or diminished with third- and fourth-degree burns because of destruction of nervous tissue.

- **Fourth-degree or char burns**—These burns affect the full-skin thickness and underlying subcutaneous tissues, have a blackened appearance, are dry and painful, and carry the danger of deep infection. Third- and fourth-degree burns take longer than 1 month to heal and form scar tissue.

Burns greater than second degree should be evaluated by a physician to prevent infection and other complications. If the degree or severity of the burn is difficult to determine, the patient should be referred to a physician.

Infection

Infection secondary to burns is dangerous and difficult to treat since the burned dead skin provides an ideal growth medium for bacteria, and the avascular burned tissue hinders effective delivery of antimicrobials. The sequence of events leading to clinically significant infections following burn injury has been elucidated. For a very brief period after a severe burn, the wound surface is sterile. Shortly thereafter, colonization occurs by a mixed flora in which gram-positive organisms predomi-

Table 1. Depth classification of burns		
Type	**Tissue affected**	**Characteristics**
First-degree	Epidermis	Erythema, pain, no blistering
Second-degree	Epidermis, some dermis	Erythema, blisters, pain
Third-degree	Full skin thickness	No blisters, leathery white appearance, less pain
Fourth-degree and char burn	Full skin thickness and underlying tissue	Blackened appearance, dryness, pain, danger of deep infection

nate (*Staphylococci* and *Streptococci*). By the third postburn day, this bacterial population becomes dominated by gram-negative organisms (*Pseudomonas aeruginosa, Klebsiella-Enterobacter* species, *Proteus*), and the fungi *Candida* (11). By the fifth postburn day, invasion of tissue well beneath the burn surface may occur. These organisms then can proliferate and eventually invade adjacent unburned tissue, causing burn wound sepsis (12).

To prevent and treat burn wound sepsis of severe burns, mafenide, silver nitrate, and silver sulfadiazine are used (13). The agents work best in patients who have burns on less than 50% of their body surface, and they have improved the survival rates of patients with burns involving 50–70% of their body surface area. When more than 70% of the body surface area is affected, studies have shown no reduction in mortality (12–14). This decrease in mortality is attributed to the control of bacterial flora and the elimination of burn-wound sepsis.

Sunburn

Sunburn is usually self-limiting and does not require treatment by a physician unless the burn is quite severe, becomes infected, or is associated with another serious problem. Energy emissions from the sun include radiation wavelengths ranging from 200 nm to more than 18,000 nm (15). Ultraviolet radiation is in the 200–400 nm range, and this spectrum is subdivided into three bands from the longer to the shorter as follows (16):

- UV-A (320–400 nm) radiation can cause tanning of the skin, but is weak in causing mild sunburn of the skin.
- UV-B (290–320 nm) radiation causes sunburn reaction, which also stimulates pigmentation (tanning) of the skin.
- UV-C (200–290 nm) radiation from sunlight does not reach the earth's surface, but artificial UV sources can emit this radiation. It does not tan the skin, but it can burn it.

Other wavelengths of light also are absorbed and, if intense enough, produce erythema and burning. This type of burning differs from sunburn in that it is due to generated heat rather than a photochemical reaction.

The vascular changes that occur secondary to exposure to ultraviolet light are biphasic. The immediate erythema reaction is a faint, transient reddening of the skin beginning shortly after exposure to ultraviolet light and fading within 30 minutes after the exposure ends. A delayed erythema reaction appears after 2–6 hours and peaks at 10–24 hours after ultraviolet-light exposure. (See *Plate 3-13.*) This erythema gradually subsides over the next 2–4 days. Peeling follows 4–7 days after a moderate to severe sunburn. The mechanisms by which these two types of erythema are produced are not understood completely. Kinins (17, 18), histamine (19), prostaglandins (20–25), other vasoactive substances (26), hydrolytic enzymes (27), and free radicals (28) have been implicated as mediators of the erythema caused by sunlight. Although prostaglandins have received much attention in the scientific and lay press, none of these substances is universally accepted as the mediators (causes) of sunburn.

Clinically, mild sunburn is tender to the touch and the patient may complain of a hot, drawn feeling of the skin. A patient with a more severe burn may experience intense pain, inability to tolerate contact with clothing, and systemic symptoms of fever, chills, nausea, and prostration.

Photosensitization

A photosensitivity reaction should be considered in a patient who experiences sunburn in greater amounts than would be normally expected from ultraviolet light exposure or who develops a rash in areas exposed to the sun. Photosensitivity reactions can occur from topically applied or systemically administered compounds. Both types of photosensitivity reactions require the presence of drug and light. (See *Plate 3-14* and *3-15*). The first type is a photoallergic reaction, in which the drug is altered in the presence of sunlight so that it becomes antigenic or acts as a hapten (Figure 3). Photoallergic eruptions require previous exposure to the offending drug and are not dose related. These eruptions may be induced by chemically related drugs and may appear in various forms, such as eczematous, macular, or papular lesions, which may not appear for 24 hours or longer after exposure. Acute urticarial lesions may develop within minutes after exposure. The eruption is not localized exclusively at sun exposure sites but frequently extends beyond the exposure area. These types of photosensitivity eruptions are usually caused by topical agents.

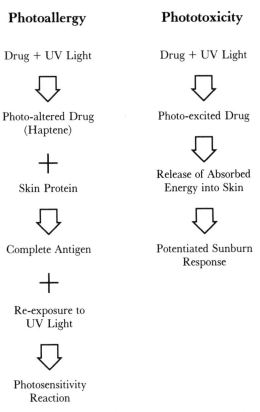

Figure 3. Comparison of photoallergy and phototoxicity reactions. Reprinted with permission from *Am. Pharm., NS21,* 296 (1981).

Table 2. Some drugs that may cause photosensitivity

Anticancer drugs
Dacarbazine
Fluorouracil
Methotrexate
Vinblastine

Antidepressants
Amitriptyline
Desipramine
Doxepin
Imipramine
Nortriptyline
Protriptyline
Trimipramine

Antihistamines
Cyproheptadine
Diphenhydramine

Antimicrobials
*Demeclocycline
Doxycycline
Griseofulvin
*Nalidixic acid
Oxytetracycline
Sulfacytine
Sulfamethazine
Sulfamethizole
Sulfamethoxazole
Trimethoprim-
  sulfamethoxazole
Sulfasalazine
Sulfathiazole
Sulfisoxazole
Tetracycline

Antipsychotic drugs
Chlorpromazine
Fluphenazine
Haloperidol
Perphenazine
Piperacetazine
Prochlorperazine
Promethazine
Thioridazine

Antipsychotic drugs
(continued)
Trifluoperazine
Triflupromazine
Trimeprazine

Diuretics
Bendroflumethiazide
Benzthiazide
Chlorothiazide
Cyclothiazide
Furosemide
Hydrochlorothiazide
Hydroflumethiazide
Methyclothiazide
Metolazone
Polythiazide
Quinethazone
Trichlormethiazide

Hypoglycemics
Acetohexamide
Chlorpropamide
Tolazamide
Tolbutamide

Sunscreens
Para-aminobenzoic acid
PABA esters

Other
*Bergamot oil, oils of citron,
  lavender, lime,
  sandalwood, cedar (used
  in many perfumes and
  cosmetics)
Carbamazepine
*Coal tar
Disopyramide
Gold salts
Hexachlorophene
*Methoxsalen
Oral contraceptives
*Trioxsalen

*Reactions occur frequently.

Reprinted with permission from *The Medical Letter on Drugs and Therapeutics, 22* (562) 64 (1980), The Medical Letter, Inc., New Rochelle, N.Y.

The second type of photosensitive eruption is known as a phototoxic reaction. In this reaction, the drug is altered by light to a toxic form which damages the skin tissue. It is independent of an allergic response. In contrast to the first type, this eruption may occur on the first exposure to the drug, is dose related, and occurs within several hours of exposure to the sun; usually no cross-sensitivity exists (Figure 3). A phototoxic reaction almost always appears as an exaggerated sunburn. In

some instances, a drug may produce both photoallergic and phototoxic reactions (photosensitivity) (see Table 2) (28, 29).

Assessment

To recommend treatment to the burn patient, the pharmacist must make an accurate assessment of the patient and the injury to determine whether the burn is amenable to self-treatment or if consultation with or referral to the patient's physician is necessary.

It is important to know the cause of the burn and when it occurred to determine what, if any, self-treatment is appropriate. Pharmacists should be able to obtain this information and arrange transportation to a medical facility if referral is indicated.

The very young and the elderly generally should be referred to a physician because they may tolerate burn trauma poorly. Also, patients in these age groups may complain less about their burn than older children or young adults.

Burn patients with chronic or debilitating conditions (diabetes, obesity, alcoholism, cardiovascular disease, and renal disease) also should be referred to a physician. Individuals with a moderate to severe chronic illness tolerate burn trauma poorly and are more susceptible to complications from burns. The burn trauma may also precipitate an exacerbation of the patient's underlying disease.

Burns of the eye, genitalia, and perineum have more serious consequences and should be evaluated by a physician. Facial burns may be associated with respiratory injuries. Burns of the hands and feet may deserve special attention because healing may be delayed in these areas and they can be quite painful.

Treatment

Initial Care

Thermal Burns

Evidence suggests that the inflammatory process secondary to thermal burns can be reduced and sometimes reversed by cold-water therapy. One study showed that when cold water was applied to a burn, the visible area of redness was observed to reduce in extent and did not reappear later, suggesting an alteration in pathological state. It has been speculated that the lowered skin temperature inhibited capillary engorgement and the resulting loss of fluids. This in turn leads to a lowered metabolic requirement of the already-damaged tissues, allowing preservation of such tissues (30). Procedures of cold-water therapy include the following:

- The burned area should be immersed immediately in water drawn from the cold tap.
- The burn should be kept in static (nonrunning) water until it is free of pain both in and when it is taken out of the water; up to ¾ of an hour may be needed.
- In the great majority of cases, there is no necessity for further treatment, since blisters, which otherwise would appear, do not form, and the injury may not even need a dressing.

- If, after treatment with cold water, the patient desires to consult a physician, he should be strongly advised not to apply anything to the burn (31).

One investigator cautions against the use of this technique for the seriously burned child. The time involved may delay the emergency treatment of shock (32).

The public should be made aware of the value of cold in controlling the intense pain of minor burns (33).

Electrical Burns

Electrical burns may appear to be quite superficial since the only area that may appear to be burned is where the current entered and exited the body. However, there may be extensive damage to underlying nervous and muscle tissue. Only very minor electrical burns should be self-medicated. If in doubt, refer the patient to a physician.

Chemical Burns

Remove clothing from the affected area. Flood with large amounts of water (at least 15 minutes for acids, and until the skin no longer feels soapy for alkalies). Chemical antidotes should not be used, since the reaction heat may cause further damage. If the eyes are involved, they should be washed immediately and irrigated with tepid water for 15-30 minutes. The eyelid(s) should be pulled apart gently while irrigating the eye from the nasal corner to the outer corner. The face and eyelids also should be washed, and care should be taken not to wash the chemical into the other eye. The eye should be covered with a clean dressing, and the patient should be transported to a medical facility as soon as possible.

Sunburn

Sunburned patients should protect the burned area from further ultraviolet light exposure as soon as possible. Generally, if sunburn on the eyes and genitalia produces second-degree burns or the patient is having severe pain, the patient should be referred to a physician. Furthermore, if the sunburn affects more than 10% of the surface area of a child's body or more than 15–20% of an adult's body, the patient should be referred to a physician.

Heat stroke is most likely to occur (but not always) with excessive exposure to sunlight in a hot environment. Because of the complications of heat stroke, patients exhibiting hyperpyrexia, confusion, weakness, or convulsions should be referred to their physicians or an appropriate medical facility.

Minor Burns

Cleansing

The goals of treating first- and second-degree burns are relieving the pain associated with the burn, protecting the area from air and preventing dryness, and providing a favorable environment for healing that minimizes the chances of infection. After applying cold moisture to the burned area, which stops the progression of the burn injury, reduces local edema, and relieves pain, the area should be cleansed with water and a bland soap (34–38). After the burn is cleansed, a nonadherent, hypoallergic burn dressing may be applied if the area is small, or a skin protectant/lubricant may be applied if the burn is extensive or in an area that cannot be dressed easily. If the burn is weeping, soaking the burn 3–6 times/day for 15–30 minutes will provide a soothing effect and diminish the weeping. Minor burns usually are benign and repair themselves without treatment.

Dressings

Sterile, nonadherent dressings are the most convenient way to treat a small burn on an area of the body that may be easily bandaged (arm or leg).

The following is the recommended sequence for dressing a small burn (normally only necessary with second-degree burns) (39).

- A nonadherent primary layer of sterile, fine-mesh gauze lightly impregnated with sterile petrolatum is recommended since it prevents the gauze from sticking to the wound and allows burn exudate to flow freely through the gauze, thus avoiding tissue maceration. Commercially prepared nonadhering petrolatum dressings, such as Xeroflo or Adaptic, incorporate wettable hydrophilic petrolatum into the gauze to aid permeability.
- An absorbent intermediate layer of piled-up gauze should be applied over the petrolatum gauze. This layer draws and stores burn exudate away from the wound, which guards against maceration. Cotton or paper products should not be used since they often stick to the burn and are painful and difficult to remove. This layer should be applied loosely to accommodate edema, should it occur.
- A supportive outer layer of rolled gauze bandage should be applied over the primary and intermediate layers to hold these layers in place and mildly restrict movement. Elastic or other expandable bandages that tighten after being applied should not be used because this restrictive outer layer could restrict circulation if edema develops.

After 48 hours, the dressing should be changed. If the dressing sticks to the wound, soaking in warm water will loosen the gauze from the burn with minimal pain and trauma. The sticking gauze should be removed slowly rather than quickly since this can destroy the regenerating epithelium and cause pain. The wound should be observed for signs of infection at each dressing change. The earliest signs of infection may appear as inflamed wound edges, new blistering, or intensification of pain. If the affected skin begins to become macerated (feels or looks wrinkled or fissured), dressing the wound should be discontinued temporarily and the wound should be exposed to air. Once the pain subsides and healing begins (in 4–10 days), wound dressings may be discontinued.

Soaks

The inflammation from first- and second-degree burns may be reduced by having the patient soak the affected area in water, normal saline, or Burow's solution di-

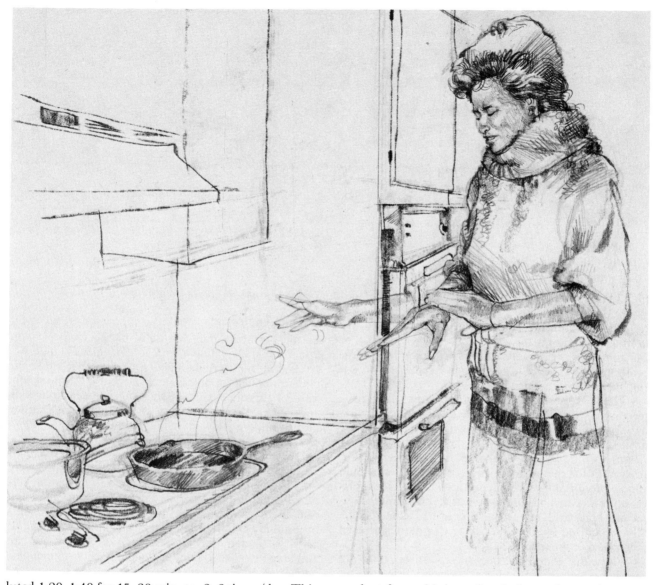

luted 1:20–1:40 for 15–30 minutes 3–6 times/day. This therapy is particularly applicable to weeping lesions because it provides a cooling, soothing treatment that promotes drying. Once weeping subsides, a skin protectant may be used. Depending on the burn size and location, the patient may immerse the affected areas directly into the soak, or apply a towel or cloth soaked in the solution (lightly wrung), or draw a bath and soak in it for the prescribed time. The temperature of the soak should be cool to warm (not cold or hot) depending on the patient's preference. If maceration occurs, soaks should be discontinued. When drying the affected areas after the soak, care must be taken not to irritate the burn by rubbing with a towel. The proper technique for drying the burned area (or other irritated areas of the skin) is patting the area gently with a dry clean towel, *not rubbing*.

Pharmacologic Agents

As previously mentioned, most minor burns heal by themselves. The major purpose of pharmacotherapy is to make the patient more comfortable and allow the burn to heal. The pharmacist should not recommend a product for a third- or fourth-degree burn, since this may cause the patient to delay appropriate treatment by his or her physician. Additionally, inappropriate applications of topical preparations to severe burns by well-meaning friends will only have to be removed (usually with considerable discomfort) when the patient seeks medical treatment. The pharmacist also should be aware that damaged skin, secondary to burns, loses some of its barrier function and that there is enhanced percutaneous absorption of drugs and chemicals (40). This factor increases the possibility of systemic side effects occurring, especially if the burn areas are large such as is seen in a patient with extensive sunburn or when the patient applies topical medicines too frequently.

Protectants

The FDA advisory review panel on nonprescription skin protectant drug products concluded that the agents in Table 3 are safe and effective (Category I) in treating first- and minor second-degree burns (41). Skin protectants benefit patients with minor burns by making the wound area more comfortable and provide their

Table 3. Skin protectants

Dryness (wetting agent)	Approved concentration	Wetness (drying agent)	Approved concentration	Lubricity	Approved concentration
Allantoin	0.5–2.0%	Aluminum hydroxide gel	0.15–5.0%	Cocoa butter	80–100%
Cocoa butter	80–100%	Calamine	1–25%	Dimethicone	1–30%
Dimethicone	1–30%	Corn starch	10–85%	Petrolatum	30–100%
Glycerin	20–45%	Dimethicone	1–30%	Shark liver oil	3%
Petrolatum	30–100%	Kaolin	4–20%	Zinc carbonate	0.2–2%
Shark liver oil	3%	Sodium bicarbonate	1–100%	Zinc oxide	1–25%
		Zinc acetate	0.1–2.0%		
		Zinc carbonate	0.2–2%		
		Zinc oxide	1–25%		

therapeutic effects by protecting the burn from mechanical irritation caused by friction and rubbing and by preventing drying of the stratum corneum. Rehydrating the stratum corneum relieves the symptoms of irritation and permits normal healing to continue. Skin protectants provide only symptomatic relief and do not stop the underlying burn process.

The FDA has additionally classified skin protectants by whether the ingredients are intended primarily to treat or relieve conditions where either dryness or wetness predominates and whether lubricity (lessening of friction) is needed. In selecting a skin protectant for the burn patient, the pharmacist should choose products that prevent dryness and provide lubrication. The panel has proposed classifying bismuth subnitrate, boric acid, sulfur, and tannic acid as not generally recognized as safe and effective or as misbranded when used as skin protectants.

The panel found no effective product or substance that "cures any irritation" or "prevents formation of blisters." Claims that certain substances contained in many skin protectants (allantoin, live yeast cell derivatives, and zinc acetate) have an effect on accelerating wound healing were not recognized by the panel. There are no controlled studies that conclusively prove that minor wounds amenable to nonprescription treatment can be healed in an accelerated fashion.

The provisional FDA-approved skin protectants are both safe and nontoxic. The panel recommended that the restriction preventing use in children under 2 be waived for most skin protectants except for products containing live yeast cell derivatives, shark liver oil, and zinc acetate where the limit applies. An additional exception was made for glycerin and aluminum hydroxide gel. The recommended labeling for these two ingredients is: "There is no recommended dosage for children under 6 months of age except under the advice and supervision of a physician." The panel made these recommendations on the basis of safety considerations. Generally, the burn patient may apply a skin protectant as often as needed, and if the burn has not improved by 7 days or worsens after treatment, the patient should consult a physician (41).

Topical Analgesics

Local Anesthetics

Local anesthetics may be useful in relieving the pain associated with minor burns. These agents should not be used to treat serious burns since they may cause the patient to delay appropriate treatment by a physician. Table 4 lists the local anesthetics concluded to be safe and effective in relieving pain associated with minor burns (42).

Local anesthetics can be divided into four classes: esters, of which benzocaine is the most commonly used agent; nonester or nonamide agents, which are rarely used; and amides and antihistamines. The antihistamines have only weak local anesthetic activity when compared to the ester and amide types (42). The antihistamine local anesthetics also can cause irritation or act as a hapten, causing sensitization (42). Thus, an amide or ester local anesthetic usually is recommended, when needed, to relieve the pain associated with minor burns.

The choice between a product containing benzocaine or lidocaine is difficult. With benzocaine or similar local anesthetics, there is a higher incidence of sensitization (43) (about 1%) than with lidocaine, but benzocaine is virtually devoid of systemic toxicities (39). Benzocaine rarely has been reported to induce reversible methemoglobinemia (44, 45). Lidocaine, while having a very low incidence of sensitization, may cause systemic side effects (CNS stimulation, CNS depression, drowsiness, nervousness, dizziness, blurred vision, nausea, tremors, convulsions, respiratory arrest, myocardial depression, and cardiac arrest) when applied over large areas of damaged skin or used for prolonged periods (42). Systemic toxicity from local anesthetics is rare because the short-term use for minor burns generally does not allow elevated toxic blood levels to occur. Cross-sensitization to local anesthetics in different classes is very rare and, thus, a patient sensitized to one class usually can use a local anesthetic in another class without problems.

Local anesthetics must penetrate the skin to produce their desired effects, and the degree of penetration is determined by the amount of damage to the skin. In general, lower concentrations of local anesthetics (Table 4) that are effective on severely damaged skin may be ineffective on intact skin or mildly damaged skin. For example, in concentrations below 20%, benzocaine fails to have beneficial effects on intact or mildly sunburned skin (46). In studies on damaged skin, however, concentrations as low as 5% are effective. To ensure effectiveness, the pharmacist should select a product containing a local anesthetic in concentrations approaching the upper limits of the FDA-recommended concentrations. Benzocaine is recommended in concentrations of 5–20% applied to the affected area; lidocaine and lidocaine hydrochloride are recommended in concentrations of 0.5–4%. However, no claim for effectiveness is made when the hydrochloride is used on intact skin in the available nonprescription concentrations (42).

The FDA advisory review panel on nonprescription topical analgesic drug products recommended that products containing local anesthetics not be applied more than 3 or 4 times/day, not be used in large quantities, and not be applied over extensive areas or on raw, blistered, or damaged skin. These recommendations were made to reduce the possibility of systemic side effects. Since the duration of action of local anesthetics is only 30–45 minutes (41), it is impossible to provide pain relief action on a continuous basis. Because of these factors, the pharmacist should recommend that products containing local anesthetics be used only when the pain may be particularly bothersome to the patient (bedtime).

Topical Hydrocortisone

Topically applied hydrocortisone, available on a nonprescription basis, is reported to be a safe and effective alternative to nonprescription anesthetics such as benzocaine, diphenhydramine, menthol, and phenol, which are currently being used for mild sunburn (48).

Counterirritants

Counterirritant agents relieve pain by stimulating cutaneous neurons to provide a feeling of warmth or coolness. Counterirritant agents may irritate the burned tissue and ultimately result in more pain for the patient. Therefore, they should not be used on burns. (See Chapter 26, *External Analgesic Products.*)

Antimicrobials

The FDA advisory review panel on nonprescription topical antimicrobial drug products, including quaternary ammonium compounds, iodophors, organic mercurials, and phenols, has created several subclasses of antimicrobial preparations that may be applicable to burn remedies (45). These new subclasses include

- **Antimicrobial soap**—a soap containing an active ingredient with both in-vitro and in-vivo activity against skin microorganisms;
- **Skin antiseptic**—a nonirritating antimicrobial-containing preparation that prevents overt skin infections;
- **Skin wound cleanser**—a nonirritating liquid preparation (or product to be used with water) that assists in removing foreign material from small superficial wounds, does not delay wound healing, and may contain an antimicrobial ingredient;
- **Skin wound protectant**—a nonirritating antimicrobial-containing preparation applied to small cleansed wounds; it provides a protective physical barrier and a chemical (antimicrobial) barrier that neither delays healing nor favors the microbial growth (49).

As previously mentioned, burn wounds are particularly susceptible to infection and, should this occur, the effects can be devastating. Because of these risks, any patient with an infected burn should be referred to a physician for evaluation and treatment.

The use of topical antibiotics is covered more fully in Chapter 28, *Topical Anti-infective Products.*

Product Formulation

Rarely will a product that is intended to treat minor burns contain only one ingredient. The FDA advisory review panel on nonprescription skin protectant drug products concluded that two or more skin protectant active ingredients may be combined provided that (42)

- Each is present in sufficient quantity to act additively or by summation to produce the claimed therapeutic effect when the ingredients are within the effective concentration range specified for each ingredient in the monograph;

Types	Approved concentrations (in %)
Ester	
Butamben[a]	1
Benzocaine	5–20
Tetracaine	1–2
Tetracaine hydrochloride	1–2
Diperodon hydrochloride	0.25–1
Amide	
Dibucaine	0.25–1
Dibucaine hydrochloride	0.25–1
Lidocaine	0.5–4
Lidocaine hydrochloride	0.5–4
Antihistamine	
Diphenhydramine hydrochloride	1–2
Methapyriline	1–2
Tripelennamine hydrochloride	0.5–2
Other	
Benzyl alcohol	10–33
Dimethisoquin hydrochloride	0.3–0.5
Dyclonine hydrochloride	0.5–1

Table 4. Local anesthetics

[a]May cause staining of the skin.

- The ingredients do not interact with each other and that one or more do not reduce the effectiveness of the other or others, by precipitation, change in acidity or alkalinity, or in some other manner that reduces the claimed therapeutic effect;
- The partition of the active ingredients between the skin and the vehicle in which they are incorporated is not impeded and that the therapeutic effectiveness of each remains as claimed or is not decreased.

Additionally, this panel recognized that skin protectants are suitable vehicles for use in delivering active ingredients classified in other categories such as topical analgesics and sunscreens. Under these circumstances, the skin protectant may serve a different purpose and is expected to meet the criteria established for this other purpose (analgesic or sunscreen).

The panel dealing with external analgesics concluded that combinations of topical analgesics listed in Table 4 may be combined with Category I counterirritants. Since the FDA has required products containing counterirritants to carry a warning label stating that this product should not be applied to wounds or damaged skin, use of these combination products on burns would be inappropriate.

Product Selection Guidelines

Once the burn has been assessed, and it is determined that nonprescription treatment is appropriate, the pharmacist should be able to recommend specific therapy once the burn has been cooled and cleansed. The pharmacist should recommend bandaging the area as outlined previously if the burn wound is small and in a location amenable to bandaging. Petrolatum-impregnated bandages are preferred, but if not available, a nonsticking gauze may be used. When using nonstick gauze, a protectant should be applied to the burn or on the gauze to provide a barrier layer to help prevent dryness and reduce the chances of infection.

If bandaging cannot be done, the pharmacist should recommend that the patient apply a protectant to prevent dryness and provide some pain relief. Protectants are available in cream, lotion, and ointment formulations. Ointments generally provide the best protection from dryness but are difficult to apply and remove. Creams are easier to apply but provide less protection from dryness. Emulsion lotion vehicles are also useful in preventing and treating dryness. Water in oil emulsions provide better efficacy than oil in water emulsions since they have a greater occlusion. Emulsions provide more protection from dryness than creams.

Shake lotions are intended to provide cooling, soothing, and drying effects. The latter effect is not desirable with a burn. They are most useful for eczematous lesions and should not be used when weeping occurs since the powder residue (left after the lotion dries) will cake and become difficult to remove. Additionally, this caked powder can allow bacteria to grow under it, which may result in infection.

In applying creams, lotions, or ointments, the pharmacist should remember to tell the patient that only a thin layer of medication is needed. If the patient can see excess cream, lotion, or ointment on the skin after application, too much has been applied. The patient should apply the protectant as often as needed with clean fingers or an applicator. To minimize the chance of contamination, the protectant should not be applied directly from its container.

To treat the pain associated with minor burns, various therapeutic modalities are available. Soaks may be particularly useful if the burn is inflamed or weeping, and they provide some pain relief. Protectants also provide some pain relief. Local anesthetics provide some short-term relief and probably are most useful with sunburn.

Aerosol dosage forms have an advantage because the patient does not have to apply the local anesthetic mechanically (causing pain). Aerosols generally are not very useful as protectants since oleaginous (occlusive) preparations are difficult to formulate into this dosage form. Aerosols should be shaken well prior to using, and the patient should be cautioned not to spray the product around the face where it could get into the eyes, nose, or could be inhaled. Generally the aerosol should be sprayed from about 6 inches above the skin in bursts of 1–3 seconds. Two disadvantages are connected with the aerosol dose form. This dosage form is costly compared with creams, lotions, etc. Moreover, when used on large areas of the body, such as the back, aerosols may produce shivering and nausea.

Aspirin or acetaminophen are valuable adjuvants in relieving burn pain. Since aspirin is an inhibitor of prostaglandin synthesis and also an anti-inflammatory agent in high doses, theoretically it should provide greater benefit than acetaminophen (44). Since prostaglandins are believed to be involved in the delayed erythema reaction in sunburn, some authorities recommend that patients experiencing sunburn should take 1,200 mg of aspirin every 4 hours for 1 day after the sunburn has begun in hopes of preventing or modifying this reaction. If GI upset or tinnitus (ringing or buzzing in the ears) occurs, the high-dose aspirin therapy should be discontinued. At this time, there is no scientific evidence to support or refute high-dose aspirin therapy. Undoubtedly high doses of aspirin provide more pain relief than standard dosages but whether aspirin actually modifies the sunburn reaction is unknown.

Nonprescription sedatives also may be useful for the burn patient since many patients with burns have trouble sleeping. Whatever the pharmacist recommends for the burn patient, the patient should be cautioned that a physician should be contacted if the condition worsens or has not improved within 7 days.

Summary

The pharmacist's understanding of burn and sunburn is important in making an accurate assessment of the burn patient and recommending appropriate treatment. The pharmacist should be able to

- Understand the etiology and pathophysiology of burns and sunburns;
- Understand the complications associated with burns and sunburns;

- Accurately assess the condition of the burn patient and refer the patient to a physician if necessary;
- Deliver initial care to the patient with a minor burn;
- Recommend appropriate nondrug therapy for the burn patient;
- Recommend appropriate pharmacotherapy for the burn patient.

In addition to providing accurate information and product recommendations to the burn patient, the pharmacist should be able to instruct the patient on how to care for the burn and how to use medications appropriately.

References

1. National Electronic Injury Surveillance System, Vol. 4, No. 2, U.S. Consumer Product Safety Commission, 1975.
2. C. A. Artz, *Med. Times, 104,* 128 (1976).
3. Department of Health, Education, and Welfare, Publication HSM 73-1763, 1973.
4. J. P. Bull, *Med. Press, 239,* 205 (1958).
5. T. Skoog, "The Surgical Treatment of Burns," Almquist and Wiksells, Stockholm, Sweden, 1963, p. 91.
6. C. Artz, J. Moncrief, and B. Pruitt, "Burns, A Team Approach," W. B. Saunders, Philadelphia, Pa., 1979, p. 19.
7. J. R. Hinshaw, *Arch. Surg., 87,* 131 (1963).
8. S. A. Order and J. A. Moncrief, "The Burn Wound," Charles C Thomas, Springfield, Ill., 1965, p. 132.
9. B. E. Zawacki, *Ann. Surg., 180,* 98 (1974).
10. T. B. Fitzpatrick, A. Z. Eisen, K. Wolff, I. M. Freedberg, and K. F. Austin, "Dermatology in General Medicine," 2nd ed., McGraw-Hill, New York, N.Y., 1979, p. 931.
11. B. C. Macmillan, *J. Infect. Dis., 124(suppl),* 278 (1971).
12. J. A. Moncrief, *J. Trauma, 4,* 233 (1964).
13. J. A. Moncrief, *Arch. Surg., 92,* 558 (1966).
14. J. A. Moncrief, *N. Engl. J. Med., 288,* 444 (1973).
15. J. R. Wuest and T. A. Gossel, *Am. Pharm., NS21,* 46 (1981).
16. *Federal Register, 43,* 38209 (1978).
17. J. H. Epstein and R. K. Winkelmann, *Arch. Dermatol., 95,* 532 (1967).
18. M. W. Greaves and J. Sondergaard, *J. Invest. Dermatol., 54,* 365 (1970).
19. E. J. Valtonen, *Acta Derm. Venerol.* [Stockh], *44,* 269 (1964).
20. G. Logan and D. L. Wilhelm, *Br. J. Exp. Pathol., 47,* 300 (1966).
21. P. Crunkhorn and A. L. Willis, *Br. J. Pharmacol., 41,* 507 (1971).
22. M. E. Goldyne, *J. Invest. Dermatol., 64,* 377 (1975).
23. J. Lord, *Br. J. Dermatol., 95,* 397 (1976).
24. D. K. Kurban et al., *J. Invest. Dermatol., 66,* 153 (1976).
25. W. L. Morrison, *J. Invest. Dermatol., 68,* 130 (1977).
26. G. Logan and D. Wilhelm, *Br. J. Exp. Pathol., 47,* 286 (1966).
27. B. E. Johnson and F. Daniels, *J. Invest. Dermatol., 53,* 85 (1969).
28. M. A. Pathak and K. Stratton, *Arch. Biochem. Biophys., 123,* 468 (1961).
29. W. P. Coleman, *Med. Clin. N. Amer., 51,* 1073 (1967).
30. E. Epstein, *Arch. Dermatol., 106,* 741 (1971).
31. A. Shulman, *J. Am. Med. Assoc., 1916,* August 27 (1980).
32. B. Sorenson, *Mod. Treatm., 4,* 1199 (1967).
33. J. S. Barnett, *Med. J. Aust., 1,* 240 (1968).
34. H. Kravitz, *Clin. Pediatr., 9,* 695 (1970).
35. H. Kravitz, *Pediatrics, 53,* 766 (1974).
36. A. Blumefield, *N. Engl. J. Med., 290,* 58 (1974).
37. J. G. Appleyard, *Lancet, 2,* 1370 (1972).
38. J. Moylan, *Postgrad. Med., 59,* 766 (1974).
39. M. F. Epstein and J. D. Crawford, *Pediatrics, 52,* 430 (1973).
40. *Patient Care,* July 1 64 (1976).
41. J. Pietsch and J. L. Meakins, *Lancet, 1,* 280 (1976).
42. *Federal Register, 43,* 4110–03 (1978).
43. *Federal Register, 44,* 234 (1979).
44. E. Epstein, *J. Am. Med. Assoc., 198,* 517 (1966).
45. H. Peterson, *N. Engl. J. Med., 263,* 454 (1960).
46. N. Goluboff and D. S. MacFayden, *J. Pediatr., 47,* 222 (1955).
47. H. Dahli and J. Adriani, *Clin. Pharmacol. Ther., 12,* 913 (1971).
48. "The Pharmacological Basis of Therapeutics," 6th ed., A. G. Gilman, L. S. Goodman, and A. Gilman, Eds., Macmillan, New York, N.Y., 1980, p. 311.
49. C. Mueller and D. West, *Am. Pharm., NS21,* 51 (1981).
50. *Federal Register, 43,* 4110–03 (1978).

Burn and Sunburn Product Table

Product (Manufacturer)	Dosage Form	Anesthetic	Antimicrobial	Other Ingredients
Americaine (American Critical Care)	aerosol ointment	benzocaine, 20%	benzethonium chloride, 0.1% (ointment)	polyethylene glycols (ointment), water-dispersible base (aerosol)
Americaine First Aid Spray (American Critical Care)	spray	benzocaine, 10%	benzethonium chloride, 0.1%	alcohol, 25%
Bactine Antiseptic/ Anesthetic First Aid Spray (Miles)	aerosol liquid	lidocaine HCl, 2.5%	benzalkonium chloride, 0.13%	
Betadine (Purdue Frederick)	aerosol ointment		povidone-iodine, 5% (aerosol) 10% (ointment)	aqueous base (aerosol), water-miscible base (ointment)
Biotres (Central)	ointment		polymyxin B sulfate, 10,000 units/g; bacitracin zinc, 500 units/g	
Burn Ointment (Pfeiffer)	ointment	benzocaine, 2%	chloroxylenol, 1%	zinc oxide, 3%
Burn Relief Spray (Rexall)	spray	benzocaine	chlorobutanol, 0.3%; benzethonium chloride	polyethylene glycol; menthol; isopropyl alcohol, 11%
Burntame Spray (Otis Clapp)	spray	benzocaine, 20%	8-hydroxyquinoline	
Butesin Picrate (Abbott)	ointment	butamben picrate, 1%		
Dermoplast (Ayerst)	aerosol	benzocaine, 20% menthol, 0.5%		methylparaben, polyethylene glycol 400 monolaurate, polysorbate 85
Foille (Carbisulphoil Blistex)	liquid ointment aerosol	benzocaine, 2%	benzyl alcohol, 4%; 8-hydroxyquinoline	sulfur (lotion, aerosol), bland vegetable oil
Gebauer's Tannic Spray (Gebauer)	pump spray	benzocaine, less than 1%	chlorobutanol, 1.3%	tannic acid, 4.5%; menthol, less than 1%
Kip for Burns (Young's)	ointment		phenol, 0.5%	spearmint oil, bay oil, zinc oxide, petrolatum, paraffin, lanolin
Lanacane (Combe)	aerosol lotion	benzocaine, 10%	benzethonium chloride, 0.165% (aerosol); 0.1% (lotion)	
Lip-Gard (Whitehall)	lip balm			live yeast derivative containing skin respiratory factor, 67 units/gm; homosalate, 5%
Medicone Dressing Cream (Medicone)	cream	benzocaine, 5 mg/g	8-hydroxyquinoline sulfate, 0.5 mg/g	cod liver oil, 125 mg/g; zinc oxide, 125 mg/g; menthol, 1.8 mg/g; petrolatum; lanolin; paraffin; talc; perfume

Burn and Sunburn Product Table, continued

Product (Manufacturer)	Dosage Form	Anesthetic	Antimicrobial	Other Ingredients
Mediconet (Medicone)	cloth wipe		benzalkonium chloride, 0.02%	hamamelis water, 50%; glycerin, 10%; ethoxylated lanolin, 0.5%; methylparaben, 0.15%; perfume
Medi-Quick (Lehn & Fink)	aerosol pump spray	lidocaine	benzalkonium chloride	isopropyl alcohol, 12% (aerosol), 79% (pump)
Noxzema Medicated (Noxell)	cream lotion		phenol, <0.5%	menthol, camphor, clove oil, eucalyptus oil, lime water, water-dispersible base
Nupercainal Cream (Ciba)	cream	dibucaine, 0.5%		acetone sodium bisulfite, 0,.37%; water-washable base
Nupercainal Ointment (Ciba)	ointment	dibucaine, 1%		acetone sodium bisulfite, 0.5%
Obtundia (Otis Clapp)	cream liquid		cresol–camphor complex	
Panthoderm (USV)	cream lotion			dexpanthenol, 2%; water-miscible base
Pontocaine (Breon)	cream ointment	tetracaine hydrochloride, 1% (cream); 0.5% (ointment)		methylparaben (cream); sodium bisulfite (cream); menthol, 0.5% (ointment); white petrolatum (ointment); white wax (ointment)
Pyribenzamine (Ciba)	cream ointment	tripelennamine, 2%		water-washable base (cream); petrolatum base (ointment)
Rexall First Aid Spray (Rexall)	spray	benzocaine	chlorothymol, methylbenzethonium chloride	isopropyl alcohol, 4% tyloxapol; camphor
Soft 'N Soothe (B. F. Ascher)	cream	benzocaine, menthol		natural oat protein, lanolin oil, mineral oil, lanolin alcohol
Solarcaine (Plough)	cream lotion	benzocaine	triclosan	menthol, camphor
Solarcaine Spray (Plough)	aerosol spray pump spray	benzocaine	triclosan, phenol	isopropyl alcohol, 31% (pump spray)
Sperti (Whitehall)	ointment			shark liver oil, 3%; live yeast cell derivative respiratory factor, 67 units/gm
Tanurol (O'Neal, Jones & Feldman)	ointment	benzocaine, 1%	phenol, 0.75%	tannic acid, 3%
Tega Caine (Ortega)	aerosol	benzocaine, 20%	benzyl alcohol, 2.3%; chloroxylenol, 0.51%	urea, 5.38%; propylene glycol

Burn and Sunburn Product Table, continued

Product (Manufacturer)	Dosage Form	Anesthetic	Antimicrobial	Other Ingredients
Unguentine (Norwich)	ointment aerosol spray	benzocaine, 3.3% (spray)	parahydracin (ointment); benzalkonium chloride (spray); chloroxylenol (spray)	phenol, 1%; aluminum hydroxide; zinc carbonate; zinc acetate; zinc oxide; eucalyptus oil; thyme oil; metacresol; mercuric chloride; alcohol, 42% (spray)
Unguentine Plus (Norwich)	cream	lidocaine hydrochloride, 2%	chloroxylenol, 2%	aluminum hydroxide; zinc carbonate; zinc acetate; zinc oxide; phenol, 1%; eucalyptus oil; thyme oil; menthol; eugenol
Vaseline First-Aid Carbolated Petroleum Jelly[a] (Chesebrough-Pond)	ointment		chloroxylenol, 0.5%; phenol, 0.2%	petroleum jelly, lanolin
Vaseline Pure Petroleum Jelly (Chesebrough-Pond)	gel			white petrolatum, 100%
Velvacain A & O (Commerce)	ointment	benzocaine, 1%	benzalkonium chloride, 0.125%	cod liver oil, 10%
Xylocaine (Astra)	ointment	lidocaine, 2.5%		polyethylene glycols, propylene glycol

[a] Not meant for use over extensive body areas (e.g., sunburn).

Questions to Ask the Patient

Do you sunburn easily?

Is it difficult for you to tan?

Do you normally spend much time in the sun? Does your job or other activities require that you spend time in the sun?

Are you currently using a sun protection product?

What products have you used in the past?

Have you ever had a growth on your skin or lip caused by sun exposure?

Have you ever had a reaction to any sunscreen products?

Are you taking any medicines such as tetracycline, diuretics, or sulfa drugs?

Will you be using the product while swimming, skiing, participating in strenuous activities, or working?

Sunbathing is a popular activity worldwide. However, for some people, hours of exposure to the sun is part of their occupation. Sunburn, with its pain, swelling, and tenderness, may occur whether the exposure is recreational or occupational. Its severity depends on the responsiveness of the individual's skin type to sun exposure and/or the effectiveness of measures taken to protect the skin.

Many people consider sunburn's effects disagreeable but relatively minor. However, the consequences of continued exposure to the sun can be significant. Long-term exposure even without severe burning causes skin to age prematurely, resulting in loss of elasticity, thinning, wrinkling, and drying. Cumulative exposure from childhood to adulthood may cause precancerous skin conditions, and skin cancer may follow.

A large number of sunscreen and suntan products exist on the market to help darken the complexion as well as to protect the skin from the harmful effects of exposure to the sun. Applied properly, they block some or all of the harmful ultraviolet rays either physically or chemically. Pharmacists need to be aware of several important factors to educate the public properly on using these products effectively.

Sunburn is caused by certain wavelengths of ultraviolet (UV) radiation striking the skin. The ultraviolet light alters the keratinocytes in the basal layer of the epidermis. A slight alteration results in erythema, and a severe alteration causes bullae to form from the fluid collected in the epidermis. To produce a suntan, ultraviolet light stimulates the melanocytes in the germinating layer to generate more melanin and oxidizes melanin already in the epidermis. Both of these processes serve as protective mechanisms by diffusing and absorbing additional UV radiation. The effects of the sun on the skin usually begin to appear anywhere from 1 to 24 hours after exposure and range from mild erythema to tenderness, pain, and edema. Severe reactions due to excessive exposure involve the development of vesicles or bullae as well as the constitutional symptoms of fever, chills, weakness, and shock. The latter, due to heat prostration or hyperpyrexia, can lead to death (1). (See Chapter 25, *Burn and Sunburn Products.*)

Ultraviolet Radiation

Ultraviolet radiation is commonly referred to as ultraviolet "light." However, "light" technically refers to the visible spectrum only. Since the correct terminology is "radiation," this will be used throughout (2).

The UV spectrum is subdivided into three bands: UV-A, UV-B, and UV-C (3).

UV-A (Longwave Radiation)

The range of the wavelength for this type of radiation is from 320 to 400 nanometers (nm). Erythrogenic activity (producing redness) is relatively weak at this wavelength. The primary action of UV-A is the development of a slow natural tan (3). At this UV level, radiation produces some immediate pigment darkening. In addition, UV-A represents the range in which most photosensitizing chemicals are active. It is also believed that UV-A may augment the effects of UV-B (4).

UV-B (Sunburn Radiation)

The wavelength of UV-B is between 290 and 320 nm. It is the most effective U-V radiation wavelength for producing erythema, which is why it is called sunburn radiation. It triggers new pigment formation as well as vitamin D production. In addition, it is thought to be responsible for inducing skin cancer (4).

UV-C (Germicidal Radiation)

This type of radiation is represented by the 200–290-nm band. UV-C radiation from the sun does not reach the surface of the earth. However, UV-C is emitted by artificial ultraviolet sources. Although it will not stimulate tanning, it causes some erythema (5).

Long-Term Hazards of Sunlight

Malignant Changes

Numerous epidemiologic studies have been conducted during the last 40 years demonstrating a strong relationship between sunlight exposure and human skin cancer (6–12). One of the most common malignancies is squamous cell epithelioma. There is also a significant relationship between sun exposure and the growth of premalignant actinic keratoses (13). The relative incidence of actinic keratosis and squamous cell carcinomas increases with increased exposure to damaging solar rays. The relationship between ultraviolet radiation and squamous cell cancer is well established. About 80% of both cancers occur on the most exposed areas of the body (14). Another common type of skin malignancy is basal cell epithelioma. However, the incidence of this type of malignancy appears to be related to factors other than ultraviolet radiation alone (15).

Although the evidence linking sun exposure to malignant changes is strong, there are several contributory factors: age, sex, skin pigmentation, and occupation. In a frequently quoted study, the incidence of skin cancer in white adults in a rural Tennessee county was a function of both age and sex. The rate ranged from 0.7/100 males under the age of 44 years to 13.6/100 males between the age of 65 and 74 years; for females, the incidence was 0.4 and 6.8/100 (16). It has also been shown that the exposed areas of the body (the hands, arms, head, and neck) are most prone to the development of skin cancer. This is borne out by the relationship between occupation and skin cancer. Some of the more susceptible groups have been identified as farmers, sailors, and construction workers. The three factors of age, sex, and occupation appear to be interrelated. The findings related to age indicate a cumulative effect from ultraviolet radiation. The findings regarding sex and occupation seem to be related because, traditionally, fewer women have held these susceptible occupations.

The fourth contributory factor is skin pigmentation. Studies have indicated that skin cancer occurs more frequently in whites than in nonwhites (17, 18). These findings support the belief that the darker pigmentation serves as a protectant against the effects of ultraviolet radiation.

Another important concept is the relationship between skin cancer and latitude. It has been shown that the incidence of skin cancer increases steadily as one lives closer to the equator. The quantity of harmful radiation that reaches the earth's surface is increased as the angle of the sun to a reference point on earth approaches 90° and the distance of the sun to the earth decreases (12, 15, 19–22). A constant rate of increase in the incidence of skin cancer was found in approaching the equator from north to south; the incidence approximately doubled for every 3°48′ reduction in latitude (23). In the United States the incidence of skin cancer increases dramatically from north to south.

Premature Aging

The second long-term hazard of ultraviolet radiation is premature aging of the skin. As with skin cancer, this is also genetically determined with whites being more susceptible than blacks. The condition is characterized by wrinkling and yellowing of the skin. It is called premature aging since the obvious physical findings are similar to those seen in natural aging. However, there are histologic and biochemical differences between these two conditions. Conclusive evidence exists that in susceptible individuals, prolonged exposure to ultraviolet radiation results in degeneration of the skin due to breakdown of the skin's elastic fibers (24). Pronounced drying, thinning, and wrinkling of the skin result (25). Other physical changes include cracking, telangiectasis (spider vessels), solar keratoses (growths), ecchymoses (subcutaneous hemorrhagic lesions), and loss of elasticity (26). These degenerative changes are not like those associated with normal aging.

Hence, although the immediate effects of ultraviolet radiation may be cosmetically and socially gratifying, the long-term effects are cumulative and potentially serious.

Sunscreens

Sunscreen agents exert their effects either through physical or chemical means. A physical sunscreen such as titanium dioxide scatters and reflects ultraviolet radiation. The majority of agents such as aminobenzoic acid are chemical sunscreens and absorb ultraviolet radiation rather than reflect or scatter it.

Indications

The primary uses of sunscreens are to prevent sunburn and aid in the development of a tan. Secondarily, they serve to protect exposed areas of the body in susceptible individuals from the long-term hazards of skin cancer and premature aging.

Photosensitivity

In addition, sunscreens can be used to protect against drug-related ultraviolet-induced photosensitivity.

Photosensitivity encompasses two types of conditions. The first and relatively uncommon condition is photoallergy (27). Drug photoallergy designates an increased reactivity of the skin to ultraviolet and/or visible radiation produced by a chemical agent on an immunologic basis. Ultraviolet radiation (typically UV-A) triggers an antigenic reaction in the skin characterized by urticaria, bullae, and/or sunburn (28). This reaction, which is not dose-related, is usually seen after at least one prior exposure to the involved agent.

Phototoxicity designates an increased reactivity of the skin to ultraviolet and/or visible radiation produced by a chemical agent on a nonimmunologic basis (27). It is often seen upon first exposure to a chemical agent (drug), is dose related, and usually exhibits no cross-sensitivity. It is most likely to appear as a sunburn (29, 30). Some of the drugs associated with phototoxicity are tetracyclines (especially demeclocycline), sulfonamides, hypoglycemics, thiazides, phenothiazines (especially chlorpromazine), and the psoralens. However, this type of reaction is not limited to drugs. It is also associated with plants, cosmetics, and soaps (31). (See Chapter 25, *Burn and Sunburn Products*).

The efficacy of sunscreens in preventing photosensitization has been questioned by some investigators (32). The issue is yet to be resolved. However, it seems reasonable to assume that since UV-A radiation is responsible for triggering a photosensitivity reaction, a sunscreen effective against UV-A would be effective in preventing photosensitivity.

Traditionally, aminobenzoic acid (formerly known as *p*-aminobenzoic acid or PABA) has been used. However, it absorbs only UV-B (290–320 nm) radiation and not UV-A (320–400 nm) radiation. One study compared the efficacy of 5% aminobenzoic acid in alcohol with a mixture of the esters of aminobenzoic acid (ABA) and benzophenone. It was demonstrated that the 5% aminobenzoic acid was ineffective. The aminobenzoic acid and benzophenone ester solution blocked the phototoxic effects of chlorpromazine, 8-methoxypsoralen, and demeclocycline (33). It seems likely that similar wide-spectrum sunscreens such as sulisobenzone, oxybenzone, and dioxybenzone could be effective either alone or in combination with aminobenzoic acid.

However, aminobenzoic acid is chemically similar to certain other drugs that have been reported to cause photosensitivity reactions in susceptible individuals. These drugs include the thiazide diuretics, sulfonamides, sulfonylureas, furosemide, and carbonic anhydrase inhibitors. Individuals who have experienced a photosensitivity reaction while taking one of these drugs should not use a sunscreen containing aminobenzoic acid or one of its derivatives such as aminobenzoate, menthyl anthranilate, or padimate A or O. A sunscreen containing oxybenzone or cinoxate may be recommended instead (25).

Sunscreen Efficacy

Minimal Erythemal Dose (MED)

It is difficult to ascertain the efficacy of these agents on humans due to the great individual variation in responsiveness to ultraviolet radiation. One measure that is used is the minimal erythemal dose (MED). This dose is defined as the "least exposure dose at a specified wavelength that will elicit a delayed erythema response. It is a dose of radiation and not a grade of erythema" (4). The MED is indicative not only of the amount of energy reaching the skin but also of the responsiveness of the skin to the radiation. For instance, 2 MED's will produce a bright erythema, 4 MED's will produce a painful sunburn, and 8 MED's will produce a blistering burn. The MED for blacks with heavy pigmentation has been estimated to be up to 33 times higher than that for whites with light pigmentation (34).

Sun Protection Factor (SPF)

Another important measure is the sun protection factor (SPF). It is derived by dividing the MED of protected skin by the MED of unprotected skin. For example, assume that an individual requires 25 millijoules/sq cm (25 units) of ultraviolet radiation to experience 1 MED on unprotected skin. If, after application of a given sunscreen, the person requires 250 units of radiation to produce 1 MED, the product would be given an SPF rating of 10. The higher the SPF, the more effective the agent in preventing sunburn. However, as the SPF goes up (and the amount of radiation striking the skin goes down), the less chance exists for the development of a slow natural tan. Table 1 illustrates the proposed classification and the relationship of skin types to SPF and product category designations (PCD) (35).

Table 1. Skin types and recommended sunscreen products

Skin type	Sunburn and tanning history	Recommended skin protection factor (SPF)	Recommended product category designation (PCD)
I	Always burns easily Never tans (sensitive)	8 or more	maximal, ultra
II	Always burns easily Tans minimally (sensitive)	6–7	extra
III	Burns moderately Tans gradually (light brown–normal)	4–5	moderate
IV	Burns minimally Always tans well (moderate brown–normal)	2–3	minimal
V	Rarely burns Tans profusely (dark brown–insensitive)	2	minimal
VI	Never burns Deeply pigmented (insensitive)		

With all of these proposed guides, a system should now exist to evaluate, with some accuracy, not only the relative effectiveness of sunscreens but also the length of time a person using a sunscreen product can spend in the sun before a burn will occur. If it normally takes 30 minutes for someone to experience 1 MED, a sunscreen with an SPF of 6 will allow that individual to stay in the sun six times longer or 3 hours before receiving 1 MED.

Molar Absorptivity

Another way of judging the efficacy of sunscreens is by looking at the molar absorptivity of each compound. Molar absorptivity is the ability of a compound to absorb ultraviolet light—the larger the value at a specified wavelength, the better the absorption. By placing each sunscreen agent in an identical solvent and subjecting each to the same ultraviolet radiation, an index of efficacy is attained. Table 2 shows the molar absorptivity of some of the more commonly used agents.

To be most effective, the range of maximum absorption for the sunscreen agent must overlap the ultraviolet range of sunlight that produces sunburn. The larger molar absorptivity value reflects the ability of that compound to absorb ultraviolet light at the indicated wavelength.

Although the pharmacist cannot control the formulation of the various commercially available sunscreen products, a knowledge of the specific active ingredients and their concentrations helps differentiate a good product from a mediocre one. The sunscreen product that contains a sunscreen with a larger molar absorptivity and is present at a higher concentration is a more efficient product, provided the sunscreen agent overlays the range of ultraviolet light that produces the sunburn. In addition, sunscreen agents that have a low or intermediate molar absorptivity may be made more effective by increasing the concentration of the active ingredient.

Ancillary Factors Affecting Efficacy

Several factors have a bearing on the efficacy of non-prescription sunscreen products. These all relate to the vehicle/solvent system.

- The partition coefficient relative to the skin should favor passage of the sunscreen to the skin.
- The pH of the solvent can vary the fraction of ionized and nonionized sunscreen agent, thereby rendering it less effective or even ineffective.
- The solvent system should provide a high degree of substantivity.
- The sunscreen must remain stable for the desired period of protection.

According to the FDA advisory review panel, "An ideal sunscreen vehicle would be stable, neutral, nongreasy, nondegreasing, nonirritating, nondehydrating, nondrying, odorless, and efficient on all kinds of human skin. It should also hold at least 50% water, be easily compounded of known chemicals, and have infinite stability during storage" (36). The panel stated that an ideal vehicle does not exist and recommended that all inactive ingredients be included on product labels. This labeling would allow evaluation by the consumer, pharmacist, and physician for several factors including sensitivity to the agent.

In addition, the vehicle and final dosage form may influence the effectiveness of the active ingredient. One study showed that ABA (5%) in ethanol was superior to ABA dissolved in methanol, propyl alcohol, acetone, *n*-butyl alcohol, and isobutyl alcohol. This study indicated that the increased effectiveness was due to the absorption of ABA by the intact epidermis and partial chemical conjugation of ABA with constituents of the horny layer. This effect prevented transmission of erythemogenic wavelengths to the underlying vulnerable cells of the viable epidermis (37).

The ability of a sunscreen to remain effective under the stress of prolonged exercise, sweating, and swimming is called substantivity. This property appears to be a function of both the absorbing agent and the vehicle. As already mentioned, ABA in ethanol is substantive, and studies have suggested that other ABA esters, such as glyceryl ABA, may be more substantive than ABA (38). Products with cream-based vehicles may in some cases be more resistant to removal than those in alcohol bases (39).

Alcohol is drying to the skin, and commercial formulas include other ingredients such as glycerin, hydroxypropyl cellulose, and fragrances to increase the cosmetic appeal and acceptability.

Table 2. Spectral parameters for selected sunscreen agents		
Compound	Molar absorptivity	nm
Aminobenzoic acid (*para*-isomer)	18,300	288.5
Cinoxate (2-ethoxyethyl *p*-methoxycinnamate)	19,400	310
Dioxybenzone (2,2'-dihydroxy-4-methoxybenzophenone)	11,951	282[a]
Glyceryl *p*-aminobenzoate	17,197	295
Homosalate (homomethyl salicylate)	6,720[b]	306
Menthyl anthranilate	941[b]	340
Oxybenzone (2-hydroxy-4-methoxy-benzophenone)	20,381	290[a]
Sulisobenzone (2-hydroxy-4-methoxy-benzophenone-5-sulfonic acid)	5,580	285[a]

All values determined in ethanol.
[a] These compounds absorb throughout the ultraviolet range.
[b] Values from A. C. Giese et al., *J. Am. Pharm. Assoc. Sci. Ed., 39*, 30 (1950).

Product Selection Guidelines

The FDA advisory review panel on nonprescription topical analgesic, antirheumatic, otic, burn, and sunburn prevention and treatment drug products has recommended three definitions for therapeutic sunscreen types (35):

- Sunscreen-sunburn preventive agent—an active ingredient that absorbs 95% or more of the radiation in the ultraviolet range at wavelengths from 290 to 320 nm and thereby removes the sunburning rays;
- Sunscreen-suntanning agent—an active ingredient that absorbs at least 85% of the radiation in the ultraviolet range at wavelengths from 290–320 nm, but transmits ultraviolet wavelengths longer than 320 nm (such agents permit tanning in the average individual and also permit some erythema without pain);
- Sunscreen-opaque sunblock agent—an opaque agent that reflects or scatters all radiation in the ultraviolet and visible range from 290 to 777 nm and thereby prevents or minimizes suntan and sunburn.

Most of the products on the market contain a combination of the first two types of agents. The primary difference between the preventive agent and the suntanning agent may only be the concentration of the active ingredient.

The opaque sunblock agents are visible when applied to the skin. They are most often used by people who cannot limit or control their exposure to the sun, (lifeguards and others whose occupations demand long, repeated exposure). The nose and the tops of the ears are often seen coated with a white substance such as zinc oxide ointment. Unfortunately, transparent agents of similar efficacy are not yet on the market.

The FDA advisory review panel on nonprescription burn and sunburn prevention and treatment drug products has recommended that 21 agents be classified as safe and efficacious for nonprescription use as topical sunscreens. These tentative recommendations are included in Table 3. Those agents that have not been judged to be both safe and efficacious are listed in Table 4.

There are a few points concerning some of the agents listed that need to be addressed.

To allow adequate diffusion of aminobenzoic acid into the horny layer of the skin, it is recommended that this agent be applied 2 hours before exposure. This approach provides a greater degree of protection as well as substantivity.

Although aminobenzoic acid is safe, there have been reports of allergic contact photodermatitis (40). The patient should be advised to try another product if sensitization develops.

Dioxybenzone has been studied in combination with several other agents including padimate A, *p*-aminobenzoate, and monoglycerol *p*-aminobenzoate. The product being evaluated against the others contained 3% dioxybenzone and 2.5% padimate A. The report concluded that the two agents in combination were more effective than either one alone or any of the combination products (41). Another report has mentioned that padimate A has photosensitizing properties (42).

Table 3. Agents recommended to be safe and effective by the FDA advisory review panel

Sunscreen	Absorbance (nm)	Maximum (nm)	Concentration
Aminobenzoic acid	260–313	288.5	5–15%
Cinoxate	270–328	310	1–3%
Diethanolamine *p*-methoxycinnamate	280–310	290	8–10%
Digalloyl trioleate	270–320	300	2–5%
Dioxybenzone	260–380[a]	282[a]	3%
Ethyl 4-[bis(hydroxypropyl)] aminobenzoate	280–330	308–311	1–5%
2-Ethylhexyl 2-cyano-3,3-diphenylacrylate			7–10%
Ethylhexyl *p*-methoxycinnamate	290–320	308–310	2–7.5%
2-Ethylhexyl salicylate	280–320	305	3–5%
Glyceryl *p*-aminobenzoate	264–315	295	3%
Homosalate	295–315	306	4–15%
Lawsone with dihydroxyacetone (DHA)	290–400		0.25% lawsone 3% DHA
Menthyl anthranilate	290–320[b]	340[b]	3.5–5%
Oxybenzone	270–350	290	2–6%
Padimate A	290–315	310	1–5%
Padimate O	290–315	310	1.4–8%
2-Phenylbenzimidazole-5-sulfonic acid	290–320	302	1–4%
Red petrolatum[c]			30–100%
Sulisobenzone[d]		285	5–10%
Titanium dioxide[e]			2–25%
Triethanolamine salicylate	260–320	298	5–12%

Adapted from the *Federal Register, 43,* 38219–38253 (1978).

[a] Values available when used in combination with other sunscreens.

[b] Values are for concentrations higher than normally found in nonprescription products.

[c] A 0.03-mm film absorbs ultraviolet below 320 nm. At 334 nm, 16% of ultraviolet radiation is transmitted while 58% is transmitted at 365 nm.

[d] Absorbs throughout the entire ultraviolet range.

[e] Scatters radiation from 290 to 700 nm rather than absorbs it.

Although ethylhexyl *p*-methoxycinnamate and menthyl anthranilate were shown to be effective as single entities, they are most often used in combination with other sunscreens.

Titanium dioxide may be so occlusive to the skin as to produce miliaria (prickly heat or heat rash) (43).

Table 4. Agents cited to lack safety and/or efficacy data by the FDA advisory review panel		
Agent	**Safe**	**Effective**
Category II		
2-Ethylhexyl 4-phenylbenzophenone-2'-carboxylic acid	Insufficient data	Insufficient data
3-(4-methylbenzylidene) camphor	Insufficient data	No data
Sodium 3,4-dimethyl-phenylglyoxylate	Insufficient data	No data
Category III		
Allantoin with aminobenzoic acid (ALPABA)	Safe	Insufficient data
5-(3,3-Dimethyl-2-norboryliden)-3-penten-2-one	Safe	Insufficient data
Dipropylene glycol salicylate	Insufficient data	Insufficient data

Adapted from the *Federal Register, 43,* 38219–38253 (1978).

Combination Products

The FDA has not recommended any limits for the number of sunscreen agents that may be used together in a nonprescription product. There are only two major recommendations from the panel:

- Any additional sunscreen agents must contribute to the efficacy of the product and not be just a marketing gimmick (44).
- Any combination of sunscreens with active nonsunscreen agents must meet the requirements for safety and efficacy.

Sunscreen Utilization

The efficacy of a product is related to its substantivity. Swimming, heat, high humidity, and sweating can reduce the substantivity (or true SPF) of a product.

Some proposed labeling guidelines for sunscreen products meeting the specific criteria are (45):

- **Sweat-resistant products**—protect for up to 30 minutes of continuous heavy perspiration;
- **Water-resistant products**—protect for up to 40 minutes of continuous water exposure;
- **Waterproof products**—protect for up to 80 minutes of continuous water exposure.

For the average person in a bathing suit, nine portions, each portion approximately one-half teaspoonful, is the amount of sunscreen needed to be applied to the skin. It is distributed as follows (34):

- Face and neck—one-half teaspoonful;
- Arm and shoulder—one-half teaspoonful to each side;
- Torso—one-half teaspoonful each to front and back;
- Leg and top of foot—one teaspoonful to each side.

Sunscreens should be applied at least 30 minutes before exposure to the sun, although aminobenzoic acid and its esters are more effective if applied 2 hours before exposure (46). This approach allows the agent to penetrate and bind with the skin. It should also be remembered that aminobenzoic acid and its esters are most apt to stain fabrics and materials. They are also responsible for producing a local sensitivity in some persons. If a reaction develops to one of these products, another product containing a chemically unrelated sunscreen can be recommended after the problem clears.

Suntan Products

Low-Efficacy Sunscreens

For cosmetic rather than therapeutic needs the patient may desire a suntan product. In many cases suntan products differ from sunscreens only by having a lower concentration of the sunscreen agent. The concentration of the active ingredient is an important factor in judging the use and effectiveness of a product. For example, SunDare Lotion, a suntan product, contains 1.75% cinoxate, while Maxafil Cream, a sunscreen product, contains 4% (about twice as much as the suntan product) and 5% menthyl anthranilate, a second sunscreen.

The activity of an agent may also be an intrinsic quality unrelated to concentration. A given agent may also work solely by absorbing radiation below 320 nm and allowing those rays above 320 nm to penetrate the skin. Aminobenzoic acid almost totally absorbs radiation in the range of 260 to 313 nm. Radiation above 313 nm is, however, transmitted to the skin (47). This effect will produce a mild short-lived tan but will protect against a burn.

Suntan products do not "promote" a tan. In addition, some suntan products, including cocoa butter and mineral oil alone or with staining materials such as iodine or tannic acid, do not contain a sunscreen agent. They mainly stain and lubricate the skin and do not reverse the aging process caused by ultraviolet radiation. The advisory review panel has stated that "claims such as 'promotes tanning' for sunlight protective agents are unsubstantiated" (36).

Pigmenting Agents

Another type of agent available is a skin-browning agent or dye such as dihydroxyacetone (DHA). For years this has been the major ingredient in products that "tan without the sun." Dihydroxyacetone produces a reddish brown color through a reaction with specific amino acids in the stratum corneum. However, the mechanism of action is not very well understood. The intensity of the "tan" is related to the thickness of the skin. One problem with this product is that if it is not washed off the hands after application, the palms will also develop this "tan." In addition, dry areas such as elbows and kneecaps will absorb the agent more readily, resulting in uneven coloration. The color fades after several weeks with desquamation of the stratum corneum. The panel has recommended that dihydroxyace-tone alone is ineffective as a sunscreen and that it should be classified as a cosmetic. However, in combination with lawsone, a major dye component of henna, the product is a sunscreen and not a cosmetic. This combination is recommended as safe and effective as a sunscreen product (Table 3).

A relatively new product is an oral "tanning" compound. Its active ingredient is the dye canthaxanthin. Canthaxanthin is a synthetic dye that the promotional literature describes as "similar to those dyes found naturally in fruits, vegetables and flowers. It has long been used in the food industry *in lower concentration* for coloring cheese, ketchup, salad dressing, and other foods." It apparently works by coloring the fat cells under the epidermal layer. Because of the variation in fat cells and epidermal thickness, the extent of the tan varies from person to person. It is dosed by body weight with a 20-day schedule necessary to achieve pigmentation. This process is followed by maintenance doses of 1–2 capsules/day to maintain the color. The literature cautions the user that if the palms are turning orange, too much of the product is being consumed. Another caution is that a normal reaction is the development of "brick red feces."

This product was not evaluated by the panel since it has been ruled as a permissible color additive for foods and drugs (a cosmetic) and is exempt from FDA certification (48). One major concern may be the color of the feces, which could mask any type of GI bleeding. A second concern may be the size of the dose, since the promotional literature states that the product is used in concentrations higher than that normally used as a food dye. There is no evidence for safe use of this agent at a high dose.

Tanning Booths

The availability of tanning booths may prompt questions from patients concerning their safety. A recent discussion of tanning booths notes that the light source commonly used provides over 95% UV-A and less than 5% UV-B radiation, a considerably different mix of UV radiation than that obtained from sunlight (49).

Ultraviolet-A radiation, while usually burning less, will produce a photosensitivity reaction in patients who have ingested or applied photosensitizing agents. In addition to a concern about photosensitivity reactions, patients should be warned to wear goggles to prevent eye burns and corneal irritations, and to eliminate increased risk of cataracts. The possibility of long-term hazards such as malignancy and premature aging have not been assessed.

As with natural sunlight, patients should understand that sunscreen agents may be used to protect part of the body customarily underexposed to the sun.

Product Selection Guidelines

Before recommending a suntan product, the pharmacist should know the identity of the active ingredient and its maximum absorption, concentration, the SPF of the product, and the tanning history of the patient. In addition, it should be remembered that the SPF's and product category designations (PCD's) are determined for the specific nonprescription product and are not based on the active ingredient alone.

The identity and concentration of the active ingredients may be supplied by the manufacturer but also should appear on the label. Without this information, recommendations can be based only on intuition or personal experience. If the information is not supplied by the manufacturer, recommendations should be limited to products that indicate the identity and concentration of the active ingredients.

The most important consideration of all in selecting a product should be the individual's skin type as defined in Table 1. Once the skin type is identified, a product with the recommended SPF should be selected. In making a recommendation to prevent sunburn, it is important to keep in mind that a product with an SPF of 15 will prevent all but the minimum of tans from occurring. This type of product should be reserved for the person who cannot tan or cannot afford any degree of sunburn. Patients who have a personal or family history of certain dermatologic problems such as excessive dryness and aging, sunburn with short exposure, and skin cancer should use a total blocking agent or a sunscreen with an SPF rating of 15 when prolonged exposure to sunlight is expected (25). Animal studies have shown that even low protective sunscreens (SPF-2) reduce the risk of tumorigenesis associated with UV

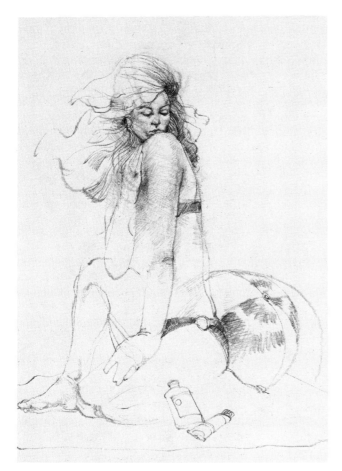

radiation by 50% (50). However, some authorities suggest that SPF-4 be the lowest allowable level (51).

Special consideration is needed when recommending a sunscreen for young children. There seems to be a consensus that the absorptive characteristics of human skin for children under the age of 6 months is different from those of adult human skin. Related to this is the belief that metabolic and excretory systems of children under the age of 6 months are not fully developed to handle any drug absorbed through the skin. Therefore, the FDA panel has recommended that persons over the age of 6 months are considered to have adult human skin.

Because of this, the panel has made two major recommendations regarding the labeling of nonprescription sunscreens with respect to the age of the person using the products (52):

- Products with an SPF of 2 to less than 4 are not to be used on children under the age of 2 years.
- Products with an SPF of 4 or more are not to be used on children under the age of 6 months.

Products in the SPF 2-4 range should not be used in children under 2 years of age since this SPF range does not supply enough protection. This age limitation is unrelated to the absorptive/metabolic characteristics.

Products with an SPF of 8–14 allow one to stay out in the sun for long periods and slowly develop a tan over several days. This assumes that the product is properly applied. It is important to remember, however, that as an individual tans, a natural protection against burning also develops. Therefore, an individual who begins the summer using a product with an SPF of 8 may need to switch to a product with an SPF of 4 as the natural tan progresses. This change will allow a more rapid deepening of the tan. The person can, however, continue to use the product with the SPF of 8. It will simply take longer to achieve the desired tan.

Studies that compare several sunscreen products in humans can also serve as a basis for professional judgment. One such study evaluated 17 sunscreen products, using a mean protection factor to evaluate each product (53). Products that contain 5% aminobenzoic acid were shown to be superior to those that contain aminobenzoic acid esters. However, aminobenzoic acid esters are generally used in a concentration of less than 5%. A study showed that alcoholic preparations of 5% aminobenzoic acid were more effective than commercial products tested (54). Another product evaluation substantiates this finding in products that contain 5% aminobenzoic acid (55). Several investigators (54, 56) agree that aminobenzoic acid is more effective as a sunscreen than popular proprietary products, but they disagree that aminobenzoic acid esters are less effective than the parent compound, aminobenzoic acid.

In addition, the sunscreen/suntan agent may damage clothing or other objects. One evaluation of commercial sunscreens found a number of products to pucker vinyl fabric, stain bathing suit material, and damage and stain fiberglass boat finish (52, 57).

Study findings revealed that none of the product labels suggested how much sunscreen should be used. The amount used by the study participants varied as much as 10-fold. It was decided that a one-half teaspoonful (2.5 ml) dose applied as described previously delivered the FDA standard test rate of 2 $\mu l/cm^2$ (57). Based on the evaluation, the recommendation followed that products within the same SPF rating group showed no advantage over one another. The cost per dose is another factor in the decision of which product to purchase. However, the staining and fabric-damaging properties should also be taken into account, as well as cosmetic properties.

One interesting finding was that all commercial products tested demonstrated an SPF several units higher than the labeled value. There appears to be a margin of safety built into the products. However, it is best to assume that the product provides at least the labeled SPF.

Several products are now on the market in "stick" or "lipstick" form. These products prevent burning of the lips (or nose) and carry the same labeling as the sunscreen lotions including the SPF. These can also differ in terms of their UV-A and UV-B spectrum. The SPF of these products is at least 15.

Products that dye the skin or fat cells can provide a false sense of security. Although one might look tanned and thereby feel protected, the fact remains that these agents provide no sunscreen protection whatsoever. The only exception to this would be if a sunscreen agent also is contained in a topical product. Otherwise there is the potential for the development of a serious burn.

In regard to product selection, several investigators have suggested using a combination of agents that protect against both UV-A and UV-B (29, 31, 33). There are several explanations for this combination. First, most photosensitive chemicals are active in the UV-A (320 nm) range. However, UV-B can also trigger such reactions. Two reports have provided preliminary evidence that repeated doses of UV-A radiation at doses less than the MED produced enhanced melanogenesis. In addition, these findings indicate that UV-A radiation may be more responsible than UV-B in producing cumulative dermal degenerative changes (aging) (58, 59). These are preliminary reports, but they may have a significant impact on the understanding of cumulative ultraviolet radiation damage to the skin. Based on these findings, it should be noted that because aminobenzoic acid and its esters are more effective sunscreens in the UV-B range than the wide spectrum agents (the benzophenones), the combination of aminobenzoic acid or one of its esters with a benzophenone (dioxybenzone, oxybenzone, and sulisobenzone) would seem to be a rational and logical choice except when the photosensitizing drug is chemically similar or crossreacts with aminobenzoic acid. Various products of this type are available.

Patient Consultation

Pharmacists can provide a great service to patients by educating them to a number of little-understood facts related to the suntanning process and the proper use of sunscreens.

The rays of the sun are the most direct and damaging between 10:00 a.m. and 2:00 p.m. It is best to avoid sunning during this period, especially at the beginning of the season before any protective tan has developed. Closely related to this is the misconception that one cannot burn on an overcast or cloudy day. While varying amounts of sunlight may not pass through the cloud cover, very little ultraviolet radiation is blocked and most will penetrate.

Another problem is the reflection of ultraviolet radiation off surfaces. Snow will reflect nearly 100% of the light and radiation that strikes it, hence the need for sunglasses while skiing on a sunny day. This reflected light is also why a skier can receive a significant sunburn even on a cloudy day. Therefore, a sunscreen is indicated for the sun-sensitive skier. Sand, while not as effective a reflective surface as snow, reflects about 4% of the radiation striking it. The person sitting in the shade of a beach umbrella is still being bombarded by the ultraviolet radiation off the sand. This contributes to the overall radiation received, and a severe sunburn may result. Water reflects only 1% of the ultraviolet radiation and allows the remaining 99% to penetrate and burn the swimmer. Therefore, time spent swimming, even if one is completely submerged, should be considered as part of the total time spent in the sun. In addition, although dry clothes reflect almost all ultraviolet radiation, wet clothes allow transmission of approximately 50% of the ultraviolet radiation.

The patient should be advised that although tanning and thickening of the skin serve as protective mechanisms against future injury, peeling of the skin removes part of this protection. The amount of exposure to the sun as well as the SPF of the product being used need to be reevaluated as tanning and/or peeling occur.

Other specific information related to the safe and effective use of sunscreen agents has been reviewed by the FDA panel, which concluded that many consumers use inadequate amounts of sunscreen. The panel recommends that the directions for use state: "Apply liberally before sun exposure and reapply after swimming or after excessive sweating" (60). The panel also recommends that labeling of all sunscreens should contain the following warnings:

- For external use only, not to be swallowed.
- Avoid contact with eyes.
- Discontinue use if signs of irritation or rash appear.

These recommendations can be emphasized during consultation.

In view of widespread use of products containing 5% aminobenzoic acid, the dosage and administration for a particular product will vary. Generally, the instructions are:

Apply liberally and evenly 1 hour before exposure. Allow time for the product to dry before dressing to avoid absorption of the agent into the garment. If used, cosmetics or emollients may usually be applied after application of the product. Mention should be made that aminobenzoic products will stain light-colored fabric and damage and/ or stain vinyl and/or fiberglass.

Summary

Tanning or burning of the skin can be the result of recreational sunbathing or outdoor activities, such as yard work or sports, or it can be an occupational hazard. Whatever the case, the long-term hazards of ultraviolet radiation are well known to the scientific and medical community and are becoming well documented. However, the public must be educated about the hazards of the sun as well as methods to minimize these hazards.

The key to proper protection is the identification by the patient of skin type. Once this is done, the product with the appropriate SPF can be selected. It would appear that within SPF rating groups, no difference exists regarding efficacy. Other considerations that may determine the selection then are: substantivity, water or perspiration resistance, ability to damage fabrics, and price.

Once a product is selected, the patient should be advised to apply it at least 30 minutes before exposure (up to 2 hours with aminobenzoic acid and its esters). The product should be applied frequently, especially after heavy sweating and swimming.

If the patient is taking photosensitizing drugs, a wide-spectrum product is preferred. Most authorities prefer to recommend a product containing aminobenzoic acid or its esters in combination with a benzophenone. However, avoidance of unnecessary exposure is the primary preventive measure.

If the ultimate goal of the patient is to develop a deep tan, the best approach is slow and cautious. Brief and gradually increasing exposures to the sun and avoidance of peak sun times allow for gradual tanning with minimal burning. This gradual tanning provides natural protection to the skin. With proper utilization of sunscreen products and judicious tanning, both the short- and long-term hazards of exposure to the sun may be minimized.

References

1. "The Merck Manual," 13th ed., R. Berkow, Ed., Merck, Rahway, N.J., 1977, p. 1716.
2. J. A. Parrish, M. B. White, and M. A. Pathak, in "Dermatology in General Medicine," T. B. Fitzpatrick et al., Eds., McGraw-Hill, New York, N.Y., 1979, p. 943.
3. *Federal Register, 43,* 38209–10 (1978).
4. J. A. Parrish, M. B. White, and M. A. Pathak, in "Dermatology in General Medicine," T. B. Fitzpatrick et al., Eds., McGraw-Hill, New York, N.Y., 1979, p. 952.
5. J. R. Wuest and T. Gossel, *Am. Pharm., NS21,* 46 (1981).
6. H. F. Blum, "Carcinogenesis by UV Light," Princeton University Press, Princeton, N.J., 1959, pp. 285–305.
7. F. Urbach, *J. Invest. Dermatol., 32,* 373 (1959).
8. F. Urbach et al., in "Environment and Cancer," Williams and Wilkins, Baltimore, Md., 1972.
9. E. A. Emmett, *CRC Crit. Rev. Toxicol., 2,* 211 (1973).
10. Monograph No. 10, F. Urbach, Ed., U.S. National Cancer Institute, Washington, D.C., 1964.
11. J. F. Dorn, *Public Health Reports, 59,* 33 (1944).
12. F. Urbach, S. O'Beirn, and P. Judge, in "Tenth International Cancer Congress" (Abstracts), Lippincott, Philadelphia, Pa., 1970, pp. 109–110.
13. J. A. Parrish, M. B. White, and M. A. Pathak, in "Dermatology in General Medicine," T. B. Fitzpatrick et al., Eds., McGraw-Hill, New York, N.Y., 1979, p. 958.
14. R. DeVorc, in "Sunbathing and Skin Cancer," *FDA Consumer* (May 1977).

15. K. V. Sanderson, in "Comparative Physiology and Pathology of the Skin," A. J. Rook and G. S. Walton, Eds., Davis, Philadelphia, Pa., 1965, p. 637.
16. Z. W. Zagula-Mally, E. W. Rosenberg, and M. Kashgarian, *Cancer, 34,* 345 (1974).
17. D. M. Pillsbury, B. Shelly, and A. M. Kligman, "Dermatology," Saunders, Philadelphia, Pa., 1956, p. 1145.
18. M. Moushovitz and B. Modan, *J. Nat. Cancer Inst., 51,* 77, (1973).
19. M. Segi, Monograph No. 10, U.S. National Cancer Institute, Washington, D.C., 1963, p. 245.
20. J. Belisario, "Cancer of the Skin," Butterworth, London, England, 1959, p. 15.
21. J. A. Elliott and D. G. Welton, *Arch. Dermatol. Syphitol., 53,* 307 (1946).
22. V. A. Belinsky and L. N. Guslitzer, in "Tenth International Cancer Congress Abstracts" (Abstracts), Lippincott, Philadelphia, Pa., 1970, p. 109.
23. H. Averbach, *Public Health Reports, 76,* 345 (1961).
24. A. M. Kligman, *J. Am. Med. Assoc., 210,* 2377 (1969).
25. J. R. Wuest and T. A. Gossell, *Am. Pharm., NS21,* 46–49 (1981).
26. J. A. Parrish, M. B. White, and M. A. Pathak, in "Dermatology in General Medicine," T. B. Fitzpatrick et al., Eds., McGraw-Hill, New York, N.Y., 1979, p. 959.
27. K. Boudreaux and B. Davidson, *U.S. Pharmacist,* 46, (June/July 1977).
28. E. Emmett, *Int. J. Dermatol., 17,* 370 (1978).
29. "Applied Therapeutics for Clinical Pharmacists," 2nd ed., M. A. Koda-Kimble, B. S. Katcher, and L. Y. Young, Eds., Applied Therapeutics, San Francisco, Calif., 1978.
30. S. Epstein, *Medical Times* (March 1965).
31. D. A. Lopez, *J. Assoc. Military Dermatol., 4,* 19 (1979).
32. *British Medical Journal, 2,* 494 (1970).
33. F. J. Akin et al., *Toxicol. Appl. Pharmacol., 49,* 219 (1979).
34. R. L. Olson et al., *Arch. Dermatol., 108,* 541 (1973).
35. *Federal Register, 43,* 38213 (1978).
36. *Federal Register, 43,* 38218 (1978).
37. M. Pathak, T. Fitzpatrick, and E. Frenk, *N. Engl. J. Med., 280,* 1459 (1969).
38. B. Compelik, *Cosmet. Toiletr., 91,* 59 (1976).
39. R. Sayre et al., *Arch. Dermatol., 115* (1979).
40. C. Mathias, H. Maibach, and J. Epstein, *Arch. Dermatol., 114,* 46 1665 (1978).
41. *Federal Register, 43,* 38223 (1978).
42. K. H. Kaidberg et al., *Arch. Dermatol., 114,* 547 (1978).
43. A. A. Fisher, "Contact Dermatitis," Lea and Febiger, Philadelphia, Pa., 1967, p. 151.
44. *Federal Register, 43,* 38216 (1978).
45. *Federal Register, 43,* 38215 (1978).
46. *Federal Register, 43,* 38220 (1978).
47. S. Rothman and J. Rubin, *J. Invest. Dermatol., 5,* 445–454 (1952).
48. *Federal Register,* 34, 222 (1969).
49. *FDA Consumer, 21,* (Oct. 1980).
50. *Journal of the American Academy of Dermatology, 3,* 30 (1980).
51. *FDC Reports, 41,* T and G2 (Jan. 1979).
52. *Federal Register, 43,* 38217 (1978).
53. D. J. Cripps and S. Hegedus, *Arch. Dermatol., 109,* 202 (1974).
54. M. A. Pathak, T. B. Fitzpatrick, and E. Frenk, *N. Engl. J. Med., 280,* 1461 (1969).
55. "Summary Minutes of the FDA Advisory Review Panel on OTC Topical Analgesic, Antirheumatic, Otic, Burn, and Sunburn Treatment Drug Products," Meetings 1–6, Rockville, Md., March, 1973–Jan. 1975.
56. I. Willis and A. M. Kligman, *Arch. Dermatol., 102,* 405 (1970).
57. *Consumer Reports, 45,* 353 (1980).
58. K. H. Kaidberg and A. M. Kligman, *J. Invest. Dermatol., 76,* 356 (1981).
59. J. A. Parrish, S. Zaynoun, and R. R. Anderson, *J. Invest. Dermatol., 76,* 356 (1981).
60. *Federal Register, 43,* 38254 (1978).

Sunscreen and Suntan Product Table

Product (Manufacturer)	SPF Value	Sunscreen Agent	Other Ingredients
A-Fil Cream (Texas Pharmacal)		menthyl anthranilate, 5%	titanium dioxide, 5%
Block Out (Carter)	10 (clear lotion) 15 (cream lotion)	octyldimethylaminobenzoic acid, 8%; oxybenzone, 6%	
Chap Stick Sunblock (Miller-Morton)	15	padimate O, 7%; oxybenzone, 0.5%	petrolatum, 44%; lanolin, 5%; isopropyl myristate, 0.5%; cetyl alcohol, 0.5%
Coppertone Lipkote (Plough)	8	homosalate, 10%	
Coppertone Lite Oil (Plough)	2	homosalate, 4%	
Coppertone Lotion and Oil (Plough)	4 (lotion) 2 (oil)	homosalate, 8% (lotion) 4% (oil)	
Coppertone Nosekote (Plough)	8	homosalate, 8%; oxybenzone, 3%	
Dark Tanning Butter (Carter)			cocoa butter, coconut oil, mineral oil
Dark Tanning Oil (Carter)		octyldimethylaminobenzoic acid, 1.4%	mineral oil, isopropyl palmitate
Eclipse (Herbert)		glyceryl *p*-aminobenzoate, 3%; padimate O, 3%	alcohol, 5%; oleth-3 phosphate; petrolatum; synthetic spermaceti; glycerin; mineral oil; lanolin alcohol; cetyl stearyl glycol; lanolin oil; triethanolamine; carbomer 934P; benzyl alcohol, 0.5%; perfume
For Faces Only Dark Tanning Lotion (Plough)	2	padimate O, 2%	
For Faces Only Sunblocking Lotion (Plough)	15	padimate O, 7%; oxybenzone, 3%	
For Faces Only Sunscreen Lotion (Plough)	6	padimate O, 5%	
For Faces Only Suntan Lotion (Plough)	4	padimate O, 3.5%	
Golden Tan Lotion (Carter)		octyldimethylaminobenzoic acid, 4%	cocoa butter, mineral oil
Maxafil Cream (Cooper)	6–8	menthyl anthranilate, 5%; cinoxate, 4%	
Mentholatum Stick (Mentholatum)	14.7	padimate O	petrolatum, menthol, camphor, essential oils
Pabafilm (Owen)	10	padimate O, 5.5%; oxybenzone, 3%	benzyl alcohol, 0.7%

Sunscreen and Suntan Product Table, continued

Product (Manufacturer)	SPF Value	Sunscreen Agent	Other Ingredients
Pabagel (Owen)	6	aminobenzoic acid, 5%	alcohol, 57%
Pabanol (Elder)	14	aminobenzoic acid, 5%	alcohol, 70%
PreSun 4 Lotion (Westwood)	4	padimate O, 4%	SD alcohol 40, 10%; water, mineral oil, PPG-15 stearyl ether, stearyl alcohol, mono- and diglycerides, benzyl alcohol, laureth-23, carbomer 934, ceteth-10, sodium hydroxide.
PreSun 8 Creamy (Westwood)	8	aminobenzoic acid, 5%	SD alcohol 40, 15%; water, PEG-8, PPG-15 stearyl ether, glyceryl stearate/PEG-100 stearate, glycerin, mineral oil, magnesium aluminum silicate, titanium dioxide, DEA-cetyl phosphate, benzyl alcohol, mono- and diglycerides, fragrance, cetyl alcohol, cellulose gum, simethicone.
PreSun 8 Gel (Westwood)	8	aminobenzoic acid, 5%	SD alcohol 40, 55%; water, animal protein derivative, hydroxyethyl cellulose
PreSun 8 Lotion (Westwood)	8	aminobenzoic acid, 5%	SD alcohol 40, 55%; water, glycerin, choleth-24, hydroxypropylcellulose.
PreSun 15 Lotion (Westwood)	15	aminobenzoic acid, 5% padimate O, 5% oxybenzone, 3%	SD alcohol 40, 58%; water, PPG-15 stearyl ether, hydroxypropyl cellulose
PreSun Sunscreen Lip Protection (Westwood)	4	octyldimethylaminobenzoic acid, 4%	mineral oil, ozokerite, petrolatum, PEG-4 dilaurate, lanolin oil, propylparaben, flavoring
Q. T. Quick Tanning Foam and Lotion (Plough)	2	padimate O, 1.5%	dihydroxyacetone
RVP (Elder)	4	red petrolatum	hydrocarbon oil, ointment base
RVPaba Stick (Elder)	10	aminobenzoic acid; red petrolatum	
RVPaque (Elder)	10	cinoxate; red petrolatum	zinc oxide, opaque base
Sea & Ski Lotion (Carter)		octyldimethylaminobenzoic acid, 6%	cocoa butter
Shade Extra Protection Lotion (Plough)	6	homosalate, 8%; oxybenzone, 3%	
Shade Plus Water-Resistant Lotion (Plough)	8	padimate O, 7%; oxybenzone, 3%	
Snootie (Carter)		octyldimethylaminobenzoic acid, 8%	glycerin, stearic acid, dimethicone
Solar Cream (Doak)		aminobenzoic acid, 4%	titanium dioxide, 12%; water-repellent cream base, 84%

Sunscreen and Suntan Product Table, continued

Product (Manufacturer)	SPF Value	Sunscreen Agent	Other Ingredients
Solbar (Person & Covey)		dioxybenzone, 3%; oxybenzone, 3%	
Sudden Tan Foam and Lotion by Coppertone (Plough)		padimate O, 1.5%	dihydroxyacetone, caramel
SunDare Clear Lotion (Texas Pharmacal)	4–6	cinoxate, 1.75%	alcohol, 51.8%
SunDare Creamy Lotion (Texas Pharmacal)	4–6	cinoxate, 2%	lanolin derivative
SunGer Extra Protection (Plough)	6	homosalate, 8%; oxybenzone, 3%	
SunGer Sun Block (Plough)	15	padimate O, 7%; oxybenzone, 3%	
SunGer Weather and Tanning Stick (Plough)	4	homosalate, 10%	
Sunswept (Texas Pharmacal)		digalloyl trioleate, 3.5%	
Super Shade Sunblocking Lotion (Plough)	15	padimate O, 7%; oxybenzone, 3%	
Tropical Blend Dark Tanning Lotion (Plough)	2	homosalate, 4%	
Tropical Blend Dark Tanning Oil (Plough)	2	homosalate, 4%	
Tropical Blend Sunscreen Lotion (Plough)	4	padimate O, 3.5%	
Tropical Blend Maximal Sunscreen Lotion (Plough)	8	padimate O, 6%; oxybenzone, 2%	
Tropic Sun Oil (Carter)		octyldimethylaminobenzoic acid, 1.4%	cocoa butter, coconut oil, almond oil, mineral oil, lanolin

27 External Analgesic Products

Paul Skierkowski and Nancy C. Lublanezki

Questions to Ask the Patient

How long has the pain been present? How did it first appear? How often does it occur?

Can you relate the pain to any specific activity (an accident or overwork)?

Is the pain in a joint or in the muscle?

(If the pain is in a joint) Is the joint red, swollen, or warm to the touch?

Is the pain worse when you get up in the morning, and does it tend to subside as the day goes on?

Does the pain move to other areas of the body?

Do you have a fever or any "flu" symptoms?

External analgesics are topically applied substances that may have either topical analgesic, topical anesthetic, topical antipruritic, or counterirritant effects. It is important to differentiate these four groups. The topical analgesic, anesthetic, and antipruritic agents depress cutaneous sensory receptors for pain, itching, and burning and act directly to diminish or obliterate these symptoms on the skin due to burns, cuts, abrasions, insect bites, and other cutaneous lesions. (See Chapters 24, *Insect Sting and Bite Products*, and 25, *Burn and Sunburn Products*.) Topical counterirritants are included among the external analgesics because they are applied to the intact skin for the relief of pain. They differ from the analgesics, anesthetics, and antipruritic agents, however, in that the pain relief they produce results from stimulation of cutaneous receptors to induce sensations such as warmth, and sometimes itching (1). These induced sensations serve as a distraction from the deep-seated pain in areas such as muscles, joints, and tendons, which are distant from the skin surface where the ingredient is applied. In this manner, deep-seated pain is indirectly relieved. Some counterirritant agents actually depress cutaneous receptors similar in action to the topical anesthetics, analgesics, and antipruritics when present in low concentrations. For example, menthol depresses cutaneous receptors in concentrations below 1.0% and stimulates them in concentrations above 1.25%. Percutaneous absorption of active ingredients is not desired with counterirritant external analgesic products and therefore they are a distinct class of analgesic products.

Etiology of Muscular Pain

Everyone is familiar with the sensation of pain. It is a multidimensional experience that involves both a discriminative capacity and an interpretation of a stimulus in terms of present and past experience.

Pain receptors are present in most areas of the body, including skeletal muscles. Stimuli activating these receptors cause sensory impulses that are translated into a pain perception. The threshold of response varies greatly among individuals (2).

Skeletal muscle pain is quite common, especially in people who are not accustomed to strenuous exercise. When strain does occur, the muscles become sore and painful, and movement becomes difficult. Muscle pain also may occur as a result of prolonged, fixed, and stressful positions such as bending over for long periods and driving a car long distances (3).

Acute, temporary stiffness and muscle pain also may result from cold, dampness, rapid temperature changes, bruises, and air currents. In some cases, internal stimuli such as tension, constipation, GI distention, and other minor disorders may cause pain to be referred to the skeletal muscles of the shoulder. These episodes tend to be acute and self-limiting, and elimination of the cause and symptomatic treatment generally provide relief. Poor posture is also a frequent cause of skeletal muscle pain.

Because of its location and structure, the shoulder area is subject to more stress and strain than any other articulation of the body. In addition to all its other activities, its pendulum structure makes it continuously subjected to gravitational pull. A painful shoulder is more prevalent among elderly persons but frequently occurs in athletes and in people with certain occupations, such as house painting, where the arms are used vigorously and repetitively (4).

A painful condition attributed to strain or injury of tendons and their attachments to bone is often loosely described as tendonitis. Frequently tendonitis is related to a particular occupation or sport. Lumbago is a specific type of tendonitis involving the tendinous attachments of the muscles of the lumbar region.

Bursae are closed sacs that are lined with a cellular membrane resembling synovium. The bursae enable the motion of the tendons and muscles over bony prominences. Bursitis, an inflammation of a bursae of the body, is a common cause of joint pain. It may be an acute pain due to trauma, or it may be chronic, in which case other causes such as infection should be suspected. Bursitis is characterized by localized pain, tenderness, and swelling. Limited motion of adjacent joints is common (5). Symptoms of bursitis may mimic arthritic pain but can be distinguished on physical examination. For instance, in contrast to arthritis, direct pressure over the joint capsule of the shoulder in bursitis does not cause pain.

Arthritic pain may be caused by rheumatoid arthritis, which may involve almost all peripheral joints, tendons, bursae, and the cervical spine, or by osteoarthritis, which involves degeneration of cartilage with secondary changes in joints. Although both types of rheumatoid disorders are chronic systemic diseases, local treatment of painful joints coupled with rest may give temporary symptomatic relief.

Mechanism of Action of Counterirritants

Counterirritants are applied locally to produce a mild, local, inflammatory reaction with the objective of providing relief in another site, usually adjacent to or underlying the skin surface being treated. The intensity of response depends on the irritant employed, its concentration, the solvent in which it is dissolved, and the period of contact with the skin (6).

The counterirritant drug is applied to the skin where pain is experienced. Pain is only as intense as it is perceived to be, and the perception of other sensations from applications of the counterirritant, such as massage and warmth, crowds out pain perception. Several theories have been proposed to explain the mechanism of action of the irritant drugs:

- Stimulation of sensory nerve endings in the skin cause reflexive stimulation of vasomotor fibers to the viscera. These reflexes are mediated through the cerebrospinal axis and produce dilation of the visceral vasculature (7).
- Stimulation of sensory nerve endings in the skin cause axon reflexes resulting in stimulation of the nerves enervating branches of arterioles to produce vasodila-

tion in the muscles. This action produces an increase in the blood flow to the muscles (8).
- Summation of pain stimuli produces intense stimulation of the areas of pain interpretation of the brain, partly abating visceral pain stimuli. According to this theory of their action, stimuli originating in the viscera or muscles are transmitted over fibers in a common pathway, along with sensations from the skin, and are referred to the same area of the spinal cord as the stimuli from the skin (Figure 1). If the intensity of the stimulation from the skin is increased by a drug's irritant action, the character of the visceral or muscle pain becomes modified. With intense skin stimulation, the referred pain stimuli may be partly or completely obliterated insofar as the sensorium is concerned. The patient's attention is diverted from the muscular or visceral structure by the application of the counterirritant drug (6).

An additional effect of some products is to produce vasodilatation of cutaneous vasculature. These drugs, known as rubefacients, produce reactive hyperemia, and it is hypothesized that this increase in blood pooling and/or flow is accompanied by an increase in localized skin temperature. The degree of irritation must be controlled, however, as stronger irritation may cause erythema and blistering. The increase in localized skin temperature then may act by the counterirritant effect. This positive thermal response for some agents has been documented by thermography (9).

Undoubtedly, the action of counterirritants in relieving pain has a strong psychological component and indeed they may exert a placebo effect through pleasant aromatic odors or a sensation of warmth or coolness that they produce on the skin.

Some topical analgesics act by overcoming the stimulus that causes the pain. To do this they must first be percutaneously absorbed. The effects following this absorption are then systemic and the action is the same as internal analgesic. (See Chapter 11, *Internal Analgesic Products*.) Relief of any deep-seated pain will be the result of a systemic effect that may follow percutaneous absorption if the interstitial fluid drug concentration obtained is sufficiently high (10).

Patient Assessment and Treatment

The pharmacist should exercise careful judgment in the assessment of the patient's condition before recommending a nonprescription counterirritant preparation. Certain questions should be asked of the patient before deciding whether to recommend a nonprescription product. It is important for the pharmacist to ask the following questions:

- How long has the pain been apparent? What kind of pain is it? Is it debilitating? Conditions amenable to nonprescription treatment are self-limiting in nature (the condition will resolve with or without treatment in a short time). Pain that has been apparent for longer than 7 days duration may indicate a more serious underlying condition. These patients should be evaluated by a physician.

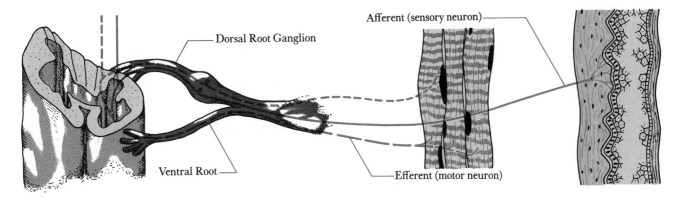

Figure 1. Reflex pathways showing the afferent (sensory) fibers, efferent (vasomotor) fibers, and their synapse in the spinal cord. Adapted from F. H. Netter, The Ciba Collection of Medical Illustrations, Ciba Pharmaceutical Company, New York, N.Y., 1962. p. 65.

- Is there any apparent cause of the pain? Often muscular or joint pain can be brought on by simple overexertion, such as exercise or other physical activity to which the patient is unaccustomed and this is a valid indication for these agents.
- Can the patient locate and describe the pain? If the pain can be specifically located and is of mild intensity, it may be appropriate to recommend a nonprescription product. If, however, the patient has difficulty in locating the origin of the pain, it may be referred pain. An example is pain in the lumbar area, which may be referred from pelvic viscera and may be an early manifestation of disease in these organs. If the pain is of severe intensity, nonprescription treatment should not be recommended.
- If the pain is in a joint, is the joint red, swollen, and tender to the touch? If so, there may be a fracture or rupture of ligaments or tendons or arthritic involvement. Nonprescription products used in this condition would delay an accurate diagnosis.
- Has the patient been diagnosed by a physician as having any type of arthritic condition? If the patient has been diagnosed and is under medical supervision for any type of arthritic condition, it may be appropriate to recommend a counterirritant preparation as adjunctive treatment only. Arthritic conditions should never be self-diagnosed or self-treated.

If the pharmacist decides that the condition is minor and that there are no serious underlying conditions, it may be appropriate to recommend a nonprescription preparation. The pharmacist should advise the patient that, if the symptoms persist or are not relieved by the preparation within 7 days, the medication should be discontinued and a physician should be consulted.

The prudent pharmacist should always arrange for a follow-up consultation with the patient to review the condition. Pharmacist follow-up may prevent the patient from prolonging ineffective self-medication while a more serious underlying disease is allowed to progress.

Pharmacologic Agents

The following ingredients have been recognized as safe and effective counterirritants by the FDA advisory review panel on nonprescription topical analgesics. Table 1 classifies these agents by their relative potencies.

Allyl Isothiocyanate

This agent, also known as volatile oil of mustard, is derived from the powdered seeds of black mustard plant and other species of mustard and can be prepared synthetically.

In high concentrations, allyl isothiocyanate is absorbed rapidly from intact skin as well as from all mucous membranes. Penetration into the skin is rapid and, if not removed soon after application, it may cause ulceration. A poultice, erroneously termed a "mustard plaster," has been used as a home remedy by many people. It is prepared by mixing equal parts of powdered mustard and flour and moistening with water to form a paste. The paste is then spread on a towel or piece of material and placed on the affected area. The continuous release of allyl isothiocyanate by the presence of water and body heat may cause the inflammatory action to go beyond erythema to vesication and, therefore, the poultice should not remain on the skin for more than a few minutes. Allyl isothiocyanate is considered to be safe and effective for nonprescription use in concentrations of 0.5–5.0%. It should be applied to the affected areas no more than 3 or 4 times/day. When preparing a mustard plaster, care should be taken to avoid inhalation of this powerful irritant. This dosage is for adults and children older than 2 years. There is no recommended dose for children less than 2 years except under the advice and supervision of a physician (11).

Stronger Ammonia Water

This agent is also known as strong ammonia solution (NF XIV). Since it is caustic and the vapors are irritating, it should be handled with care and the vapors should not be inhaled. Stronger ammonia water is an aqueous solution of ammonia containing 27–30% by weight of ammonia (NH_3). It must be diluted before use as a topical agent due to its caustic nature. The concentration considered to be safe and effective for topical use by adults and children over 2 years is a 1.0–2.5% solution of available ammonia. It should be applied to the affected area no more than 3 or 4 times/day (12).

Several liniments containing ammonia are available. They are prepared by adding diluted ammonia water to a combination of oleic acid and sesame oil. The oleic acid reacts with ammonia to form an emulsifying agent for the water and sesame oil. The concentrations of ammonia range from ~0.5–2.65%.

Aromatic ammonia spirit ("smelling salts") derived from stronger ammonia water is used for its respiratory stimulant properties. The content of available ammonia is low enough that it may be administered orally in small doses or held near the nostrils for inhalation of volatile vapor.

Methyl Salicylate

Methyl salicylate, occurring naturally as wintergreen oil or sweet birch oil, or prepared synthetically, is the most widely used counterirritant and has been categorized as safe and effective for use as a nonprescription analgesic when used in the specified dosage (13). At very low concentrations, methyl salicylate is used in oral preparations for its pleasant flavor and aroma. Ingestion of more than small amounts of the substance is hazardous due to the high salicylate content. Although the average lethal dose of methyl salicylate is estimated to be 10 ml for children and 30 ml for adults (14), as little as 4 ml has caused death in children (15).

A survey by the FDA advisory review panel considering methyl salicylate found that oral ingestion of this ingredient from products formulated as ointments caused no deaths and there were few cases manifesting severe symptoms (16). However, regulations require the use of child-resistant containers for liquid preparations containing more than 5% methyl salicylate (17). There is little evidence to suggest that these toxicity hazards restrict the rational use of topical application of the drug as a counterirritant. The agent possesses a high degree of safety for topical use and has had a long marketing history.

The recommended topical dosage range for adults and children 2 years of age or older of methyl salicylate is a 10–60% concentration applied to the affected area no more than 3–4 times/day (18). Because of the possibility of percutaneous absorption, this product should be used with caution in individuals who are sensitive to aspirin.

Turpentine Oil

Turpentine oil is commonly misnamed "turpentine." Turpentine oil for medicinal use must be of higher quality than commercial turpentine oil; it should be rectified turpentine oil. It is prepared by steam distillation of turpentine oleoresin collected from various species of pine trees.

Several human fatalities from the ingestion of turpentine oil have been reported. An oral dose of 140 ml in adults (15 ml in children) may be fatal. Turpentine oil is both a primary irritant and a sensitizer. As an irritant, it usually acts by defatting the skin, causing dryness and fissuring. It is often used as a cleanser for removing paints and waxes and is thus one of the most common causes of hand eczema.

Turpentine oil has been used as an ingredient in counterirritant preparations with a long history of safety and efficacy. The recommended dosage range for adults and children over 2 years is a 6–50% concentration applied to the affected area no more than 3 or 4 times/day (19). Application of turpentine liniments to the skin may cause vesicular eruption, urticaria, and vomiting in susceptible individuals.

Menthol

Menthol is extraced from peppermint oil or prepared synthetically. The fatal dose of menthol in humans is approximately 1 g/kg (20). It may be used safely in small quantities as a flavoring agent and has found wide acceptance in candy, chewing gum, and cigarettes. Menthol has had extensive use in inhalant preparations for the relief of nasal congestion.

Menthol causes sensitization in certain individuals, although the sensitization index is low (21). Symptoms include urticaria, erythema, and other cutaneous lesions.

When menthol is used in topical preparations in concentrations of 0.1–1.0%, it depresses sensory cutaneous receptors and acts as an antipruritic. When used in higher concentrations of 1.25–16%, it acts as a counterirritant. When applied to the skin, menthol stimulates the nerves for the perception of cold, while depressing those that perceive pain. Topical application of counterirritant concentrations of menthol initially produce a feeling of coolness that is soon followed by a sensation of warmth.

Table 1. Relative potencies of counterirritants

Group	Characteristics	Ingredients
A	Cause redness, irritation; are relatively more potent than other counterirritants	Allyl isothiocyanate, stronger ammonia water, methyl salicylate, turpentine oil
B	Produce cooling sensation; have organoleptic properties	Menthol, camphor, eucalyptus oil
C	Vasoactive substances, vasodilator	Histamine dihydrochloride, methyl nicotinate
D	Produce irritation without rubefaction, although approximately equal in potency to Group A	Capsaicin, capsicum, capsicum oleoresin

Reprinted from the *Federal Register*, 44, 69784 (1979).

Menthol is usually combined with other ingredients with antipruritic or analgesic properties, such as camphor.

The recommended dosage range for adults and children over 2 years for menthol when used as a counterirritant is 1.26–16% applied to the affected area no more than 3–4 times/day (22).

Camphor

Although camphor is naturally occurring and is obtained from the camphor tree, approximately three-fourths of the camphor used is prepared synthetically. In concentrations exceeding 3%, particularly when combined with other ingredients that produce counterirritation, camphor stimulates the nerve endings in the skin and induces relief of pain and discomfort in muscle joints and other subcutaneous structures at a site distal to the application site. When applied vigorously, it produces a rubefacient reaction.

The recommended concentration for external use as a counterirritant for adults and children 2 years of age and older is 3–11%. In concentrations of 0.1–3.0%, camphor depresses cutaneous receptors and is used as a topical analgesic, anesthetic, and antipruritic. Application should be made no more than 3 or 4 times/day. In children under 2 years of age, there is no recommended dosage except under the advice and supervision of a physician.

Because of its systemic toxicity in high concentrations and when taken internally, preparations with camphor concentrations in excess of 11%—such as camphorated oil (camphor liniment) which is a solution of 20% camphor in cottonseed oil—are not considered to be safe for nonprescription use. In 1980, an FDA advisory panel recommended the removal of camphorated oil from the over-the-counter market because it is too often confused with castor oil and has been frequently implicated in accidental poisonings in children. The panel stated that "the dangers of poisoning associated with the use of camphorated oil far outweigh the minimal therapeutic value of the product." The panel also found no evidence to support the effectiveness of camphorated oil when applied to the skin.

Camphor is highly toxic and once ingested is very difficult to treat (23, 24). The National Clearinghouse for Poison Control Centers reported that from 1974 to 1978 there were 706 poisonings due to ingestion of camphor, 421 of them occurring in children (less than 2 teaspoonfuls can be fatal in adults) (25).

The symptoms of camphorated oil poisoning are severe; their onset occurs within 5–90 minutes after ingestion (26). Nausea and vomiting may be the first to occur; headache, a feeling of warmth, vertigo, mental confusion, delirium, clonic convulsions, coma, and finally respiratory arrest lead to death (27, 28, 29). Other symptoms include epileptiform convulsions, apnea, asystole, and neuronal necrosis (28). If death does not occur, mental retardation can be a sequel (30). If the patient lives, recovery is usually complete within 48 hours; however, a 19-month-old infant died 5 days after the ingestion of 1 teaspoonful of camphorated oil (31, 32).

Treatment of camphorated oil poisoning is by no means simple. Most toxicology texts recommend symptomatic and supportive treatment. Treatment is complicated by the fact that camphorated oil is so highly soluble in lipid deposits. Lipid hemodialysis has proved an effective treatment, but the value of this procedure is constrained by its limited availability (32).

Histamine Dihydrochloride

Histamine dihydrochloride when used in a 0.025–0.10% concentration is considered to be a safe and effective counterirritant when applied no more than 3 or 4 times/day. Application of products containing histamine dihydrochloride results in vasodilatation and causes percutaneous absorption of histamine from an ointment vehicle containing other medicinal agents. Aqueous vehicles seem to be superior to ointments for percutaneous absorption (33).

Methyl Nicotinate

Methyl nicotinate when used in a 0.25–1.0% concentration is a safe and effective counterirritant when applied no more than 3 or 4 times/day. Although nicotinic acid is inactive topically, this ester possesses a marked power of diffusion and readily penetrates the cutaneous barrier. Vasodilation and elevation of skin temperature results from very low concentrations. Susceptible persons who apply methyl nicotinate over large areas may experience a drop in blood pressure and pulse rate and syncope due to generalized vascular dilatation (18).

Capsicum Preparations

Capsicum preparations (capsaicin, capsicum, and capsicum oleoresin), derived from an irritant product of cayenne pepper, produce a feeling of warmth and redness without vesicant action when they are applied to intact skin. They do not cause blistering, even in high concentrations, due to their lack of action upon capillary or other blood vessels.

The recommended dosage range for adults and children over 2 years is a concentration of capsicum preparation that yields 0.025–0.25% capsaicin, applied to the affected area no more than 3 or 4 times/day (34). It should be noted that because of variations between lots of capsicum, the concentration range for this drug cannot be expressed as a percentage, and must be calculated for each lot.

Eucalyptus Oil

This agent seems to be safe for nonprescription use, but there are insufficient data available to permit final classification of its effectiveness as a counterirritant. It may continue to be marketed in preparations when used in concentrations of 0.5–3.0% to be used not more than 3–4 times/day except in children under 2 years of age, until a final classification may be made (35).

Other Agents

The following ingredients are external analgesic agents that act by depressing cutaneous sensory receptors. All are considered safe in the concentrations normally employed for nonprescription products. However, all are presently classified in Category III for efficacy as available data are insufficient to permit final classification.

Triethanolamine Salicylate

Triethanolamine salicylate, although a salicylate ester, is not a counterirritant analgesic. The exact mechanism by which salicylates produce their analgesic effect is not known, but it is generally conceded that they act in part centrally, and in part peripherally as anti-inflammatories by inhibition of prostaglandins with subsequent relief of pain. Although data exist to show that triethanolamine salicylate is absorbed from the skin, insufficient data exist to show that the quantity absorbed is enough to produce effective analgesia (36).

Glycol Salicylate

Glycol salicylate is believed to act like other salicylates in producing analgesia. It is usually used in concentration of 1–10% in combination with counterirritants (combination products are discussed later in this chapter). At present, there is insufficient evidence to permit final classification of its effectiveness for use as a nonprescription external analgesic (37).

Salicylamide

Salicylamide is the amide of salicylic acid. However, it is not metabolized to free salicylates nor does it have any anti-inflammatory activity. Because it is poorly water soluble, the amount available for absorption through the skin will be limited. Clinical use has confirmed that salicylamide is safe in the dosage range used as a nonprescription external analgesic, but there are insufficient data available to permit final classification of its effectiveness (38). Patients sensitive to aspirin are not sensitized to salicylamide because it is not converted to salicylic acid.

Rationale for Combinations of Ingredients

A nonprescription product may combine two or more safe and effective active ingredients when each active ingredient makes a contribution to the claimed effect and when the combination does not decrease the safety or effectiveness of any of the individual active ingredients. There are four separate chemical and/or pharmacologic groups of counterirritants that provide four qualitatively different types of irritation. Many preparations marketed utilize at least two different such effects when greater potency is desired. Table 1 lists the individual ingredients and classifies them according to their relative potency. Many products will combine active ingredients from one group of counterirritants with one, two, or three other active ingredients provided that each active ingredient is from a different group. Menthol (Group B) is often combined together with one, two, or three active ingredients from different groups.

It is irrational to combine counterirritants with local anesthetics, topical antipruritics, or topical analgesics. These agents depress sensory cutaneous receptors and their effects would be opposed by the counterirritants, which stimulate cutaneous sensory receptors. It is also irrational to combine counterirritants with skin pro-

tectants since the protectants act in opposition to the counterirritants and may nullify their effects (39).

Dosage Forms

The types of vehicles used to formulate the finished product containing counterirritants are important as percutaneous absorption of counterirritant drugs is generally undesirable. The finished product should consist of ingredients and vehicles that keep skin penetration at or near zero. The nonprescription counterirritant preparations are usually available as liniments, gels, lotions, and ointments.

Liniments

Solutions or mixtures of various substances in oil, alcoholic solutions of soap, or emulsions are called liniments. They are intended for external application and should be so labeled. They are applied to the affected area with friction and rubbing of the skin, the oil or soap base providing ease of application and massage. Liniments with an alcoholic or hydroalcoholic vehicle are useful in instances in which rubefacient or counterirritant action is desired; oleaginous liniments are used primarily when massage is desired. By their nature, oleaginous liniments are less irritating to the skin than alcoholic liniments (40).

Liniments should not be applied to skin areas that are broken or bruised. The vehicle for a liniment is selected on the basis of the kind of action of the desired components in the various vehicles (40).

Gels

Gels used for the delivery of counterirritants are more appropriately called jellies because they are generally clear and are of a more uniform, semisolid consistency. A greater sensation of warmth is experienced with a gel than with equal quantities of the same product in a different dosage form such as a lotion or an ointment. Products formulated as gels promote a more rapid and extensive penetration of the medication into the skin and hair follicles. Patients should be advised against using excessive amounts of gels since increased penetration may cause an unpleasant burning sensation (40).

Lotions

These liquid suspensions or dispersions are used for external application to the skin for the protective or therapeutic value of their constituents. Depending on the ingredients, they may be alcoholic or aqueous and are often emulsions. Their fluidity allows rapid and uniform application over a wide surface area. Lotions are intended to dry on the skin soon after application, leaving a thin coat of their active ingredients on the skin's surface.

Ointments

Ointments are semisolid preparations intended for external application to the skin or mucous membranes. Ointments are applied to the skin to elicit one of these general effects: a surface activity, an effect within the stratum corneum, or a more deep-seated activity requiring penetration into the epidermis and dermis. These semisolid dosage forms are particularly desirable for counterirritants since these agents are applied with massage (40).

Clinical Considerations

The dosage forms referred to as "greaseless" are oil-in-water formulations, are therefore "water washable," and are usually preferred for daytime use. Many formulations contain lanolin or anhydrous lanolin as a vehicle. Because both of these are obtained from wool fat, many individuals are allergic to them, which should be considered when choosing the appropriate formulation.

The longer any dosage form remains in contact with the skin, the longer the duration of action. There seems to be little agreement on how long the preparations should be left in contact with the skin for optimal results, although a practical guideline is that preparations should be used no more than 3 or 4 times/day.

Labeling of Counterirritant Preparations

Labeling approved by the FDA may not necessarily be similar to advertising claims (41). The pharmacist can do much to educate the patient by providing accurate information.

Labeling of counterirritant preparations must include a list of active ingredients. The concentrations of

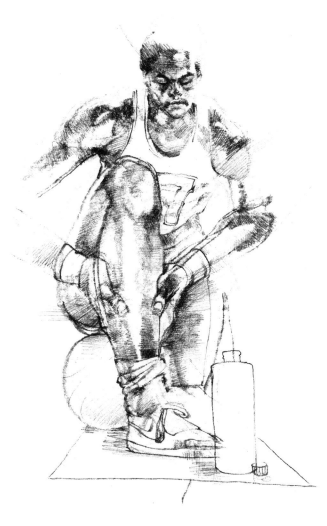

the active ingredients must be listed and the officially recognized established name of the ingredients used. The manner of usage and the frequency of applications should also be indicated (41).

The labeling for indications states that these preparations should be used "for the temporary relief of minor aches and pains of muscles and joints." In addition, the labeling recommended by the majority of the panel includes claims for simple backache, strains, bruises, and sprains (42). These terms were selected on the basis that they would be readily and easily understood by the general population.

It is acceptable to use terms describing certain physical or chemical qualities of the counterirritant preparations, as long as these terms do not imply that any therapeutic effects occur. Terms such as "nongreasy," "soothing," "cooling action," "penetrating relief," "provides warming relief," and "for cool comforting relief" are considered acceptable in labeling.

Claims related to product performance are unacceptable unless they can be substantiated by scientific data. Claims such as "fast," "quick," and "remarkable" are misleading and may be confusing to the patient unless they can be supported by adequate scientific data.

Warnings on counterirritant preparations are as follows:

- For external use only.
- Avoid contact with the eyes.
- If condition worsens, or if symptoms persist for more than 7 days, discontinue use of this product and consult a physician.
- Do not use on children under 2 years of age except under the advice and supervision of a physician.
- Do not apply to wounds or damaged skin.
- Do not bandage.

Safety of Counterirritants

The oral toxicity of the counterirritant preparations is variable; some agents such as the capsicum preparations have a low oral toxicity while other agents, such as methyl salicylate and camphor, are highly toxic when ingested orally. Although some percutaneous absorption occurs with the topical application of the counterirritants, the amounts absorbed are insignificant when the ingredients do not exceed the maximum recommended effective concentrations.

Self-medication with nonprescription counterirritant preparations may result in harm if directions are not followed exactly. Some individuals overreact to the irritant properties of counterirritants and develop rashes and blisters. In addition to irritation, counterirritants also may produce sensitization, in which case immunologic phenomena are involved. It may be difficult to distinguish between direct topical irritation and topical sensitization. Therefore, the labeling of preparations must indicate prompt discontinuation if excessive skin irritation develops.

Physical Methods of Counterirritation

Although the nonprescription preparations do have merit of their own as therapeutic agents, there are simple physical methods of inducing counterirritation. Perhaps the most frequently employed method is heat applied by means of a heat lamp, a hot-water bottle, a heating pad, or a moist steam pack. Heat helps to restore the elastic property of collagen by increasing the viscous flow. Under normal conditions, collagen recoils like a spring once the load is released. After a stretching injury, the collagen tissue does not return to its resting length. Heat also acts selectively on free nerve endings in the tissue and on peripheral nerve fibers to increase the pain threshold. This results in an analgesic effect (43). The application of heat should be used with extreme caution if it is to be used in conjunction with a counterirritant preparation. Severe burning or blistering of skin areas has resulted from the simultaneous use of a counterirritant preparation and heat.

Massaging the painful area is another method of producing counterirritation. The therapeutic benefits of massage have been known for centuries. It is possible that the beneficial effects of some counterirritants used in treating musculoskeletal disorders may be due largely to the rubbing and massage involved in the application of the medication. Massage causes an increase in the flow of blood and lymph in the skin and underlying structures.

Studies comparing massage with other modalities are virtually nonexistent because it is difficult to prepare protocols for conducting controlled objective clinical studies on the therapeutic effectiveness of massage techniques. Many clinicians have found that massage is therapeutically beneficial in select situations and use it extensively.

Summary

Counterirritant external analgesic agents provide a method of decreasing the pain and discomfort associated with many minor aches and pains of muscles and joints. They must be used correctly to be safe.

The pharmacist can play an important role in patient education by instructing patients on the proper use of these agents. It is also important that patients be educated as to the level of relief that can reasonably be expected from these agents and when self-medication is not indicated.

References

1. "The Pharmacological Basis of Therapeutics," A. Gilman, L. Goodman, and A. Gilman, Eds., MacMillan, New York, N.Y., 1980, p. 955.
2. T. S. Szasz, *Arch. Neurol. Psychiatry, 74*, 174 (1955).
3. "Cecil-Loeb Textbook of Medicine," 15th ed., P. B. Beeson and W. McDermott, Eds., W. B. Saunders, Philadelphia, Pa., 1979, p. 184.
4. J. L. Hollander, "Arthritis and Allied Conditions," Lea and Febiger, Philadelphia, Pa., 1966, p. 1233.
5. "Current Medical Diagnosis and Treatment," M. A. Krupp and M. J. Chatton, Eds., Lange Medical, Los Altos, Calif., 1981, p. 508.
6. "Krantz and Carr's Pharmacological Principles of Medical Practice," 8th ed., D. M. Aviado, Ed., Williams and Wilkins, Baltimore, Md., 1972, p. 891.
7. "The Pharmacological Basis of Therapeutics," 6th ed., A. G. Gilman, L. S. Goodman, and A. Gilman, Eds., Macmillan, New York, N.Y., 1980, p. 955.
8. B. S. Post, *Arch. Phys. Med. Rehabil., 42*, 791 (1961).
9. D. W. Lewis and P. J. Verhonick, *Appl. Radiol., 6*, 114 (1977).
10. *Federal Register, 44*, 69784 (1979).
11. *Federal Register, 44*, 69791–2 (1979).
12. *Federal Register, 44*, 69792–3 (1979).
13. *Federal Register, 44*, 68930 (1979).
14. W. B. Deichman and H. W. Gerarde, "Toxicology of Drugs and Chemicals," Academic Press, New York, N.Y., 1969, p. 662.
15. C. H. Thienes and T. J. Haley, "Clinical Toxicology," 5th ed., Lea and Febiger, Philadelphia, Pa., 1972, p. 80.
16. *Federal Register, 44*, 68831 (1979).
17. K. Trapnell, *J. Am. Pharm. Assoc., NS16*, 147 (1976).
18. *Federal Register, 44*, 69830–31 (1979).
19. *Federal Register, 44*, 69840–41 (1979).
20. *Federal Register, 44*, 69827 (1979).
21. C. Papa and W. Shelley, *J. Am. Med. Assoc., 547*, 189 (1964).
22. *Federal Register, 44*, 69828 (1979).
23. *Federal Register, 44*, 69802–3 (1979).
24. Statement of the American Pharmaceutical Association, September 27, 1978.
25. *Apharmacy Weekly, 19*, 154, (1980).
26. R. Aronow and R. W. Spiegel, *Drug Intell. Clin. Pharm., 10*, 631–634 (1976).
27. "The United States Dispensatory," 27th ed., A. Osol and R. Pratt, Eds., J. B. Lippincott, Philadelphia, Pa., 1973, p. 220.
28. R. E. Gosselin et al., "Clinical Toxicology of Commercial Products," 4th ed., Williams and Wilkins, Baltimore, Md., 1976, p. 77.
29. "The Merck Index," 9th ed., M. Windholtz, S. Budavari, L. Y. Stroumtsos, and M. N. Fertig, Eds., Merck, Rahway, N.J., 1976, p. 220.
30. J. M. Arena, "Poisoning," 3rd ed., Charles C Thomas, Springfield, Ill., 1974, p. 368.
31. H. E. Ginn et al., *J. Am. Med. Assoc., 203*, 230–231 (1968).
32. A. G. Smith and G. Margolis, *Am. J. Pathol., 30*, 857–869 (1954).
33. *Federal Register, 44*, 69812–13 (1979).
34. *Federal Register, 44*, 69804–5 (1979).
35. *Federal Register, 44*, 69850 (1979).
36. *Federal Register, 44*, 69856 (1979).
37. *Federal Register, 44*, 69852 (1979).
38. *Federal Register, 44*, 69853–5 (1979).
39. *Federal Register, 44*, 69786–87 (1979).
40. "Remington's Pharmaceutical Sciences," 16th ed., Mack, Easton, Pa., 1980, pp. 1448, 1451, 1518.
41. *Federal Register, 44*, 69784 (1979).
42. *Federal Register, 44*, 69841 (1979).
43. M. Sherman, *Am. Pharm., NS20*, 46 (1980).

External Analgesic Product Table

Product (Manufacturer)	Application Form	Counterirritant	Other Ingredients
Absorbent Rub (DeWitt)	lotion	camphor, 1.6%; menthol, 1.6%; methyl salicylate, 0.7%; wormwood oil, 0.6%; sassafras oil, 0.5%; capsicum, 0.03%	isopropyl alcohol, 69%; green soap, 11.6%; pine tar soap, 0.9%; o-phenylphenol, 0.5%; benzocaine, 0.5%
Absorbine Arthritic (W. F. Young)	lotion	methyl salicylate, menthol, methyl nicotinate	isopropyl alcohol, 3%; cetyl alcohol, 1%
Absorbine Jr. (W. F. Young)	lotion	wormwood oil, thymol, menthol, chloroxylenol	acetone
Act-On Rub (Keystone)	lotion	methyl salicylate, 10.4%; menthol, 1.5%; camphor, 1.5%; eucalyptus oil, 1.4%; mustard oil, 0.4%	isopropyl myristate, balm base, lanolin
Analbalm (Central)	lotion	methyl salicylate, 5%; camphor, 2.5%; menthol, 0.5%	greaseless nonstaining emulsion base
Analgesic Balm (Lilly)	ointment	methyl salicylate, 15%; menthol, 15%	hydrocarbon waxes, lanolin, petrolatum, sorbitan sesquioleate, water-soluble base
Aspercreme (Thompson Medical)	lotion cream		triethanolamine salicylate, 10% greaseless base
Banalg (O'Neal, Jones & Feldman)	lotion	menthol, methyl salicylate, camphor, eucalyptus oil	greaseless base
Banalg Hospital Strength (O'Neal, Jones & Feldman)	lotion	methyl salicylate, menthol	greaseless base
Baumodyne (North American)	gel	menthol, 1.5%; methyl salicylate, 11.35%; eucalyptus oil	methylparaben, propylparaben
Baumodyne (North American)	ointment	methyl salicylate, 15.2%; menthol, 3.12% eucalyptus oil	methylparaben, propylparaben
Ben-Gay (Leeming)	lotion	methyl salicylate, 15%; menthol, 7%	greaseless base
Ben-Gay Extra Strength Balm (Leeming)	ointment	methyl salicylate, 30%; menthol, 8%	greaseless base
Ben-Gay Gel (Leeming)	gel	methyl salicylate, 15%; menthol, 7%	hydroalcoholic gel base
Ben-Gay Greaseless/ Stainless Ointment (Leeming)	ointment	methyl salicylate, 15%; menthol, 10%	greaseless base
Ben-Gay Original (Leeming)	ointment	methyl salicylate, 18.3%; menthol, 16%	oleaginous base
Braska (Keystone)	lotion	methyl salicylate, 5%; menthol, 0.5%; camphor, 1%; monoglycol salicylate, 1.2%; methyl nicotinate, 0.5%	isopropyl alcohol; salicylamide, 1.2%
Counterpain Rub (Squibb)	ointment	methyl salicylate, 10.2%; menthol, 5.4%; eugenol, 1.4%	
Dencorub (Roberts)	lotion	methyl salicylate, menthol, camphor, eucalyptus oil, salicylic acid	lanolin
Doan's Rub (Jeffrey Martin)	cream	methyl salicylate, 15%; menthol, 10%	

External Analgesic Products Table, continued

Product (Manufacturer)	Application Form	Counterirritant	Other Ingredients
Emul-O-Balm (Pennwalt)	lotion	menthol, 2.2%; methyl salicylate, 2.2%; camphor, 1.1%	non-greasy base
End-Ake Cream (Columbia Medical)	cream	methyl nicotinate, 0.5%; capsicum oleoresin; dipropylene glycol salicylate	salicylamide, histamine dihydrochloride, 0.05%
Exocaine Medicated Rub (Kirk)	cream	methyl salicylate, 2.5%; clove oil, 1%; menthol, 0.9%; eucalyptus oil	
Exocaine Plus (Kirk)	cream	methyl salicylate, 27.5%; menthol, 0.9%; clove oil, 1%; eucalyptus oil	
Heet (Whitehall)	lotion spray	methyl salicylate, 15%; capsicum, 0.025%; camphor, 3.6%; menthol, 3%, (spray); methyl nicotinate, 1.0% (spray)	alcohol, 70% (lotion)
Icy Hot (Searle)	balm	methyl salicylate, 29%; menthol, 8%	lanolin
Icy Hot (Searle)	rub	methyl salicylate, 12%; menthol, 9%	
Infra-Rub (Whitehall)	cream	histamine dihydrochloride, 0.1%; capsicum oleoresin, 0.4%	glycol monosalicylate, lanolin
Mentholatum (Mentholatum)	rub cream	camphor, 9%; menthol, 1.35%	aromatic oils, petrolatum base
Mentholatum Deep Heating (Mentholatum)	rub lotion	methyl salicylate, 12.7% (rub); 20% (lotion); menthol, 6%; eucalyptus oil (rub); turpentine oil (rub)	lanolin, greaseless base
Minit-Rub (Bristol-Myers)	ointment	methyl salicylate, 15%; menthol, 3.54%; camphor, 2.3%	anhydrous lanolin, 4.5%
Mobisyl (B.F. Asctier)	cream		triethanolamine salicylate, 10%
Musterole Deep Strength (Plough)	ointment	methyl salicylate, 30%; menthol, 3%; methyl nicotinate, 0.5%	
Musterole Regular, Extra, and Children's Strength (Plough)	ointment	camphor, menthol, methyl salicylate, mustard oil, glycol monosalicylate	
Omega Oil (Block)	lotion	methyl salicylate, 23%; methyl nicotinate, 0.3%; capsicum oleoresin, 0.25%; histamine dihydrochloride, 0.02%	isopropyl alcohol, 50%
Panalgesic (Poythress)	lotion	methyl salicylate, 55%; camphor, 2%; menthol, 0.95%	emollient oils, 19%; alcohol, 17%; aspirin, 5%
Pronto Gel (Commerce)	gel	methyl salicylate, 27.5%; menthol, 1%; camphor, 1%; methyl nicotinate, 0.25%	isopropyl alcohol, 46.5%
Rid-A-Pain (Pfeiffer)	liniment	methyl nicotinate, 0.4%; methyl salicylate, 4.8%	washable base
Sloan's (Warner-Lambert)	liniment	turpentine oil, 46.76%; pine oil, 6.74%; camphor, 3.35%; methyl salicylate, 2.66%; capsicum oleoresin, 0.62%	kerosene, 39.88%
Soltice Hi-Therm (Chattem)	cream	eucalyptus oil, 10 mg/g; methyl salicylate, 50 mg/g; menthol, 70 mg/g; camphor, 70 mg/g	greaseless base

External Analgesic Products Table, continued

Product (Manufacturer)	Application Form	Counterirritant	Other Ingredients
Soltice Quick Rub (Chattem)	cream	eucalyptus oil, 10 mg/g; methyl salicylate, 50 mg/g; menthol, 50 mg/g; camphor, 50 mg/g	greaseless base
Stimurub (Otis Clapp)	ointment	menthol, methyl salicylate, capsicum oleoresin	
Surin (McKesson)	ointment	methyl salicylate, 1.14%; menthol, 0.285%; camphor, 0.475%; methacholine chloride, 0.25%	greaseless base
Yager's Liniment (Yager)	liniment	turpentine oil, camphor	aqua ammonia, 0.5%; ammonium oleate base
Zemo Liquid (Plough)	lotion	methyl salicylate, thymol, eucalyptol, menthol, phenol	sodium salicylate; sodium borate; benzoic acid; boric acid; alcohol, 41%
Zemo Liquid Extra Strength (Plough)	lotion	methyl salicylate, phenol menthol; thymol	alcohol, 40%
Zemo Ointment (Plough)	ointment	methyl salicylate, menthol	triclosan, zinc oxide, boric acid, benzoic acid, bismuth subnitrate

28 Topical Anti-infective Products

Paul Zanowiak and Michael R. Jacobs

Questions to Ask the Patient

What area of the skin is affected? How extensive is the area involved?

Is the skin broken? Is there any pus? Is it painful?

How long have you had this condition? Have you ever had it before? Are any other members of your family also affected?

Has the condition developed as the result of a previous rash or skin problem?

Has the condition worsened?

Do you have a fever or any flu-like symptoms?

Do you have diabetes? Do you have any other medical conditions?

Do you have any allergies to topical medications?

What treatments have you tried for this condition? Were they effective?

What oral or topical medications are you presently using? Have they been effective?

Topical anti-infectives are products used to counteract local infection of tissue (mucous-membranes and the skin). The active ingredients of these products are antimicrobials; most are antibacterial or antifungal. Because this product classification is so broad, discussion is limited to antimicrobial products for use in prevention and self-treatment of skin infections.

Skin Anatomy and Physiology

Normal skin thickness is 3–5 mm, the thickest skin being on the palms and soles and the thinnest skin on the eyelids and parts of the genitals. The skin is divided into three main layers (Figure 1). The outermost layer (epidermis), which is quite compact and nonvascular, consists of stratified squamous epithelial cells. The next layer (the dermis or corium) is formed of vascular connective tissue. These two layers are not similar in composition but adhere firmly to each other. The hypodermis is the innermost layer.

The epidermis is composed of several distinct sublayers. The innermost, in close association with the dermis, is the stratum germinativum, which consists of columnar/cuboidal epithelial cells. Above this is the prickle cell unit (stratum spinosum) composed of polygonal epithelial cells. This is thicker in the palms than in hairy skin. These two epidermal sublayers are in-

volved in mitotic processes of epidermal regeneration and repair. The prickle cells contain keratinocytes, the pigment-forming melanocytes that contain melanin precursors and melanin granules, and are produced by cellular division. As the keratinocytes migrate to the skin surface, they change from living cells to dead, thickwalled, flat, nonnucleated cells containing keratin, a fibrous protein.

Above the prickle cells is the granular sublayer (stratum granulosum), which is actually several thicknesses of flattened polygonal cells. These cells contain granules of keratohyaline, which are changed to keratin in the outermost portion (stratum corneum, or horny outer layer of the epidermis). The clear area (stratum lucidum), present only in thick skin, is between the granular unit and the stratum corneum. It is a narrow band of flattened, closely packed cells believed to contain eleidin, a possible derivative of keratohyaline. The stratum corneum is composed of flat, scaly dead (keratinized) tissue. Its outermost cells are flat (squamous) plates that are constantly shed (desquamated).

The dead cells lost from the outer surface of the epidermis are replaced by new cells generated by the mitotic processes of the stratum spinosum and stratum germinativum. The newer cells push older ones closer to the surface. In the process they become flattened, lose their water content, fill with keratin, and gradually die, taking their place on the skin surface.

The dermis, which supports the epidermis and separates it from the lower fatty layer, consists mainly of collagen and elastin embedded in a mucopolysaccharide substance. Fibroblasts and mast cells are found throughout. The dermis also contains a network of nerves and capillaries that are the neurovascular supply to the dermal appendages (hair follicles, sebaceous glands, and sweat glands). The main sublayers of the dermis are the papillary and reticular units. The papillary sublayer, adjacent to the epidermis, is very rich in blood vessels, and the papillae probably act as conduits to bring blood nutrients near the avascular epidermis. The reticular sublayer, below the papillae, contains coarser tissue that connects the dermis with the hypodermis.

The hypodermis, composed of relatively loose connective tissue of varying thicknesses, provides necessary pliability for the skin. In most areas, this layer also includes a fatty unit (panniculus adiposus), which facilitates thermal control, food reserve, and cushioning or padding.

Skin Appendages

Hair Follicle

A hair shaft is generated by a hair germ at the base of a follicle. The follicle is basically an inward tubular folding of the epidermis into the dermis. The hair within the follicle is a fiber of keratinized epithelial cells that grow as a result of multiplication of cells in the hair germ.

Sebaceous Glands

Most sebaceous or sebum producing-glands are located in the same area as the hair since they are usually appendages of the follicles. Sebaceous glands not associated with hair follicles may be found in the genital areas, around the nipples of the breast, and on the edge of the lips. The ducts of the glands are lined with epithelial cells that are continuous with the basal layers of the epidermis. The sebaceous glands are holocrine, because the gland cells from which the sebum is derived are destroyed in its production. Sebum covers the hair and skin surface and is a mixture of free fatty acids (mainly palmitic and oleic), triglycerides, waxes, cholesterol, squalene, other hydrocarbons, and traces of fat-soluble vitamins. With sweat it forms an emulsion that includes surface waste products of cutaneous cells.

Sweat Glands

Two types of sweat glands are identified in association with dermal anatomy: the eccrine and apocrine glands. Both are considered exocrine, since their secretions (sweat) reach the skin surface through distinct ducts. They are not holocrine, but do differ anatomically in their distribution over body surface and in the character of their secretions.

Eccrine Glands
These glands are independent of hair follicles and develop from the epithelium of the skin surface, extending in a coil fashion to the dermis. The secretory epithelium is located in the hypodermis, and the ducts ascend through the epidermis as wavy or curved channels. Except for the genital areas and the legs, they are present over most of the body surface, being especially numerous on the palms and soles.

Eccrine glands are cholinergically innervated, although the nerve fibers are sympathetic. Eccrine sweat production is controlled by the heat regulatory centers of the hypothalamus. Emotional stress and cholinergic drugs also can trigger eccrine sweating. Eccrine sweat is basically an electrolyte solution with a pH of approximately 5. It is devoid of fats, carbohydrates, and proteins. The volume produced (several liters/day) is much greater than that of apocrine sweat.

Apocrine Glands
An apocrine sweat gland generally is attached to a hair follicle by a duct, leading down into a coiled, secretory glandular tubule. These tubules are covered with myoepithelium, allowing contraction to adrenergic stimulation. Such stimulation, as in stress, releases a milky secretion that contains proteins, sugars, and lipids. This secretion is odorless until skin bacteria act upon its contents, producing the characteristic pungent odor of apocrine sweat.

Apocrine glands are present around the nipples, in the axillae, and in the anogenital region. They are much larger than eccrine glands but produce much less volume of sweat. They do not function in body temperature regulation but are responsive to hormone secretion. Consequently, the onset of action of these glands is associated with puberty.

Nails

The nails are modifications of the keratinized layer of the epidermis. The nail bed on which the nail plate lies derives from the basal epidermal layers. The body of the plate, at its periphery, is surrounded by the nail root. The root is derived from the nail groove, which is a process of the basal epidermal unit. The white area at the base is called the lunula, and the part of the nail groove that enfolds the plate at its margin is the eponychium. The hyponychium is a thick layer of stratum corneum immediately beneath the plate of the nail's distal tip.

Skin Surface

The secretions that accumulate at the skin surface are weakly acidic with a pH of 4.5–5.5 (the acid mantle) (1). The pH varies slightly from individual to individual and among different areas of the body; it is somewhat higher in areas where perspiration evaporates slowly (2).

Various microorganisms live on the surface of intact skin. The individual species that make up the flora exist in a normal ecologic balance. The flora of the various skin areas are diverse, including aerobic and anaerobic microorganisms, *Staphylococci, Corynebacteria,* and *Sarcinae* species, and occasional gram-negative rods. The number of organisms on various areas of the skin differs. Changes in the kind and number of organisms occur during different periods of life and during different seasons. Flora population varies among individuals, some having a constantly high microbial population.

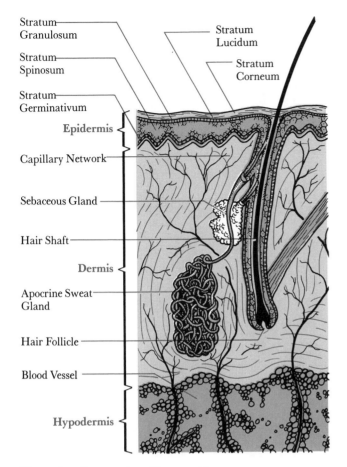

Stratum Granulosum
Stratum Spinosum
Stratum Germinativum
Stratum Lucidum
Stratum Corneum
Epidermis
Capillary Network
Sebaceous Gland
Hair Shaft
Dermis
Apocrine Sweat Gland
Hair Follicle
Blood Vessel
Hypodermis

Figure 1. Cross section of human skin.

Normal Skin Function

The skin acts as a barrier between the environment and the body, protecting the body from harmful external agents, such as pathogenic organisms and chemicals (3). The skin also contributes to sensory experiences and is involved in temperature control, development of pigment, and synthesis of some vitamins. It is important in hydroregulation because it controls moisture loss from the body and moisture penetration into the body.

Except for the stratum corneum, the cells of all layers use nutrients and oxygen and excrete water and carbon dioxide. Most oxygen is supplied from the blood, although a small amount is supplied from the external environment. Similarly, carbon dioxide is removed from the tissues mainly by the blood, but small amounts are "exhaled" directly to the atmosphere.

An important function of sebum, the secretion of sebaceous glands, is to lubricate the skin surface to ensure suppleness and prevent moisture loss, thus maintaining adequate dermal hydration. Chemically, sebum prevents penetration by other substances and has some antiseptic and antifungal properties.

Dermal hydration is important to the health and normal function of the skin. If the corneal layer becomes dehydrated, it loses elasticity, and permeation characteristics become altered. Returning water to the skin is the only means by which dryness can be reversed. The

stratum corneum can be hydrated by water transfer from the lower layers or by water accumulation (perspiration) induced by occlusive coverings, such as tight, impervious bandages (plastic wrap), or oleaginous pharmaceutical vehicles (petrolatum). Generally, such moisture accumulation seems to "open" the compactness of the stratum corneum for renewed suppleness and more effective penetration by drug molecules.

The acid mantle has been postulated to be a protective mechanism because microbes tend to grow better at pH 6–7.5. Infected areas have higher pH values than those of normal skin. Several fatty acids found in sweat and sebum (propionic, caproic, and caprylic) inhibit microbial and fungal growths (4). Thus, the importance of the acid mantle concept is not solely in the inherent pH, but more likely in the specific compounds responsible for the acidity.

The buffer capacity of skin surface secretions is another protective mechanism. When the pH is raised or lowered, the skin readjusts to a normal pH. Moreover, the normal skin flora act as a defense mechanism by controlling the growth of potential pathogenic organisms and their possible invasion of the skin and body.

Percutaneous Absorption Factors

A drug must be released from its vehicle if it is to exert an effect at the desired site of activity (either the skin surface, the epidermis, or the dermis). The release of a topical drug from its base occurs at the interface between the skin surface and the applied layer of product. The physical-chemical relationship between the drug and the base determines the rate and amount of drug released. Considerations such as the solubility of the drug in the base, its diffusion coefficient in the base, and its partition coefficient into sebum and the stratum corneum are significant to its efficacy. A drug with a strong affinity for the base is released less readily than one whose solubility in the base is lower. Likewise, a drug with a proper balance of polar and hydrocarbon moieties (a partition coefficient approaching 1), penetrates the stratum corneum more readily than drugs that are either highly polar or highly lipoidal, since that portion of the skin possesses both hydrated proteins and lipids. Other factors influencing drug release include the degree of hydration of the stratum corneum, the pKa of the drug, the pH of the base and of the skin surface, the drug concentration, the thickness of the applied layer, and the temperature. These factors are applicable to drug release from all topical dosage forms: medicated powders, ointments, pastes, emulsified cream or lotion bases, gels, suspensions, and solutions.

Substances are transported from the skin surface to the general circulation through percutaneous absorption. Minor routes of such transport involve passage between the keratinized units of the stratum corneum and through the skin's appendages (hair follicles and sweat and sebaceous glands). The major route is by direct penetration through the stratum corneum, followed successively by transfer through the deeper epidermal layers and the papillary dermis.

After application of a topical drug product, transport of the drug cannot begin until the surface of the

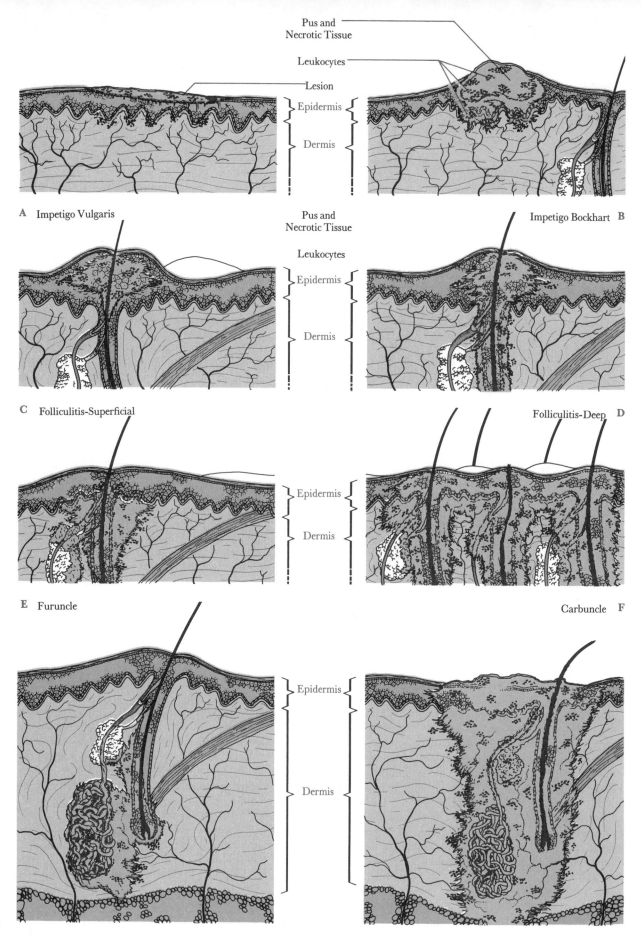

Pus and
Necrotic Tissue

Leukocytes

Lesion

Epidermis

Dermis

A Impetigo Vulgaris

Impetigo Bockhart **B**

Pus and
Necrotic Tissue

Leukocytes

Epidermis

Dermis

C Folliculitis-Superficial

Folliculitis-Deep **D**

Epidermis

Dermis

E Furuncle

Carbuncle **F**

Epidermis

Dermis

G Sweat Gland Infection

Echthyma **H**

Figure 2. Cross section of common pyodermas.

stratum corneum is "charged" with the drug. A delay period occurs while a drug is transferring from its vehicle or base into and through the sebum, and then to the stratum corneum.

Depending on the physical-chemical properties of a drug and those of sebum and the various skin layers, the drug movement into and through the skin meets with varying degrees of resistance. The sebum, when present, is a minor barrier to drug transfer. The stratum corneum provides the greatest resistance and therefore is the rate-limiting barrier to percutaneous absorption. Since it is nonliving tissue, the stratum corneum may be viewed as having the general characteristics of an artificial and semipermeable membrane, and molecular passage through it is completely passive (bulk diffusion). Once a molecule has crossed the stratum corneum, there is much less resistance to its transfer across the rest of the epidermis into the dermis.

When the corneum is hydrated extensively, drug diffusion in general is accelerated. Since occlusion (with a plastic covering) increases the hydration of the stratum corneum from within the skin, it fosters the transfer of all drugs. This occurs because the hydration swells the stratum corneum, loosening its normally tight, densely packed arrangement, thereby making such diffusion easier. Likewise, the increased amount of water present under such conditions probably further enhances the transfer of polar molecules.

Greasy, hydrocarbon bases such as petrolatum are occlusive, promote hydration, and generally increase molecular transport. Hydrous emulsion bases are less occlusive; water-soluble bases (polyethylene glycols) are nonocclusive. The latter, in fact, may attract water from the stratum corneum, thereby decreasing drug transport. Powders with hydrophilic ingredients also decrease hydration, since they promote evaporation from the skin by absorbing available water and increasing its surface area.

Wounds, burns, chafed areas and extensive lesions of various dermatoses alter the integrity of the stratum corneum and result in artificial shunts of the percutaneous absorption process. Drug absorption in such instances essentially is uncontrolled and could lead to potentially dangerous systemic concentrations. Extreme care must be used in applying topical medication to damaged skin, especially when large areas are involved.

Cutaneous Infections

Cutaneous infections may be caused by bacteria, fungi, viruses, or parasites. (See Chapter 23, *Oral Health Products,* Chapter 24, *Insect Sting and Bite Products,* and Chapter 29, *Acne Products.*) Many, but not all, bacterial and fungal infections are amenable to topical therapy. Careful assessment of the condition must be made before appropriate treatment can be recommended.

Bacterial Infections

Bacterial skin infections are classified as pyodermas since pus is usually present (Figure 2). They are caused principally by beta-hemolytic *Streptococcus* and hemolytic *Staphylococcus* species (5). The lesions result from external infection or reinfection and may be superficial or involve deeper dermal tissue. These pyodermic infections may be either primary (in which no previous dermatoses exist) or secondary (in which a predisposing dermal problem preceded the infection). Other organisms may be present in secondary pyodermas, including gram-negative bacteria (*Pseudomonas aeruginosa*), which are especially prevalent on warm moist skin such as the axillae, ear canals, and interdigital spaces.

Infections by pathogenic organisms are related to the breakdown of the skin's "disinfecting" protective mechanisms or to the development of an abundance of colonies of pathogenic organisms (1). A breakdown of the normal ecological balance may be enhanced by alterations in the skin's other defense mechanisms.

Normally, the stratum corneum has only about 10% water content, which ensures elasticity but is generally below that needed to support luxuriant microbial growth (1). An increase in moisture content may allow microbial growth, leading to infection.

A break in the intact surface has a deleterious effect on the skin's defensive properties, allowing large numbers of pathogenic organisms to be introduced into the inner layers.

In addition, infection may be caused by excessive scrubbing of the skin (especially with strong detergents), excessive exposure to water, occlusion, increasing the skin temperature, excessive sweating or bathing, and injury (1, 6–8). Thus the presence and severity of microbial skin infection generally is dependent on the condition of the skin's defense mechanisms, the number of pathogenic organisms present, and the supportive nutrient environment for those organisms.

The main pyodermic infections are impetigo, folliculitis, furuncles (boils), carbuncles, erysipelas, sweat gland infections, ecthyma, and pyonychia.

Impetigo

Impetigo vulgaris, caused by *Streptococcus* and/or *Staphylococcus* species, probably is the most superficial of the pyodermas, mainly involving the surface areas. Direct contact with the lesions or infected exudate generally is required for its transmission. The lesions initially are small red spots that rapidly evolve into characteristic vesicles (tiny sacs or blisters) filled with amber fluid (9). Exudate collects and forms yellow or brown crusts on the skin surface. The eruptions may be circular with clear central areas and may occur in groups. The exposed parts of the body are most easily affected, but no area of the skin is immune if autogenous reinfection is not controlled. (See *Plate 4-16.*) Impetigo is most common in children and highly contagious.

Furfuraceous impetigo (pityriasis simplex) is a superficial streptococcal infection found almost exclusively in children. These scaly, red, round lesions of varying sizes occur most often on the face. This impetigo seems to occur most often in cold weather, and depigmentation of the patchy areas may occur in previously affected areas.

Generally, in primary impetigo (impetigo vulgaris) the responsible bacteria cause the infection directly. Some forms, however, occur secondarily to the presence of other infections, injury, or the general breakdown of skin defenses. Bockhart's impetigo usually occurs as a secondary infection to another condition (furuncles, discharging ears, or wounds). Lesions characteristically are tiny follicular pustules around hair shafts and may be encircled by narrow red rings (areolae).

Ecthyma

Ecthyma is similar to impetigo in that the same organisms are involved, but the lesion is much deeper. In contrast to facial impetigo, the legs most commonly are affected, and the lesions occur singularly and tend to be localized. The lesion begins as an erythematous pustule that rapidly erodes and becomes crusted. This condition often occurs as a secondary infection to mild trauma or injury to the skin. In humid tropical environments, the lesions may become quite destructive.

Erysipelas

This infection, caused by beta-hemolytic *Streptococcus* species, is a cellulitis characterized by a rapidly spreading, red and edematous plaque. This superficial infection has sharply established borders and a glistening surface (9). It occurs most often on the scalp and face, and the organisms enter through a break in the skin. (See *Plate 4-17.*) It is usually accompanied by fever, chills, and malaise.

Folliculitis

Follicular pustules may be superficial or deep, depending on the pathogen or the site involved. They involve only the hair shafts; surrounding tissue is not affected. Usually the superficial forms are very similar to Bockhart's impetigo and may be secondary infections. Skin areas regularly exposed to water, grease, oils, tars, and other contaminants seem most easily affected.

Furuncles and Carbuncles

These pyodermas generally are staphylococcal infections located in or around hair follicles. The lesion may start as a superficial folliculitis but develops into a deep nodule. (See *Plate 4-18.*) The fully established furuncle has elevated swelling, is erythematous, and is very painful. Furuncles are most common in males. Hairy areas and areas subject to maceration and friction (collar, waist, buttocks, and thighs) seem most vulnerable. The initial erythema and swelling stage is followed by thinning of the skin around the primary follicle, centralized pustulation, destruction of the pilosebaceous structure, discharge of the core (plug), and central ulceration. Scarring often occurs. Chronic furunculosis is common, with new lesions appearing intermittently for months or years.

Furuncles may be secondary infections to other dermatoses or diseases. Diabetes mellitus or agammaglobulinemia may predispose an individual to furuncles or carbuncles. Chronic cases of these pyodermas should be referred to a physician for evaluation of a possible underlying disease.

Carbuncles begin in a manner similar to furuncles and may have similar etiologies. Carbuncles involve clusters of follicles with deeper and broader penetration over a larger area than furuncles. Furuncles may develop into carbuncles by infiltration or infection of adjacent follicles.

Sweat Gland Infections

These staphylococcal infections originate in eccrine and apocrine sweat glands and may resemble furuncles. Axillary apocrine sweat glands are the most common site, but other apocrine glands (perianal, perimammary, and genital) are also vulnerable. A sweat gland infection may result as a secondary infection to an irritant, especially deodorant/antiperspirant products, which may produce an initial dermatitis. (See Chapter 19, *Personal Care Products.*) Persons with chronic skin conditions such as acne or folliculitis may be predisposed to sweat gland infections (10).

Infants are subject to superficial infections (periporitis) and deeper, multiple abscesses of these glands. Infants in poor health are more prone to such infections, which occur mainly as secondary infections. Sweat gland abscesses in the axillae (hidradenitis axillaris) occur in adolescents and adults with endocrine disorders.

Sweat gland infections are manifested as small, superficial, very tender pustules. They rapidly develop into hard, tender, bluish-red elevated swellings. Within several days, softening usually occurs and the abscess ruptures, exuding pus, blood, and serous fluid.

Paronychia

Paronychia is a pyogenic infection of the nails with swelling and tenderness of the surrounding tissue caused primarily by beta-hemolytic *Streptococcus* and *Staphylococcus* species. Moderate pressure may force a pus exudate, and the nail may develop with irregularities. (See *Plate 4-19.*) It is important that this condition be differentiated from candidal or other fungal infections.

Otitis Externa

This inflammation of the external ear may be a secondary infection and is frequently associated with seborrheic scaling of the scalp. Increase in the moisture content of the external ear over long periods gradually leads to changes in the types of organisms present. External heat, humidity, or swimming may play a role in the development of this condition. The most common initial complaint is itching. With increasing severity, however, edema, crusting, and oozing may occur. (See Chapter 20, *Otic Products.*)

Fungal Infections

Fungal infections, often called dermatomycoses, are among the most common cutaneous disorders (10, 11). Characteristically, they exhibit single or multiple lesions that may have mild scaling or deep granulomas (inflamed nodules). Superficial infections affect the hair, nails, and skin and are generally caused by three genera of fungi: *Trichophyton, Microsporum,* and *Epidermophyton* species. *Candida* species may also be involved (12). Fungal infections of hairless skin are generally superficial, and the organisms are found in or on the uppermost skin layers. In fungal infections of areas covered with heavy hair, the infections are much deeper because of hair follicle penetration.

Tinea Pedis

This infection, known popularly as athlete's foot or ringworm of the feet, is caused by several species of fungi. (See Chapter 33, *Foot Care Products.*)

Tinea Capitis

Transmitted by direct contact with infected persons or animals, this infection is caused by *Microsporum* and *Trichophyton* species. Most cases of tinea capitis occur in children. The clinical presentation varies depending on the causative organism from noninflamed areas of hair loss to deep, crusted lesions, which may lead to scarring and permanent hair loss. (See *Plate 4-20.*) These large lesions, similar to carbuncles in appearance, are called kerions.

Tinea Cruris

This infection (also called jock itch) is caused by *Epidermophyton floccosum, Trichophyton rubrum,* and *Trichophyton mentagrophytes.* It occurs on the medial and upper parts of the thighs and the pubic area, and is more common in males. The lesions have specific margins that are slightly elevated and more inflamed than the central parts; small vesicles are found at the margins. Acute lesions are bright red and turn brown in chronic cases, and they may scale. This condition is generally bilateral with severe pruritus.

Tinea Corporis

Trichophyton and *Microsporum* species are the causative organisms of this condition. There is a higher incidence of tinea corporis among persons living in humid climates. The lesions involve glabrous (smooth and bare) skin and begin as small, circular, erythematous scaly areas. They spread peripherally and the borders may contain vesicles or pustules. However, tinea corporis should be differentiated from noninfectious dermatitis because the lesions may be similar in appearance.

Other Fungal Infections

Moniliasis, caused mainly by *Candida albicans,* usually occurs in intertriginous areas such as the groin, axillae, and interdigitial spaces, under breasts, and corners of the mouth. Involvement of the mucous membranes is known as thrush, vaginal candidiasis, and pruritus ani, depending on the organ affected. Candidal paronychia is most common in people whose activities involve routine immersion of the hands in water. Systemic diseases such as diabetes, infection, and malignancy may lower general resistance and allow *C. albicans* infections to flourish. Certain drugs, including oral antibiotics and steroids, may also contribute to infection. Pregnancy is often a predisposing cause of vaginal candidiasis because of changes in vaginal pH and flora.

Other fungal skin infections include tinea barbae (barber's itch or ring worm of the beard); tinea manuum (hands); tinea versicolor, where the lesions are brown; tinea circinata, generally ringed, red lesions that can agglomerate into polycyclic configurations; and tinea unguium (onychomycosis), in which the nail may become hypertrophic, discolored, and scaly (12). (See *Plate 5-21A and B.*)

Viral Infections

Viral infections may occur directly in or on the skin and present as warts, molluscum contagiosum, or herpes simplex (13). (See Chapter 23, *Oral Health Products,* and Chapter 33, *Foot Care Products.*) Herpes zoster infections present with cutaneous manifestations and affect a nerve or group of nerves of the same area.

Chicken pox and measles are systemic viral diseases that also have important diagnostic dermatologic manifestations.

Herpes Simplex

Herpes simplex is a viral infection of the skin and mucous membranes. The causative agent is a fairly large virus, *Herpesvirus hominis* (HVH). (See *Plate 5-22.*) There are two strains: herpesvirus type 1 (herpes labialis or cold sores) is commonly found on the lips, and herpesvirus type 2, which generally occurs as genital lesions and is sexually transmitted.

Herpes Zoster

This viral infection, neurotropic in humans, is caused by the zoster-varicella virus, which is the same virus that causes chicken pox. The highly contagious, generalized, and usually benign chicken pox will develop in the nonimmune host, while the localized and painful zoster (shingles) will develop in the partially immune host. Children with leukemia or on long-term therapy with corticosteroids and patients who are immunosuppressed because of disease or medications are extremely vulnerable to the zoster virus. The different clinical manifestations of these two diseases reflect the interaction between this virus and the host immune mechanisms.

Shingles probably results from reactivation of latent virus, which resides in the dorsal root or cranial nerve ganglion cells. It is mainly a disease of adults who have usually had chicken pox. Lesions appear suddenly and acutely along the course of a nerve or group of nerves on one side of the body as reddened, swollen, round plaques ranging in size from about 5 mm to areas larger than a hand; the spinal ganglia seem to be the primary site. The plaques may be painful after lesions form, and it is possible for them to appear as successive "showers" or crops over several days. The lesions develop into fairly large blisters that become crusty in 1–2 weeks. (See *Plate 5-23A and B.*) The regional lymph nodes generally are tender. An episode is followed by a lasting immunity; recurrent cases are extremely rare.

Molluscum Contagiosum

Molluscum contagiosum is a viral tumor caused by a DNA-containing poxvirus. The disease is contracted by direct contact with an infected person, fomites, or autoinoculation.

The virus is manifested by small (3–5 mm), pink, slightly raised lesions usually found on the abdomen, inner thigh, or perianal areas. The mature lesion has a slight depression on the top and has a soft core that can easily be expressed. They may occur in groups or as a single lesion. Erythema does not usually accompany the lesion unless there is a secondary bacterial infection.

Evaluation

Before recommending a topical product for self-medication of various cutaneous infections, the pharmacist should ascertain what type of infection exists. In addition the pharmacist should also be aware of noninfectious processes such as contact dermatitis, psoriasis, or drug-induced eruptions (14). Antimicrobial agents generally should be considered only in the case of an infectious etiology.

The pharmacist can play an important role by preventing erroneous self-medication and by advising the patient to seek medical attention if the condition calls for it. Incorrect self-medication may cause a delay in healing, possible progression of the disease, toxicity, obvious discomfort, and unnecessary cost. Immediate medical attention should be sought if the following circumstances exist:

- There is doubt as to the causative factor or organism (organic or some other process; bacteria or fungi).
- The condition has lasted for more than a few days.
- Appropriate treatment has not been successful and the condition is getting worse.
- Applications of drug products have been used for several days over large areas, especially on denuded skin (potential for systemic toxicity).
- Drainage is excessive and has occurred for several days.
- Improper cleaning of infectious exudate has led to widespread infection.
- There is predisposing illness, such as diabetes or systemic infection, or symptoms of such illness.
- Fever and/or malaise occurs.
- A primary dermatitis (allergic dermatitis, psoriasis, or seborrhea) exists and has developed a secondary infection that is difficult to treat with nonprescription products.
- Lesions are deep and extensive.
- Lancing is needed to aid drainage.

The use of nonprescription topical antimicrobial products should be limited to superficial conditions that involve minimal areas, when no predisposing illnesses exist. Self-administered topical products should be viewed as extensions of supportive treatment (proper cleaning, proper hygiene, and clean bandaging), and not as "miracle" treatments. Medical attention should be sought in all but the most superficial, uncomplicated skin infections, especially if it appears that systemic medication is needed. Deep-seated and complicated secondary infections require medical attention. Improper lancing as self-treatment may cause scarring and spreading of the infected exudate.

As has been noted, only the most superficial, minor cutaneous infections are amenable to topical anti-infective therapy. In more severe cases of bacterial infection, widespread fungal infection, or infections of the nails, systemic therapy is required. Medical treatment will be directed by the patient's clinical presentation and when necessary cultures of the lesion to determine the infecting organism. Minor surgical procedures such as debridement, curettage, and liquid nitrogen are indicated in the treatment of some dermatoses.

Pharmacologic Agents

The major drugs used in the prevention and treatment of various skin infections include antibiotics, antifungals, and antiseptics.

Dosage Forms

Antimicrobial agents are available in many forms for specific uses including antimicrobial soaps, antimicrobial handwashes for health-care personnel, patient preoperative skin preparations, skin antiseptics, skin-wound cleansers, and skin-wound protectants. These products are under study by the FDA advisory review panel on nonprescription antimicrobial drug products (I). The panel is studying antimicrobial soaps, health-care personnel handwashes, patient preoperative skin preparations, skin antiseptics, skin-wound cleansers, skin-wound protectants, and surgical hand scrubs. The recommendations of this panel have been published as a "Tentative Final Monograph." These recommendations are summarized in Table 1. This chapter covers antimicrobial soaps, skin antiseptics, skin-wound cleansers, and skin-wound protectants defined as follows (15):

Antimicrobial Soap

This is a soap containing an active ingredient with both in-vitro and in-vivo activity against skin microorganisms. Although by chemical definition, a soap is a metallic salt of an organic fatty acid, the FDA has indicated that soap formulations that also contain synthetic detergents are within the scope of the antimicrobial soap definition as long as they contain an antimicrobial ingredient as well.

Skin Antiseptic

A skin antiseptic is a nonirritating, antimicrobial-containing preparation that prevents overt skin infection.

Skin-Wound Cleanser

A skin-wound cleanser is a nonirritating, liquid preparation (or product to be used with water) that assists in the removal of foreign material from small superficial wounds, does not delay wound healing, and that may contain an antimicrobial ingredient.

Skin-Wound Protectant

This is a nonirritating antimicrobial-containing preparation applied to small cleansed wounds; it provides a protective physical barrier and a chemical (antimicrobial) barrier that neither delays healing nor favors the growth of microorganisms.

The FDA advisory review panel on nonprescription antimicrobial drug products (II) is studying antibiotic, antifungal, and antiacne agents specifically. These

Table 1. FDA-classified compounds

Use	Compound	Category
Antimicrobial soap	Benzalkonium chloride[a]	II
	Benzethonium chloride[a]	II
	Parachlorometaxylenol	III
	Cloflucarban	III
	Hexylresorcinol[a]	II
	Iodine complexed with phosphate ester of alkylaryloxypolyethylene glycol[a]	II
	Iodine tincture[a]	II
	Methylbenzethonium chloride[a]	II
	Nonylphenoxypoly (ethyleneoxy) ethanol-iodine[a]	II
	Phenol >1.5% aqueous/alcoholic	II
	Phenol ≤1.5% aqueous/alcoholic	III
	Poloxamer-iodine complex[a]	II
	Povidone-iodine complex	III
	Triclocarban[b]	III
	Triclosan[b]	III
	Triple dye[a]	II
	Undecoylium chloride-iodine complex[a]	II
Health care personnel handwash	Benzalkonium chloride	III
	Benzethonium chloride	III
	Parachlorometaxylenol	III
	Cloflucarban	II[c],III[b]
	Hexylresorcinol	III
	Iodine complexed with phosphate ester of alkylaryloxypolyethylene glycol	III
	Iodine tincture	II
	Methylbenzethonium chloride	III
	Nonylphenoxypoly (ethyleneoxy) ethanol-iodine	III
	Phenol >1.5% aqueous/alcoholic	II
	Phenol ≤1.5% aqueous/alcoholic	III
	Poloxamer-iodine complex	III
	Povidone-iodine complex	III
	Triclocarban[b]	III
	Triclosan	II
	Triple dye[a]	II
	Undecoylium chloride-iodine complex	III
Patient preoperative skin preparation	Benzalkonium chloride	III
	Benzethonium chloride	III
	Parachlorometaxylenol	III
	Cloflucarban	II
	Hexylresorcinol	III
	Iodine complexed with phosphate ester of alkylaryloxypolyethylene glycol	III
	Iodine tincture[d]	I
	Methylbenzethonium chloride	III
	Nonylphenoxypoly(ethyleneoxy) ethanol-iodine	III
	Phenol >1.5% aqueous/alcoholic	II
	Phenol ≤1.5% aqueous/alcoholic	III
	Poloxamer-iodine complex	III
	Povidone-iodine complex	III
	Triclocarban	II
	Triclosan	II
	Triple dye[a]	II
	Undecoylium chloride-iodine complex	III
Skin antiseptic	Benzalkonium chloride	III
	Benzethonium chloride	III
	Parachlorometaxylenol	III
	Cloflucarban	II
	Hexylresorcinol	III

Table 1. continued

Use	Compound	Category
Skin antiseptic (continued)	Iodine complexed with phosphate ester of alkylaryloxypolyethylene glycol	III
	Iodine tincture	III
	Methylbenzethonium chloride	III
	Nonylphenoxypoly(ethyleneoxy) ethanol-iodine	III
	Phenol >1.5% aqueous/alcoholic	II
	Phenol ≤1.5% aqueous/alcoholic	III
	Poloxamer-iodine complex	III
	Povidone-iodine complex	III
	Triclocarban	II
	Triclosan	III
	Triple dye[d]	II[e],III[f]
	Undecoylium chloride-iodine complex	III
Skin wound cleanser	Cloflucarban	II[c],III[b]
	Parachlorometaxylenol	II[c],III[b]
	Hexylresorcinol[g]	I
	Iodine complexed with phosphate ester of alkylaryloxypolyethylene glycol	III
	Iodine tincture	III
	Nonylphenoxypoly(ethyleneoxy) ethanol-iodine	III
	Phenol >1.5% aqueous/alcoholic	II
	Phenol ≤1.5% aqueous/alcoholic	III
	Poloxamer-iodine complex	III
	Poloxamer 188[h]	I
	Povidone-iodine complex	III
	Quaternary ammonium compounds[i]	I
	Triclocarban	II[c],III[b]
	Triclosan	III
	Triple dye[a]	II
	Undecoylium chloride-iodine complex	III
Skin wound protectant	Benzalkonium chloride	III
	Benzethonium chloride	III
	Parachlorometaxylenol	III
	Cloflucarban	II
	Hexylresorcinol	III
	Iodine complexed with phosphate ester of alkylaryloxypolyethylene glycol	III
	Iodine tincture	III
	Methylbenzethonium chloride	III
	Nonylphenoxypoly(ethyleneoxy) ethanol-iodine	III
	Phenol >1.5% aqueous/alcoholic	II
	Phenol ≤1.5% aqueous/alcoholic	III
	Poloxamer-iodine complex	III
	Povidone-iodine complex	III
	Triclocarban	II
	Triclosan	III
	Triple dye[a]	II
	Undecoylium chloride-iodine complex	III
Surgical hand scrub	Benzalkonium chloride	III
	Benzethonium chloride	III
	Parachlorometaxylenol	III
	Cloflucarban	II
	Hexylresorcinol	III
	Iodine complexed with phosphate ester of alkylaryloxypolyethylene glycol	III
	Iodine tincture	II
	Methylbenzethonium chloride	III
	Nonylphenoxypoly(ethyleneoxy) ethanol-iodine	III
	Phenol >1.5% aqueous/alcoholic	II
	Phenol ≤1.5% aqueous/alcoholic	III

Table 1. continued

Use	Compound	Category
Surgical hand scrub (continued)	Poloxamer-iodine complex	III
	Povidone-iodine complex	III
	Triclocarban	II
	Triclosan	II
	Triple dye[a]	II
	Undecoylium chloride-iodine complex	III

Reprinted from Federal Register, 43, 1210 (1978).

[a]Placed in Category II due to a physical and/or chemical incompatibility in formulation.
[b]Category III only when formulated in a bar soap to be used with water.
[c]Category II when formulated in any manner other than as a bar soap.
[d]2% iodine, 2.5% sodium iodide, 50% ethanol.
[e]Category II for use outside the neonatal nursery.
[f]Restricted to use only in neonatal nursery.
[g]N1/1000.
[h]In aqueous 20–40% solution.
[i]E.g., methylbenzethonium chloride, benzethonium chloride, and benzalkonium chloride, N1/750 in water.

Chlorhexidine gluconate has not been reviewed by the antimicrobial panels, but has received NDA clearance for use.

agents are used to prevent or treat overt skin infections and are available as creams, lotions, and ointments. (This chapter discusses the antibiotic and antifungal agents; see also Chapter 9, *Acne Products.*)

Antibiotics

The major topical nonprescription antibiotics are bacitracin, gramicidin, neomycin, and polymyxin-B sulfate, alone or in combination. The rationale for their use in combination is to ensure a broad spectrum of activity.

Bacitracin

Bacitracin is a polypeptide antibiotic that may be bactericidal or bacteriostatic depending upon the drug concentration. Specifically, bacitracin acts to inhibit cell-wall synthesis. Topically, the drug is not absorbed to any significant extent, whether applied to wounds, mucous membranes, or denuded or intact skin; systemic toxicity is rare. However, hypersensitivity reactions, ranging from localized itching and swelling to anaphylactic reactions, may occur. The drug is most active against gram-positive organisms, although some gram-negative organisms are also susceptible. The development of resistance in previously sensitive organisms is rare. Topical nonprescription preparations usually contain 400–500 units/g of ointment and are applied 1–3 times/day. Bacitracin may be used topically in both infants and children (16).

Gramicidin

Gramicidin is a polypeptide antibiotic that is active against gram-positive bacteria. Due to this limited spectrum of activity, it is never used alone but in combination with other antimicrobial agents. The drug is poorly absorbed percutaneously. However, local reactions may occur. Gramicidin is a potent hemolytic agent and, therefore, the antibiotic should not be applied to fresh traumatic wounds since hemolysis and even renewed bleeding could occur (17). The usual concentration is 0.25 mg/g of ointment, applied 1–3 times/day. This agent is currently classified in Category III since sufficient data about its safety and efficacy have not been provided (16).

Neomycin

This aminoglycoside antibiotic is effective against many gram-negative organisms and some gram-positive organisms. The mechanism of action appears to be that of inhibiting protein synthesis by irreversibly binding to the 30S ribosomal subunit. It is considered to be bactericidal. Neomycin has the highest rate of development of hypersensitivity, with reactions occurring in 5–8% of patients (18). Although not absorbed when applied to intact skin, application to large areas of denuded skin has been known to cause systemic toxicity (ototoxicity and nephrotoxicity) (18).

For topical use, neomycin is available in cream and ointment forms. Used alone or in combination with other antimicrobials, the concentrations commonly employed in nonprescription products range from 3.5–5 mg/g and applications are made 1–3 times/day. Neomycin is most frequently used in combination with polymyxin and bacitracin to prevent the development of neomycin-resistant organisms.

Polymyxin-B Sulfate

Polymyxin-B sulfate is effective against gram-negative bacteria but not against gram-positive bacteria or fungi. It is presumed to produce its antibacterial property by altering the permeability of the bacterial membrane. Toxicity rarely occurs with topical therapy. Concentrations of 5,000 units and 10,000 units/g are available in nonprescription preparations. Applications are usually made 1–2 times/day.

Tetracyclines

Tetracycline and chlortetracycline are broad-spectrum antibiotics that have been used in the treatment of cutaneous infections due to susceptible organisms. They are presumed to exert their bacteriostatic effect by binding to the 30S ribosomal subunit and thus inhibiting protein synthesis. Three-percent ointments are available and toxicity is rare when applied topically. Long-term use may lead to overgrowth of nonsusceptible bacteria or fungi. Applications of a 1-mg/g preparation of chlortetracycline hydrochloride or a preparation containing not less than 15 mg/g of tetracycline hydrochloride are made 1–3 times/day (16).

Antifungal Agents

Agents used for cutaneous skin infections are found in ointments, creams, powders, and aerosols.

Benzoic Acid and Salicylic Acid Ointment

Benzoic acid is known to exert fungistatic effects when applied topically. Additionally, salicylic acid acts as a keratolytic agent. The combined effect is to inhibit fungal growth until the tissue can be desquamated. The usual concentrations of benzoic and salicylic acids are 6% and 3%, respectively, although there may be some variation among preparations. Applications are made 2–3 times/day.

Fatty Acids

Sweat has antifungal properties probably related to its fatty acid content. Sodium propionate, a fatty acid derivative, used as a topical antiseptic, has mild fungistatic activity. It has been used in topical products in concentrations as great as 10% and sometimes with undecylenic acid. Undecylenic acid has the greatest antifungal activity of the fatty acids. It may cause irritation and sensitization and should be discontinued if these side effects occur. It is basically a fungistatic agent, requiring long exposure at high concentrations to be effective. It is used with its zinc salt in ointment, cream, powder, and aerosol forms (2–5% acid, 20% salt) for an additive antifungal effect.

Selenium Sulfide

Selenium sulfide is effective in the treatment of tinea versicolor and seborrheic dermatitis of the scalp. It is used in nonprescription topical products to control dandruff, usually as a detergent-suspension. Contact with the eyes and sensitive skin areas should be avoided since it is a potential irritant. Although not absorbed significantly when applied to the skin, it is hazardous if swallowed, producing CNS effects and respiratory and vasomotor depression. In the treatment of tinea versicolor, the agent should be applied to the affected areas, allowed to stand overnight, and washed off in the morning. This is repeated once weekly for 4 weeks.

Tolnaftate

Tolnaftate is a topical nonprescription antifungal agent effective against most species of fungi (except *C. albicans*) that cause cutaneous infections. Complete clearing of cutaneous lesions may take several months. The mechanism of action is unknown. Tolnaftate is used in the treatment of all forms of tinea, but tinea unguium responds poorly to therapy unless the infection is very superficial. Topically, tolnaftate has a low incidence of toxicity. However, if local irritation occurs, treatment should be discontinued. Tolnaftate is available as a 1% cream, powder, solution, gel, and spray. (See Chapter 33, *Foot Care Products.*)

Triacetin

Triacetin in aerosol (15%), cream (25%), or powder (33%) is used in treating superficial fungal infections. Because its activity depends upon the slow release of acetic acid, triacetin is probably best viewed as effective only in the most superficial of cutaneous fungal infections.

Antiseptics

A number of substances are used as antiseptics in nonprescription products. Not all are classified as safe and effective (Table 1) (15).

Acetic Acid

This acid has been used as a bactericide, and *Pseudomonas* species seems particularly susceptible to it. It is frequently used for surgical dressings and irrigations. Dilute solutions (1–5%) are used for otitis externa.

Boric Acid

This weak acid has been used as a topical antiseptic and eyewash. The aqueous solution (2.5%) inhibits bacterial growth but does not kill many forms of bacteria. Boric acid is an extremely dangerous systemic poison: nausea, vomiting, diarrhea, exfoliative dermatitis, kidney damage, and acute circulatory failure may result. Topical application of this agent may result in systemic absorption. The minor therapeutic value of this compound, in comparison with its potential as a poison, has led to the general recommendation that it no longer be used as a therapeutic agent.

Ethanol

Ethanol has good bactericidal activity in a 20–70% concentration and acts relatively quickly but has little residual effect. In concentrations above 80%, however, its bactericidal effect is low. It rapidly denatures cellular protein of microorganisms, lowers the surface tension of bacteria to help in their removal, and has a solvent effect on sebum. It is not an effective antiviral agent, nor does it kill spores. It is not a desirable wound antiseptic because it irritates already damaged tissue. The coagulum formed may, in fact, protect the bacteria.

Ethanol may contain denaturants. Although not recognized as a skin sensitizer, excessive exposure in high concentrations can dehydrate the corneum. Systemic ingestion produces usual alcoholic intoxication and severe GI distress. The GI symptoms may be exacerbated if denatured alcohol is ingested.

Isopropyl Alcohol

Isopropyl alcohol has somewhat stronger bactericidal activity and lower surface tension than ethanol. In general, it is used like ethanol solutions for cleaning and for its antiseptic effect on the skin. It can be used undiluted or as a 70% aqueous solution. Denaturants are not added because isopropyl alcohol itself is not potable. Isopropyl alcohol has a greater potential for drying the skin because its lipid solvent effects are stronger than those of ethanol.

Iodine

Solutions of elemental iodine or those that release iodine from chemical complexes are used as presurgical skin antiseptics and as wound antiseptics. Their antimicrobial effect is attributed to their ability to oxidize microbial protoplasm. Caution must be taken that strong iodine solution (Lugol's) not be used as an antiseptic. Iodine solution USP (2% iodine, 2.5% sodium iodide) is used as an antiseptic for superficial wounds. Iodine tincture USP (2% iodine, 2.5% sodium iodide, and about 50% alcohol) is less preferable than the aqueous solution since it is irritating to the tissue.

In general, bandaging should be discouraged after iodine applications to avoid tissue irritation. Iodine solutions stain skin, may be irritating to tissue, and may cause sensitization in some people.

Iodophors

Iodophors are organic complexes of iodine. Two of these complexes are povidone-iodine and poloxamer iodine. Free iodine is released slowly from these preparations and is probably responsible for the antiseptic effects of these agents. The percentage of active ingredient varies according to the product type from 1% in ointments to 0.75% in shampoos and skin antiseptics. Although less effective than iodine solutions, iodophors are less irritating, nonstaining, and less sensitizing.

Sodium Hypochlorite Solutions

The antimicrobial effect of sodium hypochlorite results from liberation of elemental chlorine. Concentrated solutions [Sodium Hypochlorite Solution, N.F. (5%)] are very irritating to tissue and are used as disinfectants and bleaches, and they should not be used topically. Dilute solutions [Modified Dakin's solution (0.5%)], have been used as topical antiseptics with varying degrees of success.

Chlorhexidine Gluconate

Recognized as an effective antimicrobial agent for over 20 years, chlorhexidine has been used in Europe, England, and Canada as a preservative, disinfectant, and topical antiseptic. Approval for topical antiseptic use in the United States was granted in 1976, when the FDA concluded that chlorhexidine gluconate was safe and effective as a surgical scrub, health care personnel handwash, and skin-wound cleanser (19). From 1978 to 1981, subsequent approval was granted through NDA procedures for tinted and nontinted tinctures as patient preoperative preparations, a germicidal hand rinse, and revised labeling of the original skin cleanser to include the term "antiseptic." This compound did not fall within the purview of the FDA's advisory review antimicrobial I and II panels, since it was not in use in the United States at the onset of the overall review process. Hence, the reported recommendations of these panels (Tables 1 and 2) do not include chlorhexidine gluconate.

Although similar in name to hexachlorophene, chlorhexidine gluconate is unrelated to that compound, being structurally a biguanide and resembling quaternary ammonium salts (19). It is a relatively rapid-acting antiseptic that is effective against both gram-positive

Table 2. FDA-classified antibiotic compounds

Use	Compound	Category
Skin wound antibiotic	Bacitracin	III
	Chlortetracycline hydrochloride	III
	Gramicidin D	III
	Neomycin sulfate	III
	Oxytetracycline hydrochloride	III
	Polymyxin B sulfate	III
	Tetracycline hydrochloride	III
Skin wound protectant	Bacitracin	I
	Chlortetracycline hydrochloride	I
	Gramicidin D	III
	Neomycin sulfate	III
	Oxytetracycline hydrochloride	I
	Polymyxin B sulfate[a]	I
	Tetracycline hydrochloride	I

Reprinted from *Federal Register*, 42, 17642(1977).

[a]Only when used in combination with bacitracin, tetracycline hydrochloride, chlortetracycline hydrochloride, or oxytetracycline hydrochloride.

and gram-negative bacteria and some fungi. It exhibits residual adherence to skin surfaces. Thus, when used as a surgical scrub, it appears to combine the surface adherence characteristics and relatively long duration of activity of hexachlorophene with the potential for quick reduction of microorganisms displayed by the iodophors.

Although some surfactants and serum protein can reduce the antiseptic potential of chlorhexidine gluconate, it exhibits low potential for sensitization and irritation (19). It is very slightly absorbed through intact skin. A prominent warning against use in the ear appears on the labeling of nonprescription products containing this compound.

The development of resistance of certain microorganisms to chlorhexidine has been broached in the literature. Some clinical isolates previously exposed to chlorhexidine gluconate have shown decreased sensitivity to the drug (20, 21, 22). In-vitro development of resistance by various microorganisms has been reported (defined as a 10-fold or greater increase in the minimum inhibitory concentration for the test organism) (23). However, another study submitted as part of the initial NDA proposal for chlorhexidine showed no such in-vitro resistance development (19). The clinical implications of these findings are unclear. It should be cautioned, however, that dilution of the product or failure to follow the manufacturer's directions may impair the efficacy of this agent.

Overall, chlorhexidine appears to be a promising topical antimicrobial agent. Its quick activity, residual adherence, low potential for irritation and sensitization, and poor absorption through intact skin makes it an attractive candidate for those seeking a nonprescription alternative to hexachlorophene.

Mercurial Compounds

Several mercurial compounds have antiseptic/disinfectant properties. In general, however, they are considered poor antiseptics for wounded skin because serum and tissue proteins reduce their antimicrobial potency. If these compounds are used extensively or on large areas of abraded skin, mercury may be absorbed and may become a systemic poison. Their use should be discouraged in such conditions.

Inorganic salts of mercury are tissue irritants. Such toxic properties are reduced when the mercury is incorporated into an organic compound. Some investigators believe that the alcoholic component of mercurial tinctures has greater antimicrobial effect than the mercurial component (24).

- **Merbromin**—Merbromin is less effective as a skin antiseptic than the other organic mercurials. However, it is used in some cases as a preoperative germicide (2%, aqueous). Serous fluids reduce its antimicrobial potency.
- **Nitromersol**—This compound is more effective as an antiseptic than soluble inorganic compounds of mercury but less effective than ethanol. It is not a serious tissue irritant, and it is available as a tincture in a dilution of 1:200.
- **Thimerosal**—Thimerosal has antibacterial and antifungal properties, but it is less effective than ethanol. It is found in several types of topical products, including aqueous solutions, tinctures, ointments, creams, and aerosols. Systemic toxicity occurs less frequently with thimerosal than with other mercurials because the mercury in thimerosal is tightly bound to the organic configuration. The usual concentration is 0.1%.

Hydrogen Peroxide

Hydrogen peroxide (3% solution) is the most widely used oxidizing agent; sodium and zinc peroxides also are used. Enzymatic release of oxygen from hydrogen peroxide occurs when it comes into contact with blood and tissue fluids. The mechanical (fizzing) release of the oxygen has a cleansing effect on a wound, but organic matter reduces its effectiveness. The duration of action is only as long as the period of active oxygen release. Using peroxide on the intact skin is of doubtful value, because release of the nascent oxygen is too slow.

This compound must be used only where the released gas can escape; therefore it should never be used in abscesses, nor should bandages be applied too soon after its use.

Phenolic Compounds

Phenol   In very dilute solutions, this compound is an antiseptic and disinfectant. It has local anesthetic activity and is claimed to be an antipruritic in concentrations of 1:100 to 1:200, as in phenolated calamine lotion. In aqueous solutions of more than 1%, it is a tissue irritant and should not be used on skin, except as a keratolytic or peeling agent.

Liquified Phenol, USP   This preparation is a very concentrated solution of phenol in water (90% w/w). It is used locally like trichloroacetic acid to cause peeling of lesions. As such, it must be used carefully to protect healthy intact skin from its caustic effects. This can be done by applying a coating of petrolatum on the area to be protected.

Oleaginous Phenolic Solutions   Oily solutions of phenol and camphor are often used as nonprescription antiseptics in the treatment of minor cuts, insect bites, athlete's foot, fever blisters, and cold sores. Such products contain relatively high concentrations of phenol (4%) and must be used with caution. If applied to moist areas, partitioning of the phenol out of the oleaginous vehicle into the water present results in caustic concentrations of phenol on the skin. To avoid such damaging effects, these products should be applied to dry skin only.

Substituted Phenols   Substituted phenols, including the halogenated phenols (hexachlorophene), and the alkyl-substituted phenols (cresols and resorcinol) have greater bactericidal effect than phenol. Halogenation of a phenolic compound increases antiseptic properties. Dihalogenated and trihalogenated forms have greater potency but are less water soluble than monohalogenated phenols.

- **Hexachlorophene**—This compound previously had wide success as a topical antiseptic. It became restricted to prescription use when it was shown that the agent was absorbed through the skin of infants, causing neural damage. Emulsions that contain 3% hexachlorophene are effective antiseptic/cleansing products used for hand washing of hospital personnel, surgical hand scrubs, and preoperative skin preparations. It has a substantive binding property so that repeated use leaves an antimicrobial residual film on the skin.

- **Triclosan**—This is a halogenated salicylanilide that also can be regarded as a substituted phenol. It is used in deodorant soap/detergent bars at concentrations up to 1% (24). It has been placed by the FDA advisory review panel on nonprescription antimicrobial durg products (I) in Category III for such use, as well as for use as a skin antiseptic, skin-wound protectant (Table 1). However, the panel has found it is ineffective for use as a health care personnel handwash, patient handwash, patient preoperative skin preparation, and surgical hand scrub. It is not recommended for infants less than 6 months old, since effects of precutaneous absorption have not been evaluated satisfactorily (15, 24).
- **Cresols**—Cresols are alkyl derivatives of phenol. These isomers (*ortho, meta,* and *para*) have disinfectant properties. Due to irritation of the skin, use is limited to disinfection of inanimate objects and surfaces. The isomers are more potent bactericides than phenol but are at least as toxic.
- **Resorcinol**—Resorcinol is much less potent than phenol as an antimicrobial agent, but its systemic effects are similar. As an ointment (2% or more) it has been used in other treatment (ringworm). However, other topical agents, such as tolnaftate, are more effective.
- **Resorcinol monoacetate**—This agent exerts an even milder antibacterial effect than resorcinol, but it has a longer duration of action, since it releases resorcinol slowly. Both resorcinol and the monacetate are used in acne preparations mainly for their keratolytic effect. (See Chapter 29, *Acne Products.*)
- **Hexylresorcinol**—Hexylresorcinol is more effective than phenol as an antibacterial agent and is less toxic. It has been used in mouthwashes. The FDA advisory review panel on nonprescription antimicrobial drug products (I) has judged it safe and effective (Category I) as a skin-wound cleanser (15). It is used in low concentrations (0.1%) and may be irritating, however.
- **Thymol and chlorothymol**—These compounds are also alkyl derivatives of phenol with minor antimicrobial and antifungal properties.
- **Parachlorometaxylenol**—In 2% concentration, this agent is more effective than phenol. It is an ingredient in nonprescription products used for seborrhea and acne. However, more information relative to its percutaneous absorption is needed before it can be assigned Category I status (15, 24).

Carbanilides and Salicylanilides

Some of these halogenated compounds have been used as antimicrobial agents in deodorant soap/detergent bars. Several salicylanilides, however, have been found to be potent photosensitizers that can cause serious skin disorders (25). In 1975, the FDA proposed a regulation that any drug or cosmetic product with the following ingredients would be considered a new drug or adulterated cosmetic product: tribromsalan, dibromsalan, metabromsalan, fluorosalan, and tetrachlorosalicylanilide (26). This regulation went into effect on December 1, 1975, and virtually removed these agents from use in nonprescription products.

Triclosan, another salicylanilide, is being used in several deodorant soap/detergent bars, but has been recommended by the FDA advisory review panel on nonprescription antimicrobial drug products (I) as a Category III ingredient for such use in its tentative final order (Table 1) (15). Two carbanilide compounds, cloflucarban and triclocarban, have been evaluated by the antimicrobial I panel as topical antimicrobial agents. They have been placed in Category III for use in antimicrobial soaps, skin-wound cleansers, and health care personnel handwashes, pending publication of a final regulation by FDA (Table 1) (15). More data concerning substantivity, absorption, excretion, and safety are needed. Triclocarban is used in several deodorant soap/detergent bars. Tentative concentration limit is 1.5% (24).

Silver Compounds

The silver ion has an antiseptic effect because of its ability to precipitate the protein of cellular components of microorganisms. Soluble inorganic silver salts and organic silver compounds have been used as topical antiseptics. Except for silver nitrate and silver sulfadiazine, however, most silver compounds are used less and less with the advent of more effective antiseptic agents. In general, silver salts are precipitated relatively quickly by chloride in cell components. The organic silver compounds are less irritating to tissue than the inorganic salts but are less effective as antimicrobial agents.

Silver nitrate is a fairly potent bactericide at a concentration of 1:1,000; at 1:10,000 it is bacteriostatic. Aqueous solutions (0.5%) are used on dressings for second- and third-degree burns to prevent infection. Extensive use, however, may deplete chloride ions and cause electrolyte imbalance. Toughened silver nitrate pencils may be used to cauterize minor wounds (shaving). Mild silver protein and colloidal silver iodide are other nonprescription forms of silver. However, they have minimal antiseptic efficacy.

Surfactants

Soaps and quaternary ammonium compounds are sometimes included in topical anti-infective products. In addition to their antiseptic properties, these agents are used for their cleansing properties.

Quaternary Ammonium Compounds   These compounds are cationic surfactants that have antimicrobial activity on gram-positive and gram-negative bacteria but not on spores. Gram-negative bacteria are more resistant than gram-positive ones; thus they need a longer period of exposure. Quaternary ammonium compounds emulsify sebum and have a detergent effect to remove dirt, bacteria, and desquamated epithelial cells. Their antimicrobial activity is caused by disrupting membranes and denaturing lipoproteins. These compounds are inactivated by anionic ones (soaps and base/vehicle ingredients such as some viscosity builders).

Nonprescription quaternary ammonium compound products include benzalkonium chloride, benzethonium chloride, and methylbenzethonium chloride. These compounds are formulated as creams, dusting powder, and aqueous or alcoholic solutions. Concentrates are available for dilution to proper concentration for topical use.

If used undiluted, these concentrates may cause serious irritation. Quaternary compounds are irritating to the eyes, and caution must be used in this regard. For use on broken or diseased skin, concentrations of 1:5,000 to 1:20,000 may be used. For use on intact skin and minor abrasions a concentration of 1:750 is recommended.

Methylbenzethonium chloride is effective against microorganisms that split urea to form ammonia. It is used as a diaper rinse and for applications to areas subject to irritation from ammonia formation (groin, thighs, and buttocks).

Soaps   Since soaps are metallic salts of fatty acids, they are anionic surfactants (sodium or potassium stearate or oleate). They are used as supportive treatment (cleansing) in preventing infection of minor wounds. Their actual antiseptic properties are minimal.

Antimicrobial Soaps

Some antimicrobial agents are added to soap/detergent bars to increase their antiseptic properties for use as general skin deodorants. Some of these have been removed from products because of potent photosensitivity properties. Two such compounds, however, have wide use in deodorant soap/detergent bars: triclosan and triclocarban. Individuals with potential or actual sensitivity to carbanilides and/or salicylinilides should be warned to read the labels of such products carefully for explicit statement of their presence.

The FDA advisory review panel on nonprescription antimicrobial drug products (I) has expressed some concern that such soap products could upset the normal flora on the skin surface leading to infection by surviving pathogenic organisms. However, the panel did acknowledge that more data on the relationships of concentration, contact time of antimicrobial agents with the skin, number of exposures, and the total microbial population were needed (27). Under such circumstances, the panel recommended caution in the use of these compounds/products and advised the use of concentrations that reduce the flora only enough to produce a deodorant effect. The tentative final order of 1978 concerning such products indicated the FDA's belief that claims of effectiveness as deodorants should demonstrate odor reduction correlated with a reduction in total microbial count of one log unit ($\log^{10}$) or with a significant inhibition of microbial species that are known to be responsible for production of odor (15).

The FDA Advisory Review Panels for Antimicrobial Drug Products

Since the onset of the FDA review project, two panels have made recommendations concerning topical antimicrobial products. Initially, the antimicrobial I panel's recommendations were published by FDA in September 1974, as a proposal to establish a monograph for the safety and efficacy of topical drugs used in the seven types of nonprescription products outlined previously (27). The proposal generated significant comment and additional data that necessitated further deliberation.

The antimicrobial II panel was formed initially to make evaluations of safety and efficacy of topical antibiotics in nonprescription products. Its initial "proposal" was published in April 1977 (16). Table 2 summarizes the recommendations of that proposal concerning the use of nonprescription products of this type as skin-wound protectants and skin-wound antibiotics. The panel's definition of antibiotics as skin-wound protectants includes those added to increase the product's effectiveness by "preventing the contamination of a wound with organisms introduced from the environment or by preventing the growth of organisms in the formulation;" skin-wound antibiotics includes those used to "prevent or treat overt skin infections" (16).

In January 1978, the FDA published a "tentative final" monograph for the antimicrobials reviewed by the antimicrobial I panel (Table 1) (15). This document represented the second step in the system established by the FDA for development of eventual regulations pursuant to panel recommendations (proposal to establish monograph, tentative final monograph, and final monograph). It also generated considerable new comment, submission of data, objections, and petitions to reopen the administrative record of the panel.

The record was reopened several times between 1978 and 1980 to accommodate review and consideration of the new comments and submissions (28). In March 1980, the FDA reopened the administrative record of 12 of the review panels to allow further submissions and comments. The antimicrobial I panel was included in the group (29). Nothing more definitive or "final" regarding the regulatory status of the antimicrobial I panel's recommendations has occurred since then. The recommendations of the "tentative final" monograph of 1978 (Table 1) still represents the latest evaluative statements from FDA concerning topical antimicrobial agents in nonprescription products (15). It is anticipated that a new "tentative final" monograph, which will carry the status of regulation, will be published by 1983.

Neither a final nor tentative final monograph for the antimicrobial II panel have been published. Its initial proposal was published in 1977 (16). The panel is proceeding toward publication of a tentative final monograph (28). The recommendations, as outlined in Table 2, represent the most recent FDA evaluations of topical nonprescription antibiotics. In addition, the antimicrobial II panel has the responsibility for review of topical, nonprescription antifungal and antiacne drug products (28).

Though a large number of topical antimicrobial drugs are being evaluated by the FDA panels for ultimate approval as safe and effective, it should be remembered that compounds can gain such FDA approval through the new drug application procedures as well. This was the case for chlorhexidine gluconate in 1976.

Product Selection Guidelines

Once the pharmacist has evaluated the patient's condition, medical referral or appropriate self-medication should be recommended. Topical self-medication with anti-infective products must be reserved for superficial, uncomplicated infections. More serious infections should be referred to a physician for systemic therapy. Additionally, although many anti-infective nonprescription products are available, few have been studied under controlled conditions. Studies comparing agents within a class are also limited in number. It is difficult, therefore, to recommend one product over another in the treatment of superficial infections.

For the treatment of impetigo, the compounds most studied are neomycin, bacitracin, and polymyxin, either alone or in combination. Although the topical preparations are effective, they lead to delayed clearing of lesions compared with systemic antibiotics. Topical agents seem to be most effective when the lesions are not extensive (30). Cleaning the area with soap and water and gently removing loose crusts should improve response to topical therapy. While less objective information is available for other bacterial skin infections (erysipelas, ecthyma, and folliculitis), treatment with the medications listed above may be effective as long as the infection is not extensive. Furuncles and carbuncles may require lancing, which should be done only under the direction of a physician. Bacterial infections of the nails (pyonychia) must be treated with systemic antibiotics, due to poor topical penetration.

Some superficial fungal infections, such as tinea corporis or tinea cruris, respond well to topical antifungal agents. However, success of therapy increases when the lesions are small. If the lesions are extensive, or involve scalp or nails, topical therapy is generally ineffective, and systemic therapy should be considered. As with the antibacterial agents, a relative paucity of information exists comparing topical antifungals. The short chain fatty acids have been shown to be effective in treating tinea pedis and tinea cruris (31). When compared with tolnaftate cream in the treatment of tinea pedis, undecylenic acid ointment was shown to be equally effective as demonstrated by negative fungal cultures at 4 and 6 weeks of treatment (32, 33). In the case of tinea pedis, product selection may be guided by patient preference and cost to the patient.

The use of topical antibiotics has been frequently recommended for the prevention of infection secondary to minor cuts and abrasions. Although in theory the use of topical antimicrobials seems desirable, there is little evidence to support their routine use in such cases. Cleaning the wound with soap and water or with hydrogen peroxide, followed by an appropriate dressing may be the only "treatment" necessary. Should the area become inflamed, painful, or should pus develop, a physician should be consulted immediately.

Patient Consultation

The pharmacist should advise the patient on the proper use of the suggested product. For infections, intermittent applications are considered poor therapy; regular applications are preferable. If increased irritation occurs, the patient should be instructed to contact a physician. The appropriate "thickness" of applications should be suggested to avoid over- or under-medication. The pharmacist must make sure that the patient understands that none of these topical anti-infectives are to be used internally.

In addition to the information the pharmacist provides the patient in regard to nonprescription drug usage, the pharmacist may also provide information that will help eradicate the infection and possibly prevent future infections. This information would include proper cleansing of the infected area, avoiding the use of tight fitting or "occlusive" clothing, and avoiding situations that could lead to recurring infections.

Moreover, the patient should be informed of the expected duration of therapy and those conditions that, if they occur, would result in the need for physician-directed care (the development of a secondary bacterial infection). Recurring skin infections may be a sign of undiagnosed diabetes. A pharmacist that is aware of recurring infections should refer the patient to a physician.

Summary

Topical antimicrobials are used to treat and prevent cutaneous infections caused by bacteria, fungi, and viruses. Knowledge of design and formulation aspects of topical antimicrobial products is important in selecting appropriate therapeutic agents and products. The patient interview is essential in ascertaining whether self-medication or medical attention is indicated. If self-medication is appropriate, the pharmacist should instruct the patient in the use of nonprescription drugs and other supportive procedures.

References

1. F. G. Weissmann, *Drug Intell. Clin. Pharm., 8,* 535 (1974).
2. J. S. Jellinek, "Formulation and Function of Cosmetics," 2nd ed., Wiley, New York, N.Y., 1970, pp. 4–14.
3. W. D. Stewart et al., "Dermatology: Diagnosis and Treatment of Cutaneous Disorders," 4th ed., C. V. Mosby, St. Louis, Mo., 1978, p. 3.
4. S. M. Peck and W. R. Russ, *Arch. Dermatol. Syphilol. 56,* 601 (1947).
5. W. D. Stewart et al., "Dermatology: Diagnosis and Treatment of Cutaneous Disorders," 4th ed., C. V. Mosby, St. Louis, Mo., 1978, p. 240.
6. M. T. Hojyo-Tomoka, R. R. Marples, and A. M. Kligman, *Arch. Dermatol., 107,* 723 (1973).
7. L. F. Montes and W. H. Wilborn, *Br. J. Dermatol., 81,* 23 (1969).
8. R. R. Marples, "Skin Bacteria and Their Role in Infection," H. I. Maibach and G. Hildrick-Smith, Eds., McGraw-Hill, New York, N.Y., 1965, pp. 33–42.
9. B. M. Barker and F. Prescott, "Antimicrobial Agents in

Medicine," Blackwell Scientific Publications, London, England, 1973, pp. 18–149.

10. E. L. Laden, "Modern Dermatologic Therapy," T. H. Sternberg and V. D. Newcomer, Eds., McGraw-Hill, New York, N.Y., 1959, pp. 374–377, 386–403.

11. M. B. Sulzberger and J. Wolfe, "Dermatology: Diagnosis and Treatment," 2nd ed., Year Book Medical, Chicago, Ill., 1961, pp. 277–356.

12. J. T. Scrafani, *U.S. Pharm.,* April, p. 26 (1978).

13. W. D. Stewart et al., "Dermatology: Diagnosis and Treatment of Cutaneous Disorders," 4th ed., C. V. Mosby, St. Louis, Mo., 1978, p. 293.

14. W. Bruinsma, "A Guide to Drug Eruptions," Excerpta Medica, Amsterdam, The Netherlands, 1973, pp. 45–48, 87–103.

15. *Federal Register, 43,* 1210–49 (1978).

16. *Federal Register, 42,* 17642–681 (1977).

17. L. Weinstein, "The Pharmacological Basis of Therapeutics," 5th ed., L. S. Goodman and A. Gilman, Eds., MacMillan, New York, N.Y., 1975, p. 1235.

18. M. A. Sande and G. L. Mandell, "The Pharmacological Basis of Therapeutics," 6th ed., A. G. Gilman, L. S. Goodman, and A. Gilman, Eds., MacMillan, New York, N.Y., 1980, p. 1177.

19. D. R. Ward, personal communication, Stuart Pharmaceuticals, Div. of ICI Americas Inc., Wilmington, Del.; FDA's Summary for Basis of Approval, NDA 17-768 (Hibiclens), and laboratory data developed as part of NDA requirements.

20. W. A. Gillespie, G. G. Lennon, K. B. Linton, and G. A. Phipper, *Br. Med. J., 3,* 90 (1967).

21. D. J. Stickler, C. B. Wilmont, J. D. O'Flynn, *Paraplegia, 8,* 243 (1971).

22. D. J. Stickler, *J. Clin. Pathol., 27,* 284 (1974).

23. H. N. Prince, W. S. Nonemaker, R. C. Norgard, and D. L. Prince, *J. Pharm. Sci., 67,* 1629–1631 (1978).

24. "AMA Drug Evaluations," 4th ed., Wiley, New York, N.Y., 1980, p. 1017–1026.

25. *Federal Register, 39,* 33102–103 (1974).

26. *Federal Register, 40,* 50527–531 (1975).

27. *Federal Register, 39,* 33103–141 (1974).

28. J. S. Walsh, *Am. Pharm.,* NS20, 11 (1980).

29. *Federal Register, 45,* 18398–404 (1980).

30. H. C. Dillon, *Int. J. Dermatol., 19,* 443 (1980).

31. F. E. Lyddon, K. Gundersen, and H. I. Maibach, *Int. J. Dermatol., 19,* 24, (1980).

32. J. F. Fuerst, G. F. Cox, S. M. Weaver, and W. C. Duncan, *Cutis, 25,* 544 (1980).

33. E. H. Tschen, L. E. Becker, J. A. Ulrich, W. K. Hoge, and E. B. Smith, *Cutis, 23,* 696 (1979).

Topical Anti-infective Product Table

Product (Manufacturer)	Antiseptic	Antifungal Agent	Antibiotic	Other Ingredients
Achromycin Ointment (Lederle)			tetracycline hydrochloride, 3%	
Aftate Spray Powder, Powder, and Gel for Jock Itch (Plough)		tolnaftate, 1%		alcohol, 14% (spray powder) talc (powder)
AluWets (Stiefel)	aluminum chloride hexahydrate			
Argyrol Stabilized Solution (Cooper-Vision Pharmaceuticals, Inc.)	mild silver protein, 10%			edetate calcium disodium, 1.1%
Aureomycin Ointment (Lederle)			chlortetracycline, 3%	
Baciguent Ointment (Upjohn)			bacitracin, 500 units/g	
Bacimycin (Merrell-Dow)			bacitracin, 500 units/g neomycin, 3.5 mg/g	petrolatum base
Bactine (Miles)	benzalkonium chloride, 0.13%			lidocaine hydrochloride, 2.5%
Barc Cream (Commerce)	isobornyl thiocyanate, 4.1%			
Barc Liquid (Commerce)	pyrethrins, 0.18% piperonyl butoxide, 1.76%			
Baximin Ointment (Columbia Medical)			polymyxin B sulfate, 5,000 units/g bacitracin, 400 units/g neomycin sulfate, 5 mg/g	
Betadine Solution, Microbicidal Applicator, Swab Aid, Swab Sticks, Gauze Pads, and Whirlpool Concentrate (Purdue Frederick)	povidone-iodine, 10%			
Betadine Surgical Scrub, Surgi-Prep Sponge Brush, and Shampoo (Purdue Frederick)	povidone-iodine, 7.5%			
B.F.I. Powder (Beecham Products)	bismuth formic iodide			zinc phenolsulfonate bismuth subgallate aluminum potassium sulfate boric acid eucalyptol menthol thymol
BPN (Norwich-Eaton)			bacitracin, 500 units/g polymyxin B sulfate 5,000 units/g neomycin base (as sulfate), 3.5 mg/g	

Topical Anti-infective Product Table, continued

Product (Manufacturer)	Antiseptic	Antifungal Agent	Antibiotic	Other Ingredients
Clorpactin WCS 90 Powder (Guardian)	available chlorine, 3–4%			
Clorpactin XCB (Guardian)	available chlorine, 4–4.9%			
Cruex Medicated Cream (Pharmacraft)		undecylenic acid, 3% zinc undecylenate, 20%		
Cruex Powder (Pharmacraft)		calcium undecylenate, 10%		
Cruex Spray Powder (Pharmacraft)		zinc undecylenate, 20% undecylenic acid, 2%		
Cuprex (Beecham Products)				copper oleate, 0.3% tetrahydronaphthalene, 30.97%
Desenex Antifungal Foam (Pharmacraft)		undecylenic acid, 10%		alcohol, 29%
Desenex Liquid (Pharmacraft)		undecylenic acid, 10%		alcohol, 40%
Desenex Powder and Ointment (Pharmacraft)		zinc undecylenate, 20% undecylenic acid, 5% (ointment) 2% (powder)		
Drest (Dermik)	alkylisoquinolinium bromide, 0.15% benzalkonium chloride, 0.125%			alcohol, 14.1% protein greaseless gel povidone
Ergophene (Upjohn)	phenol, 16.3 mg/g			sodium borate, 3.6 mg/g fluidextract ergot, 0.09 ml/g zinc oxide, 49 mg/g
Isodine Antiseptic Skin Cleanser (Blair)	povidone-iodine, 7.5%			
Isodine Antiseptic Solution and Ointment (Blair)	povidone-iodine, 10%			
Lubraseptic Jelly (Guardian)	o-phenylphenol, 0.1% p-*tert*-pentylphenol, 0.02% phenylmercuric nitrate, 0.007%			
Mercresin (Upjohn)	secondary amytricresols, 0.1%			o-hydroxyphenyl-mercuric chloride, 0.1% acetone, 0.1% alcohol, 0.1%

Topical Anti-infective Product Table, continued

Product (Manufacturer)	Antiseptic	Antifungal Agent	Antibiotic	Other Ingredients
Mercurochrome (Becton Dickinson)	merbromin, 2%			
Mercurochrome II (Becton Dickinson)	benzalkonium chloride, 0.13%			ethyl alcohol, 3.2%
Merlenate Ointment (North American)	phenylmercuric nitrate, 1.15%	undecylenic acid, 5%		
Myciguent Cream and Ointment (Upjohn)			neomycin sulfate, 5 mg/g	
Mycitracin (Upjohn)			polymyxin B sulfate, 5,000 units/g bacitracin, 500 units/g neomycin sulfate, 5 mg/g	
Neo-Polycin Ointment (Dow)			polymyxin B sulfate, 5,000 units/g bacitracin zinc, 400 units/g neomycin (as sulfate), 3.5 mg/g	fuzene base polyethylene glycol dilaurate polyethylene glycol distearate light liquid petrolatum synthetic glyceride wax white petrolatum
Neosporin Ointment (Burroughs Wellcome)			polymyxin B sulfate, 5,000 units/g bacitracin zinc, 400 units/g neomycin sulfate, 5 mg/g	white petrolatum
Neo-Thrycex (Commerce)			bacitracin neomycin sulfate polymixin B sulfate	
New Skin (Medtech)	8-hydroxyquinoline, 1%			clove oil, 1% pyroxylin (collodion), 98%
Norwich-Bacitracin (Norwich-Eaton)			bacitracin, 500 U/gm	
Obtundia (Otis Clapp)	cresol–camphor complex			
Obtundia First Aid Spray (Otis Clapp)	cresol–camphor complex			
Oil-O-Sol (Mosso Division of Health Care Industries)	hexylresorcinol, 0.1%			corn oil castor oil camphor oil
Polysporin Ointment (Burroughs Wellcome)			polymyxin B sulfate, 10,000 units/g bacitracin zinc, 500 units/g	white petrolatum
Poviderm Ointment, Solution (North American Pharmacal)	povidone iodine, 10% (ointment) povidone iodine, 7.5% (solution)			
Pro Comfort Jock Itch Spray Powder (Scholl)		tolnaftate, 1%		alcohol, 14%; talc

Topical Anti-infective Product Table, continued

Product (Manufacturer)	Antiseptic	Antifungal Agent	Antibiotic	Other Ingredients
Prophyllin (Rystan)		sodium propionate, 1% (solution) 5% (ointment)		chlorophyll, 0.0025% (solution) 0.0125% (ointment)
Quin III (Pfeiffer)	iodochlorhydroxyquin, 3%			
Quinolor Compound Ointment (Squibb)	halquinols, 0.5% benzoyl peroxide, 10%			methyl salicylate polyethylene mineral oil eugenol menthol
Salicylic Acid Soap (Stiefel)		salicylic acid, 3–5%		
Salicylic Acid and Sulfur Soap (Stiefel)		salicylic acid, 3% sulfur, 10%		
Sea Breeze (Sea Breeze)		benzoic acid		alcohol, 43% peppermint oil clove oil eucalyptus oil eugenol boric acid camphor
Spectrocin Ointment (Squibb)			neomycin, 2.5 mg/g gramicidin, 0.25 mg/g	polyethylene mineral oil
S.T. 37 (Beecham Products)	hexylresorcinol, 0.1%			glycerin
Terramycin Ointment with Polymyxin B Sulfate (Pfipharmecs)			oxytetracycline hydrochloride, 30 mg/g polymyxin B sulfate, 10,000 units/g	
Ting Powder and Spray Powder (Pharmacraft)		zinc undecylenate, 20% undecylenic acid, 2%		
Triple Antibiotic Ointment (North American)			polymyxin B sulfate, 5,000 units/g bacitracin, 400 units/g neomycin sulfate, 5 mg/g	
Vaseline First Aid Carbolated Petroleum Jelly (Chesebrough-Pond)	chloroxylenol, 0.5%			petroleum jelly lanolin phenol, 0.2%
Vioform Ointment and Cream (Ciba)	iodochlorhydroxyquin, 3%			petrolatum base (ointment) water-washable base (cream)
Zea Sorb Powder (Stiefel)	chloroxylenol, 0.5%			microporous cellulose, 45% aluminum dihydroxy-allantoinate, 0.2%
Zephiran Chloride Solution and Spray (Winthrop)	benzalkonium chloride, 0.13%			
Zephiran Towelettes (Winthrop)	benzalkonium chloride chlorothymol			alcohol, 20% perfume

Acne Products

Joye A. Billow and Raymond E. Hopponen

Questions to Ask the Patient

How long have you had acne?

Are the blemishes whiteheads and blackheads? Are there also swollen lumps under the skin?

Does the problem seem to be only in areas where your clothes rub, e.g., hats, headgear, shoulder pads, etc.?

Have you recently been in a hot and humid environment?

Does the sunlight in summer help to clear the acne?

What type of cosmetics, including after-shave lotions, do you use?

Do you use any hair oils or creams? How often do you shampoo your hair?

Are you currently using any prescription or nonprescription medications? If so, what are they?

Have you already tried any medications, scrubs, diets, or other treatments? How effective were they?

Have you been to a physician for treatment of this condition?

How long ago? What did he or she suggest? How long did you follow the treatment?

Acne vulgaris is a chronic skin condition characterized mainly by comedones (whiteheads and blackheads) and papules. In severe cases, inflammation, pustules, cysts, and scarring may occur. Acne occurs most commonly on the face, back, and chest. Although it does not pose a severe physical threat, acne should not be ignored since it may cause a great deal of emotional stress and anguish. The condition occurs most often in adolescence, a period in which many physiologic, social, and psychological adjustments are made and when self-image and peer acceptance are extremely important. Acne may also occur in prepubertal children and in older persons.

Studies of the incidence of acne in adolescents indicate that it is nearly universal in this group. In one study, of 1,555 young people 8–18 years old, 100% had recognizable acne at the ages of maximal incidence—14 years for girls and 16 years for boys (1). Moreover, 50% of the girls and 78% of the boys had acne severe enough to be termed clinical. Subclinical lesions were noted in about one-third of the 8–9-year-old age group. Other findings revealed that only 10–11% of a studied group of high school students had sought medical help for acne, but about 60% were self-medicating (2).

The widespread incidence of acne in adolescence, its remissions and recurrences, and its variability in response to treatment have prompted many theories implicating personal habits, diet, personality, and physiol-

ogy as contributing factors. There is little information available that supports a relationship between diet and acne (3). Although several studies demonstrated that chocolate does not affect acne (4), some clinicians remain unconvinced and suggest that it be removed from the diet. Other clinicians feel that dietary restrictions for individuals with acne are unwarranted since no convincing evidence has been presented to implicate nuts, fats, colas, or carbohydrates. Iodides and bromides are secreted in the sweat and may cause acne-like eruptions if they are ingested in substantial amounts, as in the therapeutic agents containing these ions. However, the amount of iodine in seafoods or iodized salt is not significant.

Etiology

Acne vulgaris has its origin in the pilosebaceous units in the dermis (Figure 1). These units, consisting of a hair follicle and the associated sebaceous glands, are connected to the skin surface by a duct (the infundibulum) through which the hair shaft passes. On the smooth skin of the body, the hair may be very fine or entirely absent. Because the sebaceous glands are most common on the face, back, and chest, acne tends to occur most often in these areas. The sebaceous glands produce sebum, a mixture of fats and waxes, which maintains hydration of skin and hair. The sebum passes to the skin surface through the infundibulum and then spreads over the skin surface to retard water loss.

At puberty there is an increase in the production of androgenic hormones in both sexes. The increasing influx of circulatory testosterone is taken up by the sebaceous gland and converted by an enzyme, 5-α-reductase, to dihydrotestosterone, which is considered to be the tissue androgen responsible for the acne problem. The sebaceous glands, under the influence of increased androgen levels, increase in size and activity producing larger amounts of sebum. At the same time there is increased keratinization of the follicular walls. This increased keratinization causes mechanical blockage of the sebum flow, resulting in dilation of the follicle and entrapment of sebum and cellular debris. This lesion is a microcomedo, the initial pathologic change (Figure 2).

Androgens are the major stimulus to sebaceous gland development and sebum secretion. However, patients with acne do not necessarily have higher androgen levels. It is theorized that acne-prone patients have increased end-organ sensitivity to normal level of androgens, facilitating the hypertrophic changes discussed previously (5, 6).

Exogenous sources of corticosteroids, both systemic and topical (prescription and nonprescription), may also induce the hypertrophic changes by sensitizing the follicle and producing "steroid acne." These lesions are characterized by uniform red papules succeeded by closed comedones and finally open comedones (5).

Oral contraceptives with high androgenic acitivity also have been implicated in the production of acne.

Various drugs are known to precipitate acne eruptions, especially in individuals over age 25. These include bromides, ethionamide, haloperidol, halothane, iodides, isoniazid, lithium, phenytoin, and trimethadione. Cobalt irradiation and hyperalimentation therapy also have been implicated (5, 7).

Noninflammatory Acne

The cause of acne is increased activity of the sebaceous glands and of the epithelial tissue lining the infundibulum. This increase is induced by the greater production of hormones, especially androgenic hormones, as puberty approaches. Sebum consists of free and esterified fatty acids as well as unsaponifiable lipid components. The glands produce more sebum, causing increased skin oiliness.

The epithelial tissue, an extension of the surface epidermis, forms the lining of the infundibulum and becomes thinner as it extends into the deeper portions of the duct. Normally, it continually sheds cells that are carried to the skin surface by the flow of sebum. However, in acne, the shed epithelial cells are more distinct and durable, sticking together to form a coherent horny layer that blocks the follicular channel (8). This impaction plugs and distends the follicle to form a microcomedo (Figure 2).

As more cells and sebum are added, the microcomedo enlarges and becomes visible (whitehead) and is called a closed comedo (its contents do not reach the surface of the skin) (Figure 2). If the plug enlarges and protrudes from the orifice of the follicular canal, it is called an open comedo (its contents open to the surface) (Figure 2). The tip of the plug may darken (blackhead) due to melanin produced by the epithelial cells lining the infundibulum (not dirt or oxidized fat) (9). Open comedones may be expressed carefully with a comedo extractor. Care should be taken to avoid dirty fingers or extractor, sources of secondary infection. Although sebum still is produced, the sebaceous glands tend to shrink during comedo formation. Acne characterized by the presence of closed and open comedones is called noninflammatory acne. (See *Plate 6-24*.)

The hair in the follicle may play an important role in comedo development. If the hair shaft is thin and small, it may not be able to maintain an open channel, and it then becomes entrapped in the plug. The heavier hair of the scalp and beard typically pushes the developing plug to the surface, thus preventing comedo formation. In adult life, acne may disappear spontaneously. This may be due to the cells lining the follicles becoming less susceptible to comedogenic materials (5).

Inflammatory Acne

Inflammatory acne is characterized by inflammation (surrounding the comedones), papules, pustules, and nodulocystic lesions (Figure 2). Papules are inflammatory lesions having the appearance of a raised, reddened area on the skin. A nodule is a papule with a more extensive penetration into surrounding tissue. Pustules are inflammatory lesions having the appearance of a raised, reddened area, filled with pus, and these may rupture spontaneously. This type of acne is more likely to cause permanent scarring than noninflammatory acne. (See *Plate 6-25*.) Inflammatory acne typically be-

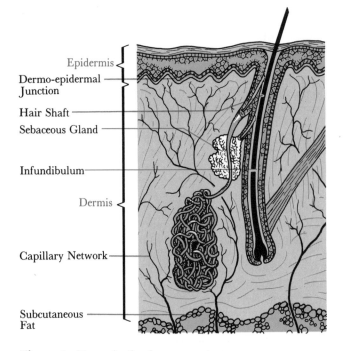

Epidermis

Dermo-epidermal Junction

Hair Shaft

Sebaceous Gland

Infundibulum

Dermis

Capillary Network

Subcutaneous Fat

Figure 1. Normal pilosebaceous unit.

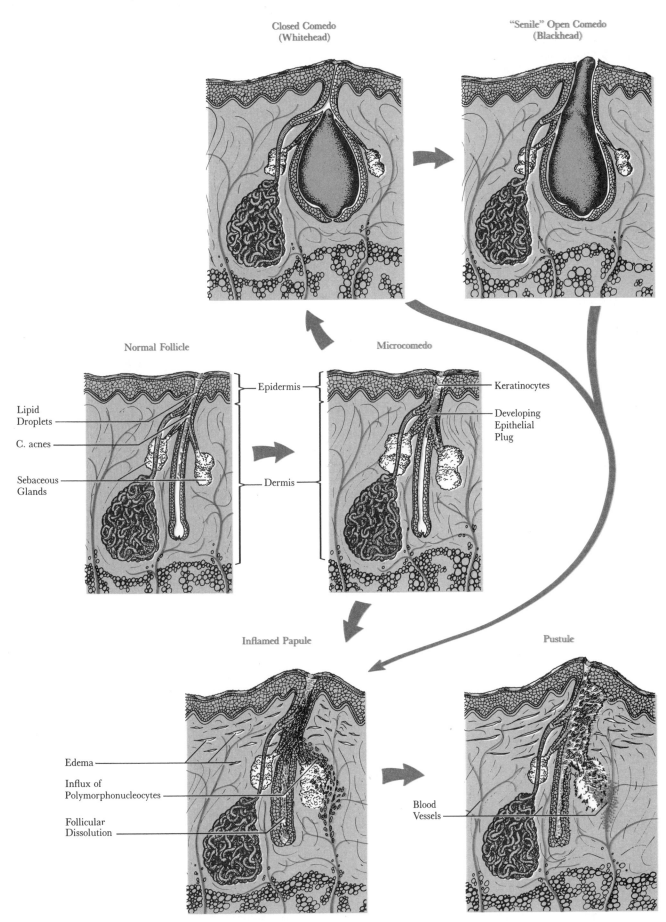

Closed Comedo
(Whitehead)

"Senile" Open Comedo
(Blackhead)

Normal Follicle

Microcomedo

Epidermis

Keratinocytes

Lipid
Droplets

Developing
Epithelial
Plug

C. acnes

Sebaceous
Glands

Dermis

Inflamed Papule

Pustule

Edema

Influx of
Polymorphonucleocytes

Follicular
Dissolution

Blood
Vessels

Figure 2. Pathogenesis of acne. Adapted with permission from J. E. Fulton and S. Bradley, *Cutis, 17,* 560 (1976).

gins in closed comedones, rarely in open comedones. As the microcomedo develops, it distends the follicle so that the cellular lining of the walls is spread apart and therefore thinner. At this stage, primary inflammation of the follicle wall may develop, with disruption of the epithelial lining and lymphocyte infiltration into and around the follicular wall (10).

However, if the follicle wall ruptures and the contents are discharged into the surrounding tissue, a more severe inflammatory reaction results. The epithelial cells, the sebum, and any microorganisms present represent foreign substances capable of eliciting an inflammatory reaction. The result may be an abscess, which, in the process of healing, may cause scars or pits. Fingering or picking at inflamed follicles or attempting to express closed comedones may produce inflammatory lesions by rupturing the follicle wall.

Current theories explaining the development of inflammatory acne suggest that the initial inflammation of the follicle wall results from the presence of free fatty acids derived from the sebum (10). In the presence of bacterial lipolytic enzymes, triglycerides of the sebum are split, releasing the fatty acids. The normal bacterial flora in the sebaceous duct produce the enzymes responsible for splitting the triglycerides.

The main microorganisms found in the sebaceous duct are an anaerobic rod, *Propionibacterium acnes* (*Corynebacterium acnes*) and one or two species of *Staphylococci.* These organisms are the predominant flora that normally inhabit the skin. They are not considered to be pathogens and die rapidly if the follicle wall is ruptured and they are released into the surrounding tissues. *Propionibacterium acnes* generally is regarded as the source of the lipolytic enzymes responsible for free fatty acid formation in the sebum. The effectiveness of oral tetracyline and topical antibiotics in treating inflammatory acne is due to their ability to suppress the normal bacterial population of the sebaceous duct, thus reducing free fatty acid concentration (11).

The presence of pustules or cysts indicates inflammatory acne, a type that should be treated by a physician. Treatment requires prescribed medication and possibly excision and drainage of lesions. Because of the danger of permanent scarring in this type of acne, medical help should be sought.

Aggravating Factors

Many women with acne experience a flare-up of symptoms during the premenstrual part of their cycle. The flare-up cannot be explained on the basis of hormone levels alone, although the change in the progesterone level has been implicated. Changes in sebaceous activity also have been claimed to be responsible. It also has been suggested that the premenstrual flare-up, seen in 60–70% of women with acne, is caused by a reduction in the size of the orifice of the pilosebaceous duct resulting in obstruction. Measurements of orifice diameters during the complete cycle showed that the size was reduced markedly during the premenstrual phase (12).

Hydration also decreases the size of the pilosebaceous duct orifice, a change that is reversible (13). This reduction explains the exacerbation of acne in conditions of high humidity or in situations where frequent and prolonged sweating occurs.

Local irritation or friction may increase the incidence of acne symptoms. Rough or occlusive clothing, headgear straps, and pieces of equipment used in athletics often aggravate acne. Resting the chin or cheek on the hand frequently for long periods creates localized conditions conducive to lesion formation in acne-prone individuals.

Acne cosmetica is a low-grade form of acne, characterized by a variable number of closed comedones on the face, cheek, and chin. In some instances, an occasional inflammatory lesion is seen. This form of acne was found in about one-third of adult women who were examined, but not in adult men (14). The lesions of acne cosmetica typically are closed, noninflammatory comedones and cannot be distinguished from similar lesions of acne vulgaris. Furthermore, half of the cosmetic cream bases used by these women were comedogenic in rabbit ear tests and on the skin of human volunteers. The condition responded readily to treatment with tretinoin. Pomade acne, manifested by comedones on the forehead and temples, was reported to be caused directly by the long-term use of hair dressings that contain petrolatum or liquid petrolatum (15).

Treatment

Acne cannot be cured. In most cases, however, with available therapeutic regimens, symptoms may be reduced, and permanent scarring minimized. Because acne persists for long periods, frequently from adolescence to the early twenties, treatment must be long-term and consistent. Remission or reduction in severity of lesions may occur, especially in summer, but treatment should be resumed when necessary. Patients should be warned not to self-medicate with topical steroids.

Treatment of acne with nonprescription products includes the following:

- Removing excess sebum from the skin;
- Preventing closure of the pilosebaceous orifice and unblocking ducts;
- Minimizing conditions conducive to acne;
- Avoiding contact of lesions with oily cosmetics.

Controlling inflammation and infection, suppressing or altering hormonal activity, and correcting destructive effects should be left to a physician (16).

Management of Acne
Removal of Excess Sebum

The preferred method for removing excess sebum from the skin is a conscientious program of daily washing. The affected areas should be washed thoroughly at least 2 times/day with warm water, soap, and a soft washcloth. Scrubbing should be gentle and excessive massaging should be avoided. This should be done for several minutes to work the lather thoroughly into the skin. The purpose of the washing is to produce a mild drying of the skin and, perhaps, mild erythema (17). Washing causes barely visible peeling that can loosen comedones.

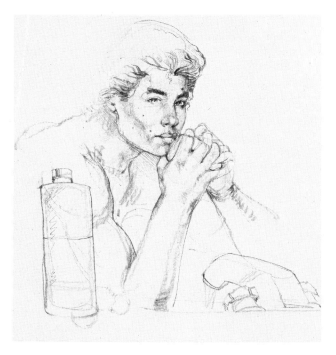

If washing produces a feeling of tautness in the skin, the intensity and frequency of washings should be reduced.

Ordinarily facial soaps are usually satisfactory. Soaps containing antibacterial agents have been suggested for controlling acne, but no conclusive evidence has been presented to indicate their value over nonmedicated soap. There is little rationale for using soaps containing sulfur, salicylic acid, or resorcinol. If the affected area is rinsed properly, these added medications will be washed away.

Soap substitutes containing surfactants (ionic or nonionic) have been suggested for acne because they are less drying to the skin. However, because a mild degree of drying is desirable, an ordinary facial soap should be tried first. Some cleansing preparations contain pumice, polyethylene, or aluminum oxide particles to add abrasive action to the cleansing effect. Used gently, they may be helpful in comedonal acne. They should be avoided in inflammatory acne. Buf-Puf is a nonmedicated cleansing sponge made of polyester fibers which, according to product information, assists in the removal of the top outer layer of dead skin cells by gentle abrasion. It is questionable whether these abrasive products are any more effective than a mild soap used with a soft washcloth. Care must be taken to avoid overzealous abrasion since this may be irritating and possibly damaging. If it is inconvenient to wash during the day, a cleansing pad that contains alcohol, acetone, and a surfactant may be used.

Because acne treatment is aimed at removing excess sebum from the skin, other topically applied fats and oils (particularly cosmetics that contain oils) should not be used. Hair dressings in excessive amounts should be avoided; those that are used should contain a minimum of oil. Frequent hair shampooing should be encouraged because acne usually is accompanied by an oily scalp.

Preventing Pilosebaceous Orifice Closure

Topical agents that cause irritation and desquamation are used to prevent closure of the pilosebaceous orifice. The irritant effect of these peeling agents causes an increased turnover rate of the epithelial cells lining the follicular duct, which increases sloughing (17). Peeling agents also cause keratolysis, which reduces the cohesiveness of the follicular lining. The net effect is to reduce the tendency to form new comedones and to loosen the structure of formed comedones and aid in their extrusion.

Ingredients in Nonprescription Products

Sulfur

Sulfur generally is used in the precipitated or colloidal form at 2–10% concentrations. The higher concentrations produce a more intense effect. Other forms of sulfur such as zinc sulfide and sodium thiosulfate are milder. Although sulfur helps resolve comedones, some evidence suggests that it also may promote the development of new ones (18). Sulfur (but not thiosulfate or sulfide) was found to be comedogenic in rabbit ear tests and, on long exposure, on the backs of human subjects (18), although recent evidence refutes this observation (19). Sulfur has met the criteria of the FDA advisory review panel on OTC antimicrobial products, allowing use of claims of antibacterial activity: "Helps prevent blackheads/whiteheads; helps prevent development of new acne lesions; helps prevent erythema/redness/inflammation associated with acne; helps reduce the bacteria *P. acnes*, a major factor/organism/microorganism associated with acne." Sulfur generally is accepted as being an effective agent for promoting the resolution of acne lesions, and its overall effect is one of improving the condition. Sulfur lotions are applied in a thin film to the affected area 1–2 times/day.

Resorcinol

Resorcinol usually is used in concentrations of 1–2%. Resorcinol monoacetate is milder and may be used at higher concentrations (up to 3%). Resorcinol may produce a dark brown scale on some darker-skinned individuals, who should be forewarned (19). The reaction is reversible when the medication is discontinued. There is some question as to whether resorcinol absorption may precipitate systemic toxicity. It is advisable to caution patients to apply resorcinol-containing products only to affected areas and not over extensive areas of the body. Resorcinol alone is classified as a Category I ingredient for safety and Category II for efficacy. Combination active ingredient, sulfur/resorcinol, was placed in Category I for safety and effectiveness.

Salicylic Acid

Salicylic acid is available in nonprescription products in concentrations of 0.5–2%. Its pharmacological action is dependent on the concentration: deep keratolytic (sloughing) action at concentrations greater than 5%, a surface keratolytic action at 1–4%, and an acidifying effect at 0.1% and greater. The keratolytic effect and possible enhanced absorption of other agents provide the rationale for the topical use of salicylic acid (20). Salicylic acid will not prevent acne but it may shorten the course of mild inflammatory lesions (6). Salicylic acid alone in concentrations of 0.5–5% is of questionable effectiveness according to the FDA advisory review panel, and has been placed in Category III. Salicylic acid and resorcinol often are added to sulfur-containing products.

Benzoyl Peroxide

Benzoyl peroxide is one of the most effective topical nonprescription medications available for acne (21). It is possible that benzoyl peroxide acts in several different ways. It is a primary irritant that increases the epithelial cell growth rate, leading to an increased sloughing rate. This increase results in a looser structure of the follicular plug and promotes resolution of comedones (22). Its oxidizing potential may contribute to bacteriostatic and bacteriocidal activity, suppressing the local population of *P. acnes* and reducing the skin surface free fatty acids. Benzoyl peroxide is an irritant, drying, peeling, and comedolytic agent in addition to its ability to suppress *P. acnes.*

Benzoyl peroxide is generally available in concentrations of 2.5–5.0% and 10%, and is formulated as a lotion, gel, cream, and ointment. The irritant ability of the various concentrations and formulations (particularly gels) are not equivalent and some products are available by prescription only, which ensures physician supervision.

Patient instructions for use of topical nonprescription benzoyl peroxide suggest applying a small quantity to affected areas with light massaging 1 or 2 times/day. Since some patients are sensitive to benzoyl peroxide, the initial applications may be limited to one or two small areas to determine if discomfort or reaction occurs. Gentle cleansing of the affected area with a nonmedicated soap followed by drying the skin with gentle patting prior to application of the product may be beneficial. Patient warnings include avoidance of use around the eyes, mouth, lips, and inside the nose, for external use only, and the possibility of stinging and burning. If stinging and burning are excessive after application, the preparation should be removed with soap and water and not reapplied until the next day. Other sources of irritation, such as sunlamps, should be avoided. Most patients tolerate benzoyl peroxide lotions, but about 1–3% are hypersensitive to the ingredient.

Benzoyl peroxide is an oxidizing agent and may bleach colored fabric.

Antibacterials

Acne is not an infection. The inflammation found in some cases is the result of a foreign body reaction to follicular contents. The only microorganisms involved are the nonpathogenic normal flora found deep within the follicles and out of the reach of the usual antibacterial agents applied to the skin surface. Therefore, most topically applied antibacterial agents generally have not been of value in treating acne.

An exception is the use of fat-soluble derivatives of erythromycin, tetracycline, and clindamycin (23, 24).

These derivatives, available by prescription, are applied as dilute solutions in organic solvents or as creams. Their effectivenss is due to their ability to diffuse through the fatty contents of the sebaceous follicle to reach the *P. acnes* located in the lower segments of the follicle. There they suppress the activity of these organisms and so reduce the production of comedogenic free fatty acids from the sebum.

Oral tetracycline, erythromycin, minocycline, and clindamycin, which require a prescription, are effective in treating inflammatory acne. An ad hoc study committee of the American Academy of Dermatology recognized oral tetracycline as a rational, effective, and relatively safe drug for use in this condition (25). However, it is not effective for the resolution of noninflammatory comedones.

These drugs suppress the growth of normal cutaneous flora (*P. acnes*), which results in decreased formation of free fatty acids (FFA) and consequently in decreased inflammation.

Oral antibiotic therapy may produce some adverse effects; however, these are usually minor. Gastrointestinal upset is the most common problem. Monilial vaginitis may occur, particularly in debilitated patients. Less common is the occurrence of a gram-negative folliculitis due to *Klebsiella* or *Proteus* species. A particular and serious disadvantage associated with clindamycin is pseudomembranous colitis, secondary to clindamycin treatment of acne (26).

Oral tetracycline is the drug of choice because it is the least costly and exhibits the fewest side effects. It is effective in low doses because high concentrations are achieved in the sebaceous follicle.

Tretinoin

Tretinoin (vitamin A acid or retinoic acid), a prescription drug, is a topical medication proven to be effective in treating acne characterized primarily by the presence of comedones. Tretinoin, which acts as an irritant to increase epithelial cell proliferation, apparently is more irritating than benzoyl peroxide, particularly in the early stages of treatment (26). Tretinoin not only changes follicular keratinization but decreases the number of normal cell layers of the stratum corneum from 14 to 5. This decreased depth of the barrier layer may allow other topical agents to penetrate the skin more readily. Patients using tretinoin for the first time should be informed that a temporary exacerbation of the condition may occur when treatment is initiated.

The pharmacist or physician should instruct the patient in the proper use of tretinoin as follows:

- Concomitant topical medication should be used with caution unless otherwise directed by the physician.
- Mild, gentle soaps should be used to cleanse the skin no more than twice daily.
- Tretinoin should be lightly applied once daily to all affected areas (except around the eyes and lips), preferably 1 hour before bedtime. The skin must be thoroughly dry before application, approximately 15 minutes after washing.
- Prolonged, excessive exposure to the sun should be

avoided. An effective sunscreen may be used if exposure cannot be avoided.

- The skin will become red and peel, usually within a week of initiating therapy. This condition will last approximately 3–4 weeks. An exacerbation of the acne can be expected to occur during the initial 4–6 weeks.
- Three months of therapy are required for clearing of comedones to take place. Inflammatory lesions will improve more rapidly. Eight to twelve weeks are required before the effectiveness of therapy can be assessed.

Ultraviolet Light

Exposure to sunlight often is beneficial in acne; consequently, improvement often is noted during the summer. The improvement is believed to result from the irritant properties of the ultraviolet wavelengths of sunlight, which stimulate increased proliferation of the epithelium. Ultraviolet lamps produce the same effect, but they generally are not recommended because of the difficulty in determining and regulating the amount of limited exposure necessary to produce the required mild erythema. If a sunlamp is used, care must be taken to protect the eyes adequately from the light's damaging effect. It also may be wise to time the exposure to avoid the danger of falling asleep under the lamp. In general, however, the use of artificial UV-light should be avoided.

Zinc Sulfate

The treatment of acne with oral zinc sulfate has been suggested by work reported in Sweden (28). Other studies, however, have not noted any significant differences between patients given zinc or placebo (29, 30).

Estrogen Therapy

Very severe or otherwise unresponsive cases of acne in young women may be treated by estrogen therapy. The effectiveness of estrogen in this case is due to its inhibition of androgens at the adrenal gland. Oral contraceptives with high estrogenic and low androgenic activities are the most common sources of estrogens for this purpose.

Other Treatments

Treatments that have been abandoned as not being effective include oral vitamin A, laxatives, bacterial vaccines, and digestive aids such as pancreatin, pepsin, bile salts, and acidophilus bacterial cultures.

Secondary Formulation Factors

Suspensions, lotions, creams, and gels are the vehicles generally used to carry antiacne medications to the skin. Lotions and creams should have a low fat content so that they do not counteract drying and peeling. Ethyl or isopropyl alcohol added to liquid preparations and gels hastens their drying to a film. Nonfatty gels, in particular, are slow drying if formulated in a completely aqueous base.

Thickening agents in preparations should not dry to a sticky film. The solids of most preparations leave a film that is not noticeably visible and does not need coloring to blend with the skin. However, some products are intended to hide blemishes by depositing an opaque film of insoluble masking agents such as zinc oxide on the skin. These products are tinted to improve their cosmetic effect.

Product Selection Guidelines

Comedonal and mild papular acne can usually be successfully self-medicated. Individuals exhibiting characteristics of moderately severe papular acne and pustular and cystic acne should be referred to a physician. The pharmacist should examine the patient's medication history, including previous measures taken to control the acne, which medications were used, when, for how long, and the degree of success and personal acceptance of the preparation tried. Subjective data on a person's attitude toward treatment and willingness to participate actively in a skin care program should be determined.

The success of a program to control acne depends on patient willingness to devote the time and effort required to carry out a continued daily regimen of washing the affected areas and applying medication. The treatment program and acne process should be explained clearly, and misconceptions should be corrected. The pharmacist should advise on scalp and hair care, the use of cosmetics, and, above all, the need for long-term, conscientious care. Positive moral support often is necessary to reduce patient concern. The pharmacist can provide a valuable service by educating the patient about the following considerations:

- Patients should avoid picking at or squeezing comedones. This increases the likelihood of infection, inflammation, and scarring. Opening or extraction of comedones should only be done under the supervision or advice of a physician.
- The skin should be kept clean to remove excess sebum and cellular debris. However, overzealous scrubbing may exacerbate the condition.
- Patients who use make-up and cosmetics should be instructed to use only noncomedogenic (oil-free or nongreasy) preparations.
- Patients using a moisturizer should be instructed to use a noncomedogenic preparation. Most acne patients have oily skin and will experience dryness as the desired effect of therapy.
- Diet plays an important role in maintaining health; however, certain foods are no longer implicated in acne exacerbations. Thus, broad dietary restrictions are ineffective in acne treatment.
- Stressful situations may play a role in acute exacerbation of acne. However, stress does not cause acne.
- There is no evidence that sexual activity plays a role in the occurrence or exacerbation of acne.
- Patients should understand that treatment only controls acne, it does not cure it. Treatment must continue even after acute exacerbations have cleared.

Claims made for nonprescription products for acne relief must be studied carefully for their accuracy. Various creams, lotions, antiseptics, and skin peels are available, and formulas should be examined carefully before judgment is made. Patients should carefully follow instructions on the product package.

If a previous medication has not been used regularly, one of the milder peeling agents should be recommended. Resorcinol, salicylic acid, or sulfur preparations have been suggested; however, the present trend is toward benzoyl peroxide as the first treatment choice. The cautions on its irritating properties should be observed. If the lower concentration has been tried conscientiously without success, treatment should progress to the next stronger product. The area should first be washed gently with soap and water and allowed to dry thoroughly before application. Cases of acne that continue to be resistant to control should be referred to a physician.

Summary

Acne vulgaris occurs almost universally in young adults from early teens to middle twenties and occasionally appears in prepubertal and older people. Acne, generally, cannot be cured, but it may be controlled to improve appearance and to prevent the development of severe acne with its resulting scarring. With understanding and reassurance, acne patients may understand that the condition is not irreparable and that care must be given to the affected areas for a long time for improvement to occur.

References

1. J. L. Burton, W. J. Cunliffe, I. Stafford, and S. Shuster, *Br. J. Dermatol., 85,* 119 (1971).
2. R. J. Schachter, E. S. Pantel, G. M. Glassman, and I. Zweibelson, *N.Y. State J. Med., 71,* 2886 (1971).
3. J. E. Rasmussen, "Diet and Acne," *Int. J. Dermatol., 16,* 488 (1977).
4. J. E. Fulton, G. Plewig, and A. M. Kligman, *J. Am. Med. Assoc., 210,* 2071 (1969).
5. "Manual of Dermatologic Therapeutics with Essentials of Diagnosis," 2nd ed., K. A. Arndt, Ed., Little, Brown, Boston, Mass., 1978, pp. 3–15.
6. M. A. Quan, et al., *J. Fam. Pract., 11,* 1041 (1980).
7. L. E. Cluff, G. J. Caranasos, and R. B. Stewart, "Clinical Problems with Drugs," Vol. V, W. B. Saunders, Philadelphia, Pa., 1975.
8. A. M. Kligman, *J. Invest. Dermatol., 62,* 268 (1974).
9. D. Blair and C. A. Lewis, *Br. J. Dermatol., 82,* 572 (1970).
10. R. K. Frienkel, *N. Engl. J. Med., 280,* 1161 (1969).
11. R. K. Frienkel, J. S. Strauss, S. Y. Yip, and P. E. Pochi, *N. Engl. J. Med., 273,* 850 (1965).
12. W. J. Cunliffe and M. Williams, *Lancet, 2,* 1055 (1973).
13. M. Williams, W. J. Cunliffe, and D. Gould, *Br. J. Dermatol., 90,* 631 (1974).
14. A. M. Kligman and O. H. Mills, *Arch. Dermatol., 106,* 843 (1972).
15. G. Plewig, J. E. Fulton, and A. M. Kligman, *Arch. Dermatol., 101,* 580 (1970).
16. S. B. Frank, "Acne Vulgaris," Charles C Thomas, Springfield, Ill., 1971, p. 175.
17. R. M. Reisner, *Pediatr. Clin. N. Am., 20,* 851 (1973).
18. O. H. Mills and A. M. Kligman, *Br. J. Dermatol., 86,* 620 (1972).
19. J. S. Strauss, P. H. Goldman, S. Nacht, and E. H. Gans, *Arch. Dermatol., 114,* 1340 (1978).
20. Panel Recommendations: FDA OTC Panel on Topical Antimicrobials, Information Copy.
21. J. Fulton, et al., *J. Cutan. Pathol., 1,* 191 (1974)
22. P. Vasarenish, *Arch. Dermatol., 98,* 183 (1968).
23. J. E. Fulton, *Arch. Dermatol., 110,* 83 (1974).
24. S. B. Frank, *Postgrad. Med., 61,* 92 (1977).
25. Ad Hoc Committee on the Use of Antibiotics in Dermatology, *Arch. Dermatol., 111,* 1630 (1975).
26. P. Dantzig, *Arch. Dermatol., 112,* 53 (1976).
27. B. S. Belnap, *Cutis, 23,* 856 (1979).
28. G. Michaelsson, I. Juklin, and A. Vahlquist, *Arch. Dermatol., 113,* 31 (1977).
29. I. Orris, A. R. Shalita, D. Sibulkin, S. J. London, and E. H. Gans, *Arch. Dermatol., 114,* 1018 (1978).
30. V. M. Weimar, S. C. Puhl, W. H. Smith, and J. E. tenBroeke, *Arch. Dermatol., 114,* 1776 (1978).

Acne Product Table

Product (Manufacturer)	Application Form	Benzoyl Peroxide	Sulfur	Resorcinol/ Salicylic Acid	Other Ingredients
Acnaveen (Cooper Care)	bar		2%	salicylic acid, 2%	colloidal oatmeal, 50%
Acne-Aid (Stiefel)	cream lotion		2.5% (cream) 10% (lotion)	resorcinol, 1.25% (cream)	alcohol, 10% (lotion) chloroxylenol, 0.375% (cream)
Acne-Aid Detergent Soap (Stiefel)	cleanser				sulfated surfactants hydrocarbon hydrotropes, 6.3%
Acnomel (Menley & James Labs)	cream cleanser		8% (cream) 4% (cleanser)	resorcinol, 2% (cream) 1% (cleanser)	
Benoxyl (Stiefel)	lotion	5 and 10%			
Bensulfoid (Poythress)	lotion		colloidal, 2%	resorcinol, 2%	alcohol, 12% zinc oxide, 6% thymol, 0.5% hexachlorophene, 0.1% perfume
Betadine Skin Cleanser (Purdue Frederick)	cleanser				povidone-iodine, 7.5%
Brasivol (Stiefel)	cleanser				aluminum oxide neutral soap detergents (fine, medium, rough)
Clearasil Acne Treatment Stick (Vicks)	stick		8%	resorcinol, 1%	
Clearasil Antibacterial Soap (Vicks)	soap				triclosan, 0.75%
Clearasil Benzoyl Peroxide Lotion (Vicks)	lotion	5%			
Clearasil BP Acne Treatment (Vicks)	cream	10%			
Clearasil Pore Deep Cleanser (Vicks)	liquid			salicylic acid, 0.5%	alcohol, 43%
Cuticura (Jeffrey Martin)	ointment		precipitated		8-hydroxyquinoline petrolatum mineral oil mineral wax isopropyl palmitate synthetic beeswax phenol pine oil rose geranium oil
Cuticura Acne Cream (Jeffrey Martin)	cream	5%			alcohol, 1%

Acne Product Table, continued

Product (Manufacturer)	Application Form	Benzoyl Peroxide	Sulfur	Resorcinol/ Salicylic Acid	Other Ingredients
Cuticura Medicated Soap (Jeffrey Martin)	soap		not stated		triclocarban, 1% oxyquinoline soap base
Dry and Clear Acne Cream (Whitehall)	cream	10%			
Dry and Clear Acne Medication (Whitehall)	lotion	5%			
Dry and Clear Cleanser (Whitehall)	liquid			salicylic acid, 0.5%	benzethonium chloride, 0.1% benzoic acid, 0.5% alcohol, 50%
Fostex (Westwood)	cream cleanser soap		2%	salicylic acid, 2%	
Fostex (Westwood)	gel	5%			
Fostex (Westwood)	cake		2%		
Fostril (Westwood)	lotion		2%		laureth-4 zinc oxide talc
Ionax Foam (Owen)	aerosol foam				benzalkonium chloride, 0.2% polyoxyethylene ethers soapless surfactant
Ionax Scrub (Owen)	paste				benzalkonium chloride, 0.2% granular polyethylene polyoxyethylene ethers alcohol, 10%
Klaron (Dermik)	lotion		colloidal, 5%	salicylic acid, 2%	alcohol, 13.1%
Komed (Barnes-Hind)	lotion			salicylic acid, 2%	isopropyl alcohol, 22% sodium thiosulfate, 8% menthol camphor colloidal alumina
Komex (Barnes-Hind)	cleanser				sodium borate tetrahydrate decahydrate granules
Liquimat (Owen)	lotion		5%		alcohol, 22% tinted bases
Listerex Golden Lotion (Warner-Lambert)	cleanser			salicylic acid, 2%	polyethylene granules surface-active cleansers
Listerex Herbal Lotion (Warner-Lambert)	cleanser			salicylic acid, 2%	polyethylene granules surface-active cleansers
Loroxide (Dermik)	lotion	5.5%			

Acne Product Table, continued

Product (Manufacturer)	Application Form	Benzoyl Peroxide	Sulfur	Resorcinol/ Salicylic Acid	Other Ingredients
Lotio Alsulfa (Doak)	lotion		colloidal, 5%		colloidal clays, 95%
Lowila (Westwood)	soap				dextrin sodium lauryl sulfoacetate water boric acid urea sorbitol mineral oil DEG–14M lactic acid docusate sodium cellulose gum
Medicated Face Conditioner (MFC) (Mennen)	liquid			salicylic acid, 1%	alcohol, 55%
Microsyn (Syntex)	lotion			resorcinol, 2% salicylic acid, 2%	sodium thiosulfate, 8% colloidal alumina menthol camphor isopropyl alcohol, 25%
Multiscrub (Bristol-Myers)	cream		2%	salicylic acid, 1.5%	soapless detergents polyethylene resin granules, 26%
Noxzema Antiseptic Skin Cleanser (Noxell)	cleanser				alcohol, 65% aluminum chlorhydroxy allantoinate
Noxzema 12-hour Acne Medicine (Noxell)	lotion		10%		
Oxy-5 (Norcliff Thayer)	lotion	5%			
Oxy-10 (Norcliff Thayer)	lotion	10%			
Oxy Wash (Norcliff Thayer)	liquid	10%			
Pan Oxyl Bar (Norcliff Thayer)	cleanser	5%			
Pernox Lotion (Westwood)	lotion		2%	salicylic acid, 1.5%	surfactants polyethylene granules
Pernox Regular and Lemon (Westwood)	cleanser		2%	salicylic acid, 1.5%	surfactants polyethylene granules
Persadox (Owen)	lotion cream	5%			
Persadox HP (Owen)	cream lotion	10%			
pHisoAc (Winthrop)	cream		colloidal, 6%	resorcinol, 1.5%	alcohol, 10%

Acne Product Table, continued

Product (Manufacturer)	Application Form	Benzoyl Peroxide	Sulfur	Resorcinol/ Salicylic Acid	Other Ingredients
pHisoDerm (Winthrop)	cleanser				sodium octoxynol-3 sulfonate white petrolatum water lanolin lanolin alcohol sodium benzoate octoxynol-1 methylcellulose lactic acid
Postacne (Dermik)	lotion		microsize, 2%		alcohol, 29%
Quinolor Compound (Squibb)	ointment	10%			halquinols, 0.5% menthol methyl salicylate polyethylene mineral oil eugenol
Rezamid (Dermik)	lotion		microsize, 5%	resorcinol, 2%	alcohol, 28.5% chloroxylenol, 0.5%
Saligel (Stiefel)	gel			salicylic acid, 5%	hydroalcoholic gel alcohol, 40%
Sastid AL (Stiefel)	cleanser		1.6%	salicylic acid, 1.6%	aluminum oxide, 20% surfactants
Sastid Plain (Stiefel)	cleanser		1.6%	salicylic acid, 1.6%	soapless surfactants
Sastid Soap (Stiefel)	cleanser		10%	salicylic acid, 3%	
Seba-Nil (Owen)	solution				alcohol, 49.7% polysorbate 80
Seba-Nil Cleansing Mask (Owen)	cleanser				polyethylene granules
Spectro-Jel (Recsei)	gel				isopropyl alcohol, 15% methylcellulose, 1.5% glycol–polysiloxane, 1% cetylpyridinium chloride, 0.1%
Stri-Dex Medicated Pads (Lehn & Fink)	medicated pads			salicylic acid, 0.5%	sulfonated alkylbenzenes citric acid alcohol, 28%
Sulforcin (Owen)	lotion		5%	resorcinol, 2%	alcohol, 11.65%
Sulfur Soap (Stiefel)	cleanser		precipitated, 10%		
Sulpho-Lac (Alvin Last)	cream		not stated		sulfurated lime zinc sulphate
Sulpho-Lac (Alvin Last)	soap		9%		zinc oxide, 1%

Acne Product Table, continued

Product (Manufacturer)	Application Form	Benzoyl Peroxide	Sulfur	Resorcinol/ Salicylic Acid	Other Ingredients
Topex (Vicks)	lotion	10%			
Transact (Westwood)	gel		2%		laureth-4, 6% alcohol, 37%
Tyrosum Packets (Summers)	cleanser				alcohol acetone polysorbate
Vanoxide (Dermik)	lotion	5%			
Vlemasque (Dermik)	solution				sulfurated lime solution, 6% alcohol, 7%
Xerac BP (Person & Covey)	gel				laureth-4
Zinc Sulfide Compound Lotion (Upjohn)	lotion		22 gr		zinc, 12.3 gr boric acid, 2 mg/ml sodium borate, 11.6 mg/ml aluminum hydroxide, 18.2 mg/ml

30

Dermatitis, Dry Skin, Dandruff, Seborrhea, and Psoriasis Products

Joseph R. Robinson and Laura J. Gauger

Questions to Ask the Patient

How long have you had this condition?

Which area of the skin is affected? Is the condition patchy or uniformly distributed?

Do you have the condition all the time or does it come and go?

What seems to make the condition worse?

Is your skin exposed to detergents or chemicals at home or at work? What types of cosmetics do you use?

Have you recently made any changes in products for personal use (soap, deodorant, or shampoo)?

Do you have a family history of skin disease, asthma, or hay fever?

Are you taking any medicines?

Have you consulted a dermatologist? What was recommended?

What treatments have you used? How effective were they?

Considering the skin's exposure to a wide variety of chemicals and environmental insults, it demonstrates remarkable resiliency and recuperative ability. (See Chapter 28, *Topical Anti-infective Products.*) However, under certain conditions the skin's defenses break down and drug therapy may be beneficial. Conditions such as dermatitis, dry skin, dandruff, seborrhea, and psoriasis must be considered from both the cosmetic and pathologic points of view so that the pharmacist can advise patients on the appropriate use of nonprescription products.

Dermatitis

Dermatitis is a noninfectious, inflammatory dermatosis in which the affected skin is erythematous. It is a pattern of skin manifestations rather than a specific disease and can be either acute or chronic.

The term "eczema" was used formerly for a large group of inflammatory skin disorders of unknown etiology, many of which are now called by more specific names, such as seborrhea and psoriasis. When the cause of a particular skin condition was elucidated, the disease was given a different name, and the eczema nomenclature was dropped or modified. Today most dermatologists use the more current term "dermatitis" and define it as "skin inflammation from whatever cause." Dermatitis may be precipitated by external (exogenous) or internal (endogenous) sources.

Symptoms

The main symptoms of dermatitis are pruritus and weeping of the skin. The itching may convert to pain over time, and the weeping may diminish, giving way to a dry, scaly condition; at no time does the epidermal tissue appear normal. Symptoms may include redness, papules, vesicles, and edema. (See Table 1 for a definition of selected dermatologic terms.) The lesions may be patchy in distribution. In the acute stages, there is a uniform pattern of papular vesicles on an erythematous base.

In the chronic form of the condition, weeping may be absent, but epidermal thickening and scaling are present. Excoriations, crusting, and secondary infections may occur as sequelae to the pruritus (1).

Exogenously Induced Dermatitis

The conditions of exogenously induced dermatitis are grouped under the general heading of contact dermatitis (Table 2). They include irritant dermatitis, due to primary or secondary irritants, and allergic dermatitis. Skin diseases are the most common of all reported occupational diseases, and the majority of these cases are due to contact dermatitis. Agricultural and manufacturing workers face the greatest risk (2). The offending substance irritates the skin on first or multiple exposure or may generate an allergic response. In either case the result is skin inflammation.

Table 1. Definition of selected dermatologic terms

Term	Definition
Crust (scab)	Dried remains of exudate from erosive or ulcerated skin lesions
Erythema	A reddening of the skin caused by congestion of the dermal vasculature
Ulceration	An erosion of the epidermis extending into the dermis
Necrosis	Death of a cell or group of cells that form part of the living body
Papule	A solid, circumscribed elevation of the skin, varying roughly from 1 mm to 1 cm in size
Pustule (superficial abscess)	A circumscribed collection of free pus in the skin
Scale	Accumulation of loose, horny fragments of stratum corneum
Vesicle (blister)	A sharply circumscribed collection of free fluid in the skin
Plaque	A papular lesion greater than 1 cm in size

Adapted from S. L. Moschella, D. M. Pillsbury, and H. J. Hurley, Jr., "Dermatology," W. B. Saunders, Philadelphia, Pa., 1975.

Irritant Dermatitis

A primary irritant, such as a strong acid, generally elicits a response on first exposure; secondary irritants such as soaps, cosmetics, topical medications, and detergents cause an inflammatory response only if the agent is repeatedly applied or if certain ancillary circumstances are met.

The symptoms of irritant dermatitis range from mild erythema accompanied by pruritus to actual necrosis and skin ulceration. Primary irritants cause pruritic erythema or perhaps ulceration; secondary irritants, which frequently generate a low-grade inflammation for a long period, tend to produce symptoms more closely related to chronic dermatitis (Table 2).

Generally, the factors influencing skin irritation are the chemical itself, the climate, and biologic variation in the host. The degree of skin irritation from an applied substance is a function of the intrinsic irritation potential of the test material, its concentration, and its ability to remain bound to the skin.

Applying a strong acid or base to the cutaneous skin surface causes irritation and a subsequent inflammatory reaction. Similarly, the irritant properties of topical drugs such as camphor, coal tar, menthol, and resor-cinol are well known, but classification of these agents as primary or secondary irritants is a function of their concentration. Very high camphor concentrations are needed to produce the same degree of irritation as that achieved with relatively low coal tar levels. Agents such as bithionol and hexachlorophene, which are bound to the epidermal layer, cause irritation with repeated application. Some substances used to treat certain skin conditions, such as psoriasis, may be irritating to the affected skin.

Environmental conditions play a role in skin texture and its resistance to irritant substances. High humidity allows greater skin hydration and thus faster penetration. Occlusion also keeps the skin hydrated.

Factors such as age and skin color also are influential in irritant dermatitis. Aged skin is less prone to irritation than youthful skin, presumably because penetration is more difficult. Darker skinned races seem to be less susceptible than lighter skinned individuals, although the evidence to prove this observation is scant.

Concomitant administration of more than one substance may induce skin irritation. A secondary irritant that is not irritating to the skin when applied alone may cause irritation in combination with an agent that promotes absorption, such as a surfactant or keratolytic. Damaged skin also encourages skin irritation.

One of the most common forms of irritant dermatitis that the pharmacist will confront is hand dermatitis or "dishpan hands." This condition often is due to repeated exposure to mild primary irritants such as soap and water. It is marked by erythema, dryness, chapping, and pruritus of the dorsa.

Allergic Dermatitis

Allergic reactions are classified as immediate (anaphylactic), intermediate (Arthus), cytotoxic, and delayed (tuberculin) (Table 3). Most cases of allergic contact dermatitis fall into the category of delayed hypersensitivity reactions. Common contact allergens include nickel, chromate, the catechols of poison ivy and poison oak, synthetic chemicals, and topical drugs such as antibiotics, antihistamines, and "caine" types of local anesthetics (3). (See Chapter 31, *Poison Ivy and Poison Oak Products,* and Chapter 28, *Topical Anti-infective Products.*) Components of cosmetics may also serve as contact allergens; the most common offenders include lanolin, parabens, perfumes, and dyes.

True allergic reactions cannot occur on first exposure to an allergen. Some individuals react abnormally, with appropriate skin manifestations, to common substances such as mushrooms, strawberries, or shellfish, but the changes do not appear to be mediated by antibodies or delayed sensitivity mechanisms, and they usually occur on first exposure. Thus they are not allergies but rather idiosyncrasies caused by an intrinsic factor or defect in the tissues. (See *Plate 6-26.*)

- **Immediate (anaphylactic) reaction**—In this case the antibody sensitizes tissue cells passively. Subsequent administration of exogenous antigen reaches the sensitized cells, causing cell injury and release of endogenous agents such as histamine, kinins, and

Table 2. Exogenously induced dermatitis

Characteristic	Weak or secondary irritant dermatitis[a]	Irritant dermatitis[b]	Allergic dermatitis[c]
Mechanism	Abrasion, desiccation, trauma, dryness, soreness, and fissures precede eruption	Direct insult to tissue, no preceding dryness or fissuring	Immunologic, initial contact sensitizes, subsequent contact elicits a response, no preceding eruption
Onset	Slow; over days, months, or years	Sudden; response in 30 minutes to several days after exposure	Sudden; response in 24–48 hours after exposure
Symptoms	Hyperkeratosis, erythema, vesicles, and fissuring	Erythema, vesicles, exudation, and sometimes necrosis	Erythema, vesicles, edema, and necrosis
Usual location	Hands	Hands	Hands and face
Patch test	Negative	Positive	Positive

[a]Cumulative insults are required.
[b]Single exposure to an offending agent is sufficient.
[c]Multiple exposures are usually required.

Table 3. Types of allergic reactions in the skin

	Anaphylaxis	Arthus reaction	Cytotoxic reaction	Delayed reaction
Response mediator	Sensitizing antibody	Precipitating antibody	Antibody or cell	Cell
Skin test	Immediate wheal or flare	Arthus reaction with polymorph infiltration, appearing in 2–4 hours but may progress to necrosis for hours or days	Immediate wheal and flare, granulomatous lesions with or without polymorphs, first appearing in 2–6 hours	Delayed, tuberculin response
Clinical manifestation	Erythema	Serum sickness	Eczema	Eczema
Skin or vascular changes	Urticaria; angioneurotic edema	Allergic vasculitis; nodular vasculitis	Purpura; homograft rejection	Contact dermatitis; homograft rejection

Adapted from W. E. Parrish, "An Introduction to the Biology of the Skin," Blackwell Scientific, Oxford, England, 1970.

prostaglandins. These agents cause further local changes, which usually include contraction of smooth muscle, increased vascular permeability, and edema. The cell injury from this type of reaction is transient, and most of the cells recover. However, cell death may occur. Antihistamines suppress or modify the tissue changes in species of animals in which histamine is the most active agent. They do not prevent the antigen-antibody reaction but rather occupy the histamine receptor sites on the effector cells.

- **Intermediate (arthus) reaction**—In this reaction the antigen combines with the antibody in tissue spaces or in the circulation to produce a type of complex, which causes secondary changes to the tissue, depending on concentration and composition. The primary change is massive infiltration of the extra-vascular tissue; this usually occurs 2–4 hours after exposure to the antigen. Corticosteroid administration suppresses full development of the Arthus reaction.

- **Cytotoxic reaction**—A cytotoxic reaction is one in which cells are damaged. In the allergic classification, it is restricted to cell damage caused by delayed sensitivity specific for the antigen in the susceptible target cell. The lysis of red blood cells by antibodies specific for the red cells is an example of the reaction of an antibody with an antigen acquired by the cell. The cell that has adsorbed the antigen usually is damaged.

- **Delayed (tuberculin) reaction**—This type of reaction may take 24–48 hours to reach a maximum response and occurs in the absence of demonstrable globulin antibody. The lesion produced is a diffuse reaction characterized by erythema and accumulation of fluid (edema). The allergic response may be inhibited by corticosteroids but is not altered by antihistamines. The essential features of the delayed sensitivity reaction are its mediation by cells only and its passive transfer to normal subjects by cells only.

Delayed hypersensitivity is the major mechanism involved in allergic contact dermatitis. Contact sensitization may occur 7–10 days after the first contact with a potent allergen, or it may develop after several years of repeated exposure to weaker allergens. Once the reaction is initiated, it builds in severity for 4–7 days and healing may occur in several weeks to a month. Susceptibility to allergic contact dermatitis may last a lifetime, although in certain cases hypersensitivity is lost.

Infective Dermatitis

Infective dermatitis is a skin condition caused by the presence of microorganism toxins, not by the organism's specific pathogenic activity. The mechanism of action for this type of dermatitis has not been established, but it is known that inoculating the skin of susceptible individuals with a bacterial culture or filtrate causes the condition. It is presumed that bacterial toxins or antigens elicit the unfavorable response. The condition responds favorably to systemic antibiotics.

Endogenously Induced Dermatitis

Atopic dermatitis and neurodermatitis are conditions due to unknown internal causes. Symptoms generally last longer (years) than those of exogenously induced dermatitis.

Atopic Dermatitis

This skin disease occurs primarily during childhood and early adulthood, usually in the folds of the arms or knees, and is one of the most common dermatologic problems seen in children. It may begin shortly after birth and last many years, or it may disappear after 1–2 years. The symptoms are erythema, scaling, and weeping, accompanied by severe pruritus. Patients are often intolerant to sudden changes and extremes of temperature and humidity. Unfortunately, secondary or associated infections are common, making diagnosis and treatment difficult. The etiology of the condition is unknown, but patients often have associated asthma or hay fever. Because skin sensitivity to a wide range of agents is common, skin tests are not very good diagnostic aids.

Atopic dermatitis sometimes is associated incorrectly with anaphylactic allergy. In both cases affected individuals show positive skin tests and develop allergic signs after exposure. However, normal treatment for allergy such as avoiding contact with allergens and administration of antihistamines seldom brings relief to the patient with atopic dermatitis.

Neurodermatitis

This chronic form of eczema is found more often in women and is generally localized in the nape of the neck, legs, genitoanal region, and forearms (4). The areas of involvement are highly lichenified (the skin thickens and hardens, and normal markings are exag-gerated) and become worse when continually rubbed or scratched. Since lichenified skin is more itchy than normal skin, a vicious cycle develops. Emotional stress plays a role in this disorder (5). Scratching actually becomes a conditioned response, leading to the development of the scratch-lichenification cycle. Minor tranquilizers, sedatives, and especially counseling are useful in treating this disorder.

Assessment

Because treatment of dermatitis is often different from that of other cutaneous disorders, assessment of the condition is important before initiating therapy. By noting the location and distribution of the lesions and taking a careful history of the patient's occupational and leisure activities, the pharmacist may be able to diagnose contact dermatitis. Atopic dermatitis should be considered in light of the patient's age, family history of atopy, and duration of the eruption.

Contact Dermatitis

In most cases of contact dermatitis, an accurate assessment is made readily on the basis of the eczematous character, configuration, and location of the rash and itching. Lesions are often asymmetric in distribution, reflecting where contact with the offending substance occurred. A rash on the backs and sides of the fingers and hands, eyelids, groin, wrists, and feet often suggests contact dermatitis. Seborrhea, however, also must be considered in cases of genitoanal or eyelid involvement. Tinea cruris (jock itch) and tinea pedis (athlete's foot) are other possibilities. (See Chapter 28, *Topical Anti-infective Products,* and Chapter 33, *Foot Care Products*.)

By questioning the patient about his or her environment (home, work, medications, and clothes), the pharmacist may be able to identify a possible irritant or allergen. Patch testing by a physician also is useful in diagnosis of allergic reactions. It is important to identify the offending substance, for its removal will result in improvement of the condition (6–8).

In some cases of dermatitis (especially eruptions of the hands) there is a mixture of infectious eczematoid, atopic, and contact dermatitis. With contact dermatitis, once the skin reacts to one substance, it may be more vulnerable to other substances, making diagnosis and treatment more complicated. Allergic or primary irritant dermatitis may be a secondary eruption caused by an agent used in therapy, complicating one of the other forms of dermatitis. Common offenders include benzocaine, neomycin, and ethylenediamine.

Atopic Dermatitis

Since atopic dermatitis is primarily a disease of the young, the age of the patient is important in diagnosis. By taking a medical history, the pharmacist may proceed to determine if the patient has a history of atopic disorders. The possibility of contact dermatitis must also be explored. Inquiries should be made regarding the onset and duration of the eruption. Atopic dermatitis is marked by remissions and exacerbations and, unlike contact dermatitis, single eruptions may last for months or years. Finally, the location and distribution of the lesions should be taken into account. The classic case of childhood atopic dermatitis involves the cheeks and extensor surfaces of the forearms and legs. (See *Plates 6-27A, B, and C.*) Unlike seborrhea and psoriasis, the disease generally does not involve the groin, and scalp involvement is limited to infants (9). Lesions are typically symmetric in distribution. If atopic dermatitis is suspected, a physician should be consulted.

Treatment

Dermatitis therapy must be approached cautiously to prevent deterioration of the condition. In some forms of dermatitis the patient is sensitive to a wide variety of agents, and therapeutic entities may aggravate inflamed skin. In atopic dermatitis, therapy is needed for long periods. In contact dermatitis, however, the duration of therapy is much shorter, because withdrawal of the allergen or irritant improves the condition. Before recommending any product for the treatment of contact dermatitis, the pharmacist should help the patient identify the offending substance(s). Prevention of further exposure is the key to effective therapy.

General Measures

For most forms of dermatitis, it is worthwhile to protect the lesions from clothing and fingernails, especially in small children. Clothing worn next to the skin should be absorbent, light, and nonirritating (such as cotton), laundered with bland soaps, and thoroughly rinsed (10). Wool, silk, and any rough clothing should be avoided. It may be necessary to loosely bandage the area and cut the patient's fingernails short to prevent scratching. Oral antihistamines may be useful to alleviate itching.

The patient should be instructed to avoid known irritants and allergens and self-testing to identify a suspected allergen, particularly in acute dermatitis. If repeated exposure to the substance occurs, the area should be irrigated immediately and thoroughly with water. The use of ordinary soaps containing fragrances and dyes also should be discouraged (11, 12). Cetaphil lotion, Lowila, or Neutrogena soap are suitable alternatives. Occlusive agents or covers should not be applied when weeping is present. Rather, during the acute weeping stage, saline, tap water, or Burow's solution compresses may be applied.

As an alternative to applying compresses, the patient may bathe 2 or 3 times/day using saline or tap

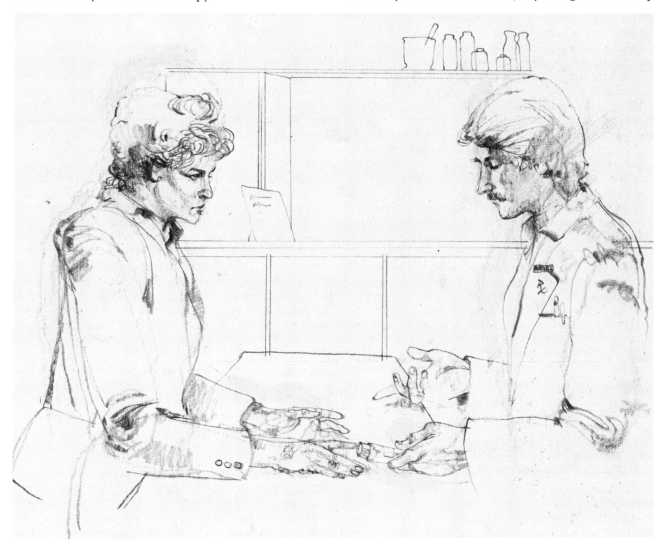

water. Exposure should be limited to 30 minutes. Oatmeal-based products such as Aveeno may be added to the bath for cleansing. Oatmeal contains 50% starch (a demulcent) with about 25% protein and 9% oil (13). It is claimed to be soothing and antipruritic, but controlled studies are lacking. If the use of compresses or bathing does not improve the weeping in 1–3 days, a physician should be consulted.

Once vesiculation subsides, topical hydrocortisone (0.5%) may be useful to decrease inflammation. The pharmacist may instruct the patient to apply the preparation every 4 hours. Improvement should be seen in several days. If not, a physician should be consulted.

The eczematous lesion may progress to a dry, scaly stage. In such a case, the patient should be instructed to soak the affected area in warm water for 5–10 minutes 3 times/day and then immediately apply an emollient such as petrolatum. This may help to moisturize the skin and alleviate attendant pruritus. Topical hydrocortisone ointment may be useful for acute flare-ups during this stage.

The pharmacist often will be confronted with cases of "dishpan hands." To aid the patient with mild hand dermatitis, the following instructions may be given (14).

- Wear vinyl gloves when doing dishes and handling fresh fruits. (Rubber gloves may be sensitizing.) Remember that wearing a glove with a hole in it will trap irritants next to the skin and is worse than wearing no gloves at all. Thin white cotton liners worn under the vinyl gloves may prevent irritation by the vinyl and absorb perspiration.
- When washing the hands, use lukewarm water and a minimal amount of soap.
- Apply a bland moisturizer such as white petrolatum or Eucerin after each hand washing and at numerous other times during the day. Do not use a wide variety of nonprescription hand creams and lotions. These may irritate the skin.
- Use a topical hydrocortisone ointment if the condition does not respond to moisturizers, barring the presence of an infection. (An ointment should be selected because of its emollient effect.) Apply the medication after each handwashing and frequently throughout the day. It should be applied thinly and massaged in thoroughly. If the skin is very dry, a thin layer of white petrolatum may be applied *after* rubbing in the hydrocortisone ointment, or cosmetic gloves may be worn.
- After the condition subsides, continue to apply a bland moisturizer or hydrocortisone ointment at least 4 times/day until the skin has healed completely.

Pharmacologic Agents

Ingredients in nonprescription products for dermatitis include antiseptics, astringents, cooling agents, antihistamines, keratolytics, protectants, and hydrocortisone. Dimers of linoleic acid represent an investigational approach.

Antiseptics

Antiseptics are necessary in infective dermatitis but should be used cautiously in the more general forms of dermatitis. Many of these agents have considerable sensitizing potential, particularly when they are used chronically. For example, neomycin should not be used for maintenance treatment of hypostatic or genitoanal dermatitis (8).

Astringents

Astringents are sometimes needed to reduce the extent of weeping. Local compresses applied 2–4 times/day for 15–30 minutes help dry weeping areas. Compresses can be made with isotonic saline solution, tap water, 1:40 or 1:20 Burow's solution, or diluted vinegar (¼ cup/pint of water). The dressings consist of washcloths or small towels soaked in the astringent solution. The dressing should be rewetted with solution throughout the period of application (15). To avoid aggravating the condition, more potent astringents should be reserved until the erythemal inflammation of the acute phase subsides. Soaks consisting of water (isotonic saline solution) or 0.25% aluminum acetate solution may be used for larger areas.

Calamine lotion and other powder-based substances that dry weeping through water adsorption or astringency should be avoided. These agents have a tendency to crust, and removing the crusts causes bleeding and potential infections.

Cooling Agents

Cooling the skin surface reduces the extent of pruritus. In the acute phase of dermatitis, soothing lotions applied as wet compresses are helpful, but aromatic substances such as menthol and camphor should be used cautiously because of their irritant potential. The cooling effect of an infrequently applied lotion or emulsion is only transitory.

Antihistamines

Orally administered antihistamines have been used for their sedative and alleged antipruritic effects. They may be useful if urticaria is present. However, the cause of itching in many other conditions such as atopic dermatitis is poorly understood, and the role of histamine has not been established. Therefore, the efficacy of systemic and topical antihistamine therapy must be questioned (16). Topical antihistamines may have an anesthetic effect on the skin but should not be recommended or used routinely because of their tendency to become skin sensitizers.

Keratolytics

Keratolytics usually are avoided in dermatitis unless extensive lichenification has occurred. These agents and those that reduce the mitotic activity of the epidermis, such as tars and anthralin, should be used cautiously.

Protectants

To protect small areas of eczematous skin, zinc oxide (Lassar's) paste, zinc oxide ointment, or paste-impregnated bandages may be used. Some of these topical products are astringents as well as protectants. Covering the lesions or applying a drug with an occlusive barrier may increase the degree of tissue maceration and prevent heat loss. This effect may contribute to discomfort of the affected area.

Bismuth subnitrate is a substance that has been used as a nonprescription skin protectant. Its efficacy has been challenged, and fatalities in infants have been reported due to oral ingestion. Therefore, the FDA advisory review panel on nonprescription skin protectant drug products tentatively recommended that bismuth subnitrate not be considered safe and effective as a skin protectant. (See Table 4 for a list of the other tentative recommendations of the panel.)

Topical Hydrocortisone

Hydrocortisone (0.5%) is one of the newer agents available for nonprescription treatment of dermatitis. Its activity stems from a generalized anti-inflammatory effect. The official indications for its use include temporary relief of minor skin irritations, itching, and rashes due to dermatitis, insect bites, poison ivy, poison oak, poison sumac, soaps, detergents, cosmetics, and jewelry, and for itchy genital or anal areas. Hydrocortisone acts prophylactically to prevent further inflammation. It does not reverse existing inflammation.

Hydrocortisone generally should be applied 3 or 4 times/day. If the emollient effect of the steroid vehicle is desired, or the agent is likely to be washed off, such as in hand dermatitis, more frequent applications may be necessary. Application to the scalp may be once a day, for the drug usually is not rubbed off (17).

Many patients do not use topical steroid preparations properly; they tend to apply far too much. Therefore, the pharmacist should instruct the patient to apply only a thin film and to massage it into the skin thoroughly. Washing or soaking the area just before application may help promote drug absorption.

Before recommending a hydrocortisone product, the pharmacist must be certain that the area of application is not infected. Signs of bacterial infection include redness, heat, pus, and crusting. Fungal infections may be marked by erythema and scaling. Topical hydrocortisone may mask the symptoms of these dermatologic infections while the infection progresses in severity.

Use of systemic steroids has been associated with many adverse effects. Topical hydrocortisone, however, generally will not produce systemic complications, because absorption is minimal. Approximately 1% of a hydrocortisone solution applied to normal skin on the forearm is absorbed systemically (18). Absorption increases in the presence of skin inflammation or with the use of occlusive agents. Certain adverse local effects such as skin atrophy may arise with prolonged use because of the antimitotic/antisynthetic effect of hydrocortisone on cells. In practice, however, clinically detectable atrophy hardly ever occurs with hydrocortisone in the concentrations available without a prescription. This problem occurs with the newer, fluorinated products. Nevertheless, continued and frequent use of topical hydrocortisone products should be discouraged. If the patient's condition worsens, or if symptoms persist for more than 7 days, therapy should be stopped and a physician consulted.

Dimers of Linoleic Acid

Dimers of linoleic acid are being investigated as prophylactic agents to reduce irritation from various detergents and allergens such as poison ivy (19). Encouraging results have been obtained after topical application of these agents, but they are not available for use in the United States.

Product Selection Guidelines

When deciding on which product to recommend for the control of dermatitis, the pharmacist must not only evaluate the various active ingredients found in nonprescription products, but also the vehicle itself. The type of vehicle (ointment, cream, lotion, gel, solution, or aerosol) has a significant effect on dermatitis. The following simple guidelines may be used to choose an appropriate vehicle (20):

- If a drying effect is desired, solutions and gels should be recommended.
- If slight lubrication is needed, creams and lotions are adequate.
- If the lesion is very dry and fissured, ointments are the vehicle of choice.
- In an acute process, ointments may cause further irritation due to their occlusive effect.
- Aerosols, gels, or lotions may be recommended when the dermatitis affects a hair-covered area of the body.

Topical nonprescription products come in various package sizes. The pharmacist must be able to recommend an appropriate amount of drug to treat a given condition. Table 5 lists the amount of drug needed to cover a given area of the body. By being aware of details such as this, the pharmacist can serve the patient economically as well as therapeutically.

Table 4. Tentative FDA classifications of nonprescription skin protectants

Compound	Category
Allantoin	I
Aluminum hydroxide gel	I
Bismuth subnitrate	II
Boric acid	II
Calamine	I
Cocoa butter	I
Corn starch	I
Dimethicone	I
Glycerin	I
Kaolin	I
Petrolatum preparations	I
Shark liver oil	I
Sodium bicarbonate	I
Sulfur	II
Tannic acid	II
Zinc acetate	I
Zinc carbonate	I
Zinc oxide	I

Table 5. Grams of cream or ointment required for four sparing applications for one day	
Part of the body	**Grams**
Face and ears	5
Neck	5
Upper extremity	10
Lower extremity	20
Anterior trunk	15
Posterior trunk	15

Excerpted from E. Epstein, "Common Skin Disorders—A Manual for Physicians and Patients," Medical Economics Company, Oradell, N.J., 07649, 1979, p. 5.

Dry Skin

Almost everyone has had dry or chapped skin. In some people it is a seasonal occurrence; in others the condition is chronic. Although dry skin is not life threatening, it is annoying and uncomfortable because of the attendant pruritus and, in some cases, pain and inflammation. In addition, dry skin is more prone to bacterial invasion than normal skin.

Symptoms

Dry skin is characterized by one or more of the following:

- Roughness and flaking;
- Loss of flexibility;
- Fissures;
- Hyperkeratosis;
- Inflammation;
- Pruritus.

The condition has a predilection for the lower legs, the back of the hands, and the forearms. Dry skin is especially prevalent during the winter months. It is known to be secondary to other disease states, prolonged detergent use, malnutrition, and physical damage to the stratum corneum.

Factors in Skin Hydration

The cardinal characteristic of a dry skin condition is inadequate moisture content in the stratum corneum. It is a common misconception that dry skin is due to a lack of natural skin oils. Rather, dry skin is due to a lack of water. The pathophysiology of dry skin therefore can be described by examining the factors involved in skin hydration.

Age

Dry skin occurs commonly in elderly individuals. As skin ages, the entire epidermal layer thins and the skin's hygroscopic substances decrease in quantity, so that ability to retain moisture decreases. Hormonal changes that accompany aging result in lowered sebum output and therefore lowered skin lubrication (21). In addition, keratin cross-linking induced by long-term exposure to ultraviolet radiation causes skin to harden. This cross-linking also is associated with increased surface dryness and general pruritus.

Other Disease States

A number of systemic and dermatologic disorders may lead to a dry skin condition. Examples of such systemic disorders include hypothyroidism and dehydration.

Dermatologic conditions marked by scaling and dryness include contact dermatitis, atopic dermatitis, and psoriasis. In psoriatic lesions, transepidermal water loss may be as high as 0.48 mg/cm²/hr as compared with 0.18 mg/cm²/hr in control subjects (22). Neighboring skin, however, is not affected (23). These dermatologic disorders may be differentiated from a simple dry skin condition on the basis of other attendant symptoms.

Two dermatologic conditions difficult to differentiate from simple dry skin are asteatotic eczema and dominant ichthyosis vulgaris. Asteatotic eczema is characterized by dry and fissured skin, inflammation, and pruritus. Sebaceous secretions are scanty or absent. It is more common during dry winter weather and in elderly individuals and apparently is an extension of the dry skin condition.

Dominant ichthyosis vulgaris affects 0.3–1.0% of the population. It is a genetic disorder that should be suspected when a patient complains of a familial tendency to excessive dryness and chapping. Patients also may have an associated history of atopic disease. Symptoms include dryness and roughness of the skin, accompanied by small, fine, white scales. The condition has a predilection for the extensor aspects of the arms and legs. Dryness of the cheeks, heels, and palms also may be noted. In severe forms of the disease, a classic fish scale-like appearance of the stratum corneum arises (22, 24).

Weather Conditions

Relative humidity is important in maintaining normal skin hydration. Keratin (the horny skin layer) softens when the stratum corneum's moisture content is about 10%. This level occurs at 60% relative humidity. In a normal indoor climate, moisture content is 10–15%; at 95% relative humidity, the stratum corneum's moisture content increases to 65%. With low temperature and relative humidity, however, the outer skin layer dries out (25, 26), becomes less flexible, and may crack when flexed, increasing the rate of moisture loss. High wind velocity also causes this condition.

Integrity of Stratum Corneum Cell Membranes

One theory states that water retention in the stratum corneum depends on the presence of hygroscopic substances within the corneum cells (27). These substances are contained by cell membranes permeable to water but not to electrolytes. Physical disruption, extraction of lipids with solvents, or prolonged detergent use may damage cell membranes, allowing the hygroscopic substances to be lost and reducing the ability of the stratum corneum to retain water (28–31).

Natural Moisturizing Factor

Moisture is diffused rapidly to the keratin layer from lower skin layers, about 50–100 times faster than it is lost from the epidermal surface to the environment. However, water movement through the keratin itself is relatively slow. A hydrophilic substance called natural moisturizing factor may influence keratin moisture retention (32). Several components of this substance, including lactate, polypeptides, hexosamines, pentoses, urea, pyrrolidine, carboxylic acids, and inorganic ions, have been isolated and identified (33–35). However, when they are applied to the skin surface, only temporary hydration results. It is thought that natural moisturizing factor, due to its natural hygroscopicity, increases the amount of water the stratum corneum absorbs at any given relative humidity but that it does not interact significantly with the protein itself in the horny layer (36).

Many of the components of natural moisturizing factor are water soluble and easily removed from the skin. Perhaps this is why excessive bathing may lead to a dry skin condition; hygroscopic substances may be leached from the skin, especially if soaps are present to disrupt stratum corneum cell membranes.

Integrity of the Stratum Corneum

To maintain normal skin hydration, the water content of the stratum corneum must remain at approximately 10%. Water is lost from the skin through perspiration (as much as 2 liters/hour under extreme thermal stress) and transepidermal diffusion, a relatively constant process. Because human skin is such an effective barrier, only about 120 ml of water/day is lost from the average adult skin surface (2 m²) through transepidermal diffusion (37). Removal of the stratum corneum barrier increases the water loss rate about 50 times (38, 39).

Physical damage to the stratum corneum dramatically increases the transepidermal water loss, but within 1–2 days a temporary parakeratotic barrier (a barrier consisting of incompletely keratinized, nucleated cells) provides 50% of the normal function, and total function is restored in 2–3 weeks.

Assessment

When assessing a dry skin condition, the pharmacist should take several factors into account before suggesting a therapeutic program that will eliminate or counteract any causative factors. Arndt outlined a series of such measures in the *Manual of Dermatologic Therapeutics* (40). The temperature and relative humidity of the home and work environment should be considered; keeping room temperatures low and using humidifiers may be beneficial. A history of the work environment also is useful to determine whether the problem may be due to repeated exposure to detergents; "dishpan hands" may be aided by the use of vinyl gloves. Frequency of bathing also should be considered. Excessive bathing (more than once every 1–2 days) may have a drying effect on the skin.

Dry skin may be the manifestation of another disease state. By obtaining a medical history, the pharmacist may be able to uncover a primary disorder triggering the dry skin condition such as hypothyroidism or atopic disease. Psoriasis and contact dermatitis are other possibilities. A drug history should be taken to investigate the possibility of a drug eruption or dehydration secondary to diuretic use. If any of these primary events is suspected or if signs of an infection are present (redness, heat, and pus), a physician should be consulted.

Asteatotic eczema and dominant ichthyosis vulgaris are difficult to differentiate from a simple dry skin condition. If the condition is severe enough to be associated with inflammation and pruritus, asteatotic eczema may be the correct diagnosis. If the pharmacist elicits a positive history of atopic disease or a familial tendency toward dry skin, or if the normal markings in the patient's palms and soles are clearly accentuated, dominant ichthyosis vulgaris is a possibility. Fortunately, misdiagnosis is not of great consequence, because simple dry skin, asteatotoic eczema, and dominant ichthyosis vulgaris are treated similarly.

Treatment

The main objectives in treating dry skin are to raise the stratum corneum's moisture level and to re-establish its integrity. Water is the only true plasticizer for human stratum corneum, but simply adding water to the skin is not a useful approach, unless the stratum corneum can retain it (32). If hydrated skin is not covered immediately with an occlusive substance, such as petrolatum or with a plastic covering, it dehydrates quickly. Several approaches in treating a dry skin condition are available (41):

- Lubricating the skin;
- Moisturizing (hydrating and thickening) the skin;
- Chemically softening the keratinous epidermal layer;
- Using topical hydrocortisone if inflammation is present.

Lubricating the Skin

A lubricant is any substance that lessens friction. It does not necessarily raise the stratum corneum moisture level. Rather, the use of a lubricant is more psychological—the skin feels smooth. Various nonprescription cosmetic products in an assortment of vehicles serve as lubricants. Those most heavily promoted in advertisements include bath oils and products containing natural vegetable and animal oils.

Bath Oils

Bath oils generally consist of a mineral or vegetable oil plus a surfactant. Mineral oil products are adsorbed better than vegetable oil products (42). Adsorption onto and absorption into the skin increases with increases in temperature and oil concentration. Bath oils, which are applied at a high temperature but unfortunately at a low oil concentration, are moderately effective in improving a dry skin condition. Part of their effect is due to the slip or lubricity they impart to the skin, which may be more important to the patient than the occlusive properties. When applied as wet compresses, however, bath oils are effective in treating dry skin (43). Patients may also be instructed to mix 1 tsp of bath oil per ¼ cup warm water and use this as a rubdown. In this way, excessive bathing may be avoided.

Natural Products

Attempts have been made to formulate products that duplicate the normal oil mantle of the skin as a means of treating dry skin. Because sebum and skin surface lipids contain a relatively high concentration of fatty acid glycerides, vegetable and animal oils, such as avocado, cucumber, mink, peanut, safflower, sesame, and turtle, have been used. The inclusion of these oils in dry skin products is presumably due to their unsaturated fatty acid content. However, sebum is not an effective barrier against moisture loss from the skin. Though the use of these oils contributes to skin flexibility and lubricity, their occlusive effect is less than that of petrolatum. There is a great psychological appeal to products containing these oils. However, their actual value in treating a dry skin condition is not documented. Squalene, another ingredient that has been utilized, is a normal component of skin lipids and serves as a reasonably effective barrier against moisture loss.

Moisturizing Agents

An ideal moisturizer should fulfill certain conditions (35). It should regulate and maintain the stratum corneum water level above the critical level (10%) but not to such a degree as to induce superhydration or maceration. Superhydration of the stratum corneum reduces its barrier efficiency, making it more susceptible to invasion by microorganisms, irritants, and allergens. In addition to this most important characteristic, the effectiveness of a moisturizing agent should be independent of environmental changes, and continued application should not cause damage to the stratum corneum by the removal of or interference with its natural moisturizers. The product should be nonirritating and nonsensitizing, and stable in cosmetic formulations. The agents used most commonly as nonprescription moisturizers are humectants and occlusives.

Humectants

Humectants are defined as substances that promote retention of water due to their hygroscopicity. The most commonly used humectants in dermatology include glycerin and propylene glycol. Theoretically, the humectant acts by being absorbed into the skin to help replace any missing hygroscopic substances, or, if absorption does not occur, the humectant on the skin surface attracts water from the atmosphere and serves as a reservoir for the stratum corneum. In the case of glycerin, however, these theoretical mechanisms of action do not apply.

Products containing 50% glycerin (glycerin and rose water) often are used to treat a dry skin condition. Glycerin does not penetrate into the skin, and high humidity is needed for it to attract water from the environment. (The incidence of dry skin is lowest when relative humidity is high.) Glycerin also increases the transepidermal moisture loss rate, an effect opposite to what is usually desirable. Despite these limitations, glycerin is effective in treating dry skin.

A partial explanation for glycerin's mechanism of action is that it accelerates moisture diffusion from the dermal tissue to the surface and holds water in intimate contact with the skin. Through this mechanism it brings moisture from the dermal region to the parched stratum corneum. In addition, glycerin provides lubrication to the skin surface. The FDA advisory review panel on nonprescription skin protectant drug products tentatively has recommended that diluted glycerin (20–45%) be given Category I status as a skin protectant. Undiluted glycerin, however, may have a dehydrating effect on the skin and is not considered by the panel to be an effective skin protectant.

Occlusive Agents

Occlusives are substances that promote retention of water due to their hydrophobicity; moisture in the skin cannot pass through the occlusive barrier. These agents, also known as emollients, often are used in combination with a humectant in dry skin formulations. The most commonly used occlusives include petrolatum, lanolin, mineral oil, and silicones.

Occlusives have several mechanisms of action in correcting a dry skin condition. First, they prevent moisture evaporation from the skin surface. Some researchers believe that the prevention of normal transepidermal water loss is not sufficient to maintain normal hydration (35). Therefore, the pharmacist should instruct the patient to soak the affected area in water for 5–10 minutes and then immediately apply the occlusive agent (44). In this way, more moisture will be trapped in the skin.

Occlusives also may act by re-establishing the integrity of the stratum corneum. It is felt that prolonged occlusion (a plastic film used 6–14 nights) enhances the metabolic rate in the epidermis, thereby increasing production of protein and low molecular weight, water-soluble materials that become part of the stratum corneum (45). Substances that restore damaged keratin quickly are preferable to occlusives with long-term action.

Frequency of application depends on the severity of the dry skin condition as well as the hydration efficiency of the occlusive agent. In the case of dry hands, the patient may need to apply the occlusive agent after each hand washing and at numerous other times during the day. Care must be exercised to avoid excessive hydration or maceration. In addition, although most commercial formulations generally are bland, contact with the eye or with broken or abraded skin should be avoided because irritation from formulation ingredients is possible in these cases. This is especially true with emulsion systems because the surfactants in these systems may denature protein. Moreover, recent studies imply that so-called "inert" vehicles may have an effect on wound healing, either accelerating or retarding it, depending on the vehicle used (46, 47).

Petrolatum seems to be the most effective occlusive agent and tentatively has been given Category I status as a skin protectant. Unfortunately, it is not well accepted by the consumer because of its greasiness and staining properties. Mineral oil is not as effective a barrier as petrolatum, and silicones are even less effective than mineral oil (48, 49). Because of its high occlusive ability, petrolatum should not be applied over puncture wounds, infections, or lacerations, since maceration and further inflammation may occur under the seal.

Lanolin is found in many nonprescription moisturizing products. It is a natural product, derived from sheep wool. Some patients develop an allergic reaction to this substance, presumably due to its wool wax fraction. For this reason, lanolin has been omitted from inclusion in many ointment preparations. Patients with a previous history of allergic reactions to topical medicaments apparently have a greater risk of developing an allergic reaction to lanolin. Through examining the patient's medication history, the pharmacist may identify such patients and advise accordingly.

There is a general lack of consumer appeal for oleaginous products because of the greasy texture and difficulty of spreading. In most cases, the less effective but more esthetic oil-in-water emulsions are preferred. These agents help alleviate the pruritus associated with dry skin by virtue of their cooling effect as the water evaporates from the skin surface. Moreover, there is sufficient oil in most oil-in-water emulsions to form a continuous occlusive film on the skin surface with the aid of waxes, gums, and other formulating agents (50). This film forms after the water has evaporated.

The second type of emulsion system is the water-in-oil emulsion. These products feel greasier than oil-in-water emulsions. Whether one emulsion form is safer and more effective than the other has not been determined. The thickness of the oil film on the skin from an oil-in-water emulsion is less than that from a water-in-oil emulsion because the former product contains less oil. However, other ingredients in the product may contribute to correcting the dry skin condition (28, 51).

Topical application of estrogenic creams improves the water retention capacity, proliferation of cells, plumpness, and overall appearance of the skin. However, the FDA limits the amount of hormone in cosmetic hormone products, and such products have no reported beneficial effect on a dry skin condition over and above that of the vehicle containing the hormone. Since most hormone-containing products are in oleaginous or semioleaginous vehicles, it is difficult to separate the contributions of the base from that of the hormone. Most, if not all, of the effects of cosmetic hormone creams (plumping of the skin, disappearance of the tiny crow's feet lines, and alleviation of the dry skin condition), are due to the vehicle rather than the hormone.

Keratin-Softening Agents

Chemically altering the keratin layer softens the skin and cosmetically improves its appearance. This treatment approach does not need substantial addition of water, but all of the attendant dry skin symptoms may not be alleviated unless water is added to the keratin layer. Agents used as softeners in nonprescription dry skin products are urea, lactic acid, and allantoin (41).

Urea (Carbamide)

Urea (10–30%) is mildly keratolytic and increases water uptake in the corneum, giving it a high water-binding capacity (52, 53). Moreover, this small molecule apparently has a direct effect on stratum corneum elasticity by virtue of its ability to bind to skin protein (54). Urea accelerates fibrin digestion at about 15% concentration and is proteolytic at 40%. It is considered safe and has been recommended for use on crusted necrotic tissue. Concentrations of 10% have been used on simple dry skin and 20–30% systems have been used for treating difficult dry skin conditions, such as those seen in podiatric practice. Urea-containing creams are claimed to produce good hydration and help remove scales and crusts (44). They also have the advantage of being less greasy than some occlusive preparations. In some instances, urea preparations cause stinging and burning and may be irritating to sensitive patients. Animal or human urine has been used for centuries in treating dry skin, presumably because of the urea content.

Lactic Acid

Lactic acid (2–5%) is an alpha-hydroxy acid that has been useful in the treatment of dry skin conditions. It is found in products such as LactiCare and Purpose Dry Skin Cream. It apparently increases the hydration of human skin and may act as a modulator of epidermal keratinization rather than as a keratolytic agent (55). The carboxyl group of the molecule seems to be indispensible for keratinization control, and structure-activity relationships for various alpha-hydroxy acids have been established (56). It is thought that alpha-hydroxy acids may serve as natural regulators of epithelial function and therefore have the potential of being ideal pharmacologic agents (19).

Allantoin

Allantoin (0.5–2.0%) and allantoin complexes are claimed to soften keratin by disrupting its structure. Allantoin is a product of purine metabolism and is considered a relatively safe compound but apparently less effective than urea. It may be useful for individuals sensitive to various topical preparations, for it is purported to form complexes with a variety of sensitizing agents, rendering them nonsensitizing (57). The FDA advisory review panel on nonprescription skin protectant drug products has tentatively recommended that allantoin be considered safe and effective as a skin protectant for adults, children, and infants when applied in concentrations of 0.5–2.0%.

Topical Hydrocortisone

Topical hydrocortisone (0.5%) may be used in the treatment of dry skin if inflammation and its attendant pruritus are present. An ointment should be selected because of its emollient effect. However, the inflammation and pruritus associated with dry skin is best treated by alleviating its cause (restoring normal skin hydration). Therefore, a more direct approach to the problem is to use moisturizers and keratin-softening agents.

Secondary Formulation Ingredients

The main active ingredients contained in nonprescription dry skin products are simply water and oil. However, an overwhelming number of secondary ingredients are added to enhance product elegance and stability:

- **Emulsifiers**
  Cholesterol
  Magnesium aluminum silicate
  Polyoxyethylene lauryl ether (Brij)
  Polyoxyethylene monostearate (Myrj)
  Polyoxyethylene sorbitan monolaurate (Tween)
  Propylene glycol monostearate
  Sodium borate plus fatty acid
  Sodium lauryl sulfate
  Sorbitan monopalmitate (Span)
  Triethanolamine plus fatty acid

- **Emulsion stabilizers (thickening agents)**
  Carbomer
  Cetyl alcohol
  Glyceryl monostearate
  Methylcellulose
  Spermaceti
  Stearyl alcohol

- **Preservatives**
  Cresol
  Parabens

Many secondary formulation ingredients have the potential for producing contact dermatitis, either through an irritant or sensitizing effect. For example, sodium lauryl sulfate, polysorbates, and sorbitan esters may serve as dermal irritants; ethylenediamine, parabens, or naturally occurring fatty substances may generate allergic reactions. From a toxicity standpoint, these ingredients cannot be assumed inert.

Product Selection Guidelines

When deciding on which product to recommend for a dry skin condition, the pharmacist should take three factors into account: the efficacy of individual products, the area to which the agent will be applied, and patient acceptance. One of the most efficacious products for dry skin care is petrolatum. Moreover, many elderly patients seem to tolerate it better than some of the more elegant preparations (44). Other effective alternatives include Eucerin, Nivea cream, Purpose Dry Skin Cream, and urea-containing products such as Aquacare/HP. Urea products not only are effective, but have the advantage of being less greasy than many of the occlusive agents.

A large number of cosmetic dry skin formulations are available on the market. These may contain natural oils, vitamins, or a variety of fragrances that have a great psychologic appeal. However, the fragrances and dyes found in many of these formulations may be irritating to sensitive dry skin.

Efficacy may need to be sacrificed to achieve patient acceptance of a product. Greasy products may be unacceptable if the area of application is the face, hands, feet, or intertriginous (skin fold) areas. In such cases, gels or oil-in-water emulsions may be useful. Gels and lotions also may be used if the area of application is quite hairy. The pharmacist should recommend the most efficacious product that the patient will accept.

Dandruff

Dandruff is a chronic, noninflammatory scalp condition characterized by excessive scaling of scalp tissue (58). Subjective estimates of its incidence range widely (2.5–70% of the population) (59, 60). However, on the basis of visual observation and objective corneocyte count, about 18% of the population has moderately severe dandruff or worse, and another 18% has mild dandruff (61, 62).

Dandruff is not a disease but rather a normal physiologic event much like growth of hair and nails, except that the end product is visible on the scalp and thus has substantial cosmetic and social impact. It appears at puberty, when many skin activities are altered, reaches a peak in early adulthood, levels off in middle age, and declines in advancing years. The process correlates very well with the proliferative activity of the epidermis.

Symptoms

Dandruff is characterized by accelerated epidermal cell turnover (epidermopoiesis), an irregular keratin break-up pattern, and the shedding of cells in large flakes. Pruritus may also occur. It is normal for epidermal cells on the scalp to slough off continually just as on other parts of the body. However, the epidermal cell turnover rate in normal individuals is greater on the scalp than on other parts of the body and involves the infundibulum of the hair follicle (63, 64). In dandruff patients, the epidermal cell turnover rate is about twice that in individuals without dandruff.

Flaking seems to be the only visible manifestation of dandruff. This is a result of an increased rate of horny substance production on the scalp and the sloughing of large scales (squamae). Dandruff flakes often appear around a hair shaft due to the epithelial growth at the base of the hair, which restricts elimination of sloughed keratin. The flakes appear white because of air in the clefts between the cellular fragments. This phenomenon does not occur in the normal condition, because the horny substance breaks up in a much more uniform fashion (58). Scalp horny layer in normal individuals consists of 25–35 fully keratinized, closely coherent cells per square millimeter arranged in an orderly fashion. However, in dandruff, the intact horny layer has fewer than 10 normal cells per square millimeter and nonkeratinized cells are common. With dandruff, crevices occur deep in the stratum corneum, resulting in cracking, which generates large flakes. If the large clumps or flakes can be broken down to smaller units, the visibility of dandruff decreases.

As the rate of keratin cell turnover increases, the number of incompletely keratinized cells (parakeratotic cells) increases. Parakeratosis is characterized by retention of nuclei in keratin layer cells. The number of these cells helps distinguish dandruff from psoriasis or seborrhea; there are more cells in psoriasis and seborrhea than in the dandruff condition. Parakeratotic cells in dandruff appear in clusters, possibly as a result of tiny inflammation foci that are incited when capillaries squirt a load of inflammatory cells into the epidermis, causing accelerated epidermal growth in a small area

(65). These microfoci are found in all scalps but are increased proportionately in dandruff.

The specific cause of the accelerated cell growth seen in dandruff is unknown. It is not due, as had been earlier theorized, to microorganisms. For many years it was assumed that dandruff was a result of elevated microorganism levels, particularly of the yeast, *Pityrosporum ovale,* on the scalp (60, 66). However, the presence of these organisms does not lead to dandruff, nor does their elimination influence the condition (67). Their accelerated growth occurs as a result of the dandruff condition, which provides a favorable growth medium. Despite the absence of a causative link between micro-organisms and dandruff, certain antidandruff products contain antimicrobial ingredients such as benzalkonium chloride, povidone iodine, and diiodohydroxyquin. The questionable statement, "to prevent secondary infections," is not altogether acceptable as a rationale for inclusion of these agents.

Assessment

Dandruff is a trivial medical problem, and treatment is fairly straightforward. Some characteristic features may help the pharmacist in distinguishing dandruff from other, more serious skin conditions such as seborrhea and psoriasis (61):

- Dandruff is seasonal; it is mild in the summer months and most severe from October through December.
- Unlike seborrhea and psoriasis, dandruff is considered noninflammatory and is limited to the scalp.
- Dandruff is uniform and diffuse in its distribution. Patchiness occurs only as a result of brushing the hair, which dislodges adherent flakes.
- Dandruff is a very stable process and is not subject to sudden shifts in severity from week to week. It is less subject to outside stress than psoriasis and seborrhea.

- Poor hygiene does not cause dandruff in a nondandruff patient, but it can exacerbate existing symptoms.

Table 6 lists distinguishing features of dandruff, seborrhea, and psoriasis. In addition to these rather general differences, there are more elaborate cytologic differences (68). For the pharmacist without access to extensive laboratory diagnostic aids, the site of the condition, the influence of external factors, and the overall severity of the condition are often useful in distinguishing the conditions.

Treatment

There is no cure for dandruff, only control of the condition. Total removal of hair eliminates the dandruff condition, but this approach is obviously rather drastic and generally unacceptable. Cleaning the hair and scalp frequently, perhaps daily, often is sufficient to control dandruff. Nonprescription dandruff products contain specific ingredients to reduce epidermal turnover rate, dissolve keratin flakes, and disperse the scales into smaller subunits. Dandruff is not a type of scalp dermatitis. Therefore, the use of nonprescription hydrocortisone products is not indicated.

To control a dandruff condition, patients may change from one antidandruff product to another. This is rational as long as the patient changes to a product with a different mechanism of action.

Cytostatic Agents

Using cytostatic agents is the most direct approach to controlling dandruff. By increasing the time necessary for epidermal turnover, it is possible to bring about a dramatic decline in visible scurf. Selenium sulfide (Selsun Blue) and zinc pyrithione (Head and Shoulders) at concentrations of 1–2% reduce cell turnover rate

Table 6. Distinguishing features of dandruff, seborrhea, and psoriasis			
Characteristic	**Dandruff**	**Seborrhea**	**Psoriasis**
Location	Scalp	Scalp and other areas of the body, e.g., axilla	Scalp and other areas of the body, particularly those prone to stress (elbows, knees, scalp, and face)
Influence of external factors	Generally a stable condition, does not fluctuate from week to week	Influenced by many external factors, notably stress	Influenced by irritation and other external stress
Inflammation	Absent	Present	Present
Epidermal hyperplasia	Absent	Present	Present
Epidermal kinetics	Turnover rate is two times faster than normal[a]	Turnover rate is about five to six times faster than normal[a]	Turnover rate is about five to six times faster than normal[a]
Percentage of parakeratotic cells	Rarely exceeds 5% of total corneocyte count[b]	Commonly makes up 15–25% of corneocyte count[b]	Commonly makes up 40–60% of corneocyte count[a]

[a]Adapted from K. J. McGinley et al., *J. Invest. Dermatol., 53,* 107 (1969)
[b]Adapted from A. M. Kligman et al., *J. Soc. Cosmet. Chem., 25,* 73 (1974)

significantly. This cytostatic activity is not restricted to conditions where the rate of epidermal turnover is great, but also is observed in normal skin, where application of these compounds proportionately lengthens turnover time. Each product has its own mechanism of action for accomplishing this. Selenium sulfide is thought to have a direct antimitotic effect on epidermal cells whereas zinc pyrithione's action is more likely due to a nonspecific toxicity for epidermal cells. The pyrithione moiety is apparently the active part of the molecule (69). Zinc pyrithione is considered by some to be slower acting than selenium sulfide, but this suggestion has not been proven (61, 64). At nonprescription concentrations, both products are effective in controlling dandruff.

Their effectiveness is influenced by several factors. Zinc pyrithione is strongly bound to both hair and the external skin layers, and the extent of binding correlates with clinical performance (70). The drug does not penetrate into the dermal region. Its absorption increases with contact time, temperature, concentration, and frequency of application. Before using one of these products, the patient may be advised to shampoo with a cleansing agent to remove dirt and scale. This may be followed by a zinc pyrithione shampoo, worked into the scalp vigorously for 5–10 minutes, and repeated 2–3 times weekly.

Long-term use of 1–2% zinc pyrithione shampoos has not been associated with toxicity. Nevertheless, pharmacists should caution against using this agent on broken or abraded skin. Rare cases of contact dermatitis have been reported.

Selenium sulfide, like zinc pyrithione, is more effective with longer contact time and should be applied in a similar manner. This product must be rinsed from the hair thoroughly or discoloration may result. Frequent use of selenium sulfide tends to leave a residual odor and make the scalp oily. The pharmacist may advise the patient to follow the selenium sulfide shampoo with a cream rinse or conditioner to help counteract any undesirable effects. This, however, may reduce the efficacy of the therapeutic shampoo (71, 72).

In general, cytostatic toxicity is minimal. Selenium sulfide, however, has been associated with several adverse effects; skin burns, particularly under the fingernails, and some cases of conjunctivitis have been reported. Pharmacists should caution the patient to avoid contact with the eyes and broken skin. Selenium sulfide is highly toxic if ingested orally.

Keratolytic Agents

Keratolytic agents are used in dandruff products to dissolve or lyse keratin and facilitate its removal from the scalp in smaller particles. There are many types of keratolytics, with distinctly different modes of action. Resorcinol is presumed to act as a keratolytic by its irritant effect, which causes vesicle formation in the stratum corneum. Sulfur is believed to function by an inflammatory process, causing increased sloughing of cells. Salicylic acid lowers skin pH, causing increased hydration of keratin and thus facilitating its loosening and removal.

Vehicle composition, contact time, and concentration are important considerations to the success of a keratolytic. Salicylic acid functions best as a keratolytic when used in an oil-in-water emulsion base (73–76), whereas sulfur shows its best activity in a nonemulsion base. Contact time is minimal in a shampoo. Therefore, significant absorption/adsorption of the agent by the skin cannot occur. Ointments applied a few times per day and left on are naturally much more effective. However, ointments and pastes are difficult to use on the hairy scalp, and thus aqueous and alcoholic preparations are preferred.

The keratolytic concentrations in nonprescription scalp products are not sufficient to impair the normal skin barrier but do affect the abnormal parakeratotic stratum corneum (77). Salicylic acid at a concentration of 10–15% shows a keratolytic effect in 2–3 days; 3–5% concentrations take 7 days; and 1% concentrations (the usual concentration in nonprescription shampoos is 1–2%) take 10 days. Sulfur acts similarly. A 10–20% concentration is keratolytic after 1–2 days, 5% in 7 days, 3% in 8–9 days, and 1% in 14 days. The *Medical Letter* has classified antidandruff keratolytic products as being moderately effective in controlling dandruff (72).

Keratolytic agents are associated with several adverse side effects, and the pharmacist should counsel the patient accordingly. These agents have a primary irritant effect, particularly on mucous membranes and the conjunctiva of the eye. Toxic manifestations after application of resorcinol to broken or abraded skin have been reported (78, 79). These agents also have the potential of acting on hair keratin as well as skin keratin, and hair appearance may suffer as a result.

The FDA advisory review panel on nonprescription miscellaneous external drug products has recommended that salicylic acid (2–3%) and sulfur (2–5%) be placed in Category I for dandruff treatment. This rating also applies to products containing both ingredients.

Scale-Dispersing Agents

Dispersing the scales into smaller subunits decreases their visibility and may be accomplished by several means. Agitation of the scalp during shampooing provides an immediate dispersion of scales. Components of both nonmedicated and medicated shampoos may contribute to maintaining this effect.

For mild forms of dandruff, vigorous washing with a nonmedicated shampoo at frequent intervals (every 1–3 days) may help control excess scaling. This beneficial effect may be due to the detergent found in the shampoo. Many nonmedicated shampoos leave a detergent residue on the scalp that perhaps interrupts the lipid-horny cell layer structure at the keratin layer surface, causing subsequent sloughing of keratin in smaller, less-visible subunits. (See Chapter 19, *Personal Care Products*.)

Medicated dandruff shampoos that contain various detergents, antiseptics, and coal tars also are available. These products are not to be confused with the cytostatic and keratolytic agents mentioned earlier. Rather, their primary effect may be due to scale dispersion. Because their activity increases with longer contact time, medicated shampoos should be left on the scalp for 5–10 minutes before rinsing. It is important to rinse the hair thoroughly after shampooing: Although a detergent residue may be beneficial to a point, soaps and other components of medicated products sometimes act as a "glue," joining together small flakes to make larger, more visible ones.

Detergents found in dandruff shampoos include sodium lauryl sulfate, polyoxyethylene ethers, triethanolamine, and quaternary ammonium compounds. Due to their surfactant activity, these agents may function to reduce the size of the horny scale. The value of antiseptics such as benzalkonium chloride (a quaternary ammonium compound) may be due more to dispersion of the flakes than to other activity.

Coal tars may have been used since ancient times for their antidandruff properties. Their activity seems to be dependent on dispersion of scales (61). Although traditional dermatologic agents, coal tars have undesirable side effects such as retardation of wound healing and photosensitivity. The active photosensitizers of coal tar include acridine, anthracene, and pyridine. Its color, odor, and staining properties tend to make it cosmetically unacceptable. In general, coal tar products should not be recommended for dandruff unless the condition is refractory.

Product Selection Guidelines

When deciding on which product to recommend for dandruff, the pharmacist may follow these simple guidelines:

- The patient first should increase the frequency of shampooing to once every 1–3 days using his or her usual product. The hair should be rinsed thoroughly after shampooing.
- If increased frequency of shampooing does not control the condition, a zinc pyrithione-containing product may be used 2–3 times per week. Selenium sulfide is a suitable alternative. Improvement may be noted within several weeks.
- Keratolytic agents and medicated shampoos may be utilized, but do not appear to have any advantage over the more effective cytostatic agents.

Dandruff is a normal physiologic event, and total control using therapeutic agents may not be possible. The patient must be reassured that the condition eventually runs its course and will decline in severity.

Seborrhea

Seborrheic dermatitis is a general term for a group of eruptions that occur predominantly in the areas of greatest sebaceous gland activity (the scalp, face, and trunk). Nonprescription therapy is effective in many cases. Through an understanding of the symptoms of seborrhea and the appropriate therapy, the pharmacist may play a key role in its management.

Symptoms

Seborrhea is marked by accelerated epidermal proliferation and sebaceous gland activity. The distinctive characteristics of the disorder are its common occurrence in hairy areas (especially the scalp), the appearance of well demarcated, dull yellowish-red lesions, and the associated presence of greasy or dry scales (80). Pruritus is not uncommon. Seborrhea may occur in children, but it is more common in middle-age groups and the elderly, particularly males. The most common form is seborrheic capitis, which is characterized by greasy scales on the scalp, frequently extending to the middle one-third of the face with subsequent eye involvement. (See *Plate 7-28.*) Lesions also may appear in the external auditory canal and around the ear.

Etiology

The cause of seborrhea is unknown. A constitutional predisposition seems to exist, and emotional or physical stress may serve as aggravating factors (81). Proposed etiologic factors have included vitamin B deficiency, food allergies, autoimmunity, and climate changes (82). The characteristic accelerated cell turnover and enhanced sebaceous gland activity give rise to the prominent scale displayed in the condition, although there is no quantitative relationship between the degree of sebaceous gland activity and susceptibility to seborrhea. Hence, predisposing factors are complex.

It is almost universally accepted that seborrhea is merely an extension of dandruff. Some researchers, however, dissent from this view, offering evidence that seborrhea is a separate condition from simple dandruff (61). Nucleocytes (parakeratotic cells) commonly make up 15–25% of the corneocyte count in seborrheic dermatitis but rarely exceed 5% in dandruff. This evidence and other distinguishing features of the two conditions are shown in Table 6.

Assessment

The differential diagnosis of seborrheic dermatitis is not always simple. Other disorders that need to be considered include dandruff, psoriasis, atopic dermatitis, and fungal infections. Fortunately, misdiagnosis of the seborrheic condition as dandruff is not of great consequence because both involve accelerated epidermal turnover with scaling as the principal manifestation. Therefore, treatment is generally the same in both cases. However, some unique aspects of seborrheic capitis are worth noting. Dandruff is considered a relatively stable condition, whereas seborrhea fluctuates in severity, often as a result of stress. Involvement of eyebrows and eyelashes with associated eyelid problems, such as blepharitis, is common in seborrhea but not in dandruff. Another distinguishing feature is the fact that dandruff is a noninflammatory condition whereas seborrhea is accompanied by erythema and sometimes by crusting (83).

The best distinguishing characteristic to differentiate seborrhea from psoriasis is the location of the lesions. Seborrhea commonly involves the face and generally is not found on the extremities, whereas psoriasis is rarely found on the face and has a predilection for the elbows and knees. The scalp generally is involved in both conditions, and if this is the only site of involvement, differential diagnosis is difficult. The term "seborrhiasis" has been coined to describe this condition. The appearance of the scales may help to distinguish the two disorders; seborrhea usually is marked by greasy, thick yellow scales where psoriatic scales are generally dry and silvery in appearance.

Atopic dermatitis, like psoriasis, may be distinguished from seborrhea on the basis of scale appearance and location of the lesions; atopic dermatitis commonly occurs in the folds of the arms or knees and itching is generally more intense than in seborrhea. Moreover, patients presenting with atopic dermatitis often have a history of atopic disease, such as asthma or hayfever. Thus, by taking a medical history, the pharmacist may help determine the probable etiology of the condition.

Fungal infections constitute a fourth condition that may be mistaken for seborrhea. Proper diagnosis is important, for seborrheic therapy utilizing hydrocortisone may worsen fungal infections. If the lesion is located in the groin, tinea cruris (jock itch) must be considered, especially during warm weather. Scalp lesions must be evaluated for the possibility of tinea capitis (ringworm of the scalp). Tinea capitis spreads peripherally and leads to partial alopecia.

Treatment

The treatment of seborrhea capitis is generally the same as the treatment of dandruff. Both respond to keratolytic preparations, tars, selenium sulfide (1–2%), and zinc pyrithione (1–2%). After an initial cleansing shampoo to remove scale, one of these agents may be applied to the scalp vigorously for 5–10 minutes. This may be repeated 2–3 times/week for best results.

Frequent use of selenium sulfide tends to make the scalp oily and may actually aggravate the seborrheic condition. If the patient has a very oily scalp, a more drying shampoo such as Sebulex (2% salicylic acid and 2% sulfur) may be beneficial (82). The FDA advisory review panel on nonprescription miscellaneous external drug products has recommended that salicylic acid (1.8–3%) be placed in Category I for treatment of seborrheic dermatitis. Combination products containing salicylic acid and sulfur have been placed in Category III.

If the seborrhea spreads to include the ear canal or the eyelids, a physician should be consulted for appropriate therapy. Control of the scalp condition as well as the use of specific otic and ophthalmic agents is warranted.

The main difference between the treatment of dandruff and seborrhea is the use of topical steroids in the latter. Hydrocortisone lotions for scalp dermatitis are now available without a prescription. These products are not indicated for the dandruff condition, but they may play a useful role in seborrhea management.

The use of topical hydrocortisone in seborrhea capitis should be reserved for those cases that have not responded to therapy with shampoos. The patient may be instructed to apply the hydrocortisone product once a day at the onset of therapy and then intermittently to control acute exacerbations of the disease.

The pharmacist should instruct the patient in the proper technique of applying the hydrocortisone lotion to the scalp. The hair should be parted and the product applied directly to the scalp and massaged in thoroughly. This process is repeated until desired coverage is achieved. The absorption of medication into the scalp will be enhanced if the lotion is applied after shampooing, for skin hydration will promote drug absorption.

Frequent and continued use of hydrocortisone in the treatment of seborrhea capitis is to be discouraged, for topical steroids are capable of producing a rebound dermatitis when therapy is discontinued. If the condition worsens or if symptoms persist for more than 7 days, a physician should be consulted. The patient should be instructed to rely primarily on shampooing to control the disease, and to use hydrocortisone only when necessary (82).

Product Selection Guidelines

Seborrhea capitis often can be controlled with nonprescription products. When deciding on which product to recommend to the patient, the pharmacist may follow these simple guidelines:

- To initiate therapy, a zinc pyrithione-containing product may be used 2–3 times/week. Selenium sulfide and keratolytic preparations are suitable alternatives. Improvement should be seen within 2 weeks.
- If the condition fails to respond to the above agents, a tar-containing shampoo may be utilized. Alternatively, a coal tar gel or a tar-oil bath additive may be applied sparingly to the lesions 3–8 hours before shampooing (83).
- If the condition still is refractory, a hydrocortisone lotion, spray, or gel may be applied sparingly once a day and worked into the scalp thoroughly. Improvement should be seen within 7 days.
- Recalcitrant cases should be referred to a physician for evaluation.

Psoriasis

Psoriasis accounts for approximately 5% of all visits to dermatologists in the United States (80). Its annual cost to Americans is estimated at $248 million (84). Of particular interest to pharmacists is the fact that nonprescription drug products represent $100 million of this total figure. A thorough understanding of the symptoms of psoriasis as well as its pathophysiology, assessment, and treatment is therefore warranted.

Symptoms

Psoriasis is a papulosquamous skin disease marked by the presence of small elevations of the skin as well as scaling. Lesions are flat-topped, pink or dull red in color, and covered with silvery scales. The edge of the lesion is sharply delineated, and individual diameters may vary from a few mm to 20 cm or more (85). When psoriatic scales are removed mechanically, small bleeding points appear (Auspitz sign). Psoriatic skin is more permeable to many substances than normal skin. For example, it may lose water 8–10 times faster than normal skin. In fact, when large areas of the body surface are involved, whole body skin water loss may be as much as 2–3 liters/day, in addition to normal perspiration loss. Evaporation of this volume of water requires over 1,000 calories. For this reason, psoriatic patients may show increased metabolic rates at the expense of tissue catabolism and muscle wasting (86).

Psoriatic lesions have a marked predilection for certain areas of the body such as the scalp, elbows, knees, fingernails, and the genitoanal region. Lesions frequently develop in sites of vaccination or skin tests, scratch marks, or surgical incisions, and have been reported to be produced by shock and noise. In fact, the response to skin trauma is so predictable (Koebner's phenomenon) that it can be used in diagnosis. For example, when scaling is not evident, diagnosis is difficult. However, scales may be induced by light scratching. It has been shown that both the epidermis and dermis must be damaged before the reaction occurs, and the response generally occurs in 6–18 days following injury (87, 88).

Psoriasis assumes several different pathologic forms. Acute guttate psoriasis accounts for about 17% of psoriatic cases. It is characterized by many small lesions distributed more or less evenly over the body. These lesions may later coalesce to form large characteristic plaques. (See *Plate 7-29A, B, and C.*) Psoriasis in children is usually of the guttate variety and may be precipitated by various systemic diseases such as streptococcal tonsillitis. Acute attacks of guttate psoriasis also have been noted to occur at puberty and following childbirth. When the psoriatic condition is initiated by a guttate attack, the disease carries a better prognosis than that of a slower and more diffuse onset.

A second type of psoriasis is known as "pustular psoriasis." This type may or may not be a true form of psoriasis. It is marked by localized pustules on the palms and soles.

Psoriasis is basically a disease of the skin. The only tissues besides skin known to be clinically involved are the synovium and nails. In many patients with coexisting joint disease and psoriasis, the arthritic component is not easily distinguishable from rheumatoid arthritis. Certain psoriatic patients, however, have a unique form of arthritis, which has been dubbed psoriatic arthritis. Psoriatic arthritis is distinguished from rheumatoid arthritis in several respects. First, its onset is often in the distal rather than the proximal joints of the fingers or toes, and this involvement is almost always associated with psoriasis of the nails. Second, psoriatic arthritis is often asymmetric in its joint involvement and generally affects a fewer number of joints (89).

The duration of psoriasis is variable. A lesion may last a lifetime, or it may disappear quickly. When lesions disappear, they may leave the skin either hypopigmented or hyperpigmented. The disease course is marked by spontaneous exacerbations and remissions and tends to be chronic and relapsing.

Pathophysiology

When one examines the natural history of psoriasis in patients, several points of interest emerge. For example, there seems to be an inherited predisposition to psoriasis, because about 40% of psoriatic patients show an associated family history (90). Evidence supports an autosomal dominant mode of inheritance, and genetic markers as determined by the major histocompatibility locus antigen (HLA) system have been identified (91). In the case of psoriasis, HLA-B17 has been associated with the disease (92). Environmental factors, however, are not to be downplayed. Hot weather and sunlight have been noted to improve the condition; cold weather worsens it. Many investigators agree that emotional stress also affects psoriasis adversely (93). Another factor involved in the pathogenesis of psoriasis is endocrine function. For example, psoriasis has been noted to improve or clear during pregnancy and reappear after parturition. The bulk of information supports a multifactorial inheritance of psoriasis, since both genetic and environmental components play a role in the disease.

A natural history of psoriasis goes on to reveal that no age is exempt from the condition; most cases develop in individuals 10–50 years old. Psoriasis is approximately three times more prevalent in white people than it is in nonwhites, rarely being found in Afro-Americans, Japanese, and American Indians. It is distributed almost equally between men and women.

The pathophysiology of the psoriatic lesion is very complex, involving not only the epidermis, but also the dermis and the body's immune system. The major pathophysiologic events involved in the disease process are accelerated epidermal proliferation and metabolic activity, proliferation of capillaries in the dermal region, and invasion of the dermis and epidermis by inflammatory cells. An understanding of these three basic processes is fundamental to an appreciation of psoriasis therapy.

Accelerated epidermal proliferation is one of the hallmarks of psoriasis, leading to excessive scaling of the skin. Normal epidermal turnover is 25–30 days; in psoriatic plaque skin it is $\leq$ 3–4 days (94). There are two schools of thought to explain this phenomenon; both deal with cell cycle kinetics. The first theory is that the accelerated epidermal proliferation is due to a shortening of cell division cycle time. Data have been collected showing that the germinative cell cycle of the psoriatic cell is 12 times faster than normal (37.5 versus 457 hours) (95). These data, however, have been disputed (96). The second theory is that the germinative layer in human epidermis is composed of three distinct populations of epidermal cells. In normal skin, only one of these populations is actively cycling, whereas in psoriasis all three populations are recruited into active proliferation (97).

Accelerated epidermal proliferation is aided by the fact that the psoriatic lesion demonstrates extensive infolding of the dermal-epidermal junction. The greatly expanded surface area that results and the presence of 2–3 basal cell layers lead to a greatly exaggerated mitotic growth and epidermal thickness. The keratin produced has many parakeratotic cells, and the granular layer is absent in severe cases.

When one considers the extent of epidermal proliferation present in psoriasis, it logically follows that an expanded vascular system is needed to satisfy increasing metabolic requirements. In psoriasis, proliferation of capillaries in the dermal region occurs. The resultant capillary loops are arranged vertically at the center of the plaque and are responsible for the bleeding of the Auspitz sign. It has been postulated that the psoriatic plaque may generate an angiotactic substance responsible for this capillary proliferation, enabling the lesion to expand (98, 99).

The third major pathophysiologic event in psoriasis is invasion of the dermis and epidermis by inflammatory cells. Mononuclear cells and polymorphonuclear (PMN) leukocytes can be found in the dermis; PMN leukocytes also tend to infiltrate the epidermis (100). Extracts of psoriatic scale have been shown to contain factors that can induce directed migration (chemotaxis) of these inflammatory cells (100). Moreover, mononuclear cells and PMN leukocytes from psoriatic patients have been shown to exhibit enhanced responsiveness to chemoattractants (101, 102). Lithium carbonate increases the total mass of circulating PMN leukocytes in patients and also has been associated with an induction or exacerbation of psoriatic symptoms (103, 104). The presence of inflammatory cells in psoriatic skin may induce epidermal proliferation and has led to many postulations about the possible role of the immune system in the pathogenesis of psoriasis.

The mononuclear infiltrate found in psoriatic dermal tissue is largely composed of T-lymphocytes and macrophages (105). The T-lymphocytes are thought to be responsible for cell-mediated immunity and also can suppress or assist the stimulation of antibody production. It has been postulated that there is a T-cell defect in psoriasis. More specifically, there may be a lack of suppression of the humoral immune system, leading to autoantibody production against skin antigens (106). Various data have been collected in support of an autoimmune theory of psoriasis (107).

Although much research has been done recently on the causes of psoriasis (107–112), the specific biochemical event triggering psoriatic skin formation remains unknown. Prostaglandins and polyamines as well as cyclic nucleotides are being investigated as having a possible role. It is possible that cyclic adenosine 3′: 5′-monophosphate (cyclic AMP) mediates the regulation of epidermal proliferation and that there is a defect in the adenylcyclase–cyclic AMP system in psoriatic skin (113–118). It originally was thought that cyclic AMP levels were lowered in the psoriatic lesion and that this contributed to enhanced epidermal proliferation. Conflicting data, however, have been obtained, and the precise role of cyclic AMP in the pathogenesis of psoriasis has yet to be clarified (117).

Assessment

Diagnosis usually is straightforward for simple psoriasis. Sites of involvement, the dry silvery appearance of the scale, and a small area of bleeding (Auspitz sign) after scale removal are characteristic. Pruritus and joint involvement also may be present. Precipitating factors such as a recent vaccination, disease, pregnancy, or trauma are useful evidence in a preliminary diagnosis.

It is important not to confuse psoriasis with other diseases that may have similar symptoms but call for different treatment. When the scalp or the flexural and intertriginous areas are involved, psoriasis must not be mistaken for moniliasis or seborrhea. Identifying the fungal organism from lesion scrapings proves the presence or absence of moniliasis. Seborrhea and psoriasis sometimes are distinguished by their scale appearance and color. Psoriasis of the scalp generally produces silvery, dry, patchy, adherent scales; seborrhea usually is manifested as a yellowish, oily scale (seborrhea oleosa) and tends to be more diffuse. Moreover, in psoriasis the plaque has a full, rich, red color with a particular depth of hue and opacity not normally seen in seborrhea or dermatitis. In dark-skinned races this quality is lost. If lesions are present in the groin, axilla, and inframammary region, diagnosis based on visual inspection may be difficult. More elaborate histologic and pathologic diagnosis may be done by a physician (119–121).

Other skin diseases whose symptoms resemble those of psoriasis are localized neurodermatitis, particularly in the genitoanal region, and fungal conditions with circular or annular lesions. When psoriasis alternates with or is complicated by other diseases, such as seborrhea, diagnosis is much more difficult.

Treatment

There is no cure for psoriasis, only a reduction in severity. Different stages of the disease are treated by different methods. Acute psoriatic onset characterized by severely erythematous lesions calls for soothing local therapy such as a bland, nonmedicated cream. Tars, salicylic acid, and aggressive ultraviolet light therapy must be avoided at this stage, because of their potential irritant effect. As the acute process subsides and the usual thickscaled plaques appear, more potent therapy with agents such as keratolytics may be used. Many patients respond well to simple measures, whereas others are refractory to the most formidable treatment.

There is consensus that "guerilla tactics are better than a frontal assault," with the more powerful agents held in reserve (79). In eruptive or unstable forms of the disease, even mild sunlight may provoke a Koebner-type exacerbation. In general, psoriatic patients should be under a physician's care. Nonprescription drugs may be an efficacious part of the physician's armamentarium, and the pharmacist must be a knowledgeable consultant. Nonprescription therapy may take the following approach:

- Discussion with the patient as to the nature of the condition (acceptance of the disease may reduce stress or emotional instability);
- Simple local measures such as bland emollients or creams, and mild keratolytic products;
- Sunlight (ultraviolet light in suberythemal doses) and tar products;
- Topical hydrocortisone.

In addition to nonprescription products, several prescription-only medications are available. The use of these medications sometimes necessitates day-care or hospitalization of the patient.

Topical Agents

Drug penetration of diseased skin is facilitated if a portion of the psoriatic plaque is removed before therapy, the area is first soaked in water, or an occlusive bandage is used after the drug is applied. Occlusion with a plastic film also alters the skin cell metabolic rate and allows reformation of the granular layer in the psoriatic plaque. Daily baths containing oil emulsions and use of bland emollients are helpful in removing scale (122). Psoriatic skin is more permeable to many substances than normal skin, resulting in rapid drug entrance. Thus, in the early stage, the disorder responds rapidly to local treatment, and then the improvement rate slows as the skin barrier approaches normalcy.

The nonprescription agents most commonly found in topical products for treatment of psoriasis are coal tar, keratolytics, and bland emollients either individually or in combination. In general, combination therapy consists of applying coal tar at night and using a keratolytic during the day. A new addition to the nonprescription armamentarium is topical hydrocortisone.

Tar Products

Tar products have been a very popular treatment for psoriasis over the years, and many nonprescription products are available. Crude coal tar consists of a heterogeneous mixture of many different compounds. Its mechanism of action is not known, but coal tar has been attributed with being antiseptic, antipruritic, keratoplastic (capable of building up horny substance), and possibly photosensitizing (123).

Crude coal tar (1–5%) and ultraviolet light therapy have been used in the treatment of psoriasis since 1925 in a method known as the Goeckerman regimen (124). A therapeutic benefit of both the tar alone and the irradiation alone has been demonstrated, but the combination is more effective than either agent by itself, and remissions lasting up to 12 months have been reported after 2–4 weeks of therapy (125, 126). The coal tar is removed from the skin before irradiation takes place. Otherwise, the ultraviolet light will not reach the skin. For many years, the therapeutic response with this form of therapy was believed to be caused by phototoxicity, but this theory has been challenged (127–130). Now it is thought that the mechanism of coal tar may lie in its ability to cross-link with DNA (84). Coal tar in combination with ultraviolet light also may increase prostaglandin synthesis in the skin, which may be related to its beneficial effect (84). Combinations of 1% crude coal tar with long-wavelength ultraviolet light and of 6% crude coal tar with ultraviolet light have been shown to be equally effective (131). Hence, only modest levels of coal tar are needed. Moreover, crude coal tar from high- and low-temperature sources seems equally effective (132).

Coal tar is available in many different kinds of pharmaceutical vehicles. Creams, ointments, pastes, lotions, bath oils, shampoos, soaps, and gels are available. This wide variety of products has in part resulted from an attempt to develop a cosmetically acceptable product, one that masks the unpleasant odor, color, and staining properties of crude coal tar. Liquor carbonis detergens (LCD) is a 20% tincture of coal tar that has been useful in the development of cosmetically acceptable tar products. It is used in concentrations of 3–15%.

Tar gels (Estar and psoriGel) represent a unique dosage form that appears to deliver the beneficial elements of crude coal tar in a form both convenient to apply and cosmetically acceptable (84). These gels are nongreasy and nonstaining, since they do not rub off on clothing. They also have the advantage of being nearly colorless. The pharmacist should caution the patient, however, that these gels may have a drying effect on the skin, necessitating use of an emollient (123).

Certain side effects are associated with the use of coal tar. These include folliculitis, photosensitization, and dermatitis due to irritation (133). Certain patients may even show a worsening of the condition when exposed to coal tar products. If the patient is currently using other photosensitizing drugs such as tetracyclines, phenothiazines, or sulfonamides, the pharmacist should give appropriate warnings. Moreover, the patient should not utilize extensive exposure to sunlight or sunlamps to simulate the Goeckerman regimen. This procedure requires careful monitoring of ultraviolet light exposure by a physician.

Crude coal tar and ultraviolet light both are thought to have carcinogenic potential. However, Watson states that there have been no reports of an increased frequency of skin cancer in psoriatic patients treated for many years with coal tar and ultraviolet light (122). Nevertheless, the FDA advisory review panel on nonprescription miscellaneous external drug products has recommended that topical coal tar products be placed in Category III for safety considerations. An exception was made for coal tar shampoos. Since contact time with the skin is minimal, coal tar shampoos were deemed safe enough to be placed in Category I.

Anthralin (Dithranol)

Anthralin is an effective topical agent that may cause a more rapid resolution of psoriatic plaques than crude coal tar. Remissions may last for weeks to as long as 2 years. Anthralin is structurally related to acridine and is thought to act by reducing DNA synthesis due to its intercalation between DNA base pairs (122).

Anthralin (0.2–0.8%) is used in combination with a daily coal tar bath and ultraviolet light exposure in a procedure known as the Ingram technique (133). Anthralin is most effective when incorporated into a stiff paste allowing prolonged adherence to the skin. These pastes, however, can be difficult to apply and have the disadvantage of not being water soluble, thereby making removal from the skin difficult (122).

Anthralin is irritating to the skin and therefore should not be applied to normal skin, the face, genitalia, or areas of acute eruption. It also has a propensity to stain clothing and skin a purple-brown color (133). A derivative of anthralin, triacetoxyanthracene, lacks the burning and staining effects of anthralin but is less effective.

Keratolytics

Keratolytics, by definition, are chemical substances that loosen keratin, thereby facilitating desquamation. They are useful in psoriasis when very thick scales are present. One of the most commonly used nonprescription keratolytics is salicylic acid (2–10%). It has been suggested that salicylic acid acts by decreasing corneocyte to corneocyte cohesion in the abnormal honry layer found in psoriatic lesions (134). Salicylic acid also has been classified as being antiseptic, photoprotective, astringent, antipruritic, anti-inflammatory, and antiepidermoplastic (135, 136). Other nonprescription keratolytics include sulfur, allantoin, and resorcinol. Salicylic acid, however, has emerged as the most effective and least toxic of the keratolytics (133). Many patients respond to salicylic acid in cream or ointment form, applied several times per day. The FDA advisory review panel on nonprescription miscellaneous external drug products has recommended that salicylic acid (1.8–3%) be placed in Category I for treatment of psoriasis. Combination products containing salicylic acid and sulfur have been placed in Category III.

Proper therapy with salicylic acid calls for consultation by the pharmacist. The patient should be told that salicylic acid is more effective if the psoriatic area is first soaked in warm water for 10–20 minutes (122). An occlusive dressing may be employed. Extensive body application of concentrated salicylic acid preparations (>5%) must be avoided, or systemic toxicity may occur (84). The patient should be warned that the initial signs of systemic toxicity include nausea, vomiting, hearing changes, or mental confusion (133). Since salicylic acid is an irritant, there is concern about worsening of the psoriatic condition. Keratolytics therefore should be applied at a low concentration initially, and the dose should be increased as patient tolerance develops.

Salicylic acid is useful in the treatment of psoriasis when combined with other agents. Since it has a keratin-softening effect, it may aid the penetration of these agents into the skin (135). It has been suggested that the efficacy of salicylic acid could be improved if it were available in a slow-release vehicle or one maintaining close proximity of the compound to the skin (19).

Antipruritics

Pruritus associated with psoriasis may be related to the dry skin condition that accompanies the disease. Bland emollients such as petrolatum and Aquaphor are effective hydrating agents. Moreover, the use of white petrolatum may inhibit the development of Koebner's phenomenon (88). Since many occlusives are greasy, patients may prefer the less effective, more esthetic oil-in-water emulsion creams or lotions such as Nivea cream, Albolene, and Lubriderm (122).

It has been suggested that the attendant pruritus of psoriasis may be alleviated with systemically administered antihistamines. However, it has yet to be established whether the itching of psoriasis is histamine mediated. Perhaps antihistamines are serving as no more than sedatives in these patients. Although sedation may be beneficial, a more direct therapy for pruritus should be sought.

Antihistamines also have been used topically to alleviate pruritus. This type of therapy should be discouraged, because of its questionable efficacy and the possibility of producing an allergic contact dermatits.

Topical Corticosteroids

Topical corticosteroids play an important role in the management of psoriasis. These agents have several effects on cellular activity, including anti-inflammatory, antimitotic/antisynthetic, vasoconstrictor, and immunosuppressive effects (137). Efficacy may be enhanced by the use of fluorinated compounds or an occlusive dressing. Continued use of topical steroids beyond 2–3 weeks may render the drug less effective in psoriasis (tachyphylaxis may occur) (133).

Certain adverse effects are associated with the use of topical steroids. These include local atrophy of the skin after prolonged use and the aggravation of certain cutaneous infections. The possibility of systemic sequelae exists and is enhanced by the use of fluorinated compounds, occlusive dressings, or application to large areas of the body (133). Since children have a greater surface area to body mass ratio, they are at greater risk of developing systemic complications. In general, however, systemic sequelae are unlikely with the concentrations of hydrocortisone available without a prescription.

Another problem with hydrocortisone is that there is usually a prompt rebound of psoriasis when topical steroid therapy is discontinued. The psoriasis may reappear as the more severe pustular form (122). Relapse occurs more quickly after topical corticosteroids than after tar or anthralin therapy.

Topical hydrocortisone preparations are available on a nonprescription basis. Pharmacists may play a vital role in patient care by prudently advising patients about the use of these products. The patient may be instructed to apply the hydrocortisone as a thin film 2–4 times a day at the onset of therapy, and intermittently thereafter to control exacerbations. The medication should be massaged into the skin thoroughly. Continued and frequent use of topical hydrocortisone is to be discouraged, since topical steroids may become less effective with prolonged use, promote local rebound, have potentially adverse local effects, and, most importantly, do not induce remissions of psoriasis (122). The patient should be instructed to rely primarily on other treatments, such as tars and keratolytics, for psoriasis and to use topical hydrocortisone only when necessary.

The FDA advisory review panel on nonprescription miscellaneous external drug products has recommended that hydrocortisone (up to 0.5%) be placed in Category III for treatment of psoriasis and seborrheic dermatitis. This rating is due to a lack of submissions of efficacy data. Concentrations of 0.5–1.0% also have been placed in Category III.

Ammoniated Mercury

Ammoniated mercury (5–10%) with or without a keratolytic has been used in the treatment of psoriasis. Its beneficial effect is doubtful, and its propensity toward causing sensitivity and potential nephrotoxicity should restrict its use.

Colchicine

Application of colchicine (1%) in hydrophilic ointment for several weeks has been tried. This approach is still experimental, and the possibility of toxic side effects such as tissue necrosis may limit its usefulness (138, 139).

Systemic Agents

PUVA Therapy

An increasingly important mode of therapy is the use of systemic or topical psoralens in combination with ultraviolet light (140–146). This photochemotherapeutic process has the acronym, PUVA, which stands for psoralen (P) and long-wave ultraviolet light (UVA) (320–340 nm). The most common psoralen employed in this process is 8-methoxypsoralen (8-MOP, methoxsalen), which is used in oral doses of 0.65 mg/kg, followed 2 hours later by carefully monitored exposure to long-wave ultraviolet light (122). This timing corresponds with the attainment of peak serum levels of the psoralen (133). Treatments are repeated 2–3 times weekly until clearing of the lesion occurs (an average of 20 treatments). Patients then receive weekly or biweekly maintenance therapy. Remissions averaging 22 weeks, however, have been reported even without the use of maintenance therapy (147).

Instead of oral administration, methoxsalen may be used as a 0.15–1% topical suspension applied to lesions 1–2 hours before ultraviolet exposure (133). Topical application, however, enhances the risk of blistering, and patients must be cautioned to avoid any sun exposure after application of the product. The topical preparation has the advantage of being clean, nonstaining, and odorless.

The mechanism of action of PUVA therapy remains elusive. It has been suggested that, under the influence of long-wave ultraviolet light, psoralens bind to thymidine in DNA and form interstrand cross-links, thereby inhibiting DNA replication and cell multiplication (133, 148). Another theory is that PUVA inhibits the chemotactic activity of psoriatic scale, suppressing the migration of PMN leukocytes into the lesion (149).

PUVA therapy has demonstrated its efficacy in the treatment of psoriasis. However, the safety of the procedure must also be considered. Immediate side effects that may occur include nausea, pruritus, erythema, and occasional blistering. Concomitant use of other dermal irritants may aggravate dermal toxicity, and special cautions have been called for in the treatment of patients who are using other photoactive drugs such as sulfonamide-based diuretics. A prospective study of patients receiving PUVA therapy failed to demonstrate a significantly increased rate of severe, acute toxicity in patients concomitantly using other photoactive drugs (150). However, this study was not tightly controlled, and the photoactive drugs being used by many of the patients were diuretics. Controlled studies utilizing a balanced cross-sampling of photoactive drugs are needed to draw a general conclusion about the safety of using such drugs during PUVA therapy. Until that time, it is prudent for the pharmacist to give appropriate warnings to these patients.

PUVA therapy must be considered experimental until long-term safety is established. Long-range side effects that may occur include the development of cataracts or cutaneous carcinoma. One study demonstrated that PUVA-treated patients had an observed incidence of cutaneous carcinoma 2.6 times that expected for an age, sex, and geographically matched population (151). This increased incidence, however, may be due to other carcinogens to which this population had been exposed, and the relative importance of PUVA for the development of these tumors is difficult to assess. Nevertheless, PUVA therapy has a potential for serious long-range side effects and must be studied further before it is put to general use.

Retinoids

Retinoids consist of a group of compounds including vitamin A and its analogs. Vitamin A is believed to be involved in epidermal activity, particularly the physiologic control of keratinization. Consensus, however, is that it is ineffective in treating psoriasis. Preliminary results on topically applied tretinoin (vitamin A acid) are encouraging, but additional work is needed. Tretinoin has the disadvantage of producing considerable irritation when applied topically.

Vitamin A analogs represent a new frontier in the management of psoriasis (152–155). These agents may act by helping to normalize cell differentiation in the psoriatic lesion. An investigational oral retinoid, RO 10-9359, has been shown to be a potent antipsoriatic agent and has been used in combination with PUVA therapy (152). Combination therapy decreases the total energy of ultraviolet light required for PUVA alone, accelerates the response of psoriasis to PUVA, and is effective in certain patients who have been considered PUVA failures (154).

Side effects associated with the use of RO 10-9359 include dryness of the lips, mouth, and nose, alopecia, and elevated serum transaminase levels (153). Combination therapy employing lower doses of RO 10-9359 may decrease the incidence of such side effects.

Methotrexate

Accelerated epidermal proliferation has been cited as one pathophysiologic event of psoriasis. Methotrexate has been employed in the therapy of psoriasis because it serves as an antimitotic agent. Specifically, it is thought to inhibit DNA synthesis by blocking dihydrofolate reductase. The serious potential side effects and toxicity of systemic methotrexate are well known. Strict supervision of patients receiving methotrexate, including frequent blood analysis and regular liver biopsy, is essential (156). Results of a recent survey of dermatologists showed that methotrexate, hydroxyurea, and azaribine were used in chemotherapy for psoriasis by 50%, 10%, and 2% of the dermatologists polled (157). Despite this relatively high usage of methotrexate, only a small percentage of the patients were given liver biopsy and creatinine tests.

It has been postulated that topical administration of methotrexate could perhaps minimize the undesirable side effects associated with systemic therapy. Topical therapy, however, has proven ineffective. One study suggests that methotrexate acts directly on psoriatic plaque rather than systemically at some distant site (158). Therefore topical therapy is potentially efficacious, therapeutic failures up to this point may be related to slow partitioning of the active form of the drug from experimental vehicle formulations.

Systemic Corticosteroids

The systemic use of corticosteroids is contraindicated in all but the most severe forms of psoriasis. This restricted use is due to the undesirable side effects accompanying systemic use of steroids as well as the fact that after therapy is stopped, the disease is almost certain to be worse than it was initially (159).

Product Selection Guidelines

When deciding on which product to recommend for a psoriatic condition, the pharmacist must consider the area to which the agent is going to be applied. The response to topical medications shows striking regional variation. The following guidelines may be utilized by the pharmacist to choose an appropriate product (160):

Scalp Psoriasis

Elaborate psoriasis shampoos are not necessary to control psoriasis of the scalp. Frequency of shampooing rather than the product itself is the key to effective therapy. The patient may be instructed to shampoo using any type of product. The resultant removal of scales is the goal of therapy. Tar-oil bath additives such as Balnetar and Doak oil or coal-tar solutions may be painted sparingly to the lesions 3–12 hours before each shampoo. Tar gels also may be useful in this approach. Hydrocortisone has been claimed to have little impact on psoriasis of the scalp.

Psoriasis of the Body, Arms, and Legs

Coal tar products may be applied to the body, arms, and legs at bedtime. Since coal tar often stains clothing, the pharmacist should advise the patient to use old sheets and bed clothing. This therapy may be followed by a bath in the morning to help remove the coal tar as well as psoriatic scale.

Topical hydrocortisone may be applied to the lesions 2–3 times during the day. The medication should be applied sparingly and massaged into the skin thoroughly. Continued and frequent use of hydrocortisone is to be discouraged.

A product containing salicylic acid may be useful if thick scales are present. It may be applied several times during the day. The pharmacist may instruct the patient to soak the area of application in warm water for 10–20 minutes before application of the medication.

Intertriginous Psoriasis

Intertriginous areas such as the armpits and genitoanal region are sensitive to irritants such as coal tar and salicylic acid. Therefore, these agents should not be used to treat psoriasis in these areas. Rather, hydrocortisone cream may be applied sparingly 2–3 times/day and used less frequently as improvement occurs.

It must be remembered that psoriasis is not a trivial medical problem, and psoriatic patients should be under a physician's care. The pharmacist's role in the management of psoriasis is that of a knowledgeable consultant.

Summary

Many patients are afflicted with dermatitis, dry skin, dandruff, seborrhea, and psoriasis. It is important that patients suffering from these dermatologic problems be assessed properly before self-medication is recommended. Therapy effective in one disorder may exacerbate another. The pharmacist can perform a valuable service by helping patients determine the nature of their problem and the most effective therapy to alleviate it.

References

1. "Textbook of Dermatology," 3rd ed., Vol. 1, A. Rook, D. S. Wilkinson, and F. J. G. Ebling, Eds., Blackwell Scientific Publications, London, England, 1979, pp. 299–349.
2. C. L. Wang, *Lab. Rev.*, Feb., 1979, p. 17.
3. *Journal of Investigative Dermatology, 73,* 414 (1979).
4. "Textbook of Dermatology," 2nd ed., Vol. 2, A. Rook, D. S. Wilkinson, and F. J. G. Ebling, Eds., Blackwell Scientific Publications, Oxford, England, 1975, pp. 289–290.
5. H. Baker, *Br. Med. J., 4,* 544 (1973).
6. D. Munro-Ashman, *Br. J. Clin. Pract., 17,* 537 (1963).
7. L. Fry, *Update Int., 1,* 113 (1974).
8. D. G. C. Presbury, *Update Int., 1,* 334 (1974).
9. A. M. Margileth, *Ped. Ann., 8,* 495 (1979).
10. K. A. Arndt, "Manual of Dermatologic Therapeutics with Essentials of Diagnosis," Little, Brown, Boston, Mass., 1978, p. 53.
11. R. B. Stoughton, *Arch. Dermatol., 92,* 281 (1965).
12. I. Sarkany, *Nurs. Times, 1211,* 1212 (1971).
13. K. A. Arndt, "Manual of Dermatologic Therapeutics with Essentials of Diagnosis," Little, Brown, Boston, Mass., 1978, p. 333.
14. E. Epstein, *Med. Times, 108,* 36 (1980).
15. S. A. Davis, *Med. Times, 108,* 54 (1980).
16. *British Journal of Dermatology, 102,* 113 (1980).
17. E. Epstein, "Common Skin Disorders—A Manual for Physicians and Patients," Medical Economics, Oradell, N.J., 1979, p. 5.
18. K. A. Arndt, "Manual of Dermatologic Therapeutics with Essentials of Diagnosis," Little, Brown, Boston, Mass., 1978, p. 293.
19. *Journal of Investigative Dermatology, 73,* 473 (1979).
20. E. Epstein, "Common Skin Disorders—A Manual for Physicians and Patients," Medical Economics, Oradell, N.J., 1979, pp. 3–4.
21. R. M. Handjani-Vila, B. Rondot, and F. Lachampt, *Cosmet. Perfum., 90,* 39 (1975).
22. "Dermatology," Vol. 2, S. L. Moschella, D. M. Pillsbury, and H. J. Hurley, Jr., W. B. Saunders, Philadelphia, Pa., 1975, pp. 1062–1064.
23. G. Rajka and P. Thune, *Br. J. Dermatol., 94,* 253 (1976).
24. "Textbook of Dermatology," 3rd ed., Vol. 2, A. Rook, D. S. Wilkinson, and F. J. G. Ebling, Eds., Blackwell Scientific Publications, London, England, 1979, pp. 1273–1275.
25. R. H. Wildnaur, J. W. Bothwell, and A. B. Douglass, *J. Invest. Dermatol., 56,* 72 (1971).
26. J. D. Middleton and B. M. Allen, *J. Soc. Cosmet. Chem., 24,* 239 (1973).
27. J. D. Middleton, *Br. J. Dermatol., 80,* 437 (1968).
28. M. Mezei, W. Sager, W. D. Stewart, and A. L. DeRuyters, *J. Pharm. Sci., 55,* 584 (1966).
29. H. Baker, *J. Invest. Dermatol., 50,* 283 (1968).
30. J. D. Middleton, *J. Soc. Cosmet. Chem., 20,* 399 (1969).
31. I. H. Blank and E. B. Shapiro, *J. Invest. Dermatol., 25,* 391 (1975).
32. I. H. Blank, *J. Invest. Dermatol., 18,* 433 (1952).

33. O. K. Jacobi, *Proc. Sci. Sect. Toilet Goods Assoc., 31,* 22 (1959).

34. K. Laden, *Am. Perfum. Cosmet., 82,* 77 (1967).

35. S. J. Stianse, *Cosmet. Perfum., 89,* 57 (1974).

36. B. F. VanDuzee, *J. Invest. Dermatol., 71,* 140 (1978).

37. A. M. Kligman, in "The Epidermis," W. Montagna and W. C. Lobitz, Jr., Eds., Academic, New York, N.Y., 1964.

38. D. Spruit and K. W. Malton, *J. Invest. Dermatol., 45,* 6 (1952).

39. D. Monash and I. H. Blank, *Arch. Dermatol., 78,* 710 (1958).

40. K. A. Arndt, "Manual of Dermatologic Therapeutics with Essentials of Diagnosis," Little, Brown, Boston, Mass., 1978, p. 76.

41. R. L. Goldenberg, *Skin Allerg. News, 5,* 20 (1974).

42. E. A. Taylor, *J. Invest. Dermatol., 37,* 69 (1961).

43. I. I. Lubowe, *West. J. Med., 1,* 45 (1960).

44. K. A. Arndt, "Manual of Dermatologic Therapeutics with Essentials of Diagnosis," Little, Brown, Boston, Mass., 1978, p. 77.

45. R. L. Anderson, J. M. Cassidy, J. R. Hansen, and W. Yellin, *J. Invest. Dermatol., 61,* 375 (1974).

46. W. H. Eaglstein and P. M. Mertz, *J. Invest. Dermatol., 74,* 90 (1980).

47. N. S. Penneys, W. Eaglstein, and V. Ziboh, *Br. J. Dermatol., 103,* 257 (1980).

48. G. Barnett, in "Cosmetics: Science and Technology," 2nd ed., M. S. Balsam and E. Sagarin, Eds., Wiley, New York, N.Y., 1972.

49. G. K. Steigleder and W. P. Raab, *J. Invest. Dermatol., 38,* 129 (1962).

50. E. M. Seiner, S. Bieser, R. Guidice, I. O. Kawat, E. Kaplan, B. Kauth, and D. Stone, *J. Am. Podiatr. Assoc., 63,* 571 (1973).

51. S. Rothman, "Physiology and Biochemistry of the Skin," University of Chicago Press, Chicago, Ill., 1954, p. 26.

52. H. Ashton, E. Frank, and C. J. Stevenson, *Br. J. Dermatol., 84,* 194 (1971).

53. D. P. Nash, *J. Am. Podiatr. Assoc., 61,* 382 (1971).

54. B. F. VanDuzee, *J. Invest. Dermatol., 71,* 140 (1978).

55. E. J. Van Scott and R. J. Yu, *Arch. Dermatol., 110,* 586 (1974).

56. E. J. Van Scott and R. J. Yu, in "The Ichthyoses," R. Marks and P. J. Dykes, Eds., Spectrum Publications, Inc., New York, N.Y., 1978, p. 3.

57. *Federal Register, 43,* 34634 (1978).

58. A. B. Ackerman and A. M. Kligman, *J. Soc. Cosmet. Chem., 20,* 81 (1969).

59. S. Bourne and A. Jacobs, *Br. Med. J., 1,* 1268 (1956).

60. F. C. Roia and R. W. Vanderwyk, *J. Soc. Cosmet. Chem., 20,* 113 (1969).

61. A. M. Kligman, R. R. Marples, L. R. Lantis, and K. J. McGinley, *J. Soc. Cosmet. Chem., 25,* 73 (1974).

62. K. J. McGinley, R. R. Marples, and G. Plewig, *J. Invest. Dermatol., 53,* 107 (1969).

63. H. Goldschmidt and A. M. Kligman, *Arch. Dermatol., 88,* 709 (1963).

64. G. Plewig and A. M. Kligman, *J. Soc. Cosmet. Chem., 20,* 767 (1969).

65. A. M. Kligman, *Cosmet. Perfum., 90,* 16 (1975).

66. F. C. Roia and R. W. Vanderwyk, *J. Soc. Cosmet. Chem., 15,* 761 (1964).

67. J. J. Leyden, K. J. McGinley, and A. M. Kligman, *Arch. Dermatol., 112,* 333 (1976).

68. H. Goldschmidt and M. A. Thew, *Arch. Dermatol., 106,* 476 (1972).

69. G. C. Priestly and J. C. Brown, *Acta Dermatovener. (Stockholm), 60,* 145 (1980).

70. T. Okumura, S. Hayashi, F. Tokiwa, and S. Horin, *Cosmet. Perfum., 90,* 101 (1975).

71. C. A. Bond, in "Applied Therapeutics for Clinical Pharmacists," 2nd ed., M. A. Koda-Kimble, B. S. Katcher, and L. Y. Young, Eds., Applied Therapeutics, San Francisco, Calif., 1978, p. 857.

72. *Medical Letter on Drugs and Therapeutics, 19,* 63 (1977).

73. E. Strokosch, *Arch. Dermatol. Syphilol., 47,* 16 (1943).

74. E. Strokosch, *Arch. Dermatol. Syphilol., 47,* 216 (1943).

75. E. Strokosch, *Arch. Dermatol. Syphilol., 48,* 384 (1943).

76. E. Strokosch, *Arch. Dermatol. Syphilol., 48,* 393 (1943).

77. "Textbook of Dermatology," 3rd ed., Vol. 2, A. Rook, D. S. Wilkinson, and F. J. G. Ebling, Eds., Blackwell Scientific Publications, London, England, 1979, p. 2310.

78. "The United States Dispensatory," 27th ed., Lippincott, Philadelphia, Pa., 1973, p. 1018.

79. K. W. Chesterman, *J. Am. Pharm. Assoc., NS12,* 576 (1972).

80. "Textbook of Dermatology," 3rd ed., Vol. 1, A. Rook, D. S. Wilkinson, and F. J. G. Ebling, Eds., Blackwell Scientific Publications, London, England, 1979, pp. 308–312.

81. K. A. Arndt, "Manual of Dermatologic Therapeutics with Essentials of Diagnosis," Little, Brown, Boston, Mass., 1978, p. 173.

82. D. L. Cram, *Medical Times, 108,* 74 (1980).

83. E. Epstein, "Common Skin Disorders—A Manual for Physicians and Patients," Medical Economics, Oradell, N.J., 1979, p. 86.

84. *Journal of Investigative Dermatology, 73,* 402 (1979).

85. J. W. Burnett and H. M. Robinson, Jr., "Clinical Dermatology for Students and Practitioners," Yorke Medical, New York, N.Y., 1978, p. 178.

86. "Textbook of Dermatology," 3rd ed., Vol. 2, A. Rook, D. S. Wilkinson, and F. J. G. Ebling, Eds., Blackwell Scientific Publications, London, England, 1979, p. 1333.

87. L. Stankler, *Br. J. Dermatol., 81,* 534 (1969).

88. J. S. Comaish and J. S. Greener, *Br. J. Dermatol., 94,* 195 (1976).

89. M. A. Krupp and M. J. Chatton, "Current Medical Diagnosis and Treatment," Lange Medical, Los Altos, Calif., 1981, p. 499.

90. E. M. Farber and M. L. Nall, *Dermatologica, 148,* 7 (1974).

91. L. E. Cutler, J. E. Bernstein, and K. Soltani, *Arch. Dermatol., 116,* 718 (1980).

92. R. C. Williams, A. W. McKenzie, J. H. Roger, and V. C. Joysey, *Br. J. Dermatol., 95,* 163 (1976).

93. R. H. Seville, *Br. J. Dermatol., 97,* 301 (1977).

94. G. Weinstein, *Br. J. Dermatol., 92,* 229 (1975).

95. G. Weinstein and P. Frost, *J. Invest. Dermatol., 50,* 254 (1968).

96. M. Duffill, N. Wright, and S. Shuster, *Br. J. Dermatol., 94,* 355 (1976).

97. S. Gelfant, *Br. J. Dermatol., 95,* 577 (1976).

98. F. S. Glickman and Y. Rapp, *Arch. Dermatol., 112,* 1789 (1976).

99. J. E. Wolf, Jr. and W. R. Hubler, Jr., *Arch. Dermatol., 113,* 1458 (1977).

100. M. V. Dahl, W. E. Lindroos, and R. D. Nelson, *J. Invest. Dermatol., 71,* 402 (1978).

101. G. G. Krueger, W. W. Jederberg, B. E. Ogden, and D. L. Reese, *J. Invest. Dermatol., 71,* 195 (1978).

102. A. Wahba, H. Cohen, M. Bar-Eli, and R. Callily, *Acta Dermatovener. (Stockholm), 59,* 441 (1979).

103. I. Skoven and J. Thormann, *Arch. Dermatol., 115,* 1185 (1979).

104. G. Lazarus and R. Gilgor, *Arch. Dermatol., 115,* 1183 (1979).

105. J. R. Bjerke, H. Krogh, and R. Matre, *J. Invest. Dermatol., 71,* 340 (1978).

106. D. N. Sauder, P. L. Bailin, J. Sundeen, and R. S. Krakauer, *Arch Dermatol., 116,* 51 (1980).

107. J. J. Guilhou, J. Meynadier, J. Clot, E. Charmasson, W. Dardenne, and J. Brochier, *Br. J. Dermatol., 95,* 295 (1976).

108. K. Aso, E. K. Orenberg, and E. M. Farber, *J. Invest. Dermatol., 63,* 375 (1975).

109. G. Mahrle and C. E. Orfanos, *Br. J. Dermatol., 93,* 495 (1975).

110. P. D. Mier and J. Van Den Hurk, *Br. J. Dermatol., 94,* 219 (1976).

111. J. J. Guilhou, J. Clot, J. Meynadier, and H. Lapinski, *Br. J. Dermatol., 94,* 501 (1976).

112. G. Mahrle and C. E. Orfanos, *Br. J. Dermatol., 95,* 591 (1976).

113. J. J. Voorhees and E. A. Duell, *Arch. Dermatol., 104,* 352 (1971).

114. R. K. Wright, S. H. Mandy, K. M. Halprin, and S. L. Hsia, *Arch. Dermatol. 107,* 47 (1973).

115. M. M. Mui, S. L. Hsia, and K. M. Halprin, *Br. J. Dermatol., 92,* 255 (1975).

116. S. Wadskov, V. Kassis, and J. Sondergaard, *Acta Dermatovener. (Stockholm), 59,* 525 (1979).

117. K. Adachi, H. Iizuka, K. M. Halprin, and V. Levine, *J. Invest. Dermatol., 74,* 74 (1980).

118. C. L. Marcelo, E. A. Duell, M. A. Stawiski, T. F. Anderson, and J. J. Voorhees, *J. Invest. Dermatol., 72,* 20 (1979).

119. "Dermal Pathology," J. H. Graham, W. C. Johnson, and E. B. Helwig, Eds., Harper and Row, New York, N.Y., 1972, pp. 325–332.

120. M. Gordon, W. C. Johnson, and C. F. Brugoon, Jr., *Arch. Dermatol., 95,* 402 (1967).

121. E. J. Van Scott and T. M. Ekel, *Arch. Dermatol., 88,* 373 (1963).

122. W. Watson, *Rat. Drug Ther. 13,* 4 (1979).

123. C. Grupper, in "Psoriasis"—Proceedings of the International Symposium at Stanford University, 1971, E. M. Farber and A. J. Cox, Eds., Stanford University Press, Stanford, Calif., 1971, p. 354.

124. W. H. Goeckerman, *Northwest Med., 24,* 299 (1925).

125. P. Frost, S. N. Horwitz, R. V. Caputo, and S. M. Berger, *Arch. Dermatol., 115,* 840 (1979).

126. D. L. Cram, *Hospital Formulary, 11,* 596 (1976).

127. L. Tanenbaum, J. A. Parrish, M. A. Pathak, R. R. Anderson, and T. B. Fitzpatrick, *Arch. Dermatol., 111,* 467 (1975).

128. L. Tanenbaum, M. A. Pathak, and J. A. Parrish, *Arch. Dermatol., 111,* 395 (1975).

129. J. A. Parrish, W. L. Morison, E. Gonzalez, T. M. Krop, H. A. D. White, and R. Rosario, *J. Invest. Dermatol., 70,* 111 (1978).

130. P. Frost, S. N. Horwitz, R. V. Caputo, and S. M. Berger, *Arch. Dermatol., 115,* 840 (1979).

131. A. R. Marisco, W. H. Eaglstein, and G. D. Weinstein, *Arch. Dermatol., 112,* 1249 (1976).

132. R. S. Chapman and O. A. Finn, *Br. J. Dermatol., 94,* 71 (1976).

133. B. G. Bryant, *Am. J. Hosp. Pharm., 37,* 814 (1980).

134. D. L. Roberts, R. Marshall, and R. Marks, *Br. J. Dermatol., 103,* 191 (1980).

135. E. G. Weirich, *Dermatologica, 151,* 268 (1975).

136. E. G. Weirich, J. K. Longauer, and A. H. Kirkwood, *Dermatologica, 151,* 321 (1975).

137. *British Journal of Dermatology, 101,* 599 (1979).

138. K. H. Kaidbey, J. W. Petrozzi, and A. M. Kligman, *Arch. Dermatol., 111,* 33 (1975).

139. P. M. Gaylarde and I. Sarkany, *Arch. Dermatol., 112* (1976).

140. H. Schaefer, K. Vivell, V. Kentsch, W. Schella, and S. Jenny, *Br. J. Dermatol., 94,* 363 (1976).

141. J. W. Petrozzi, K. M. Kaidbey, and A. M. Kligman, *Arch. Dermatol., 113,* 292 (1977).

142. *Archives of Dermatology, 112,* 35 (1976).

143. T. Lakshmipathi, P. W. Gould, L. A. Machenzie, B. E. Johnson, and W. Frain-Bell, *Br. J. Dermatol., 96,* 587 (1977).

144. K. W. Wolff, T. B. Fitzpatrick, J. A. Parrish, F. Gschnait, B. Gilchrest, H. Honigsmann, M. A. Pathak, and L. Tanenbaum, *Arch. Dermatol., 112,* 943 (1976).

145. J. W. Melski, L. Tanenbaum, J. A. Parrish, T. B. Fitzpatrick, and H. L. Bleich, *J. Invest. Dermatol., 68,* 328 (1977).

146. J. W. Petrozzi and J. O. Barton, *Arch. Dermatol., 115,* 1061 (1979).

147. A. H. Siddiqui and R. H. Cormane, *Br. J. Dermatol., 100,* 247 (1979).

148. R. S. Cole, *Biochem. Biophys. Acta, 217,* 30 (1970).

149. N. Mizuno, H. Enami, and K. Esaki, *J. Invest. Dermatol., 72,* 64 (1979).

150. R. S. Stern, R. A. Kleinerman, J. A. Parrish, T. B. Fitzpatrick, and H. L. Bleich, *Arch. Dermatol., 116,* 1269 (1980).

151. R. S. Stern, L. A. Thibodeau, R. A. Kleinerman, J. A. Parrish, T. B. Fitzpatrick, and 22 participating investigators, *N. Engl. J. Med., 300,* 809 (1979).

152. A. Lassus, *Br. J. Dermatol., 102,* 195 (1980).

153. H. J. Van Der Rhee, J. G. P. Tijssen, W. A. Herrmann, A. H. Waterman, and M. K. Polano, *Br. J. Dermatol., 102,* 203 (1980).

154. P. O. Fritsch, H. Honigsmann, E. Jaschke, and K. Wolff, *J. Invest. Dermatol., 70,* 178 (1978).

155. G. Heidbreder and E. Christophers, *Arch. Dermatol. Res., 264,* 331 (1979).

156. L. E. King, Jr., *Arch Dermatol., 111,* 131 (1975).

157. R. G. Bergstresser, S. H. Schreiber, and G. D. Weinstein, *Arch. Dermatol., 112,* 977 (1976).

158. A. E. Newburger, G. D. Weinstein, and J. L. McCullough, *J. Invest. Dermatol., 70,* 183 (1978).

159. G. M. Lewis and C. E. Wheeler, "Practical Dermatology," 3rd ed., W. B. Saunders, Philadelphia, Pa., 1967, pp. 207–218.

160. E. Epstein, "Common Skin Disorders–A Manual for Physicians and Patients," Medical Economics, Oradell, N.J., 1979, p. 133.

Dandruff and Seborrhea Product Table

Product (Manufacturer)	Application Form	Keratolytic	Cytostatic Agent	Other Ingredients
Aeroseb-HC (Herbert)	spray			hydrocortisone, 0.5%; alcohol, 47.2%
Anti-Dandruff Brylcreem (Beecham Products)	shampoo		zinc pyrithione, 1%	mineral oil, propylene glycol, paraffin wax, water, excipients
Breck One (Breck)	cream lotion shampoo		zinc pyrithione, 1%	anionic surfactants, 15.6%
Cuticura Anti-Dandruff Shampoo (Jeffrey Martin)	shampoo	sulfur, 2%; salicylic acid, 2%		protein, surfactants
Danex (Herbert)	shampoo		zinc pyrithione, 1%	sodium methyl cocoyl taurate, magnesium aluminum silicate, sodium cocoyl isethionate, citric acid, fragrance
Diasporal (Doak)	cream	colloidal sulfur, 3%; salicylic acid, 2%		isopropyl alcohol, 95%
Duponol Shampoo with 10% LCD (C&M)	shampoo			sodium lauryl sulfate, 15%; coal tar, 10%
Glover's Medicated Ointment (Glover)	ointment	salicylic acid, 3%; sulfur, 5%		petrolatum, mineral oil, cetyl alcohol, quaternium-18, hectorite, propylene carbonate, fragrance, polysorbate-20, propylparaben, iron oxides, talc
Head & Shoulders Cream (Procter & Gamble)	shampoo		zinc pyrithione, 2%	anionic detergent
Head & Shoulders Lotion (Procter & Gamble)	shampoo		zinc pyrithione, 2%	lauryl sulfate, cocamide, ethanolamine, triethanolamine, magnesium aluminum silicate, hydroxypropyl methylcellulose
Ionil (Owen)	shampoo	salicylic acid, 2%		polyoxyethylene ethers (nonionic); benzalkonium chloride, 0.2%; alcohol, 12%
Klaron (Dermik)	lotion	colloidal sulfur, 5%; salicylic acid, 2%		greaseless, hydroalcoholic vehicle; alcohol, 13.1%
Meted (Coopercare)	shampoo	sulfur, 3%; salicylic acid, 2%		highly concentrated detergents
Meted 2 (Coopercare)	shampoo	colloidal sulfur, 2.3%; salicylic acid, 1%		mild detergent blend
Neomark (C&M)	lotion	salicylic acid, 1.6%; resorcinol monoacetate, 1%		coal tar solution, 2%; betanaphthol, 1%; castor oil; isopropyl alcohol, 68%; purified water
Ogilvie (Ogilvie)	shampoo			monoundecylenamido MEA-sulfosuccinate disodium
Pernox (Westwood)	shampoo			sodium laureth sulfate, lauramide DEA, quaternium 22, lanate 25, sodium chloride, lactic acid

Dandruff and Seborrhea Product Table, continued

Product (Manufacturer)	Application Form	Keratolytic	Cytostatic Agent	Other Ingredients
pHisoDan (Winthrop)	shampoo	precipitated sulfur, 5%; sodium salicylate, 0.5%		entsufon sodium, lanolin cholesterols, petrolatum
Rezamid Tinted (Dermik)	lotion	microsize sulfur, 5%; resorcinol, 2%		chloroxylenol, 0.5%; alcohol, 28.5%
Rinse Away (Alberto Culver)	liquid			benzalkonium chloride, 0.05%; laurylisoquinolinium bromide, 0.05%
Sebaquin (Summers)	shampoo			diiodohydroxyquin, 3%
Sebaveen (Coopercare)	shampoo	salicylic acid, 2%; sulfur, 2%		colloidal oatmeal, 5%; emollients, 4%
Sebisol (C&M)	shampoo	salicylic acid, 2%		clorophene, 0.1%; betanaphthol, 1%; alkyl aryl surfactant base (biodegradable); aliphatic alcoholamide conditioner; purified water
Sebucare (Westwood)	lotion	salicylic acid, 1.8%		laureth-4, 4.5%; alcohol, 61%; water; butyl ether; dihydroabietyl alcohol
Sebulex Conditioning Shampoo with Protein (Westwood)	shampoo	salicylic acid, 2%; sulfur, 2%		water, sodium octoxynol-3 sulfonate, sodium lauryl sulfate, lauramide DEA, acetamide MEA, amphoteric-2, hydrolyzed animal protein, magnesium aluminum silicate, propylene glycol, methylcellulose, PEG-14M, fragrance, disodium EDTA, dioctyl sodium sulfosuccinate, FD & C blue 1, D & C yellow 10
Sebulex Medicated Shampoo (Westwood)	shampoo	sulfur, 2%; salicylic acid, 2%		surfactants
Sebutone (Westwood)	shampoo	sulfur, 2%; salicylic acid, 2%		tar, 0.5%; surfactants; cleansers; wetting agents
Selsun Blue (Abbott)	shampoo		selenium sulfide, 1%	surfactants
Soltex (C&M)	shampoo			clorophene, 0.1%; alkyl aryl surfactant base (biodegradable); aliphatic alcoholamide conditioner; purified water
Sul-Blue (Columbia Medical)	shampoo		selenium sulfide, 1%	
Sulfoam (Alvin Last)	shampoo	sulfur		sodium lauryl sulfate, lauramide DEA, glycol stearate, lanolin, citric acid, fragrance, formaldehyde

Dandruff and Seborrhea Product Table, continued

Product (Manufacturer)	Application Form	Keratolytic	Cytostatic Agent	Other Ingredients
Sulfur-8 Hair and Scalp Conditioner (Plough)	ointment	sulfur, 2%		menthol, triclosan
Sulfur-8 Shampoo (Plough)	shampoo			triclosan
Sulpho-Lac (Alvin Last)	cream	microfine sulfur		sulfurated lime, zinc sulfate
Sulpho-Lac Soap (Alvin Last)	soap	sulfur, 9%		zinc oxide, 1%
Vanseb (Herbert)	cream lotion shampoo	sulfur, 2%; salicylic acid, 1%		proteins, surfactants
Zincon (Lederle)	shampoo		zinc pyrithione, 1%	surfactants

Dry Skin Product Table

Product (Manufacturer)	Application Form	Keratin Softener	Humectant	Other Ingredients
Acid Mantle (Dorsey)	cream lotion		glycerin	aluminum acetate, water, cetearyl alcohol, sodium lauryl sulfate, petrolatum (cream), synthetic beeswax (cream), mineral oil (cream), methylparaben
Alpha Keri (Westwood)	bath oil			mineral oil, lanolin oil, polyethylene glycol-4-dilaurate, benzophenone-3, fragrance, D&C Green 6
Alpha Keri Soap (Westwood)	soap			nondetergent soap
Aquacare (Herbert)	cream lotion	urea, 2%	glycerin	oleth-3 phosphate, petrolatum, triethanolamine, synthetic spermaceti, carbomer 934P, mineral oil, lanolin alcohol, cetyl stearyl glycol, lanolin oil, benzyl alcohol, perfume
Aquacare/HP (Herbert)	cream lotion	urea, 10%	glycerin	oleth-3 phosphate, cetyl stearyl glycol, petrolatum, triethanolamine, synthetic spermaceti, carbomer 934P, mineral oil, lanolin alcohol, lanolin oil, benzyl alcohol, perfume
Carmol 20 (Syntex)	cream	urea, 20%		nonlipid base
Carmol 10 (Syntex)	cream	urea, 10%		nonlipid base
Clocream Ointment (Upjohn)	ointment			vitamins A and D, vanishing cream base
Corn Huskers Lotion (Warner-Lambert)			glycerin, 6.7%	water, 5 D alcohol 40 (5.7%), algin, TEA-oleoyl sarcosinate, methylparaben, guar gum, calcium sulfate, calcium chloride
Emulave (Coopercare)	soap		glycerin	vegetable oils and dewaxed lanolin, 25%; colloidal oatmeal, 30%

Dry Skin Product Table, continued

Product (Manufacturer)	Application Form	Keratin Softener	Humectant	Other Ingredients
Esoterica (Norcliff Thayer)	lotion			water, propylene glycol dicaprylate/dicaprate, propylene glycol, TEA stearate, mineral oil, isocetyl stearate, glyceryl stearate, cetyl esters wax, hydrolyzed animal protein, dimethicone, TEA carbomer-941, fragrance, methylparaben, propylparaben, quaternium-15
Extra Strength Vaseline Intensive Care (Chesebrough-Pond's)	lotion		glycerin	white petrolatum, zinc oxide
Italian Balm (Jeffrey Martin)	lotion		glycerin, sorbitol, propylene glycol	SD alcohol 40, water, tragacanth gum, fragrance, PEG-8 stearate, methylparaben, benzoic acid, butylparaben
Jeri-Bath (Dermik)	oil			dewaxed oil-soluble fraction of lanolin, mineral oil, nonionic emulsifier
Jeri-Lotion (Dermik)	lotion			dewaxed oil-soluble fraction of lanolin, mineral oil, nonionic emulsifier
Keri Creme (Westwood)	cream			water, mineral oil, talc, sorbitol, lanolin alcohol, magnesium stearate, glycerol oleate, methylparaben, propylparaben, fragrance
Keri Facial Cleanser (Westwood)	lotion			water, glycerin, squalane, propylene glycol, glyceryl stearate/PEG-100 stearate, stearic acid, steareth-20, lanolin alcohol, magnesium aluminum silicate, cetyl alcohol, beeswax, PEG-20-sorbitan beeswax, methylparaben, propylparaben, quaternium-15, fragrance
Keri Facial Soap (Westwood)	soap			sodium tallowate, sodium cocoate, water, mineral oil, octyl hydroxystearate, fragrance, glycerin, titanium dioxide, PEG-75, lanolin oil, dioctyl sodium sulfosuccinate, PEG-4 dilaurate, propylparaben, PEG-40 stearate, glyceryl monostearate, PEG-100 stearate, sodium chloride, BHT, EDTA
Keri Lotion (Westwood)	lotion (scented and unscented)			mineral oil, water, propylene glycol, glyceryl stearate, polyethylene glycol 40 stearate, polyethylene glycol 100 stearate, polyethylene glycol 4 dilaurate, laureth-4, lanolin oil, methylparaben, propylparaben, carbomer 934, triethanolamine, dioctyl sodium sulfosuccinate, quaternium-15
Keri Light Lotion (Westwood)	lotion			water, stearyl alcohol/ceteareth-20, cetearyl octanoate, glycerin, stearyl heptanoate, stearyl alcohol, squalane, carbomer 934, fragrance, sodium hydroxide, methylparaben, propylparaben, quaternium-15
Lacti Care (Stiefel)	lotion		lactic acid sodium PCA	
Lowila Cake (Westwood)	cleanser bar	urea	lactic acid	dextrin, sodium lauryl sulfoacetate, water, boric acid, sorbitol, mineral oil, polyethylene glycol 14-M, dioctyl sodium sulfosuccinate, cellulose gum, fragrance
Lubriderm (Warner Lambert)	cream		glycerin	lanolin derivatives, cetyl alcohol, petrolatum blend
Lubriderm Lotion (Warner Lambert)	lotion			lanolin derivatives, mineral oil, sorbitol, cetyl alcohol, triethanolamine stearate

Dry Skin Product Table, continued

Product (Manufacturer)	Application Form	Keratin Softener	Humectant	Other Ingredients
Mammol (Abbott)	ointment			bismuth subnitrate, 40%
Nutraderm (Owen)	lotion cream			water, mineral oil, sorbitan stearate, stearyl alcohol, sodium lauryl sulfate, cetyl alcohol, carbomer 940, methylparaben, triethanolamine, propylparaben, fragrance
Nutraplus (Owen)	cream lotion	urea		water, glyceryl stearate, acetylated lanolin alcohol, isopropyl palmitate, stearic acid, ceteareth-5, petrolatum, methylparaben, prypylparaben, carbomer 940
NutraSpa (Owen)	liquid			mineral oil, PEG-4, dilaurate, lanolin oil, butylparaben, benzophenone-3, fragrance, D&C Green #6
Oilatum Soap (Stiefel)	soap			polyunsaturated vegetable oil, 7.5%
Plexolan (Alvin Last)	cream			lanolin, 15%, zinc oxide
Pretty Feet & Hands (Norcliff Thayer)	lotion			water, paraffin, TEA-palmitate, TEA-stearate, magnesium aluminum silicate, fragrance, palmitic acid, stearic acid, methylparaben, propylparaben
Saratoga Ointment (Blair)	ointment			zinc oxide, 14%; boric acid, 1.75%; eucalyptol, 1.1%; servum preparatum; white petrolatum
Sardo (Plough)	bath oil			mineral oil, isopropyl palmitate
Sardoettes (Plough)	towelettes			mineral oil, isopropyl palmitate
Sayman Salve (Goody's)	ointment	propylene glycol		petrolatum, zinc oxide, camphor, lanolin
Shepard's (Dermik)	lotion			sesame oil
Sofenol (C&M)	lotion		glycerin	peanut oil, lanolin, cetyl alcohol, stearyl alcohol, purified water, perfume, triethanolamine stearate, sorbic acid
Soft 'N Soothe (B. F. Ascher)	cream			benzocaine, menthol, natural oat protein, lanolin oil, mineral oil, lanolin alcohol
Surfol (Stiefel)	bath oil			mineral oil, isopropyl myristate, isostearic acid, PEG-40 sorbitan peroleate
Triapon (Spirt)	liquid			olive oil, vegetable oils, nonionic surfactant
Vaseline Dermatology Formula (Chesebrough-Pond's)	cream lotion		glycerin	white petrolatum, mineral oil, dimethicone
Vaseline Pure Petroleum Jelly (Chesebrough-Pond's)	gel			white petrolatum
Wibi (Owen)	lotion			water, SD alcohol 40, glycerin, PEG-4, PEG-6-32, stearate, PEG-6-32, glycol stearate, carbomer 940, PEG-75, methylparaben, triethanolamine, menthol, fragrance

Dermatitis and Psoriasis Product Table

Product (Manufacturer)	Application Form	Keratolytic/ Keratin Softener	Tar Product	Other Ingredients
Alma Tar (Schieffelin)	bath shampoo		juniper tar, 35% (bath), 4% (shampoo)	polyoxyethylene ether, edetate sodium, sulfonated castor oil, coconut oil, triethanolamine (all in shampoo only)
Alphosyl (Reed & Carnrick)	lotion cream	allantoin, 1.7%	coal tar extract, 5%	greaseless, vanishing cream base
Bactine Hydrocortisone Skin Cream (Miles)	cream			hydrocortisone, 0.5%
Balentar (Westwood)	bath oil		tar equiv. to 5% coal tar	mineral oil, lanolin oil
CaldeCORT (Pharmacraft)	cream spray			hydrocortisone, 0.5%
ClearAid (E. R. Squibb)	cream			hydrocortisone, 0.5%
Cortaid (Upjohn)	cream			hydrocortisone, 0.5%
Denorex (Whitehall)	shampoo (plain & herbal)		coal tar solution	menthol; alcohol, 7.5%
Dermolate (Schering)	cream spray			hydrocortisone, 0.5%
Dermtex HC (Pfeiffer)	cream lotion			hydrocortisone, 0.5%
DHS Tar (Person & Covey)	shampoo		coal tar, 0.5%	cleansing agents
Diasporal-Tar (Doak)	cream	colloidal sulfur, 3% salicylic acid, 2%	tar distillate, 5%	isopropyl alcohol, 90%
Estar (Westwood)	gel		tar equiv. to 5% coal tar	hydroalcoholic gel
Hycort (Elder)	cream	allantoin		hydrocortisone, 0.5%
Ichthyol (Stiefel)	ointment		ichthyol, 10%	
Ionil T (Owen)	shampoo	salicylic acid, 2%	coal tar solution, 5% (equivalent)	polyoxyethylene ethers (nonionic); benzalkonium chloride, 0.2%; alcohol, 12%
Kay-San (Commerce)	cream	allantoin, 0.5% resorcinol, 0.4%	coal tar, 0.5%	sodium salicylate, 0.6%; parachlorometaxylenol, 0.25%
Lanacort (Combe)	cream			hydrocortisone, 0.5%
Lavatar (Doak)	bath oil		tar distillate, 25%	
L.C.D. (Schieffelin)	cream		coal tar solution, 5.8%	

Dermatitis and Psoriasis Product Table, continued

Product (Manufacturer)	Application Form	Keratolytic/ Keratin Softener	Tar Product	Other Ingredients
Lipoderm (Spirt)	capsule			pancreas, 500 mg; pyridoxine hydrochloride, 3 mg
Mazon Cream (Norcliff Thayer)	cream	salicylic acid, 1% resorcinol, 1%	coal tar, 0.18%	benzoic acid, 0.5%
Neutrogena T/Derm (Neutrogena Dermatologics)	body oil		coal tar, 2% (equivalent)	2-ethylhexyloxystearate, PEG 40 sorbitan peroleate, benzoic acid
Neutrogena T/Gel (Neutrogena Dermatologics)	shampoo		coal tar, 2%	bland, shampoo base
Oxipor VHC (Whitehall)	lotion	salicylic acid, 1.0%	coal tar solution, 48.5%	benzocaine, 2.0%; alcohol, 81%
Packer's Pine Tar (Cooper Care)	soap		pine tar, 6%	soap chips, 93%
Packer's Pine Tar Shampoo (Cooper Care)	shampoo		pine tar, 0.82%	isopropyl alcohol, 2.175%
Pentrax (Texas Pharmacal)	shampoo		coal tar, 8.75%	highly concentrated detergents
Polytar (Stiefel)	soap bath oil shampoo		juniper, pine, and coal tars, 1% (soap, shampoo); 25% (bath oil)	surfactant base (soap, shampoo)
Pragmatar (Menley & James Labs)	cream	salicylic acid, 3% colloidal sulfur, 3%	cetyl alcohol–coal tar, 4%	emulsion base
Prepcort (Whitehall)	cream			hydrocortisone, 0.5%
Psorex (Jeffrey Martin)	shampoo		coal tar, 1%	surfactants
Psorex Medicated (Jeffrey Martin)	cream shampoo	allantoin, 0.25% (cream), 0.20% (shampoo)	coal tar, 0.50%	silicone base (cream), lanolin and protein base (shampoo), surfactants
Riasol (also known as Dermoil) (Blair)	lotion			phenol, 0.5%; mercury, 0.45% (as coconut oil soap); cresol, 0.75%
Sulfur-8 (Plough)	ointment	sulfur, 2%		menthol, 1%; triclosan, 0.1%; mineral oil
Supertah (Purdue Frederick)	ointment		coal tar fraction, 1.25%	zinc oxide, starch
Tarbonis (Reed & Carnrick)	cream		coal tar extract, 5%	hydrophilic base
Tar-Doak (Doak)	lotion		tar distillate	
Tarpaste (Doak)	paste		tar distillate, 5%	zinc oxide
Tarsum (Summers)	shampoo	salicylic acid, 5%	coal tar solution, 10%	

Dermatitis and Psoriasis Product Table, continued

Product (Manufacturer)	Application Form	Keratolytic/ Keratin Softener	Tar Product	Other Ingredients
Tegrin (Block)	cream lotion shampoo	allantoin, 0.2% (cream and lotion)	coal tar extract, 5%	
Tersa-Tar (Doak)	shampoo		tar distillate, 3%	
Vanseb-T (Herbert)	shampoo	sulfur, 2% salicyclic acid, 1%	coal tar, 5%	sodium lauryl sulfate, sodium stearate, fatty alkylolamide condensate, hydrolyzed animal protein, polyethylene glycol 75, lanolin, silicone–glycol copolymer, imidazolidinyl-urea, perfume
Vaseline Pure Petroleum Jelly (Chesebrough-Pond)	gel			petrolatum, 100%
Wellcortin (Burroughs Wellcome)	cream lotion ointment			hydrocortisone, 0.5%
Zetar (Dermik)	shampoo		crude colloidal coal tar, 1%	chloroxylenol, 0.5%

31

Poison Ivy and Poison Oak Products

Henry Wormser

Questions to Ask the Patient

Have you been exposed to any poisonous plants recently?

Have you been walking in the woods, camping, or working in the garden recently?

Have you ever had a poison ivy/oak/sumac rash before?

How long have you had the rash?

Where is the rash located? How extensive is it?

Are the skin lesions oozing?

What treatments have you tried? Were they effective?

Are you allergic to any medicine or product?

Poison ivy, poison oak, or poison sumac dermatitis is a common, seasonal, allergic contact dermatitis. It may be acute or chronic depending on the extent of exposure and the degree of sensitivity to the allergens. Symptoms range from transient redness to severe swelling and the formation of bullae (blisters); itching and vesiculation nearly always occur. (See Chapter 30, *Dermatitis, Dry Skin, Dandruff, Seborrhea, and Psoriasis Products.*)

Etiology

Causative Plants

Various plants and parts of plants—trees, grasses, flowers, vegetables, fruits, weeds, and airborne pollen—may produce allergic responses (1). Among the 60 or more plants that frequently cause contact dermatitis, those most commonly encountered and responsible for the more severe lesions are poison ivy (*Toxicodendron radicans*), western poison oak (*Toxicodendron diversilobum*), eastern poison oak (*Toxicodendron quercifolium*), and poison sumac, or poison dogwood (*Toxicodendron vernix*) (2). Formerly the species were assigned to the genus *Rhus*; hence, the term rhus dermatitis is used to describe the topical reactions resulting from exposure to these plants. These plants belong to the Anacardiaceae family, members of which often are both noxious and useful and are found in many parts of the world. Members include the Japanese lacquer tree (*Rhus verniciflua*), which grows in Japan, China, and Indochina and from which a rich furniture lacquer is obtained; the cashew nut tree (*Anacardium occidentale*), found in India and Pakistan, the East Indies, Africa, and Central and South America; and the mango tree (*Mangifera indica*), found in tropical areas. Cross-sensitivity may occur on contact of skin with cashew nut shells, mango rinds, and furniture painted with natural lacquer.

Poison ivy and poison oak are the main causes of rhus dermatitis in the United States. Poison ivy is particularly abundant in the eastern United States and southeastern Canada. It may be either a shrub or a vine and is identified readily by its characteristic leaves with leaflets arranged in a cluster of three per stalk; by white berries produced in the fall; and by its usual climbing nature (when it is a vine) (Figure 1). Western poison oak is found along the Pacific coast area from New Mexico to Canada. It commonly grows as a bush without support, and the center leaf of the three-leaflet cluster resembles an oak leaf (Figure 2). Eastern poison oak is found from New Jersey to Florida and from central Texas to Kansas. Poison sumac is a coarse, woody shrub or small tree commonly found in swamps of the southern and eastern United States. It differs from the other two plants by having 7 to 13 leaflets per leaf arranged in two stalks (3) (Figure 3).

In England and western Europe, primrose dermatitis, due to the sensitizing agent primulin, is more common than poison ivy dermatitis (4). A few isolated cases have been reported from France and Australia (5–7). Dark-skinned people seem somewhat less susceptible to these dermatitides than others. Young people are more susceptible than the elderly, and newborns may be sensitized readily by applying the sap of the plant to the body (8). Development of the dermatitis requires that the individual be sensitized to the toxic agent by a previous exposure; therefore, not everyone who is exposed to the plants has an allergic reaction. However, it is estimated that at least 70% of the U.S. population could react after casual exposure to the plants (8).

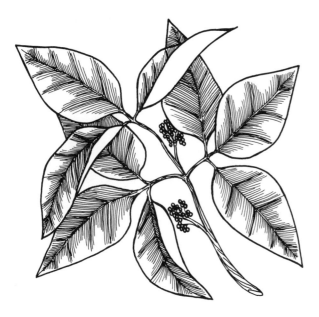

Figure 1. Poison ivy.

Allergenic Constituents

Toxicodendrol, a phenolic oily resin, is present in all of the poisonous species and contains a complex active principle, urushiol. Urushiol is distributed widely in the roots, stems, leaves, and fruit of the plant but not in the flower, pollen, or epidermis (9). Therefore, contact with the intact epidermis of the plant is harmless; dermatitis occurs only if contact is made with a bruised or injured plant or its juice. The dermatitis cannot be contracted through the air because neither toxicodendrol nor urushiol are volatile. However, smoke from burning plants can carry a substantial amount of the oleoresin and may cause serious reactions in susceptible individuals.

The identification and structure elucidation of poison ivy's allergenic constituents are credited mainly to research at Columbia University (10–12). Investigators found four allergens, all possessing a 1,2-dihydroxybenzene or catechol nucleus with a 15-carbon atom side chain at position 3. The only difference among the allergens is the degree of unsaturation of the side chain. There is a saturated component (3-pentadecylcatechol or 3-PDC), a mono-olefin (unsaturated at C-8), a diolefin (unsaturated at C-8 and C-11), and a triolefin (unsaturated at C-8, C-11, and C-14). Certain individuals hypersensitive to 3-pentadecylcatechol show cross-reactivity with other compounds such as resorcinol, hexylresorcinol, and the hydroquinones but not with phenol itself (13).

As little as 1 μg of crude urushiol causes dermatitis in sensitive individuals (14). Direct contact with the plant is not necessary in a sensitive person; contact with the allergens may be made from an article that injured the plant or from soot particles that contain allergenic material from the plant. Stroking a dog whose fur is contaminated also is a common source of allergenic material. The oleoresin may be active for months on tools,

shoes, and clothing. Contaminated clothing, a frequent source of allergens, is rendered harmless by machine laundering with commercial detergent (8).

Although the highest incidence of the dermatitis occurs in the spring and summer months when the leaves are young, soft, and easily bruised, it also may occur in the fall and winter. In the fall, yellow leaves still have allergenic properties, but they are more resistant to injury than earlier in the season. Once they wither and fall, the leaves are much less allergenic. Winter dermatitis, which occurs most often around Christmas in tree nursery employees and in those who cut their own trees, is due to contact with the plant's roots.

Mechanism of Contact Dermatitis

The natural course of contact dermatitis is divided into two phases: a sensitization phase, during which a specific hypersensitivity to the allergen is acquired and an elicitation phase, during which subsequent contact with the allergen elicits a visible dermatologic response (15). In the sensitization phase, urushiol components (catechols) are oxidized to the *o*-quinone derivatives, which then can react readily with epidermal proteins by nucleophilic addition to form complete antigens. Each conjugate leaves the skin through the lymphatic system. The conjugate is then carried to the reticuloendothelial system, where special globulins and antibodies are synthesized and lymphocytes are sensitized in response to the antigenic stimulus. In the elicitation phase, repeated contact with the allergen again produces the antigenic conjugate, this time causing a noticeable reaction. The

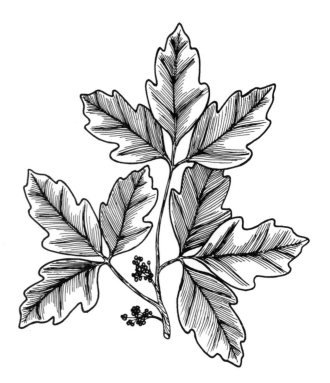

Figure 2. Poison oak.

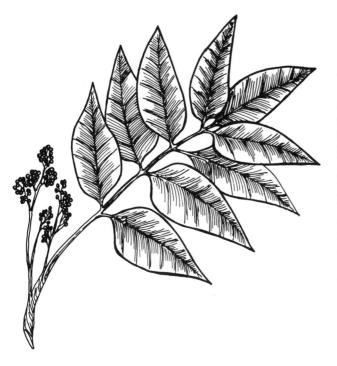

Figure 3. Poison sumac.

reaction appears to be triggered by the association of specific immunologic elements carried by the blood to the skin.

The interval between contact with the allergen and the appearance of the rash varies with the degree of sensitivity and the amount of allergen contacted. Reaction time, the time between contact of sensitized skin with the allergen and the first sign of reaction, is usually 2–3 days, but not less than 12 hours. This interval is characteristic of delayed hypersensitivity reactions involving cell-mediated immunity.

Lesions vary from simple macules to vesicles and bullae. Contrary to popular belief, fluids in the vesicles and bullae are not antigenic, and patch tests with the fluids give negative reactions. Histologically, nonspecific inflammatory changes occur in the dermis, and spongiosis (edema) followed by intraepidermal vesicles is seen in the epidermis in the acute stage of the disease. Bursting of the vesicles may be a problem, because it may lead to secondary infection.

Symptoms

Although the limbs, face, and neck are common sites of the dermatitis, all skin areas that come in contact with the sensitizing substance may be affected. Sometimes distribution of the lesions is bizarre, especially if the antigenic agent is in the clothes or is transferred to various parts of the body by the fingers. The dermatitis may appear in one area and later in another. The phenomenon is often called "spreading." Thorough washing of the skin and laundering of clothes may help prevent this phenomenon by removing the oleoresin before it contacts other areas of the body. Different parts of the body may not have the same sensitivity. Often, parts of the body may sustain a heavy concentration of the antigen with more severe reactions and remain "hypersensitive" for several years.

The type of eruption produced by poison ivy is an allergic eczematous contact dermatitis. Following exposure to the antigen, the initial reaction is erythema or rash. The development of raised lesions (erythematous macules and papules) follows, and finally, vesicles and bullae form, caused by fluid accumulation in the epidermis. (See *Plate 7-30A and B*.) The initial lesions usually are marked by mild to intensive itching and burning. The affected area, often hot and swollen, oozes and eventually dries and crusts (16). Secondary bacterial infections may occur. Very rare complications include eosinophilia, kidney damage, urticaria, erythema multiforme, dyshidrosis, marked pigmentation, and leukoderma (loss of melanin pigmentation occurring in patches). Most cases of the dermatitis are self-limiting and disappear in 14–20 days. Again, disappearance depends on the degree of sensitization and frequency of re-exposure to the allergen.

Rhus dermatitis may be diagnosed not only from the morphologic appearance of the lesions but also from their distribution—linear streaking is common and occurs naturally as the result of "brushing" the skin against the poisonous plant. A history of exposure facilitates the diagnosis. *Toxicodendron* plants are not photosensitizers. The dermatitis occurs on covered and uncovered parts of the body and does not require sunlight to develop.

Diagnostic patch testing is a valuable tool in investigating allergic contact dermatitis (17). However, it should be employed only by individuals thoroughly familiar with accepted techniques. Patch testing should not be done during the acute phase of any dermatitis. It must be understood that substances used for patch testing may sensitize the patient during testing. Positive and negative results of patch testing are not diagnostic in themselves but are interpreted properly in light of the history, the physical findings, and the practitioner's clinical experience.

Treatment

Prophylaxis

The poison ivy antigen enters the skin very rapidly and early washing of the skin with soap (within 10 minutes of exposure) is necessary in any attempt to remove the antigen. Topical prophylactic measures used for poison ivy and poison oak dermatitis include removal of the antigen by washing with soap and water or organic solvents, prior use of barrier creams, and/or use of detoxicants (oxidizing and complexing agents that chemically inactivate the antigen) (13). However, many investigators have shown that the benefits derived from these measures are questionable (18–20).

Thirty-four barrier preparations were tested on a group of highly sensitive people over a 2-year period (13). The preparations were detoxicants that contained substances such as potassium permanganate, hydrogen peroxide, sodium perborate, iodine, and iron and silver salts. The investigator concluded that all preparations were incapable of preventing the dermatitis. It is inferred by this conclusion that the antigen reacts rapidly and quite selectively with the skin and that irreversible damage occurs before preventive action can be taken. Enthusiastic claims have been made for zirconium oxide, an agent used in many nonprescription products. However, tests found it to be completely ineffective (13). In addition, several researchers found extensive, sarcoid-like granulomas of glabrous skin that develops because of allergic hypersensitivity to insoluble zirconium oxide (21–23).

The best prophylaxis for allergic contact dermatitis is complete avoidance of the allergen. People should be taught to recognize and avoid poison ivy and related plants and to observe and search surrounding terrain carefully before choosing a picnic area or campsite. Susceptible individuals should be advised to wear protective clothing such as long sleeves, long pants, socks, and shoes when exposure to the offending agents is probable (e.g., on a picnic or hike). These individuals should be instructed also to dispose of or carefully launder their clothing after the outing. Any object that may have come in contact with the plants should be washed to remove the oleoresin, which will remain potent on the objects' surface for a considerable time.

A black, enamel-like deposit is frequently present on injured areas of poison ivy, poison oak, and poison sumac plants. This finding can be reproduced by crushing leaves onto a sheet of paper. The resulting stain should darken on exposure to air if it came from a *Toxicodendron* plant (24).

When a poisonous plant is in a garden or cannot be avoided, it should be removed physically or destroyed chemically. The latter method is easier and less dangerous, but there are areas where chemicals cannot be used, e.g., around hedges and shrubbery, where the poison ivy is mixed closely with valuable plants. In such situations, digging and pulling (wear gloves) are the only satisfactory methods. The chemicals most effective against poison ivy include amitrole (aminotriazole), ammonium sulfamate, (2,4-dichlorophenoxy)acetic acid (2,4-D), (2,4,5-trichlorophenoxy)acetic acid (2,4,5-T), ammonium thiocyanate, borax, carbon disulfide, coal tar creosote oils, fuel oil and similar petroleum distillates, sodium chlorate, and sodium arsenite. Individuals using these chemicals should wear appropriate protective gear. Chemical sprays may be used at any time when poison ivy is in full leaf, June and July being perhaps the best months. Ordinarily, treatments should begin no later than mid-August, because poison ivy begins to go dormant then and sprays are ineffective. At least three to four treatments at an interval of 2–8 weeks are necessary before all plants are dead (25).

Hyposensitization Therapy

Specific hyposensitization may be tried by administering repeated doses of *Rhus toxicodendron* antigens, but such prophylaxis is neither complete nor permanent; the original sensitivity returns approximately 6 months after the treatment is stopped (26, 27). Various forms of the plant antigens and several routes of administration have been used. Antigens can be administered orally or by intramuscular injection. For equivalent effects, larger amounts of the oleoresin are required orally than parenterally. Orally, there may be partial inactivation and imperfect absorption. Sustained release is probably the major factor in the superior efficacy of the intramuscular route. The maximal hyposensitization can be achieved with approximately 2–2.5 g IM or 2.5–3 g orally of poison ivy oleoresin antigen. Pure pentadecylcatechol may be administered in doses of 2.5–3 g IM or 3.5–4 g orally (26).

Hyposensitization by administering crude extracts or oleoresins from plants usually has been ineffective because extract potency varies and recommended dosages are usually far below those required. Three or four injections cannot provide clinical protection for moderately or extremely sensitive persons. An alum-precipitated pyridine extract has been used with some success. The outlook for successful hyposensitization has been improved by the availability of intramuscularly administered 3-pentadecylcatechol. Large amounts (1–3 g) may be needed in a course of 8–20 injections to provide clinical protection. The greater the sensitivity, the larger the amount needed. Administering an antigenic substance to sensitive individuals involves a certain degree of risk. The exact course of treatment must be individualized and geared to the particular sensitivity level and the person's capacity to tolerate the antigen without serious allergic reactions. If the dermatitis appears during prophylactic treatment, the treatment should be stopped for the duration of the eruption. Chewing poison ivy leaves may result in edematous swelling and pain of the tongue, cheeks, palate, pharynx, and anal region (28).

Hyposensitization is temporary, and maintenance doses of the antigen should be administered at predetermined intervals. Hyposensitization generally results in milder and shorter reactions and lessens the reaction's tendency to "spread" to other parts of the body. It is important that the dermatitis be diagnosed properly by a qualified dermatologist before hyposensitization because prophylactic administration of *Toxicodendron* antigens has no effect on contact dermatitis due to other causes. The only objective proof of successful hyposensitization is a negative or weakly positive patch test reaction to the antigens at a previously strong positive reaction site.

Dermatitides

The initial symptoms of the reaction may be alarming, and the temptation to treat is strong. Simplicity and safety are keynotes of treatment. Many claims for products used for self-medication take credit for the body's own natural reparative processes; in most cases, contact dermatitis is self-resolving. The major treatment objectives are

- To provide protection to the damaged tissue until the acute reaction has subsided;
- To prevent excessive accumulation of debris resulting from oozing, scaling, and crusting without disturbing normal tissue;

- To relieve itching and prevent scratching and excoriation.

Mild Dermatitis

Linear streaks of papules and vesicles often characterize a mild poison ivy or poison oak dermatitis. These lesions and the accompanying pain and itching can be treated by an antipruritic "shake lotion" such as calamine or zinc oxide lotion. A combination of menthol (1%) and equal parts of calamine or zinc oxide lotion and rubbing alcohol can be very soothing (29).

Soaks, baths, or wet dressings also can be effective in soothing pain and itch. Dilute aluminum acetate solution (Burow's solution), saline, or sodium bicarbonate solution can be used in this manner for 30 minutes, 3 or 4 times/day. (Aluminum acetate solution for topical use is usually a 1:10 or 1:40 dilution of aluminum acetate solution USP in water.) In addition, the application of either very cold or moderately hot water may provide relief.

Topical preparations containing local anesthetics and/or antihistamines are available; their use is controversial due to their sensitizing capabilities. Topical steroids such as hydrocortisone also are available for self-medication; however, efficacy of these products has been disputed.

Greasy ointments should not be used during active vesiculation and oozing.

Moderately Severe Dermatitis

Moderately severe poison ivy dermatitis may be characterized by the presence of bullae and edematous swelling of body parts in addition to the papules and vesicles present in milder cases. Large bullae may be drained, by puncturing at the edge, to reduce discomfort; aseptic technique should be used. The tops of the lesions should be kept intact because they protect the underlying, denuded epidermis of the lesions as they dry. The patient should be reassured that the fluid from the lesions will not lead to spreading of the dermatitis, nor will touching someone with the dermatitis transmit the dermatitis. Application of cool compresses of aluminum acetate solution (1:10) to edematous areas may be useful. If the eyelids are affected, cold compresses of boric acid solution can be used (8). During the healing phase, application of a neutral soothing cream, e.g., cold cream, helps prevent crusting, scaling, and lichenification (thickening) of the lesions.

Involvement of the face can be treated by application of wet dressings. Lotions tend to cake, causing discomfort, and should be avoided. Men may find that shaving, although uncomfortable, is less uncomfortable than the accumulation of crust and debris in the beard.

Tub baths using potassium permanganate, oatmeal, or a commercially available colloidal preparation such as Aveeno may be soothing and aid drying of lesions. Potassium permanganate is especially useful after vesicles or bullae are opened. It will aid drying of the lesions and help prevent secondary infection. The patient should be instructed to sit for approximately 15–20 minutes in a tubful of lukewarm water to which 1 teaspoonful of potassium permanganate has been added (8). The crystals should be completely dissolved before the patient gets into the tub to avoid possible caustic skin burns.

Oatmeal or colloidal baths may be very soothing; however, the patient should be warned that these preparations can make the tub surface very slick, and a nonskid mat should be used.

Severe Dermatitis

When the reaction is spread over the body and/or is associated with major swelling or involvement on or around the eyes, systemic treatment is necessary and the patient should be referred to a physician.

Systemic treatment always involves prescription drugs such as anti-inflammatory steroids. Corticosteroids commonly are administered orally over 7 days to 3 weeks in a gradually descending dosage schedule. This type of treatment is relatively safe, since it does not lead to hypercorticism or depress adrenal cortical function significantly, as is inevitably the case in more chronic conditions.

Oral antihistamines may be useful for their antipruritic and sedative effects (8, 30).

Topical treatment of severe poison ivy dermatitis is similar to that recommended for moderately severe dermatitis (8).

Pharmacologic Agents

Four major types of pharmacologic agents—local anesthetics, antipruritics, antiseptics, and astringents—are used in topical nonprescription products for poison ivy and poison oak dermatitis.

Local Anesthetics

Local anesthetics affect sensation by interfering with the transmission of impulse along the sensory nerve fiber. Many nerve fibers, specialized endings or receptors, and free nerve endings are in the epidermis. The superficially applied anesthetic acts very near the application site. However, it is questionable whether the agent can reach the nerve endings when applied to unbroken skin. Benzocaine, diperodon hydrochloride, pramoxine hydrochloride, dibucaine, tetracaine hydrochloride, and cyclomethycaine are the most common agents found in poison ivy/poison oak products. The advantage of the poorly soluble anesthetics, such as benzocaine, over the soluble ones (tetracaine hydrochloride) is the lessened danger of absorption to produce systemic toxicity. These toxic effects, however, occur at relatively high serum concentrations. Fortunately, these high levels are difficult to achieve by applying available topical products. Undesirable effects include dermatitis, characterized by cutaneous lesions, urticaria, and edema; and anaphylactic reactions. Topically applied "caine" anesthetics can be strong sensitizers in susceptible individuals. (See Chapter 25, *Burn and Sunburn Products*.)

Antipruritics

Topically applied antipruritics, including antihistamines, counterirritants, and hydrocortisone, are agents that can help alleviate itching.

Antihistamines

Antihistamines such as diphenhydramine, pyrilamine, tripelennamine, and phenyltoloxamine relieve the discomfort of itching by competing with histamine at the H_1 receptor (one of two broad classes of histamine receptors) and also by their topical anesthetic effect. The anticholinergic action and systemic toxicity of these drugs is of no consequence in considering topical use. However, like the "caine" anesthetics, they may act as sensitizers. Antihistamines are more effective orally than topically as antipruritics, particularly when itching is generalized. For topical products, application of a 1–2% concentration of the drugs to the affected area 3 times/day will bring about relief from itching. (See Chapter 24, *Insect Sting and Bite Products.*)

Counterirritants

Counterirritants such as menthol, phenol, and camphor produce a sensation of coolness and reduce the irritation of the dermatitis. The sensation is difficult to explain because these chemicals produce local hyperemia. However, the counterirritants in low concentrations have an analgesic effect due to a depression of cutaneous receptors. Care must be exercised when these agents are applied to damaged skin since they may be irritating. (See Chapter 27, *External Analgesic Products.*)

Hydrocortisone

Hydrocortisone is a naturally occurring steroidal hormone manufactured endogenously in the adrenal cortex. It has been marketed in the United States as a prescription drug since 1952.

Although useful for a variety of dermatitides, there is some controversy as to whether topical corticosteroids are effective for poison ivy and poison oak dermatitis. Steroids previously were implicated in the exacerbation of bacterial infections. However, the FDA review panel on nonprescription external analgesic drug products re-

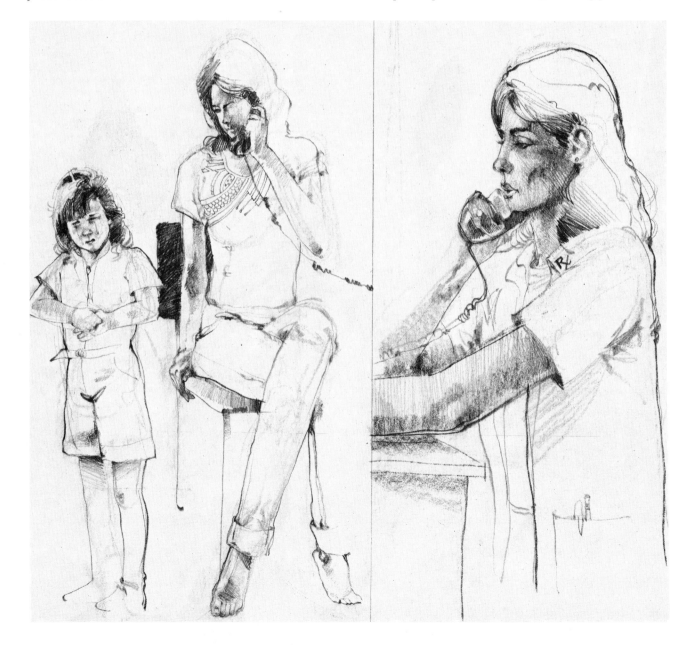

ported that there seems to be no danger of exacerbation of cutaneous bacterial, fungal, or viral infections by topical application of 0.25–0.5% hydrocortisone. The panel also reported that allergic reactions to hydrocortisone at these concentrations were rare. Additionally, the panel found evidence that prolonged administration of 0.25–0.5% hydrocortisone did not appear to cause toxic effects by systemic absorption even when applied to large areas of damaged or abraded skin (31).

One of the FDA-approved uses of hydrocortisone-containing products available for nonprescription sale must carry specific labeling as follows: "For the temporary relief of minor skin irritations, itching, and rashes due to eczema, dermatitis, insect bites, poison ivy, poison oak, poison sumac, soaps, detergents, cosmetics, and jewelry and for itchy genital and anal areas but not for ophthalmic use."

The dosage for adults and children 2 years of age and older is 0.25–0.5% hydrocortisone applied to the affected area 3 or 4 times/day. There is no recommended dosage for children under 2 except under the advice and supervision of a physician. Contact with the eyes should be avoided.

Antiseptics

Antiseptics used in poison ivy and poison oak products probably are intended for prophylaxis against secondary infections, but their effectiveness is questionable. Of the available antiseptics (phenols, alcohols, and oxidizing agents) and quaternary ammonium compounds such as benzalkonium chloride, the quaternary ammonium agents seem to be more effective. Unfortunately, their action is antagonized by anionic compounds such as soap (6).

Astringents

Astringents are mild protein precipitants that form a thick coagulum on the surface of lesions or coagulate and remove overlying debris. The astringent action is accompanied by contraction and wrinkling of tissue and by blanching. The cement substance of the capillary endothelium is hardened so that pathologic transcapillary movement of plasma proteins is inhibited and local edema, inflammation, and exudation is thereby reduced. These substances, including aluminum acetate, tannic acid, zinc and iron oxides, and potassium permanganate, are used to stop oozing, reduce inflammation, and promote healing. Astringents also have mild antiseptic properties.

Aluminum acetate solution (Burow's solution) is usually used as a wet dressing up to 3 times/day and is generally diluted with about 10 to 40 parts of water. Therapy may be continued for approximately 5–7 days. Continuous or prolonged use for extended periods may produce necrosis.

Zinc oxide may be used as a 15–25% lotion or ointment as it is insoluble in water. It has mild astringent, protective, and antiseptic action. Calamine, a mixture of zinc oxide and 1% ferric oxide, is often preferred to plain zinc oxide because of its tan color.

Potassium permanganate may not be desirable because it leaves an objectionable purple stain. It is most useful after the vesicles or bullae are opened and is used as a 0.01% solution (29).

Product Selection Guidelines

Selection of products depends on the severity of the dermatitis. Mild to moderately severe cases of poison ivy or poison oak dermatitis usually can be treated with local or topical products. Preparations that contain benzocaine or other local anesthetics should be used with caution, and zirconium oxide products should be avoided. Hydrocortisone products may or may not be effective; other effective treatments should be recommended first. In severe cases of poison ivy dermatitis a physician should be consulted.

Individuals sensitive to *Toxicodendron* plants should be informed of certain cosmetics, hair dyes, bleaches, and other commercial products that contain compounds related to 3-pentadecylcatechol, which could exhibit cross-allergenicity. Shake lotions, which may contain phenol or menthol, provide immediate relief due to the cooling effect of water evaporation. Phenol and menthol increase the antipruritic activity. However, consultation should include cautioning against the frequent use of shake lotions, which pile on the skin masses of plaster-like material that are difficult and painful to remove.

Summary

Poison ivy, poison oak, and poison sumac cause contact dermatitides in many people every year. Prophylaxis and therapy of this allergy are still in the early stages of study, although much research is being conducted and progress is being made. Better understanding of the mechanism of the allergic reaction, cross-sensitivity, and hyposensitization will help in designing better products to alleviate and possibly eradicate this annoying and often serious disorder.

References

1. A. A. Fisher, "Contact Dermatitis," 2nd ed., Lea and Febiger, Philadelphia, Pa., 1973, p. 1.
2. M. A. Lesser, *Drug Cosmet. Ind., 70,* 610 (1952).
3. C. R. Dawson, *Trans. N.Y. Acad. Sci. Sect. Phys. Chem., 18,* 427 (1956).
4. A. Rook and H. T. H. Wilson, *Br. Med. J., 1,* 220 (1965).
5. J. Beurey, J.-M. Mougeolle, M. Weber, and J. Mazet, *Ann. Dermatol. Venerol., 107,* 65 (1980).
6. J. H. Apted, *Austral. J. Dermatol., 19,* 35 (1978).
7. J. H. Apted, *Int. J. Dermatol., 19,* 81 (1980).
8. A. A. Fisher, "Contact Dermatitis," 2nd ed., Lea and Febiger, Philadelphia, Pa., 1973, pp. 260-266.
9. J. H. Doyle, *Pediatr. Clin. North Am., 8,* 259 (1961).
10. S. V. Sunthankar and C. R. Dawson, *J. Am. Chem. Soc., 76,* 5070 (1954).
11. W. E. Symes and C. R. Dawson, *J. Am. Chem. Soc., 76,* 2959 (1954).
12. B. Love and C. R. Dawson, *J. Am. Chem. Soc., 78,* 1180 (1956).
13. A. M. Kligman, *Arch. Dermatol., 77,* 149 (1958).
14. F. A. Stevens, *J. Am. Med. Assoc., 127,* 192 (1945).
15. A. L. deWeek, in "Dermatology in General Medicine," T. B. Fitzpatrick, K. A. Arndt, W. H. Clark, Jr., A. Z. Isen, E. J. Van Scott, and J. J. Vaughan, Eds., McGraw-Hill, New York, N.Y., 1971, p. 669.
16. P. M. Selfon, *Milit. Med., 128,* 895 (1963).

17. A. M. Kligman, *J. Invest. Dermatol., 47,* 369, 375, 393 (1966).
18. B. Shelmire, *J. Am. Med. Assoc., 113,* 1085 (1939).
19. O. Gisvold, *J. Am. Pharm. Assoc. Sci. Ed., 30,* 17 (1941).
20. J. B. Howell, *Arch. Dermatol. Syphilol., 48,* 373 (1943).
21. P. J. LoPresti and G. W. Hambrick, Jr., *Arch. Dermatol., 92,* 188 (1965).
22. W. L. Epstein and J. R. Allen, *J. Am. Med. Assoc., 190,* 940 (1963).
23. N. A. Hall, *J. Am. Pharm. Assoc., NS12,* 576 (1972).
24. J. D. Guin, *J. Am. Acad. Dermatol., 2,* 332 (1980).
25. D. M. Crooks and L. W. Kephart, "Farmers' Bulletin," Publication No. 1972, U.S. Department of Agriculture, Washington, D.C., 1951, 30 pp.
26. A. M. Kligman, *Arch. Dermatol., 78,* 47 (1958).
27. A. M. Kligman, *Arch. Dermatol., 78,* 359 (1958).
28. S. H. Silvers, *J. Am. Med. Assoc., 116,* 2257 (1941).
29. "Current Therapy," H. F. Conn, Ed., W. B. Saunders, Philadelphia, Pa., 1979, p. 588.
30. "Applied Therapeutics for Clinical Pharmacists," 2nd ed., M. A. Koda-Kimble, B. S. Katcher, and L. Y. Young, Eds., Applied Therapeutics, San Francisco, Calif., 1978, p. 860.
31. *Federal Register, 44,* 69822 (1979).

Poison Ivy and Poison Oak Product Table

Product (Manufacturer)	Application Form	Anesthetic	Antipruritic/ Antihistamine	Antiseptic	Astringent	Other Ingredients
Americaine (American Critical Care)	spray	benzocaine, 10%		benzethonium chloride, 0.1%		alcohol, 25%
Caladryl (Parke-Davis)	cream lotion		diphenhydramine hydrochloride, 1% camphor, 0.1%		calamine, 8%	alcohol, 2% (lotion)
Calamatum (Blair)	ointment lotion spray	benzocaine, 3%	camphor	phenol	zinc oxide calamine	
Calamox (Mallard)	ointment		camphor, 0.5% pyrilamine maleate, 1%	phenol, 0.5%	calamine, 20% zinc oxide, 10%	
Dalicote (Dalin)	lotion	diperodon hydrochloride, 0.25%	pyrilamine maleate camphor		zinc oxide	dimethyl polysiloxane silicone greaseless base
Dermapax (Recsei)	lotion		pyrilamine maleate, 0.22% chlorpheniramine maleate, 0.06%	chlorobutanol, 1% benzyl alcohol, 1%		isopropyl alcohol, 40%
Didelamine (Commerce)	gel		tripelennamine hydrochloride, 0.5% diphenhydramine hydrochloride, 1% menthol, 0.1%	benzalkonium chloride, 0.25%		clear gel
Hista-Calma Lotion (Rexall)	lotion	benzocaine, 1%	phenyltoloxamine citrate, 1%		calamine, 5%	
Ivarest (Carbisulphoil-Blistex)	cream lotion	benzocaine, 1%	pyrilamine maleate, 1.5% menthol, 0.7% camphor, 0.3%		calamine, 14%	
Ivy Dry Cream (Ivy)	cream	benzocaine, 5 mg/ml	menthol, 4 mg/ml camphor, 6 mg/ml		tannic acid, 8%	methylparaben, 2.5 mg/ml propylparaben, 0.3 mg/ml isopropyl alcohol, 7.5%
Ivy Dry Liquid (Ivy)	liquid				tannic acid	isopropyl alcohol, 12.5%
Ivy SupEz Dry (Ivy)	liquid	benzocaine, 5 mg/ml	menthol, 2 mg/ml camphor, 4 mg/ml		tannic acid, 100 mg/ml	isopropyl alcohol, 35% methylparaben, 0.01 mg/ml propylparaben, 0.1 mg/ml
Ivy-Chex (Bowman)	non-spray aerosol			benzalkonium chloride, 1:1000		alcohol, 89.5% acetone polyvinyl-pyrrolidone-vinyl acetate copolymers

Poison Ivy and Poison Oak Product Table, continued

Product (Manufacturer)	Application Form	Anesthetic	Antipruritic/ Antihistamine	Antiseptic	Astringent	Other Ingredients
Ivy-Rid (Mallard)	aerosol			benzalkonium chloride		alcohol acetone isobutane methylene chloride polyvinyl-pyrrolidone-vinyl acetate copolymers
Nupercainal Cream (Ciba)	cream	dibucaine, 0.5%				acetone sodium bisulfite, 0.37% water-washable base
Nupercainal Ointment (Ciba)	ointment	dibucaine, 1%				acetone sodium bisulfite, 0.5%
Obtundia Calamine Cream (Otis Clapp)	cream			cresol–camphor complex	calamine zinc oxide	
Poison Ivy Cream (McKesson)	cream	benzocaine, 2.5%	pyrilamine maleate, 15 mg/g		zirconium oxide, 4% (as carbonated hydrous zirconia)	
Poison Ivy Spray (McKesson)	aerosol	benzocaine, 0.5%	menthol camphor		calamine, 2% zinc oxide, 1%	isopropyl alcohol, 9.44%
Pontocaine (Breon)	cream ointment	tetracaine hydrochloride, 1% (cream); 0.5% (ointment)	menthol, 0.5% (ointment)			methylparaben (cream) sodium bisulfite (cream) white petrolatum (ointment) white wax (ointment)
Pyribenzamine (Ciba)	cream ointment		tripelennamine, 2%			water-washable base (cream) petrolatum base (ointment)
Rhuli Cream (Lederle)	cream	benzocaine, 1%	menthol, 0.7% camphor, 0.3%		zirconium oxide, 1%	isopropyl alcohol, 8.8%
Rhuli Spray (Lederle)	spray	benzocaine, 0.98%	camphor, 0.098% menthol, 0.009%		zirconium oxide, 1% calamine, 0.98%	isopropyl alcohol, 9.5%
Rhuligel (Lederle)	gel		menthol, 0.3% camphor, 0.3%	benzyl alcohol, 2%		alcohol, 31%
Rhulihist (Lederle)	lotion	benzocaine, 1.153%	camphor, 0.253% menthol, 0.025%	benzyl alcohol, 0.674%	calamine, 4.710%	alcohol, 28.76%
Surfadil (Lilly)	cream lotion	cyclomethy-caine, 0.5%	diphenhydramine hydrochloride, 1%			titanium dioxide, 5% (lotion)

Poison Ivy and Poison Oak Product Table, continued

Product (Manufacturer)	Application Form	Anesthetic	Antipruritic/ Antihistamine	Antiseptic	Astringent	Other Ingredients
Topic (Syntex)	gel		camphor menthol	benzyl alcohol, 5%		isopropyl alcohol, 30% greaseless base
Tronothane Hydrochloride (Abbott)	cream jelly	pramoxine hydrochloride, 1%				water-miscible base water-soluble base
Tyrohist Cream (Columbia Medical)	cream	benzocaine	pyrilamine maleate, 1% camphor menthol	benzalkonium chloride	neocalamine	
Ziradryl (Parke-Davis)	lotion		diphenhydramine hydrochloride, 2% camphor, 0.1%		zinc oxide, 2%	alcohol, 2%
Zotox (Commerce)	spray				zirconium hydrate, 8.36%	

32 Diaper Rash and Prickly Heat Products

Gary H. Smith

Questions to Ask the Parent

Diaper Rash

Do you use disposable diapers or a diaper service?

Do you use cloth diapers? How do you launder them?

Where does the rash occur and what does it look like?

Do you use double diapers or plastic pants?

How often do you change the baby's diapers?

How do you clean the baby's skin during a diaper change?

What products have you already tried using for the rash?

Does the baby have a fever?

Has the baby had diarrhea recently?

Has the baby ever had a yeast infection?

Prickly Heat

Where is the rash located and what does it look like?

How long has the rash been present?

Does the baby sleep in a very warm and humid room?

How much clothing do you put on the baby during the day and night?

What products have you already tried for the rash?

Diaper rash and prickly heat (miliaria rubra) are acute, transient, inflammatory skin conditions that occur in many infants and young children. Both conditions cause burning and itching that can result in restlessness, irritability, and sleep interruption. Most cases can be reversed easily by simple home remedies; however, prevention is the best treatment.

The skin of most adults is about 2 mm thick, but infant skin is about 1 mm thick and therefore more delicate. The epidermis (the outermost skin layer) represents about 5% of the total skin thickness; therefore, the external barrier that protects the infant from the environment is very thin (1). (See Chapter 28, *Topical Antiinfective Products,* for a discussion of skin anatomy.) For the skin to function most efficiently, it should remain dry and smooth and maintain a slightly acidic pH.

Diaper Rash

Diaper rash, or diaper dermatitis, is one of the most common dermatitides in infants. One study reported an incidence of 17% in 1-week-old infants (2). Diaper rash is an acute, inflammatory reaction of the skin in the diaper area caused by one or more factors and is probably best viewed as a group of disorders rather than as a specific diagnosis (3).

Etiology

Urine or urine contents and feces have long been implicated as being the cause of diaper rash. Normal newborns begin urinating within 24 hours after birth. Urination occurs up to 20 times/day until 2 months of age and as many as 8 times/day from 2 months to 8 years of age. Defecation also occurs several times/day in infants (4). Breast-fed infants tend to urinate less frequently and have a lower incidence of dermatitis than bottle-fed infants. Furthermore, the urine and feces tend to be less alkaline and therefore less irritating than that of bottle-fed infants (5, 6).

The distribution of diaper rash may be positional: If the baby lies on his or her stomach, the rash may be dorsal; if the baby lies on his or her back, the rash may be ventrally located. It may spread to the entire diaper area, depending on the promptness of therapy and what causes the rash. The diaper area is vulnerable to inflammation because the skin is often warm and moist and is exposed to irritants and bacteria. Ammonia probably plays a role in irritating a previously existent condition, but it is also possible that high-protein foods (excluding milk) in the diet of the baby may be a contributing factor. High-protein foods may make the urine and stools more acidic and produce an "acid scald" (7). Secondary infections caused by various microorganisms and other complications may occur.

The histopathologic changes vary with the causative factors and the severity of the dermatitis. Diaper rash may range from superficial conditions such as mild erythema with or without maceration and chafing, progressing to vesicles, pustules, or bullae. Deeper nodular and infiltrated lesions may develop depending on the primary cause of the dermatitis. Seborrhea, psoriasis, and atopic diathesis, or frequent bowel movements may lower skin resistance to irritation and infection.

Ammonia

Until recently, the most widely accepted theory of the etiology of diaper rash was the presence of ammonia and other irritating end products of the enzymatic breakdown of urine. Ammoniacal dermatitis was first described in 1886 (8), and other reports followed in the early 1900's (9, 10). It was later learned that ammonia in the diaper area is produced by urea-splitting bacteria found in the stool (11). The causative organism, *Brevibacterium ammoniagenes*, was isolated from stool samples of 31 children with diaper rash. Other ammonia-liberating organisms include Micrococcaceae, the aerobic diphtheroids, lactose-fermenting gram-negative rods, and *Proteus* and *Pseudomonas* species. These organisms are saprophytic and can ferment urea to produce ammonia as follows:

$$CO(NH_2)_2 + 2H_2O \rightleftharpoons (NH_4)_2CO_3$$
$$\rightleftharpoons 2NH_3 + H_2O + CO_2$$

Ammonia may cause diaper rash by raising the skin pH. Moreover, it may form soaps after combining with constituents of natural skin oils.

One study found a close correlation between urine's odor and its ability to produce erythema, regardless of the urinary pH (12). This study showed that malodorous, putrescent materials, in the absence of ammonia and high pH, may cause erythema. These materials also are produced by enzymatic degradation of urine.

Some investigators (13) failed to demonstrate erythema or other changes in the skin of the buttocks of 10 infants after a 24-hour occlusive dressing containing 1.6% ammonia in urine was applied. This ammonia concentration was five times the mean concentration found in 26 infants with diaper rash. It was further noted that in the 26 infants with diaper dermatitis, 44.4% had organisms capable of liberating ammonia in 4–6 hours; 52.3% of 82 control infants without diaper rash had ammonia-liberating organisms present. *Brevibacterium ammoniagenes* was isolated in a total of 5 of the 26 infants, of which only three had diaper rash. This study casts doubt on the importance of this organism and ammonia as a causative factor in diaper dermatitis.

Sweat Retention

If a soiled diaper is not changed promptly, the stratum corneum in the diaper area becomes waterlogged. This saturation causes keratotic plugging of the sweat glands (plugging with loose protein material on the skin),

which results in perspiration retention and may cause erythematous papules (14).

Mechanical and Chemical Irritants

Tightly fitting diapers covered with plastic pants increase the humidity and temperature in the diaper area and prevent air from circulating around the skin, producing an environment conducive to irritation and causing secondary infection. Irritation results from the diaper's constant rubbing against the skin. Broken skin is more susceptible to infection. If diapers are changed frequently, irritation may be prevented.

Chemical irritants from various sources may precipitate a rash in the diaper area. Feces remaining in contact with the skin cause irritation, especially if the infant's diet promotes the elimination of irritating substances, such as alkaline material, unabsorbed foodstuffs, and diarrhea. (See *Plate 8-31.*). Preparations commonly applied to the diaper area, such as proprietary antiseptic agents and harsh soaps containing mercury, phenol, tars, salicylic acid, or sulfur, also may cause diaper rash. Diapers rinsed inadequately after washing may retain residues from detergents or bleach that can irritate the diaper area or cause allergic reactions. Precautions should be taken to avoid exposing the sensitive skin of infants and young children to these irritating substances (14, 15).

Complications

Yeast and bacterial infections are the most common complications of diaper rash. These cutaneous infections are often secondary to untreated or improperly treated diaper dermatitis. The moist, warm, alkaline environment created by unchanged diapers is conducive to the development and multiplication of many pathogenic bacteria and yeast (13). Most bacteria and yeast do not produce lesions on normal skin. However, if the skin is broken or macerated or the normal balance of the skin's bacterial flora is disturbed, these organisms may become pathogenic and cause a serious infection in the diaper area (5).

Yeast infections are caused most commonly by *Candida albicans*, an organism that is part of the normal colonic flora. Infections due to *C. albicans* represent the most frequent cause of diaper rash complications. The feces are the most common source of this organism (13, 16). Because candidal infections of the diaper area are a secondary complication of diaper dermatitis, the clinical picture is often obscure, and the only precise method of diagnosis is culturing *C. albicans* from scrapings of the skin lesions (14, 17). In newborns less than 2 weeks old, candidal diaper dermatitis usually is accompanied by oral thrush. Both conditions probably result from the presence in the mother of a candidal vaginal infection before and during delivery. The lesions are usually erythematous and are surrounded by characteristic satellite pustules. They may become eroded and weeping. A physician should be consulted for appropriate treatment of this condition.

Bacterial infection of the diaper area is caused most commonly by *Staphylococcus aureus* and is often a form of folliculitis. Classic lesions are follicular micropustules that enlarge with those adjacent to form lakes or pustules. These may coalesce to form an area of secondarily infected dermatitis. Occasionally, bullous or encrusted impetigo, characterized by large blister-like lesions or honeycomb crusting, respectively, may occur. In some cases, group A *Streptococcus* species may be the pathogen. Glomerulonephritis rarely may develop as a tertiary complication. An infant with a suspected bacterial infection in the diaper area should be referred to a physician for appropriate diagnosis and therapy (3, 13, 18).

Ulceration of the penile meatus may be a painful complication of diaper rash in circumcised babies. The pain associated with this condition may lead to reflex inhibition of micturition and secondary distention of the bladder (19, 20).

Prickly Heat (Miliaria)

The lesions associated with this acute dermatitis result from obstruction of the sweat gland pores. Retained sweat causes the dilation and rupture of the epidermal sweat pores, producing swelling and inflammation. (See *Plate 8-32.*) The term "prickly heat" was coined because the lesions usually produce itching and stinging. Prickly heat occurs primarily during hot, humid weather or during a febrile illness with heavy sweating. It also may occur as a result of excessive clothing and overcovering, especially at night in warm, humid rooms. Prickly heat may occur at any time during infancy as well as in adulthood.

The lesions appear in intertriginous areas of maceration and under plastic pants, diapers, and adhesive tape. The lesions, which are erythematous papules, may become pustular and are usually localized to the sites of occlusion (8, 21, 22).

Patient Assessment

In general, if the diaper dermatitis is confined to the diaper area and does not present symptoms of fungal or bacterial infections, the pharmacist may recommend a nonprescription product. If the infant has had diaper rash for only a few days, self-treatment may be recommended. The pharmacist should determine whether laundry detergents containing irritants are being used. If diaper rash persists 1 week or more after the infant has been treated with protectants and has been changed frequently, or the rash recurs frequently, the rash may be caused by a problem other than the diaper, and a physician should be consulted. If the infant has had persistent diarrhea, appears irritable, has a fever, or the rash is resistant to nonprescription treatment, a physician should be consulted because the problem may be more serious than simple diaper rash.

If the rash is more widespread than the diaper area (groin, intergluteal fold, or lower abdomen), a condition such as atopic dermatitis or seborrheic dermatitis may be present and these infants should be diagnosed by a physician for appropriate treatment. Candidal and bacterial infections also require a definitive diagnosis by a physician. If the lesions are follicular micropustules, bullous, or look like impetigo, a bacterial infection may be the cause.

The pharmacist may be able to recognize the cause of many conditions by questioning the parents. In addition to explaining the steps that must be taken to prevent diaper rash and prickly heat, the pharmacist may recommend several products suited to the child's condition. If the pharmacist ascertains that the dermatitis has persisted and appears to be complicated by infection or another process, it should be suggested that the child be taken to a physician.

Treatment

The treatments for diaper rash and prickly heat may be considered together, but modifications and additional measures may be required for each entity. The active treatment of diaper rash involves removing the source of irritation, reducing the immediate skin reaction, relieving discomfort, and preventing secondary infection and other complications. The treatment plan should be individualized for both diaper rash and prickly heat. The area should be kept as dry and clean as possible. The diaper should be loose, well ventilated, dry, and changed as quickly as possible after becoming soiled. Plastic pants should be avoided. Products helpful in treatment include protectants, agents to promote healing, antiseptics, and anticandidal and anti-inflammatory agents. The pharmacist should be able to advise parents about which products should be used for a particular kind of dermatitis and the specific care required. As with most forms of therapy, the simplest regimen is the one most likely to be followed consistently. A baby's skin is sensitive, and many babies may be irritated by or allergic to some available products.

In treating mild forms of diaper rash the best remedy is changing diapers as soon as they are soiled and completely drying the diaper area before a new diaper is used. The parent should be advised to place the infant on an opened diaper during the nap to avoid soiling bed clothes. The condition of infants with ammoniacal dermatitis can improve when they are exposed to air as often as possible. Cornstarch as a dusting powder should be avoided since it may be metabolized by microorganisms and encourage bacterial overgrowth (23). Use of an incandescent lamp as a heat source may speed healing (24, 25). The use of a good protective agent such as zinc oxide paste (Lassar's paste) or white petrolatum provides a barrier to protect the skin from moisture.

In the treatment of prickly heat, the primary goal is to reduce further sweating. The clothing should be made of light material and should not cause any rubbing of the skin. Light clothing and covering are recommended to allow air to reach the skin. Air conditioning the environment helps lower humidity and temperature. Maceration and irritants may be reduced by frequent bathing or sponge baths at least 2 times/day and the use of a bland talc dusting powder. Oatmeal (1 cup of Aveeno Colloidal Oatmeal in a tub of warm water) and soy protein (1 packet of protein colloidal bath powder in a tub of warm water) may help in treating prickly heat. Frequent diaper changes and the elimination of any excessive soap or chemical irritants help reduce discomfort associated with prickly heat.

Treatment of diaper dermatitis with a light application of 0.5–1% topical hydrocortisone after each diaper change for a limited time period has been recommended (27, 28). One investigator has recommended application of 2.5% hydrocortisone in highly inflammatory diaper rash. However, it should be noted that corticosteroids may alleviate symptoms of diaper rash but not eliminate the cause.

Because occlusive dressings facilitate the absorption of topically applied steroids through normal (not inflamed) skin, they should not be used in the diaper area (27). When steroids are applied topically to inflamed or abraded skin, systemic levels may be higher than when they are applied to normal skin, due to increased absorption (29).

Recognition of the value of topical hydrocortisone for diaper dermatitis by the medical community does not warrant its use for infants on a nonprescription basis. Now that 0.5% hydrocortisone cream is available for nonprescription use, pharmacists should caution parents concerning the use of this product for diaper rash. Hydrocortisone is not recommended for use on children under 2 years of age except under the advice and supervision of a physician. Furthermore, comments have been made that hydrocortisone should be reserved for cases in which zinc oxide ointment or similar products, along with standard preventive measures, have not been sufficient (30). With this in mind, advice to use hydrocortisone topically for the infant patient without physician intervention does not appear warranted. (See Chapter 31, *Poison Ivy and Poison Oak Products*, for a more complete discussion of hydrocortisone.)

Secondary Complications

Secondary infections caused by bacteria or *Candida* species should be diagnosed and treated by a physician. Various antiseptic agents have been used to treat staphylococcal- and streptococcal-induced infections. Topical antibiotics available without prescription have an adjunct role at best in the treatment of these bacterial infections. Systemic antibiotics are the treatment of choice for impetigo (31). Quaternary ammonium compounds are included as antibacterial agents in commercial products; however, their effectiveness has been questioned. In addition, these compounds may act as irritants in some cases, exacerbating the inflammation, and causing discomfort when applied (33). Antibiotic ointments, especially neomycin, should be used only when clearly indicated because they may cause hypersensitivity reactions (34).

In candidal diaper rash, the use of anticandidal agents may be necessary. Aluminum acetate (Burow's) solution soaks may be used for severe dermatitis followed by the application of nystatin dusting powder or ointment at a concentration of 100,000 units/g (17, 35). A 2% amphotericin B ointment also is effective (36). More recently, topical 2% miconazole nitrate cream and 1% haloprogin cream have been shown to be effective in treating candidal diaper rash (37, 38). Hydroxyquinoline can be applied topically for its antibacterial and antifungal activity. Calcium undecylenate is used for its antifungal activity. Nystatin, amphotericin B, micona-

zole nitrate, clotrimazole, haloprogin cream, and hydroxyquinoline are prescription-only products; aluminum acetate solution and calcium undecylenate are available without prescriptions.

Avoidance of Dietary Irritants

The theory that various foods and food additives cause a higher incidence of diaper rash has not been substantiated. In a study of 1,184 infants, there was no significant difference in diaper rash between infants fed an iron-fortified formula and those fed formulas without iron (39). If a certain food appears to cause problems, it may be discontinued for a trial period. The nutrients provided by the food, however, should be provided by another food.

Prophylaxis

Good prophylactic practices depend on parental cooperation and responsibility. Common sense is perhaps the best guide for preventive therapy.

A diaper should be changed as soon as it is soiled; leaving a wet diaper on for several hours increases the chances of diaper rash. The apparently unsoiled part of the diaper should never be used to wipe the baby. This spreads millions of microorganisms over the skin that will proliferate when the child next urinates. If frequent changes are impossible, the infant should be kept belly down to reduce the tendency for feces and urine to become compressed under the gluteal area. Diapers should be made of soft material and fastened loosely to prevent rubbing. Plastic pants should be used as seldom as possible, since they are occlusive and impede the passage of air through the diaper. The use of plastic pants at night and for extended periods should be discouraged.

Infants often urinate soon after they are put to bed for the night. Parents can reduce the time a child is exposed to a wet diaper and the amount of urine accumulated at night by changing the diaper within several hours after putting the child to bed.

The diaper area should be cleaned at each diaper change. Mild soap (Oilatum or a commercial baby soap) should be used for cleaning the diaper area and for bathing. It is important that skin folds that entrap perspiration and feces be cleaned thoroughly and rinsed well with clean water. The diaper area should be completely dry before a clean diaper is put on. Exposing the diaper area to warm, dry air for a few minutes between changes helps to keep the skin dry. A bland ointment or dusting powder (such as zinc oxide ointment or talcum powder) may be recommended after washing.

Several reports have dealt with the use of antibacterial compounds in laundering diapers. If home-laundered diapers are used, they can be soaked in a solution of Borax (½ cup Borax/gallon of water) before washing (25). Another antibacterial compound that can be used for presoaking, to reduce odor, and to disinfect diapers is a diluted sodium hypochlorite solution, provided the infant is not sensitive to bleach. Diapers should be washed with mild soap. The use of harsh detergents and water softeners should be avoided. After they are washed, the diapers should be rinsed thoroughly.

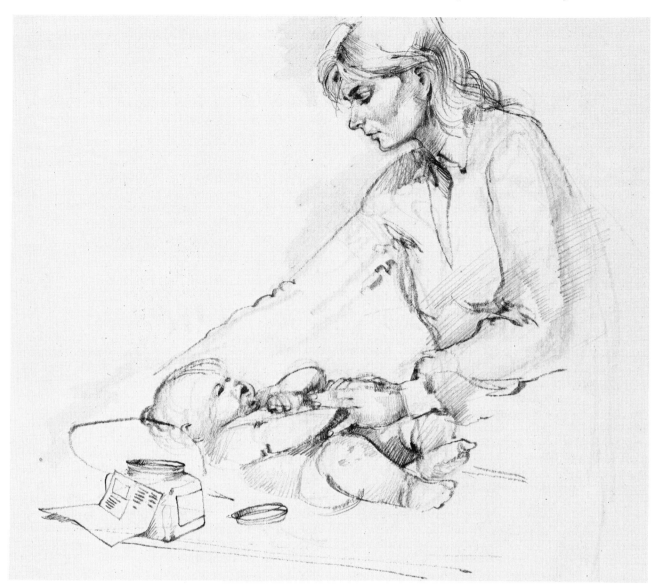

The addition of a disinfectant during the washing process is an effective means of reducing bacterial count. A 5.25% sodium hypochlorite bleach (Clorox) properly diluted, reduced the number of organisms from 277/in² to 2/in² (40). The use of clorophene (*o*-benzyl-*p*-chlorophenol) in the first rinse of diapers in a concentration of 1 part clorophene to 2,500 parts water also is effective in treating and preventing ammoniacal diaper dermatitis (41). Acidification of diapers may also be helpful. This effect can be accomplished by a final rinsing of diapers in a solution made by adding 1 cup of vinegar to a half-filled washing machine tub. The diapers are then added and soaked for ½ hour. This is a more economical alternative (42).

One study found that diapers cleaned by a diaper service were associated with the lowest incidence of diaper rash (24.4%), disposable diapers showed a similar low incidence (25%), and home-laundered diapers were associated with the greatest incidence (35.6%) (43). The home-laundered diapers were not rinsed with a bacteriostatic agent. These reports show the necessity of using a bacteriostatic agent either in the rinse water or in the diaper pail. Diapers containing fecal material

should be rinsed well in the toilet before they are placed in the diaper pail. Commercial diaper services provide essentially sterile diapers. The only disposable diapers that are occlusive are those with elasticized sides.

Another study (44) compared home-laundered diapers with a commercial paper diaper in 146 1-month-old infants. The incidence of severe rash was greater (16.1%) with the commercial disposable diaper than that seen with home-laundered cloth diapers (3.3%). The manufacturer of the disposable diaper has responded with evidence that "types and severity of rash do not differ significantly" between infants diapered in cloth or commercial disposable diapers (45). It seems that the prompt changing of diapers when soiled or wet is the best prevention of diaper rash irrespective of the type of diaper used.

Prophylaxis with powders and ointments is not necessary for all babies. Just because an infant wears diapers does not mean that powders and ointments should be applied. If a problem occurs, it should be treated. If it recurs, then prophylaxis is warranted. However, most babies who develop diaper rash will respond to treatment and not need prophylaxis. Babies who require continued prohylaxis should have it stopped periodically to determine if it is still necessary.

Pharmacologic Agents

Nonprescription products for diaper rash and prickly heat treatment include protectants, powders, and antiseptics.

Protectants

The following compounds are classified as safe and effective in the proposed rules of the FDA advisory review panel on nonprescription skin protectant drug products (46): allantoin, aluminum hydroxide gel, calamine, cocoa butter, cornstarch, simethicone, glycerin, kaolin, petrolatum preparations (petrolatum and white petrolatum), shark liver oil, sodium bicarbonate, zinc acetate, zinc carbonate, and zinc oxide. Petrolatum, zinc oxide, calamine, and simethicone are the agents most commonly found in diaper rash products. It can be seen from the product table that other protectants are also included in various products. Benzoin, compound tincture of benzoin, bismuth subnitrate, titanium dioxide, and magnesium carbonate are listed as protectants in these products. No evidence has been found that establishes the value of these compounds in the treatment of diaper rash. Although they may have protectant action, it seems reasonable to assume that since the FDA advisory review panel did not include them in their evaluation, their use is of questionable value (46). Zinc oxide, an excellent protectant found in many products used to treat diaper rash, is a mild astringent with weak antiseptic properties. Many properties contain various concentrations of zinc oxide and petrolatum. Zinc oxide paste USP, the simplest of these formulations, contains 25% zinc oxide, 25% cornstarch, and 50% white petrolatum. Parents should be informed that this is most easily removed with mineral oil. This combination serves as a highly water-immiscible base. Many commercial preparations contain zinc oxide, in some cases at a higher concentration than Lassar's paste (Desitin contains 40% zinc oxide). Most of the preparations also contain one or more of various other medicaments such as cod liver oil, vitamins A and D, lanolin, peruvian balsam, and silicone.

The FDA advisory review panel on nonprescription skin protectant drug products has recommended that the 2-year lower age limit applicable for most nonprescription ingredients be waived for the majority of skin protectants. This waiver does not refer to zinc acetate, shark liver oil, and live yeast cell derivative, for which the 2-year age limit will continue to apply. Additionally, glycerin and aluminum hydroxide gel are not recommended for use on infants less than 6 months of age (47).

In general, these various products are popular and are promoted primarily for the treatment of diaper rash. Only recently have there been controlled studies with these products (48, 49). Reports from Leeming/Pacquin (48, 49) showed Desitin Ointment to be superior to bland soap and unmedicated talcum powder in the treatment of diaper rash. Only one report has been published that compares one product with the other (48). In this report, Lantiseptic Ointment (Corona) [*p*-chloromercuriphenol (1:1,500) in a lanolin and petrolatum base] in a controlled study was shown to be equal or superior to vitamin A and D ointment in the treatment of diaper rash. Although several anecdotal reports indicate that vitamin A and D ointment or cod liver oil–containing ointments may be beneficial in preventing and treating diaper rash (50–53), no evidence exists that indicates any of these products are superior to zinc oxide paste or white petrolatum. Therefore, zinc oxide paste or white petrolatum should be recommended as a protectant and as initial treatment for diaper rash. Use of these products avoids subjecting the infant to compounds that may cause skin sensitization, such as peruvian balsam.

Powders

The powdered agents used in treating diaper rash and prickly heat are talc, calcium carbonate, kaolin, zinc stearate, microporous cellulose and magnesium stearate. Talc is a natural hydrous magnesium silicate that allays irritation, prevents chafing, and absorbs sweat. Talc is similar to ointments and creams in that it adheres well to the skin. It is a finely milled powder that will not cake in the folds and cause maceration by friction. Magnesium stearate is included in some dusting powders promoted for infant use because of its ability to adhere to the skin and to serve as a mechanical barrier to irritants. Calcium carbonate, kaolin, zinc stearate, and microporous cellulose are also included in products for their moisture-absorbing properties. When applied after each changing, these products serve primarily to keep the diaper area dry. They should be used cautiously because inhalation of the dust by the infant may be harmful and could lead to chemical pneumonia. They should be applied with a cotton fluff to spread evenly. Powders should never be applied to an acute oozing dermatitis since they may promote secondary crusting and infection.

Antiseptics

Boric acid has been used extensively in the past for its bacteriostatic and fungistatic activity in diaper dermatitis and prickly heat treatment. It has been incorporated into ointments in concentrations of as much as 3% and into dusting powders. However, there have been reports of toxicity and, in two instances, death associated with boric acid use (54, 55). In one quantitative study of 16 infants, boron levels were significantly high in infants treated with 3% boric acid/borate ointments (56). Concern about boron toxicity has prompted the American Academy of Pediatrics Committee on Drugs to recommend to the FDA that products containing boric acid be reformulated, eliminating boric acid as an ingredient. The FDA advisory review panel on nonprescription topical antiseptic drug products concluded that boric acid is not safe for nonprescription use due to the possibility of systemic absorption and toxicity (57).

Other antiseptic compounds are found in diaper rash products. Quaternary ammonium compounds such as benzalkonium chloride, benzethonium chloride, methyl benzethonium chloride, and cetylpyridium chloride are included in several products. As mentioned previously, these compounds have not been shown to be of any benefit in the treatment of diaper rash. Their inclusion in products is primarily aimed at reducing bacterial flora and preventing infection. However, they are irritating substances and may aggravate or even induce a rash. Since the presence of ammonium-producing bacteria have not been shown to correlate with diaper rash and there is questionable efficacy of the quaternary ammonium compounds, it is suggested that products containing these substances be avoided (58).

Product Selection Guidelines

Pharmacists should advise parents about the correct use of any product recommended. Some general precautions should be mentioned, such as expiration dates and the possibility of stinging and irritation when the topical preparation is applied. If powders are recommended, parents should be instructed to apply them carefully to prevent the infant from inhaling the powder, which could lead to chemical pneumonia. When soaks and solutions (such as aluminum acetate solution) are used, the unused portion should be discarded after each use; i.e., only fresh preparations should be used each time.

Above all, pharmacists should caution parents about the general use of any medication for a baby's skin. The best therapy for diaper dermatitis is to keep the skin clean and dry.

Few infants escape diaper rash. The pharmacist may help by teaching parents the proper procedures for preventing diaper rash and prickly heat. Parents should understand that using medications indiscriminately is not the proper way to treat either condition and is ill advised. Drugs alone cannot stop or prevent diaper rash or prickly heat. Many newborns, infants, and young children may be hypersensitive to various medicaments, and more harm than good can result from their use.

Summary

Pharmacists should be prepared to offer sound advice on a good prophylactic program and to recommend therapy for uncomplicated, uninfected cases. They also should be prepared to assess the severity of the rash and be able to recommend appropriate action, either referral to a physician or a treatment plan.

Diaper dermatitis and prickly heat are the two most common afflictions of newborns, infants, and young children, but the incidence and severity may be reduced by following the proper procedures. If the dermatitis does not respond to frequent diaper changes, frequent exposure to air, and application of a good protectant, such as zinc oxide paste, within 1 week, a physician should be consulted.

References

1. W. L. Weston, "Practical Pediatric Dermatology," Little, Brown, Boston, Mass., 1979, pp. 1–2.
2. G. Weipole, *Klin. Paediatr., 186,* 259 (1974).
3. J. J. Leyden and A. M. Kligman, *Arch. Dermatol., 114,* 56 (1978).
4. K. S. Shepard, "Care of the Well Baby," Lippincott, Philadelphia, Pa., 1968, p. 2310.
5. D. R. Marlow, "Textbook of Pediatric Nursing," W. B. Saunders, Philadelphia, Pa., 1973, pp. 136–137.
6. P. J. Koblenzer, *Clin. Pediatr., 12,* 386 (1973).
7. *Clinical Pediatrics, 3,* 409 (1964).
8. L. Jacquet, *Rev. Mens. Mal. Enf., 4,* 208 (1886).
9. T. S. Southworth, *Arch. Pediatr., 30,* 730 (1913).
10. J. Zahorsky, *Am. J. Dis. Child., 10,* 436 (1915).
11. J. V. Cooke, *Am. J. Dis. Child., 22,* 481 (1921).
12. G. W. Rapp, *Arch. Pediatr., 72,* 113 (1955).
13. J. L. Leyden, S. Katz, R. Stewart, and A. M. Kligman, *Arch. Dermatol., 113,* 1678 (1977).
14. L. M. Solomon and N. E. Esterly, "Neonatal Dermatology: Major Problems in Clinical Pediatrics," Vol. 9, W. B. Saunders, Philadelphia, Pa., 1973.
15. M. D. Lewis, *Med. J. Aust., 2,* 83 (1976).
16. R. F. Pittillo, *J. Dermatol., 12,* 245 (1973).
17. P. J. Kozinn, *Antibiot. Annu.,* 910 (1958/1959).
18. L. F. Montes, R. F. Pittillo, D. Hunt, A. J. Narketes, and M. D. Dillon, *Arch. Dermatol., 103,* 400 (1971).
19. S. Swift, *Pediatr. Clin. N. Am., 3,* 759 (1956).
20. J. Brennemann, *Am. J. Dis. Child., 21,* 38 (1921).
21. H. L. Barnett, "Pediatrics," Appleton-Century-Crofts, New York, N.Y., 1968, pp. 1808–1809.
22. E. Holzle and A. M. Kligman, *Br. J. Dermatol., 99,* 117 (1978).
23. K. Arndt, "Manual of Dermatologic Therapeutics," 2nd ed., Little, Brown, Boston, Mass., 1978, p. 68.
24. M. M. Alexander and M. S. Brown, "Pediatric Physical Diagnosis for Nurses," McGraw-Hill, New York, N.Y., 1974, pp. 22–23.
25. D. A. Humphries, Master of Nursing Thesis, University of Washington, Seattle, Wash., 1966.
26. W. E. Nelson, "Textbook of Pediatrics," 2nd ed., W. B. Saunders, Philadelphia, Pa., 1979, p. 1885.
27. R. D. Carr and W. M. Tarnowski, *Acta Derm. Venereol., 48,* 417 (1968).
28. R. B. Scoggins and B. Kliman, *N. Engl. J. Med., 273,* 831 (1965).
29. R. J. Feldman and H. I. Maibach, *Arch. Dermatol., 91,* 661 (1965).
30. A. Kligman and A. Kaidberg, *Cutis, 22,* 232 (1978).
31. T. Mochizuki, *Hosp. Pharm., 12,* 260 (1977).
32. E. Shmunes and E. J. Levy, *Arch. Dermatol., 105,* 91 (1972).
33. J. Patrick, J. D. Panzer, and V. J. Darbes, *Arch. Dermatol., 102,* 532 (1970).
34. P. J. Kozinn, *J. Pediatr., 59,* 76 (1961).
35. P. J. Kozinn, *Antibiot. Annu.,* 128 (1956/1957).
36. R. M. Mackie and E. Scott, *Practitioner, 222,* 124 (1979).
37. L. F. Montes and H. W. Hermann, *Cutis, 21,* 410 (1978).
38. W. W. Grant, L. Street, and R. G. Fearnow, *J. Pediatr., 81,* 973 (1972).
39. H. S. Whitehouse and N. W. Ryan, *Am. J. Dis. Child., 112,* 225 (1967).
40. W. Friend, *Calif. Med., 87,* 56 (1962).
41. A. H. Jacobs, *Pediatr. Clin. N. Am., 25,* 209 (1978).
42. W. W. Grant, L. Street, and R. G. Fearnow, *Clin. Pediatr., 12,* 714 (1973).
43. F. Wiener, *J. Pediatr., 95,* 422 (1979).
44. W. E. Jordan, *J. Pediatr., 96,* 957 (1980).
45. *Federal Register, 43,* 34628 (1978).
46. *Federal Register, 43,* 34632 (1978).
47. Leeming/Pacquin Pharmaceutical Co., research report, 1974.
48. W. S. James, *J. Med. Assoc. Ga., 64,* 133 (1975).
49. H. T. Behram, F. C. Combes, A. Bobroff, and R. Leviticus, *Ind. Med. Surg., 18,* 512 (1949).
50. C. B. Heimer, H. G. Grayzel, and B. Kramer, *Arch. Pediatr., 68,* 382 (1951).
51. P. M. Kruschner, H. F. Cohen, H. R. Moskow, and A. Snyder, *J. Am. Osteopath. Assoc., 53,* 215 (1953).
52. H. G. Grayzel, C. B. Heimer, and R. B. Grayzel, *N.Y. State J. Med., 53,* 2233 (1953).
53. W. T. Maxon, *J. Ky. Med. Assoc., 52,* 423 (1954).
54. *Brit. Med. J., 2,* 603 (1970).
55. P. Jensen, *Nord. Med., 86,* 1425 (1971).
56. *Federal Register, 45,* 34642 (1978).
57. *Federal Register, 43,* 1237 (1978).

Diaper Rash and Prickly Heat Product Table

Product (Manufacturer)	Application Form	Protectant	Powdered Agent	Antimicrobial	Other Ingredients
A and D Ointment (Schering)	ointment				cod liver oil petrolatum anhydrous lanolin base
Ammens Medicated Powder (Bristol-Myers)	powder	zinc oxide, 9.10%	talc, 45.06% starch, 41%	boric acid, 4.55% 8-hydroxyquinoline, 0.1% 8-hydroxyquinoline sulfate, 0.05%	aromatic oils, 0.14%
Ammorid Dermatologic Ointment (Kinney)	ointment	zinc oxide		benzethonium chloride	lanolin
Ammorid Diaper Rinse (Kinney)	powder			methylbenzethonium chloride	edetate disodium
Aveeno Bar (Cooper Care)	cleanser				colloidal oatmeal, 50% mild sudsing agent (soap free) lanolin
Aveeno Colloidal Oatmeal (Cooper Care)	powder				oatmeal derivatives
Aveeno Lotion (Cooper Care)	lotion				colloidal oatmeal, 10% nonionic surfactants emollients
Aveeno Oilated (Cooper Care)	liquid				colloidal oatmeal, 43% lanolin fraction liquid petrolatum
Bab-Eze Diaper Rash Cream (A.V.P.)	cream	zinc oxide	starch		cod liver oil diperodon hydrochloride, 0.25% aluminum acetate peruvian balsam
Baby Magic Lotion (Mennen)	lotion			benzalkonium chloride, 0.1%	lanolin refined sterols
Baby Magic Oil (Mennen)	oil				mineral oil lanolin
Baby Magic Powder (Mennen)	powder			methylbenzethonium chloride, 0.1%	
Bagbalm (Dairy Associates)	ointment			8-hydroxyquinoline sulfate, 0.3%	petrolatum and lanolin base
Balmex Baby Powder (Macsil)	powder	zinc oxide	talc starch calcium carbonate		peruvian balsam
Balmex Emollient Lotion (Macsil)	lotion				peruvian balsam purified silicone lanolin fraction
Balmex Ointment (Macsil)	ointment	zinc oxide bismuth subnitrate			vitamins A and D peruvian balsam base containing silicone

Diaper Rash and Prickly Heat Product Table, continued

Product (Manufacturer)	Application Form	Protectant	Powdered Agent	Antimicrobial	Other Ingredients
B-Balm Baby Ointment (North American)	ointment	zinc oxide, 10% compound benzoin tincture, 0.005 ml/g			phenol, 2.17 mg/g methyl salicylate, 0.67 mg/g
Biotres (Central)	ointment			polymyxin B sulfate, 10,000 units/g bacitracin zinc, 500 units/g	
Borofax (Burroughs Wellcome)	ointment			boric acid, 5%	lanolin
Caldesene Medicated Ointment (Pharmacraft)	ointment	zinc oxide	talc		cod liver oil lanolin petrolatum
Comfortine (Dermik)	ointment	zinc oxide, 12%			lanolin vitamins A and D
Dalicreme (Dalin)	cream			methylbenzethonium chloride, 0.1%	vitamins A and D diperodon hydrochloride, 0.25% scented greaseless base
Dalisept (Dalin)	ointment			methylbenzethonium chloride, 0.1% hexachlorophene, 1%	vitamin A, 750 units/g vitamin D, 75 units/g diperodon hydrochloride, 1% petrolatum–lanolin base
Desitin Ointment (Leeming)	ointment	zinc oxide, 40%	talc		cod liver oil petrolatum lanolin
Diapa-Care Baby Powder (Paddock)	powder		corn starch	benzethonium chloride	sodium bicarbonate
Diaparene Baby Powder (Glenbrook)	powder	magnesium carbonate, 3.5%	corn starch, 96.0%		
Diaparene Medicated Cream (Glenbrook)	cream			methylbenzethonium chloride, 1:1,000	petrolatum glycerin
Diaparene Peri-Anal Medicated Ointment (Glenbrook)	ointment	zinc oxide, 20%		methylbenzethonium chloride, 1:1,000	cod liver oil, 5% water-repellent base
Johnson & Johnson Medicated Powder (Johnson & Johnson)	powder	zinc oxide	talc		menthol fragrance
Johnson's Baby Cream (Johnson & Johnson)	cream				water mineral oil paraffin sodium borate lanolin white beeswax ceresin glyceryl stearate
Johnson's Baby Powder (Johnson & Johnson)	powder		talc		fragrance

Diaper Rash and Prickly Heat Product Table, continued

Product (Manufacturer)	Application Form	Protectant	Powdered Agent	Antimicrobial	Other Ingredients
Mediconet (Medicone)	cloth wipe			benzalkonium chloride, 0.02%	hamamelis water, 50% glycerin, 10% ethoxylated lanolin, 0.5% methylparaben, 0.15% perfume
Methakote Pediatric Cream (Syntex)	cream		talc	benzethonium chloride, 0.2%	protein hydrolysate
Mexsana Medicated Powder (Plough)	powder	zinc oxide, 10.8%	corn starch kaolin	triclosan, 0.1%	camphor eucalyptus oil
Oilatum Soap (Stiefel)	cleanser				polyunsaturated vegetable oil, 7.5%
Panthoderm (USV)	lotion				dexpanthenol, 2% water-miscible base
Plexolan Cream (Alvin Last)	cream				lanolin, 15% zinc oxide
Rexall Baby Powder (Rexall)	powder		talc		fragrance
Spectro-Jel (Recsei)	gel			cetylpyridinium chloride, 0.1%	glycol-polysiloxane, 1% isopropyl alcohol, 15% methylcellulose, 1.5%
Taloin (Warren-Teed)	ointment	calamine, 3.6%		methylbenzethonium chloride, 0.13%	eucalyptol, 0.3% silicone base, 1.0%
Vaseline Pure Petroleum Jelly (Chesebrough-Pond)	gel				white petrolatum, 100%
ZeaSorb (Stiefel)	powder		microporous cellulose carbohydrate acrylic copolymer talc		
Zincofax Cream (Burroughs Wellcome)	cream	zinc oxide, 15%			petrolatum-lanolin base

33   Foot Care Products

Nicholas G. Popovich

Questions to Ask the Patient

Where is the lesion located (on or between the toes or on the sole of the foot)? Is the toenail involved?

Is there any redness, itching, blistering, oozing, scaling, or bleeding from the lesion?

Is a physician treating you for any other medical condition, such as diabetes, heart trouble, or problems with your circulation?

Do you take insulin? What other medicines do you take?

Is the condition painful? Is it too uncomfortable to walk?

Have you tried to treat this problem yourself? If so, how?

Did you see your physician about this problem? If so, what did he or she tell you to do? What have you done? Did it help?

How long have you had the problem?

Did the problem begin with the use of new shoes (sandals or enclosed shoes, flat or high heels), socks, or soaps?

Do you have any allergies, asthma, or skin problems?

Is there any history of trauma to the foot?

Do your feet sweat a lot?

How often and in what manner do you trim your toenails? (When appropriate)

What is your occupation?

Although foot conditions generally are not life-threatening, except perhaps in diabetic patients, they may cause some measure of discomfort and impaired mobility—from a limitation of activity to a serious disease condition (1). Corns, calluses, and ingrown toenails are common and may contribute to impairment.

Pain usually is associated with corns and warts. The pain from corns may be severe and sharp (when downward pressure is applied) or dull and discomforting. Calluses usually are asymptomatic, causing pain only when pressure is applied (2). Individuals who suffer from calluses on the sole of the foot frequently draw a parallel of their discomfort to that of a person walking with a pebble in the shoe. Another important sign with foot problems is hardening of the skin, signaling a biochemical problem and causing abnormal weight distribution in that particular area of the foot. This hardening, which can be identified physically by the physician and the patient, is an objective sign, as opposed to pain, which is subjective. A podiatric examination is warranted to determine whether an imbalance is present.

Human mycotic (fungal) infections that have cutaneous manifestation may be subdivided conveniently into five categories based on site of invasion (Table 1) (3). The superficial and cutaneous types usually warrant the pharmacist's advice.

The primary lesions of athlete's foot often consist of macerated tissues, slight scaling, occasional vesiculation, and fissuring between and under the toes (4). Any or all of the interdigital webs of the foot may be affected, although usually the skin beneath the fourth and fifth toes of each foot is involved. A relapse of the disease is inevitable if there is nail involvement (unless treated with griseofulvin or ketoconazole), or if the infection is present on the soles of the feet and treatment has not been adequate (5, 6).

Corns and Calluses

Pressure commonly resulting from tightly fitting shoes is the most frequent cause of pain from corns. Narrow-toed or high-heeled shoes crowd the toes into the narrow

Table 1. Classification of mycotic infections of man that possess cutaneous manifestation according to site of invasion

Mycotic infection type	Site(s) of invasion	Example
Superficial	Outermost layer of skin and appendages	Tinea versicolor (caused by *Malassezia furfur*)
Cutaneous	Skin lesion and/or nail	Tinea pedis (caused by *Trichophyton rubrum*)
Subcutaneous	Cutaneous and subcutaneous tissue	Sporotrichosis (caused by *Sporotrichum schenkii*)
Intermediate	Skin, mucous membranes, internal viscera	Vaginal candidiasis (caused by *Candida albicans*)
Deep systemic	Viscera, bone, nerve, skin	Blastomycosis (caused by *Blastomyces dermatitidis*)

Reprinted with permission from J. Raskin, in "Current Therapy," H. F. Conn, Ed., W. B. Saunders, Philadelphia, Pa., 1976, pp. 611–614.

toe box. The most lateral toe, the fifth, experiences the most pressure and friction and is the usual site of a corn. Friction (caused by loosely fitting shoes), walking barefoot, and orthopedic biomechanical problems contribute to the development of calluses. Orthopedic problems include improper weight distribution, pressure, and the development of bunions with age (7). Tight-fitting hosiery and nonlubricated friction in hosiery may cause blisters, calluses, and corns.

Symptoms

Corns and calluses are strikingly similar in one respect: each has a marked hyperkeratosis of the stratum corneum. (See Chapter 28, *Topical Anti-infective Products.*) Beyond this feature, however, there are marked differences.

A corn (clavus) is a small, sharply demarcated, hyperkeratotic lesion having a central core (Figure 1) (8). It is raised, has a yellowish gray color, and ranges from a few mm to 1 cm or more in diameter. The base of the corn is on the skin surface. The apex of the corn points inward and presses on the nerve endings in the dermis, causing pain.

Corns may be either hard or soft. Hard corns occur on the surfaces of the toes and are shiny and polished. Soft corns are whitish thickenings of the skin unusually found on the webs between the fourth and fifth toes. Accumulated perspiration macerates the epidermis and gives the corn a soft appearance. This situation occurs because the fifth metatarsal is much shorter than the fourth, and the web between these toes is deeper and extends more proximally than the webs between other toes.

Hard corns (usually) and soft corns (less frequently) are caused by underlying bony prominences. A bony spur, or exostosis (a bony tumor in the form of an ossified muscular attachment to the bone surface), nearly always exists beneath long-lasting hard and soft corns. A lesion located over non-weight-bearing bony prominences or joints, such as metatarsal heads, the bulb of the large toe, the dorsum of the fifth toe, or the tips of the middle toes, is usually a corn (9).

A callus differs from a corn in that it has no central core and has more diffuse thickening of the skin (Figure 1) (7, 8). It has indefinite borders and ranges from a few millimeters to several centimeters in diameter. It is usually raised, yellow, and has a normal pattern of skin ridges on its surface. Besides joints, calluses form on weight-bearing areas, such as the palms of the hands and the sides and soles of the feet. (See *Plate 8-33.*)

During corn or callus development, the cells in the basal cell layer undergo mitotic division, leading to the migration of maturing cells through the prickle cell (stratum spinosum) and the granular (stratum granulosum) skin layer. The rate is equal to the continual surface cellular desquamation. Normal mitotic activity and subsequent desquamation lead to complete replacement of the epidermis in about 1 month (10). In the case of a callus, friction and pressure cause faster mitotic activity of the basal cell layer (10). This activity produces a thicker stratum corneum as more cells reach the outer skin surface. When the friction or pressure is relieved, mitotic activity returns to normal, causing remission and disappearance of the callus.

Treatment

The success of treatment of corns and calluses with nonprescription products depends on eliminating the causes: pressure and friction. This process entails the use of well-fitting, nonbinding footwear that distributes body weight evenly. For anatomical foot deformities, orthopedic corrections must be made. These measures relieve pressure and friction to allow the resumption of normal mitosis of the basal cell layer, the normalization of the stratum corneum after total desquamation of the hyperkeratotic tissue, and the action of efficacious topical products. Before instituting a self-treatment program, it may be wise to secure a medical opinion.

Experiments have been made to treat corns by injecting fluid silicone subdermally (11). The injected silicone seems to augment digital and plantar tissues, using a cushioning effect, reducing pain and decreasing the need for regular palliative treatment.

Bunions

Bunions are swellings of the bursae and can be caused by various conditions. Pressure from a tightly fitting shoe over a period of time generally causes the condition, but pressure may result from the manner in which a person sits, walks, or stands. Friction on the toes from bone malformations (wide heads or lateral bending) also causes bunions.

Symptoms

The hallux, or great toe, along with the inner side of the foot provides the elasticity and mobility needed to walk or run. Thus, the hallux is a dynamic organ (12). However, this mobility causes several anatomical disorders associated with the foot, such as hallux valgus, the deviation of the great toe toward the lateral (outer) side of the foot (13). Prolonged pressure caused by hallux valgus may result in pressure over the angulation of the metatarsophalangeal joint of the great toe, causing inflammatory swelling of the bursa over the metatarsophalangeal joint (Figures 2A and B). This may result in bunion formation (Figure 1) (14).

Treatment

Corrective steps to alleviate bunions often depend on the degree of discomfort. Bunions may be asymptomatic but usually become quite painful, swollen, and tender. The bunion itself usually is covered by an extensive keratinous overgrowth. Topical nonprescription drugs do provide some relief; however, surgery may be indicated.

Bunions are not amenable to topical drug therapy. The patient should correct the condition by wearing properly fitting shoes or seek the advice of a podiatrist or orthopedist. If the condition is not severe, shielding the bunion with protective pads (moleskin) may be all that is necessary. However, if the manifestation is severe or particularly unsightly, surgical correction is usually indicated.

Larger footwear may be necessary to compensate for the space taken up by the pad; not increasing shoe size may cause pressure in other areas. Also, protective pads should not be used on bunions when the skin is broken or blistered. Before pads are applied, palliative treatment first should involve treatment of the abraded skin. If these conditions persist, particularly in diabetic patients, the pharmacist should recommend that the patient see a podiatrist or orthopedist. Surgical treatment may be necessary.

Warts (Verrucae)

Warts, or intraepidermal tumors of the skin, are the most common viral skin infection; warts are caused by specific DNA viruses of the papova group (15). Although there are several kinds of warts, it is presumed that several types of human papilloma viruses are responsible for a majority of them. At least six types of cutaneous human papilloma viruses have been identified and isolated (16). Biochemical and immunologic characterization of viruses in different types of wart lesions has been difficult and impeded by the lack of a cell system that allows replication of these viruses in vitro (17). In addition, these viruses possess variable viral content (nucleic acids and proteins) according to clinical type (17). Studies have shown that the virus responsible for genital condyloma (HPV-6) demonstrates serologic, molecular hybridization; epidemiologic data suggest that it is a type of virus that may be different from skin wart viruses (18, 19). Information in humans is based upon observation of existing infections since for ethical reasons it has not been possible to innoculate the human subject with typical human papilloma virus isolates (17).

Common virogenic warts are defined according to their location. Common warts (verruca vulgaris) are located on the hands and fingers, although they may occur on the face. (See *Plate 8-34*.) Periungal and subungual verrucae occur around and underneath the nail beds, especially in nail-biters and cuticle pickers (20).

Juvenile, or flat, warts (verruca plana) usually occur in groups on the face, neck, and dorsa or the hands, wrists, and knees. Venereal warts (condyloma lata and condyloma acuminata), occur near the genitalia and anus. Plantar warts (verruca plantaris) are common on the soles of the feet (21). (See *Plate 8-35*.)

Symptoms

Warts begin as minute, smooth-surfaced, skin-colored lesions that enlarge over time. Repeated irritation causes the wart to continue enlarging. Plantar warts (on the soles of the feet) usually are asymptomatic and may not be noticed. However, if the plantar warts are large or occur on the heel or ball of the foot, the limitation of function and the discomfort may be bothersome to the point where professional advice is sought.

Three criteria must be met for an individual to develop a wart. The papovavirus must be present; there must be an open avenue for the virus to enter through the skin, such as abraded skin, and the individual immune response of the patient must be susceptible to the virus (probably the key reason certain individuals develop warts and others do not). Indeed, immunodeficient patients (those maintained on systemic or topical glucocorticoids), once infected, develop widespread and highly resistant warts (22).

Warts are most common in children and young adults and usually appear on exposed areas of the fin-

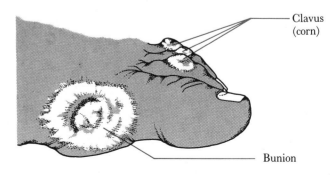

Figure 1. Conditions affecting the top of the foot.

gers, hands, face, and soles of the feet. The peak incidence of warts occurs between 12 and 16 years of age, and as many as 10% of the school children under 16 years of age have one or more warts (20). In addition, the incidence of warts is significantly higher in butchers and meat-cutters than in the general population (16). Whether this is the result of bovine papilloma viruses or human papilloma viruses remains unresolved at present (16).

Warts may spread by direct person-to-person contact, by autoinoculation to another body area, or indirectly through public shower floors or swimming pools. The incubation period after inoculation is 1–20 months, with an average of 3–4 months. An increase in plantar warts in England may have been due to an increase in the number and use of swimming pools (23). The hypothesis was that swimming, especially in warm water with a pH greater than 5, produced swelling and softening of the horny skin layer cells on the sole of the foot. The surrounding surface area of the pool and diving board is abrasive enough to contribute to tissue debridement, and inoculation in the area of heavy foot traffic around the pool (the diving board) is likely, especially when running and springing contribute to stress on the soles of the feet. Scrapings of the horny layer of plantar warts contain virus particles; therefore, it is conceivable that an area of heavy traffic of a pool can be contaminated easily by one person with a plantar wart.

Warts are not necessarily permanent; approximately 30% clear spontaneously in 6 months, 65% in 2 years, and most warts in 5 years (24, 25). The mechanism of spontaneous resolution is not fully understood. Acquired immunity may account for the remission (26). The wart virus stimulates production of two immunoglobulins, IgM and IgG (27). The cure of warts in one population sample seemed to correlate with the presence of complement-fixation antibodies (IgG) (28). The rapid occurrence of complement-fixation antibodies was associated with rapid healing; 75% of these patients were cured during the first 2 months of the observation period. In contrast, in patients with antibodies measurable only by immuodiffusion (IgM and/or low titers of IgG), only 16% were cured during the first month.

The development of immunity is directly related to the amount of virus present. This amount may vary among the different types of warts and their duration (28). Plane and mosaic warts and those of long duration, which are all clinically difficult to cure, are those in which little virus is found (22). In one study, 65% of patients treated topically for plantar warts for 12 weeks had wart antibodies (29). These results demonstrate that topical therapy will not prevent the formation of protective antibodies, as would be the case if the antigenic stimulus was removed by early curettage of the wart. Destroying a wart too early by curettage may lead to reinfection, because protective immunity seems to require about 6 months to develop. Insufficient immunity development may be correlated with the relatively low rate of cure by electrodestruction and curettage (24).

Electron microscopy demonstrates that warts contain their highest concentration of virus particles when they are about 6 months old. Peak antibody titers in the body are reached 6–12 months after inoculation (20). In light of this finding, it is questionable whether warts should be treated at all. The determination can be made only after making appropriate differential diagnosis

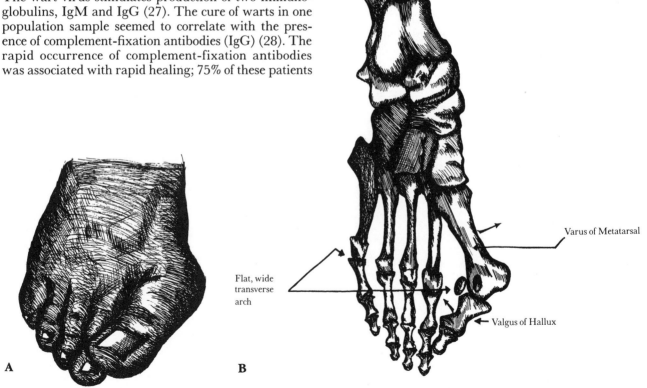

Flat, wide transverse arch

Varus of Metatarsal

Valgus of Hallux

A

B

Figure 2A and B. Two views of hallux of valgus. **A**, gross representation of hallux of valgus. **B**, bone structure of hallux of valgus.

and weighing the advantages and disadvantages of therapy predicated on patient circumstance. Indeed, when tests for wart antibody become routine, it will be possible to predict which patients are likely to enjoy early spontaneous remission.

Many practitioners, however, believe that because of the contagious nature of plantar warts, early and vigorous treatment provides the best results. Prolonged treatment with nonprescription products may increase the chance of autoinoculation. In addition, the urgency for treatment will also include such considerations as the desired cosmetic effect, such as facial warts, the number of warts present in an area, the site of the wart (weight-bearing area of the foot), and the age of the patient (30).

Plantar warts, hyperkeratotic lesions resulting from pressure, are more common in older children and adolescents but also occur in adults (31). They may be confined to the weight-bearing areas of the foot (the sole of the heel, the big toe, the areas below the heads of the metatarsal bones, and the ball), or they may occur in non-weight-bearing areas of the sole of the foot (Figure 3A). Calluses are also more commonly found under weight-bearing areas of the foot. Isolated solitary plantar warts may have a smooth keratotic surface, making the distinction between a wart and a corn or callus difficult (20). Thus, a differential diagnosis by a podiatrist should be made.

Plantar warts demonstrate marked hypertrophy of the horny skin layer, thickening of the prickle cell layer (acanthosis), formation of minute spaces (vacuolization) in the granular layer, and development of many papillomas (circumscribed overgrowth of a small nipple-like process) (26). The warts are circumscribed lesions under constant pressure and usually are not raised above the skin surface unless they are on non-weight-bearing surfaces. The wart itself is in the center of the lesion. It is roughly circular with a diameter of 0.5–1.0 cm. The surface is grayish and friable, and the surrounding skin is thick and heaped. The entire area forms a uniform, slight swelling (31, 32). The plantar wart surface may contain small black points that are the result of hypertrophied papillae that contain highly distended blood vessels. Rupture of the vessels allows coagulated blood into the epidermis which eventually is carried to the outer surface of the epidermis (20).

Plantar warts may occur in clusters (Figure 3B), or several contiguous warts are fused, giving the appearance of one wart (mosaic wart) (12). They often are confused with corns and calluses, which are mainly thickened areas of the corneous layer (31).

Treatment

Warts are a result of viral infection. No specific effective medication is available, but topical agents and procedures help in their removal and relief of pain. Treatment is extremely difficult. Warts may reappear several months after they have been "cured."

Multiple flat warts, facial warts, painful plantar warts, periungual warts, and venereal warts should all be treated by a physician. Topical therapy might not be indicated at all. For instance, periungual warts will not

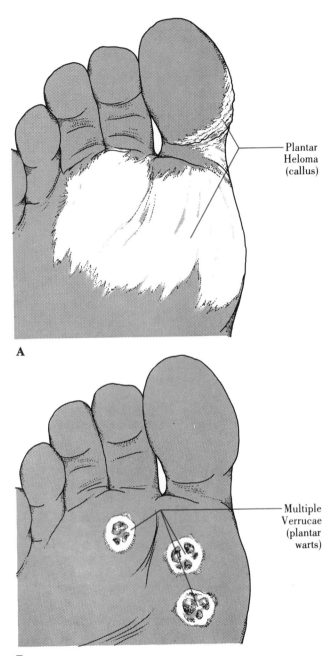

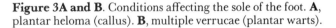

Figure 3A and B. Conditions affecting the sole of the foot. **A**, plantar heloma (callus). **B**, multiple verrucae (plantar warts).

be resolved until nail-biting is stopped. The FDA advisory review panel on nonprescription miscellaneous external drug products recommended that these products be labeled for treating only common and plantar warts (33).

Simple, localized warts may be self-treated depending on how the products are used and on the use of ancillary procedures (foot baths for 5 minutes and debridement with an emory board or a wash cloth) that make the treatment effective. Nonprescription products should be applied once daily to the wart only. The patient should use the product until the wart disappears, not to exceed 12 weeks (33). If the wart is still present after 12 weeks, the patient should consult a physician.

Evaluation of Corns, Calluses, and Warts

Many foot conditions require a physician's attention, especially those accompanying chronic, debilitating diseases, such as diabetes mellitus or arteriosclerosis. Without proper supervision, nonprescription products may induce more ulceration and possibly gangrene, particularly in cases of vascular insufficiency in the foot (1). In addition, simple lesions may mask more serious abscesses or ulcerations. If exostoses associated with corns are not excised by a physician, the corns will persist. Sites with many corns, many calluses, or lesions that ooze purulent material (a sign of secondary infection) should be examined by a physician.

Most patients with rheumatoid arthritis eventually have foot involvement (34). Painful metatarsal heads, hallux valgus, and clawtoes are the major forefoot deformities in patients with rheumatoid arthritis. Corrective surgical procedures often are indicated to reduce pain and improve function. There is little evidence to support the effectiveness of conventional nonoperative therapy (orthopedic shoes, metatarsal inserts, conventional arch supports, or metatarsal bars) (34).

The medical history and medication profile are extremely valuable, particularly in cases where self-medication has been tried. Warts, calluses, and corns can mask more serious abscesses and ulcerations; if left medically unattended, they may lead to conditions, such as osteomyelitis, requiring hospitalization. Because circulation is impaired in chronic, debilitating diseases, injury to normal skin inadvertently treated with nonprescription products may require a long time to heal. Diabetics and those not properly screened for ischemic changes are susceptible to disastrous gangrene. (See Chapter 13, *Diabetes Care Products.*)

The pharmacist must be cognizant that warts occasionally can be indicators of more serious conditions, such as squamous cell carcinoma and deep fungal infections (35). Squamous cell carcinomas may develop rapidly, attaining a diameter of 1 cm within 2 weeks. The lesion appears as a small, red, conical, hard nodule that quickly ulcerates (36). Subungual verrucae, which occur under the nail plate, may exist in conjunction with periungual verruca. The long-standing subungual verruca may be difficult to differentiate from a squamous cell carcinoma, especially in elderly patients (35). Condyloma acuminata are venereal warts that are moist and are often cauliflower-like in appearance. They must be differentiated from condyloma lata (secondary syphilis), which have a smooth, whitish surface (37).

The medical history and medication profile should include the following:

- Characteristics (particularly oozing and bleeding of warts) and duration of the condition;
- Whether similar problems have occurred in other family members;
- Any medical treatment being given for the problem or other conditions (e.g., immunosuppressive therapy, diabetes mellitus, rheumatoid arthritis);
- Any drug allergies.

Medical referral is indicated if

- A peripheral circulatory disease, diabetes mellitus, or a condition already under a physician's care exists.
- Hemorrhaging or oozing of purulent material occurs.
- Corns and calluses indicate an anatomical defect or fault in body weight distribution.
- Corns or calluses are extensive on the foot and can be painful and debilitating.
- Facial warts, plantar warts on weight-bearing areas, periungual warts, perianal or venereal warts, or extensive warts at one site exist.
- Proper self-medication for warts has been tried for an adequate period with no beneficial results.

Self-treatment is appropriate if

- Chronic, debilitating diseases do not contraindicate the use of these products.
- The patient is not a diabetic.
- The directions for use of the products can be followed with no difficulty.
- No concurrent medication (immunosuppressives) is being taken that contraindicates the use of these products.
- Corns and calluses are minor.
- Predisposing factors (ill-fitting footwear and hosiery) of corns and calluses are removed.
- Neither an anatomical defect nor faulty weight distribution is indicated by corns or calluses.
- Plantar warts are not spread extensively over the sole of the foot.

Pharmacologic Agents

Drugs with enough keratolytic activity for use in products intended for the treatment of corns, calluses, and warts include ascorbic acid, calcium pantothenate, castor oil, glacial acetic acid, lactic acid, podophyllum resin, salicylic acid, and zinc chloride. Certain drug products, such as castor oil, are included in proprietary drug products as emollients. Several topical products contain a local anesthetic, such as diperodon hydrochloride, to help alleviate the pain of corns or calluses. Salicylic acid is the most common ingredient in nonprescription drug products intended for corns, calluses, and warts.

There are several prescription products that might serve the patient better. For example, injection of a small amount of a corticosteroid beneath a painful corn results in a dramatic relief of symptoms (2). Table 2 illustrates the current status of ingredients in wart remover products (33).

Agents Used to Treat Corns, Calluses, and Warts

Glacial Acetic Acid and Lactic Acid   Glacial acetic acid and lactic acid are organic acids included in nonprescription formulations for corns, calluses, and warts because of their corrosive properties. They should be applied only on the affected area, not on surrounding healthy skin. Usually moderate concentrations of glacial acetic acid (11%) or lactic acid (5–17%) are in formulations that also include salicylic acid.

Table 2. FDA OTC review panel decisions relative to foot products

FDA OTC Review Panel	Category assignment		
	Category I	Category II	Category III
Miscellaneous external drug products (*Federal Register,* 10/3/80)	Salicylic acid (5–17%)	Benzocaine	Glacial acetic acid (up to 11%)
		Camphor	Ascorbic acid
		Castor oil	Calcium pantothenate
		Iodine	Lactic acid (5–17%)
		Menthol	Salicylic acid (5–17%) Lactic acid (5–17%) Collodion base qs
			Salicylic acid (5–17%) Glacial acetic acid (11%) Collodion base qs
			Ascorbic acid (0.16%) Calcium pantothenate (0.20%) Starch base qs
Ingrown toenail relief products (*Federal Register,* 10/17/80)	None	None	Sodium sulfide (1%) Tannic acid (up to 25%)

Reprinted from the *Federal Register, 45,* 65609 (1980).

These acids are contraindicated in cases involving debilitating illness. Overuse may cause skin irritation and ulceration. Used appropriately, these agents are safe for adults and children. However, the efficacy of these agents for wart removal is unsubstantiated and, for this reason, these agents have been classified by the FDA advisory review panel on nonprescription miscellaneous external drug products as Category III (33).

Salicylic Acid Salicylic acid (5–10% and higher) softens and destroys the stratum corneum by increasing endogenous hydration, probably the result of lowering the pH, which causes the cornified epithelium to swell, soften, macerate, and then desquamate (38). This concentration is advantageous in hyperkeratotic conditions such as corns and calluses.

The presence of moisture is important for therapeutic efficacy of salicylic acid in corn and callus therapy. If not well hydrated, tolerable amounts of salicylic acid will not soften cornified epithelium. Salicylic acid usually is incorporated in dosage forms (such as plasters, flexible collodions, and occlusive ointments) that occlude the area and promote moisture buildup, causing maceration and sloughing of tissues (38). These occlusive dosage forms may cause percutaneous absorption of salicylic acid (39). One study demonstrated the effect of various ointment bases on the percutaneous absorption of salicylic acid using rabbits as the animal model (40). The amount of salicylic acid absorbed through the skin from hydrophilic ointment was greater than that obtained from either hydrophilic petrolatum, petrolatum, or polyethylene glycol ointment (40). Rarely, however, for the treatment of corns, calluses, and warts would

enough salicylic acid be absorbed to cause salicylism. However, this condition may develop when a salicylic acid preparation is used frequently over an extensive area of the foot. Three adults with extensive psoriasis (scalp, trunk, and extremities) experienced percutaneous salicylic acid intoxication when either a 3% or a 6% salicylic acid ointment was applied (41). The patients applied these ointments 6 times/day and the symptoms of intoxication developed between the second and the fourth days of therapy. This salicylate intoxication abated when the use of the ointment was discontinued. Absorbed salicylic acid is metabolized in the liver to a degree and excreted in urine; patients with impaired liver and/or kidney function are therefore predisposed to systemic salicylate buildup. These patients cannot tolerate absorbed salicylate because toxic serum levels may develop (39, 42).

Salicylic acid is keratolytic at 3–6%. However, salicylic acid preparations of 10–40%, in appropriate dosage forms applied only to the affected area, are needed to soften hyperkeratotic tissue. Thus, large amounts of salicylic acid preparations should be applied carefully to avoid skin destruction, particularly of adjacent healthy skin. Patients with diabetes mellitus or peripheral vascular disease, where acute inflammation or ulcer formation from topical salicylic acid would be difficult to treat, should not use salicylic acid products except under direct physician supervision.

A plaster provides direct and prolonged contact of drugs with corns, calluses, and warts. Salicylic acid plaster (USP XIX) is a uniform solid or semisolid adhesive mixture of salicylic acid in a suitable base, spread on appropriate backing material (felt, moleskin, cotton, or plastic) and applied to the affected area. The usual concentration of salicylic acid in the base is 40%. A small piece of the 40% plaster may be cut to the size of the wart and held in place by waterproof tape, which is replaced every 3 days until the wart turns white (43). This material is preferably pared away with a sharp blade every week by a podiatrist or a physician. Plasters are occlusive and prevent the dissipation of moisture (44).

Salicylic acid is used most often with lactic acid or glacial acetic acid in the following classic prescription for corns and warts (6): one part each of salicylic and lactic acids to up to 10 parts with flexible collodion. One-percent formalin also may be included for its disinfectant effect against the pathogenic virus. This product can be applied every day to the corn or twice daily to the wart. The macerated tissue then is removed daily by washing. Although this combination is favored by dermatologists for common warts, especially in pediatric patients, a case of permanent scarring with inappropriate use of the product has been reported (45). Seemingly appropriate instructions were misinterpreted, resulting in overapplication of the material.

This type of treatment for warts with salicylic acid is the easiest to use. However, this modality requires patience and persistence on the patient's part. The therapy is long; however, the healing process is rapid once the wart is eliminated and the treatment is discontinued (30). The diseased area should be kept dry and cleaned with hydrogen peroxide to enhance this therapy (30). It is suggested that the collodion film be peeled away every 2–3 days to remove keratotic debris (20).

Based on current literature and wide clinical use, the FDA advisory review panel on nonprescription miscellaneous external drug products concluded that salicylic acid in a collodion vehicle is safe and effective as a keratolytic agent for the treatment of warts at concentrations of 5–17%. Salicylic acid was placed in Category I (33).

Collodions   Topical keratolytics used in treating corns, calluses, and warts generally are formulated in flexible collodion delivery systems containing pyroxylin, volatile solvents, such as ether or alcohol, and a plasticizer, usually castor oil. Pyroxylin is a nitrocellulose derivative that, after evaporation of the volatile solvents, remains on the skin as a water-repellent film (46). Collodion drug delivery systems are advantageous because they form an adherent flexible or rigid film (47). They also prevent moisture evaporation and thus facilitate penetration of the active ingredient into the affected tissue, resulting in sustained local action of the drug. The systems are water insoluble, as are most of their active ingredients, such as salicylic acid. They are less apt to run than aqueous solutions.

The disadvantages of collodions are that they are extremely flammable and volatile, and they may be mechanically irritating by occluding normal water transport through the skin. Also, the collodions favor systemic absorption of some drugs by their occlusive nature, and their aromatic odors make them vehicles that children or adults might abuse by sniffing their contents (48).

Additional Agents Used to Treat Corns and Calluses

Castor Oil   Castor oil is included in several corn and callus products for its emollient properties; it also may be used by itself.

It forms an occlusive film, which prevents water loss and sweat evaporation from the surface of the corn or callus and allows the keratinous tissue to remain soft and pliable. The oil usually is applied at bedtime, and the foot is covered by a sock. The sock serves a dual purpose in that it prevents oil stains on bed linens and helps occlude the affected area for better drug penetration.

Since data demonstrating the safety and effectiveness of castor oil in these products were not available, the panel classified it as Category II (33).

Local Anesthetics   To ease the pain of a corn or callus, several topical products contain a local anesthetic used with the keratolytic agents. Diperodon hydrochloride, usually incorporated into preparations at 1%, is as potent as cocaine and has a longer duration of action. It should not be applied to abraded or denuded areas where systemic absorption is possible. Diperodon hydrochloride is contraindicated in patients hypersensitive to other local anesthetic agents, such as benzocaine.

Menthol, benzocaine, and camphor are included in several nonprescription products for wart removal as counterirritants or as mild, local anesthetics. However, since data demonstrating the safety and effectiveness of benzocaine, camphor, and menthol in these products were not available, the drugs have been placed in Category II (33).

Zinc Chloride   Zinc chloride is included in several formulations of topical nonprescription products as an escharotic for corns and calluses. It owes its astringent activity to the zinc ion, which precipitates protein (zinc chloride is used as an astringent in solutions of 0.2–2%). Because it is irritating and caustic, its concentration is low, usually less than 3%. Zinc chloride is very soluble in water and ether. Because zinc chloride is extremely corrosive and irritating, it should not come into contact with mucous membranes or healthy skin and should not be used for long periods of time (49).

Agents Used to Treat Warts

Ascorbic Acid   Although ascorbic acid is essential to the development of supporting tissue (collagen and intracellular ground substance) and healing, there are insufficient data available to establish its efficacy in topical wart therapy (33). The panel has recommended further study of ascorbic acid before it can be considered both safe and effective for nonprescription use (33).

Calcium Pantothenate   Application of the alcohol derivative pantothenol in various ulcerative and pyogenic dermatoses stimulates epithelialization and allays itching. There have been no reports of sensitization or allergic reaction to topical therapy with pantothenic acid or its derivatives (50). The use of these drugs in adults and children seems safe. Topical formulations contain 2–5% of the active pantothenic acid derivative. However, there are insufficient data available on the effectiveness of this agent. Thus, the panel classified calcium pantothenate as Category III (33).

Cantharidin   Cantharidin is a potent vesicant available by prescription only as an ingredient of Cantharone. For wart therapy, this liquid is applied lightly with a stick or swab, allowed to dry, and then covered by a piece of waterproof adhesive tape slightly larger than the wart (35). Depending on the physician's directions, the bandage is left in place between 24 hours and 1 week and then removed. The drug effects a separation at the dermal-epidermal junction and therefore the removal of the epidermal-residing wart (30). Following the blister formation, minor inflammation can be resolved with tap water soaks (30).

In approximately 7–14 days, a blister, often hemorrhagic, which has formed will break, crust, and fall off. At this time, the physician debrides the dead material with fine-curved iris scissors (43). Since the effect of cantharidin is entirely intraepidermal, no scarring ensues.

A disadvantage of cantharidin is that, on occasion, annular warts may develop at the blister periphery (22). In addition, since this method is considered dangerous, it should be performed only by the physician and never by the patient at home (43). However, a successful trial of cantharidin treatment of warts at home has been reported (51). Application of the occlusive tape was omitted from the instruction to simplify the process and produce fewer reactions. This mode demonstrated an easy, safe, and reasonably effective means of treating warts. To help facilitate correct application of this product, some investigators advocate that the product be colored by the addition of some green food coloring dye (30).

Podophyllum   Podophyllum resin (in concentrations of up to 25%) dispensed in compound benzoin tincture or as a solution in alcohol is effective in the treatment of condyloma acuminatum (genital warts). It is a cytotoxic agent that arrests mitosis in metaphase. This caustic and powerful skin irritant is available by prescription only for short-term use. It may be reapplied every 4–7 days, generally for 2–4 weeks, depending on individual response and any residual chemical irritation (20). In 24–48 hours after application, lesions become necrotic, and in the following days, begin to slough off and gradually disappear.

The primary toxicologic problem associated with the use of podophyllum resin, aside from its topical irritant qualities, is peripheral neuropathy when it is absorbed percutaneously into the systemic circulation (52). Podophyllum should be applied only in small amounts by the physician. The patient should be instructed to wash off the podophyllum preparation with soap and water within 8–12 hours of its application. Because the usual delivery system is a low-viscosity suspension (compound tincture of benzoin) or tincture (alcohol), the solution tends to run onto adjacent tissue, causing damage. This risk may be minimized if white petrolatum or talc is applied to the healthy surrounding skin before the podophyllum preparation is applied to the wart (20, 30).

Podophyllum resin for vulvar warts in pregnant women should be used cautiously, if at all. The topical application of podophyllum applied five times for 4 hours each from the 23rd to the 29th week of pregnancy was suspected of causing teratogenic effects (53). Podophyllum should not be used on hemorrhaging skin or where an extensive skin surface area is involved. These conditions increase the possibility of percutaneous absorption. Because podophyllum is a potent corrosive, it should not be used with other keratolytic agents, such as salicylic acid.

Miscellaneous Prescription Drugs Used to Treat Warts   Other prescription drugs used fairly successfully in treating warts are the antibiotic bleomycin sulfate (Blenoxane) for recurrent or recalcitrant plantar warts, tretinoin (retinoic acid) for flat warts and plantar warts (43, 54, 55), and fluorouracil (56). Bleomycin has not been approved by the FDA for wart treatment. Theoretical objection to the local use of bleomycin is that it may interfere with DNA metabolism and induce skin cancer (57). Results with tretinoin and fluorouracil therapy are variable and, in those cases that do respond, it has not been determined whether the disease is simply taking its natural course (35).

Adjunctive Therapy

In addition to nonprescription products, self-therapy measures include daily soaking of the affected area throughout treatment for at least 5 minutes in very warm (not hot) water to remove dead tissue (22). Dead tissue should be removed gently after normal washing. Skin should not be removed forcibly because further damage could result. Sharp knives or razor blades that have not been properly sterilized should not be used to cut dead tissue because they may cause bacterial infection. A rough towel, callus file, or pumice stone effectively removes dead tissue of corns and calluses. Petroleum jelly should be applied to the healthy skin surrounding the affected area to avoid accidental application of corrosive products. This precaution is especially important in cases where poor eyesight increases the chances of misapplication.

To relieve painful pressure emanating from inflamed underlying tissue and irritated or hypertrophied bones directly underneath a corn or callus, patients may use a pad such as, Dr. Scholl's with an aperture for the corn or callus. If the skin can tolerate the pads, they may be used up to 1 week or longer (58). To prevent the pads from adhering to hosiery, patients may wax the pads with paraffin or a candle and powder them daily with a hygienic foot powder. If, despite these measures, friction causes the pads to peel up at the edge and stick to hosiery, the pharmacist may recommend that patients cover their toes with the forefoot of an old stocking or pantyhose before putting on hosiery (58).

Patients should be advised that if at any time the pad begins to cause itching, burning, or pain, it should be removed and a podiatrist should be consulted. The pharmacist also should advise the patient that these pads will provide only temporary relief and rarely cure a corn or a callus.

To avoid the spread of warts, which are contagious, patients should wash their hands before and after treating or touching wart tissue, and a specific towel should be used only for drying the affected area after cleaning. Patients should not probe or poke the wart tissue. Footwear should be worn in the case of plantar warts. If warts are present on the sole of the foot, patients should not walk in bare feet unless the wart is securely covered.

Product Selection Guidelines
Corns and Calluses

There are no clinical studies to indicate whether prescription-only products are superior to nonprescription products. Conclusions are based only on subjective physician evaluation reports (2, 9). Salicylic acid in a plaster or collodion dosage form appears to be the most effective treatment for corns and calluses. Some studies advocate the use of a 50% silver nitrate solution, applied by the physician, followed by weekly applications of 40% salicylic acid plasters for corns (7, 9).

Bunions

If the pharmacist recommends the use of topical adhesive cushioning to alleviate the pressure on a bunion, instructions should be given on proper use. Before the protective pad is applied, the foot should be bathed and dried thoroughly. The pad then is cut into a shape that conforms to the bunion. If the intent is to relieve the pressure from the center of the bunion area, the pad can be cut to surround the bunion. Precut pads are available for immediate patient use. Constant skin contact with adhesive-backed pads should be avoided, unless under a physician's recommendation.

Warts

Opinions about the best wart treatment vary from nitric acid for plantar warts to cantharidin preparations for common warts (35, 59). The findings of the FDA advisory review panel on nonprescription miscellaneous external drug products clarified the effectiveness and safety of nonprescription drugs (33).

In an evaluation of four plantar wart products, a dimethylbenzylammonium dibromide solution (Callusolve paint) was less effective than either a 50% podophyllum resin–liquid paraffin preparation or an established salicylic paint [salicylic acid–lactic acid–collodion preparation (1:1:4)] (29). A flexible collodion was used as the control preparation. The study also showed that the basic treatment for simple plantar warts takes about 6 weeks, and the cure rate was fastest with the salicylic paint. It was concluded that the treatment of plantar warts with a salicylic acid–lactic acid–flexible collodion mixture was enhanced when the application method was understood and was carried out under a physician's supervision.

The salicylic acid–lactic acid–flexible collodion preparation used in this study was safe and effective in children and adults; no incidences of hypersensitivity or systemic involvement were reported. Podophyllum also was used with no acute reactions, but it was under the direct supervision of a physician, and the therapy was for plantar, not genital warts. Podophyllum toxicity, associated with treatment of genital warts, has been reported (52, 60, 61).

Patient Consultation

Remission of corns, calluses, and warts does not happen quickly; it can take several days to several months. Usually, nonprescription treatment lasts 3–7 days for corns and calluses and up to 12 weeks for warts; if the wart remains, a physician should be consulted. Adherence to the dosage regimen and selection of a convenient time to apply the product are important. The pain and lack of mobility associated with corns, calluses, or warts is a strict reminder to adhere to the medication. Topical products should be applied no more than twice daily; the most convenient times are generally in the morning and at bedtime for a majority of patients.

The pharmacist should explain clearly how to use the medication. Because many products contain corrosive materials, the product should be applied only to the corn, callus, or wart. If a plaster or pad is used, the process of trimming the pad to follow the contours of the corn or callus should be explained.

If a solution is used, one drop at a time is applied directly to the corn, callus, or wart and is allowed to dry and harden to avoid running; the procedure continues until the entire area is covered. Adjacent areas of normal healthy skin should not come in contact with the product. If the solution touches healthy skin, it should be washed off immediately with soap and water. If the solution is intended for a soft corn between the toes, the toes should be held apart comfortably until the solution is applied and allowed to dry. This procedure should be followed for 3–6 days. The solution should solidify before a dressing is applied.

A plaster should be cut to the size of the lesion, applied to the skin, and covered with adhesive occlusive tape. The next day, the dressing is removed and the foot is soaked in warm water. The macerated, soft white skin of the corn or callus then is removed by scrubbing gently with a rough towel, pumice stone, or callus file, and the plaster is reapplied. Patients must be careful not to debride healthy skin when using a pumice stone or callus file.

A cream should be applied after washing the wart with soap and water. Then an occlusive dressing generally is placed over the wart.

Because nonprescription preparations contain volatile and irritating ingredients, precautions should be taken in using them. After use, the container should be tightly capped, avoiding evaporation and preventing the active ingredients from assuming a greater concentration. The volatile delivery systems are quite flammable, and the product should be stored away from direct sunlight or heat in amber or light-resistant containers.

The products that contain collodions are poisonous when they are taken orally, and they should be stored out of children's reach. They have an odor similar to that of airplane glue and may be subject to abuse by inhaling the vapors (48).

Nonprescription products are not recommended for patients with diabetes or circulatory problems. Contraindications should be pointed out to all patients to avoid inadvertent use of these products by other family members who have such conditions. These products are keratolytic and cause skin tissue to slough off, leaving an unsightly pinkish tinge to the skin; nevertheless, they should continue being used. They should be discontinued only when a severe inflammatory response (swelling or reddening) or irritation occurs.

Ingrown Toenails

An ingrown toenail occurs when a section of nail presses into the soft tissue of the nail groove. The nail curves into the flesh of the toe corners and becomes imbedded in the surrounding soft tissue of the toe, causing pain. Swelling, inflammation, and ulceration are some secondary complications that can arise from this condition.

Etiology

The frequent cause of ingrown toenails is incorrect trimming of the nails. The correct method of cutting the toenail is to cut the nail straight across without tapering the corners in any way. Wearing pointed-toe or too tight shoes, as well as wearing hosiery which is too tight, also have been implicated. In these instances, direct pressure can force the lateral edge of the nail into the soft tissue. Bedridden patients may develop ingrown toenails due to tight bed covers that create pressure of the soft skin tissue against the nails. Those people who have toenails that naturally curl also are predisposed to this malady.

Treatment

Prevention through education is probably the best mode to offset the development of ingrown toenails. In the early stages of development of an ingrown toenail, therapy is directed at providing adequate room for the nail to resume its normal position adjacent to soft tissue. This is accomplished by relieving the external source of pressure and applying medications that will harden the nail groove or help shrink the soft tissue.

Pharmacologic Agents

The FDA advisory review panel on nonprescription miscellaneous external drug products has classified two active ingredients in these products, sodium sulfide and tannic acid, into Category III. [There are no drugs in either Category I or II (Table 2.)] (62). At present, there are insufficient data to determine their effectiveness for this condition. In theory, sodium sulfide is intended to soften the keratin in the nail and the calloused skin surrounding the nail, thereby providing relief of pressure and pain caused by the imbedded nail (62). The claimed effect of tannic acid is that it hardens the skin surrounding the imbedded nail and shrinks the soft tissue adjacent to the nail, providing enough room for the nail to resume its normal position adjacent to soft tissue (62).

Ingrown toenail products with these active ingredients should not be used for more than 7 days. If there is no improvement within this time, a physician should be consulted. These products should not be applied to open sores, and use of the product should be stopped and a physician should be consulted if swelling and redness increase, or if a discharge is present around the nail. Patients with circulatory disease, such as diabetes mellitus, should not use these products without the knowledge of their physician.

To enhance the effectiveness of these products, the panel recommended that the directions for use include the statement, "Cleanse affected toes thoroughly. Place a small piece of cotton in the nail groove (the side of the nail where the pain is) and wet cotton thoroughly with the solution. Repeat several times daily until nail discomfort is relieved but do not use more than 7 days" (62).

To provide temporary protection of the toe while the ingrown nail is being treated, a patient may use a soft foam toe cap. However, continual use of a toe cap without removing the source of the problem merely forestalls the inevitable.

Frostbite

Frostbite is defined as the actual freezing of tissues by excessive exposure to low temperatures. Although it is not amenable to therapy with nonprescription drug products, it is a condition that can involve the foot and other extremities. This is a result of the fact that frostbite usually involves areas of the body that are the farthest from deep organs or large muscles (ear lobes, nose, cheeks, hands, and feet) (63). To maintain normal core temperature in cold weather, the body reduces reflexly the flow of blood to the skin surface and the extremities. The condition may range from minor blanching of the skin to the severe—gangrene resulting in the loss of toes and/or fingers (63).

Etiology

Predisposing factors to the development of frostbite include the following:

- Low temperatures (especially with high winds);
- Long periods of exposure to cold;
- Lack of proper clothing;
- Wet clothing;
- Poor nutrition, exhaustion, or dehydration;
- Circulatory disease;
- Immobility;
- Direct contact with metal or petroleum products at low temperatures;
- Individual susceptibility to cold.

Treatment

The frostbitten part should be promptly and thoroughly rewarmed in warm water (between 104° and 108°F) (63). The water should not be hot to a normal hand at room temperature and should not be tested with the frozen part. The container with this water should be large enough to allow free movement of the frozen part without it bumping against the sides. Rewarming should be continued until a flush returns to the most distal tip of the thawed part (64). This usually takes about 20–30 minutes (63). Dry heat is not advocated for treatment since it is difficult to control the temperature and re-warm the part evenly (63). The injured part should be soaked for about 20 minutes in a whirlpool bath once or twice daily until the healing process is complete (63).

The best treatment for frostbite is prevention and there are a few simple rules that one can follow (65). The most important rule is to direct people to dress to maintain body warmth, including areas of the face, the neck, and the head. Other simple rules include the following:

- Avoid exposure to cold during times of sickness or exhaustion.
- Do not exceed one's tolerance to cold exposure.
- Avoid tight-fitting garments; dress with layered clothing.
- Wear clothing that allows ventilation and avoids perspiration buildup (water enhances heat loss).
- Wear insulated boots or shoes and socks (wool preferable) that fit snugly but not tight in spots.
- Wear mittens instead of gloves in severe cold (the thumb should be with the rest of the fingers and not by itself).
- Never touch objects (especially cold metal or petroleum products) that facilitate heat loss.

There are a few misconceptions that the pharmacist should seek to correct when given the opportunity. It is dangerous to rub the affected limb with ice or snow even though it seems to provide warmth (63). This can result in prolonged contact with the cold and may cause lacerations of the cells from the ice crystals. In addition, a person should refrain from drinking alcohol for anti-freeze purposes at least until he or she is in a warm place. Alcohol can induce a loss of body heat even though it may give the person a feeling of warmth when ingested. Lastly, smoking should be avoided by frostbite victims. Nicotine can induce peripheral vasoconstriction and effect a further decrease of blood supply to the frostbitten extremity (63, 65).

Athlete's Foot

The most prevalent cutaneous fungal infection in humans is athlete's foot (dermatophytosis of the foot or tinea pedis), the itchy, scaling lesions between the toes. Tinea pedis has a prevalence rate of 38.7 per 1,000 people (66). It is more common in males with a prevalence of 68.4/1,000 compared with 10.7/1,000 for females (66). Since ringworm fungi (dermatophytes) generally are the causative or initiating organisms responsible, athlete's foot often is synonymous with a ringworm infection (4).

The clinical spectrum of athlete's foot ranges from mild scaling to a severe, exudative inflammatory process characterized by fissuring and denudation. The prevalent type of athlete's foot, midway between these two extremes, is characterized by maceration, hyperkeratosis, pruritus, malodor, and a stinging sensation of the feet.

Etiology

Species of the genera *Trichophyton, Microsporum,* and *Epidermophyton* are common fungal pathogens found in cutaneous infections of the skin, nails, and hair. The most commonly implicated pathogens of tinea pedis are the *Trichophyton* species, specifically, *T. mentagrophytes* and *T. rubrum* (67). It is perplexing, however, to note that the recovery rates of fungi have been low in cases clinically diagnosed as athlete's foot (6, 8), especially of the symptomatic, macerated, hyperkeratotic type with erosions, exudation, and intense inflammation (69). Recent evidence supports the theory that normal resident skin aerobic diphtheroids and gram-negative organisms, such as *Proteus* and *Pseudomonas* species, also may play a role in the manifestations of the disease (4, 5, 69). Thus, athlete's foot exhibits a continuum from a relatively asymptomatic condition (slight scaling) produced by fungi to a symptomatic condition (soggy, hyperkeratotic skin) that is an ultimate result of secondary bacterial overgrowth. (See *Plate 8-36.*)

In addition to microorganisms, other predisposing factors contribute to the disease's development. Overhydration of the skin may be due to exercise, emotional hyperhidrosis, tightly fitting occlusive footwear, and/or hot, humid weather (5). These conditions may be accentuated by debilitating disease (diabetes), poor nutrition, and/or poor body hygiene.

Although tinea pedis may occur at all ages, it is more common in adults. However, it should not be ignored as a diagnostic possibility in children just because of infrequent occurrence (70). This infection is acquired most often by walking barefoot on infected floors, such as those in hotel bathrooms and locker rooms of clubs, schools, and camps. Tinea pedis may be present among several family members, presumably due to the spread of the fungi from the bathroom floor, floor mats, or rugs. Pathogenic fungi and bacteria also may be found in contaminated shoes and socks.

Tinea pedis is not thought to be transmitted simply by exposure to the fungal infection. Trauma to the skin, especially blister-producing trauma (wearing ill-fitting footwear), may contribute significantly to the occurrence of human fungal infections (71).

Susceptibility

Although there are many pathogenic fungi in the environment, the overall incidence of actual superficial fungal infections is remarkably low. Many degrees of susceptibility produce a clinical infection—from instantaneous "takes" by as few as one spore to severe trauma with massive exposure (72). One of the most important determinants of susceptibility to clinical fungal infection may be undefined host-resistant factors (73). Acquired protective immunity occurs in most infected patients. Reinfection requires a greater exposure to fungi, and lesions appear to heal more rapidly. About 20% of those afflicted with an acute superficial fungal infection develop a chronic fungal infection. An adequate immune response is not acquired by these patients (74). They seem to have a fungus infection "that comes and goes and that no one can cure" (75).

Pathophysiology

Superficial fungi, such as dermatophytes, attach to, proliferate, and live in the horny skin layer. These fungi produce keratinase, an enzyme that digests keratin, causing the outermost skin layer to disintegrate and scale (76, 77). Dermatophytic fungi grow only in keratinous tissue because a potent antifungal factor protects living tissue from deep penetration by fungal elements (78). However, after initial invasion of the horny layer by dermatophytes, enough moisture may accumulate to trigger a bacterial overgrowth (4). Large numbers of normally resident aerobic diphtheroids may become involved. Increased moisture and temperature then lead to bacterial proliferation and release of products that diffuse easily through the underlying horny layer already damaged by fungal invasion. In the more severe cases, gram-negative organisms intrude and may exacerbate the condition.

Experimental manipulation of the microflora supports the concept that bacterial overgrowth in an interspace already damaged by dermatophyte invasion results in the symptomatic types of athlete's foot (4). When occlusive dressings were applied to feet harboring the dermatophytes, the interdigital spaces became macerated and symptomatic within 7–10 days. These changes, however, did not occur when antibiotics (0.1% gentamicin sulfate cream) were added daily to the dressings to prevent bacterial overgrowth (4). A combination of an antibiotic and an antifungal (either two separate agents or one of the newer broad-spectrum agents, such as miconazole nitrate or clotrimazole) produced faster and more complete resolution of symptoms (4).

There are two main clinical types of tinea pedis: vesicular and intertriginous. Vesicular tinea pedis is an acute, inflammatory condition caused predominantly by *T. mentagrophytes* (67). Vesicles 2–3 mm wide appear on the soles or sides of the feet or between the toes. They may be sparse or closely grouped into areas 2.5–5 cm wide. Erythema may be extensive or absent altogether. Burning and itching usually are present, along with hyperhidrosis (excessive sweating). After a few days, vesicles may become yellowish and purulent; they may rupture, causing a weeping surface open to infection by pathogenic cocci, or they may simply dry up as the acute stage subsides, leaving yellowish-brown crusts.

Intertriginous tinea pedia, a chronic dermatophytosis, is caused primarily by *Trichophyton rubrum*. This type is divided into two subclassifications (4). Dermatophytosis simplex, characterized by dry, scaly lesions, is relatively asymptomatic except for periodic low-grade pruritus. Dermatophytosis complex, characterized by soggy scaling, has symptoms of itching, malodor, and discomfort between the toes. Manifestations of this condition may range from hyperkeratotic, leukokeratotic plaques to erosions and fissures. The horny skin layer becomes white and macerated and usually peels off in large friable scales. Beneath the scales, the epidermis may be reddened, swollen, and tender. The most severe form of dermatophytosis complex occurs when there is an overgrowth of gram-negative bacteria (*Proteus* and *Pseudomonas* species). This form produces an extremely painful, erosive, purulent interspace that can be disabling and is known synonymously as gram-negative athlete's foot (69).

Intertriginous tinea pedis may be restricted to a small patch adjacent to a fungus-infected toenail (usually caused by *T. rubrum*) or to a patch between or under the toes (78). The absence of vesiculation is characteristic. *T. rubrum* infections are often unilateral (involving only one foot) and remain localized for years (72).

Evaluation

The most common complaint of patients suffering from tinea pedis is pruritus. However, if fissures are present, particularly between the toes, painful burning and stinging may occur. If the foot area is abraded, denuded, or inflamed, weeping or oozing may occur in addition to frank pain. Some patients may merely remark on the bothersome scaling of dry skin, particularly if it has progressed to the soles of the feet. Small vesicular lesions may combine to form a larger bullous eruption marked by pain and irritation. The only symptoms may be brittleness and discoloration of a hypertrophied toenail.

The only true determinant of a fungal foot infection is clinical laboratory evaluation of tissue scrapings from the foot. This process involves a potassium hydroxide mount preparation of the scrapings and cuttings on a special growth medium to show the actual presence and specific identity of fungi (79). The procedure can be ordered and performed only at the direction of a physician. However, microscopic confirmation probably will be possible only in the dry, scaly type. The recovery of fungi for diagnosis decreases as athlete's foot becomes progressively more severe (69). In typical cases of dermatophytosis complex, fungus recovery rates are only about 25–50% (5).

The pharmacist should question the patient thoroughly as to the condition and its characteristics to obtain a description of the condition and determine the extent of disease, and any mitigating circumstances, such as diabetes or obesity, that would render the patient susceptible, and previous patient compliance with medications.

The pharmacist should seek to distinguish tinea pedis from diseases with similar symptoms. Dermatitis, allergic contact dermatitis, and atopic dermatitis also may occur on the feet and should be treated by a physician. In addition, hyperhidrosis of the sole of the foot and infection of toe webs by gram-negative bacteria are common. In hyperhidrosis, tender vesicles cover the sole of the foot and toes and may be quite painful. The skin generally turns white, erodes, and becomes macerated. This condition is accompanied by a foul foot odor.

Infection by gram-negative bacteria is characterized by a soggy wetness of the toe webs and immediately adjacent skin (80). The affected tissue is damp, softened, and soggy. The last or next to last (adjacent to the little toe) toe webs are the most common types of primary or initial involvement (80). The web between the fourth and fifth toes is deeper and extends more proximally than the web between the other toes. Furthermore, a semiocclusive anatomical setting, abundant exocrine sweat glands, and the added occlusion provided by footwear enhance development of the disease at this site. Severe forms of this disease may progress to disintegration and denudation of the affected skin and profuse, serous, or purulent discharge. Denudation may involve all of the toe webs, the dorsal and plantar surfaces of the toes, and an area about 1 cm wide beyond the base of the toes on the plantar surface of the foot. When the disease is out of control, its progression is observed on the dorsum of the foot and the calf in the form of tiny red follicular crusts. This condition paradoxically may be caused by use of reputed germicidal soaps such as pHisoHex, Dial, and Safeguard (80). It was hypothesized that these soaps reduce harmless saprophytes and thus promote resistant pathogens (such as *Pseudomonas aeruginosa* and *Proteus mirabilis*) by removing their competitors.

If the patient has used a nonprescription antifungal product appropriately for several weeks without relief, a disease other than tinea pedis may be involved. Therapeutic failure may be due to gram-negative athlete's foot; no nonprescription antifungal product will ameliorate the condition. Patients suffering from hyperhidrosis, allergic contact dermatitis, or atopic dermatitis, or from a possible gram-negative infection of the toe should see a podiatrist or family physician for treatment.

Treatment

Before self-medication can be effective, the correct type of tinea pedis as well as correct treatment must be evaluated. Treatment of an acute, superficial tinea foot infection may be effective if certain conditions are met. In acute, inflammatory tinea pedis, characterized by reddened, oozing, and vesicular eruptions, the inflammation must be counteracted before antifungal therapy can be instituted. This step is especially important if the eruptions are caused by a secondary bacterial infection (72).

Hydrocortisone, in conjunction with iodochlorhydroxyquin, demonstrated favorable results toward a resolution of uncomplicated cutaneous fungal infections (tinea cruris, tinea pedis, and moniliasis) (81). Erythema and itching were relieved more with the combination of these two drugs than by either drug itself or the placebo cream. However, with the availability of topical hydrocortisone products on a nonprescription basis, it is conceivable that the indiscriminate use of one of these products for the relief of the itching and redness of athlete's foot could complicate and delay appropriate medical care (82). Topical hydrocortisone by itself is contraindicated in the presence of fungal infections.

Self-treatment is effective only if the patient understands the importance of compliance with all facets of the treatment plan. Specific antifungal products must be used appropriately in conjunction with other treatment measures, including general hygienic measures and local drying. Some clinical studies have demonstrated efficacy in the placebo groupings with local hygienic measures alone (66, 83).

The pharmacist should recommend that the patient consult a physician in the following circumstances:

- If the toenail is involved, topical treatment is ineffective and does not allay the condition until the disease's primary focus is treated with oral griseofulvin or ketoconazole or until other preventive measures are instituted (surgical avulsion, or tearing away of the nail).
- If vesicular eruptions are oozing, including purulent material that could indicate a secondary bacterial infection, topical astringent therapy and/or antibiotic therapy may be appropriate.
- If the interspace between the toes is foul smelling, whitish, painful, very soggy, characterized with erosions, oozing, and/or serious inflammation, and especially if the condition is disabling, the patient should be referred. Fortunately, this variety is not too common (69).
- If the foot is seriously inflamed and/or swollen and a major portion is involved, supportive therapy must be instituted before an antifungal agent may be applied.
- If the patient is under a physician's supervision for a disease, such as diabetes or asthma, where the normal defense mechanism may be deficient, nonprescription products should not be used.

Pharmacologic Agents

The pharmacologic agents used to treat athlete's foot have been evaluated for safety and efficacy by the FDA advisory review panel on antimicrobial drug products (II) (84). However, to date the recommendations of this panel have not been published in the *Federal Register*. The Bureau of Drugs (FDA) has kindly shared the findings of this panel through the Freedom of Information Act. Table 3 summarizes the assignment of each agent categorically.

Carbol-Fuchsin Solution   Basic fuchsin (NF XIII) dye is a mixture of rosaniline and pararosaniline hydrochlorides. It is used only in superficial fungal foot infections in the form of carbol-fuchsin solution (NF XIII) or Castellani's paint. The solution is dark purple but appears red when painted onto the affected area in a fine film. It has local anesthetic, drying, and antimicrobial properties.

The use of carbol-fuchsin solution in tinea pedis is indicated in the subacute or chronic stages of infection when there is little or no inflammation. The solution should not be applied to inflamed or denuded skin.

In one study, carbol-fuchsin solution demonstrated equivalent efficacy to a 30% aluminum chloride solution for interdigital dermatophytosis (5). The drying and antimicrobial properties of carbol-fuchsin are well suited for the ultrasoggy, steaming athlete's foot. However, its staining properties and poisonous nature limit this medication's usefulness.

Before the solution is applied, the affected area should be cleaned thoroughly with soap and water and dried. The solution then is applied to the area with an applicator and reapplied once or twice daily for 1 week. After this time, if the condition has not improved, choice of medication as well as assessment of the actual condition should be re-evaluated.

The efficacy of carbol-fuchsin solution must be questioned, especially if an infected toenail is involved. Because the preparation contains several volatile com-

Table 3. FDA Advisory Review Panel on OTC Antimicrobial Drug Products (II) Panel decisions relative to nonprescription athlete's foot drug products

Classification	Classification
Category I Tolnaftate (for treatment and prophylaxis of athlete's foot), 1% Undecylenic acid and derivatives (for treatment of athlete's foot, 10–25% (undecylenate content)	**Category III** Alcloxa, 0.25–10.0% Aluminum sulfate, 1.5–10.0% Basic fuchsin, 0.3% Benzethonium chloride, 0.13% Benzoic acid, 0.75–12.0% Boric acid/sodium borate, 0.5–5.0% (borate content) Chlorothymol, 0.2–1.0% Chloroxylenol, 0.5–3.75%
Category II Camphor Coal tar Menthol Phenol Phenolate sodium Resorcinol Tannic acid Thymol	Oxyquinoline sulfate, 0.06–0.25% (oxyquinoline content) Sodium caprylate/zinc caprylate, 10–20% Salicylic acid, up to 3.0% Triacetin, 15–33.3%

Unpublished Report of FDA Advisory Review Panel on OTC Antimicrobial Drug Products (II), February 23, 1981.

ponents, the patient should tighten the cap securely to avoid evaporation. Otherwise, volatile ingredients escape, causing other nonvolatile components (resorcinol) to become more concentrated, and irritation may result with subsequent applications.

Although carbol-fuchsin solution is an effective agent, it should not be applied to an area greater than 10% of the foot or to a severely inflamed foot because of systemic toxicity if percutaneously absorbed. This limitation, its staining properties, and possible patient sensitivity to the product ingredients limit the usefulness of carbol-fuchsin solution for tinea pedis. This is unfortunate since carbol-fuchsin solution possesses all facets necessary for effective athlete's foot therapy. The solution suppresses fungi and bacteria and simultaneously produces a local drying or astringent effect. Testimonial evidence indicates that the extemporaneous preparation and use of the paint without the fuchsin dye may be just as effective and more esthetically acceptable (85, 86). The FDA advisory panel on nonprescription antimicrobial drug products (II) has classified basic fuchsin into Category III (84).

Tolnaftate Tolnaftate is the only ingredient approved by the FDA advisory panel on nonprescription antimicrobial drug products (II) for both therapeutic and prophylactic use in athlete's foot (84). The most notable naphthol derivative synthesized for antifungal activity is tolnaftate (87). Its spectrum of action encompasses typical fungi responsible for tinea pedis, including *T. mentagrophytes* and *T. rubrum*. Also, it is effective against *E. floccosum* and *Microsporum* species. Although the exact mechanism of action of tolnaftate has not been reported, it is believed that it distorts the hyphae and stunts the mycelial growth of the fungi species. Tolnaftate is more effective in tinea pedis than in onychomycosis or tinea capitis. For onychomycosis and tinea capitis, concomitant administration of oral griseofulvin is necessary, unless the condition is superficial.

Tolnaftate is well tolerated when applied to intact or broken skin in either exposed or intertriginous areas. Tolnaftate usually stings slightly when applied. Although there has been one report of a developed delayed-hypersensitivity reaction to tolnaftate, there have been no references to hypersensitivity associated with its use (88). As with all topical medicaments, irritation, sensitization, or worsening of the skin condition warrants discontinuance of the product.

Tolnaftate (1% solution or 1% cream) is applied sparingly twice daily after the affected area is cleansed thoroughly. Effective therapy usually takes 2–4 weeks, although treatment lasting 4–6 weeks may be necessary with some individuals (patients with lesions between the toes or on pressure areas of the foot). When medication is applied to pressure areas of the foot, where the horny skin layer is thicker than normal, concomitant use of a keratolytic agent may be advisable. Neither keratolytic agents nor wet compresses, such as aluminum acetate (Burow's) solution, which promote the healing of oozing lesions, interfere with the efficacy of tolnaftate. If weeping lesions are present, the inflammation should be treated before tolnaftate is applied.

The cream dosage form of tolnaftate is formulated in a polyethylene glycol 400–propylene glycol vehicle; the solution is formulated in polyethylene glycol 400. The solution may be more effective than the cream. These vehicles are particularly advantageous in superficial antifungal therapy because they are nonocclusive, nontoxic, nonsensitizing, water miscible, anhydrous, easy to apply, and efficient in delivering the drug to the affected area.

High molecular weight polyethylene glycol bases have been reported to form associated complexes with some medicaments, such as benzoic and salicylic acids. Although diffusion of the medicament to the skin is adequate with polyethylene glycol bases, little percutaneous absorption occurs (89, 90). In regard to topical antifungal therapy, however, complex formation seems inconsequential because the role of the vehicle in this instance is to supply drug to the horny skin layer.

Tolnaftate solution solidifies when exposed to cold. However, if the preparation is allowed to warm, it will liquefy with no loss in potency.

The topical powder formulation of tolnaftate uses cornstarch-talc as the vehicle. This vehicle not only is an effective drug delivery system but also offers therapeutic advantage due to the water-retaining nature of the two agents. The topical aerosol formulation of tolnaftate includes talc and the propellant vehicle.

Tolnaftate has demonstrated marked clinical efficacy since its commercial introduction into the United States in 1965, and it has become the standard topical antifungal medicament (91, 92). In addition, there has been a consistent absence of irritation and hypersensitivity to tolnaftate in cream, solution, or powder form, thus enabling its approval for nonprescription use.

Tolnaftate is valuable primarily in the dry, scaly type of athlete's foot. Superficial fungal infection relapse has occurred after tolnaftate therapy was discontinued (93). However, the relapse may have been caused by an inadequate treatment time, patient noncompliance with the medication, or the use of tolnaftate where oral griseofulvin should have been instituted. Since tolnaftate does not possess antibacterial properties, its value in the soggy, macerated type of athlete's foot must be viewed with skepticism, if indeed bacteria are involved (4, 69).

Organic Fatty Acids   Studies of the antifungal effect of various fatty acids and their salts on dermatophytes reported encouraging clinical results with sodium propionate, a constituent of sweat (94). The sodium salt of caprylic acid (an eight-carbon fatty acid) was more effective than sodium undecylenate in treating dermatophytosis of the foot (95). However, both propionic and undecylenic acids are weakly fungistatic (96).

Whether organic fatty acids are more effective than sulfur and/or iodine preparations in treating superficial fungal infections is questionable. Organic acid preparations should be used, if at all, only for very mild or chronic forms of tinea pedis.

These organic fatty acids and/or their salts are available in various dosage forms. The cream or ointment form usually is used at bedtime; solutions should be used for their soothing effects after a footbath. The powder usually is sprinkled into the socks and shoes in the morning.

Acetic Acid   Acetic acid is delivered to the infected area as triacetin. The fungistatic activity of triacetin is based on the fact that at the neutral or alkaline pH of infected skin, fungal esterase enzymes cleave triacetin into acetic acid and glycerin (97). The acetic acid then effects antifungal activity by lowering the pH at the infection site. As the pH increases after the initial release of acetic acid, more acetic acid is generated by the enzymes, and the process is repeated. The efficacy of products containing triacetin has not been proven by controlled clinical trials (84). Since the ultimate efficacy of triacetin will depend upon the presence of moisture for conversion to the active acetic acid, the FDA advisory panel on nonprescription antimicrobial drug products (II) placed this drug in Category III with the proviso it be recommended and used only for the soggy, wet form of athlete's foot (84).

Used topically, triacetin is relatively colorless and odorless. In the concentrations used, the small amount of acetic acid liberated is probably nonirritating to the skin in most cases. The corresponding incidence of sensitization also is low. However, the acetic acid formed may damage rayon fabrics, so the treated areas should be covered with a clean bandage. Triacetin must not come into contact with the eyes.

Triacetin is available as a cream and an ointment (25% in each). Both should be applied every morning and evening after thorough cleansing. The product should be used until the infection has cleared entirely, then once a week as a preventive measure.

Undecylenic Acid–Zinc Undecylenate   This combination is widely used and may be effective for various mild superficial fungal infections excluding those involving nails and/or hairy parts of the body. It is fungistatic and is effective in mild chronic cases of tinea pedis. Compound undecylenic acid ointment (USP XX) contains 5% undecylenic acid and 20% zinc undecylenate in a polyethylene glycol vehicle. It is believed that zinc undecylenate liberates undecylenic acid (the active antifungal entity) on contact with moisture (perspiration). In addition, zinc undecylenate has astringent properties due to the presence of zinc ion (98). This astringent activity decreases the irritation and inflammation of the infection.

Applied to the skin as an ointment, diluted solution, or dusting powder, the combination undecylenic acid–zinc undecylenate, is relatively nonirritating, and hypersensitivity reactions are not common. The undiluted solution, however, may cause transient stinging when applied to broken skin, due to its alcohol content. Caution must be exercised to ensure that these ingredients do not come into contact with the eye or that the powder is not inhaled.

The vehicle in compound undecylenic acid ointment has a water-miscible base, making it nonocclusive, removable with water, and easy to apply. The powder uses talc as its vehicle and absorbent. The aerosol contains menthol, which serves as a counterirritant and antipruritic. The solution contains 10% undecylenic acid in an isopropyl alcohol vehicle with either an applicator or spray pump container. The product is applied twice daily after the affected area is cleansed. The usual period for therapeutic results depends on the patient. However, improvement should occur in 2–4 weeks, after which time the condition should be re-evaluated and an alternative medication tried.

When the solution is sprayed or applied onto the affected area, the area should be allowed to air dry. Otherwise, the possibility of water accumulation and further tissue maceration could exist. The relatively high alcohol concentration in these solutions could cause some burning with application. The rancid odor of undecylenic acid may be objectionable to some patients and may promote patient noncompliance.

A comparison study of two 20% zinc undecylenate–2% undecylenic acid powder formulations used in the treatment of tinea pedis demonstrated no difference in clinical efficacy between products (99). However, these two formulations collectively effected clinical and mycologic cures in 53% of the patients treated as compared with 7% of those treated with the talc vehicle or left untreated (using daily foot washings or changes or socks). There was no indication whether patients failing to respond to either formulation possessed the more severe forms of tinea pedis. Another study (100) with a powder containing the same active ingredients reported similar results. In this study, 88% of patients treated with the active powder had negative cultures after 4 weeks compared with 17% of those treated with placebo powder ($p < 0.001$).

Two studies demonstrated the comparable effectiveness of undecylenic acid to tolnaftate in clinical studies (83, 101). One study demonstrated indistinguishable clinical and mycologic effects between undecylenic acid ointment and tolnaftate cream (83). Both formulations were superior to placebo (ointment base of the undecylenic acid) although the gross improvement toward erythema, fissuring, and vesiculation was slow. These medications seem best suited for the mild forms of athlete's foot characterized by dry scaling of tissue. In light of the prior studies, undecylenic acid and/or its derivatives (between 10–25% total undecylenate content) have been classified into Category I by the FDA advisory review panel on nonprescription antimicrobial drug products (II) for the treatment of athlete's foot (84).

Other preparations, such as ointments, powders, and tinctures, incorporate undecylenic acid (10%) by itself in the vehicle. This concentration has minor irritant effects on the skin.

Phenolic Compounds and Derivatives

Phenol and resorcinol have been included in many topical antifungal products for their keratolytic or fungicidal effects. The fungicidal potency of resorcinol is about one-third that of phenol. Phenol is reported to be more effective in aqueous solutions than in glycerin or fats; it is relatively ineffective when incorporated into soaps (102).

Applied to unabraded skin in low concentrations, phenol causes warmth and a tingling sensation. Its irritant qualities usually restrict its effectiveness in athlete's foot remedies. To be fungicidal in these preparations, concentrations irritating to human skin generally must be used.

Resorcinol, in concentration usually applied topically ($< 10\%$), is nonirritating; higher concentrations may be irritating. Rarely does resorcinol produce allergic reactions.

Phenol and resorcinol resemble each other with regard to systemic action, particularly on the CNS. Thus, preparations containing either agent should never be applied to large areas or to irritated or denuded skin because of possible absorption and systemic toxicity. In the future, nonprescription phenol products will be limited to concentrations of 1.5% or less (103). Because local and systemic toxicity may occur following the use of phenol-containing products covered with bandages or occlusive dressings, one must be concerned with its use in athlete's foot. In this instance, occlusive footwear could enhance absorption after its application. This percutaneous absorption would seem to be more favorable from the top of the foot rather than beneath the foot where the thick outer layer of skin would seem to inhibit any penetration. With the inherent safety problems associated with the use of phenol and the fact that sufficient data were lacking about phenol's efficacy for athlete's foot in concentrations equal to or less than 1.5%, the FDA advisory review panel on nonprescription antimicrobial drug products (II) classified phenol into Category II (84).

Chloroxylenol, a substituted phenol, is a nonirritating antiseptic agent. Chloroxylenol (0.5% solution) was reported to be effective in treating and preventing athlete's foot (104). It is included in some topical preparations in liquid, cream, and powder forms. Chloroxylenol's limited water solubility makes its efficacy in powder drug delivery systems questionable. If the inert agents of the vehicle are effective in adsorbing moisture, the effect of the chloroxylenol may be diminished. Chloroxylenol causes no cutaneous irritation up to concentrations of 5% (105). It is less toxic than phenol, but eczematous reactions have followed its use (106). Since efficacy data is lacking, chloroxylenol was placed in Category III by the FDA advisory panel on nonprescription antimicrobial drug products (II) (84).

Salicylic Acid

In high concentrations, salicylic acid is a keratolytic agent, causing the keratin layer of the skin to shed and facilitating penetration of other drugs. Lower concentrations ($< 2\%$) are keratoplastic; they aid normal keratinization. Salicylic acid (5–10%) softens the stratum corneum by increasing the endogenous hydration of this layer. This effect probably results from lowering the pH, which causes the cornified epithelium to swell, soften, macerate, and then desquamate (38). If no moisture is present, cornified epithelium is not softened significantly by tolerable amounts of salicylic acid. Because salicylic acid accelerates exfoliation of the infected keratin tissue, its use in conjunction with topical antifungals may be very beneficial in appropriate conditions (93).

Salicylic acid alone has little or no antifungal activity. It usually is applied to the skin as a combination of 3% salicylic acid and 6% benzoic acid in a polyethylene glycol base (Whitfield's ointment). Benzoic acid alone is alleged to have some fungistatic activity, but this claim is debatable. This ointment is available in double strength and half strength. The half-strength formula (1.5% salicylic acid) does not have the keratolytic properties of the regular or double strength and therefore should never be used when keratolytic activity is necessary. The basic criterion for evaluating the efficacy of salicylic acid products as keratolytic agents is the concentration of salicylic acid. Thus, on the basis of current literature, these products should contain concentrations of more than 2% salicylic acid. Since there was insufficient evidence in support of either salicylic or benzoic acid for the treatment of athlete's foot these agents were classified as Category III by the FDA advisory review panel on nonprescription antimicrobial drug products (II) (84).

The pharmacist should be aware of the irritant properties of topically applied salicylic acid. Many skin irritations have been reported following unsupervised self-medication.

Quaternary Ammonium Compounds Quaternary ammonium compounds (benzethonium chloride and methylbenzethonium chloride) are used in several antifungal aids for their skin antiseptic and detergent properties. Solutions of these agents have emulsifying properties that favor wetting and penetration of surfaces to which they are applied. The fungicidal activity of quaternary ammonium compounds is generally less than their bactericidal activities (107). (See Chapter 28, *Topical Anti-infective Products*.)

The disinfectant action of these compounds may not be as great as expected. Gram-positive microorganisms generally are more susceptible to the effect of quaternary ammonium compounds than are gram-negative pathogens. A concern with quaternary ammonium compounds is that their misuse or overuse could lead to *Pseudomonas* species or other gram-negative pathogen overgrowth, especially in debilitated patients. This possibility should be kept in mind with nonprescription antifungal products, although realistically this occurrence would be expected to be rare with the use of low concentrations of quaternary ammonium compounds. These agents are cationic and have a chemical incompatibility with anionic compounds such as soaps. Thus, any residual soap or soap film on the skin may inactivate them (108). In athlete's foot, where patients are told to clean their feet thoroughly daily, patients also must be instructed to rinse the affected area thoroughly before drying it. Otherwise, if the nonprescription product contains a quaternary ammonium compound, any beneficial effects may be negated. This thought also should bring to mind any formulations of these compounds that contain anionic compounds (zinc undecylenate and sodium propionate) (107). Predictably, the germicide would be rendered ineffective.

A tincture delivery system of these cationic compounds is more effective as a skin disinfectant and is less affected by soap than an aqueous solution (109). Accordingly, tincture forms of these agents are used in more dilute concentrations than aqueous solutions.

Therefore, in a liquid form, especially a tincture, quaternary compounds should be effective if appropriate concentrations are used. However, when applied topically in powder form with adsorbent agents included in the formulation, their efficacy is doubtful. If all moisture is removed effectively by the adsorbing material, the quaternary compound may be unable to dissolve and exert its germicidal activity, although these compounds dissolve in a minimal amount of water.

Quaternary ammonium compounds generally are safe when applied topically. However, the assignment of quaternary ammonium compounds (most notably benzethonium chloride) to Category III indicates a need for substantive data relevant to efficacy (84). However, each compound has its own sensitization index and its own ability to produce contact dermatitis resulting from widespread usage and multiple exposures to these chemicals.

Quinoline Derivatives Of 24 quinoline derivatives investigated in vitro, only benzoxiquine (8-hydroxyquinoline benzoate) was active in fungistatic and fungicidal testing (110). It has been postulated that the activity of 8-hydroxyquinoline is due to chelation of trace metals, essential for the growth of fungi, in either the nutritive media or the cell of the fungus (111). A 3% benzoxiquine preparation in a vanishing cream base was fungicidal in vitro when compared to other antifungal ointments (96). Subsequently, an antifungal preparation containing 2.5% benzoxiquine was used successfully in the treatment of dermatophytosis (112).

Several proprietary powder antifungals use 8-hydroxyquinoline sulfate in their formulations. This compound is fungicidal. Because the sulfate salt is fairly water soluble and forms an acidic solution in the presence of moisture, it may enhance the antifungal effect of 8-hydroxyquinoline. However, there is no clinical evidence to support the hypothesis; these agents have been classified into Category III (84).

Salts of Aluminum Historically, the foremost astringent used for the acute inflammatory stage of tinea pedis and the wet, soggy type of tinea pedis has been aluminum acetate (Burow's solution). However, recent evidence also supports the use of aluminum chloride in treating the wet, soggy type (5).

The action and efficacy of these aluminum salts appear to be two-pronged. First, these compounds act as astringents. Their drying ability probably involves the complexing of the astringent agent with proteins, thereby altering the proteins' ability to swell and hold water (5). These astringents decrease edema, exudation, and inflammation by reducing the cell membrane permeability and hardening the cement substance of the capillary epithelium. Second, in concentrations greater than 20%, aluminum chloride, for instance, possesses antibacterial activity. Aluminum chloride (20%) may exhibit its antibacterial activity in two ways: by directly killing bacteria and by drying the interspaces (5). Solutions of 20% aluminum acetate and 20% aluminum chloride demonstrated equal in-vitro antibacterial efficacy (5).

Aluminum acetate solution for use in tinea pedis generally is diluted with about 10–40 parts of water. Depending on the situation, the patient either immerses the whole foot in the solution for 20 minutes up to 3 times/day (every 6–8 hours) or merely applies the solution to the area in the form of a wet dressing. In a recent trial, 10 subjects compared undiluted aluminum acetate solution (5%) to the recommended 1:20 dilution (of the 5% solution) on the macerated, soggy type of athlete's foot (5). After 7 days, the 5% solution produced moderate drying and symptomatic improvement in five subjects; the 1:20 dilution was ineffective.

For patient convenience aluminum acetate solution (Burow's solution) or modified Burow's solution products are available in a number of dosage forms for immediate use (in solution) or for preparation before use with water (powder packets, powder, and effervescent tablets). These products are intended for external use only, are not to be ingested, and should be kept away from contact with the eyes. Prolonged or continuous use of aluminum acetate solution for extended periods may produce necrosis (113). However, in the acute inflammatory stage of tinea pedis, this solution should be used less than 1 week. The pharmacist should instruct the patient to discontinue use of the solution if extensive inflammatory lesions appear to worsen or if irritation becomes more apparent.

Concentrations of 20–30% aluminum chloride have been the most beneficial for the wet, soggy type of athlete's foot (5). Twice-daily applications of aluminum chloride generally are used until the signs and symptoms, such as odor, wetness, and whiteness, abate. Once-daily applications control the symptoms after that time (114). In hot, humid weather, the original condition returns within 7–10 days after the application is stopped (114).

The application of aluminum salts does not entirely cure athlete's foot. This treatment merely shifts the disease process back to the simple dry type of athlete's foot, which then can be controlled with other agents such as tolnaftate. Safety and efficacy data were submitted for only two aluminum compounds, alcloxa (aluminum chlorhydroxyallantoinate) and aluminum sulfate, to the FDA advisory review panel on nonprescription antimicrobial drug products (II). Due to a lack of sufficient data available on the effectiveness of these agents, both were classified as Category III (84).

Since aluminum salts penetrate skin poorly, the toxicity of salts like aluminum chloride is rather low. However, one study demonstrated a few cases of irritation in patients where deep fissures were present (5), so that the aluminum salt was able to come in contact with living skin. Thus, a contraindication to the use of concentrated aluminum salt solutions would be severely eroded or deeply fissured skin. In these cases, dilution of the salts to a lower concentration (10% aluminum chloride) is necessary for initial treatment.

Used appropriately, aluminum acetate solution or aluminum chloride solution is valuable in the wet, soggy, macerated form of athlete's foot and in the acute inflammatory stages of athlete's foot. However, each solution has potential for misuse (accidental childhood poisoning by ingesting the solutions or ingesting the solid tablets). The problem is real, and precautions must be taken to prevent this occurence.

Benzoyl Peroxide A 5% or 10% gel of benzoyl peroxide has been suggested for use in the symptomatic interdigital treatment of athlete's foot (115). The drying or astringent effect of this formulation coupled with the antimicrobial activity of the benzoyl peroxide offers the advantage of rapid clinical improvement of this form of tinea pedis. However, this product must be used with caution, since it may be irritating, particularly to denuded areas or deep fissures. Prolonged use of benzoyl peroxide on inflamed or ulcerated skin should be avoided because of its strong sensitizing ability.

Other Ingredients and Dosage Forms The primary drug delivery systems used for treatment of tinea pedis are creams, solutions, and powders. Powders, including those in aerosol dosage forms, generally are indicated for adjunctive use with solutions and creams. In very mild conditions, powders may suffice as the only therapy.

The vehicle of the solution or cream forms should be

- Nonocclusive (it should not retain moisture or sweat, which exacerbates the condition);
- Water miscible or water washable (removable with minimal cleansing efforts, since hard scrubbing of the affected area further abrades the skin);
- Anhydrous, since including water in the formulation introduces a variable that is one of the primary causes of the condition;
- Spreadable with minimal effort and without waste;
- Capable of efficient drug delivery (it must not interact with the active ingredient, but allow it to penetrate to the seat of the fungal infection);
- Nonsensitizing and nontoxic when applied to intact or denuded skin, especially if it is absorbed into the systemic circulation.

Most vehicles used to deliver topical solutions and creams are essentially polyethylene glycol and alcohols, which meet these criteria. Polyethylene glycol bases deliver water-insoluble drugs topically more efficiently than water-soluble agents. This feature is an added advantage because most topical antifungal drugs are basically water insoluble (tolnaftate, for example).

The criteria for the powder dosage form (shaker or aerosol) are basically the same as those for creams or solutions. Certain agents in powder forms are therapeutic and also serve as vehicles (talc and/or cornstarch). Powders inhibit the propagation of fungi by adsorbing moisture and preventing skin maceration. Thus, they actually alter the ecologic conditions of the fungi, but the actual effective agent in these formulations is unknown (91). For example, the adsorbing material within the powder might be responsible for the remission of the disease instead of the intended active ingredient.

Many authorities consider cornstarch superior to talc for these formulations, since it is virtually free of chemical contamination and it does not tend to produce granulomatous reactions in wounds as readily as talc (116). Moreover, a study comparing adsorbance showed that cornstarch adsorbed 25 times more moisture from moisture-saturated air than talc (117).

Product Selection Guidelines

Since the product chosen may influence patient compliance, the pharmacist should recommend an appropriate dosage form designed to cause the least interference with daily habits and activities without sacrificing efficacy. Product selection should be geared to the particular patient. For example, elderly patients may require a preparation that is easier than normal to use, and obese patients, in whom excessive sweating may contribute to the disease, should use topical talcum powders as adjunctive therapy.

Before recommending a nonprescription product, the pharmacist should review the patient's medical history. In patients with diabetes, for example, the glucose level, which as a normal constituent of sweat provides an excellent growth medium for fungi, must be under control (104). Patients with allergic dermatitides are extremely sensitive to most oral and topical agents. Such patients usually have a history of asthma, hay fever, or atopic dermatitis, which is indicated on the medication profile. Thus, the pharmacist can distinguish a tinea infection from atopic dermatitis and avoid recommending a product that may cause skin irritation.

The concentration of organic fatty acids and/or their salt forms usually is too low to be irritating to the skin. Although these products are nonsensitizing, treatment should be discontinued if irritation or sensitivity develops with their use.

The pharmacist should bear in mind that prescription-only drugs may be more beneficial in some cases than nonprescription products (118, 119). In the soggy, macerated athlete's foot complicated by bacteria, the broad-spectrum antifungal agents miconazole nitrate and clotrimazole are preferable to both tolnaftate and the prescription drug haloprogin (4).

Patient Consultation

The pharmacist should advise patients not to expect dramatic remission of the condition initially. The onset of symptomatic relief may take several days because healing generally is gradual. Patients should be advised that depending on certain factors (extent of the affected area and patient variability to medication), the medication may have to be used a minimum of 2–4 weeks. The patient should be told of the necessity to adhere to the physician-prescribed dosage regimen or the suggested directions on the product label. Although patient noncompliance is not documented, it probably contributes to the failure of topical products in treating tinea pedis. The pharmacist should ask the patient to continue the medication for a few days after the recommended time period to help prevent relapse.

All topical antifungal products may induce various hypersensitivity reactions. Although the incidence is small, patients should be advised to discontinue the product if itching, swelling, or further exacerbation of the disease occurs. In addition, patients should avoid contact of the product with the eyes. After applying the product, patients should wash their hands thoroughly with soap and water.

Before effective drug therapy for athlete's foot can be instituted, the pharmacist should emphasize the need for proper hygiene. The feet should be cleaned and dried thoroughly each day. Even though transmission of the disease to other individuals may be rare, patients should have their own washcloth and towels. The affected area should be patted thoroughly dry. After bathing, the feet should be dried last so as not to spread the infection with the towel to other sites.

General measures should be taken to eliminate the predisposing factors, heat and perspiration. Shoes and light cotton socks that allow ventilation should be worn. Wool and some newer synthetic fabrics interfere with foot moisture dissipation. Occlusive footwear, including canvas rubber-soled athletic shoes, should not be worn. Shoes should be alternated as often as possible so that the insides can adequately dry. Socks should be changed daily and washed thoroughly after use. Shoes should be dusted with drying powders. Interestingly, there was a mycologic improvement in 25% of the test population who used a topical placebo formulation with preventive hygienic measures (83).

Clothing and towels should be changed frequently and laundered well in hot water. The feet, particularly the area between the toes, should be dusted with a drying powder at every change of socks. Whenever possible, the feet should be aired to prevent moisture buildup. Nonocclusive protective footwear (e.g., rubber or wooden sandals) should be worn in areas of family or public use such as the home bathroom, community showers, or bathing areas.

The pharmacist should inform the patient of the need for protective measures that aid the topical antifungal product in eradicating the fungal infection. However, patients should be cautioned against overzealous cleansing with soap and water and vigorous drying between the toes; this practice may irritate the area further.

Since dermatophytes enjoy living on moist warm wood, public baths and shower areas should not be constructed with wooden grills (75).

Summary

The nonprescription drug of choice in the treatment of corns, calluses, and warts is salicyclic acid in a flexible collodion (10%) or plaster (40%) form, whichever is more convenient. However, it is ineffective if predisposing factors responsible for corns and calluses are not corrected. (Surgical excision of corns associated with exostoses prevents development of corns only in that area.) The effectiveness of salicylic acid in treating warts is increased if the wart is pared to the point of bleeding or pain. This procedure should be performed only by a podiatrist or other physician. Plantar warts should be treated with a higher concentration (20–40% of salicylic acid); warts on thin epidermis require a lower concentration (10–20%). Because warts are usually self-limiting, treatment should be conservative; vigorous therapy with salicylic acid may scar tissue.

The nonprescription drug of choice in treating the dry, scaly type of athlete's foot is tolnaftate. However, recent clinical trials have demonstrated comparable efficacy between tolnaftate and its strongest challenger, undecylenic acid (66, 83). Nevertheless, other predisposing factors to tinea pedis must be eliminated by the patient for tolnaftate or undecylenic acid to be effective. These drugs are effective in all their drug delivery systems, but the powder form should be reserved only for extremely mild conditions or as adjunctive therapy.

When recommended for suspected or actual dermatophytosis of the foot, these drugs should be used twice daily, morning and night. Because the vehicle forms of the solution and cream are spreadable, they should be used sparingly. Treatment should be continued 2–4 weeks, depending on the symptoms. After this time, effectiveness should be evaluated by the patient and pharmacist.

The value of any topical nonprescription product for the treatment of the soggy, macerated type of athlete's foot is dubious. The complex nature of the topical flora (resident aerobic diphtheroids) superimposed on the fungal infection dictates rigorous therapy with broader spectrum antifungals (miconazole nitrate or clotrimazole). Otherwise, soaks and compresses of astringent agents (aluminum chloride) may be indicated to dry the soggy, macerated tissue. Once this step is accomplished, tolnaftate therapy may be instituted.

Alleviation of the symptoms does not occur overnight. Patients should be made aware of this fact to minimize noncompliance associated with a product believed to be ineffective. Furthermore, patients should be cautioned that frequent recurrence of any of these problems is indication for consultation with a podiatrist or physician.

References

1. S. Rosen, *J. Med. Assoc. St. Ala.*, *43*, 617 (1974).
2. K. A. Arndt, "Manual of Dermatological Therapeutics," Little, Brown, Boston, Mass., 1974, pp. 23–25.
3. J. Raskin, in "Current Therapy, 1976," H. F. Conn, Ed., W. B. Saunders, Philadelphia, Pa, 1976, pp. 611–614.
4. J. J. Leyden and A. M. Kligman, *Postgrad. Med.*, *61*, 113 (1977).
5. J. J. Leyden and A. M. Kligman, *Arch. Dermatol.*, *111*, 1004 (1975).
6. H. T. Behrmann, T. A. Labow, and J. H. Rozen, "Common Skin Diseases: Diagnosis and Treatment," 3rd ed., Grune and Stratton, New York, N.Y., 1978, p. 39.
7. A. N. Domonkos, "Andrews' Diseases of the Skin," 6th ed., W. B. Saunders, Philadelphia, Pa., 1971, pp. 54–58.
8. G. K. Potter, *J. Am. Podiat. Assoc.*, *63*, 57 (1973).
9. J. W. Burnett and H. M. Robinson, Jr., "Clinical Dermatology for Students and Practitioners," 2nd ed., Yorke, New York, N.Y., p. 143.
10. W. D. Stewart, J. L. Danto, and S. Maddin, "Dermatology: Diagnosis and Treatment of Cutaneous Disorders," 4th ed., C. V. Mosby, St. Louis, Mo., 1978, p. 129.
11. S. W. Balkin, *Arch. Dermatol.*, *111*, 1143 (1975).
12. N. J. Giannestras, "Foot Disorders: Medical and Surgical Management," 2nd ed., Lea and Febiger, Philadelphia, Pa., 1973, pp. 24–26.
13. I. Yale, "Podiatric Medicine," Williams and Wilkins, Baltimore, Md., 1974, pp. 244–246.
14. "DuVries' Surgery of the Foot," 3rd ed., V. T. Inman, Ed., C. V. Mosby, St. Louis, Mo., 1973, pp. 206–223.
15. E. Jawetz, J. L. Melnick, and E. A. Adelberg, "Review of Medical Microbiology," 11th ed., Lange Medical, Los Altos, Calif., 1974, pp. 449–450.
16. G. Orth, S. Jablonski, M. Favre, O. Croissant, S. Obalek, M. Jarzabek-Chorzelska, and N. Jibard, *J. Invest. Dermatol.*, *76*, 97 (1981).
17. J. R. Coggin, Jr., and H. zur Hausen, *Cancer Res.*, *39*, 545 (1979).
18. G. Orth, M. Favre, and O. Croissant, *J. Virol.*, *24*, 108 (1977).
19. L. Gissmann and H. zur Hausen, *Int. J. Cancer*, *25*, 605 (1980).
20. M. Jarratt, *Pediatr. Clin. N. Am.*, *25*, 339 (1978).
21. "Dermal Pathology," J. H. Graham, W. C. Johnson, and E. B. Helwig, Eds., Harper and Row, Hagerstown, Md., 1972, pp. 533–535.
22. M. H. Bunney, *Drugs*, *13*, 445 (1977).
23. J. S. Pegum, *Practitioner*, *209*, 453 (1972).
24. F. A. Ive, *Br. Med. J.*, *4*, 475 (1973).
25. K. A. Arndt, "Manual of Dermatological Therapeutics," Little, Brown, Boston, Mass., 1974, pp. 167–173.
26. W. D. Stewart, J. L. Danto, and S. Maddin, "Dermatology: Diagnosis and Treatment of Cutaneous Disorders," 4th ed., C. V. Mosby, St. Louis, Mo., 1978, pp. 316–321.
27. A. P. Goffe, J. D. Almeida, and F. Brown, *Lancet*, *2*, 607 (1966).
28. S. Pyrhonen and E. Johansson, *Lancet*, *1*, 592 (1975).
29. M. H. Bunney, J. A. A. Hunter, M. M. Ogilvie, and D. A. Williams, *Practitioner*, *207*, 197 (1971).
30. W. B. Harwell, R. N. Buchanan, Jr., and J. R. Hamilton, *J. Tennessee Med. Assoc.*, *71*, 830 (1978).
31. F. R. Bettley, "Skin Diseases in General Practice," Charles C Thomas, Springfield, Ill., 1965, pp. 243–253.
32. H. T. Behrman, T. A. Labow, and J. H. Rozen, "Common Skin Diseases: Diagnosis and Treatment," 3rd ed., Grune and Stratton, New York, N.Y., 1978, pp. 139–142.
33. *Federal Register*, *45*, 65609 (1980).
34. J. P. Barrett, Jr., *J. Am. Med. Assoc.*, *235*, 1138 (1976).
35. B. B. Sanders, Jr., and G. S. Stretcher, *J. Am. Med. Assoc.*, *235*, 2859 (1976).
36. R. B. Rees, Jr., in "Current Diagnosis and Treatment," M. A. Krupp and M. J. Chatton, Eds., Lange Medical, Los Altos, Calif., 1979, p. 73.
37. A. S. Wigfield, *Br. Med. J.*, *3*, 585 (1972).
38. "Drug Design," Vol. 4, E. J. Ariens, Ed., Academic, New York, N.Y., 1973, p. 134.
39. "Drug Design," Vol. 4, E. J. Ariens, Ed., Academic, New York, N.Y., 1973, p. 178.
40. M. E. Stolar, G. V. Rossi, and M. Barr, *J. Am. Pharm. Assoc., Sci. Ed.*, *49*, 144 (1960).
41. J. F. vonWeiss and W. F. Lever, *Arch. Dermatol.*, *90*, 614 (1964).
42. J. A. Mills, *N. Engl. J. Med.*, *290*, 781 (1974).
43. A. L. Norins, in "Current Therapy, 1976," H. F. Conn, Ed., W. B. Saunders, Philadelphia, Pa., 1976, pp. 667–670.
44. H. C. Ansel, "Introduction to Pharmaceutical Dosage Forms," 3rd ed., Lea and Febiger, Philadelphia, Pa., 1981, p. 306.
45. A. Gaisin, *Arch. Dermatol.*, *112*, 1791 (1976).
46. "Sprowls' American Pharmacy," 7th ed., L. W. Dittert, Ed., Lippincott, Philadelphia, Pa., 1974, p. 167.
47. H. C. Ansel, "Introduction to Pharmaceutical Dosage Forms," 3rd ed., Lea and Febiger, Philadelphia, Pa., 1981, p. 305.
48. E. M. Brecher, and Editors of Consumer Reports, "Licit and Illicit Drugs," Little, Brown, Boston, Mass., 1972, pp. 309–320.
49. R. E. Gosselin, H. C. Hodge, R. P. Smith, and M. N. Gleason, "Clinical Toxicology of Commercial Products, Acute Poisoning," 4th ed., Section II, Williams and Wilkins, Baltimore, Md., 1976, p. 99.
50. "AMA Drug Evaluations," 3rd ed., Publishing Sciences Group, Acton, Mass., 1977, pp. 188–189.
51. E. W. Rosenberg, R. A. Amonette, and J. H. Gardner, *Arch. Dermatol.*, *113*, 1134 (1977).
52. M. J. Chamberlain, *Br. Med. J.*, *3*, 391 (1972).
53. M. D. Karol, C. S. Conner, A. S. Watanabe, and K. J. Murphrey, *Clinical Toxicology*, *16(3)*, 282 (1980).
54. R. R. M. McLaughlin, *Arch. Dermatol.*, *106*, 129 (1972).
55. R. Lester and D. Rosenthal, *Arch. Dermatol.*, *104*, 330 (1971).
56. M. W. Hursthouse, *Br. J. Dermatol.*, *92*, 93 (1975).
57. Medical News, *J. Am. Med. Assoc.*, *237*, 940 (1977).
58. L. Hymes and G. S. Hymes, *J. Am. Podiat. Assoc.*, *65*, 1023 (1975).
59. D. F. Tutunji, *Br. Med. J.*, *4*, 241 (1972).
60. C. G. Schirren, *Hautarzt*, *17*, 321 (1966).
61. M. P. Adams and J. Elenbaas, *Drug Intell. Clin. Pharm.*, *15*, 279 (1981).
62. *Federal Register*, *45*, 69128 (1980).
63. *Medical Letter on Drugs and Therapeutics*, *18 (25)*, 105 (1976).
64. W. J. Mills, Jr., *Emergency Med.*, *8*, 134 (1976).

65. T. Schwinghammer, *U.S. Pharm.*, *3 (#1)*, 48 (1978).
66. E. H. Tschen, L. E. Becker, J. A. Ulrich, W. H. Hoge, and E. B. Smith, *Cutis*, *23*, 696 (1979).
67. G. C. Sauer, "Manual of Skin Diseases," 3rd ed., Lippincott, Philadelphia, Pa., 1973, pp. 159–181.
68. C. M. Davis, R. L. Garcia, J. P. Riordan, and D. Taplin, *Arch. Dermatol.*, *105*, 558 (1972).
69. J. J. Leyden and A. M. Kligman, *Arch. Dermatol.*, *114*, 1466 (1978).
70. C. M. Caravati, Jr., E. M. Hudgins, and L. W. Kelly, Jr., *Cutis*, *17*, 313 (1976).
71. R. L. Baer and S. A. Rosenthal, *J. Am. Med. Assoc.*, *197*, 187 (1966).
72. W. D. Stewart, J. L. Danto, and S. Maddin, "Dermatology: Diagnosis and Treatment of Cutaneous Disorders," 4th ed., C. V. Mosby, St. Louis, Mo., 1978, pp. 265–280.
73. "An Introduction to the Biology of the Skin," R. H. Champion, T. Gillman, A. J. Rook, and R. T. Sims, Eds., Davis, Philadelphia, Pa., 1970, pp. 206–221.
74. K. A. Arndt, "Manual of Dermatologic Therapeutics," Little, Brown, Boston, Mass., 1974, pp. 61–77.
75. J. H. S. Pettit, *Drugs*, *10*, 130 (1975).
76. A. Jarrett, "The Physiology and Pathophysiology of the Skin: The Epidermis," Vol. 1, Academic, New York, N.Y., 1973, p. 155.
77. R. J. Yu, S. R. Harmon, and F. Blank, *J. Bacteriol.*, *96*, 1435 (1968).
78. "Dermal Pathology," J. H. Graham, W. C. Johnson, and E. B. Helwig, Eds., Harper and Row, Hagerstown, Md., 1972, pp. 137–253.
79. J. W. Burnett and H. M. Robinson, Jr., "Clinical Dermatology for Students and Practitioners," 2nd ed., Yorke, New York, N.Y., 1978.
80. R. A. Amonette and E. W. Rosenberg, *Arch. Dermatol.*, *107*, 71 (1973).
81. H. I. Maibach, *Arch. Dermatol.*, *114*, 1773 (1978).
82. C. E. Mueller and D. P. West, *Amer. Pharm.*, *NS21*, 299 (1981).
83. J. F. Fuerst, G. F. Cox, S. M. Weaver, and W. C. Duncan, *Cutis*, *25*, 544 (1980).
84. FDA Advisory Panel on OTC Antimicrobial Drug Products (II) Findings, Adopted 2/23/81, in press, Bureau of Drugs, FDA, Rockville, Md.
85. H. L. Arnold, Jr., *Arch. Dermatol.*, *115*, 1287 (1979).
86. L. M. Field, *Arch. Dermatol.*, *115*, 1287 (1979).
87. T. Noguchi, A. Kaji, Y. Igarashi, A. Shigematsu, and K. Taniguchi, "Antitrichopyton Activity of Naphthiomates in Antimicrobial Agents and Chemotherapy," American Society for Microbiology, Ann Arbor, Mich., 1962, p. 259.
88. G. A. Gellin, H. I. Maibach, and G. N. Wachs, *Arch. Dermatol.*, *106*, 715 (1972).
89. J. B. Shelmire, Jr., *J. Invest. Dermatol.*, *26*, 105 (1956).
90. K. H. Kaidbey and A. M. Kligman, *Arch. Dermatol.*, *110*, 868 (1974).
91. E. B. Smith, J. E. Dickson, and J. M. Know, *S. Med. J.*, *67*, 776 (1974).
92. A. H. Gould, *Dermatologica Tropica et Ecologica Geographica*, *3*, 255 (1964).
93. "AMA Drug Evaluations," 4th ed., Publishing Sciences Group, Acton, Mass., 1980, p. 1366.
94. S. M. Peck and H. Rosenfeld, *J. Invest. Dermatol.*, *1*, 237 (1938).
95. E. L. Keeney, L. Ajello, E. Lankford, and L. Mary, *Bull. Johns Hopkins Hosp.*, *17*, 422 (1945).
96. M. J. Golden and K. A. Oster, *J. Am. Pharm. Assoc., Sci. Ed.*, *39*, 47 (1950).
97. W. C. Cutting, "Handbook of Pharmacology," 5th ed., Meredith, New York, N.Y., 1972, p. 56.
98. F. Sadik, *PharmIndex*, *15(7A)*, 5 (1973).
99. E. B. Smith, R. F. Powell, J. L. Graham, and J. A. Ulrich, *Int. J. Dermatol.*, *16*, 52 (1977).
100. J. H. Chretien, J. G. Esswein, L. M. Sharpe, J. J. Kiely, and F. E. Lyddon, *Int. J. Dermatol.*, *19*, 51 (1980).
101. F. E. Lyddon, K. Gundersen, and H. I. Maibach, *Int. J. Dermatol.*, *19*, 24 (1980).
102. "The Pharmacological Basis of Therapeutics," 6th ed., A. G. Gilman, L. S. Goodman, and A. Gilman, Eds., Macmillan, New York, N.Y., 1980, p. 967.
103. *Federal Register*, *43*, 1238 (1978).
104. M. H. Walker, *J. Am. Podiatr. Assoc.*, *52*, 737 (1962).
105. R. E. Gosselin, H. C. Hodge, R. P. Smith, and M. N. Gleason, "Clinical Toxicology of Commercial Products, Acute Poisoning," 4th ed., Williams and Wilkins, Baltimore, Md., 1976, Section II, p. 131.
106. J. K. Morgan, *Br. J. Clin. Pract.*, *22*, 261 (1968).
107. *Federal Register*, *3*, 1236 (1978).
108. "Sprowls' American Pharmacy," 7th ed., L. W. Dittert, Ed., Lippincott, Philadelphia, Pa., 1974, p. 49.
109. P. B. Price, *Arch. Surg.*, *61*, 23 (1950).
110. K. A. Oster and M. J. Golden, *J. Am. Pharm. Assoc., Sci. Ed.*, *37*, 429 (1948).
111. G. A. Zentmyer, *Science*, *100*, 294 (1944).
112. K. A. Oster and M. J. Golden, *Exp. Med. Surg.*, *1*, 37 (1949).
113. R. E. Gosselin, H. C. Hodge, R. P. Smith, and M. N. Gleason, "Clinical Toxicology of Commercial Products, Acute Poisoning," 4th ed., Williams and Wilkins, Baltimore, Md., 1976, Section II, p. 89.
114. L. Goldman, in "Current Therapy, 1972," H. F. Conn, Ed., W. B. Saunders, Philadelphia, Pa., 1972, p. 585.
115. A. M. Kligman, J. J. Leyden, and R. Stewart, *Int. J. Dermatol.*, *16*, 413 (1977).
116. H. Myllarniemi, M. Frilauder, M. Turunen, and L. Saxen, *Acta Chirurgica Scand.*, *131*, 312 (1966).
117. *Federal Register*, *43*, 34636 (1978).
118. E. B. Smith, J. L. Graham, and J. A. Ulrich, *S. Med. J.*, *70*, 47 (1977).
119. H. E. Jones, J. G. Simpson, and W. M. Artis, *Arch. Dermatol.*, *117*, 129 (1981).

Athlete's Foot Product Table

Product (Manufacturer)	Application Form	Antifungal	Keratolytic	Other Ingredients
Aftate (Plough)	spray liquid spray powder powder gel	tolnaftate, 1%		
Bevill's Lotion (Bevill)	lotion		salicylic acid	alcohol, 68% ether, 8% methyl salicylate, 1%
Blis Foot Bath (Commerce)	powder		salicylic acid, 17%	boric acid, 47.5% epsom salt, 10.7%
Blis-To-Sol (Chattem)	liquid aerosol powder powder	undecylenic acid, 5% (gel) 50 mg/g (liquid) zinc stearate, 10 mg/g (aerosol, powder) benzoic acid, 10 mg/g (aerosol) 19 mg/g (powder)	salicylic acid, 90 mg/g (liquid) 10 mg/g (aerosol) 19 mg/g (powder)	
Bluboro (Herbert Labs)	liquid[a]			aluminum sulfate calcium acetate boric acid
Buro-Sol (Doak)	powder cream			aluminum acetate
Caldesene Medicated Powder (Pharmacraft)	powder	calcium undecylenate, 10%		
Desenex (Pharmacraft)	ointment powder aerosol powder soap	zinc undecylenate, 20% (not in soap) undecylenic acid, 5% (ointment) 2% (powder, soap)		
Desenex Antifungal Foam (Pharmacraft)	foam	undecylenic acid, 10%		isopropyl alcohol, 29%
Desenex Liquid (Pharmacraft)	solution	undecylenic acid, 10%		isopropyl alcohol, 40% propylene glycol triethanolamine
Deso-Creme (Columbia Medical)	cream	zinc undecylenate, 20% caprylic acid, 5% sodium propionate, 2%		
Domeboro (Dome)	liquid[a]			aluminum sulfate, 47.4% calcium acetate, 44.3%
Dr. Gordshell's Salve (Thomas & Thompson)	ointment	benzoic acid		lard, tallow, beeswax, resin, elder flowers, bayberry, sassafras
Dr. Scholl's Athlete's Foot Gel (Scholl)	gel	tolnaftate, 1%		
Dr. Scholl's Athlete's Foot Powder (Scholl)	powder	tolnaftate, 1%		talc, corn starch

Athlete's Foot Product Table, continued

Product (Manufacturer)	Application Form	Antifungal	Keratolytic	Other Ingredients
Dr. Scholl's Athlete's Foot Spray (Scholl)	aerosol spray	tolnaftate, 1%		alcohol, 14%
Dr. Scholl's Athlete's Foot Spray (Scholl)	aerosol powder	tolnaftate, 1%		alcohol, 36%
Enzactin (Ayerst)	cream	triacetin, 250 mg/g		
Fungacetin (Blair)	liquid ointment powder	triacetin, 30% (liquid) 25% (ointment) 33.3% (powder)		
Medicated Foot Powder (Upjohn)	powder	benzoic acid, 2.5% chlorothymol, 0.04%	salicylic acid, 2.5%	boric acid, 10% zinc oxide, 2% camphor oil, 0.1% cinnamaldehyde, 0.08%
NP 27 Aerosol (Norwich-Eaton)	aerosol	zinc undecylenate		alcohol, 20.5% by weight
NP 27 Cream (Norwich)	cream	8-hydroxyquinoline benzoate, 2.5% benzoic acid	salicylic acid	methylparaben propylparaben
NP 27 Liquid (Norwich)	liquid	undecylenic acid, 10% w/w benzoic acid		
NP 27 Powder (Norwich)	powder	benzoic acid	salicylic acid, 1.5%	eucalyptol menthol
Pro Comfort (Scholl)	spray	tolnaftate, 1%		alcohol, 36%
Quin III (Pfeiffer)	cream	iodochlorhydroxyquin, 3%		
Quinsana Plus Medicated Foot Powder (Mennen)	powder	zinc undecylenate, 20% undecylenic acid, 2%		talc silica fragrance
Rid-Itch Cream (Thomas & Thompson)	cream	zinc undecylenate, 20% undecylenic acid, 5%		emulsion base
Rid-Itch Liquid (Thomas & Thompson)	liquid	resorcinol, 1% benzoic acid, 2% chlorothymol, 1%	salicylic acid, 7%	boric acid, 5% alcohol glycerin
Salicresen (Upjohn)	liquid	secondary amyltricresols, 0.1% *o*-hydroxyphenylmercuric chloride, 0.1%	salicylic acid, 2%	acetone, 10% benzoic acid, 2% alcohol, 50%
Sopronol (Wyeth)	liquid ointment powder	sodium propionate, 12.3% (liquid, ointment) 5% (powder) sodium caprylate, 10% zinc caprylate, 5% (ointment) zinc propionate, 5% (powder)		

Athlete's Foot Product Table, continued

Product (Manufacturer)	Application Form	Antifungal	Keratolytic	Other Ingredients
Tinactin Cream and Solution (Schering)	cream solution	tolnaftate, 1%		polyethylene glycol 400 propylene glycol (cream) butylated hydroxytoluene titanium dioxide (cream)
Tinactin Powder (Schering)	powder aerosol powder	tolnaftate, 1%		corn starch (powder) talc propellants (aerosol) butylated hydroxytoluene (aerosol)
Ting (Pharmacraft)	cream	zinc stearate benzoic acid		boric acid zinc oxide alcohol, 16% (cream)
Ting (Pharmacraft)	powder	zinc undecylenate, 20% undecylenic acid, 2%		
Verdefam Cream (Owen)	cream	propionic acid, 3% undecylenic acid, 2% sodium propionate, 1% sodium caprylate, 1% copper undecylenate, 0.5%	salicylic acid, 3%	
Verdefam Solution (Owen)	solution	undecylenic acid, 5% propionic acid, 3% sodium propionate, 2% sodium caprylate, 2% copper undecylenate, 0.5%	salicylic acid, 5%	

[a]Product is diluted or reconstituted and then applied to the skin.

Callus/Corn/Wart Product Table

Product (Manufacturer)	Application Form	Active Ingredients	Other Ingredients
Bevill's Corn Remedy (Bevill)	lotion	salicylic acid ferric chloride tincture	alcohol, 70% ether methyl salicylate
Compound W Wart Remover (Whitehall)	liquid	salicylic acid, 14% glacial acetic acid, 9%	ether, 57%
Corn Fix (Alvin Last)	liquid	phenol	soap turpentine oil
Derma-Soft Creme (Creighton)	cream	salicylic acid, 2.5%	cream base
Dr. Scholl's Corn/Callus Salve (Scholl)	ointment	salicylic acid, 15%	eucalyptus oil petrolatum lanolin mineral oil
Dr. Scholl's Fixo Corn Plaster (Scholl)	unmedicated pads medicated discs	salicylic acid, 40% (medicated discs)	

Callus/Corn/Wart Product Table, continued

Product (Manufacturer)	Application Form	Active Ingredients	Other Ingredients
Dr. Scholl's Onixol (Scholl)	liquid	sodium sulfide, 1%	
Dr. Scholl's Waterproof Corn Pads (Scholl)	unmedicated pads medicated discs	salicylic acid, 40% (medicated discs)	
Dr. Scholl's Zino-Pads (Scholl)	unmedicated pads medicated discs	salicylic acid, 12% (for soft corns); 40% (for hard corns)	
Dr. Scholl's "2" Drop Corn-Callus Remover (Scholl)	liquid	salicylic acid, 12.6%	alcohol, 15% ether, 0.321 g/ml
Freezone Corn and Callus Remover (Whitehall)	liquid	salicylic acid, 13.6% zinc chloride, 2.18%	alcohol, 20.5% ether, 64.8%
Gets-It Liquid (Oakhurst)	liquid	salicylic acid, 13.9% zinc chloride, 2.7%	ether alcohol collodion
Johnson's Foot Soap (Combe)	powder[a]		borax iodide bran
Mosco (Moss)	ointment	salicylic acid	methyl salicylate
Nail-A-Cain (Medtech)	liquid	benzocaine, 15% tannic acid, 4%	isopropyl alcohol, 61% diethyl ether, 20%
Off Ezy (Commerce)	liquid	salicylic acid, 17%	flexible collodion
Outgro (Whitehall)	liquid	chlorobutanol, 5% tannic acid, 25%	isopropyl alcohol, 83%
Vergo (Daywell)	ointment-cream	calcium pantothenate ascorbic acid	starch
Wart Fix (Alvin Last)	liquid	castor oil	

[a]Product is diluted or reconstituted and then applied to the skin.

34 Hemorrhoidal Products

Benjamin Hodes

Questions to Ask the Patient

What is the nature of the symptoms?

How long have the symptoms been present? Do they recur? Are they associated with straining at a bowel movement?

Have you noticed any bleeding? Describe the bleeding.

Have you treated the symptoms without the use of medicine?

Have you previously used any nonprescription or prescription drugs for these symptoms?

Do you take laxatives regularly? If so, which ones and how frequently?

What other medicines do you take?

Are you pregnant or have you recently been pregnant?

Do you frequently suffer from constipation or diarrhea?

Do you have any other medical conditions such as heart failure, liver disease, or inflammatory disease of the intestine?

Anorectal disease, including hemorrhoids, is one of the most annoying and uncomfortable disorders. Several diseases affecting the anorectal area are not amenable to self-treatment; however, many symptoms of anorectal disease may be self-treated. Numerous nonprescription products are available for relief of the burning, pain, itching, inflammation, irritation, swelling, and the general discomfort of hemorrhoids.

Clinical Considerations

In addition to hemorrhoids, anorectal disease encompasses other disorders, some of which may be serious.

The pharmacist should evaluate symptoms reported by the patient carefully before recommending a product for self-medication. Some anorectal disorders require immediate medical attention.

Anatomy and Physiology

Three parts of the body are of concern with respect to anorectal diseases. These are the perianal area, the anal canal, and the lower portion of the rectum (Figure 1).

Perianal Area

The perianal area (about 7 cm in diameter) is the portion of the skin and buttocks immediately surrounding the anus. The skin is more likely to be moist than exposed skin in other areas of the body. The presence of sensory nerve endings make the perianal area very sensitive to pain.

Anal Canal

The anal canal (about 3 cm long) is the channel connecting the end of the GI tract (rectum) with the outside of the body. The lower two-thirds of the canal is covered by modified anal skin, which is structurally similar to the skin covering other parts of the body. The canal contains sensory nerve endings as well as pressure receptors that allow the perception of distention pain.

The point in the upper canal at which the skin lining changes to mucous membrane is the anorectal or pectinate line.

Two sphincters encircling the anal canal control passage of fecal material. The external (anal) sphincter, located at the bottom of the anal canal, is a voluntary muscle. The internal sphincter, which allows passage into the anal canal, is an involuntary muscle. Both sphincters lie under the tissues of the anal canal and extend downward. Under normal conditions the external sphincter is closed and prevents the involuntary passage of feces and/or discharges.

In healthy individuals, the skin covering the anal canal serves as a barrier against absorption of substances into the body. Therefore, treatment applied to this area of the anal canal can be expected to manifest only local effects. If disease is present, the character of the skin covering the canal may be altered due to the loss of protective oils or breaks in the surface; consequently, the ability of the skin to serve as a protective barrier is diminished.

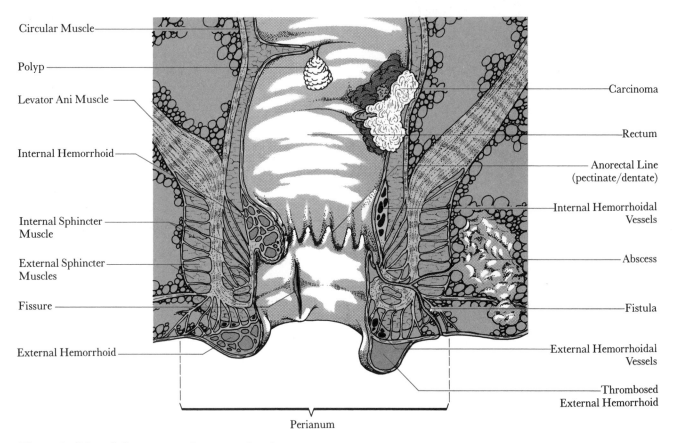

Circular Muscle

Polyp

Levator Ani Muscle

Internal Hemorrhoid

Internal Sphincter
Muscle

External Sphincter
Muscles

Fissure

External Hemorrhoid

Carcinoma

Rectum

Anorectal Line
(pectinate/dentate)

Internal Hemorrhoidal
Vessels

Abscess

Fistula

External Hemorrhoidal
Vessels

Thrombosed
External Hemorrhoid

Perianum

Figure 1. Selected disease states in anorectal region.

Anal crypts are normal pocket-like formations located at the internal side of the anorectal line. They face upward and, because of their position, sometimes retain small amounts of fecal material that may cause irritation. This irritation may lead to subsequent infections and stimulate the development of anorectal disease. Some investigators distinguish between rectal mucosa and anal mucosa and consider the anorectal ring to be the end of the anal canal (1). For the purposes of this discussion, the appearance of the mucosal region will mark the beginning of the rectal area.

Rectum

The rectum (about 12–15 cm long) is the lower end of the GI tract that extends from the anorectal line up to the sigmoid colon. It is lined with semipermeable mucous membranes, is highly vascularized, and contains no sensory pain fibers. Like the anal canal, it contains pressure receptors. The skin of the anal canal and the mucous membrane in the rectum in individuals without anorectal disease protect the body from invasion by the bacteria present in the feces.

Substances absorbed through the mucous membrane may exert systemic effects due to the plexus of hemorrhoidal vessels beneath the mucosa and the paths followed by the blood returning to the heart through the hemorrhoidal veins. This process may allow some substances to enter the systemic circulation without passing through the liver. This effect is important in evaluating the potential systemic toxicity of locally applied drugs. The rectal pH, ranging from neutral to basic, is important in determining the extent to which substances in the rectum are absorbed.

The most prominent parts of the vasculature in the region above and below the pectinate line are the three hemorrhoidal arteries along with the accompanying veins. Veins and arteries above the pectinate line are referred to as internal, and those below are external.

Etiology

Hemorrhoidal disease appears with greatest frequency in subjects 20–50 years of age (2). Numerous etiologic factors give rise to the considerable confusion regarding the cause or causes or hemorrhoidal disease. Etiologic factors may be divided into predisposing and precipitating causes (3). The causes of hemorrhoids include (2)

Predisposing causes:
- Erect posture;
- Heredity;
- Occupation;
- Diet.

Precipitating causes:
- Constipation;
- Diarrhea;
- Pregnancy;
- Anal infection;
- Rectal carcinoma;

- Pelvic tumors;
- Cardiac failure;
- Portal hypertension;
- Coughing, sneezing, vomiting;
- Physical exertion.

Predisposing Causes

The main predisposing causes are the human upright position, heredity, and occupation. The human upright position causes increased hydrostatic pressure within the hemorrhoidal vessels. Because the portal venous system contains no valves, the veins are unable to counteract the weight of the blood column impinging upon them. Continuous anorectal pressure may contribute to distention of the vessels. Heredity also is considered important to hemorrhoid formation, although this is controversial (4). Occupations involving severe muscular strain, prolonged sitting, or prolonged standing also are believed to be predisposing factors.

Dietary and cultural patterns may also predispose persons to hemorrhoids (5). Low-fiber diets and inadequate fluid intake contribute to hard and stiff stools. This in turn may lead to constipation, an important precipitating cause of hemorrhoids caused by excessive straining in defecation.

Precipitating Causes

Hemorrhoids may be precipitated by constipation, diarrhea, cathartic abuse, heart failure, portal hypertension, coughing, sneezing, vomiting, pregnancy, pelvic tumors, carcinoma of the rectum, physical exertion, and anal infection. Constipation leads to straining at defecation, which in turn leads to greatly increased pressure within the hemorrhoidal vessels. Diarrhea, coughing, sneezing, vomiting, heart failure, portal hypertension, and physical exertion all increase the pressure within the hemorrhoidal vessels and thereby may precipitate hemorrhoids.

Pregnancy is by far the most common cause of hemorrhoids in young women. The gravid uterus causes increased pressure in the middle and inferior hemorrhoidal vessels. Labor also may intensify the hemorrhoidal condition and produce intense symptoms after delivery. Pelvic tumors may give rise to hemorrhoids by a similar process.

Another possible cause of anorectal disorders is an infection occurring initially in the anal crypts that spread to the tissue nearby, causing inflammation that may result in a thrombosed hemorrhoid.

Description

Hemorrhoids (also known as piles) are abnormally large or symptomatic conglomerates of vessels, supporting tissues, and overlying mucous membrane or skin of the anorectal area. They may be classified according to degree of severity or location (6) (Figure 1).

External Hemorrhoids

External hemorrhoids occur below the anorectal line.

Thrombotic A thrombotic hemorrhoid is a hemorrhoidal vessel in either the anal canal or adjacent to the anus, that has ruptured and formed a blood clot or hematoma. The clot may vary in size from a pea to a walnut.

Cutaneous (Skin Tags) These consist of fibrous connective tissue covered by anal skin and are located outside the anal sphincter at any point on the circumference of the anus. They may result from a previously thrombosed external hemorrhoid in which the clot has become organized and replaced by connective tissue (7) or from uneven skin healing after hemorrhoidectomy.

Internal Hemorrhoids

Internal hemorrhoids occur above the anorectal line. Occasionally, because of its size and distention, an internal hemorrhoid descends below the anorectal line and outside the anal sphincter. It is then referred to as a prolapsed hemorrhoid.

Internal-External Hemorrhoids

Also known as mixed hemorrhoids, these are a combination of external and internal hemorrhoids in continuity with one another that appear as baggy swellings. The following types occur:

- **Prolapsed**—characterized by pain until the prolapse is reduced; bleeding, which would be bright red, may or may not be present;
- **Without prolapse**—bleeding may be present, but no pain;
- **Strangulated**—hemorrhoid that has prolapsed to such a degree and for so long that its blood supply is occluded by the anal sphincter's constricting action; very painful and usually becomes thrombosed.

Other Anorectal Disorders

Some potentially serious disorders may also present hemorrhoidal symptoms, including fissures and fistulas, and should not be self-medicated. Patients should be referred to a physician if any of the following conditions are suspected:

- **Abscess**—a painful swelling in the perianal or anal canal area due to a bacterial infection and resulting in the formation of a localized area of pus. Usually, *Staphylococcus* is the primary genus involved;
- **Anal fistula**—a channel-like lesion near the anus with swelling, pain, and pruritus; anorectal abscess or cryptitis usually results in an anal fistula;
- **Anal fissure**—a slit-like ulcer in the anal canal lining; this common condition may exist alone or in conjunction with hemorrhoids;
- **Condyloma latumi**—one of the secondary lesions of syphilis; its symptoms are similar to those of external hemorrhoid;
- **Condyloma acuminata**—venereal warts that appear as multiple, polymorphic lesions in the genital and/or perianal region; they are believed to be sexually transmitted;
- **Cryptitis**—inflammation and hypertrophy of the semilunar anal valve; the main symptom is anal discomfort aggravated by walking and defecation; the condition probably originates in an anal gland;

- **Malignant neoplasm**—a serious disease often characterized by a progressively enlarging "lump" beside the anus; bleeding and pain may be associated with malignant anal tumors, the most common of which is squamous cell carcinoma;
- **Polyps**—benign tumors of the large bowel that are often characterized by bleeding, protrusion of a mass through the anus, and a feeling of fullness or pressure in the rectum.

Symptoms

Itching, burning, pain, inflammation, irritation, swelling, and discomfort are common symptoms of anorectal disease that may be relieved by self-medication if they are not manifestations of more serious anorectal disease. Bleeding, seepage, protrusion, prolapse, and thrombosis are more serious symptoms of anorectal disease. These symptoms should not be self-medicated because a more serious disorder may be masked and there is no appropriate nonprescription therapy available.

Itching

Itching, or pruritus, occurs as a manifestation of mild inflammation associated with many anorectal disorders. Pruritus ani refers to persistent itching in the anal and perianal area that may occur even with good hygiene.

Itching is one of the most common symptoms of anorectal disease and may be secondary to swelling, irritation due to dietary factors, or moisture in the anal area.

Itching is not always symptomatic of hemorrhoidal disease. Sensitivity to fabrics, dyes and perfumes in toilet tissue, detergents, and fecal contents may precipitate itching. Fungal infections, parasites, allergies, and associated anorectal pathologic lesions may also cause itching. Broad-spectrum antibiotic therapy may trigger itching as a result of infection secondary to overgrowth of nonsusceptible organisms. Chronic use of mineral oil can lead to pruritus ani. Sometimes itching may be attributed to some psychologic cause.

Burning

Burning, a common symptom of anorectal disease, represents a somewhat greater degree of irritation of the anorectal sensory nerves than itching. The burning sensation may range from a feeling of warmth to a feeling of intense heat.

Pain

Acute inflammation of the anal tissue can cause pain. Hemorrhoidal pain has a steady and aching character that is usually not relieved by defecation. Pain is experienced in acute external hemorrhoids. Chronic external hemorrhoids often exhibit no pain. In view of the absence of sensory nerve endings above the anorectal line, uncomplicated internal hemorrhoids rarely cause pain. When strangulation, thrombosis, or ulceration occur, however, the pain may be severe (7). Patients with severe persistent pain should be referred to a physician.

Inflammation

Tissue reaction distinguished by heat, redness, pain, and swelling characterizes inflammation. Inflammation often is caused by trauma, allergy, or infection. The inflammation itself, but not the underlying cause, may be relieved by self-medication.

Irritation, Swelling, and Discomfort

Irritation is a response to stimulation of the nerve ending, and is characterized by the appearance of burning, itching, pain, or swelling. Swelling represents accumulation of excess fluid associated with engorged hemorrhoids or hemorrhoidal tissue. Discomfort, a vague and generalized uneasiness, may result from any or all of these symptoms.

Bleeding

Bleeding is almost always associated with internal hemorrhoids and may occur before, during, or after defecation. The amount of bleeding experienced is often variable and is not related to the amount of hemorrhoidal tissue present. When bleeding occurs from an external hemorrhoid, it is due to an acute thrombosis accompanied by rupture. Pain often accompanies the bleeding in this case, although a patient may experience some relief of the pain with the onset of the bleeding. Blood from hemorrhoids is usually bright red and covers the fecal matter. Bleeding is stimulated by defecation but may occur as an "oozing," soiling underclothes. Minor blood spots appearing on toilet tissue are likely to be due to anal fissures rather than hemorrhoids.

Bleeding hemorrhoids infrequently produce severe anemias due to the chronic blood loss. Bleeding may indicate the presence of serious anorectal disease and should not be self-medicated.

Seepage

Seepage is caused by an anal sphincter that cannot close completely and involves the involuntary passing of fecal material or mucus. This symptom cannot be self-medicated and the patient should be referred to a physician.

Protrusion

Protrusion is an early symptom of uncomplicated internal and external hemorrhoids and is defined as the projection of hemorrhoidal or rectal tissue outside the anal canal. The rectal protrusion may vary in size and usually appears after defecation, prolonged standing, or unusual physical exertion. It is painless except when thrombosis, infection, or ulceration is present. Strangulation of a protruding hemorrhoid by the sphincter may occur and may lead to thrombosis. Self-treatment is not appropriate.

A prolapsed hemorrhoid is an internal hemorrhoid that, because of distention, is located below the anorectal line and outside the anal sphincter.

A painful lump may develop when the anal sphincter contraction interferes with blood flow from a prolapsed internal or mixed hemorrhoid, resulting in thrombosis. If this prolapsed hemorrhoid returns to above the anal sphincter before thrombosis occurs, the pain and lump usually disappear. However, when defecation occurs at some later time, both lump and pain are likely to recur. Permanently prolapsing internal hemorrhoids cause a mucoid discharge, which in turn may lead to perianal irritation.

Thrombosis

Thrombosis, or blood clotting, within a hemorrhoid is a common complication. An abrupt onset of severe, constant pain in the anal area is a sign that thrombosis of a mixed or external hemorrhoid may have occurred. If untreated, the burning pain persists about 5–7 days, diminishing in intensity after the first day. A hard, tender lump at the site of the pain also appears; after the second day this lump slowly dissipates and eventually leaves a skin tag.

If the thrombosed hemorrhoid resides entirely above the anorectal line (pure internal hemorrhoid), there probably is no pain because of the lack of sensory nerve supply. Patients are likely to be unaware of the presence of this type of hemorrhoid unless there are sudden changes in bowel habits.

If thrombosed hemorrhoids do not disappear, gangrene and ulcers may develop on the hemorrhoid surface. This condition may lead to an oozing of blood as well as hemorrhaging, particularly at the time of defecation or if the patient is standing. If the clot remains exposed, infection may occur, and an abscess or fistula may result.

Assessment

Questioning the patient should enable the pharmacist to determine whether self-medication is desirable and, if so, which nonprescription product is suitable.

The pharmacist should recommend an appropriate nonprescription product for treatment of minor anorectal symptoms (itching, burning, pain, swelling, or discomfort). The patient should be referred to a physician if there is bleeding, seepage, prolapse, or severe and persistent pain or if symptoms do not improve after 7 days of self-treatment.

Treatment

Nonprescription products for symptomatic treatment of anorectal disease are available in many dosage forms.

Pharmacologic Agents

The main pharmacologic agents used for relief of anorectal disease symptoms are local anesthetics, vasoconstrictors, protectants, counterirritants, astringents, wound-healing agents, antiseptics, keratolytics, and anticholinergics. Products containing an excessive number of agents may not be optimally effective because of potential interaction among ingredients.

Local Anesthetics

Topical anesthetics temporarily relieve pain, burning, itching, discomfort, and irritation by preventing the transmission of nerve impulses. They should be used in the perianal region or the lower anal canal; symptoms within the rectum generally are not relieved by topical anesthetics because there are no rectal sensory nerve fibers (8–9).

Since absorption of local anesthetics through the rectal mucosa may be quite rapid and cause potentially toxic systemic effects, their application should be limited to the area below the rectum (10, 11). Absorption through the perianal skin, even if abraded, would not be particularly rapid.

Local anesthetics may produce allergic reactions, both locally and systemically (12, 13). Such reactions may cause burning and itching that are indistinguishable from symptoms of the anorectal disease being treated. If symptoms return after cessation of therapy, a physician should be contacted.

Recommended Anesthetics Of the local anesthetics used in hemorrhoidal preparations, only benzocaine and pramoxine hydrochloride are recommended, if used in appropriate doses.

- **Benzocaine**—In the base form, benzocaine, when used externally, is effective in concentrations of 5–20% applied up to 6 times/day. Dose should not exceed 2.4 g/24 hours (14, 16). Since absorption through the skin is poor, the possible systemic effects are minimized. The most common adverse reaction to topical benzocaine is sensitization (17, 18). Polyethylene glycol ointment is the recommended vehicle; other vehicles may not release benzocaine as well (19).
- **Pramoxine hydrochloride**—Pramoxine hydrochloride, when used externally, is effective in a cream or jelly water-miscible base at a 1% concentration applied up to 5 times/day not to exceed 100 mg/24 hours. Adverse effects are rare, and pramoxine hydrochloride exhibits less cross-sensitivity than other local anesthetics due to its distinct chemical structure (20).

Anesthetics Not Recommended Other local anesthetics used in hemorrhoidal preparations are not recommended because they are not generally recognized as safe and effective. Studies have shown that diperodon is not effective, and phenacaine is considered unsafe because of the possibility of absorption leading to systemic toxicity (21, 22). Additional evidence is required to show that the following anesthetics are effective either intrarectally or externally: benzyl alcohol, dibucaine, dibucaine hydrochloride, dyclonine hydrochloride, lidocaine, tetracaine, and tetracaine hydrochloride (21).

Vasoconstrictors

Vasoconstrictors are chemical agents structurally related to the naturally occurring catecholamines, epinephrine and norepinephrine, that function as transmitters of messages from nerves to receptors. Applied locally in the anorectal area, they stimulate the alpha-adrenergic receptors in the vascular beds, causing constriction of the arterioles. Although it has been demonstrated that there is a prompt altering of the blood supply to the mucosa when vasoconstrictors are applied locally, the FDA advisory review panel does not recognize or approve the use of vasoconstrictors for the control of minor bleeding (23, 24). In view of the fact that rectal bleeding may be a sign of more serious disease, a physician should be consulted in case of bleeding.

Vasoconstrictors relieve local itching because they also produce a slight anesthetic effect by an unknown mechanism (25). Conclusive evidence that vasoconstrictors reduce swollen hemorrhoids is lacking, even though they constrict arterioles in skin and mucous membranes in other parts of the body.

Adverse Effects   The FDA advisory review panel concluded that potentially serious side effects, including elevation of blood pressure, cardiac arrhythmia, nervousness, tremor, sleeplessness, and aggravation of symptoms of hyperthyroidism can be avoided when vasoconstrictors are used locally in recommended safe dosages (24). Because of the possibility of systemic adverse reactions, vasoconstrictors should not be used in patients who have diabetes, hyperthyroidism, hypertension, and cardiovascular disease and in those who are taking monoamine oxidase inhibitors.

Recommended Vasoconstrictors   Three vasoconstrictors are recommended for external use: aqueous solutions of ephedrine sulfate, epinephrine hydrochloride, and phenylephrine hydrochloride. Ephedrine sulfate and phenylephrine hydrochloride solutions are also recommended for internal use (intrarectal). These agents are not available for anorectal use in a solution dosage form. Other drugs used in hemorrhoidal preparations, such as epinephrine undecylenate and epinephrine hydrochloride, have been classified as ineffective for intrarectal use. Additional data are needed to establish the safety and effectiveness of epinephrine base for external and intrarectal use and epinephrine undecylenate for external use. Phenylephrine hydrochloride suppositories are considered safe although their effectiveness remains to be established.

- **Ephedrine sulfate (aqueous solution)**—This drug, which is readily absorbed through mucous membranes in the rectum, has a more prolonged effect than epinephrine and acts on both alpha- and beta-adrenergic receptors. Because ephedrine antagonizes the effects of phenothiazines, it is contraindicated in patients receiving such therapy (26). The hypertensive effects of ephedrine are potentiated by monoamine oxidase inhibitors, as well as tricyclic antidepressants. Combined use through the oral route can lead to serious, even lethal effects (27). Its onset of action ranges from a few seconds to 1 minute, its duration of action is 2–3 hours, and it is effective in the relief of itching and swelling. The recommended dose is 2–25 mg/dosage unit applied up to 4 times/day and not to exceed 100 mg/24 hours (28).

- **Epinephrine hydrochloride (aqueous solution)**—This drug is effective in the relief of itching and swelling only when used externally because epinephrine is inactivated at the pH of the rectum (29). Epinephrine is absorbed from the mucous membrane and acts on both alpha- and beta-adrenergic receptors. In a solution dosage form, epinephrine hydrochloride applied externally is effective for the temporary relief of itching and swelling (28). The recommended dose is 0.1–0.2 mg/dosage unit applied up to 4 times/day and not to exceed 0.8 mg/24 hours.

- **Phenylephrine hydrochloride (aqueous solution)**—This drug is believed to relieve itching due to histamine release and reduces congestion in the anorectal area (28, 30). It acts primarily on the alpha-adrenergic receptors and produces vasoconstriction by a direct effect on receptors rather than by norepinephrine displacement. The recommended dosage is 0.5 mg/dosage unit applied up to 4 times/day and not to exceed 2 mg/24 hours (28).

Protectants

Protectants act to prevent irritation of the anorectal area and water loss from the stratum corneum skin layer by forming a physical barrier on the skin. Little or no absorption is expected from protectants. Protection of the perianal area from irritants such as fecal matter and air leads to a reduction in irritation and concomitant itching.

Absorbents, adsorbents, demulcents, and emollients are included in the protectant classification. Many substances classified as protectants also are used as vehicles, bases, and carriers of pharmacologically active substances.

Adverse reactions are minimal with protectants as a class. Wool alcohols do cause allergies and are probably responsible for most cases of lanolin allergy (31).

Recommended Protectants   The protectants recommended for use are aluminum hydroxide gel (in moist conditions only), calamine, cocoa butter, cod liver oil, glycerin in aqueous solution, kaolin, lanolin, mineral oil, shark liver oil, starch, white petrolatum, wool alcohols, and zinc oxide. All of these protectants are recommended for external and internal (intrarectal) use, with the exception of glycerin, which is recommended for external use only. Of the recommended protectants, petrolatum is probably the most effective (32).

If a protectant is used in a nonprescription preparation, it should comprise at least 50% of the dosage unit; if two to four protectants are used, their total concentration should be at least 50%. These dosages were arrived at by determining the amount of protectant required to provide adequate thickness to prevent water loss from the epidermis (33).

Protectants Not Recommended   The bismuth salts found in some hemorrhoidal products are not recommended as protectants. Bismuth subnitrate is not considered safe because it may be absorbed, producing toxic symptoms from the bismuth ion as well as the nitrate ion (34). The effectiveness of bismuth oxide, bismuth subcarbonate, and bismuth subgallate as protectants in the anorectal area has not been established.

Counterirritants

Counterirritants distract from the perception of pain and itching by stimulating cutaneous receptors to evoke a feeling of comfort, warmth, cooling, or tingling. Because the rectal mucosa contains no sensory nerve endings, counterirritants exert no effect in this area and are recommended for external use only and not for intrarectal use. (See Chapter 27, *External Analgesic Products.*)

Recommended Counterirritant   Menthol, in aqueous solution, is the only recommended counterirritant but it is not available. It is effective in concentrations of 0.25–2.0%, used externally (35). The FDA advisory review panel recommends that menthol be applied externally in concentrations of 0.25–1.0% no more than 6 times/day (36). The primary adverse effect of menthol is the possibility of sensitivity reactions (37).

Counterirritants Not Recommended Camphor, hydrastis (golden seal), juniper tar, and oil of turpentine are not recommended for use as counterirritants in the anorectal area. Because of camphor's rapid absorption due to its high lipid solubility, toxic concentrations may be reached (38). Both hydrastis and oil of turpentine are not considered safe and lack demonstrated effectiveness (39, 40). Juniper tar has neither been proven safe nor effective.

Astringents

Applied to the skin or mucous membranes for a local and limited effect, astringents coagulate the protein in the skin cells, thereby protecting the underlying tissue and producing a decrease in the cell volume. When appropriately used, astringents lessen mucus and other secretions and help relieve local anorectal irritation and inflammation (41).

Calamine and zinc oxide in concentrations of 5–25% are recommended as astringents for both external and internal use. The heavy metal zinc in these compounds acts as a protein precipitant and provides an astringent effect. Witch hazel (hamamelis water) 10–50% is recommended as an astringent for external use in anorectal disorders; its effectiveness is probably due to its alcohol content. The FDA advisory review panel concluded that hamamelis water provides temporary relief of itching and burning and is safe and effective for external use (42). Witch hazel is incorporated in pads or wipes that are commercially available and are advertised as being useful for hemorrhoids.

Tannic acid is not safe for anorectal use because it is well absorbed and may cause liver damage (43).

Wound-Healing Agents

Several ingredients in nonprescription hemorrhoidal products are claimed to be effective in promoting wound healing or tissue repair in anorectal disease. In particular, considerable controversy surrounds the substance skin respiratory factor (SRF), a water-soluble extract of Brewer's yeast also referred to as live yeast cell derivative. Although some tests have supported manufacturer claims, there is no conclusive evidence that products containing skin respiratory factor promote the healing of diseased anorectal tissue (44). The FDA advisory review panel on nonprescription hemorrhoidal drug products studied data on live yeast cell derivative as well as cod liver oil, peruvian balsam, shark liver oil, vitamin A, and vitamin D and found them lacking in demonstrated effectiveness as wound healers (45). Well-designed and well-controlled studies are still needed to determine the efficacy of wound healers in anorectal disease.

Antiseptics

Antiseptics generally inhibit the growth of microorganisms. Some nonprescription anorectal products contain compounds intended for use as antiseptics. However, because of the large numbers of microorganisms in feces, it is unlikely that the use of antiseptics in the anorectal area will provide a degree of antisepsis greater than that achieved by washing with soap and water. There is no convincing evidence that using antiseptics prevents infection in the anorectal area.

Specific compounds claimed to have antiseptic properties are boric acid, boric acid glycerite, hydrastis, phenol, resorcinol, and sodium salicylic acid phenolate. Boric acid and boric acid glycerite are not considered safe because of boric acid toxicity (46). Hydrastis, phenol, resorcinol (when used intrarectally), and sodium salicylic acid phenolate (46) are not considered safe for use in the anorectal area (39, 40, 47). Evidence is lacking to clearly demonstrate the effectiveness of resorcinol as an antiseptic used externally, although it is considered safe at concentrations of 0.5–2.5%/dosage unit (48). Benzethonium, 8-quinolinol benzoate, secondary amyl tricresols, 8-hydroxyquinoline sulfate, cetylpyridinium, and chlorothymol have been used as antiseptics in products intended for use in the anorectal area. The safety and efficacy of these compounds remain to be evaluated for use in treating the symptoms of anorectal disease.

Keratolytics

Keratolytics cause desquamation and debridement or sloughing of the epidermal surface cells. By loosening surface cells, keratolytics may help to expose underlying skin tissue to therapeutic agents. Used externally, they are useful in reducing itching, although their mechanism of action is unknown. Since mucous membranes contain no keratin layer, the use of keratolytics intrarectally is not justified.

The two keratolytics recommended for external use only are aluminum chlorhydroxy allantoinate (alcloxa) and resorcinol. The dosage ranges established by the FDA advisory review panel are up to six 2-g applications/day of a 0.2–2.0% ointment for alcloxa and of a 1.0–3.0% ointment for resorcinol (49). Precipitated and sublimed sulfur are not effective for intrarectal use as keratolytics.

Resorcinol is not safe when used intrarectally as a keratolytic. Additional evidence is required to determine if either precipitated and sublimed sulfur are effective as keratolytics when used externally. Although evidence exists that allantoin is effective as a keratolytic and protectant, the safety and effectiveness of allantoin in treating the symptoms of anorectal disease remains to be evaluated (50).

Anticholinergics

Anticholinergics inhibit or prevent the action of acetylcholine, the transmitter of cholinergic nerve impulses. Since anticholinergics produce their action systemically, they are not effective in ameliorating the local symptoms of anorectal disease.

Atropine, which is included in some products designed for anorectal use, is not safe because systemic poisoning may result from the absorption of the alkaloid through diseased skin and through the rectal mucosa if the product is applied intrarectally (50).

Hydrocortisone

Topically applied hydrocortisone-containing products have the potential to reduce itching, inflammation, and discomfort by vasoconstriction, lysosomal membrane stabilization, and antimitotic activity (51). However, complete and rigorous evaluations of these products for use in treating most symptoms of anorectal disease are needed before definitive statements can be made concerning their effectiveness.

Hydrocortisone and hydrocortisone acetate, 0.5%, for topical application are available on a nonprescription basis and are indicated for temporary relief of itching genital and anal areas.

Bulk-Forming Laxatives

Since constipation is a precipitating factor in hemorrhoidal disease, patients may be advised to consider the use of bulk-forming laxatives. (See Chapter 6, *Laxative Products*.) Ingredients commonly found in these products include barley malt extract, methylcellulose, and psyllium hydrocolloid. Adequate fluid intake in general should be encouraged and patients must follow directions with each product for proper fluid intake to prevent impaction and increase efficacy.

Miscellaneous

Collinsonia (stoneroot), *Escherichia coli* vaccines, lappa (burdock), leptandra (culver's root), and mullein are ingredients in nonprescription products that do not fall within the previously discussed pharmacologic classifications. With the exception of *E. coli* vaccines, these compounds are remnants of herbal medicine. There is no evidence that they are effective in treating symptoms of anorectal disease. The safety and effectiveness of *E. coli* vaccines also are unproven (52).

Dosage Forms

Drugs for treatment of anorectal disease symptoms are available in many dosage forms. For intrarectal use, suppositories, creams, ointments, gels, and foams are used. Applicators, one's fingers, and pile pipes are used to facilitate their application. Creams, ointments, gels, pastes, pads, liquids, and foam are used externally.

Ointments

Although there are considerable pharmaceutical differences among ointments, creams, pastes, and gels, the therapeutic differences are not significant. "Ointment" will be used to refer to all semisolid preparations designed for external or intrarectal use in the anorectal area.

Ointments may serve as vehicles for drugs used in treating anorectal disease symptoms and also possess inherent protectant and emollient properties. The primary function of an ointment base is the efficient delivery of the active ingredient(s). Applying an ointment may have a beneficial psychologic effect on patients with anorectal disorders (53). When used externally, ointments should be applied to the perianal area and the anal canal as a thin covering.

For intrarectal use, pile pipes and one's fingers have been used to apply ointments. Pile pipes have the advantage over fingers in that the drug product may be introduced into the rectal mucosa where a finger cannot reach. For most efficient use, the pile pipe should have lateral openings, as well as a hole in the end, to allow the drug product to cover the greatest area of rectal mucosa and should be lubricated prior to insertion. The potential for systemic absorption is greatest from the rectal mucosa.

Suppositories

A suppository may ease straining at the stool by a lubricating effect. Also, the insertion of a suppository may provide a beneficial psychologic effect. However, because of their many disadvantages, suppositories are not recommended as a dosage form in treating anorectal disease symptoms. In prone patients, suppositories may leave the affected region and ascend into the rectum and lower colon (54). If the patient remains prone after inserting a suppository, the active ingredients may not be evenly distributed over the rectal mucosa. Suppositories are relatively slow acting because they must melt to release the active ingredient.

Foams

Foam products present no proven advantage over ointments. Their disadvantages are that there is difficulty in establishing that the foam will remain in the affected area and that the size of the foam bubbles determines the concentration of active ingredient available (55).

Anal Hygiene

Cleansing the anorectal area with mild soap and water on a regular basis and after each bowel movement is helpful in relieving hemorrhoidal symptoms and may prevent recurrence of perianal itching. Practical means of cleansing after a bowel movement include the use of commercially available hygienic wipes or pads. Patients should be advised to blot or pat rather than rub the irritated perianal area with these wipes (this advice also applies to the use of toilet tissue).

Sitz baths are also useful in relieving hemorrhoidal symptoms and promoting good hygiene. A sitz bath is accomplished by sitting in warm water (110°–115° F) 2–3 times/day for 15 minutes (56). Plastic sitz baths, which fit over the toilet rim for convenient patient use, are easily cleaned and commonly available from pharmacies.

Surgical Treatment

Modern methods of treating hemorrhoids surgically include injection of sclerosing agents, rubber band ligation, dilatation of anal canal and lower rectum, cryosurgery, and hemorrhoidectomy (57).

Product Selection Guidelines
Patient Considerations

Knowledge of a patient's present condition, medical history, and medication profile obtained from a patient interview is necessary to determine how an individual patient may respond to self-medication. Of prime importance is to determine if the patient has symptoms amenable to self-medication.

Conditions such as diarrhea and/or constipation will complicate, if not render impossible, the self-treatment of anorectal disease symptoms. If a patient is confined to bed, a suppository dosage form is probably not appropriate. Patients with cardiovascular disease, diabetes, hypertension, and hyperthyroidism should not use a product containing a vasoconstrictor. Patients experiencing difficulty in urination and/or taking monoamine oxidase inhibitors should also not use an anorectal product containing a vasoconstrictor. Patients taking phenothiazines should avoid anorectal products containing ephedrine. Individuals with a tendency toward skin allergies should avoid ingredients such as wool alcohols and benzocaine in anorectal products.

With respect to pregnant and nursing women, any recommended ingredient should be used externally. For internal/intrarectal use, only the recommended protectants should be used. Children with hemorrhoids should be referred to a physician (58).

Product Considerations

Nonprescription anorectal preparations are intended to provide symptomatic relief for the burning, itching, pain, swelling, irritation, and discomfort of anorectal disorders. The prescription-only products available for treating symptoms of anorectal disease generally contain the same concentration of steroid as nonprescription products. The superiority of prescription-only over nonprescription products has not been established.

In recommending an appropriate nonprescription product, the pharmacist should consider ingredients and dosage form. A product containing recommended ingredients in appropriate combination should be offered. For intrarectal use the only recommended ingredients are vasoconstrictors, protectants, and astringents. A pile pipe of appropriate length and with a well-lubricated and flexible tip, with holes on the sides, may be used to apply an ointment-type of product. Suppositories are not recommended for use as a dosage form to treat anorectal conditions.

As a general rule, the products containing the least number of recommended ingredients in combination are the ones that should be suggested to a patient. These products minimize undesirable interactions and maximize effectiveness.

Biopharmaceutical Considerations

The bioavailability of drugs from anorectal dosage forms is a result of complex interplay among physicochemical, physiologic, manufacturing, dosage form, dosage, and application variables. Absorption from anorectal dosage forms involves release from the vehicle, dissolution into surrounding medium, diffusion to a membrane, and penetration of the membranes. For oleaginous bases, diffusion from the base is the rate-limiting step in the release of a drug from its vehicle (59). Most drugs used in hemorrhoidal products are basic amines (local anesthetics and vasoconstrictors). The un-ionized base is soluble in lipid ointment bases; the salt form is not soluble in lipid ointment bases. The un-ionized form penetrates the lipid tissue barriers such as

nerve membranes. Salt forms from weak bases are converted to the un-ionized base at tissue pH.

The solubility of the drug and its partitioning in a vehicle determines to a large extent its release rate from that vehicle.

If a drug has a greater affinity for the vehicle than the surrounding medium, a relatively slow release rate is expected. Conversely, if a drug has a greater affinity for the surrounding medium than the vehicle, a relatively rapid release rate occurs. Ephedrine sulfate dissolved in an oleaginous base such as cocoa butter is released relatively rapidly into a surrounding aqueous medium.

In the case of oleaginous bases, the rate-limiting step in absorption seems to be the rate at which the drug leaves the vehicle and dissolves in the surrounding fluid (60). The rate at which a drug diffuses from its base depends on a number of factors, including the vehicle pH, the drug concentration, the dissociation constant of the drug, the presence of surfactants, and the drug's particle size (61, 62).

For a water-soluble or water-miscible base (polyethylene glycol), a water-soluble drug form is preferred to facilitate absorption, because the absorption rate appears to be controlled by the transfer of the drug through the mucosa.

In ointments, creams, and suppositories, additives such as viscosity-increasing agents and/or surfactants are often required to achieve a high-quality product. Surfactants may increase or decrease drug absorption (63).

The absorption of an anorectal product may be affected by the manufacturing process. For example, the release rates associated with cocoa butter may vary according to the temperature at which the cocoa butter was melted. This effect may be explained by the polymorphic nature of cocoa butter.

Patient Consultation

The pharmacist should emphasize the importance of good anal hygiene in helping to prevent and alleviate symptoms. Specific advice to the patient should include the following reminders:
- For maximum effect, nonprescription anorectal products should be used after bowel movements rather than before.
- If seepage, bleeding, and/or protrusion occurs, a physician should be contacted as soon as possible.
- Products designed for external use only should not be inserted into the rectum.
- If insertion of a product in the rectum causes pain, use of the product should be discontinued and a physician consulted.
- Products to be used externally should be applied sparingly.
- Pile pipes may be too long and may deliver medication well beyond the hemorrhoidal problem area.
- If possible, the anorectal area should be washed with warm water before any nonprescription anorectal product is applied.
- If symptoms do not improve after 7 days, a physician should be consulted.

Cleansing the anorectal area with a moistened toilet tissue or cotton ball after defecation is recommended. Sitz baths are an alternative nondrug therapy for symptoms of uncomplicated anorectal disease. Moreover, the importance of maintaining normal bowel function by eating properly, drinking adequate amounts of fluid, and avoiding excessive laxative use should be emphasized as a means of preventing anorectal disease. A diet high in bulk and fluid will promote the formation of large, easily passed stools, thereby preventing constipation and accompanying straining. Stool softeners may be useful to prevent straining which may lead to hemorrhoids. (See Chapter 5, *Antidiarrheal Products*, and Chapter 6, *Laxative Products*.)

Summary

For external use, an ideal formulation would contain, in addition to one or two protectants totaling at least 50% of the formulation composition, three recommended ingredients, each from a separate pharmacologic category chosen from the following: local anesthetics, counterirritants, astringents, vasoconstrictors, and keratolytics. A combination containing a suitable local anesthetic, protectant, and astringent should be effective in relieving the itching, irritation, burning, discomfort, and pain associated with anorectal disease.

For internal/intrarectal use a model product would contain one or two protectants totaling at least 50% of the dose and an appropriate astringent. An ointment-type dosage form applied with the suitable pile pipe is recommended. This product should relieve the itching, swelling, discomfort, irritation, and pain of anorectal disease.

Products containing benzocaine (20%) in a polyethylene glycol base would be expected, when used externally, to be effective in treating itching, burning, and pain. For intrarectal use, a product consisting of 100% petrolatum is appropriate to recommend and is safe for use by pregnant women.

The pharmacist should make clear to the patient that if symptoms do not improve after 7 days or if bleeding, protrusion, and/or seepage occurs, a physician should be consulted as soon as possible.

References

1. R. L. Holt, "A Cure and Preventative: Hemorrhoids," California Health, Laguna Beach, Calif., 1977, p. 22.
2. D. Driscoll, M. DeFelice, R. Baptista, and P. Silverman, *U. S. Pharmacist*, 5, 43–44, 50 (May 1981).
3. R. T. Shackelford, in "Diseases of Colon and Anorectum," R. Turell, Ed., W. B. Saunders, Philadelphia, Pa., 1969, pp. 899–904.
4. E. Granet, "Manual of Proctology," Yearbook, Chicago, Ill., 1954, p. 115.
5. R. L. Holt, "A Cure and Preventative: Hemorrhoids," California Health, Laguna Beach, Calif., 1977, pp. 50–69.
6. H. Dodd, *Am. J. Surg.*, 79, 55 (1950).
7. R. T. Shackelford, in "Diseases of Colon and Anorectum," R. Turell, Ed., W. B. Saunders, Philadelphia, Pa., 1969, p. 896.
8. L. Van Dam, Statement to FDA Advisory Review Panel on OTC Hemorrhoidal Drug Products, May 1, 1976.
9. J. C. White, Statement to FDA Advisory Review Panel on OTC Hemorrhoidal Drug Products, May 1, 1976.
10. "The Pharmacological Basis of Therapeutics," 6th ed., A. G. Gilman, L. S. Goodman, and A. Gilman, Eds., Macmillan, New York, N.Y., 1980, p. 311.
11. J. Adriani and D. Campbell, *J. Am. Med. Assoc.*, 162, 1527 (1956).
12. E. Epstein, *J. Am. Med. Assoc.*, 198, 517 (1966).
13. C. G. Lange and R. Luifart, *J. Am. Med. Assoc.*, 146, 717 (1951).
14. H. Dalili and J. Adriani, *Clin. Pharmacol. Ther.*, 12, 913 (1971).
15. J. Adriani and P. Zipernich, *J. Am. Med. Assoc.*, 188, 711 (1964).
16. J. Adriani and H. Dalili, *Curr. Res. Anesth. Analg.*, 50, 834 (1971).
17. H. Wilson, *Practitioner*, 197, 673 (1966).
18. *The Medical Letter on Drugs and Therapeutics*, 11, 70 (1969).
19. *Federal Register*, 45, 35609–10 (1980).
20. "The Pharmacological Basis of Therapeutics," 6th ed., A. G. Gilman, L. S. Goodman, and A. Gilman, Eds., Macmillan, New York, N.Y., 1980, p. 310.
21. *Federal Register*, 45, 35613 (1980).
22. "The United States Dispensatory," 27th ed., A. Osol and R. Pratt, Eds., J. B. Lippincott, Philadelphia, Pa., 1973, p. 889.
23. O. Thulesius and J. E. Gjores, *Acta Chir. Scand.*, 139, 476 (1973).
24. *Federal Register*, 45, 35621 (1980).
25. F. M. Melton and W. B. Shelly, *J. Invest. Dermatol.*, 15, 325 (1950).
26. "The Pharmacological Basis of Therapeutics," 6th ed., A. G. Gilman, L. S. Goodman, and A. Gilman, Eds., Macmillan, New York, N.Y., 1980, p. 414.
27. "The Pharmacological Basis of Therapeutics," 6th ed., A. G. Gilman, L. S. Goodman, and A. Gilman, Eds., Macmillan, New York, N.Y., 1980, pp. 427 and 430.
28. *Federal Register*, 45, 35623–25 (1980).
29. E. Granet, "Manual of Proctology," Yearbook, Chicago, Ill., 1954, p. 59.
30. F. M. Melton and W. B. Shelley, *J. Invest. Dermatol.*, 15, 325 (1950).
31. *Federal Register*, 45, 35635 (1980).
32. G. K. Steigleder and W. P. Raab, *J. Invest. Dermatol.*, 38, 129 (1962).
33. *Federal Register*, 45, 35627 (1980).
34. J. M. Arena, "Poisoning," Charles C Thomas, Springfield, Ill., 1979, p. 391.
35. J. Adriani, R. Zepernick, J. Arens, and E. Authermont, *Clin. Pharmacol. Ther.*, 5, 49 (1963).
36. *Federal Register*, 45, 35641 (1980).
37. W. C. Carey and T. G. Randolph, *J. Am. Med. Assoc.*, 175, 539 (1961).
38. *Journal of the American Medical Association*, 234, 145 (1975).
39. K. Genest and D. W. Hughes, *Can. J. Pharm. Sci.*, 4, 4145 (1969).
40. W. B. Deichman and H. W. Gerarde, "Toxicology of Drugs and Chemicals," Academic, New York, N.Y., 1969, p. 448.
41. E. M. Boyd, in "Pharmacology in Medicine," 4th ed., V. A. Drill, Ed., McGraw-Hill, New York, N.Y., 1971, p. 1034.
42. *Federal Register*, 45, 35646 (1980).
43. B. Korpassy and K. Kovacs, *Br. J. Exp. Pathol.*, 30, 266 (1949).
44. W. Goodson, D. Hohn, T. K. Hunt, and D. Y. K. Leung, *J. Surg. Res.*, 21, 125 (1976).
45. *Federal Register*, 45, 35650 (1980).
46. M. A. Valdes-Dapena and J. B. Arey, *J. Pediatr.*, 61, 531 (1962).
47. "AMA Drug Evaluations—1973," 2nd ed., American Medical Association, Chicago, Ill., 1973, p. 893.
48. *Federal Register*, 45, 35663 (1980).
49. *Federal Register*, 45, 35665 (1980).
50. D. W. Melxell and S. B. Mecca, *J. Am. Pod. Assoc.*, 56, 357 (1966).
51. "AMA Drug Evaluations—1980," 4th ed., John Wiley and Sons, New York, N.Y., 1980, pp. 1009–1052.
52. "The Pharmacological Basis of Therapeutics," 6th ed., A. G. Gilman, L. S. Goodman, and A. Gilman, Eds., Macmillan, New York, N.Y., 1980, p. 126.
53. *Federal Register*, 45, 35669 (1980).
54. *Federal Register*, 45, 35589 (1980).

55. L. Augsberger and R. T. Shangraw, *J. Pharm. Sci.*, *57*, 624 (1968).
56. E. W. Martin, "Techniques of Medication," J. B. Lippincott, Philadelphia, Pa., 1969, p. 181.
57. *The Medical Letter on Drugs and Therapeutics*, *17*, 5 (1975).
58. *Federal Register*, *45*, 35599 (1980).
59. "Evaluations of Drug Interactions," 2nd ed., American Pharmaceutical Association, Washington, D.C., 1976.
60. W. A. Ritschel, "Biopharmaceutical Development and Evaluation of Rectal Dosage Forms, Applied Biopharmaceutics II,"
University of Cincinnati, College of Pharmacy, Cincinnati, Ohio, 1973, p. 1160.
61. N. A. Allawalla and S. Riegelman, *J. Am. Pharm. Assoc. Sci. Ed.*, *42*, 267 (1953).
62. J. Anschel and H. A. Lieberman, in "The Theory and Practice of Industrial Pharmacy," 2nd ed., L. Lachman, H. A. Lieberman, and J. L. Kanig, Eds., Lea and Febiger, Philadelphia, Pa., 1976, pp. 245–269.
63. S. Riegelman and W. J. Crowell, *J. Am. Pharm. Assoc. Sci. Ed.*, *47*, 115 (1958).

Hemorrhoidal Product Table

Product (Manufacturer)	Application Form	Anesthetic	Antiseptic	Astringent	Protectant	Other Ingredients
A-Caine (A.V.P.)	ointment	benzocaine, 2% diperodon hydrochloride, 0.25%		zinc oxide, 5% bismuth subcarbonate, 0.2%	cod liver oil base	phenylephrine, 0.255% pyrilamine maleate, 0.1%
Americaine (Arnar-Stone)	ointment	benzocaine, 20%	benzethonium chloride, 0.1%		polyethylene glycol base	
Anusol (Parke-Davis)	suppository ointment	pramoxine hydrochloride, 1% (ointment)		zinc oxide, 11% (ointment) peruvian balsam, 1.8% (ointment) bismuth subgallate, 2.25% (suppository) bismuth–resorcinol compound, 1.75% (suppository)	vegetable oil base (suppository)	benzyl benzoate, 1.2% kaolin, liquid petrolatum, cocoa butter, polyethylene wax, glyceryl monooleate, glyceryl stearate (ointment)
Balneol (Rowell)	cleansing lotion					water, mineral oil, propylene glycol, glyceryl stearate/PEG-100 stearate, laureth-4, PEG-4 dilaurate, lanolin oil, sodium acetate, carbomer-934, triethanolamine, sorbic acid, docusate sodium, fragrance, acetic acid
BiCozene (Creighton)	cream	benzocaine, 6%			cream base	resorcinol, 1.67%
Blue-Gray (Columbia Medical)	suppository	benzocaine, 50 mg	boric acid, 20 mg	bismuth subgallate, 47 mg bismuth–resorcinol compound, 16 mg zinc oxide, 40 mg peruvian balsam, 12 mg		
Calmol 4 (Leeming)	suppository			zinc oxide, 15%	Norwegian cod liver oil cocoa butter	
Cortef Rectal Itch Ointment (Upjohn)	ointment					hydrocortisone, 0.5%
Diothane (Merrell-National)	ointment	diperodon, 1%	8-quinolinol benzoate (salt), 0.1%		propylene glycol	sorbitan sesquioleate
Epinephricaine Ointment (Upjohn)	ointment	benzocaine, 2.5%	secondary amyltricresols, 1%	zinc oxide, 2%	petrolatum white wax	epinephrine, 0.2% vitamin A, 88 μg/g vitamin D, 1.35 μg/g

Hemorrhoidal Product Table, continued

Product (Manufacturer)	Application Form	Anesthetic	Antiseptic	Astringent	Protectant	Other Ingredients
Gentz Wipes (Philips Roxane)	medical pad	pramoxine hydrochloride, 1%	cetylpyridinium chloride, 0.5%	hamamelis water, 50% aluminum chlorhydroxy allantoinate, 0.2%	propylene glycol, 10%	fragrance
Hemorrin (Jeffrey Martin)	ointment suppository			bismuth subgallate, 2.25% bismuth resorcin compound, 1.75% peruvian balsam, 1.8% zinc oxide, 11%		
HTO Ointment (DeWitt)	ointment	benzocaine, 1%	phenol, 0.5% menthol, 0.2%	tannic acid, 1.5%	lanolin, 2.5%	allantoin, 0.5% ephedrine hydrochloride, 0.2%
HTO Stainless (DeWitt)	ointment	benzocaine, 1%	phenol, 0.5%	zinc oxide, 10%	lanolin, 3%	allantoin, 0.5% ephedrine hydrochloride, 0.2%
Lanacane (Combe)	cream	benzocaine, 6%	chlorothymol		water-washable base	resorcinol, 2%
Mediconet (Medicone)	medical pad		benzalkonium chloride, 0.02%	hamamelis water, 50%	ethoxylated lanolin, 0.5% glycerin, 10%	methylparaben, 0.15% perfume
Non-Steroid Proctofoam (Reed & Carnrick)	foam	pramoxine hydrochloride, 1%			mineral oil, 40%	
Nupercainal Ointment (Ciba)	ointment	dibucaine, 1%				acetone sodium bisulfite, 0.5%
Nupercainal Suppositories (Ciba)	suppository	dibucaine, 2.5 mg		zinc oxide bismuth subgallate	cocoa butter	acetone sodium bisulfite, 0.05%
Pazo (Bristol-Myers)	ointment suppository	benzocaine, 0.8%	camphor, 2.18%	zinc oxide, 4%	petrolatum, 87.78% (ointment) lanolin, 5% (ointment) hydrogenated vegetable oil (suppository)	ephedrine sulfate, 0.24%
Perifoam (Rowell)	foam	pramoxine hydrochloride, 1.0%	benzalkonium chloride, 0.1%	hamamelis water, 35%	lanolin	allantoin, 0.3% methylparaben, 0.15% propylparaben, 0.05% alcohol, 5%
Peterson's Ointment (Peterson)	ointment	camphor, 4.86% phenol, 3.16%		tannic acid, 2.16% zinc oxide, 6.5%	petrolatum beeswax	

Hemorrhoidal Product Table, continued

Product (Manufacturer)	Application Form	Anesthetic	Antiseptic	Astringent	Protectant	Other Ingredients
Pontocaine (Breon)	cream ointment	tetracaine hydrochloride (equivalent to 1% base) (cream) base, 0.5% (ointment)	menthol, 0.5% (ointment)		white petrolatum (ointment) white wax (ointment)	methylparaben (cream) sodium bisulfite (cream)
Preparation H (Whitehall)	ointment suppository				shark liver oil, 3%	live yeast cell derivative (supplying 2000 units of skin respiratory factor)/oz. phenylmercuric nitrate, 0.01%
Preparation H Cleansing Pads (Whitehall)	pads			hamamelis water, 30%	glycerin, 10%	
Proctodon (Rowell)	cream	diperodon hydrochloride, 1%				
Rantex (Holland-Rantos)	medical pad		benzalkonium chloride	hamamelis water, 50%	lanolin	methylparaben alcohol, 7%
Rectal Medicone Suppositories (Medicone)	suppository	benzocaine, 50.4 mg/g	8-hydroxy-quinoline sulfate, 5.55 mg/g menthol, 3.75 mg/g	zinc oxide, 75 mg/g peruvian balsam, 24 mg/g	cocoa butter vegetable and petroleum oils	
Rectal Medicone Unguent (Medicone)	ointment	benzocaine, 20 mg	8-hydroxy-quinoline sulfate, 5 mg menthol, 4 mg	zinc oxide, 100 mg peruvian balsam, 12.5 mg	petrolatum, 625 mg lanolin, 210 mg	
Tanicaine Ointment (Upjohn)	ointment	phenacaine hydrochloride, 10.8 mg/ml	camphor, 15.1 mg/ml phenol, 13 mg/ml menthol, 4.3 mg/ml	zinc oxide, 0.17 g/ml tannic acid, 0.053 g/ml		atropine, 0.54 mg/ml
Tanicaine Suppositories (Upjohn)	suppository	phenacaine hydrochloride, 22 mg	phenol, 13 mg	zinc oxide, 390 mg tannic acid, 110 mg		atropine, 1 mg
Tronolane (Abbott)	cream suppository	pramoxine hydrochloride, 1%			water miscible base (cream) vegetable oil triglyceride (suppository)	
Tucks Cream and Ointment (Parke-Davis)	cream ointment			hamamelis water, 50%	lanolin petrolatum	
Tucks Pads (Parke-Davis)	medical pad			hamamelis water, 50%	glycerin, 10%	methylparaben, 0.1% benzalkonium chloride, 0.003%

Hemorrhoidal Product Table, continued

Product (Manufacturer)	Application Form	Anesthetic	Antiseptic	Astringent	Protectant	Other Ingredients
Vaseline Pure Petroleum Jelly (Chesebrough-Ponds)	ointment				white petrolatum, 100%	
Wyanoid Ointment (Wyeth)	ointment	benzocaine, 2%	boric acid, 18%	zinc oxide, 5% peruvian balsam, 1%	castor oil, 2% petrolatum, 58%	ephedrine sulfate, 0.1%
Wyanoid Suppositories (Wyeth)	suppository		boric acid, 543 mg	zinc oxide, 176 mg bismuth subcarbonate, 146 mg bismuth oxyiodide, 30 mg peruvian balsam, 30 mg	cocoa butter	belladonna extract, 15 mg ephedrine sulfate, 3 mg

Index

Trade names of products included in the product tables appear in italics. Page numbers referring to products and ingredients listed in the product tables are also italicized. Generic names and all other main entries appear in bold face type.